Textbook of

Respiratory Disease in Dogs and Cats

Lesley G. King, MVB, MRCVS, DACVECC, DACVIM, DECVIM-CA
Associate Professor of Critical Care
Department of Clinical Studies
School of Veterinary Medicine
University of Pennsylvania
Philadelphia, Pennsylvania

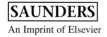

SAUNDERS
An Imprint of Elsevier

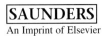

An Imprint of Elsevier

11830 Westline Industrial Drive
St. Louis, Missouri 63146

Textbook of Respiratory Disease in Dogs and Cats   ISBN 0-7216-8706-7
Copyright © 2004, Elsevier (USA). All rights reserved.

NOTICE

Veterinary Medicine is an ever-changing field. Standard safety precautions must be followed, but as new research and clinical experience broaden our knowledge, changes in treatment and drug therapy may become necessary or appropriate. Readers are advised to check the most current product information provided by the manufacturer of each drug to be administered to verify the recommended dose, the method and duration of administration, and contraindications. It is the responsibility of the licensed veterinarian, relying on experience and knowledge of the patient, to determine dosages and the best treatment for each individual patient. Neither the publisher nor the author assumes any liability for any injury and/or damage to persons or property arising from this publication.

International Standard Book Number 0-7216-8706-7

Executive Editor: Ray Kersey
Senior Developmental Editor: Denise LeMelledo
Publishing Services Manager: John Rogers
Senior Project Manager: Cheryl A. Abbott
Designer and Cover Art: Kathi Gosche

Printed in the United States of America

Last digit is the print number: 9 8 7 6 5 4 3 2 1

For my parents, Violet and Gerald,
with much love and gratitude.
And in honor of my godparents,
Noreen Pollock and Dr. Philip Davis.

Preface

Dogs and cats are frequently presented to the small animal practitioner with clinical signs of respiratory tract disease, such as coughing, sneezing, and exercise intolerance. In addition, animals that present in respiratory distress pose difficult and sometimes stressful management challenges because of their inherent fragility. The frequency with which respiratory tract disease occurs, the impetus from client demands for more advanced health care for pets, the increasing availability of sophisticated diagnostic and monitoring tools, and our own medical curiosity have all combined to produce dramatic advances in knowledge and expertise in the discipline of respiratory medicine for dogs and cats over the last 20 years. Much remains to be learned, however.

This book is intended, therefore, as a state-of-the-art clinical resource for diagnosis and management of dogs and cats with respiratory tract disease. The first sections of this book are organized to facilitate rapid use by presenting a problem-based approach and describing techniques for diagnostic testing and general support of patients with respiratory tract disease. The last section provides an in-depth description of specific respiratory disorders, including pathophysiology, diagnostics, expected clinical course, and management.

This textbook represents a collaboration by numerous specialists throughout the world who manage dogs and cats with respiratory tract disease every day as part of their clinical practice. I am profoundly grateful to the many experts in specific respiratory disciplines who were willing to share their expertise by contributing chapters. I am also grateful to Ray Kersey at Elsevier for his recognition of the need for a textbook of respiratory disease in dogs and cats, for his invitation to me to act as Editor, and for his dedicated support and encouragement along the way. Finally, I'd like to express my respect and gratitude for two special mentors who sadly are no longer with us. Dr. Joan O'Brien and Dr. David Knight taught us, challenged us, inspired us, and laid the early foundations for development of this discipline. We remember their personalities fondly, and we hold their contributions and achievements in the utmost esteem.

Lesley G. King

Contributors

Janet J. Aldrich, DVM
Staff Veterinarian, Emergency/Critical Care Service
School of Veterinary Medicine
University of California
Davis, California

Lillian R. Aronson, VMD, DACVS
Assistant Professor of Surgery
Department of Clinical Studies
School of Veterinary Medicine
University of Pennsylvania
Philadelphia, Pennsylvania

Jennifer L. Baez, VMD, DACVIM
Assistant Professor of Oncology
Department of Clinical Studies
School of Veterinary Medicine
University of Pennsylvania
Philadelphia, Pennsylvania

Linda Barton, DVM, DACVECC
The Animal Medical Center
New York, New York

Jeff D. Bay, DVM, DACVIM
Specialty of Internal Medicine
Rowley Memorial Animal Hospital
Springfield, Massachusetts

Clifford R. Berry, DVM, DACVR
Central Florida Veterinary Radiology, P.A.
Veterinary Specialist Center
Maitland, Florida

Dale E. Bjorling, DVM, MS, DACVS
Professor and Chairman
Department of Surgical Sciences
School of Veterinary Medicine
University of Wisconsin
Madison, Wisconsin

Dawn Merton Boothe, DVM, PhD, DACVIM, DACVCP
Professor
Department of Physiology and Pharmacology
College of Veterinary Medicine
Texas A&M University
College Station, Texas

Colleen A. Brady, DVM, DACVECC
Pacific Veterinary Specialists and Emergency Service
Capitola, California

Daniel J. Brockman, BVSc, CVR, CSAO, MRCVS, DACVS, DECVS
Senior Lecturer in Small Animal Surgery
Royal Veterinary College, University of London
Hatfield, Hertfordshire
United Kingdom

Mary Beth Callan, VMD, DACVIM
Assistant Professor of Medicine
Department of Clinical Studies
School of Veterinary Medicine
University of Pennsylvania
Philadelphia, Pennsylvania

Vicki L. Campbell, DVM
Assistant Professor, Department of Clinical Sciences
College of Veterinary Medicine and Biomedical Sciences
Colorado State University
Fort Collins, Colorado

Janet K. Carreras, VMD, DACVIM (Oncology)
Gulf Coast Veterinary Oncology
Houston, Texas

Daniel L. Chan, DVM
Resident in Emergency and Critical Care
Department of Clinical Sciences
School of Veterinary Medicine
Tufts University
North Grafton, Massachusetts

Craig A. Clifford, DVM, MS
Section of Oncology
Red Bank Veterinary Hospital
Red Bank, New Jersey

Steven G. Cole, DVM
Lecturer, Section of Critical Care
Department of Clinical Studies
School of Veterinary Medicine
University of Pennsylvania
Philadelphia, Pennsylvania

Brendan M. Corcoran, MVB, DipPharm, PhD, MRCVS
Senior Lecturer
Head of Cardiopulmonary Service
Hospital for Small Animals
Division of Veterinary Clinical Studies
College of Medicine and Veterinary Medicine
The University of Edinburgh
Easter Bush Veterinary Centre
Roslin, Midlothian, Scotland

Daniel L. Costa, ScD, DABT
Pulmonary Toxicology Branch, Experimental Toxicology
  Division
National Health and Environmental Effects Research
  Laboratory,
United States Environmental Protection Agency
Research Triangle Park, North Carolina

Merilee Costello, DVM, ACVECC
Lecturer, Section of Emergency and Critical Care
Department of Clinical Studies
School of Veterinary Medicine
University of Pennsylvania
Philadelphia, Pennsylvania

Michael S. Davis, DVM, PhD, DACVIM
Assistant Professor, Physiology
Department of Physiologic Sciences
College of Veterinary Medicine
Oklahoma State University
Stillwater, Oklahoma

Susan Dawson, BVMS, PhD
Department of Veterinary Clinical Science and Animal
Husbandry
University of Liverpool Veterinary Teaching Hospital
Leahurst, Neston
United Kingdom

Ross Doust, BVSc Cert SAS, MRCVS
Division of Small Animal Clinical Studies
Faculty of Veterinary Medicine
Glasgow University Veterinary School
Bearsden, Glasgow
Scotland

Kenneth J. Drobatz, DVM, MSCE, DACVECC, DACVIM
Associate Professor of Critical Care
Department of Clinical Studies
School of Veterinary Medicine
University of Pennsylvania
Philadelphia, Pennsylvania

Janice A. Dye, DVM, MS, PhD, DACVIM
Pulmonary Toxicology Branch, Experimental Toxicology
Division
National Health and Environmental Effects Research
Laboratory,
United States Environmental Protection Agency
Research Triangle Park, North Carolina

Richard B. Ford, DVM, MS, DACVIM
Professor of Medicine
College of Veterinary Medicine
North Carolina State University
Raleigh, North Carolina

Theresa W. Fossum, DVM, MS, PhD, DACVS
Professor and Chief of Surgery
Department of Small Animal Medicine and Surgery
College of Veterinary Medicine
Texas A&M University
College Station, Texas

Rosalind M. Gaskell, BVSc, PhD
Professor
Department of Veterinary Pathology
University of Liverpool Veterinary Teaching Hospital
Leahurst, Neston
United Kingdom

Greg M. Griffin, MVB, MRCVS, DACVS, DECVS
Regional Veterinary Referral Center
Springfield, Virginia

Susan G. Hackner, BVSc, MRCVS, DACVIM, DACVECC
VCA Veterinary Referral Associates
Gaithersburg, Maryland

Neil K. Harpster, VMD, DACVIM
Department of Cardiology
Angell Memorial Animal Hospital
Boston, Massachusetts

Steve C. Haskins, DVM, MS, DACVA, DACVECC
Professor of Anesthesia and Intensive Care
Department of Surgery and Radiology
University of California
School of Veterinary Medicine
Davis, California

Eleanor C. Hawkins, DVM, DACVIM
Professor, Internal Medicine
Department of Clinical Sciences
College of Veterinary Medicine
North Carolina State University
Raleigh, North Carolina

Joan C. Hendricks, VMD, PhD, DACVIM
Bower Professor of Small Animal Medicine
Chief, Section of Critical Care
Department of Clinical Studies
School of Veterinary Medicine
University of Pennsylvania
Philadelphia, Pennsylvania

Rosemary A. Henik, DVM, MS, DACVIM
Clinical Associate Professor
Department of Medical Sciences
School of Veterinary Medicine
University of Wisconsin—Madison
Madison, Wisconsin

Rebecka S. Hess, DVM, DACVIM
Assistant Professor of Medicine
Department of Clinical Studies .
School of Veterinary Medicine
University of Pennsylvania
Philadelphia, Pennsylvania

Andrew M. Hoffman, DVM, DVSc, DACVIM
Department of Clinical Sciences
School of Veterinary Medicine
Tufts University
North Grafton, Massachusetts

David E. Holt, BVSc, DACVS
Associate Professor of Surgery
Department of Clinical Studies
School of Veterinary Medicine
University of Pennsylvania
Philadelphia, Pennsylvania

John P. Hoover, MS, DVM, DAVBP, DACVIM
Professor, Small Animal Internal Medicine
Department of Veterinary Clinical Sciences
Oklahoma State University
Stillwater, Oklahoma

Dez Hughes, BVSc, MRCVS, DACVECC
Senior Lecturer, Veterinary Emergency and Critical Care
Department of Veterinary Clinical Sciences
Royal Veterinary College, University of London
Hatfield, Hertfordshire
United Kingdom

C. Bisque Jackson, VMD
Philadelphia, Pennsylvania

Lynelle R. Johnson, DVM, PhD, DACVIM
Assistant Professor of Veterinary Medicine and
Epidemiology
School of Veterinary Medicine
University of California
Davis, California

Dennis Keith, DVM, DACVR
Radiology Department
Mesa Veterinary Hospital
Mesa, Arizona

†David H. Knight, DVM, MMedSc, DACVIM
Emeritus Professor of Cardiology
Department of Clinical Studies
School of Veterinary Medicine
University of Pennsylvania
Philadelphia, Pennsylvania

Lesley G. King, MVB, MRCVS, DACVECC, DACVIM, DECVIM-CA
Associate Professor of Critical Care
Department of Clinical Studies
School of Veterinary Medicine
University of Pennsylvania
Philadelphia, Pennsylvania

Ned F. Kuehn, DVM, MS, DACVIM
Internal Medicine
Michigan Veterinary Specialists
Southfield, Michigan

Michael R. Lappin, DVM, PhD, DACVIM
Professor, Department of Clinical Sciences
College of Veterinary Medicine and Biomedical Sciences
Colorado State University
Fort Collins, Colorado

Justine A. Lee, DVM
Department of Small Animal Clinical Sciences
College of Veterinary Medicine
University of Minnesota
St. Paul, Minnesota

Andrew J. Mackin, BSc, BVMS, MVS, DVSc, FACVSc, DSAM, MRCVS, DACVIM
Associate Professor, Small Animal Medicine
College of Veterinary Medicine
Mississippi State University
Mississippi State, Mississippi

Deborah C. Mandell, VMD, DACVECC
Staff Veterinarian, Section of Critical Care
Department of Clinical Studies
School of Veterinary Medicine
University of Pennsylvania
Philadelphia, Pennsylvania

F. A. Mann, DVM, MS, DACVS, DACVECC
Associate Professor
Director of Small Animal Emergency and Critical Care
Services
Veterinary Medical Teaching Hospital
University of Missouri
Columbia, Missouri

Robert A. Mason, DVM, DVSc, DABVP, DACVIM
Oceanview Veterinary Specialists
Poulsbo, Washington

Kyle G. Mathews, DVM, MS, DACVS
Assistant Professor of Surgery
Department of Clinical Science
College of Veterinary Medicine
North Carolina State University
Raleigh, North Carolina

Jonathan F. McAnulty, DVM, MS, PhD
Associate Professor of Surgery
School of Veterinary Medicine
University of Wisconsin
Madison, Wisconsin

†Deceased.

Margaret C. McEntee, DVM, DACVIM (Oncology), DACVR (Radiation Oncology)
Associate Professor of Oncology
Department of Clinical Sciences
College of Veterinary Medicine
Cornell University
Ithaca, New York

Patricia M. McManus, VMD, PhD, DACVP
Associate Professor of Clinical Pathology
Department of Pathobiology
School of Veterinary Medicine
University of Pennsylvania
Philadelphia, Pennsylvania

Matthew S. Mellema, DVM
Harvard School of Public Health
Boston, Massachusetts

Eric Monnet, DVM, PhD, FAHA, DACVS, DECVS
Cardio-Thoracic and Vascular Surgery
Associate Professor, Small Animal Surgery
College of Veterinary Medicine
Colorado State University
Fort Collins, Colorado

Prudence J. Neath, BSc(Hons), BvetMed, DACVS, DECVS, MRCVS
Soft Tissue Surgeon
Animal Health Trust Lanwades Park
Suffolk, England

Carol R. Norris, DVM, DACVIM
Immunology Graduate Group
Department of Pathology, Microbiology, and Immunology
School of Veterinary Medicine
University of California
Davis, California

Sandra Z. Perkowski, VMD, PhD, DACVA
Assistant Professor of Anesthesia
Department of Clinical Studies
School of Veterinary Medicine
University of Pennsylvania
Philadelphia, Pennsylvania

Robert Poppenga, DVM, PhD, DABVT
Associate Professor of Veterinary Toxicology
Department of Pathobiology
School of Veterinary Medicine
University of Pennsylvania
Kennett Square, Pennsylvania

Lisa L. Powell, DVM, DACVECC
Assistant Clinical Specialist/ICU Director
Department of Small Animal Clinical Sciences
College of Veterinary Medicine
University of Minnesota
St. Paul, Minnesota

Jennifer Prittie, DVM, DACVIM, DACVECC
The Animal Medical Center
New York, New York

David A. Puerto, DVM, DACVS
Section of Surgery
Department of Clinical Studies
School of Veterinary Medicine
University of Pennsylvania
Philadelphia, Pennsylvania

Alan D. Radford, BSc, BVSc, PhD
Lecturer in Small Animal Studies
University of Liverpool Veterinary Teaching Hospital
Leahurst, Neston
United Kingdom

Marc R. Raffe, DVM, MS, DACVECC, DACVA
Professor, Section of Critical Care
College of Veterinary Medicine
University of Illinois
Urbana, Illinois

Elizabeth A. Rozanski, DVM, DACVECC, DACVIM
Assistant Professor
Department of Clinical Sciences
School of Veterinary Medicine
Tufts University
North Grafton, Massachusetts

John E. Rush, DVM, PhD, DACVIM (Cardiology), DACVECC
Assistant Professor
Co-Director, ICU and Emergency Services
School of Veterinary Medicine
Tufts University
North Grafton, Massachusetts

Nancy A. Sanders, DVM, DACVIM, DACVECC
VCA Veterinary Referral Associates
Gaithersburg, Maryland

Valérie Sauvé
Resident, Section of Critical Care
Department of Clinical Studies
School of Veterinary Medicine
University of Pennsylvania
Philadelphia, Pennsylvania

H. Mark Saunders, VMD, MS, DACVR
Associate Professor of Radiology
Department of Clinical Studies
School of Veterinary Medicine
University of Pennsylvania
Philadelphia, Pennsylvania

Darcy H. Shaw, DVM, MVSc, DACVIM
Associate Professor, Department of Companion Animals
Atlantic Veterinary College
University of Prince Edward Island
Charlottetown
Canada

Robert G. Sherding, DVM, DACVIM
Professor and Department Chair
Department of Veterinary Clinical Sciences
College of Veterinary Medicine
The Ohio State University
Columbus, Ohio

Gretchen K. Sicard, DVM
Assistant Professor of Surgery
College of Veterinary Medicine
Kansas State University
Manhattan, Kansas

Deborah C. Silverstein, DVM, DACVECC
Adjunct Assistant Professor
Section of Critical Care
Department of Clinical Studies
School of Veterinary Medicine
University of Pennsylvania
Philadelphia, Pennsylvania

Meg Sleeper, VMD, DACVIM (Cardiology)
Assistant Professor and Section Chief of Cardiology
Department of Clinical Studies
School of Veterinary Medicine
University of Pennsylvania
Philadelphia, Pennsylvania

Mark M. Smith, VMD, DACVS, DAVDC
Professor and Chief
Small Animal Surgery and Anesthesia
Department of Small Animal Clinical Sciences
VA-MD Regional College of Veterinary Medicine
Virginia Tech
Blacksburg, Virginia

Karin U. Sorenmo, CMV, DACVIM (Oncology)
Assistant Professor of Oncology
Department of Clinical Studies
School of Veterinary Medicine
University of Pennsylvania
Philadelphia, Pennsylvania

Jennifer L. Steele, DVM
Department of Small Animal Clinical Sciences
College of Veterinary Medicine
University of Minnesota
St. Paul, Minnesota

Martin Sullivan, BVMS, PhD, DVR, MRCVS, DipECVDI
Division of Small Animal Clinical Studies
Faculty of Veterinary Medicine
Glasgow University Veterinary School
Bearsden, Glasgow
Scotland

Rebecca S. Syring, DVM, DACVECC
Assistant Professor of Critical Care
Department of Clinical Studies
School of Veterinary Medicine
University of Pennsylvania
Philadelphia, Pennsylvania

Laura W. Tseng, DVM, DACVECC
Philadelphia, Pennsylvania

A. Reid Tyson, DVM
Radiology House Officer
Veterinary Specialist Center
Maitland, Florida

Lori S. Waddell, DVM, DACVECC
Adjunct Assistant Professor, Intensive Care Unit
Department of Clinical Studies
School of Veterinary Medicine
University of Pennsylvania
Philadelphia, Pennsylvania

Contents

†Deceased.

PART ONE

Approach to Problems in Respiratory Medicine

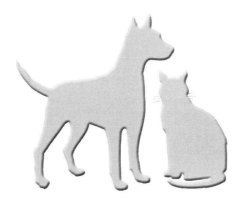

CHAPTER 1

Respiratory Distress and Cyanosis in Dogs

Justine A. Lee • Kenneth J. Drobatz

Introduction

Respiratory distress is a common presenting complaint in emergency medicine, and is diagnostically and therapeutically challenging. Prompt recognition and appropriate therapeutic intervention is essential. Delayed recognition and treatment can result in severe compromise or death of the patient. Familiarity with the clinical manifestations of respiratory distress and with the pathophysiology of hypoxemia and hypercarbia will facilitate recognition and management of this life-threatening problem (Figure 1-1).

Patients with respiratory distress are fragile, therefore, stress induced by diagnostic testing should be minimized to prevent further decompensation, which can progress to respiratory arrest. Oxygen supplementation may aid immediate stabilization. The clinician must rapidly determine the cause of respiratory distress by relying on physical examination findings, the medical history, and noninvasive diagnostic testing. Dyspneic dogs can be quickly categorized into groups defined by the probable anatomic localization of disease (e.g., large/ upper airways, pulmonary parenchyma, pleural space, or thoracic wall).[1,2]

Emergency interventional procedures may be necessary to relieve respiratory distress. Depending on the cause of respiratory distress, emergency techniques such as oxygen supplementation, pharmacological intervention, thoracocentesis, thoracostomy tube placement, tracheostomy, and positive-pressure ventilation may be required.

This chapter will define respiratory distress and cyanosis, review physical examination parameters of patients with respiratory distress, discuss stabilization of critically hypoxemic patients, categorize the anatomical locations of respiratory distress, briefly address the causes and treatment of respiratory distress, and discuss serial monitoring of the respiratory patient. The perti-

1

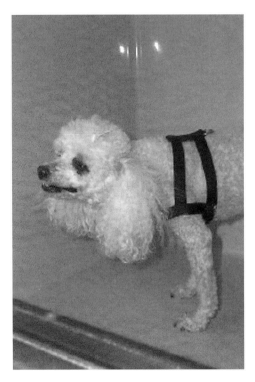

Figure 1-1. *This photo illustrates the classic posture of dogs in severe respiratory distress. This poodle with fulminant pulmonary edema prefers to stand with abducted elbows, is mouth breathing and exhibiting extension of the head and neck, and has an anxious expression.*

nent chapters regarding specific disease processes should be consulted for more detail.

Respiratory Distress

Hypoxia refers to a state in which oxygen in the blood, lung, and/or tissues is abnormally low, resulting in cellular damage or abnormal organ function.[3] *Hypoxemia* refers to insufficient oxygenation of blood necessary to meet metabolic requirements.[3] Hypercapnia drives normal respiratory stimulation; however, hypoxemia may become a significant respiratory stimulant when the arterial partial pressure of oxygen (Pao_2) is less than 50 mm Hg.[4] Respiratory distress is triggered by a Pao_2 less than 60 mm Hg, or by an arterial partial pressure of carbon dioxide ($Paco_2$) greater than 50 mm Hg.[4] These trigger levels will vary depending upon the chronicity of the respiratory problem.

The appropriate response to hypoxemia is respiratory adjustment to improve oxygenation, to assist in carbon dioxide removal, and to improve oxygen delivery to the tissues. These adjustments result in increased ventilatory drive, increased work of breathing, increased cardiac rate and contractility, and therefore in the clinical signs of respiratory distress. Although these physiologic adjustments may be initially effective in correcting hypoxemia or hypercarbia, untreated, progressive respiratory distress may lead to ventilatory failure, manifested

by gradually increased use of accessory muscles for ventilation, intercostal retraction, cyanosis, paradoxical respiration, tachycardia, or even narcosis or coma from hypercapnia. Therefore, prompt recognition and treatment of respiratory distress is imperative.

Hypoxia and Cyanosis

Cyanosis is defined as a bluish to red-purple color in the tissues due to an increased amount of deoxygenated, or reduced, hemoglobin.[5] Clinically detectable cyanosis does not occur until the amount of deoxygenated hemoglobin reaches 3 to 5 g/dl.[5] The amount of reduced hemoglobin depends on the hemoglobin concentration and on the percent hemoglobin saturation of the arterial blood (Sao_2), which is correlated to the Pao_2. An animal with a normal hematocrit must have an Sao_2 of 73% to 78% (Pao_2 of 39 to 44 mm Hg) before cyanosis can be detected.[6] Anemic animals may have severe hypoxemia and never have clinical evidence of cyanosis. The lower the total Hb concentration, the more the Sao_2 must fall before cyanosis can be clinically detected.[6]

Cyanosis and hypoxemia may also be difficult to detect in animals that are in shock, those with carbon monoxide toxicity, or those with methemoglobinemia.[1,6] Patients with polycythemia may have a normal to reduced Pao_2 and Sao_2, but an overall increase in oxygen content (Cao_2) because of the increased hemoglobin concentration.[7] Shock may result in vasoconstriction and pale mucous membranes, and thus not enough hemoglobin circulating through the periphery for cyanosis to be detectable. Carbon monoxide can result in hypoxemia due to its high affinity for hemoglobin, displacing oxygen from hemoglobin in the erythrocytes. In animals with carbon monoxide toxicity, Pao_2 may be normal despite elevated carboxyhemoglobin levels, and total oxygen content drops dramatically.[8] The mucous membranes can appear cherry-red despite significantly decreased oxygen content. Methemoglobin differs from hemoglobin only in that the iron moiety of heme has been oxidized to the ferric (+3) state, resulting in reduced oxygen carrying capacity[9] and therefore a normal Pao_2 but a reduced Sao_2 and Cao_2.[7] Animals with methemoglobinemia may appear cyanotic, and the blood may appear brown after venipuncture. It is important to reiterate that, whereas cyanotic mucous membranes indicate severe hypoxemia, one cannot assume that a patient with pink or white mucous membranes has normal oxygenation.[1,10]

Cyanosis may be classified as central or peripheral. Peripheral cyanosis is a localized increase in deoxygenated hemoglobin (e.g., due to an aortic saddle thrombus or tourniquet application). Peripheral cyanosis may reflect central cyanosis or may result from decreased local capillary perfusion or venous blood stagnation.[6] Central cyanosis is primarily associated with respiratory disease and the six major causes of arterial hypoxemia.[6] The six causes of hypoxemia include:[11] (1) decreased fraction of inspired oxygen (Fio_2) or inspired oxygen concentration; (2) alveolar hypoventilation; (3) ventilation-perfusion mismatch; (4) diffusion impairment; (5) shunt; and (6) abnormal hemoglobin.[11]

Decreased Fio_2 or inadequate inspired oxygen, most commonly occurs due to high altitude or anesthetic accidents, and responds well to oxygen supplementation. Alveolar hypoventilation occurs when oxygen flow to the alveoli is decreased. This may be due to neuromuscular failure, increased dead space, obstruction of the major airways, primary pulmonary disease, or pleural space disorders. Severe brain disorders, the effects of anesthesia on the respiratory center, or muscular fatigue are other conditions that may result in alveolar hypoventilation. Although rare, conditions such as paralysis of the respiratory muscles due to organophosphate toxicity, myasthenia gravis, myelomalacia of the cervical and thoracic spinal cord, lower motor neuron disease, and overdose of paralytic agents (e.g., cisatracurium*) can all cause alveolar hypoventilation with risk for respiratory arrest.[1]

The third cause of hypoxemia is ventilation-perfusion (V/Q) mismatch, which is seen in animals with many severe pulmonary parenchymal diseases. Due to an anatomical regional pattern, there is a small amount of ventilation-perfusion inequality in the normal lung. Although both ventilation and perfusion are greater in the ventral lung fields due to the effect of gravity, perfusion is affected more than ventilation.[11,12] Therefore, the V/Q ratio is high at the top of the lung, where blood flow is minimal, and much lower at the bottom of the lung.[13] When ventilation and blood flow are mismatched, diffusion of oxygen and carbon dioxide is impaired. Ventilation-perfusion mismatch is the most common cause of hypoxemia because an effective increase in dead space results in inadequate gas exchange.[11] Hypoxia is worsened when V/Q mismatch is combined with hypoventilation, low cardiac output, or diffusion impairment. Oxygen supplementation is beneficial for patients with V/Q mismatch because hypoventilated areas (relative to perfused areas) will then convert to normal ratios after nitrogen is washed out of the alveoli and replaced with pure oxygen.[11]

Diffusion impairment, which is due to a thickened alveolar barrier, impairs the ability of oxygen to reach the red blood cells. Normally, oxygen and carbon dioxide pass through multiple respiratory membranes (i.e., the alveolar surfactant and fluid layer, the alveolar epithelium and basement membrane, the thin interstitial space, and the capillary basement membrane and endothelium).[13] Changes in the thickness or surface area of these layers, along with alterations in the regional perfusion, alter the degree of oxygen exchange at the alveolus. Fick's law states that the rate of diffusion of gas is proportional to the tissue area and the difference in partial pressure of the gas between the two sides, while being inversely proportional to the thickness of the tissue. Thus factors that determine how rapidly a gas will pass through a membrane include: (1) the surface area of the membrane; (2) the thickness of the membrane; (3) the diffusion coefficient of the gas in the substance of the membrane; and (4) the

pressure difference of the gas between the two sides of the membrane.[13]

The surface area of the respiratory membranes can decrease gas exchange. For example, if an entire lung were removed, the total surface area for gas diffusion would decrease to one-half normal.[13] When the total surface area is decreased to one fourth of normal, exchange of gases through the membrane is impeded significantly, even under resting conditions.[13] The thickness of the respiratory membrane can be increased by pulmonary edema, fibrosis, or other lung pathology. Thus the respiratory gases must diffuse not only through the membrane, but also through the fluid, fibrosis, or neoplastic tissue. The rate of diffusion through the membrane is inversely proportional to the thickness of the membrane; therefore, any thickening of the membrane greater than two to three times normal can significantly interfere with normal gas exchange.[13] The diffusion coefficient depends upon the square root of the gas's molecular weight and the solubility of the gas in the membrane. The diffusion coefficient of carbon dioxide is 20 times that of oxygen; therefore carbon dioxide diffuses much more rapidly than oxygen. The final factor that affects the rate of gas diffusion is pressure difference, the difference between the partial pressure of the gas in the alveoli and the pressure of the gas in the pulmonary capillary blood. This is a measure of the net tendency for the gas molecules to move through the membrane.[13] Diffusion impairment is seen with severe lung pathology (e.g., chronic obstructive pulmonary disease, interstitial pneumonia, or neoplasia). Mild increases in Fio_2 should improve the gradient for oxygen transfer in patients with this condition.[11]

The fifth cause of hypoxemia is shunt, which occurs when venous blood completely bypasses oxygenation in the lungs and mixes with the arterial circulation, resulting in venous admixture and a decrease in the arterial partial pressure of oxygen. Shunting occurs in animals with cardiac disease and right to left shunting (e.g., with tetralogy of Fallot, tricuspid valve stenosis, common atrioventricular canal, transposition of the great vessels, intrapulmonary shunting, and various other arterial or vascular anatomical defects). Whereas true intrapulmonary shunts (a-v fistulas) are rare, areas of lung that are completely unventilated but still perfused can represent physiological right to left shunts. For example, lung lobes consolidated as a result of pneumonia, pulmonary edema, neoplasia, or atelectasis may result in profound degrees of intrapulmonary shunt. Primary cardiac disease that results in a right to left shunt may result in clinical signs of cyanosis, which usually does not respond to oxygen therapy, particularly if the shunt fraction is greater than 30%. However, increased quantities of dissolved oxygen may be mildly beneficial in critical situations.[11]

Finally, abnormal hemoglobin can cause hypoxemia. Hypoxia becomes evident when more than 20% to 40% of hemoglobin has been oxidized to methemoglobin. Causes of methemoglobinemia include deficiencies of methemoglobin reductase (seen in the dog) or oxidizing agents such as benzocaine or acetaminophen (in the

---

*Cisatracurium, Catalytica Pharmaceutical Inc., Greenville, N.C.

cat). As little as 1.5 g/dl of methemoglobin or 0.5 g/dl of sulfhemoglobin can produce cyanosis.[6]

Stabilization

When presented with a dyspneic dog or cat, the initial treatment for hypoxia, regardless of the anatomical location, is oxygen supplementation. Oxygen supplementation increases both the dissolved oxygen concentration and, more importantly, the oxygen saturation of hemoglobin. Once oxygen supplementation has been provided, a limited evaluation of the patient can be performed. Care must be taken because these critical patients are predisposed to respiratory arrest or collapse with manipulation. Excessive stress or struggling, or dorsal recumbency positioning for ventral-dorsal radiographs, may be life threatening.

In the event of severe respiratory distress, the first priority should be to ensure that a patent airway is available. Airway patency is evaluated by observation of the patient's breathing pattern. It is not appropriate to open the mouth and attempt to observe the pharynx and larynx because such efforts are likely to exacerbate distress in a dyspneic animal, and are unlikely to be successful even in a compliant patient. Complete airway obstruction is easily recognized by observation of exaggerated or prolonged inspiratory effort with little or no air movement. Tissue oxygenation may not occur despite oxygen supplementation if a primary airway obstruction is present; therefore, immediate invasive measures (e.g., sedation, intubation, and positive-pressure ventilation) may be indicated.

Ideally, intravenous catheter placement with ongoing oxygen supplementation should be attempted because venous access for immediate administration of emergency drugs or intravenous fluids may be necessary. If possible, blood should be collected for an emergency database (e.g., packed cell volume, total solids, dipstick estimation of blood urea nitrogen, blood glucose, a blood smear, venous blood gas, and electrolytes) while placing the catheter.[14] Even this minimal bloodwork may provide valuable information about the patient and its underlying disease, and may provide clues towards a diagnosis of the cause of respiratory distress.[14] For example, the presence of circulating lymphoblasts on a blood smear might raise suspicion of lymphosarcoma and a neoplastic pleural effusion, or the presence of a mediastinal compressive mass.

PHYSICAL EXAMINATION AND HISTORICAL FINDINGS

After ensuring airway patency, providing oxygen supplementation, and obtaining vascular access, a limited yet focused physical examination should be performed with minimal restraint and stress to the patient.[10] The posture, mental attitude, and breathing pattern of the patient are observed. Auscultation of the thorax and the neck, with evaluation of the mucous membranes and pulses, are important clues for evaluation and treatment of dyspneic animals. Observation of the respiratory pattern may help localize the anatomic region causing the respiratory distress. For example, animals with upper airway obstruction often have deep inspiratory effort with stridorous sounds. In contrast, those with pleural space or thoracic wall disease tend to have short, shallow breaths due to smaller tidal volumes and a high respiratory frequency as a result of stiff lungs or restricted lung expansion.[10]

At rest in a normal animal, the respiratory pattern should be smooth and barely noticeable. The ribs should move craniolaterally, with the abdomen moving slightly outward due to caudal movement of the diaphragm.[10] With increased work of breathing and respiratory distress, paradoxical respiration may be noted and may include: (1) inward collapse of the intercostal spaces due to a greater negative inspiratory pressure or intercostal weakness; (2) inward collapse of the abdomen during inspiration; (3) inward movement of the lower ribs due to contraction of the diaphragm and tension exerted on the caudal ribs' costal insertion of the diaphragm; and (4) inward movement of the ribs with inspiration.[10]

Other signs of respiratory distress include orthopnea, sitting with the head and neck extended, abduction of the elbows, open-mouthed breathing, a glazed expression, nasal flare, and agitation (see Figure 1-1).[1,10]

Useful information may be obtained from a thorough patient history. Inquiries about voice change, previously diagnosed cardiac disease, the presence of coughing, any history of foreign body ingestion, trauma, and ongoing systemic disease are imperative.[10] In addition, information about exercise intolerance, stertor or stridor, vomiting, difficulty swallowing, drug therapy, polyuria, polydipsia, polyphagia, and toxins are collected as part of a complete history.[10]

In summary, physical examination findings and the medical history of the patient may help identify the cause of respiratory distress or at least allow the origin to be localized to one of the following anatomical regions: (1) airway; (2) pulmonary parenchyma; (3) pleural space; or (4) thoracic wall.[2]

Prompt identification of the anatomical origin of dyspnea will aid in swift and appropriate treatment, as outlined below.

Airway Obstruction

DEFINITION AND CLINICAL SIGNS

The upper airways include the larynx and pharynx, the trachea, and the mainstem bronchi. Clinical signs of upper airway obstruction may include inspiratory and/or expiratory stridor or stertor, cyanosis, extension of the head and neck, orthopnea, exercise intolerance, choking, collapse, retching, frothing at the mouth, attempting to vomit, clawing at the face and neck, and honking sounds.[2] Animals may present with slow, pronounced inspiratory effort, but when they become distressed, rapid, stridorous effort may occur. With lower airway obstruction, forceful expiratory effort may be observed. Clinical signs may change depending on the location and the severity of the lesion.

DIFFERENTIAL DIAGNOSIS

Diseases of the upper airways include infections (e.g., viral fungal, or bacterial upper respiratory infection), inflammatory diseases (e.g., pharyngitis/laryngitis), pharyngeal edema, laryngeal paralysis, laryngeal spasm, foreign body, hematoma, nasopharyngeal polyp, neoplasia, abscesses, granulomatous disease, collapsing trachea, coagulopathies with tracheal bleeding, tracheal tears or avulsions, and tracheal stenosis.[1,2,15-25] Other examples include upper airway obstruction from trauma (e.g., facial and mandibular fractures), epistaxis, angioneurotic edema from an anaphylactic reaction, soft palate displacement, and brachycephalic disease.[1]

Laryngeal paralysis is a common cause of upper airway obstruction that can be seen in many breeds. Congenital laryngeal paralysis has been described in the Bouvier des Flandres (autosomal dominant), Siberian husky, and the English bulldog.[15] Acquired laryngeal paralysis occurs typically in middle age to older dogs, and may be bilateral or unilateral. Signs of exercise intolerance, stridor, altered vocalization, and gagging may be noted, and affected animals may have severe respiratory distress, hypoxemia, hypercapnia, and syncopal episodes.[21,23] Upper airway obstruction may cause noncardiogenic pulmonary edema or aspiration pneumonia, exacerbating the respiratory distress.[25] Auscultation reveals stridorous, referred upper airway noise, loudest over the larynx or cervical trachea on inspiration.

Another cause of upper airway respiratory distress includes tracheal foreign bodies such as foxtails, plant awns, bones, marbles, balls, parasitic infections (e.g., granulomas, *Cuterebra* spp.), and food. Foreign bodies often lodge at the bifurcation of the mainstem bronchi.[26] It is important to distinguish signs of an esophageal foreign body (e.g., pawing at the face, gagging, or retching) from those of a tracheal foreign body. Auscultation reveals exaggerated inspiration or expiration (depending on the location of the obstruction), which may be loudest over the trachea.

Tracheal stenosis, although uncommon, may be seen with neoplastic disease, previous tracheal surgery, endotracheal tube pressure necrosis, scar formation from previous trauma (blunt or penetrating), a previous tracheostomy, abscesses, vascular anomalies, or granulomas.[1,26]

Tracheal collapse is another common cause of upper airway respiratory distress, with an average age of onset at approximately 7 years. Dyspnea may be seen during either inspiration (cervical trachea) or expiration (thoracic trachea). The cartilaginous rings and/or the dorsal tracheal membrane may be involved. If the dorsal membrane is redundant or weak (grade 1or 2), the membrane will sink or fall into the cervical tracheal lumen during inspiration.[15] During expiration, the membrane results in a functional stenosis of the intrathoracic trachea.[15] If the cartilaginous rings are unable to maintain the C configuration due to hypoplasia or fibrodystrophia (grade 3 or 4), the tracheal lumen is further diminished, resulting in a smaller cross-sectional area of the functional lumen and higher airway resistance.[15] Auscultation reveals referred upper airway noises loudest over the trachea, along with a honking cough.[1]

Brachycephalic airway syndrome (most commonly seen in English bulldogs, boxers, Boston bull terriers, pugs, Chinese shar-peis, French bulldogs, Pekingese, and Shih-Tzus) is characterized by an elongated soft palate, stenotic nares, everted laryngeal saccules, a hypoplastic trachea, and laryngeal malformation.[1,2,15,27] Brachycephalic airway obstructive disease may lead to acute respiratory distress when the animal is exposed to stress, heat, anesthesia, sedation, or excitement. Hyperplastic or hypertrophied pharyngeal tissue and eversion of the lateral ventricles of the larynx may be seen due to increased negative pressure in the oropharynx during inspiration.[28]

INITIAL MANAGEMENT

Initial management of animals with dyspnea caused by an upper airway obstruction should be based on the philosophy "above all, do no harm." Emergency stabilization should begin with oxygen supplementation. Cooling the patient is imperative because adequate heat dissipation may not occur due to ineffective panting. The use of cool oxygen supplementation, administration of cool intravenous fluids, alcohol application to the foot pads, wetting the patient's hair coat, application of ice packs, and cooling fans may quickly decrease core body temperature.

Sedation or anxiolytic pharmacological therapy is often beneficial because reduction of central respiratory drive may decrease the amount of negative inspiratory pressure being generated, reducing the degree of collapse of the extrathoracic soft tissue structures. Acepromazine maleate* (0.025 to 0.1 mg/kg IV or IM) or butorphanol tartrate† (0.1 to 0.2 mg/kg IV) may be used as anxiolytic agents.[2] Corticosteroids may be beneficial at an antiinflammatory dose (e.g., dexamethasone sodium phosphate‡ 0.05 to 0.1 mg/kg IV or IM) to decrease laryngeal and pharyngeal edema, inflammation, or swelling. Judicious use of steroids is important because their use may mask a diagnosis of lymphosarcoma; however, withholding corticosteroids may jeopardize patients with severe airway inflammation.

In animals with profound or complete airway obstruction, or in those that do not respond to stabilization efforts within a short time, a secure and patent airway must be obtained as soon as possible. Initially it is appropriate to attempt orotracheal intubation, but if there is a mass or foreign body obstructing the upper airway, an emergency tracheostomy may be needed. In emergency situations, a red rubber catheter can sometimes be passed around the obstruction and oxygen bubbled into the airway to provide oxygenation until an airway is secured.

DIAGNOSTIC TESTING

Diagnosis of upper airway obstruction is based on physical examination, but distinction of the cause of the obstruction usually relies on direct visualization, which typically requires anesthesia. Radiographs may be bene-

*Acepromazine, Boehringer, St Joseph, Mo.
†Butorphanol, Fort Dodge, Fort Dodge, Iowa.
‡Dexamethasone sodium phosphate, American Regent, Shirley, N.Y.

ficial in defining tumors, tracheal disease, collapsing trachea, fractures, or radiopaque foreign bodies. However, great care must be exercised when taking radiographs in awake patients with upper airway obstruction because positioning often impedes respiration and the diagnostic benefit may not outweigh the risk to the patient. Radiographs should be taken as efficiently as possible; personnel should be gowned, the animal premeasured, and the machine pre-set to allow minimal handling time without oxygen therapy.[2] A single view in the least stressful position may be diagnostic. In many cases the safest approach is to delay radiography until the patient is anesthetized and the airway has been secured.

Sedation or anesthesia is required for a thorough oropharyngeal, laryngeal, and upper airway examination, which is an essential part of diagnosing upper airway disease. This allows assessment of the upper airway; laryngeal function; and the presence of soft tissue swellings, foreign bodies, edema, polyps, or neoplasia. While anesthetized, biopsies of any abnormal tissue should be obtained because multiple sedations should be avoided in these critically ill patients. Ideally, definitive management of the problem, by removal of the obstruction or placement of a tracheostomy tube, should occur prior to extubation.

To evaluate laryngeal function and vocal fold function, the timing and degree of movement of the larynx are assessed under light sedation. The normal palate should barely overlap the tip of the epiglottis, and should be examined for any signs of thickness, inflammation, or elongation.

Other tools necessary to diagnose upper airway disease include a dental mirror, fluoroscopy, and bronchoscopy. The dental mirror is warmed to reduce fogging, then used to evaluate the nasopharynx for polyps or foreign bodies by looking above the soft palate. Fluoroscopy may determine the presence of tracheal collapse (e.g., cervical versus intrathoracic). Bronchoscopy allows evaluation of the larynx, oropharyngeal area, trachea, and mainstem bronchi; in addition, the removal of foreign bodies, as well as biopsies from structures in the lumen of the lower airways, may also be performed.[2]

In animals with airway obstruction by foreign bodies, the Heimlich maneuver can be attempted by holding the animal in a head-down position and applying a sharp abdominal compression to the cranial abdomen; however, this is often unsuccessful, and endoscopy may be necessary to retrieve the foreign body. In rare instances, foreign bodies may be difficult to retrieve, even with endoscopy. If the animal cannot ventilate appropriately due to the foreign body, the foreign body can be pushed into a distal bronchus so that the animal can appropriately ventilate until surgery can be performed.

Pulmonary Parenchyma

DEFINITION AND CLINICAL SIGNS

Parenchymal lung disease often results in hypoxemia due to diffusion impairment, shunting, and ventilation/perfusion mismatch. Clinical signs include open mouth breathing, paradoxical respiration, cyanosis, nasal flare, coughing, gagging, dyspnea, anxiety, and orthopnea. Physical examination findings with parenchymal disease vary depending on the origin of the disease process. In animals with primary cardiac disease and congestive heart failure, crackles, heart murmurs, or arrhythmias may be present on auscultation. Clinical signs of other parenchymal diseases may include coughing, hemoptysis, fever, tachypnea, weakness, depression, anorexia, mucopurulent nasal discharge, tachycardia, dyspnea, cyanosis, and panting.[1,28,29]

DIFFERENTIAL DIAGNOSIS

Examples of common pulmonary parenchymal diseases include pneumonia (e.g., bacterial or aspiration), neoplasia, pulmonary contusions, pulmonary edema (cardiogenic versus noncardiogenic), dirofilaria infection, and pulmonary thromboembolism.[1,2] Other causes include fungal infection, smoke inhalation, toxin inhalation, uremic pneumonitis, and acute respiratory distress syndrome (ARDS).[1,2]

Pneumonia is one of the most common causes of lung parenchymal disease in dogs, occurring due to viral, bacterial, or fungal infection; aspiration; or secondary to smoke inhalation or asthma. Due to decreased airway defense mechanisms, decreased mucociliary clearance, or systemic immunosuppression, bacteria and fungi can proliferate in the moist, warm environment of the lung parenchyma. Aspirated foreign material or inflammatory/infectious exudates decrease the surface area for gas exchange, preventing carbon dioxide and oxygen transfer and resulting in life-threatening respiratory distress. Auscultation may reveal crackles; increased bronchovesicular sounds; or, rarely, decreased lung sounds due to severe consolidation.

Traumatic causes of pulmonary parenchymal disease may result from high-rise syndrome, vehicular accidents, or abuse.[1,30,31] Pulmonary contusions are sequelae of a compression-decompression injury to the thoracic body wall that occurs while the glottis is open.[32] This injury results in rupture of the alveoli and adjacent blood vessels[33-36] and hemorrhage into the intraalveolar and interstitial tissue. Progressive loss of plasma constituents into the interstitium and air spaces is accompanied by infiltration of cells, inflammatory mediators, and edema fluid.[1,32] Decreased lung compliance, ventilation/perfusion mismatch, and a gas diffusion barrier result in decreased arterial partial pressure of oxygen. Pulmonary contusions can vary in severity, causing mild to severe respiratory distress. Concurrent injuries are often present, including pneumothorax, rib fractures, or diaphragmatic hernia. In animals with pulmonary contusions, increased bronchovesicular sounds or crackles may be auscultated throughout the affected lung fields.

Pulmonary edema, or the accumulation of excessive fluid within the pulmonary interstitium and alveoli, may have cardiogenic or noncardiogenic origins. In the normal lung, alveolar fluid accumulation is prevented by a combination of the thin alveolar epithelium, alveolar-capillary interstitial space, and the pulmonary capillary endothelium.[1] Tight junctions between the alveolar epithelial cells prevent movement of fluid into the alveoli.[1] Loose junctions between endothelial cells allow movement of fluid, electrolytes, and protein. Fluid leaking from the pulmonary capillaries is absorbed by the pulmonary lymphatic vessels and returned to the venous system. When the capacity of the lymphatic system is exceeded, excessive interstitial fluid accumulates.[1] When pressure in the interstitium exceeds the alveolar pressure, fluid accumulates in the alveolar spaces and fulminant pulmonary edema is recognized in the patient.[1] Fluid accumulation therefore depends on capillary hydrostatic and oncotic pressure, interstitial hydrostatic and oncotic pressure, normal lymphatic function, and the integrity of normal capillary wall ultrastructure.[1] As alveolar fluid accumulates, ventilation-perfusion mismatching and diffusion impairment occurs, resulting in hypoxemia. In animals with pulmonary edema, crackles can be auscultated throughout the affected lung fields.

Pulmonary thromboembolism (PTE) is most commonly seen in dogs with dirofilariasis,[37,38] but it also occurs in association with hyperadrenocorticism, immune-mediated hemolytic anemia, nephrotic syndrome, protein-losing nephropathy, glomerulonephritis, neoplasia, sepsis, vasculitis, disseminated intravascular coagulation, pancreatitis, cardiac disease, hypothyroidism, bacterial endocarditis, and polycythemia.[37-43] Coughing, dyspnea, hemoptysis, fever, anorexia, and depression may be present,[38] and auscultation may reveal increased bronchovesicular sounds or crackles. PTE may be difficult to diagnose because it has no classic radiographic appearance.[44] Radiographic changes include increased alveolar densities that are usually indistinct and fluffy, but may be triangular or lobar.[1,44] Hypovascular regions may be noted in up to 50% of cases, and mild pleural effusion may be seen.[1,44] Diagnostic techniques for PTE can include computerized tomographic angiography and ventilation-perfusion scintigraphy.[45]

Acute respiratory distress syndrome is defined as life-threatening, acute, respiratory failure caused by noncardiogenic pulmonary edema and heterogeneous acute lung injury. It is characterized by normal pulmonary capillary wedge pressure, impaired pulmonary compliance, acute pulmonary arterial hypertension, refractory hypoxemia, and radiographic findings consistent with diffuse bilateral pulmonary infiltration.[46] The multifactorial pathophysiology of ARDS includes injury to the alveolar-capillary membrane by inflammatory mediators, resulting in protein exudation, inactivation of surfactant, and type II pneumocyte damage.[46] Fluid and protein may leak into the gas exchange areas of the lung, resulting in stiff lungs with low functional residual capacity, severe hypoxemia, and impaired compliance.[46] Compensatory vasoconstriction and occlusion of pulmonary microvasculature may result in pulmonary hypertension, further causing right ventricular dysfunction.[46] Clinical signs can include dyspnea, shallow breathing, hyperventilation, tachycardia, and cyanosis. Auscultation findings vary but usually reveal crackles or increased bronchovesicular sounds.

Smoke inhalation occasionally causes pulmonary parenchymal disease and cyanosis. Accumulation of microparticles of carbon in the lower airways is accompanied by decreased mucociliary clearance due to smoke or thermal damage to the mucociliary elevator. Thermal injury can cause edema and swelling of the nasal, oral, or pharyngeal tissue resulting in upper airway obstruction.[1,47,48] Hypoxemia may result from the formation of carboxyhemoglobin.[49] Auscultation may reveal increased bronchovesicular sounds and crackles, and expiratory wheezes due to small airway narrowing from mucosal swelling and bronchoconstriction.

INITIAL MANAGEMENT

Initial management of animals with dyspnea due to pulmonary parenchymal disease includes oxygen supplementation and provision of a stress-free environment. Because many of these patients have similar clinical findings (e.g., dyspnea, cyanosis, and crackles on auscultation) but are too unstable for extensive diagnostic testing, possible diagnoses may be inferred based on the history, signalment, and physical examination. The history can often provide helpful information about the possible etiology of respiratory distress. For example, pulmonary hemorrhage can be suspected in a patient that has sustained trauma or ingested a rodenticide, and aspiration pneumonia might be considered in a weak dog with a history of regurgitation. A brief physical examination, targeted towards the cardiopulmonary system, may also be very helpful, especially if a heart murmur or arrhythmia is auscultated.

Ideally, thoracic radiographs and other diagnostic tests are required in order to distinguish the various causes of pulmonary parenchymal disease. If the patient is initially too unstable to perform diagnostic testing, it is reasonable to treat empirically for the most likely diagnosis. In extremely unstable patients that do not respond to oxygen supplementation and empiric drug therapy, intubation and positive pressure ventilation may be required to overcome hypoxemia, to reduce the work of breathing, and to allow diagnostic testing. Positive end expiratory pressure may be beneficial to recruit alveoli.

In addition to oxygen supplementation, treatment for suspected cases of pneumonia includes nebulization and coupage, maintenance of hydration, and broad-spectrum antibiotic therapy pending culture and sensitivity results.[1] Treatment for cardiogenic pulmonary edema includes diuretic administration and vasodilators such as nitroglycerin.*[50] Management of PTE may include anticoagulation with heparin, administration of thrombolytics, and treatment for the underlying cause of hypercoagulability. There is no specific treatment for animals with pulmonary contusions, smoke inhalation, ARDS, or noncardiogenic pulmonary edema; supportive care, oxygen therapy, and positive pressure ventilation may be indicated, along with removal of the underlying cause.

Additional supportive care for patients with pulmonary parenchymal disease may also include careful

---

*Nitroglycerin 2%, Fougera Division of Altana, Inc., Melville, N.Y.

intravenous fluid therapy. Caution should be exercised while providing intravenous fluids because aggressive use of fluid therapy can cause fluid overload of damaged alveolar epithelium and capillary endothelium, resulting in progression of respiratory distress regardless of the etiology of the pulmonary parenchymal disease. Sedation may help to improve efficiency of gas exchange, reduce oxygen demand, and decrease anxiety. Morphine* may be used (0.04 to 0.11 mg/kg SQ, IM, or IV) to increase systemic venous capacitance, reduce sympathetic stimulation, and act as a mild venodilator and anxiolytic.

DIAGNOSTIC TESTING

Diagnostic investigation for pulmonary parenchymal disease should be pursued after initial stabilization with oxygen therapy. Radiographs are one of the most important diagnostic tests; however, they should only be obtained if the animal is deemed stable. In dogs, a caudodorsal alveolar radiographic pattern with a normal cardiac silhouette may support a tentative diagnosis of noncardiogenic or neurogenic pulmonary edema, whereas a perihilar alveolar pattern, cardiomegaly, and venous distension suggest congestive heart failure. Contusions may be radiographically evident as a patchy alveolar pattern; the location is dependent on the area and time of trauma. In animals with bronchopneumonia, the initial radiographic appearance may be a bronchointerstitial pattern that may progress to an alveolar pattern. With aspiration pneumonia, a cranioventral alveolar pattern may be evident. The radiographic appearance of PTE is variable but may include any combination from normal lung fields to pleural effusion, patchy alveolar infiltrates, hyperlucent lung fields, and truncated pulmonary arteries.[2,44] Acute respiratory distress syndrome can cause a generalized or patchy alveolar pattern.[46,51] Granulomatous disease and neoplasia may appear as multiple nodular, diffuse nodular, or miliary patterns.

Diagnostic testing for pulmonary parenchymal disease also includes obtaining samples from the airways and lungs by techniques such as transtracheal wash (TTW), endotracheal lavage (ETL), bronchoalveolar lavage (BAL), or fine needle lung aspirates. Samples are analyzed cytologically and cultured for bacteria or fungi as appropriate. Bronchoscopy and BAL may be utilized to identify lower airway disease. Ultrasound-guided (or CT-guided) lung aspirates and biopsies can be useful for ruling out neoplasia, abscesses, chronic fibrosis, granulomas, and fungal disease.

Ancillary testing may also include coagulation testing in animals with suspected coagulopathies or thrombosis, serology in animals with possible fungal pneumonia, or fecal analysis in those suspected of having lungworms. In animals suspected of neoplasia or sepsis, diagnostic tests should include evaluation of the abdomen by radiographs or ultrasound. Echocardiography may be required in animals that might have primary cardiac disease.

*Morphine, Elkins-Sinn, Cherry Hill, N.J.

Pleural Space

DEFINITION AND CLINICAL SIGNS

The pleural space is the serous membrane that lines the entire thoracic cavity. It is composed of two layers: the visceral pleura, which covers the lungs; and the parietal pleura, which covers the remaining thoracic cavity.[15] The pleura consists of a thin layer of mesothelial cells supported by elastic connective tissue. The parietal pleura contains a rich lymphatic system that drains the pleural cavity. The space between the right and left pleural membrane sacs forms the mediastinum, a median partition in the thorax where the heart and other thoracic organs lie.[52] A small amount of pleural fluid (approximately 2.4 ml in a 10 kg dog) is normal; this allows instantaneous and complete transmission of thoracic volume changes to the lung and low-friction sliding between the pleural spaces. However, as fluid or air accumulates between the pleura, the resultant loss of negative pleural pressure causes the lungs to collapse due to elastic recoil.[53,54] Pleural effusion absorption and production is controlled by Starling's forces. Effusion results when pleural fluid dynamics favor decreased fluid absorption or increased fluid formation.[15] It is still undetermined whether the left and right pleural cavities are normally completely separate or simply disrupted in the presence of pathology. Pleural air or fluid accumulation may be evident bilaterally or may occur predominantly on either the left or the right sides.

Clinical signs in animals with pleural space disease include short, shallow breaths; tachypnea; open mouth breathing; cyanosis; and signs of respiratory distress. Thoracic auscultation may reveal dull lung sounds (dorsally or ventrally), muffled heart sounds, the presence of gastrointestinal sounds, or an auscultable fluid line.

DIFFERENTIAL DIAGNOSIS

The pleural space can cause respiratory distress when occupied by air, fluid, neoplasia, or abdominal organs. Specific causes of pleural space disease include pneumothorax, heart disease, hemorrhage, pyothorax, chylothorax, neoplasia, lung lobe torsion, vascular leak syndromes, hypoalbuminemia, and diaphragmatic hernia.[1,2]

Pneumothorax may be due to rupture of the major airways or lung parenchyma as a result of thoracic trauma; penetrating wounds; perforation of the esophagus; or as a result of bullous, necrotizing, or neoplastic lung disease that allows air to freely enter the pleural space.[55,56] Iatrogenic pneumothorax may result from intrathoracic surgery, resuscitative efforts, positive pressure ventilation, or lung aspirates.[1] Auscultation reveals dull lung sounds dorsally and increased bronchovesicular sounds ventrally.

A variety of different fluids can accumulate in the pleural cavity; therefore, thoracocentesis and fluid analysis is imperative in animals with pleural space disease. Regardless of the type of pleural effusion, auscultation may reveal dull lung and heart sounds ventrally and increased bronchovesicular sounds dorsally. Chylothorax is the accumulation of chyle in the thoracic cavity as a result of disruption of the thoracic duct. It can be seen with lymphangiectasia (in breeds such as the Afghan hound and Shiba Inu[57]), cranial vena cava obstruction, neoplasia, fungal infection, dirofilariasis, diaphragmatic hernia, lung lobe torsion, heart disease, or trauma (rupture of the thoracic duct).[1] Pyothorax (empyema) is the presence of a septic exudate within the thoracic cavity. Causes of pyothorax include penetrating wounds to the thorax or esophagus; hematogenous spread of infection; migration of foreign bodies; or extension of infections from the abdomen, mediastinum, thoracic body wall, or lungs.

Pure or modified transudates may accumulate within the thoracic cavity due to increased hydrostatic pressure in animals with right-sided congestive heart failure or to decreased oncotic pressure in animals with severe hypoalbuminemia. Serosanguinous pleural effusions may occur in animals with vascular leak syndromes, PTE, neoplasia, lung lobe torsion, or diaphragmatic hernia. Hemothorax may result from trauma, coagulopathy, or neoplasia.

Diaphragmatic hernia and lung lobe torsion are two surgical emergencies that can cause severe respiratory distress. A nonseptic pleural exudate, with a high nucleated cell count and high protein count, is often observed. Auscultation may reveal focally dull lung sounds or borborygmi.

INITIAL MANAGEMENT

Initial management of animals with pleural space disease includes oxygen supplementation and immediate thoracocentesis. Thoracocentesis allows reexpansion of the lungs, which have been compressed by fluid, soft tissue, or air. Therefore thoracocentesis is recommended prior to radiography in order to stabilize the patient and to allow better radiographic interpretation. Any fluid collected by thoracocentesis should be submitted for diagnostic purposes (e.g., cytology, cell counts and protein determination, and microbiologic culture including both aerobic and anaerobic bacterial cultures).

In most cases thoracocentesis results in rapid stabilization of the patient and further testing can then follow. Diagnostics can include thoracic radiographs (e.g., horizontal beam studies), echocardiography, thoracic ultrasonography, or computerized tomography. These tests may allow identification of the cause of pleural space disease (e.g., intrathoracic masses, underlying heart disease, or other pathologic processes).

If negative pressure is not reached at the end of the thoracocentesis (tension pneumothorax) or if the patient deteriorates again and repeated thoracocentesis is necessary (e.g., in animals with a rapidly forming pleural effusion), thoracostomy tube placement is recommended.[58,59]

Although rare, reexpansion pulmonary edema can occur when chronically compressed lungs are suddenly reexpanded.[2] It has been reported in humans within 24 hours of pleural evacuation and in dogs and cats within 2 hours after surgical repair of pectus excavatum and diaphragmatic hernia.[60-63] Reexpansion pulmonary edema

results in accumulation of protein-rich fluid in the alveoli due to free radical-induced injury to the pulmonary vasculature. It may also be associated with decreased surfactant concentration and a rapid increase in negative interstitial pressure that causes a rapid increase in pulmonary blood flow and capillary pressure.[60-63]

Definitive management depends on the cause of the pleural effusion. Animals with chylothorax may require surgical treatment (e.g., thoracic duct ligation, partial pericardectomy, or omentalization) to be implemented following stabilization. Those with pyothorax may require resuscitation for septic shock and endotoxemia using intravenous fluid therapy and broad-spectrum antibiotics. Thoracostomy tube placement, to lavage and effectively drain the pleural space, is indicated once the patient is stable. A thoracotomy may be necessary if abscessation of the lung is present or if severe pulmonary parenchymal disease does not respond to medical management. Antibiotic therapy should be based on gram-stain results, pending culture results.[64]

In animals with hemothorax or coagulopathies, unless severe dyspnea is occurring as a result of the effusion, the hemorrhagic fluid should be allowed to passively absorb from the pleural cavity. Treatment may include surgery for a diaphragmatic hernia or lung lobe torsion, or administration of plasma and vitamin K* for animals with coagulopathies.

THORACIC TUBE PLACEMENT

Thoracostomy tubes should be placed in animals that require multiple thoracocentesis attempts over a short time; those in which negative pressure is not reached; or animals that require repeated effective thoracic drainage (e.g., animals with pyothorax). Ideally, general anesthesia would be beneficial for full control of ventilation during thoracostomy tube placement; however, critically ill animals have a high risk for respiratory arrest with sedation. A light sedative and a local intercostal nerve block may be utilized instead if necessary. In decompensated animals, or in those with a tension pneumothorax, an assistant can continue to aspirate air from the thorax to maximize oxygenation as anesthesia is induced.[2]

The size of the thoracostomy tube varies with the size of the animal. The size of the tube to be placed can be estimated by comparison with the size of the mainstem bronchus on radiographs. Designated thoracostomy tubes containing placement stylets are available; these produce good resolution of gas or pleural effusion. Other tubes*(e.g., red rubber catheters†) can also be used but may have a greater tendency to kink during use.

For placement, the lateral thorax is clipped from the point of the elbow to the last rib, extending from the dorsal spine to the ventral midline. Aseptic technique must be used to prevent iatrogenic infection. A small skin incision should be made in the dorsal third of the lateral thoracic wall at approximately the tenth intercostal space.[1,2,15] A subcutaneous tunnel can be bluntly dis-

---

*Vitamin K, Phoenix Pharmaceutical, Inc., St Joseph, Mo.
†Red rubber catheter, Kendall Co., Mansfield, Mass.

sected towards the elbow (in a cranioventral direction) over three to four intercostal spaces, and then the tube is placed into the seventh or eighth intercostal space. Alternatively, an assistant can stretch the skin forward to allow the thoracostomy tube to be placed in the seventh or eighth intercostal space, which would cause a tunnel under the skin of approximately three intercostal spaces. Using hemostatic forceps to bluntly dissect through the intercostal muscles and to hold the tip of the tube, the tube is introduced into the seventh or eighth intercostal space with a brisk but controlled thrust directed towards the opposing shoulder. Prior to introduction of the tube into the pleural cavity, manual ventilation is transiently stopped to prevent expansion of lung against the point of the tube; this decreases the incidence of iatrogenic trauma. The thoracostomy tube can then be introduced into the cranial ventral pleural space as it is being fed off the stylet. The stylet can be used as a measure of how far the tube should be advanced.

The tube is then sutured to the thoracic wall skin using a purse string suture and Chinese finger trap. A liberal amount of antiseptic ointment aids in preventing air leakage around the tube site and decreases migration of bacteria along the tube. A light bandage should then cover the chest, and radiographs should be taken to confirm the placement of the chest tube. A three-way stopcock is attached to form a closed system. Close 24-hour monitoring of the patient is imperative due to the risks of disconnection, biting the tube or collection system, iatrogenic pneumothorax, and air leaking into the chest around the tube.[2]

Pain management is imperative after thoracostomy tube placement because pain can exacerbate signs of respiratory distress and may cause reluctance to take deep breaths, resulting in atelectasis. After removing all of the effusion or air, bupivacaine* (1.5 mg/kg IP every 6 to 8 hours) can be infused into each chest tube, diluted with an equal amount of air or saline. Bupivacaine can be painful during initial injection because it is an acidic solution.

After thoracostomy tube placement, either intermittent or continuous pleural evacuation can be used. Intermittent pleural drainage is chosen when the repeated accumulation of pleural effusion or air is neither rapid nor excessive in amount. Intermittent aspiration of the chest tubes allows accurate measurement of both fluid and air volumes and allows the entire tube to be protected and incorporated in the bandage, reducing the risk of removal by the patient. However, the amount of negative pressure exerted on the pleural cavity can be difficult to control during intermittent aspiration, and excessive negative pressure may occasionally result in recurrence of pneumothorax. Continuous suction is beneficial because it creates a continuous, controlled amount of negative pressure in the pleural space, possibly aiding in sealing lung leaks and reducing the incidence of pleuropulmonary fistulas or hemorrhage by keeping the pleural surfaces consistently in contact. Continuous suction is indicated when excessive amounts of effusion or air accumulate at a life-threatening rate. Many different systems are available for continuous pleural evacuation (e.g., Thora-Seal III system*). Disadvantages of continuous suction systems include their expense and complicated nature, the fact that the animal cannot easily be moved while connected to such a system, and the risk of disconnection and iatrogenic pneumothorax.

After being in place for more than a day or two, the tubes themselves may induce formation of a pleural effusion (up to 2 to 10 ml/kg/day) until the tube is removed.[15] When air and fluid are no longer actively being evacuated in large volumes, or when the character of the effusion has become benign (in the case of animals with pyothorax), the thoracostomy tubes should be removed. After removal, antiseptic ointment and a light bandage should be used to cover the site, minimizing subcutaneous emphysema.

Thoracic Wall

DEFINITION AND CLINICAL SIGNS

Thoracic wall function must be evaluated in any animal with respiratory distress. Injury to the thoracic wall may result in rib fractures, flail chest, sucking chest wounds, and penetrating wounds. Such an injury correlates closely with both pleural space disease and parenchymal lung disease because hemothorax, pneumothorax, diaphragmatic hernia, and pulmonary contusions may also result. Nontraumatic disorders of thoracic wall function include neurological, muscular, and orthopedic disease.

Typically, animals with failure of thoracic wall function have evidence of varying degrees of hypoventilation due to failure of the bellows apparatus. Clinical signs include evidence of respiratory distress, cyanosis, decreased chest wall movement, lack of diaphragmatic and abdominal movement during respiration, and lack of intercostal muscle assistance in respiration. Animals with thoracic wall injuries may have obvious lacerations or bruising, or evidence of air movement into the wound during respiration. Flail chest may be manifested by the presence of a segment of ribs that moves independently of the rest of the ribcage, typically collapsing inwards during inspiration.

DIFFERENTIAL DIAGNOSIS

Various thoracic wall injuries can be sustained during trauma, including rib fractures, flail chest, and penetrating chest wounds. Peripheral nerve and neuromuscular junction disorders (e.g., myasthenia gravis, botulism, tick paralysis, and polyradiculoneuritis) can affect the movement of the thoracic wall, along with central neurologic disorders, anesthesia, hypoventilation, metabolic disease, spinal cord disease (in the area of C_1 to C_4 from trauma or disk disease), disease involving phrenic innervation (C_5 to C_6), and severe electrolyte abnormalities such as hypokalemia.[2]

---

*Bupivacaine, Abbott Labs, North Chicago, Ill.

*Thora-Seal III, Argyle, Sherwood Medical Company, St Louis, Mo.

INITIAL MANAGEMENT

Treatment of severe hypoventilation due to thoracic wall dysfunction involves controlling thoracic wall movement and supplementing oxygen by intubation and ventilation while the underlying disease is being identified and addressed. Stabilizing and protecting the pleural space (i.e., thoracocentesis to relieve pneumothorax) is a priority in animals with thoracic wall trauma. Animals with flail chest should be restrained with the flail side down on the table, which often results in rapid stabilization. Often the underlying lung contusion and the severity of pain is the primary cause of dyspnea, rather than the flail segment itself; therefore, stabilization of a flail segment is rarely necessary in an emergency setting.[65,66] Healthy anesthetized dogs with experimentally induced flail segments rarely had significant distortion of their normal respiratory motion; rather, pain and contusions appear to be the cause of the deleterious effects of flail chest.[66]

Monitoring Patients with Respiratory Distress

Because animals with respiratory distress can decompensate very quickly, careful monitoring is imperative. Serial physical examinations must be performed to assess respiratory rate, respiratory effort, auscultation findings, mucous membrane color, pulse quality, and capillary refill time. Both noninvasive and invasive monitoring can be used depending on the animal's stability. Options include serial measurement of pulse oximetry, end-tidal carbon dioxide monitoring, and arterial blood gas analysis.

Pulse oximetry is a noninvasive, nonpainful, and readily available tool to monitor oxygen saturation.[67,68] Hemoglobin saturation of 95% and greater is normal, but values greater than 93% are acceptable in room air.[67] Pulse oximeter values less than 90% may indicate severe hypoxemia and correlate with a Pao_2 of 60 mm Hg on the oxyhemoglobin-dissociation curve. End-tidal CO_2 ($ETco_2$) monitoring measures the exhaled alveolar carbon dioxide concentration, but is usually reserved for anesthetized animals.[69] Normal $ETco_2$ values are 35 to 45 mm Hg, and values exceeding 50 mm Hg are predictive of hypoventilation. Arterial blood gas analysis remains the most objective way to monitor oxygenation and ventilation. Normal values include a Pao_2 of greater than 85 mm Hg and a $Paco_2$ between 35 and 45 mm Hg.[14]

REFERENCES

1. Taboada J, Hoskins JD, Morgan RV: Respiratory emergencies. In Emergency medicine and critical care: The compendium collection, Trenton, NJ, 1992, WB Saunders.
2. Tseng LW, Waddell LS: Approach to the patient in respiratory distress, Clin Tech Sm An Prac 215(2):53-62, 2000.
3. McDonnell W: Respiratory system. In Thurmon JC, Tranquilli WJ, Benson GJ, editors: Lumb & Jones veterinary anesthesia, Baltimore, 1996, Williams & Wilkins.
4. Marino PL: Hypoxemia and hypercapnia. In The ICU book, ed 2, Baltimore, 1998, Williams & Wilkins.
5. Stedman's pocket medical dictionary, Baltimore, 1987, Williams & Wilkins.
6. Stepien RL: Cyanosis. In Ettinger SJ, Feldman EC, editors: Textbook of veterinary internal medicine, Philadelphia, 2000, WB Saunders.
7. Aldrich J, Haskins SC: Monitoring the critically ill patient. In Bonagura JD, editor: Kirk's current veterinary therapy, vol 12, Philadelphia, 1995, WB Saunders.
8. Dumonceaux GA: Illicit drug intoxication in dogs. In Bonagura JD, editor: Kirk's current veterinary therapy, vol 12, Philadelphia, 1995, WB Saunders.
9. Harvey JW: Methemoglobinemia and Heinz-body hemolytic anemia. In Bonagura JD, editor: Kirk's current veterinary therapy, vol 12, Philadelphia, 1995, WB Saunders.
10. Hendricks JC: Respiratory conditions in critical patients, Vet Clin North Am Small Anim Pract 19(6):1167-1188, 1989.
11. West JB: Respiratory physiology: The essentials, ed 6, Philadelphia, 2000, Williams & Wilkins.
12. West JB: Pulmonary pathophysiology, ed 5, Philadelphia, 2000, Williams & Wilkins.
13. Guyton AC: Textbook of medical physiology, ed 9, Philadelphia, 2000, WB Saunders.
14. Drobatz KJ: Respiratory distress: Initial assessment and stabilization and diagnostic evaluation. In Proceedings, Ann Meet Amer Coll Vet Int Med, pp. 810-815, 2000.
15. Slatter D: Textbook of small animal surgery, ed 2, Philadelphia, 1993, WB Saunders.
16. Meuten DJ, Calderwood-Mays MB, Dillman RC et al: Canine laryngeal rhabdomyoma, Vet Pathol 22:533-539, 1985.
17. Saik JE, Toll SL, Diters RW et al: Canine and feline laryngeal neoplasia: A 10 year survey, JAAHA 22:359-365, 1986.
18. Withrow SJ: Tumors of the respiratory tract. In Withrow SJ, MacEwen EG, editors: Clinical veterinary oncology, Philadelphia, 1989, JB Lippincott.
19. Bryan RD, Frome RW: Tracheal leiomyoma in a dog, JAVMA 178(10):1069-1070, 1981.
20. Harvey HJ, Sykes G: Tracheal mast cell tumor in a dog, JAVMA 180(9):1097-1100, 1981.
21. LaHue TR: Treatment of laryngeal paralysis in dogs by unilateral cricoarytenoid laryngoplasty, JAAHA 25:317, 1989.
22. Bjorling DE: Laryngeal paralysis. In Bonagura JD, editor: Kirk's current veterinary therapy, vol 12, Philadelphia, 1995, WB Saunders.
23. Love S, Waterman AE, Lane JG: The assessment of corrective surgery for canine laryngeal paralysis by blood gas analysis: A review of 35 cases, J Small Anim Pract 28:597, 1987.
24. Aron DN: Laryngeal paralysis. In Kirk RW, editor: Current veterinary therapy, vol 10, Philadelphia, 1989, WB Saunders.
25. Gaber CE, Amis TC, LeCouteur A: Laryngeal paralysis in dogs: A review of 23 cases, JAVMA 186:377-380, 1985.
26. Hedlund CS: Surgical disease of the trachea, Vet Clin North Am Small Anim Pract 17:301-332, 1987.
27. Hendricks JC: Recognition and treatment of congenital respiratory tract defects in brachycephalics. In Bonagura JD, editor: Kirk's current veterinary therapy, vol 12, Philadelphia, 1995, WB Saunders.
28. Tams TR: Pneumonia. In Kirk RW, editor: Current veterinary therapy, vol 10, Philadelphia, 1989, WB Saunders.
29. Thayer GW, Robinson SK: Bacterial bronchopneumonia in the dog: A review of 42 cases, JAAHA 20:731-735, 1984.
30. Spackman CJA, Caywood DD: Management of thoracic trauma and chest wall reconstruction, Vet Clin North Am Small Anim Pract 17:431-447, 1987.
31. Whitney WO, Mehlhaff CJ: High-rise syndrome in cats, JAVMA 191:1399-1403, 1987.
32. Hackner SG: Emergency management of traumatic pulmonary contusions, Compendium on Continuing Education 17(5):677-686, 1995.
33. Trinkle JK, Furman RW, Hinshaw MA et al: Pulmonary contusions: Pathogenesis and effect of various resuscitative measures, Ann Thorac Surg 16(6):568-573, 1973.
34. Jones KW: Thoracic trauma, Surg Clin North Am 60(4):957-981, 1980.
35. Trinkle JK: Pulmonary contusions, Ann Thorac Surg 16:568-573, 1973.
36. Oppenheimer L, Craven KD, Forkert L et al: Pathophysiology of pulmonary contusions in the dog, J Appl Physiol 47(4):718-728, 1979.
37. Calvert CA, Rawlings CA: Pulmonary manifestations of heartworm disease, Vet Clin North Am Small Anim Pract 15:991-1009, 1985.
38. LaRue MJ, Murtaugh RJ: Pulmonary thromboembolism in dogs: 47 cases (1986-1987), JAVMA 197:1368-1372, 1990.

39. Burns MG, Kelly AB, Hornof WJ et al: Pulmonary artery thrombosis in three dogs with hyperadrenocorticism, *JAVMA* 178:388-393, 1981.
40. Klein MK, Dow SW, Rosychuk RAW: Pulmonary thromboembolism associated with immune-mediated hemolytic anemia in dogs: 10 cases (1982-1987), *JAVMA* 195:246-250, 1989.
41. Green RA, Russo EA, Green RT et al: Hypoalbuminemia-related platelet hypersensitivity in two dogs with nephrotic syndrome, *JAVMA* 186:485-488, 1985.
42. Green RA, Kabel AL: Hypercoagulable state in three dogs with nephrotic syndrome: Role of acquired antithrombin III deficiency, *JAVMA* 181:914-917, 1982.
43. Dennis JS: The pathophysiologic sequelae of pulmonary thromboembolism, *Compend Contin Educ Pract Vet* 13(12):1811-1818, 1991.
44. Fluckiger MA, Gomez JA: Radiographic findings in dogs with spontaneous pulmonary thrombosis or embolism, *Vet Radiol* 25:124-131, 1984.
45. Koblik PD, Hornof W, Harnagel SH et al: A comparison of pulmonary angiography, digital subtraction angiography, and ^{99m}Tc-DTPA/MAA ventilation-perfusion scintigraphy for detection of experimental pulmonary emboli in the dog, *Vet Radiol* 30:159-168, 1989.
46. Parent C, King L, Walker L et al: Clinical and clinicopathologic findings in dogs with acute respiratory distress syndrome: 19 cases (1985-1993), *J Am Vet Med Assoc* 208:1419-1427, 1996.
47. Drobatz KD, Walker LM, Hendricks JC: Smoke exposure in dogs: 27 cases (1988-1997), *J Am Vet Med Assoc* 215:1306-1311, 1999.
48. Drobatz KD, Walker LM, Hendricks JC: Smoke exposure in cats: 22 cases (1986-1997), *J Am Vet Med Assoc* 215:1312-1316,1999.
49. Tams TR, Scherding RG: Smoke inhalation injury, *Compend Contin Educ Pract Vet* 3(11):986-992, 1981.
50. Keene BW, Bonagura JD: Therapy of heart failure. In Bonagura JD, editor: *Kirk's current veterinary therapy*, vol 12, Philadelphia, 1995, WB Saunders.
51. Crowe DT: Traumatic pulmonary contusions, hematomas, pseudocysts and acute respiratory distress syndrome: An update—Part I, *Compend Contin Educ* 5:396-402, 1983.
52. Cunningham JG. The respiratory apparatus. In Cunningham JG: *Textbook of veterinary physiology*, Philadelphia, 1992, WB Saunders.
53. Kagan KG, Stiff ME: Pleural disease. In Kirk RW, editor: *Current veterinary therapy*, vol 8, Philadelphia, 1983, WB Saunders.
54. Bauer T: Mediastinal, pleural, and extrapleural diseases. In Ettinger SJ, editor: *Textbook of veterinary internal medicine*, Philadelphia, 1989, WB Saunders.
55. Yoshioka MM: Management of spontaneous pneumothorax in 12 dogs, *J Am Anim Hosp Assoc* 18:57-62, 1982.
56. Holtsinger RH, Beale BS, Bellah JR et al: Spontaneous pneumothorax in the dog: A retrospective analysis of 21 cases, *J Am Anim Hosp Assoc* 29:195-210, 1993.
57. Fossum TW, Birchard SJ: Chylothorax. In Kirk RW, editor: *Current veterinary therapy*, vol 10, Philadelphia, 1989, WB Saunders.
58. Miller KS, Sahn SA: Chest tubes – indications, technique, management and complications, *Chest* 91:258-263, 1987.
59. Kagan K: Thoracic trauma, *Vet Clin North Am* 10:641-653, 1980.
60. Wingfield WE: *Veterinary emergency medicine secrets*, ed 2, Philadelphia, 2001, Hanley & Belfus.
61. Raptopoulos D, Papazoglou LG, Patsikas MN: Re-expansion pulmonary oedema after pneumothorax in a dog, *Vet Rec* 136(15):395, 1995.
62. Soderstrom MJ, Gilson SD, Gulbas N: Fatal re-expansion pulmonary edema in a kitten following surgical correction of pectus excavatum, *JAAHA* 31:133-136, 1995.
63. Stampley AR, Waldron DR: Re-expansion pulmonary edema after surgery to repair a diaphragmatic hernia in a cat, *J Am Vet Med Assoc* 203:1699-1701, 1993.
64. Roudebush P: Bacterial infections of the respiratory system. In Green CE, editor: *Infectious diseases of the dog and cat*, Philadelphia, 1990, WB Saunders.
65. Voggenreiter G, Neudeck F, Aufmkolk M et al: Operative chest wall stabilization in flail chest: outcome of patients with or without pulmonary contusion, *J Am Coll Surg* 187:130-137, 1998.
66. Cappello M, Yuehua C, De Troyer A: Rib cage distortion in a canine model of flail chest, *Am J Respir Crit Care Med* 151:1481-1485, 1995.
67. Hendricks J: Pulse oximetry. In Bonagura JD, editor: *Kirk's current veterinary therapy*, vol 12, Philadelphia, 1995, WB Saunders.
68. Fairman NB: Evaluation of pulse oximetry as a continuous monitoring technique in critically ill dogs in the small animal intensive care unit, *JVECC* 2(2):50-56, 1993.
69. Hendricks J: End tidal carbon dioxide monitoring. In Bonagura JD, editor: *Kirk's current veterinary therapy*, vol 12, Philadelphia, 1995, WB Saunders.

CHAPTER 2

Respiratory Distress in Cats

Deborah C. Mandell

Treating respiratory distress in cats can be very stressful for veterinarians. Most of the time the cat is not stable enough for diagnostic tests, yet it can seem difficult to determine how to stabilize it without a tentative diagnosis. Valuable information can be gathered from the patient history, observation of the cat, and a quick physical examination. This chapter will cover the signs of respiratory distress, physical examination findings, and the causes of hypoxemia and dyspnea in cats.

History

Historical findings can be helpful in treating dyspneic cats. Cats with a history of coughing have two major differential diagnoses: asthma, and heartworm disease.[1,2] In contrast to dogs, cats with pulmonary edema due to heart disease do not cough. Any stridor, change in meow, or recent onset of snoring might indicate nasopharyngeal disease such as polyps or neoplasms.[3,4] Weight loss, anorexia, and the presence and rate of progression of respiratory distress or exercise intolerance should be ascertained.

Signs of Respiratory Distress

It is important to recognize the signs that cats exhibit when they have respiratory distress. There can be an increase in respiratory rate, an increase in inspiratory or expiratory effort, open mouth breathing, lethargy, or depression. Cats may want to sit or lie in a sternal position (orthopnea).

Respiratory distress is associated with two breathing patterns: restrictive, and obstructive.[5] Determining which pattern the cat is exhibiting can help narrow the differential diagnosis list. Restrictive diseases prevent the lungs from fully expanding and lead to short, rapid, shallow breaths. Included are pulmonary parenchymal diseases that make the lungs stiff (e.g., pneumonia, edema, and neoplasia) and pleural space diseases (e.g., pneumothorax and pleural effusion) that mechanically prevent the lungs from expanding. Airway narrowing, as occurs in laryngeal disease or feline asthma, is termed obstructive disease; it leads to slower, deeper breaths. Upper airway narrowing or obstruction results in increased inspiratory effort, whereas lower airway disease results in increased expiratory effort.

With increasing or prolonged respiratory distress and high work of breathing, the respiratory muscles start to fatigue. If fatigue occurs, the cat may exhibit a paradoxical breathing pattern in which the caudal intercostal muscles and ribs collapse inwards during inspiration, and the abdomen collapses inwards during inspiration and outward on expiration.

Physical Examination

Physical examination findings, even if performed in less than 1 or 2 minutes, can also help narrow the differential diagnosis list and thus help determine how to stabilize the dyspneic cat. The first parameter to evaluate is mucous membrane color. Pale or white mucous membranes can signify hypoxemia, anemia, or peripheral vasoconstriction. Cyanotic or blue mucous membranes signify extreme hypoxemia. Special consideration should be given to mucous membranes that are brown or muddy in color; this signifies methemoglobinemia and acetaminophen toxicity. Cats with acetaminophen toxicity may also have facial edema and severe respiratory distress.

The next step should be thoracic auscultation to listen for crackles, wheezes, and harsh or dull lung sounds. Normal cat lungs are very quiet on auscultation. Harsh lung sounds are pronounced bronchovesicular sounds that can signify turbulent flow in the airways. Crackles, which sound like soft popping bubbles, are often heard at the end of inspiration, and are usually due to air bubbling through fluid, signifying the presence of fluid in the alveoli. The fluid can be a transudate, as in pulmonary edema secondary to left-sided congestive heart failure; an exudate, as in pneumonia; or blood, as in pulmonary contusions or hemorrhage. Alternatively, the opening and closing of small airways in cats with bronchial disease can also sound like loud popping bubbles; this is termed harsh crackles.

Wheezes are high-pitched musical sounds or squeaks that signify air moving through narrowed airways. In cats, the most common cause of wheezes is feline asthma, which is associated with bronchoconstriction, airway inflammation, and increased mucus production. Because the lower airways are constricted, wheezes and an increased respiratory effort are recognized on expiration.

When it is difficult to hear anything, dull or muffled lung sounds are present. Dull lung sounds occur when space-occupying air, fluid, or tissue in the pleural space prevents transmission of lung sounds through the interface. The most common cause of pleural space disease in cats is pleural effusion. Pneumothorax can also occur secondary to blunt trauma, endotracheal intubation,[6] or, less commonly, heartworm disease.[7,8]

Cardiac auscultation and peripheral pulse palpation should be performed simultaneously to detect heart murmurs or arrhythmias. Unfortunately, even cats with severe heart disease do not necessarily have a murmur or a gallop rhythm, therefore the absence of these does not rule out heart disease. If a murmur or gallop can be auscultated, and it is combined with crackles or harsh lung sounds, left-sided congestive heart failure and pulmonary edema should be considered. Abnormal cardiac auscultation combined with dull lung sounds may indicate heart failure and resultant pleural effusion.

Oxygen Dissociation Curve

It is important to remember the oxygen dissociation curve (Figure 2-1) when dealing with animals in respiratory distress.[9,10] This curve relates the amount of dissolved oxygen, the arterial partial pressure of oxygen, and the percent of hemoglobin saturation with oxygen. Oxygen forms an easily reversible combination with hemoglobin, which helps oxygen uptake in the lungs and its release to the tissues. The curve shows that the amount of oxygen carried by hemoglobin (saturation) rapidly increases to an arterial partial pressure of oxygen of 50 to 60 mm Hg, and above this the curve is flatter. On the steep part of the curve, a large decrease in the amount of oxyhemoglobin occurs with a small drop in arterial partial pressure of oxygen. On the flat, plateau part of the curve, a large decrease in arterial partial pressure of oxygen (from 100 to 60 mm Hg) is associated with only a small drop in oxygen hemoglobin saturation.

The sigmoid shape of the curve becomes important when disease leads to hypoxia and acts as a safety measure. Cats with respiratory distress can compensate and sit at or just above the knee of the curve when at rest, and their oxygen hemoglobin saturation is preserved. Any stress, especially a trip to the hospital, may cause decompensation, and the arterial partial pressure of oxygen and oxygen hemoglobin saturation can easily fall to the

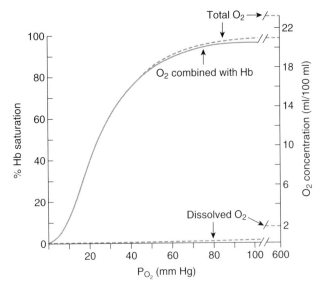

Figure 2-1. *The oxygen dissociation curve shows the relationship between the saturation of hemoglobin with oxygen and the arterial partial pressure of oxygen. The curve shows that the amount of oxygen carried by hemoglobin rapidly increases to a Pa_{O_2} of 50 to 60 mm Hg and then plateaus; therefore, the Pa_{O_2} can decrease within this range (from 100 to 60 mm Hg) without a significant decrease in saturation. Once the Pa_{O_2} drops below 60 mm Hg, the percent hemoglobin saturation drops rapidly. (From West JB: Respiratory physiology: The essentials, ed 5, Philadelphia, 1995, Williams & Wilkins.)*

steep part of the curve. Therefore by the time a cat with respiratory distress presents to a veterinarian, it is usually severely hypoxic. Thus leaving the cat alone to relax in an oxygen-enriched environment is very beneficial.

Stabilization

If there is respiratory distress, or any question of respiratory distress, oxygen supplementation should be started immediately. Methods of oxygen supplementation include face mask, nasal, flow-by, oxygen cage, intubation, and ventilation. Oxygen supplementation is provided in order to increase the inspired oxygen concentration, which will increase the arterial partial pressure of oxygen unless a shunt is present. In patients with anatomic shunts, the shunted blood is not exposed to the higher oxygen concentration, and the animal will not improve when oxygen supplementation is provided. In animals with alveolar hypoventilation, increasing the inspired oxygen concentration will result in improvement in the Pa_{O_2} but will not change the Pa_{CO_2}, for which definitive treatment requires increasing the minute ventilation, potentially by intubation and assisted ventilation.

Oxygen cages are usually the optimal method of providing oxygen for dyspneic cats. It is important to monitor the cat frequently to make sure that the respiratory status is indeed improving. It is equally as important to proceed slowly with diagnostic tests or procedures in a

dyspneic cat. Many times procedures must be performed gradually, and supplemental oxygen and rest should be instituted between each procedure. For example, the patient should be placed back in the oxygen cage after intravenous catheter placement. Then, following a period of rest, a radiograph may be obtained if the cat is stable. Again, place the cat back in the oxygen cage to rest with supplemental oxygen. Performing all procedures and diagnostic tests at once can be very detrimental and is potentially life threatening.

Severely dyspneic cats are often not stable enough for any diagnostic tests, and may have confusing thoracic auscultation findings. In this situation, empirical treatment is instituted concurrently for the major causes of respiratory distress until the cat is stable enough for diagnostic testing. Supplemental oxygen is always the first line of treatment. Because pleural effusion is a common cause of feline dyspnea, thoracocentesis should be performed in any cat with suspicious dull lung sounds. Thoracocentesis is performed prior to radiography because it is both a diagnostic and a therapeutic procedure that may result in a significant improvement in the status of the patient if it is productive. If thoracocentesis is negative, then the remaining two most common immediately treatable causes of feline respiratory distress are cardiogenic pulmonary edema and feline asthma. Therefore empirical drug therapy consists of one dose of furosemide (1 to 2 mg/kg IM, IV) *and* one dose of corticosteroids (dexamethasone 0.25 to 0.5 mg/kg IM, IV). One dose of furosemide will not harm an asthmatic, and one dose of steroids will not harm a cat with heart disease. These drugs are only given *once*, along with supplemental oxygen, to stabilize the cat until further diagnostic tests can be performed.

Common Causes of Respiratory Distress in Cats

The most common treatable causes of respiratory distress in cats fall into three major categories: heart disease, pleural space disease, and asthma (Figure 2-2). Observation and physical examination findings can help determine into which category the dyspneic cat should be placed.

HEART DISEASE

Cardiogenic pulmonary edema is one of the most common causes of feline dyspnea. The three types of heart disease in cats include hypertrophic, dilated, and restrictive cardiomyopathy. Hypertrophic and restrictive cardiomyopathy lead to diastolic failure, which is characterized by ventricular filling dysfunction.[12] Dilated cardiomyopathy leads to systolic failure, which is characterized by ventricular ejection failure. Congestive heart failure occurs when the failure of forward flow causes an increase in hydrostatic pressure in the pulmonary vessels. This increased hydrostatic pressure causes fluid to leak out into the pulmonary interstitium, causing pulmonary edema.

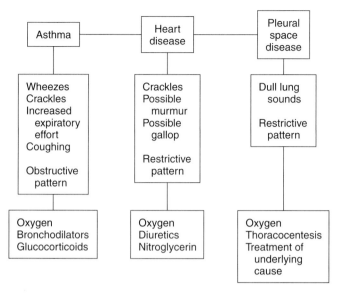

Figure 2-2. *Algorithm for diagnosis and therapy of the dyspneic cat. The most common treatable causes of respiratory distress in cats fall into three major categories: heart disease, pleural space disease, and asthma. Observation of the type of breathing pattern and physical examination findings, especially thoracic auscultation, will help determine into which category the dyspneic cat should be placed, and thus which treatment should be instituted.*

Cats with heart disease usually present with acute or progressive respiratory distress without a helpful history. Unlike dogs, cats are not asked to exercise or walk regularly, so exercise intolerance is not a presenting complaint. Likewise, cats with heart disease do not cough, and they may not have a murmur or gallop rhythm. A restrictive pattern of breathing is usually present, and thoracic auscultation reveals harsh lung sounds or crackles. Thoracic radiographs can show the classic perihilar alveolar lung pattern or a patchy pattern of alveolar disease in any part of the lung. Cardiomegaly may also be observed.

The emergency treatment of pulmonary edema secondary to heart failure in cats includes supplemental oxygen, intravenous or intramuscular administration of a diuretic such as furosemide (0.5 to 1 mg/kg), and cutaneous application of nitroglycerin ($^1/_4$ to $^1/_2$ inch) as a venodilator. Nitroprusside (0.5 to 4 µg/kg/min), a balanced vasodilator, may be used in cats with severe pulmonary edema, but the cat must be closely monitored for hypotension. In cats with dilated cardiomyopathy, dobutamine, a beta-agonist (1 to 5 µg/kg/min), can be used to increase contractility. Dobutamine can cause seizures in cats; these are self-limiting and cease once the drug is discontinued. Seizures could, however, result in acute decompensation of an unstable patient. Dobutamine should not be used in cats without a positive diagnosis of dilated cardiomyopathy because it could result in worsening of the condition of a cat with hypertrophic or restrictive cardiomyopathy. An echocardiogram should always be performed once the cat is stable to determine the type and severity of the heart disease.

PLEURAL SPACE DISEASE

The second major cause of respiratory distress in cats is pleural space disease.[13,14] Cats with pleural space disease have a restrictive respiratory pattern and muffled or dull lung sounds on thoracic auscultation. Pleural effusion is the most common cause of pleural space disease in cats; however, pneumothorax can also be seen secondary to blunt trauma, such as in high-rise syndrome,[8] heartworm disease,[7] or following endotracheal intubation.[6] Initial management of pleural disease includes supplemental oxygen, thoracocentesis, and treatment of the underlying disease. Thoracic radiographs can be obtained to confirm the presence of an effusion, but if pleural fluid is suspected, thoracocentesis should be performed sooner rather than later. Oxygen supplementation will be helpful, but thoracocentesis will be diagnostic and therapeutic.

Fluid analysis should include determination of total protein, cell counts, and cytology. Samples should also be saved for triglyceride analysis and microbiologic culture and sensitivity. Cytologic findings can often narrow the diagnosis and should be assessed in hospital in addition to laboratory submission to a cytopathologist. Additional diagnostic tests may also be appropriate (Table 2-1).

Definitive management depends on the type and underlying cause of the effusion. The treatment of pyothorax includes intravenous fluids, intravenous broad-spectrum antibiotics pending culture and sensitivity results, and chest tube placement.[15] A thoracotomy may also be needed when severe pulmonary parenchymal disease or focal abscessation is suspected. Idiopathic chylothorax is diagnosed based on effusion triglyceride level (in comparison to serum triglyceride level) and exclusion of heart disease and neoplasia.[16-18] Management of idiopathic chylothorax can be particularly frustrating, with success rates varying from 30% to 60%. Treatment for right-sided heart failure is similar to that for left-sided heart failure, but it also includes thoracocentesis. An echocardiogram should always be performed once the cat is stable. In cats with neoplastic effusions, exploratory surgery may be required to remove a thymoma, whereas cranial mediastinal lymphosarcoma may respond to chemotherapy.

FELINE ASTHMA

The last major cause of respiratory distress in cats is feline asthma.[19-21] Asthma is generally characterized by concurrent bronchoconstriction, increased mucus production, inflammatory exudate in the airways, and smooth muscle hypertrophy. Asthmatic cats typically present with a history of coughing. They tend to have an obstructive respiratory pattern, with an increased expiratory effort as they try to force air out of narrowed small airways. Thoracic auscultation classically reveals wheezes, but harsh lung sounds or crackles can also be heard.

Radiographs reveal a bronchial pattern with "doughnuts" and "railroad tracks," hyperinflation of the lungs, and flattening of the diaphragm due to air trapping. A

TABLE 2-1. **Cause, Appearance, Total Protein, and Cytology Findings of Pleural Effusions in Cats**

Cause	Appearance	Total Protein	Cytology	Other Tests
Pyothorax	Cloudy, tomato soup, malodor	>4 g/dl	Degenerative neutrophils, intracellular and extracellular bacteria, macrophages, few red blood cells	Aerobic culture and sensitivity
Idiopathic chylothorax	Milky white	≤3 g/dl	Mature lymphocytes, few red blood cells, few macrophages, few neutrophils	Triglyceride level
Right-sided heart failure	Clear	≤2 g/dl	Very few cells—red blood cells, lymphocytes	Echocardiogram
Lymphosarcoma	Clear, milky, serosanguinous	2-4 g/dl	Immature lymphoblasts, few mature lymphocytes, few red blood cells	Thoracic radiographs Thoracic ultrasound Aspirate/cytology of mass
Thymoma	Clear, milky, serosanguinous	2-4 g/dl	Mesothelial cells, mature lymphocytes, few red blood cells, few macrophages	Thoracic radiographs Thoracic ultrasound Aspirate/cytology of mass
Neoplasia (e.g., carcinoma)	Clear, cloudy, serosanguinous, bloody	2-4 g/dl	Clumps of neoplastic cells	Thoracic radiographs Thoracic ultrasound
Feline infectious peritonitis	Straw-colored cloudy	>4 g/dl	Macrophages, lymphocytes, red blood cells, fibrin	FIP-PCR on fluid Serum FIP titer

collapsed right middle lung lobe can also be seen, because the right middle lung lobe is dependent and the bronchus can become occluded with mucus, resulting in absorption atelectasis. There is no correlation between the severity of radiographic changes and the severity of clinical signs.

Emergency management of asthma includes supplemental oxygen, bronchodilators, and corticosteroids. Terbutaline, a selective β_2-agonist, causes bronchodilation. The injectable drug can be given intravenously, intramuscularly, or subcutaneously (0.01 mg/kg). This drug is very effective in cats with an acute asthma attack, and can lead to significant improvement within 15 to 30 minutes. Tachycardia rarely occurs at this dose, but terbutaline should be avoided in cats that might have hypertrophic cardiomyopathy. Glucocorticoids (e.g., dexamethasone 0.25 to 0.5 mg/kg IM, IV) are the mainstays of treatment for a cat with acute asthma because they effectively decrease airway inflammation and thereby ameliorate bronchoconstriction.

Other Causes of Respiratory Distress

Other, less common causes of respiratory distress and cyanosis in cats are also recognized. Once again, the history and physical examination can help localize the disease and determine the most common etiology.

UPPER AIRWAY DISEASE

Upper airway disease leads to stridor, which is most prominent on inspiration. Cats may also have a history of snoring, intermittent open mouth breathing, nasal dis-

charge, and decreased appetite. Nasopharyngeal and laryngeal disorders include benign polyps and malignant tumors (e.g., lymphosarcoma and squamous cell carcinoma). Diagnosis involves an upper airway examination including palpation and endoscopy dorsal to the soft palate, and treatment is usually surgical. Nasopharyngeal stenosis occurs most commonly in brachycephalic breeds, and nasopharyngeal foreign bodies can also be seen. Laryngeal paralysis is rare in cats but can occur. Other causes of upper airway disease include tracheal foreign bodies, tracheal stenosis, and tracheal masses. Thoracic radiographs can be helpful in localizing the lesion. Bronchoscopy and/or exploratory surgery are necessary to treat tracheal foreign bodies and masses.

BACTERIAL PNEUMONIA

Bacterial pneumonia can be seen in cats, although it is much less common in this species than in dogs. The history usually includes anorexia, lethargy, and respiratory distress. Physical examination can reveal harsh lung sounds, crackles, or dull lung sounds if there is lung lobe consolidation. Thoracic radiographs should be performed if the cat is stable. If the cat is stable enough, an endotracheal wash should be performed for cytological evaluation and aerobic culture and sensitivity. If the cat is sick enough to require supplemental oxygen, intravenous fluids and broad-spectrum antibiotics should be instituted. Bronchodilators can also be helpful, as well as saline nebulization and coupage.

PULMONARY THROMBOEMBOLISM

Pulmonary thromboembolic disease is very uncommon but has been reported in cats.[22] It should be suspected in any cat with respiratory distress and a known underlying cause that leads to a hypercoagulable state (e.g., cardiac disease, neoplasia, corticosteroid administration, protein losing nephropathy or enteropathy, immune mediated hemolytic anemia, sepsis, or disseminated intravascular coagulation). The history usually includes anorexia, lethargy, and respiratory distress. Thoracic radiographs can be normal or reveal pleural effusion, atelectasis, consolidated lung lobes, or pulmonary vessel abnormalities. Treatment has not been evaluated in cats but includes oxygen therapy; treatment of the underlying cause, if known; and anticoagulants.

REFERENCES

1. Padrid P: Feline asthma, *Vet Clin North Am Small Anim Pract* 30(6):1279-1293, 2000.
2. Atkins CE, DeFrancesco TC, Coats JR et al: Heartworm infection in cats: 50 cases (1985-1997), *JAVMA* 217(3):355, 2000.
3. Griffon DJ: Upper airway obstruction in cats: Pathogenesis and clinical signs, *Comp Cont Educ* 22(9):822, 2000.
4. Griffon DJ: Upper airway obstruction in cats: Diagnosis and treatment, *Comp Cont Educ* 22(10):897, 2000.
5. Turnwald GH: Dyspnea and tachypnea. In Ettinger SJ, Feldman EC, editors: *Textbook of veterinary internal medicine*, ed 4, vol 1, Philadelphia, 1995, WB Saunders.
6. Mitchell SL, McCarthy R, Rudloff E et al: Tracheal rupture associated with intubation in cats: 20 cases (1996-1998), *JAVMA* 216(10):1592, 2000.
7. Smith JW, Scott-Moncrieff C: Pneumothorax secondary to *Dirofilaria immitis* infection in two cats, *JAVMA* 213(1):91, 1998.
8. Holtsinger RH, Ellison GW: Spontaneous pneumothorax, *Comp Cont Educ* 17(2):197, 1995.
9. West JB: Gas transport to the periphery. In *Respiratory physiology: The essentials*, ed 5, Philadelphia, 1995, Williams & Wilkins.
10. West JB: Ventilation-perfusion relationships. In *Respiratory physiology: The essentials*, ed 5, Philadelphia, 1995, Williams & Wilkins.
11. Jacobs G: Cyanosis. In Ettinger SJ, Feldman EC, editors: *Textbook of veterinary internal medicine*, ed 4, vol 1, Philadelphia, 1995, WB Saunders.
12. Kittleson MD: CVT update: Feline hypertrophic cardiomyopathy. In Bonagura JD, editor: *Kirk's current veterinary therapy*, vol 12, Philadelphia, 1995, WB Saunders.
13. Hawkins EC, Fossum TW: Medical and surgical management of pleural effusion. In Bonagura JD, editor: *Kirk's current veterinary therapy*, vol 13, Philadelphia, 2000, WB Saunders.
14. Orton EC: Pleura and pleural space. In Slatter D: *Textbook of small animal surgery*, ed 2, Philadelphia, 1993, WB Saunders.
15. Walker AC, Jang SS, Hirsh DC: Bacteria associated with pyothorax of dogs and cats: 98 cases (1989-1998), *JAVMA* 216(3):359, 2000.
16. Suess RP, Flanders JA, Beck KA et al: Constrictive pleuritis in cats with chylothorax: 10 cases (1983-1991), *JAAHA* 30:70, 1994.
17. Fossum TW: Feline chylothorax, *Comp Contin Educ* 15(4):549, 1993.
18. Smeak DD, Kerpsack SJ: Management of feline chylothorax. In Bonagura JD, editor: *Kirk's current veterinary therapy*, vol 12, Philadelphia, 1995, WB Saunders.
19. Padrid P: New strategies to treat feline asthma, *Vet Forum*, pp 46-50, 1996.
20. Boothe DM, McKiernan BC: Respiratory therapeutics, *Vet Clin North Am Small Anim Pract* 22(5):1231-1258, 1992.
21. Padrid P: CVT update: Feline asthma. In Bonagura JD, editor: *Kirk's current veterinary therapy*, vol 13, Philadelphia, 2000, WB Saunders.
22. Norris CR, Griffey SM, Samii VF: Pulmonary thromboembolism in cats: 29 cases (1987-1997), *JAVMA* 215(11):1650, 1999.

CHAPTER 3

Nasal Discharge, Sneezing, and Reverse Sneezing

Ross Doust • Martin Sullivan

The upper respiratory tract provides a common pathway for the respiratory and gastrointestinal systems. It performs, or is part of, complex motor tasks such as sniffing, smelling, aspiration, suckling, swallowing, retching, vomiting, modification of breathing, pulmonary defense, arousal, and orientation. In most situations these are reflex responses, coordinated by central neural mechanisms. The nasal cavity has specific nonmotor pulmonary defense and homeostatic functions that include filtration, heat and moisture exchange, and evaporative cooling.[1-4]

The nasal cavities are symmetrical compartments divided on the midline by a septum, the vomer bone ventrad, with a cartilaginous part dorsad. Each nasal cavity is divided into four air passages: the dorsal, middle, ventral, and common nasal meati. The dorsal, middle, and ventral meati are divided by the dorsal nasal concha (dorsal nasoturbinate) and the ventral nasal concha (maxilloturbinate). The common nasal meatus is lateral to the nasal septum.

Associated with each nasal cavity are paranasal sinuses. The dog has lateral, medial, and rostral frontal sinuses, and a large maxillary recess. These are divided by osseous septa, and drain into the middle nasal meatus via distinct ostia (nasofrontal ducts) The maxillary recess is not a true sinus because it is not within the maxillary bone, lying instead between the frontal bone and the maxilloturbinate, dorsal to the roots of the upper fourth premolar, on the nasal surface of the maxilla. In the cat there is only one frontal sinus on each side, the maxillary sinus is small, and there is a sphenoidal sinus that extends caudad from the nasal cavity into the sphenoid bone, ventral to the brain.[5,6]

The delicate scrolls of the nasal and ethmoidal conchae create the large mucosal surface area of the nasal cavity. The conchae are cartilaginous rostrad, osseous caudad, and covered with a vascular ciliated pseudocolumnar mucosa. Cilia normally beat at a rate of 15 to 20 beats per second; this rate may be reduced by some drugs and airway disease. Rostrad is the smaller dorsal nasoturbinate and the larger maxilloturbinate, and caudad are the ethmoturbinates. Olfactory neuroepithelium is found on the ethmoturbinates near the cribriform plate. The cribriform plate is the fenestrated part of the ethmoid bone separating the nasal cavity and the cranial vault.[4-6]

Filtration of inspired air occurs as particles contact the nasal, pharyngeal, tracheal, and bronchial mucosae. Turbulence, created by disturbance of airflow around the conchae, increases contact with the mucosal surfaces. Most large particles (5 to 30 μm) contact the mucosae of the nostril and nasopharynx, where they are trapped in a mucus layer and transported to the nasopharynx by the cilia of mucociliary cells. Smaller particles (1 to 5 μm) usually settle in the bronchioles, where the mucociliary system moves them toward the pharynx. Very small particles (less than 1 μm) may reach the alveoli, where they remain until removed by alveolar macrophages. Particles in the nasal cavity or nasopharynx can initiate a sneeze or aspiration reflex.[1-5,7]

Countercurrent heat and moisture exchange occurs between the air and the superficial capillary network of the turbinate mucosa. Inspired air is warmed and humidified, while heat and moisture are recovered from expired air. Nonolfactory mucosa contains 30% or more of large, thin-walled veins, which act as heat exchange and capacitance vessels. Exchange is so efficient that dogs can exhale air at 16.5° C below body temperature, and in dry air at 0° C can conserve 75% of water and 80% of heat. The degree of filling of these capacitance vessels influences the degree of nasal congestion.[5,8-13]

Lateral nasal glands, found in the maxillary sinus, contribute significantly, with nasolacrimal duct excretions, to the wetness of the dog's nose. These glands, in the dog, discharge large volumes of serous fluid via a duct that opens at the rostral end of the dorsal nasal concha. This secretion is a principal source of cooling fluid. In the cat the lateral nasal glands are only visible microscopically, and produce a small volume of mucoid discharge.[4,5,13-15]

Dogs and cats preferentially nose breathe, and will resist mouth breathing even with very high nasopharyngeal airway resistance. During resting respiration the nasal cavity accounts for 79% of inspiratory resistance and 74% of expiratory resistance, and even more in brachycephalic breeds. Otherwise healthy dogs and cats are able to breathe comfortably through a single nostril. Overwhelming nasal resistance leads to mouth breathing

to avoid the increased work of breathing; this reduces olfaction, heat and moisture exchange, and filtration.[4,16] Olfaction is an important component of appetite in carnivores, particularly cats, which will often refuse food when their sense of smell is impaired. This is important when considering palliative treatment for chronic nasal discharge.[17]

Upper airway (UA) mechanosensitive reflexes (e.g., aspiration, sniff, gasp, and sigh) are an important part of the survival strategy of the body. Spasmodic inspiratory reflexes attempt to provide a patent airway and air supply under life-threatening and comatose situations. Dysfunction of the upper airway reflexes has been investigated due to potential links with perinatal asphyxia, sudden infant death syndrome, sleep apnea, aspiration pneumonia, and agonal inspiration. Upper airway stimulation reverses central apnea in experimental models of sleep apnea, a reflex that could potentially be utilized for the restitution of respiration because respiratory center reactivity may persist more than 20 minutes after cessation of spontaneous breathing.[1,15]

Stimulation of the upper airways can cause reflex constriction of the lower airways and coughing (i.e., the nasobronchial reflex). This is a pulmonary defense mechanism that limits inspiration of noxious agents. Complete apnea may result. In humans the nasobronchial reflex is an important factor in asthma, and control of upper airway disease is an important element of treatment.[18-23]

Nasal Discharge

DEFINITION AND CLINICAL SIGNS

Nasal discharge is usually, but not always, self-evident. A serous discharge may be missed or licked away before it is seen, and discharge originating caudally may drain to the nasopharynx rather than the external nares, presenting as a cough. Discharges should be described by their properties, including volume (copious or scant); frequency (continuous or intermittent); location (unilateral or bilateral); and appearance (serous, purulent, mucoid, mucopurulent, sanguineous, or epistaxis).

PATHOPHYSIOLOGY

Nasal discharges vary with type and duration of the primary lesion. Discharge may result from either local disease in the nasal cavities or paranasal sinuses, or it may be the only presenting sign of a serious extranasal disorder. Examples include a purulent nasal discharge secondary to a purulent bronchopneumonia, and epistaxis as a result of a coagulopathy. The nature of a discharge may change with progression of the disease process.

Serous discharge is clear and acellular, and usually represents a nonspecific irritation of the nasal mucosa, but may result from increased lacrimation. It is often the first sign of upper respiratory tract disease but may not be detected by the owner because the animal may lick and remove the discharge as it is produced.

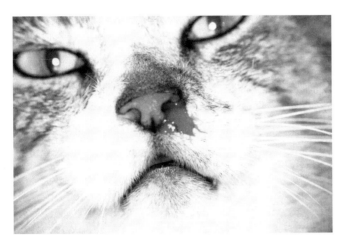

Figure 3-1. *Epistaxis caused by nasal neoplasia in a cat.*

Mucoid discharge is clear and acellular with a high protein content. It represents an exuberant production of mucus by Goblet cells in the nasal mucosa. It is a response to chronic, noninfectious nasal disease.

Purulent nasal discharge is opaque, viscous, and pale yellow to light green, containing abundant neutrophils and bacteria. A change to a purulent discharge may indicate inability of the mucociliary clearance mechanism to oppose bacterial colonization. Purulent nasal discharge may result from intra- or extranasal causes.

Mucopurulent discharge is a mixture of mucoid and purulent discharges. Bacteria are variably seen depending on the etiology. This type of discharge may be seen in patients with chronic nasal disease where there is bacterial infection or a necrotic focus.

Sanguineous discharges are seen when blood is mixed with another discharge. A sanguineous component to a discharge indicates damage to the nasal mucosa.

Epistaxis is frank hemorrhage into the nasal cavity, and consists of mainly red blood cells (Figure 3-1); it may be caused by intranasal or extranasal disease.

Sneezing

DEFINITION AND CLINICAL SIGNS

Sneezing is a protective reflex that manifests as an explosive expiratory airflow that dislodges and expels foreign particles from the nasal cavities. The onset, nature, duration, and progression may be important. An example is a possible foreign body, where sudden onset of paroxysmal sneezing with pawing at the face is highly suspicious. Sneezing tends to decrease as the disease process becomes more chronic, even if the discharge persists or increases. Any cause of nasal mucosal irritation or nasal discharge is a differential diagnosis for sneezing.[24]

PATHOPHYSIOLOGY

Irritation of the nasal mucosa stimulates subepithelial myelinated trigeminal nerve endings that act as rapidly adapting receptors, initiating the sneeze reflex. The sneeze reflex may also be initiated in humans by sudden exposure to strong light; this is known as a "photic sneeze." There are three phases of the sneeze: inspiratory, compression, and expulsion. Compression is achieved by thyroarytenoideus muscle adduction of the vocal folds and abdominal muscle contraction, abruptly increasing the subglottic pressure. Vocal fold abduction with a continuous expiratory effort results in an explosive expiratory airflow. Airflow is directed through the nasal cavities by elevation of the caudal aspect of the tongue; this is a result of styloglossus muscle contraction, under the control of the lateral branch of the hypoglossal nerve.[24-32]

Reverse Sneezing

DEFINITION AND CLINICAL SIGNS

Reverse sneezing consists of a paroxysmal, noisy, labored inspiratory effort with, in some cases, adoption of an orthopneic position with neck extension and elbow abduction. There is no obstructive dyspnea, exercise tolerance is not compromised, and patients usually behave normally between episodes of extreme inspiratory effort.[33-36]

Reverse sneezing is a mechanosensitive aspiration reflex. It has been investigated as a model for the inspiratory reflexes because it is repeatable, easily evoked, resistant to various influences (e.g., anesthetics, hyperthermia, hypothermia, hypercapnia, and hypoxia), and can be elicited in cats even when in severe hypoxic coma. The aspiration reflex can be experimentally induced in all phases of respiration because it has a marked ability for recruitment. Evocation can inhibit, transiently interrupt, or even reverse some tonic respiration–related processes (e.g., hiccup, apneusis, laryngospasm, and bronchospasm). Although reverse sneezing is clinically seen more commonly in the dog, experimentally the aspiration reflex is more expressive in cats and pigs and less so in dogs, rats, mice, and human neonates. For this reason the cat is used as the standard experimental model.[1,34,37-44]

PATHOPHYSIOLOGY

Intraepithelial and subepithelial myelinated trigeminal nerve endings, with rapidly adapting properties, act as receptors. The distribution of these nerve endings influences the threshold responsiveness of distinct areas, with the most responsive site in the lateral nasopharynx. There is significant overlap in the receptor fields with other upper airway reflexes such as sniffing and gasping. Rapidly adapting receptors are more responsive to spatial and temporal summation of stimuli (e.g., sliding a probe over the mucosa or strong air jet puffs) than gentle single spot touching, chemicals, or dust. Involvement of the gasping center, located in the lateral medulla (nucleus tractus solitorii, lateral tegmental field, and nucleus ambiguus), has been demonstrated, implying a common reflex pathway.[2,32,37,40,45-47]

Powerful contraction of inspiratory muscles and adduction of laryngeal cartilages generates negative pleural and tracheal pressure. The strong tracheal occlusion pressure with a sudden opening of the glottis produces a rapid inspiratory airflow. This rapid inhalation tends to tear off irritant particles and accumulated mucus, resulting in aspiration from the nasopharynx to the oropharynx, effectively supporting mucociliary clearance and allowing subsequent elimination by swallowing or coughing. Aspiration of irritant particles into the lower respiratory tract seems to be prevented by an immediate late and postinspiratory glottal narrowing, and by coughing.[1,36,37,48,49]

Differential Diagnosis

Nasal discharge, sneezing, and reverse sneezing are all clinical signs of nasal or nasopharyngeal disease; therefore, nasal and nasopharyngeal differential diagnoses should be considered. Reverse sneezing localizes the problem to the nasopharynx.[1,34]

FELINE UPPER RESPIRATORY TRACT INFECTION COMPLEX

The major causes of feline upper respiratory tract infection are feline herpesvirus-1 (FHV-1) also known as feline rhinotracheitis virus (FRV), feline calicivirus (FCV) and *Chlamydia psittaci.* These infections may occur independently or in combination. Bacterial infections commonly occur secondary to mucosal damage from these agents. Up to 80% of cats with acute viral upper respiratory tract disease may become chronic carriers. A variable number may intermittently or continuously demonstrate clinical signs ranging from mild to severe. Disease may spontaneously resolve in some chronic carriers. Transmission occurs by direct contact with infected animals or fomites, or by aerosol transmission. Aerosol transmission only occurs over relatively short distances. Stress, particularly overcrowding, is an important risk factor in this disease complex.[50-54]

FHV-1 survives 18 to 24 hours outside the body and is shed intermittently, often during periods of stress. Shedding may be associated with mild clinical signs and may last a couple of weeks. The incubation period for the virus is 3 to 5 days. Affected cats are often pyrexic and anorexic. FHV-1 has a particular affinity for sites of osteogenesis, resulting in necrosis and destruction of the nasal conchae. There may be a sanguineous discharge during this period of active infection, often with continued clinical signs following virus elimination due to mucosal damage and secondary bacterial infection. Affected animals usually have a marked nasal discharge with severe sneezing, ulcerated nares, turbinate necrosis, severe conjunctivitis, and ulcerative keratitis. Panophthalmitis may be seen in neonates. FHV-1 infection has been associated with abortion and neonatal death.[50,52,55,56]

FCV survives longer out of the body than FHV-1 (8 to 10 days) and may be shed persistently for months or years following recovery from acute infection. The incubation period for the disease is usually 1 to 3 days. FCV has a higher affinity for oral sites, resulting in ulceration, particularly of the tongue and the palate. Nasal signs such as

sneezing, discharge, and ulcerated nares tend to be mild and inconsistent. Other clinical signs seen variably include pyrexia, anorexia, conjunctivitis, viral pneumonia, polyarthritis, interdigital ulcers, and enteritis.[50,55-57]

C. psittaci is an obligate intracellular anaerobe that is responsible for 10% to 20% of upper respiratory tract infections in cats. Signs of rhinitis in affected cats are usually mild, although infection may progress to pneumonia if not treated. Ocular signs, with a chronic unilateral or bilateral mucopurulent ocular discharge, are common with *C. psittaci* infection.[50,52,55,56,58]

Bordetella bronchiseptica has been shown to be capable of causing primary disease, particularly in overcrowded conditions. The disease is usually self-limiting, although in young animals it may progress to bronchopneumonia if untreated.[53,54,59]

CANINE VIRAL INFECTIONS

Signs of nasal disease may be seen with canine parainfluenza (CPI), canine herpesvirus (CHV), canine distemper virus (CDV), and canine adenoviruses types 1 and 2.[50]

BACTERIAL INFECTION

Most bacterial infections of the nasal cavity are considered to be secondary. They may occur following any compromise of the nasal defense mechanism, including viral, mycotic, or mycoplasmal infection; foreign bodies or other trauma; dental disease or extensions of other oral cavity disease; neoplasia; benign nasal or nasopharyngeal polyps; immunosuppressive drug regimes; and traumatic fracture of conchae or facial bones with secondary osteomyelitis.[50,51,56]

MYCOTIC INFECTION

Canine nasal mycotic infections are most commonly caused by *Aspergillus fumigatus,* but may also be caused by *A. nidulans, A. niger, A. flavus,* a number of Penicillium species, and *Rhinosporidium seeberi. A. fumigatus* is a normal inhabitant of the nasal cavity. Unlike humans, in which nasal fungal infections usually only occur in patients with immunocompromise, there is usually no evidence of immunocompromise in dogs. In some cases an underlying cause such as neoplasia or a foreign body can be identified. Nasal mycosis can occur in dogs of any age, but it tends to be more prevalent in younger animals.[60-63]

Cryptococcus neoformans is the most common cause of nasal mycosis in cats. Immunocompromise may be important in feline nasal cryptococcosis, and all cases should be screened for feline leukemia virus (FeLV) and feline immunodeficiency virus (FIV). Fungal granulomas may form with cryptococcosis and can mimic neoplasia radiographically.[64,65]

NEOPLASIA

Neoplasia of the nasal cavities occurs more often in the dog than in the cat, and more commonly in the cat than in other domestic animals. Eighty percent of nasal masses are malignant, although nasal and nasopharyngeal polyps and fungal granulomas can occur. Sixty to seventy-five percent of malignancies are epithelial in origin. The three most common are adenocarcinoma, lymphosarcoma, and undifferentiated carcinoma. Other reported neoplasms include osteosarcoma, fibrosarcoma, chondrosarcoma, and transmissible venereal tumor. Nasal tumors tend to be locally invasive, but have low metastatic potential. Approximately 10% metastasize, the most common sites being the regional lymph node, the lung, and the brain. Tumors are more likely to invade the cranial vault by local infiltration than by distant metastasis. Disease onset and progression is usually insidious, and tumors have often been present for some time at diagnosis. The average interval from diagnosis to death is 3 to 5 months. Nasal neoplasia tends to occur in middle age and older dogs, although the reported range is 1 to 15 years. There is no sex or breed predisposition, although nasal neoplasia is reported to occur more often in dolichocephalic and mesocephalic breeds. Nasal discharge is usually initially unilateral, but it may progress to become bilateral. A majority of tumors develop in the caudal nasal cavity; therefore, the discharge may be directed caudally to the nasopharynx rather than cranially towards the external nares and can appear to stop completely. Other clinical signs associated with nasal neoplasia include sneezing, epistaxis, epiphora, exophthalmus, facial deformity, pain, and neurological signs.[66-69]

ALLERGIC RHINITIS

Allergic rhinitis is either an unusual or an underdiagnosed condition in small animals. It is the result of a type I hypersensitivity reaction to inhaled allergens. There is typically a serous to mucoid discharge, with large numbers of eosinophils on cytological examination. With prolonged exposure to an allergen, epithelial hyperplasia may occur with submucosal lymphoplasmacytological infiltration.[50,70]

LYMPHOPLASMACYTIC RHINITIS

Lymphoplasmacytic rhinitis is an uncommon condition of nasal mucosal infiltration with lymphocytes and plasma cells. The cause is unknown, but it may follow an acute rhinitis of infectious or allergic origin, or it may be immune mediated. There are no eosinophils, unlike an acute type I hypersensitivity response.[50-71]

CHRONIC HYPERPLASTIC RHINITIS

Also known as chronic inflammatory rhinitis/sinusitis or chronic idiopathic rhinitis, this is a poorly defined disease that is largely a diagnosis of exclusion in dogs and cats and can present a diagnostic and therapeutic challenge. It may be present for months or years prior to diagnosis. Cases usually present with unilateral discharge at first, progressing to bilateral. Initially serous, the discharge usually progresses to become mucoid, mucopurulent, or sanguineous as a result of secondary infection.

There may be an initial response to antibiotics, with a relapse at the cessation of therapy. Often no precipitating causes are discovered. There may be a secondary tonsillitis or pharyngitis. These animals often sneeze predominantly first thing in the morning because of overnight accumulation of discharge. Whippets and dachshunds are thought to be predisposed.[50,61,70,72]

NASOPHARYNGEAL POLYPS

Nasopharyngeal polyps are proliferations of inflammatory tissue in the nasopharynx of cats. The polyps extend via the eustachian tube from the middle ear, and may grow into the external ear canal. The etiology of these growths is uncertain. They occur most often in young cats, with the average age 3 years and a range of 4 months to 7 years. Many of these cats have a mass that is evident on digital palpation of the soft palate. Nasopharyngeal polyps must be differentiated from lymphosarcoma, which may appear grossly similar but usually occurs in older cats (average age 10 years, range 5 to 19 years).[64,73,74]

NASAL (ETHMOTURBINATE) POLYPS

Nasal polyps have been reported in the cat. They originate from the ethmoturbinates and are inflammatory in nature. A variety of terms have been used to describe them, including fibrous dysplasia, ossifying fibroma, inflammatory nasal polyps, and aneurysmal bone cysts. The etiopathogenesis is obscure, although many cases have a recent history of upper respiratory tract infection, suggesting a chronic inflammatory process. Histologically there is a prominent vascular component with bone metaplasia, which also distinguishes them from nasopharyngeal polyps.[75]

PARASITIC RHINITIS

Parasites that can cause clinical signs in the nasal cavity include *Cuterebra* spp., *Linguatala serrata*, *Pneumonyssoides caninum*, and *Capillaria aerophila*. *Syngamus ierei* has also been reported in the cat. *C. aerophila* is primarily found in the lower respiratory tract, but has been reported in the upper airways. *P. caninum* has been closely associated with reverse sneezing because of its predilection for the nasopharynx.[72,75-79]

ORAL DISEASE

Purulent nasal discharge can occur as a result of the foreign body response to food particles that enter the nasal cavity through defects in the hard or soft palate, and the concomitant secondary bacterial infection. Palate defects may be congenital, resulting from a failure of the palate to fuse during fetal development, or acquired, usually as a result of head trauma. Periapical infections of the upper teeth may result in a purulent nasal discharge if the infection extends to the nasal mucosa. Infections may result from poor oral hygiene or a fracture of the tooth that extends into the pulp cavity.[72,80]

FOREIGN BODIES

Nasal foreign bodies result in a nasal discharge, initially serous but progressing to purulent with the onset of secondary bacterial infection. Inhalation of a nasal foreign body is usually accompanied by paroxysmal sneezing and pawing at the face. Occasionally there is acute epistaxis, or a chronic sanguineous discharge following mucosal damage. Foreign bodies may be inhaled or migrate from the external nares or oral cavity.[61,70,81]

EPISTAXIS

Epistaxis may have local or systemic causes. Local causes include mycotic infection; neoplasia; foreign body; and acute trauma to the nose, including trauma to the mucosa from sneezing. Systemic causes include coagulopathies, systemic hypertension, thrombocytopenia (e.g., ehrlichiosis, Rocky Mountain spotted fever), hyperviscosity syndrome, multiple myeloma, polycythemia, and vasculitis. Any coagulopathy may result in epistaxis, but it is more commonly associated with disorders of platelet number or function. Coagulopathies may be inherited (e.g., von Willebrand's disease, factor VIII deficiency) or acquired (e.g., vitamin K antagonist ingestion, disseminated intravascular coagulation, or immune mediated thrombocytopenia).[82,83]

MISCELLANEOUS

Other causes of nasal discharge include defects of the ciliary clearance mechanism, mechanical or chemical irritation from inhaled dust or chemicals, cystic Rathke's cleft, nasopharyngeal stenosis, bronchopulmonary disease, megaesophagus, and swallowing disorders that result in nasopharyngeal reflux of food (e.g., cricopharyngeal achalasia). The ciliary clearance mechanism is an important part of the local defense system, and is responsible for removing debris. It may be overwhelmed by large amounts of discharge, or in young animals primary ciliary dyskinesia may result in reduced clearance.[20,75,84,85]

REVERSE SNEEZE

Reverse sneezing localizes the lesion to the nasopharynx and has been reported in association with nasopharyngeal foreign bodies, *Pneumonyssoides caninum* infestation, and cystic Rathke's cleft. Other historically reported causes of reverse sneezing include behavioral causes, airborne irritants, neoplasia, sinus disease, post nasal drip, soft palate flutter, nasopharyngeal foreign body, and entrapment of the epiglottis within the laryngeal opening.[24,34,36,76-79,85-88]

Diagnostic Approach

A chronic nasal discharge is defined as one that has persisted for more than 4 weeks. A thorough evaluation of nasal disease should be performed as early as possible in its course, because early diagnosis and treatment can improve the prognosis for many conditions.

The order in which investigative procedures are carried out is important. Routine hematology and biochemistry are performed before general anesthesia. Coagulation profiles should also be performed in cases with epistaxis or a sanguineous discharge. Then, unless there is evidence of thrombocytopenia, hyperglobulinemia, or coagulopathy, the patient is anesthetized for diagnostic imaging, rhinoscopy, and sample collection. Diagnostic imaging is performed prior to rhinoscopy or sample collection because the presence of blood or saline may interfere with interpretation. Rhinoscopy is performed prior to sample collection because hemorrhage impedes visualization.*

SIGNALMENT

Signalment may provide a useful guide for diagnosis. Cats have some unique diseases, including nasopharyngeal polyps and feline upper respiratory tract disease complex. Age can give an indication of the diagnosis: in young animals, congenital or developmental diseases are more likely (e.g., congenital megaesophagus, cleft palate, and nasopharyngeal polyps). Mycotic rhinitis is seen more commonly in younger animals, whereas neoplasia is seen more in older animals, though the age spectrum is wide. Idiopathic hyperplastic rhinitis is seen more commonly in some breeds, especially the whippet. Breed associations are reported in over 30 breeds for von Willebrand's disease, whereas other breeds have a predisposition for megaesophagus.[24,61]

HISTORY

A description of the clinical signs includes an indication of the duration and progression of the disease, including treatments used and response to therapy. It is important to differentiate whether the discharge has consistently been unilateral, bilateral, started unilateral and become bilateral, or unilateral but changing sides. The type of discharge is categorized. Response to an appropriate course of treatment may help to indicate etiology. Discharges that respond during a course of antibiotics, but return after the cessation of treatment, indicate a secondary bacterial infection. Purulent or mucopurulent discharges that are unresponsive to antibiotics may indicate a mycotic infection or tumor.[24,50,61]

CLINICAL EXAMINATION

Thorough clinical examination of the patient is mandatory prior to focusing on the nose. It is essential to rule out concurrent systemic disease, which may be significant in the etiopathogenesis. Following examination of the animal the ocular, oral, and nasal areas should be assessed. An ocular examination should note the presence of discharge or epiphora, exophthalmus or enophthalmus, and include a retinal examination. Epiphora may indicate a nasolacrimal duct obstruction or may be the cause of a serous nasal discharge; exophthalmus indi-

---

*References 61,64,65,70,82,89.

cates a retrobulbar lesion (abscess or tumor); and cases of systemic cryptococcosis may demonstrate retinitis. The face should be examined for symmetry or distortion, depigmentation, and carefully palpated to locate pain. Airflow through both nostrils should be assessed using a glass slide to detect condensation, hair or cotton wool to detect turbulence, or by occlusion of a single nostril. Dogs and cats should be able to breathe comfortably through a single nostril.[24,61]

The oral cavity should be examined for oronasal fistulae and dental disease; and the soft palate should be digitally palpated, under sedation or general anesthesia if necessary. A dental probe should be used to examine the gingival sulcus of each upper tooth. Easy passage into the deeper periodontal region is suspicious. Dental radiography can be used as a further assessment of this area. Digital palpation may reveal pharyngeal masses, particularly nasopharyngeal polyps in cats. If the animal is sedated or anesthetized it should be possible to retract the soft palate rostrally with a hook to examine the nasopharynx.[24,50,61,64]

Although a definitive diagnosis cannot be made from history and physical examination alone, they are useful to help guide the choice of ancillary diagnostic procedures.

HEMATOLOGY AND BIOCHEMICAL PROFILE

Neutrophilia indicates the presence of inflammation or infection, which may be localized to the nose or may be associated with distant disease (e.g., pneumonia). Eosinophilia may occur with allergic or parasitic rhinitis. Thrombocytopenia and/or elevated concentrations of fibrinogen degradation products indicate a coagulopathy. Blood typing and cross-matching with potential donor blood should be performed in cases with severe epistaxis or when a rhinotomy is anticipated. The most significant biochemical finding that relates specifically to nasal disease is hyperglobulinemia, although serum biochemistry is obviously useful to screen for concurrent disease prior to anesthesia.[70,82]

COAGULATION PROFILE

Laboratory tests include the activated clotting time (ACT), activated partial thromboplastin time (APTT), one stage prothrombin time (OSPT), and measurements of fibrinogen and fibrinogen degradation products. Atraumatic collection and the use of citrated siliconized glass or plastic tubes, with the correct ratio of blood to anticoagulant (i.e., one part 3.8% citrate to nine parts blood), are essential for accurate results. Coagulation times are compared with a normal control sample taken from a healthy animal at the same time. A buccal mucosal bleeding time (BMBT) is a useful test of platelet function. A commercial bleeding time template should be used to create a wound of standard depth and size. Blood welling up from the incision is blotted, taking care to avoid touching the wound edges. Although the normal time to cessation of bleeding is quoted as 2.6 ± 0.5 minutes in the dog and 1.9 ± 0.5 minutes in the cat, times less than 5 minutes may be considered normal.[70,90]

PREANESTHESIA DIAGNOSTICS

In cases with suspected feline viral upper respiratory tract infection, swabs may be taken from the oropharynx and placed into virus transport media for isolation of FHV-1 and FCV, and conjunctival swabs can be taken for detection of *C. psittaci* and FHV-1. *Bordetella bronchiseptica* can be isolated from oropharyngeal swabs. In chronic cases in which the initiating factor was FHV-1, however, the primary viral infection may no longer be detectable. Swabs for bacterial culture may be taken, but unless there is a pure, heavy growth of pathogenic bacteria, the results are disregarded.[51-53,64,81]

A diagnosis of ehrlichiosis is confirmed by positive titers, but serology for *Aspergillus* spp. and *Penicillium* spp. may be confusing. A positive result can be considered consistent with, but not diagnostic for, infection because normal animals may sometimes have positive titers. Affected animals can remain seropositive for a long time after successful treatment, so serial estimation of titer does not provide an accurate evaluation of response to therapy. Although there is a decline over time following treatment, most dogs will retain a positive titer. False negatives are rare with the agar gel immunodiffusion assay for *Aspergillus* spp. and *Penicillium* spp., but counter immunoelectrophoresis may yield up to 15% false negatives. An enzyme linked immunosorbent assay (ELISA) is also available for aspergillus and penicillin detection, but is considered less reliable. Confirmation of serology should be sought by culture, cytology, biopsy, or direct visualization of fungal plaques. When a diagnosis of mycotic infection is confirmed, the possibility of an underlying cause such as immunosuppression or neoplasia should be considered.[61-63,91] Feline cryptococcosis is detected by latex agglutination capsular antigen test (LCAT), which is extremely sensitive and specific and can be used to monitor response to treatment in affected animals.[65,92] Feline immunodeficiency virus (FIV) and feline leukemia virus (FeLV) should be assayed in cats with cryptococcosis because immune compromise is considered important in the pathogenesis of the disease.[65]

DIAGNOSTIC IMAGING

The nasal cavity can be imaged using conventional radiography, computed tomography (CT), or magnetic resonance imaging (MRI). Although radiography is the most widely available and least expensive, it is also the least sensitive. CT and MRI are more sensitive to early change, allow better evaluation of the extent of tumors and the integrity of the cribriform plate, and are necessary for planning radiotherapy (Figures 3-2 and 3-3). General anesthesia is essential for radiography, CT, or MRI to allow correct positioning, and for radiography to allow the use of high detail film-screen combinations.[93-99]

Radiography requires two orthogonal views: the lateral skull; and a selection of a dorsal ventral (DV), a dorsal ventral intraoral (DVIO) or occlusal, or a ventro 20° rostral-dorsocaudal oblique open mouth (V20°R-DCdO). The DVIO requires the use of a flexible cassette to allow

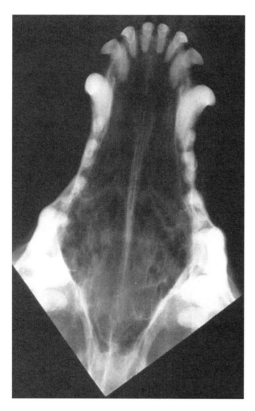

Figure 3-2. *DV/IO radiographic view of the nasal cavity of a dog with a septal nasal tumor, showing disruption of the caudal part of the nasal septum.*

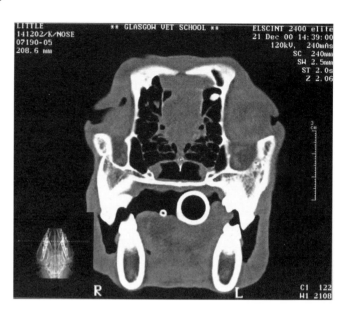

Figure 3-3. *Computed tomography view of the same dog as in Figure 3-2, showing the nasal septal tumor.*

sufficiently caudal insertion into the oral cavity. Traditionally, mammography film or nonscreen films were used for the DVIO because of their high detail and flexibility; however, flexible cassettes with screens are now widely available. When a flexible cassette is not available, or in brachycephalic dogs and all cats, the V20°R-DCdO view allows good visualization of the caudal nasal cavity and the cribriform plate. As the oblique angle increases above 20 degrees, the cribriform plate becomes less visible. The cribriform plate is a convex, domelike structure with multiple small fenestrations, so the radiographic line assessed as the cribriform plate is a tangential view. Defects in the cribriform plate need to be large (half the size or more of the cribriform plate), or must be radiographed in the correct plane before they can be visualized. In brachycephalic dogs the facial bone is superimposed onto the cribriform plate in the DV projection, so the oblique view (V20°R-DCdO) may be necessary to fully visualize the cribriform plate. A disadvantage of the oblique view is interpretation of the distorted radiographic anatomy.[100]

Radiographic evaluation should include an assessment of symmetry, bone or turbinate destruction, masses, variations of opacity, and soft tissue changes. It is important to assess the integrity of the boundaries of the nasal cavity, especially in cases where there is a destructive lesion such as neoplasia or fungal rhinitis. Interpretation of the normal radiographic anatomy of the nasal cavity and surrounding structures can be difficult due to superimposition of structures, extensive compartmentalization, intricate nasal anatomy, and wide variability of normal appearance of cat and dog skulls. The cartilaginous septum may not be visible radiographically, so any deviation or increased radiolucency of the septum may be due to destruction of the vomer bone.[50,69,100-102]

Computed tomography (CT) provides a detailed view of the nasal cavity and paranasal sinuses, with higher resolution and sensitivity than radiography. CT should be used prior to the treatment of nasal tumors to assess the full extent of the tumor for irradiation with or without prior debulking. CT allows better evaluation of areas such as the cribriform plate, and is also useful for soft tissue masses in the early stages of disease, when the mass has destroyed only the dorsal or ventral conchae. The cross-section view of the nasal cavity provided by CT removes the problems of superimposition seen with plain radiography. Using CT, nasal discharge or epistaxis may be difficult to differentiate from soft tissue opacity. Hounsfield units (HU) measure the attenuation of a field of interest. Air is −1000 HU, water 0 HU, compact bone >250 HU, spongy bone 130 ± 100 HU, and most soft tissue organs 30 to 45 ± 10 HU. In humans these measurements are used to identify different tissue types (e.g., in the nasal cavity to differentiate between a mass and epistaxis or nasal discharge). The use of intravenous contrast media to delineate tumors in the nasal cavities of dogs has not been evaluated, but it is useful when tumor invasion through the cribriform plate into the brain is suspected.[102,103]

Magnetic resonance imaging (MRI) has greater soft tissue resolution than CT and conventional radiography. It is superior to CT for detection and delineation of tumors and, unlike CT, tumors can be easily distinguished from nasal discharge and epistaxis. Contrast media can be used to increase the highlighting of tumor tissue. MRI is not useful for describing osseous changes, but is more sensitive for evaluation of tumor invasion, especially into the cranial vault. MRI is the imaging modality of choice for investigation of nasopharyngeal disease in humans, especially when neoplasia is suspected, because tumor margins, mass effects and extension to lymph nodes can be detected without contrast material or repositioning.[96-99]

ENDOSCOPY

Endoscopy allows direct evaluation of lesions and foreign bodies, and collection of biopsy samples under visual guidance. It should be performed after diagnostic imaging so that hemorrhage does not obscure or create radiographic lesions.

Rhinoscopy can be performed with an otoscope and a bright light source; a needle arthroscope or cystoscope; or, in larger breeds, a flexible fiberoptic bronchoscope, which will create less damage than a rigid arthroscope. The tip of the endoscope should be lubricated and gently inserted, never forced, through the external naris. Initially the tip of the scope should be directed medially and ventrally to gain access to the nasal cavity. Nasal mucosal bleeding is a common problem. The normal mucosa should appear shiny pink with minimal serous discharge. Mycotic lesions may appear as white or yellow to light green fluffy plaques. Turbinate destruction, such as with aspergillus infection, creates a cavernous, air-filled space.

Nasopharyngoscopy is used to evaluate the pharynx above the soft palate; it requires a flexible endoscope with a bidirectional tip. It should be possible to visualize the caudal choanae.

TISSUE BIOPSY

Final diagnosis of nasal disorders usually requires biopsy. Biopsy can be performed under direct visualization with endoscopy, or using blind techniques. Care must be taken not to penetrate the cribriform plate when using blind sampling techniques: the medial canthus of the eye is generally considered a useful guide for the maximum distance to enter the nasal cavity. Blind collection techniques include the use of a rigid polyethylene tube, to take essentially a core biopsy, or Jackson (arthroscopic) cup biopsy forceps. Samples collected should be evaluated histologically, cytologically, and cultured for fungal and bacterial growth. Histopathological diagnosis is required for definitive diagnosis of nasal tumors. Aspiration biopsy using a large-diameter rigid plastic tube can retrieve a diagnostic sample in most cases, and is a suitable method for collection where endoscopic or Jackson cup forceps are not available. A large bore tube, 5 to 7 millimeters in diameter, is inserted to the level of the area of interest, as identified by radiography, taking care not to go past the level of the medial canthus of the eye. Suction is applied and the tube

is withdrawn. Trephination may be performed for localized entry over suspected lesions, a technique particularly applicable for frontal sinus disease because it allows biopsy and placement of drains. Hemorrhage is a major complication of tissue biopsy by any method. Packing the nasal cavity temporarily with cotton buds soaked in dilute epinephrine or phenylephrine may control mild to moderate hemorrhage from closed biopsy techniques. Care should be taken to use a subtherapeutic dose of epinephrine because it is well absorbed across the mucosa.[67,83]

CYTOLOGY

Cytological examination is a useful screening test for nasal disease. Negative or nonspecific results do not exclude the presence of serious nasal diseases such as neoplasia or fungal rhinitis. Cytology may be performed on all biopsy samples collected for histopathological examination. Prior to placing the biopsy sample in formalin, a touch preparation is made. Blood is blotted off the sample, which is then touched onto the surface of a glass slide several times. This slide is then dried and stained as usual. Aspiration biopsies may provide tissue fragments that can be smeared for cytological examination. Other techniques for acquiring samples specifically for cytology include nasal flushing or a guarded brush.[89,104-106]

Nasal flushing should not be relied on to provide a sample for definitive diagnosis, but it has been shown to be diagnostic in approximately 50% of dogs with nasal tumors.[107] Various techniques are described. One technique is to pack the nasopharynx and external nares with gauze swabs, and using a urinary catheter cut at 45 degrees, inserted to the area of interest, use intermittent flushing and suction of saline to obtain tissue and fluid. The gauze swabs should also be examined at the completion of the flush for further samples. Cytological preparations should be examined for the presence of fungal elements, tumor cells, the type of inflammatory cells, and the presence of bacteria. Care should be taken in the interpretation because in severe inflammation some dysplastic cells may appear neoplastic.[50,66,67]

CULTURE

The normal canine and feline nasal cavity may contain a mixed bacterial and fungal population, which can make interpretation of culture results difficult. If bacteria are involved, they are usually considered to be secondary to another disease process (e.g., mycotic infection, viral infection, foreign body, or tumor). Bacterial culture is only considered significant if there is heavy growth of a single isolate. The diagnostic value of bacterial culture may be increased if the sample is obtained by surgical or endoscopic biopsy. Fungal culture should ideally be carried out on samples collected by direct visualization from fungal colonies. Sabaroud's dextrose agar with antibacterials should be used as the culture media. A positive fungal culture in a symptomatic dog should be considered positive unless collected with poor aseptic technique. Fungal infection may occur in up to 30% to 40% of cases with a nasal tumor. False negative fungal culture may occur with poor collection techniques, poor culture techniques, or bacterial overgrowth.[50,108]

RHINOTOMY

Rhinotomy may be performed if other attempts at diagnosis have failed. It may be possible to remove the causative factor (e.g., a foreign body); however, visualization is hindered by the inevitable hemorrhage, though temporary occlusion of the common carotids has been described.[109] Other complications of rhinotomy include persistent epistaxis, chronic nasal discharge, and subcutaneous emphysema, so careful planning and good client communication are important. Hemorrhage may be profuse and may require circulatory support and, in some cases, transfusion.[83,110]

Initial Management

Sudden onset of paroxysmal sneezing should be investigated for foreign body involvement. The initial use of corticosteroids should be avoided, because they may interfere with later diagnostic procedures.

Swallowing has been reported to be effective in terminating reverse sneezing, so owners may be encouraged to stroke the pharyngeal area to induce swallowing. Other reported methods of stopping reverse sneezing include covering the external nares, or distraction techniques, including loud noises.[35,36]

In areas in which *P. caninum* is endemic, it is common to treat empirically with ivermectin (200 to 400 μg/kg) or milbemycin oxime (1 mg/kg) before beginning investigation for other causes. The diagnosis and success of treatment are both based on the clinical response to treatment. Milbemycin is safe in all dogs and is considered to have fewer side effects than ivermectin, although animals sensitive to ivermectin may also be sensitive to an overdose of milbemycin. If milbemycin is not available, ivermectin may be titrated to a safe maximum dose by once daily dosing starting at 50 μg/kg, increasing by 50-μg/kg increments until a therapeutic dose of 300 μg/kg is reached. Signs of toxicity for both drugs are similar and include mydriasis with poor pupillary light reflex, apparent blindness, ataxia, changes in behavior, weakness, recumbency, lethargy, ptyalism, coma, and death. Reported cases of toxicosis with ivermectin have recovered spontaneously over the course of 1 to 7 days.[88,111-114]

Treatment of nasal discharge should be focused on identification and management of the primary etiology. Palliative care of animals with chronic nasal discharges is important, because a chronic viscous discharge can reduce olfaction and impair appetite, particularly in cats. Treatment involves reducing the production and aiding clearance of the discharge. The volume of discharge may be reduced by the use of decongestants. Phenylephrine and phenylpropanolamine are α₁-adrenergic agonists that by peripheral vasoconstriction act to reduce congestion and edema of the nasal mucosa. Phenylephrine 0.25% may be given intranasally; in cats the recommended dose is one drop every 4 to 6 hours. Rebound congestion and discharge may occur when the treatment is stopped. Nostrils may be treated alternately for 3 to 4 days at a time to reduce rebound. Phenylpropanolamine should also only be given for 3 to 4 days at a time to reduce rebound. Humidification and mucolytic drugs may aid clearance of discharge. Humidification may be achieved by placing the animal in a humid atmosphere (e.g., the bathroom with a hot shower running) three or four times a day for 15 to 30 minutes each time; or by administering sterile saline directly into the nasal cavity. Bromhexine can also be effective in some cases. The external nares should be cleaned regularly with moistened cotton. Cats in particular will improve if their faces are kept clean. Heating the food and the use of drugs such as intravenous diazepam or cyproheptadine *per os* can stimulate appetite in affected cats. Enteral nutritional support and intravenous fluid therapy may be required in severe cases and should be initiated promptly. Good nursing is essential in these cases.[50,55,56,74,115]

Corticosteroids can be useful in some cases, but should be avoided if possible, particularly before diagnostic procedures. Antihistamines are preferable when an allergic basis is suspected. In addition to the systemic side effects of long-term corticosteroid administration, prolonged use may predispose to mycotic rhinitis, allow mycotic infection to disseminate, increase viral shedding, or mask the presence of a tumor. However, in the presence of an untreatable neoplasm, corticosteroids may provide palliation.[71,115]

In some cases, flushing the nasal cavity with dilute povidone-iodine in a 1:10 solution may provide short-term relief from nasal congestion. Even clearing secretions from the nasal cavity with a saline flush at the time of diagnostic evaluation provides some relief.[50,115]

Severe epistaxis, especially if there is an underlying coagulopathy, may require shock doses of intravenous crystalloid or colloid administration, or blood transfusion. The patient should be cross-matched with potential donors at the earliest possible time. In traumatic cases of epistaxis, the skull and the oral cavity should be examined, and the animal cage-rested and examined for neurological deficits. Narcotic agents provide both analgesia and sedation, although morphine should be avoided because of the associated risk of vomiting, which might increase intracranial pressure. If the patient is still anxious, benzodiazepines are useful. The head should be kept low to reduce the risk of aspiration. External ice packs should be avoided because they increase anxiety and have no effect on hemostasis. Packing the external naris or nares, without concurrently packing the caudal choanae, should be avoided because this redirects hemorrhage to the nasopharynx, increasing the risk of aspiration. If the animal will tolerate placement (possibly with general or local anesthetic), the nasal cavity can be packed with gauze soaked in epinephrine (1:100000), phenylephrine, or, where available, cocaine 4%, which also has an analgesic effect. Packing material should be left in place for 24 hours. Rhinotomy is rarely required to remove damaged conchae or bone fragments and control hemorrhage. Possible sequelae to nasal trauma include bacterial or mycotic osteomyelitis, sequestra, sinusitis, and frontal mucocele.[83,110]

REFERENCES

1. Tomori Z, Benacka R, Donic V: Mechanisms and clinicophysiological implications of the sniff- and gasp-like aspiration reflex, *Respir Physiol* 114:83-98, 1998.
2. Widdecombe JG: Reflexes from the upper respiratory tract. In Cherniack NS, Widdecombe JG, editors: *Handbook of physiology, section 3: The respiratory system*, vol. 3, *Control of breathing*, part 1, Washington DC, 1986, American Physiological Society.
3. Iscoe SD: Central control of upper airway. In Mathew OP, Sant'Ambrogio G, editors: *Respiratory function of upper airway*, Basel, 1988, Marcel Deckker.
4. Tucker A: Pathophysiology of the respiratory system. In Douglas Slatter, editor: *Textbook of small animal surgery*, ed 2, London, 1993, WB Saunders.
5. Grandage G, Richardson K: Functional anatomy. In Douglas Slatter, editor: *Textbook of small animal surgery*, ed 2, London, 1993, WB Saunders.
6. Evans HE: The nasal cavity. In Evans HE, editor: *Miller's anatomy of the dog*, ed 3, Philadelphia, 1993, WB Saunders.
7. Toremalm N-G: Factors influencing the mucociliary activity in the respiratory tract, *Eur J Respir Dis* 61(suppl 107): 41, 1980.
8. Adams DR, Deyoung DW, Griffith R: The lateral nasal gland of the dog: Its structure and secretory content, *J Anat* 132:29, 1981.
9. Adams DR: *Canine anatomy: A systematic study*, Ames, IA, 1986, Iowa State University Press.
10. Adams DR, Hotchkiss DK: The canine nasal mucosa, *Anatomia Histologia Embryologia* 12:109, 1983.
11. Wolf AM: Nasal cavity and paranasal sinus disease. In Bojrab MJ, editor: *Disease mechanisms in small animal surgery*, ed 2, London, 1993, Lea & Febiger.
12. Goldberg MB, Langman VA, Taylor CR: Panting in dogs: Paths of air flow in response to heat and exercise, *Respir Physiol* 43(3):327-328, 1981.
13. Blatt CM, Taylor CR, Habal MB: Thermal panting in dogs: The lateral nasal gland, a source of water for evaporative cooling, *Science* 177:804, 1972.
14. Evans HE: The lateral nasal gland and its duct in the dog, *Anat Rec* 187:574, 1977.
15. Tomori Z, Kurpas M, Donic V et al: Reflex reversal of apneic episodes by electrical stimulation of upper airways in cats, *Respir Physiol* 102:175-185, 1995.
16. Ohnishi T, Ogura JH: Partitioning of pulmonary resistance in the dog, *Laryngoscope* 79:1847, 1969.
17. Lane JG: Feline nasal disorders. In King N, editor: *ENT and oral surgery of the dog and cat*, Bristol, 1982, John Wright and Sons.
18. Cook JR: Infection in asthma, *Sem Resp Med* 8:259-263, 1987.
19. Adinoff AD, Irvin CG: Upper respiratory tract disease and asthma, *Sem Resp Med* 8:308-314, 1987.
20. Dye JA, McKiernan BC, Rozanski EA et al: Bronchopulmonary disease in the cat: Historical, physical, radiographic, clinicopathologic, and pulmonary functional evaluation of 24 affected and 15 healthy cats, *J Vet Int Med* 10:385-400, 1996.
21. Kaufman J, Wright GW: The effect of nasal and nasopharyngeal irritation on airway resistance in man, *Am Rev Resp Dis* 100:626-630, 1969.
22. Nolte D, Berger B: On vagal bronchoconstriction in asthmatic patients by nasal irritation, *Europ J Resp Dis* 64:110-115, 1983.
23. Buckner CK, Songsiridej V, Dick EC et al: In vivo and in vitro studies on the use of the guinea pig as a model for virus-provoked airway hyperreactivity, *Am Rev Resp Dis* 132:305-310, 1985.
24. McKiernan BC: Sneezing and nasal discharge. In Ettinger SJ, Feldman EC, editors: *Textbook of veterinary internal medicine*, ed 5, Philadelphia, 2000, WB Saunders.
25. Satoh I, Shiba K, Kobayashi N et al: Upper airway motor outputs during sneezing and coughing in decerebrate cats, *Neurosci Res* 32:131-135, 1998.
26. Wallois F, Bodineau L, Macron JM et al: Role of respiratory and nonrespiratory neurones in the region of the NTS in the elaboration of the sneeze reflex in cat, *Brain Res* 768:71-85, 1997.
27. Shiba K, Satoh I, Kobayashi N et al: Multifunctional laryngeal motor neurons: An intracellular study in the cat, *J Neurosci* 19: 2717-2727, 1999.
28. Korpas J, Tomori Z: Sneezing. In Herzog HS, editor: *Progress in respiration research: Cough and other respiratory reflexes*, vol 12, Basel, 1979, Karger.
29. Wallois F, Macron JM, Duron B: Activities of vagal receptors in the different phases of sneeze in cats, *Resp Physiol* 101:239-255, 1995.
30. McKiernan BC: Sneezing and nasal discharge. In Ettinger SJ, Feldman EC, editors: *Textbook of veterinary internal medicine*, ed 5, Philadelphia, 2000, WB Saunders.
31. Whitman BW, Packer RJ: The photic sneeze reflex: Literature review and discussion, *Neurology* 43:868-871, 1993.
32. Sant'Ambrogio G, Widdicombe J: Reflexes from rapidly adapting receptors, *Respir Physiol* 125:33-45, 2001.
33. Blood DC, Studdert VP: Reverse sneeze. In Blood DC, Studdert VP, editors: *Saunders comprehensive veterinary dictionary*, London, 1999, WB Saunders.
34. McKiernan BC: Sneezing and nasal discharge. In Ettinger SJ, Feldman EC, editors: *Textbook of veterinary internal medicine*, ed 4, Philadelphia, 1995, WB Saunders.
35. Venker-van Hagen AJ: Reverse sneezing. In Ettinger SJ, Feldman EC, editors: *Textbook of veterinary internal medicine*, ed 5, Philadelphia, 2000, WB Saunders.
36. Lane JG: Reverse sneezing. In King N, editor: *ENT and oral surgery of the dog and cat*, Bristol, 1982, John Wright and Sons.
37. Korpás J, Tomori Z: *Cough and other respiratory reflexes*, Basel, 1979, Karger.
38. Tomori Z, Kurpas M, Donic V et al: Reflex reversal of apneic episodes by electrical stimulation of upper airways in cats, *Resp Physiol* 105:175-185, 1995.
39. Tomori Z, Donic V Benacka R et al: Reversal of apnea by aspiration reflex in anaesthetized cats, *Europ Respir J* 4:1117-1125, 1991.
40. Benacka R, Tomori Z: The sniff-like aspiration reflex evoked by electrical stimulation of the nasopharynx, *Respir Physiol* 102:163-174, 1995.
41. Tomori Z, Fung M-L, Donic V et al. Power spectral analysis of respiratory responses to pharyngeal stimulation in cats, *J Physiol* 485:551-559, 1995.
42. St. John WM: Medullary regions for neurogenesis of gasping: Noeud or noeuds vitals? *J Appl Physiol* 81:1865-1877, 1996.
43. Salem MR, Baraka A, Rattenborg CC et al: Treatment of hiccups by pharyngeal stimulation in anesthetized and conscious subjects, *J Am Med Assoc* 202:32-36, 1967.
44. Tomori Z, Widdecombe JG: Muscular, bronchomotor and cardiovascular reflexes elicited by mechanical stimulation of the respiratory tract, *J Physiol* 200:25-49, 1969.
45. Wallois F, Macron LJM, Jounieux V et al: Trigeminal nasal receptors related to respiration and to various stimuli in cats, *Respir Physiol* 85:111-125, 1994.
46. Fung M-L, St. John WM, Tomori Z: Reflex recruitment of medullary gasping mechanisms in eupnea by pharyngeal stimulation in cats, *J Physiol* 475:519-529, 1994.
47. Nail BS, Sterling GM, Widdecombe JG: Patterns of spontaneous and reflex-induced activity in phrenic and intercostal motor neurons, *Exp Brain Res* 15:318-332, 1972.
48. Tomori Z, Donic V, Kurpas M: Comparison of inspiratory effort in sniff-like aspiration reflex, gasping and normal breathing in cats, *Europ Respir J* 6:53-59, 1993.
49. Stránsky A: *Activity of laryngeal motorneurons and changes in laryngeal resistance induced by stimulation of pulmonary and airway receptors*, PhD Thesis, Martin, Slovakia, 1975, Medical Faculty Comenius University.
50. Kuehn NF, Roudebush P: Nasal discharge. In Allen DG, editor: *Small animal medicine*, Philadelphia, 1991, JB Lippincott.
51. Cape L: Feline idiopathic chronic rhinosinusitus: A retrospective study of 30 cases, *JAAHA* 38:149-154, 1992.
52. Sykes JE, Anderson GA, Studdert VP et al: Prevalence of feline *Chlamydia psittaci* and feline herpesvirus 1 in cats with upper respiratory tract disease, *J Vet Intern Med* 13:153-162, 1999.

53. Jacobs AAC, Chalmers WSK, Pasman J et al: Feline bordetellosis: Challenge and vaccine studies, *Vet Rec* 133:260-263, 1993.
54. Binns SH, Speakman AJ, Cuevas LE et al: Prevalence and risk factors for feline *Bordetella bronchiseptica* infection, *Vet Rec* 144:575-580, 1999.
55. Ford RB: Viral upper respiratory infection in cats, *Compend Cont Ed Pract Vet* 13:593-602, 1991.
56. Ford RB: Infectious respiratory disease, *Vet Clin North Am Small Anim Pract* 14(5):985-1006, 1984.
57. Knowles JO, McArdle F, Dawson S et al: Studies on the role of feline calicivirus in chronic stomatitis in cats, *Vet Microbiol* 27:205-219, 1991.
58. Hoover EA, Kahn DE, Langloss JM: Experimentally induced feline chlamydial infection (feline pneumonitis), *Am J Vet Res* 39:541-547, 1978.
59. Welsh R: *Bordetella bronchiseptica* infections in cats, *JAAHA* 32:153-158, 1996.
60. Caniatti M, Roccabianca P, Scanziani E et al: Nasal rhinosporidiosis in dogs: Four cases from Europe and a review of the literature, *Vet Rec* 142:334-338, 1998.
61. Sullivan M: Nasal discharge in the dog. In Gorman N, editor: *Canine medicine and therapeutics*, Oxford, 1998, Blackwell Science.
62. Lane JG, Warnock DW: The diagnosis of *Aspergillus fumigatus* infection of the nasal chambers of the dog with particular reference to the value of the double diffusion test, *J Small Anim Pract* 18:169-177, 1977.
63. Richardson M, Warnock DW, Bovey SE et al: Rapid serological diagnosis of *Aspergillus fumigatus* infection of the frontal sinuses and nasal chambers of the dog, *Res Vet Sci* 33:167-169, 1982.
64. Allen HS, Brossard J, Noone K: Nasopharyngeal diseases in cats: A retrospective study of 53 cases (1991-1998), *J Am An Hosp Assoc* 35:457-461, 1999.
65. Norsworthy GD: Finding the cause of chronic nasal discharge in cats, *Veterinary Medicine* 90:1038-1046, 1995.
66. Theisen SK, Lewis DD, Hosgood G: Intranasal tumors in dogs: Diagnosis and treatment, *Compend Cont Ed Pract Vet* 18:131-138, 1996.
67. Legendre AM: Canine nasal and paranasal sinus tumors, *J Am An Hosp Assoc* 19:115-123, 1983.
68. Bradley PA, Harvey CE: Intranasal tumors in the dog: An evaluation of prognosis, *J Small Anim Pract* 14:459-467, 1973.
69. Hayes HM, Wilson GP: Carcinomas of the nasal cavity and paranasal sinuses in dogs: Descriptive epidemiology, *Cornell Vet* 72:168-179, 1982.
70. Tasker S, Knottenbelt CM, Munro EAC et al: Aetiology and diagnosis of persistent nasal disease in the dog: A retrospective study of 42 cases, *J Small Anim Pract* 40:473-478, 1999.
71. Burgener DC, Slocombe RF, Zerbe CA: Lymphoplasmacytic rhinitis in five dogs, *JAAHA* 23:565-568, 1987.
72. Lane JG: Canine nasal disorders. In King N, editor: *ENT and oral surgery of dog and cat*, Bristol, 1982, John Wright and Sons.
73. Anderson DM, Robinson RK, White RAS: Management of inflammatory polyps in 37 cats, *Vet Rec* 147:684-687, 2000.
74. Bradley RL: Selected oral, pharyngeal, and upper respiratory conditions in the cat, *Vet Clin North Am Small Anim Pract* 14(6):1173-1184, 1984.
75. Galloway PE, Kyles A, Henderson JP: Nasal polyps in a cat, *J Small Anim Pract* 38:78-80, 1997.
76. Christensson D, Rehbinder C: *Pneumonyssus caninum:* A mite in the pneumatic cavities of the dog, *Nordisk Veterinärmedicin* 23:499-505, 1971.
77. Gunnarsson L, Zakrisson G, Lilliehöök I et al: Experimental infection of dogs with the nasal mite *Pneumonyssoides caninum*, *Vet Parasit* 77:179-186, 1998.
78. Marks SL, Moore MP, Rishniw M: *Pneumonyssoides caninum:* The canine nasal mite, *Compend Cont Ed Pract Vet* 16:577-582, 1994.
79. Bredal W: Nesemidd hos hund, *Norsk Veterinærtidsskrift* 108:11-17, 1996.
80. Bellows J: A misdiagnosed cause of chronic sneezing in a dog, *Veterinary Medicine* 96:103-104, 2001.
81. Gabor L, Price JE, Laurendet HM et al: Paroxysmal sneezing in a 7-year-old cat, *Aust Vet J* 75:320, 328, 335, 1997.
82. Littlewood JD: A practical approach to bleeding disorders in the dog, *J Small Anim Pract* 27:397-409, 1986.
83. Mahoney OM: Bleeding disorders: Epistaxis and hemoptysis. In Ettinger SJ, Feldman EC, editors: *Textbook of veterinary internal medicine*, ed 5, Philadelphia, 2000, WB Saunders.
84. Vaden SL, Breitscwerdt EB, Henrikson CK, et al: Primary ciliary dyskinesia in Bichon-frise litter mates, *J Am Anim Hosp Assoc* 27:633-640, 1991.
85. Beck JA, Hunt GB, Goldsmid SE et al: Nasopharyngeal obstruction due to cystic Rathke's clefts in two dogs, *Austral Vet J* 77:94-97, 1999.
86. Tomori Z: The function of the glottis in respiratory tract reflexes, *Folia Medica Martiniana* 4:243-258, 1979.
87. Tyler JW:. Endoscopic retrieval of a large, nasopharyngeal foreign body, *J Am Anim Hosp Assoc* 33:513-516, 1997.
88. Bredal W, Vollset I: Use of milbemycin oxime in treatment of dogs with nasal mite *(Pneumonyssoides caninum)* infection, *J Small Anim Pract* 39:233-237, 1998.
89. Andreason CB, Rakich PM, Latimer KS: Nasal exudates and masses. In Cowell RL, Tyler RD, Meinkoth JH, editors: *Diagnostic cytology of the dog and cat*, St Louis, 1999, Mosby.
90. Couto CG, Hammer AS: Hematologic and oncologic emergencies. In Murtaugh RJ, Kaplan PM, editors: *Veterinary emergency and critical care*, London, 1992, Mosby.
91. Khan ZU, Richardson MD, Warnock DW et al: Evaluation of an enzyme-linked immunosorbent assay (ELISA) for the diagnosis of *Aspergillus fumigatus* intranasal infection of the dog, *Sabouraudia* 22:251-254, 1984.
92. Medleau L, Marks AM, Brown J et al: Clinical evaluation of a cryptococcal antigen latex agglutination test for diagnosis of cryptococcosis in cats, *JAVMA* 196:1470-1473, 1990.
93. Gibbs C, Lane JG, Denny HR: Radiological features of intranasal lesions in the dog: A review of 100 cases, *J Small Anim Pract* 20:515-535, 1979.
94. Burk RL: Computed tomographic anatomy of the canine nasal passages, *Vet Radiol Ultrasound* 33:170-176, 1992.
95. Burk RL: Computed tomographic imaging of nasal disease in 100 dogs, *Vet Radiol Ultrasound* 33:177-180, 1992.
96. Voges AK, Ackerman N: MR evaluation of intra and extracranial extension of nasal adenocarcinoma in a dog and cat, *Vet Radiol Ultrasound* 36:196-200, 1995.
97. Dillon WP, Mills CM, Kjos B et al: Magnetic resonance imaging of the nasopharynx, *Radiology* 152:731-738, 1984.
98. Moore MP, Gavin PR, Kraft SL et al: MR, CT, and clinical features from four dogs with nasal tumours involving the rostra cerebrum, *Vet Rad* 32:19-25, 1991.
99. Assheur J, Sager M: Splanchnocranium. In Assheur J, Sager M, editors: *MRI and CT atlas of the dog*, London, 1997, Blackwell Science.
100. Schwarz T, Sullivan M, Hartung K: Radiographic anatomy of the cribriform plate (lamina cribosa), *Vet Radiol Ultrasound* 41:220-225, 2000.
101. Harvey CE: The nasal septum of the dog: Is it visible radiographically? *Vet Rad* 20:88-90, 1979.
102. Berry CR, Koblik PD: Evaluation of survey radiography, linear tomography and computed tomography for detecting experimental lesions of the cribriform plate in dogs, *Vet Rad* 31:146-154, 1990.
103. Assheur J, Sager M: Principles of imaging techniques. In Assheur J, Sager M, editors: *MRI and CT atlas of the dog*, London, 1997, Blackwell Science.
104. French TW: The use of cytology in the diagnosis of chronic nasal disorders, *Compend Cont Ed Pract Vet* 9:115-121, 1987.
105. Withrow SJ, Susaneck SJ, Macy DW et al: Aspiration and punch biopsy techniques for nasal tumours, *JAAHA* 21:551-554, 1985.
106. Meyer DJ: The management of cytology specimens, *Compend Cont Ed Pract Vet* 9:10-16, 1987.
107. MacEwen EG, Withrow SJ, Patnaik AK: Nasal tumours in the dog: Retrospective evaluation of diagnosis, prognosis and treatment, *JAVMA* 170:45-48, 1977.
108. Turnwald GH: Dyspnea and tachypnea. In Ettinger SJ, Feldman EC, editors: *Textbook of veterinary internal medicine*, ed 5, Philadelphia, 2000, WB Saunders.
109. Hedlund CS, Tangner CH, Elkins AD et al: Temporary bilateral carotid artery occlusion during surgical exploration of the nasal cavity of the dog, *Vet Surg* 12:83-85, 1983.

110. Hedlund CS: Rhinotomy techniques. In Bojrab MJ, Ellison GW, Slocum B, editors: *Current techniques in small animal surgery,* ed 4, Baltimore, 1997, Williams and Wilkins.
111. Stansfield DG, Hepler DI: Safety and efficacy of milbemycin oxime for parasite control, *Canine Pract* 16:11-16, 1991.
112. Mueller RS, Bettenay SV: A proposed new treatment protocol for the treatment of canine mange with ivermectin, *J Am An Hosp Assoc* 35:77-80, 1999.
113. Paradis M: Ivermectin in small animal dermatology, part I, pharmacology and toxicology, *Compend Cont Ed Pract Vet* 20:193-200, 1998.
114. Tranquilli WJ, Paul AJ, Todd KS: Assessment of toxicosis induced by high dose administration of milbemycin oxime in collies, *Am J Vet Res* 52:1170-1172, 1991.
115. Norsworthy GD: Treating chronic nasal discharge in cats, *Veterinary Medicine* 90:1048-1054, 1995.

CHAPTER 4

Epistaxis

Mary Beth Callan

Definition and Clinical Signs

Epistaxis refers to hemorrhage from the nasal cavity. Bleeding may be noted from one or both nares, and may vary in volume from a few drops to life-threatening blood loss leading to hypovolemia and severe anemia. The degree of epistaxis may appear diminished if some of the blood is swallowed; this results in melena. The presence of other clinical signs depends on the underlying cause of the epistaxis, which may result from a local or systemic disorder.

General Pathophysiology

The blood supply to the nose arises from the maxillary and facial arteries via the external carotid artery, and from the internal and external ethmoidal arteries via the internal carotid artery. These vessels branch into a fine capillary meshwork that can be readily damaged. Normal hemostasis is dependent on platelets to prevent extravasation of blood from capillaries. Due to the exposed capillaries in the nasal mucosa, primary hemostatic disorders such as thrombocytopenia, thrombopathia, and von Willebrand's disease may lead to spontaneous bleeding from the nasal cavity. Epistaxis may result from traumatic rupture of blood vessels in the nasal cavity, as well as from local processes damaging the nasal mucosal lining (e.g., neoplasia or fungal infection). Systemic hypertension results in arteriolar changes (e.g., hyalinization and degeneration of arteries/arterioles, intimal proliferation, medial hypertrophy, and atherosclerosis) that may lead to changes in capillary permeability and hemorrhage. Similarly, hyperviscosity secondary to polycythemia or hyperglobulinemia leads to decreased blood flow, distension of capillaries and small vessels, and possible rupture of blood vessels.

History and Physical Examination

The patient's signalment may be helpful in prioritizing differential diagnoses. For example, von Willebrand's disease (vWD) should be a top differential diagnosis in a young Doberman pinscher with epistaxis (and possibly other surface bleeding) as its only clinical sign. Neoplasia is more likely to occur in older animals, whereas an inflammatory lesion or nasal foreign body may be more common in younger animals.

A complete history and physical examination are essential in helping to determine if the epistaxis is due to a local or systemic disorder. A history of chronic sneezing, serous or mucoid nasal discharge, and stertorous breathing suggests a local problem involving the nasal cavity, whereas an acute onset of epistaxis without other signs of nasal disease may be more suggestive of a systemic disorder. Trauma may result in a single episode of epistaxis and may not warrant a complete diagnostic evaluation if it resolves spontaneously or with local therapy. Recurrence of epistaxis or the presence of other mucosal surface bleeding may suggest a primary hemostatic disorder. Excessive bleeding following surgery or trauma in an otherwise young healthy animal, or a family history of similar bleeding, may be suggestive of an inherited hemostatic defect. Considering the many potential causes of acquired quantitative and qualitative platelet disorders, a complete medication history is imperative. Information about recent vaccinations, tick exposure, and previous or concurrent medical problems is relevant. Also, travel history may reveal that the patient has visited an area where particular infectious diseases are endemic. In patients with hypertension or polycythemia, acute onset of blindness or seizures, respectively, may be noted in addition to epistaxis.

Whereas a complete physical examination is essential to evaluate for evidence of systemic illness, particular attention to the head is indicated in patients with epistaxis. Facial asymmetry, exophthalmos, or inability to retropulse the eyes are suggestive of neoplasia; however, facial asymmetry may also be noted with aggressive infectious and inflammatory processes. Retrobulbar hemorrhage as a result of a bleeding disorder may also cause exophthalmos. Ulceration of the nasal planum may be noted with both neoplasia and fungal infections. A complete oropharyngeal examination should be performed to evaluate for erosion of tumor through the hard palate, for a polyp, or for a penetrating foreign body, as well as for severe dental disease or an oronasal fistula, which may lead to nasal discharge and epistaxis. The regional lymph nodes may be enlarged as a result of either metastasis or a local inflammatory response, or as part of a generalized lymphadenopathy associated with a systemic disorder. Ophthalmological examination may reveal retinal detachment or hemorrhage in patients with hypertension, tortuous retinal vessels in patients with polycythemia, and uveitis or chorioretinitis in patients with various infectious diseases and neoplasia. The presence of petechiae, ecchymoses or other surface bleeding indicates a primary hemostatic disorder.

Differential Diagnosis

Epistaxis may be due to a systemic disorder or a local process within the nasal cavity. However, it should be noted that animals with disease in the nasal cavity may experience excessive bleeding as the result of a concurrent bleeding disorder. As noted above, a careful history and physical examination are essential in prioritizing differential diagnoses and in formulating an appropriate diagnostic and therapeutic plan.

SYSTEMIC DISORDERS

Bleeding Disorders

In general, disorders of secondary hemostasis (i.e., coagulopathies) tend to result in bleeding into body cavities and hematoma formation, whereas disorders of primary hemostasis typically cause mucosal surface bleeding and formation of petechiae and ecchymoses. However, epistaxis has been noted in animals with coagulopathies, whether they are hereditary (e.g., hemophilia), acquired (e.g., anticoagulant rodenticide poisoning), or combined hemostatic disorders (e.g., disseminated intravascular coagulation).

The most common disorder of primary hemostasis is thrombocytopenia, which results either from decreased platelet production by the bone marrow or from increased platelet destruction, consumption, or sequestra-tion. Often more than one mechanism is involved. For example, bone marrow suppression, consumption of platelets secondary to vasculitis, splenic sequestration, and increased destruction of platelets by both immune-mediated and nonimmunological mechanisms may contribute to thrombocytopenia in dogs and cats with infectious diseases. Spontaneous bleeding is typically not expected until the platelet count is less than $40,000/\mu l$, unless there is a concurrent coagulopathy or vasculitis. In dogs, the most common cause of severe thrombocytopenia is immune-mediated thrombocytopenia (IMT), a disorder in which antibody bound to the surface of the platelet results in premature removal by the reticuloendothelial system. In contrast, IMT occurs rarely in cats, but may be seen with infectious diseases (especially viral infections), neoplasia, and drug reactions.

vWD, the most common canine inherited bleeding disorder, results from a reduction in the amount of functional plasma von Willebrand's factor (vWF), leading to impaired platelet-vessel adhesion. vWD rarely causes petechiae, although ecchymoses may be observed in some dogs with vWD following trauma and surgical procedures. As with other primary hemostatic defects, typical signs of vWD include bleeding from mucosal surfaces (e.g., epistaxis, melena, and hematuria) and excessive bleeding following surgery or trauma. Although identified in more than 50 breeds of dogs, vWD has been documented in only a few cats.[1]

Hereditary disorders of platelet function represent aberrations of platelet adhesion, aggregation, and secretion. Glanzmann's thrombasthenia is a platelet membrane disorder characterized by an absence or deficiency of glycoprotein (GP) IIb/IIIa receptors, which are binding sites for fibrinogen and vWF. This deficiency results in defective platelet aggregation and has been identified in a Great Pyrenees dog[2] and in otter hounds.[3] Disorders of platelet secretion may be due to an abnormal secretory mechanism, as in basset hounds[4,5] and spitz dogs[6] with a signal-transduction disorder; or a deficiency in platelet dense granules or granule contents, as in δ-storage pool disease (δ-SPD) in the American cocker spaniel.[7] A combined signal-transduction disorder and δ-SPD have been described in grey collies with cyclic hematopoiesis.[8] Scott syndrome, a defect of platelet procoagulant activity, has been reported recently in a family of German shepherds in which repeated episodes of severe epistaxis were noted.[9]

In contrast to dogs, hereditary thrombopathias are rarely reported in cats. A platelet δ-SPD has been identified as part of the Chediak-Higashi syndrome in blue smoke Persian cats.[10] Recently, isolated intrinsic platelet function defects have been described in young domestic shorthair cats with persistent bleeding tendencies, including severe recurrent epistaxis with no underlying disorder, likely representing hereditary thrombopathias.[11]

In contrast to hereditary thrombopathias, in which the affected dogs and cats typically are clinically normal except for a bleeding tendency, animals with acquired platelet dysfunction may be systemically ill. Hyperglobulinemia, as seen with plasma cell tumors[12] and ehrlichiosis,[13] may be associated with platelet dysfunction because of interaction between the immunoglobulins and the platelet surface that interferes with platelet adhesion and stimulus-response coupling. In addition to platelet dysfunction, a hyperviscosity syndrome secondary to the hyperglobulinemia may also contribute to epistaxis. Antiplatelet antibodies in dogs with IMT may induce dysfunction by binding to glycoprotein receptors such as GP IIb/IIIa, interfering with fibrinogen binding and producing a thrombasthenic-like state.[14] Myeloproliferative and lymphoproliferative disorders have been associated with abnormal platelet morphologic features and reduced aggregation, secretion, and procoagulant activity. Thrombopathias associated with uremia and liver disease have been reported in the dog but have not been well characterized because they often coexist with other hemostatic defects.

Platelet dysfunction induced by many drugs has been documented in vitro, however the in vivo effects are less clear. Aspirin and other nonsteroidal antiinflammatory drugs acetylate and inactivate the enzyme cyclooxygenase, preventing production of thromboxane A_2 from arachidonic acid. Thromboxane A_2 is needed to promote platelet aggregation and vasoconstriction. Aspirin irreversibly inactivates cyclooxygenase, inhibiting thromboxane production in affected platelets for their 7- to 10-day life spans, whereas other nonsteroidal antiinflammatory drugs inactivate cyclooxygenase reversibly. In one study, administration of aspirin (10 mg/kg PO once) to dogs resulted in a significant prolongation of the buccal mucosal bleeding time (BMBT) from the baseline at 21 hours, but despite this increase the posttreatment BMBT remained in the reference range for 9 of the 10 healthy dogs tested.[15] Cephalothin[16] and acepromazine[17] have been associated with impaired platelet aggregation in the dog, yet a clinical bleeding tendency was not observed. However, in patients with known bleeding disorders, and especially those in need of surgery, it may be prudent to avoid use of such drugs.

Hypertension

Whereas acute blindness caused by retinal hemorrhage and/or detachment appears to be the most common manifestation of systemic hypertension in cats and dogs, epistaxis has also been noted.[18,19] Animals may be stressed or uncooperative, resulting in increased heart rate and blood pressure, which complicate the interpretation of blood pressure results. In general, blood pressure measurement in the awake, nonanxious cat and dog does not exceed 160/100 mm Hg.[18,20] In a retrospective evaluation of 24 cats with clinical signs associated with systemic hypertension, the mean systolic blood pressure measured indirectly by the Doppler technique was 219.4 ± 43.2 mm Hg, and the mean systolic/diastolic blood pressure measured directly by femoral arterial puncture was 233.2 ± 40.9/148.1 ± 28.7 mm Hg.[18] Primary or essential hypertension has been documented to occur in dogs.[20,21] Underlying disorders such as renal disease, hyperthyroidism, hyperadrenocorticism, and pheochromo-

cytoma may cause systemic hypertension in companion animals.[18,22]

Polycythemia

Absolute polycythemia, defined as an increase in the red blood cell (RBC) count, hemoglobin (Hb) concentration, and packed cell volume (PCV), may cause epistaxis as a result of hyperviscosity,[23] although neurological signs such as behavior changes, tremors, ataxia, and seizures have been reported as the most common clinical signs in cats.[24] Primary polycythemia, also known as polycythemia vera, is a myeloproliferative disorder in which there is clonal proliferation of erythroid cells independent of erythropoietin (EPO). Secondary polycythemia occurs in response to increased EPO production as a result of persistent, systemic tissue hypoxia due to cardiorespiratory disease with right-to-left shunting, local kidney hypoxia, or an EPO-producing mass (renal or other). Serum EPO concentrations may help to differentiate primary from secondary polycythemia, with high EPO concentrations diagnostic of secondary polycythemia and low to normal values suggestive of primary polycythemia.[24]

LOCAL PROCESSES

Whereas systemic disorders typically result in pure hemorrhage from the nasal cavity, many of the local disease processes involving the nasal cavity may result in a serous, mucoid, or mucopurulent discharge in addition to epistaxis.

Neoplasia

Nasal tumors account for only 1% to 2% of all neoplasms in the dog and cat,[25] yet represent one of the most common causes of epistaxis in middle-age to older animals. The epistaxis may be unilateral initially but may become bilateral as the tumor progresses. Other common clinical signs include sneezing, stertor, and facial deformity. Adenocarcinoma and lymphosarcoma are the most common nasal tumors in the dog and cat, respectively (see Chapter 37).

Infectious Rhinitis

Nasal aspergillosis, most commonly caused by the ubiquitous soil saprophyte *Aspergillus fumigatus,* primarily affects young to middle-age dogs of dolichocephalic and mesocephalic breeds.[26] In addition to epistaxis, other clinical signs may include mucopurulent nasal discharge, sneezing, signs of nasal pain, and nasal depigmentation or ulceration.[26] Nasal cryptococcosis, caused by *Cryptococcus neoformans,* is diagnosed much more commonly in cats than in dogs. Common clinical signs include sneezing, cutaneous lesions, nasal discharge, nasal deformity, a fleshy mass protruding from the nares, and weight loss.[27] Less common nasal fungal infections that may cause epistaxis include rhinosporidiosis, in which polyps form in the nares or nasal cavities in dogs; and phaeohyphomycosis (*Alternaria*) in dogs and cats (see Chapter 36).

Viral upper respiratory tract infections, particularly feline herpesvirus-1 and calicivirus, represent the most common cause of rhinitis in cats. Epistaxis is an infrequent finding in affected cats; instead, sneezing, oculonasal discharge, conjunctivitis, fever, and anorexia may be noted (see Chapter 35). Viral infections are an uncommon cause of rhinitis in dogs, but distemper virus, adenovirus, and parainfluenza virus have all been associated with nasal inflammation in dogs.

Secondary bacterial infections may develop in dogs and cats that have nasal epithelium damaged by a previous or concurrent viral, fungal, or parasitic infection, by a neoplasm, or by a foreign body; however, bacterial infection is not likely to be a primary cause of rhinitis. In addition, severe periodontal disease with subsequent formation of oronasal fistulae may lead to nasal discharge, including epistaxis.

Parasitic infections represent an uncommon cause of epistaxis. *Capillaria aerophila* infection, though not typically confined to the nasal cavities or frontal sinuses and more often involving the trachea and bronchi, has been associated with severe epistaxis necessitating blood transfusion in a dog.[28] *Leishmania infantum*, a protozoan parasite, has also been associated with epistaxis, the pathogenesis of which has been attributed to a combination of inflammatory and ulcerative lesions of the nasal mucosa, although dysproteinemia and thrombocytopenia may have contributed to the bleeding in some cases.[29] *Linguatula serrata*, an arthropod, and *Cuterebra*, a botfly larva, may also parasitize the nasal cavity and cause epistaxis.

Lymphoplasmacytic Rhinitis

In dogs with typical clinical signs of rhinitis (including epistaxis), the histologic finding of lymphoplasmacytic infiltrate of the nasal mucosa and submucosa in the absence of neoplasia or demonstrable infection, as well as clinical response to corticosteroid therapy, suggests that this form of rhinitis may be an immune-mediated disorder (see Chapter 39).[30]

Miscellaneous

Trauma is commonly the cause of a single episode of epistaxis that resolves spontaneously, although bleeding may be profuse and persistent and require specific measures to control hemorrhage. Nasal foreign bodies, most commonly inhaled, may lead to an acute onset of epistaxis if there is direct damage to the nasal mucosa, or may result in a secondary bacterial rhinitis (see Chapter 38). Vascular malformations in the nasal cavity are a rare cause of epistaxis.

Diagnostic Testing

The diagnostic approach for epistaxis depends on the patient's history and physical examination findings, which may indicate whether a systemic disorder or a local process is responsible for the clinical signs. In general, a complete blood cell count, serum chemistry profile, coagulation testing, and urinalysis should be performed to evaluate for an underlying systemic disorder. In an emergency situation with profuse epistaxis, determination of a PCV and total solids (TS), evaluation of a blood smear to obtain an estimate of platelet number (10 to 20 platelets per oil immersion field is deemed adequate), and measurement of an activated clotting time (ACT) may be helpful with making decisions regarding the need for blood component therapy while waiting for final laboratory results.

COMPLETE BLOOD CELL COUNT

The RBC count, Hb concentration, and PCV/TS will be helpful in assessing the severity of blood loss, as well as in evaluating the degree of hyperviscosity. The RBC indices may point towards chronic external blood loss if a hypochromic, microcytic anemia indicative of iron deficiency is noted. The finding of polychromasia or reticulocytosis ($>60,000/\mu$l) suggests that the bleeding began more than 3 days earlier and a regenerative anemia is present. Chronic reticulocytosis is noted in animals with polycythemia without evidence of blood loss.[24] Platelet count determinations are performed quickly and accurately by electronic particle counters in the dog. However, cell counting instruments that have a threshold function to separate platelets and RBC by volume may not be accurate in the cat because there is often considerable overlap between erythrocyte and platelet volumes in the cat; this results in spuriously low platelet counts. In addition, feline platelets tend to clump. A manual platelet count and evaluation of a blood smear are recommended for all cats and for dogs in which the automated platelet count is low. If thrombocytopenia is confirmed, a search for underlying disease should be performed (e.g., serology for infectious diseases, bone marrow aspirate, and thoracic and abdominal radiographs to evaluate for neoplasia). Changes in white blood cell (WBC) count may be nonspecific but may suggest diagnoses in certain cases (e.g., pancytopenia in chronic ehrlichiosis, or lymphocytosis with circulating lymphoblasts in acute lymphoblastic leukemia).

SERUM CHEMISTRY PROFILE

Azotemia due to renal failure may be associated with an acquired thrombopathia and/or hypertension. A decrease in serum albumin alone (i.e., normal globulin and no other evidence of liver dysfunction) may indicate a protein-losing nephropathy, which is often associated with hypertension. Liver failure may lead to a coagulopathy as a result of failure to synthesize coagulation factors. A complete biliary obstruction may lead to a vitamin K–dependent coagulopathy as a result of failure of intestinal absorption of this fat-soluble vitamin. Hyperglobulinemia, which may result in an acquired thrombopathia or hyperviscosity syndrome, is most marked in patients with ehrlichiosis, multiple myeloma, or feline infectious peritonitis, but may develop in response to any chronic antigenic stimulation. Elevation of serum alkaline phosphatase and cholesterol, in conjunction with appropriate clinical signs, may be suggestive of hyperadrenocorticism and associated hypertension. In addition, serologic testing for aspergillosis or cryptococcosis may be considered if fungal infection is a likely differential diagnosis.

URINALYSIS

Ideally, a urinalysis should be evaluated concurrently with a serum chemistry profile to allow differentiation between prerenal and renal azotemia. Evaluation of urine protein in light of urine specific gravity and sediment examination may suggest significant proteinuria and warrant submission of a urine protein:creatinine ratio. In addition, the finding of hematuria in a patient with epistaxis suggests that a bleeding disorder, most likely a primary hemostatic defect, is the cause of the mucosal surface bleeding.

HEMOSTATIC TESTING

In addition to the platelet count, measurement of the prothrombin time (PT) and activated partial thromboplastin time (aPTT), or ACT in an emergency situation, is indicated in the initial evaluation of a bleeding patient. If there is no evidence of thrombocytopenia or of a coagulopathy, a BMBT should be performed to evaluate primary hemostasis. The BMBT is performed using a spring-loaded device that is standardized to produce uniform incisions.[15] Simplate devices* are available with one or two blades and produce incisions approximately 5 mm long and 1 mm deep. Single blade devices are recommended for cats and small dogs. Normal BMBT in the dog is less than 3.6 minutes, and in the cat is less than 2 minutes. A prolongation of the BMBT in a patient with a normal platelet count suggests a thrombopathia, vWD, or a vascular disorder. Since vWD is much more common in the dog than intrinsic platelet function defects or vascular disorders, measurement of plasma vWF concentration is recommended prior to platelet function testing (i.e., platelet aggregation studies). In general, a bleeding tendency may be observed in dogs with plasma vWF concentration less than 35%.[31]

BLOOD PRESSURE MEASUREMENT

For patients with epistaxis and no other clinical signs or physical examination findings suggestive of a local disease process in the nasal cavity (especially if there is evidence of retinal hemorrhage or detachment), blood pressure should be measured indirectly using Doppler or oscillometric techniques. Given the potential for increased blood pressure secondary to stress or excitement, the blood pressure should be measured several times to evaluate for repeatability, and interpreted in light of the heart rate. If blood pressure is persistently elevated (>160/100 mm Hg), the patient should be evaluated for thyroid, renal, and adrenal disorders.

---

*Organon Tecknika Corp., Durham, N.C.

EVALUATION OF THE NASAL CAVITY

Complete evaluation of the nasal cavity requires general anesthesia. Once the patient is asleep, a careful examination of the mouth should be performed to evaluate for dental disease, tumor eroding through the hard palate, or evidence of a nasopharyngeal polyp or foreign body. Radiographic studies to assess changes in bone and soft tissue are performed prior to rhinoscopy or obtaining samples from the nasal cavities because hemorrhage will result in increased radiographic opacity. Similarly, ongoing hemorrhage may complicate radiographic evaluation. Computerized tomography (CT) or survey radiography of the nasal cavities and frontal sinuses aids in determining the nature and extent of the disease. In addition, CT-guided biopsies may be an option, depending on the location of the disease. Retroflexed endoscopic evaluation of the nasopharynx is helpful in visualizing tumors protruding from the choanae and in identifying foreign bodies. Passage of an endoscope through the nares to evaluate the nasal cavities may be difficult in cats and small dogs, but use of a cystoscope or bronchoscope may allow visualization in larger patients. If a lesion is identified by endoscopy, biopsies may be performed under direct visualization with forceps advanced through the endoscope. Alternatively, biopsies may be performed blindly using cup forceps. Nasal flushing may yield a foreign body or pieces of tumor that can be submitted for histopathology (see Chapter 14). Samples can also be obtained for microbiologic culture to identify fungal or bacterial organisms.

Initial Management Pending Results of Diagnostic Tests

Appropriate management of epistaxis requires identification of an underlying disorder. If, for example, systemic hypertension or polycythemia is recognized during the initial evaluation, specific therapy (i.e., antihypertensive medications or phlebotomy, respectively) should be initiated.

In most cases with a less apparent cause, mild epistaxis may be controlled with cage rest pending the results of diagnostic tests. If the patient is anxious or distressed, a sedative (e.g., butorphanol) may be helpful. Acepromazine may not be a good choice as a sedative given its potential to cause or exacerbate hypotension in a bleeding animal as well as adversely affect platelet function. If the patient is cooperative, a topical solution of phenylephrine or epinephrine (diluted 1:100,000) may be squirted into the nasal cavities to cause vasoconstriction.

In cases with severe epistaxis, general anesthesia with tracheal intubation to protect the airway may be necessary to allow gauze packing of the nasal cavities and/or nasopharynx, depending on the site of bleeding. Endoscopic cauterization and placement of balloon catheters in the nasal cavities or nasopharynx to exert pressure at the site of bleeding are techniques often used to control epistaxis in humans[32] but have not been reported in animals. Temporary ligation of both carotid arteries has been described as an effective means to reduce hemorrhage during intranasal surgery.[33] Permanent ligation of the carotid artery on the side of the epistaxis has been utilized when all other measures to control spontaneous bleeding have failed.[34] More recently, percutaneous arterial embolization has been used to treat intractable epistaxis in humans[35] and dogs.[36]

While efforts are made to locally control the bleeding, the patient may also require intravenous fluids to treat hypovolemia and transfusion of packed RBC (10 ml/kg initially) to provide additional oxygen-carrying support if the bleeding is severe. If the initial hemostatic tests reveal severe thrombocytopenia <40,000 μl) or are suggestive of a thrombopathia, transfusion of fresh whole blood (10 to 20 ml/kg initially) should be considered in patients with uncontrolled bleeding. In all cases, only blood-typed compatible blood should be administered. Fresh frozen plasma transfusion (6 to 10 ml/kg q 8 to 12 hours) is indicated in patients with coagulopathies, and cryoprecipitate (1 unit/10 kg q 12 hours) is the blood component of choice in managing severe bleeding due to vWD and hemophilia A. In addition, patients with coagulopathies and suspected or confirmed anticoagulant rodenticide poisoning should also be treated with vitamin K$_1$ (2.5 mg/kg PO BID).

In addition to local control of bleeding and blood component therapy, administration of desmopressin (DDAVP) may be considered in dogs with vWD and either acquired or inherited thrombopathias. The recommended formulation and dose of DDAVP for dogs is the intranasal preparation* at 1 μg/kg SC or IV. In humans, administration of DDAVP results in a two- to fivefold increase in plasma vWF concentration in normal individuals as well as those with type 1 vWD.[37] The effect of DDAVP on plasma vWF concentration in normal dogs and dogs with type 1 vWD is much less dramatic, with an approximate 50% increase above baseline in some but not all dogs.[38-40] Despite minimal, if any, change in plasma vWF, DDAVP has resulted in a significant shortening of the BMBT in vWF-deficient dogs 30 and 120 minutes postadministration, as well as control of excessive surgical bleeding.[40] However, as in humans, the hemostatic response to DDAVP in dogs with vWD is variable.

Conclusion

In summary, epistaxis may pose a significant diagnostic and therapeutic challenge. Successful management depends on identification of the underlying cause. A careful history and physical examination aid in differentiating between a local process and a systemic disorder. Treatment of a specific underlying disorder, cage rest, sedation, topical vasoconstrictors, and blood component therapy may be successful in controlling bleeding in most patients, but surgical intervention or arterial embolization may be required in cases with uncontrollable epistaxis.

*Desmopressin Acetate Rhinal Tube, Ferring Pharmaceuticals Inc., Tarrytown, N.Y.

REFERENCES

1. French TW, Fox LE, Randolph JF et al: A bleeding disorder (von Willebrand's disease) in a Himalayan cat, J Am Vet Med Assoc 190:437-439, 1987.
2. Boudreaux MK, Kvam K, Dillon AR et al: Type I Glanzmann's thrombasthenia in a Great Pyrenees dog, Vet Pathol 33:503-511, 1996.
3. Dodds WJ: Familial canine thrombocytopathy, Thromb Diath Haemorrh 26:241-247, 1967.
4. Catalfamo JL, Raymond SL, White JG et al: Defective platelet-fibrinogen interaction in hereditary canine thrombopathia, Blood 67:1568-1577, 1986.
5. Boudreaux MK, Dodds WJ, Slauson DO et al: Impaired camp metabolism associated with abnormal function of thrombopathic canine platelets, Biochem Biophys Res Commun 140:595-601, 1986.
6. Boudreaux MK, Crager C, Dillon AR et al: Identification of an intrinsic platelet function defect in Spitz dogs, J Vet Intern Med 8:93-98, 1994.
7. Callan MB, Bennett JS, Phillips DK et al: Inherited platelet δ-storage pool disease in dogs causing severe bleeding: An animal model for a specific ADP deficiency, Thromb Haemost 74:949-953, 1995.
8. Lothrop CD, Candler RV, Pratt HL et al: Characterization of platelet function in cyclic hematopoietic dogs, Exp Hematol 19:916-922, 1992.
9. Brooks MB, Catalfamo JL, Brown HA et al: A hereditary bleeding disorder of dogs caused by a lack of platelet procoagulant activity, Blood 99:2434-2442, 2002.
10. Meyers KM, Seachord CL, Holmsen H et al: Evaluation of the platelet storage pool deficiency in the feline counterpart of the Chediak-Higashi syndrome, Am J Hematol 11:241-253, 1981.
11. Callan MB, Griot-Wenk ME, Hackner SG et al: Persistent thrombopathy causing bleeding in two domestic shorthaired cats, J Vet Intern Med 14:217-220, 2000.
12. Ward DA, McEntee MF, Weddle DL: Orbital plasmacytoma in a cat, J Sm Anim Pract 38:576-578, 1997.
13. Varela F, Font X, Valladares JE et al: Thrombocytopathia and light-chain proteinuria in a dog naturally infected with Ehrlichia canis, J Vet Intern Med 11:309-311, 1997.
14. Kristensen AT, Weiss DJ, Klausner JS: Platelet dysfunction associated with canine immune-mediated thrombocytopenia (ITP), J Vet Intern Med 8:323-327, 1994.
15. Jergens AE, Turrentine MA, Kraus KH et al: Buccal mucosal bleeding times of healthy dogs and of dogs in various pathologic states, including thrombocytopenia, uremia, and von Willebrand's disease, Am J Vet Res 48:1337-1342, 1987.
16. Schermerhorn T, Barr SC, Stoffregen DA et al: Whole blood platelet aggregation, buccal mucosa bleeding time, and serum cephalothin concentration in dogs receiving a pre-surgical antibiotic protocol, Am J Vet Res 55:1602-1608, 1994.
17. Barr SC, Ludders JW, Looney AL et al: Platelet aggregation in dogs after sedation with acepromazine and atropine and during subsequent general anesthesia and surgery, Am J Vet Res 53:2067-2070, 1992.
18. Littman MP: Spontaneous systemic hypertension in 24 cats, J Vet Intern Med 8:79-86, 1994.
19. Dhupa N, Littman MP: Epistaxis, Compend Contin Educ Pract Vet 14:1033-1041, 1992.
20. Bovee KC, Littman MP, Crabtree BJ et al: Essential hypertension in a dog, J Am Vet Med Assoc 195:81-86, 1989.
21. Bovee KC, Littman MP, Saleh F et al: Essential hereditary hypertension in dogs: A new animal model, J Hypertens (Suppl 5) 4:S172-S173, 1986.
22. Littman MP, Robertson JL, Bovee KC: Spontaneous systemic hypertension in dogs: Five cases (1981-1983), J Am Vet Med Assoc 193:486-494, 1988.
23. McGrath CJ: Polycythemia vera in dogs, J Am Vet Med Assoc 164:1117-1122, 1974.
24. Hasler AH, Giger U: Serum erythropoietin values in polycythemic cats, J Am Anim Hosp Assoc 32:294-301, 1996.
25. Madewell BR, Priester WA, Gillette EL et al: Neoplasms of the nasal passages and paranasal sinuses in domesticated animals as reported by 13 veterinary colleges, Am J Vet Res 37:851-856, 1976.

26. Mathews KG, Davidson AP, Koblik PD et al: Comparison of topical administration of clotrimazole through surgically placed versus nonsurgically placed catheters for treatment of nasal aspergillosis in dogs: 60 cases (1990-1996), *J Am Vet Med Assoc* 213:501-506, 1998.
27. Flatland B, Greene RT, Lappin MR: Clinical and serologic evaluation of cats with cryptococcosis, *J Am Vet Med Assoc* 209:1110-1113, 1996.
28. King RR, Greiner EC, Ackerman N et al: Nasal capillariasis in a dog, *J Am Anim Hosp Assoc* 26:381-385, 1990.
29. Koutinas AF, Polizopoulou ZS, Saridomichalakis MN et al: Clinical considerations on canine visceral leishmaniasis in Greece: A retrospective study of 158 cases (1989-1996), *J Am Anim Hosp Assoc* 35:376-383, 1999.
30. Burgener DC, Slocombe RF, Zerbe CA: Lymphoplasmacytic rhinitis in five dogs, *J Am Anim Hosp Assoc* 23:565-568, 1987.
31. Giger U, Brooks M, Dodds WJ et al: Advances in canine von Willebrand disease, *Proceedings 18th Ann Meet Vet Med Forum* 481-482, 2000.
32. Tan LKS, Calhoun KH: Epistaxis, *Med Clin North Am* 83:43-56, 1999.
33. Hedlund CS, Tangner CH, Elkins AD et al: Temporary bilateral carotid artery occlusion during surgical exploration of the nasal cavity of the dog, *Vet Surg* 12:83-85, 1983.
34. Bistner SI, Ford RB: *Kirk and Bistner's handbook of veterinary procedures and emergency treatment,* ed 6, Philadelphia, 1995, WB Saunders.
35. Elahi MM, Parnes LS, Fox AJ et al: Therapeutic embolization in the treatment of intractable epistaxis, *Arch Otolaryngol Head Neck Surg* 121:65-69, 1995.
36. Weisse WC: Personal communication, October 2002.
37. Mannucci PM: Desmopressin: A nontransfusional form of treatment for congenital and acquired bleeding disorders, *Blood* 72:1449-1455, 1988.
38. Giger U, Dodds WJ: Effect of desmopressin in normal dogs and dogs with von Willebrand's disease, *Vet Clin Pathol* 18:39-42, 1989.
39. Meyers KM, Wardrop KJ, Dodds WJ et al: Effect of exercise, DDAVP, and epinephrine on the factor VIII:C/von Willebrand factor complex in normal dogs and von Willebrand factor deficient Doberman Pinscher dogs, *Thromb Res* 57:97-108; 1990.
40. Kraus KH, Turrentine MA, Jergens AE et al: Effect of desmopressin acetate on bleeding times and plasma von Willebrand factor in Doberman pinscher dogs with von Willebrand's disease, *Vet Surg* 18:103-109, 1989.

CHAPTER 5

Upper Airway Obstruction, Stertor, and Stridor

David E. Holt

Definition and Clinical Signs

Mild to marked upper airway obstruction is seen often in small animal practice. For the purposes of this chapter, the upper airway is defined as the nasal passages, choanae, nasopharynx, mouth, oropharynx, larynx, and trachea. Many diverse conditions can affect the anatomic structures of the upper airway and cause obstruction and respiratory compromise. Stertor is defined as a noise similar to snoring in humans. Cats breathe predominantly through their noses, as do dogs when they are not exercising or panting. During nasal breathing, stertorous respiration may be associated with partial obstruction of the nasal passages, choanae, or nasopharynx. Stridor is a harsh, high-pitched respiratory sound usually heard on inspiration. Stridorous respiration often indicates conditions affecting the larynx and trachea (e.g., laryngeal paralysis in dogs).

The nature and magnitude of clinical signs is determined by the site and severity of the respiratory obstruction. In animals with minimal obstruction, a slightly stertorous or stridorous noise on inspiration is often the only detectable abnormality. Even with marked obstruction of the nasal passages in some dogs with nasal neoplasia, clinical signs of respiratory obstruction may not be apparent. These dogs simply mouth breathe, and this is not recognized as abnormal by the owner. In cases of worsening respiratory obstruction, inspiratory and sometimes expiratory muscles contract more forcefully. Usually the inspiratory phase of respiration is prolonged and associated with a loud stertorous or stridorous noise. Affected dogs adopt a characteristic posture, standing with neck extended and elbows abducted in an attempt to reduce airway resistance. Cats sit with their necks extended and may open-mouth breathe. In severe cases, the tongue can appear cyanotic. Hyperthermia may occur because of poor airflow over the surface of the tongue. Severely affected animals are often extremely distressed. Animals with prolonged, severe dyspnea may appear exhausted and collapsed or occasionally seizure secondary to hyperthermia.

Other clinical signs may be present depending on the nature and location of the respiratory obstruction. Obstruction of the caudal nasal passages, choanae, or cranial nasopharynx by neoplasms, foreign bodies or polyps can cause nasal discharge that varies from serous to mucopurulent. Fungal or neoplastic lesions of the nose often cause intermittent epistaxis. Nasal neoplasia in dogs and cats and *Cryptococcus* infection in cats may result in distortion of the nasal, maxillary, and frontal bones. Some nasal or frontal sinus tumors erode the frontal, palatine, and lacrimal bones and invade the retrobulbar space, causing exophthalmos. Pharyngeal neoplasms and mucoceles can cause visible swellings and difficulty swallowing. In some dogs, laryngeal paralysis is just one manifestation of a more generalized peripheral neuropathy, and on close examination proprioceptive deficits may be apparent.

General Pathophysiology

In normal dogs, the nose contributes 80% of the total airway resistance during inspiration.[1] This is understandable, because the majority of the nasal cavity is filled with scrolled conchae covered with an extremely vascular epithelium.[2] Resistance to airflow in the nose creates turbulence needed for effective olfaction and heat exchange. In contrast, the remainder of the upper airway contributes minimally to airway resistance during inspiration in a normal dog.[1] Hence dogs that are dyspneic because of nasal or nasopharyngeal obstructions simply mouth breathe to minimize airway resistance. Obstructive lesions in the upper airway increase resistance to airflow primarily by decreasing the radius of the affected air passage(s). The importance of the radius of the airway in obstruction can be seen from Poiseuille's law[3]:

$$Q = \frac{\pi \times \Delta P \times r^4}{8 \times L \times N}$$

where the rate of air flow (Q) is proportional to the radius of the airway to the fourth power (r^4). P = Pressure difference between the ends of the airway; N = viscosity of the gas; L = length of the airway. It is clear that if the radius of a section of the airway, such as the larynx or trachea, decreases by half, flow through the airway decreases by a factor of 16 (i.e., $1/2^4 = 1/16$).

In response to increasing resistance, the inspiratory muscles contract for a longer time during each breath cycle, prolonging inspiration. This response appears to be mediated by the Hering-Breuer reflex.[4] The force of inspiratory muscle contraction increases, possibly due to the conscious sensation of dyspnea and stimulation of muscle spindles. Strong chemical feedback through increases in Pa_{CO_2} and decreases in Pa_{O_2} stimulates increased respiratory effort when compensation by other mechanisms is inadequate. If the upper airway obstruction decreases ventilation, even small increases in Pa_{CO_2} will stimulate the animal to attempt to make large changes in respiratory minute volume (e.g., 2.5 L/min increase for a 1 Torr increase in Pa_{CO_2} in humans).[5]

Even in upper airway obstructions where the primary problem is inspiratory difficulty, expiratory muscles are recruited to restore tidal volume.[5] Expiratory muscles force end-expiratory volume below the passive functional residual capacity and thereby store elastic energy

in the chest wall for inspiration.[5] This allows substantial inspiratory airflow before the onset of inspiratory muscle contraction.

As the intercostal muscles and diaphragm contract with increased force over time, muscle fatigue and failure can occur. This is a well-recognized problem in human medicine.[6] Extra muscles are recruited to aid inspiration. As the diaphragm contracts forcefully, the caudal ribs are drawn inward, especially if the force of the diaphragmatic contraction is unopposed by the intercostal muscles. The diaphragm contracts towards the cranial abdominal cavity, pushing the abdominal contents caudally. The chest wall appears to move inward on inspiration while the abdomen moves outwards. Abdominal muscles that are recruited to aid expiration contract and the abdomen moves inwards on expiration while the chest appears to move outwards. This clinical finding is termed paradoxical respiration because the chest and abdominal wall move paradoxically during the different phases of respiration. Paradoxical respiration is a clear indication of severe dyspnea, increased work of breathing, and respiratory muscle fatigue.

Compensatory mechanisms usually maintain ventilation in animals with upper airway obstruction for some time; however, substantial hypoxia can occur. In dogs with moderate and severe laryngeal paralysis, Pa_{O_2} values were 80 ± 3 and 51 ± 7 mm Hg, respectively, compared to a control population reference value of 91 mm Hg.[8] Values for Pa_{CO_2} were within the normal range for both groups. The increased work performed by the inspiratory and expiratory muscles generates substantial heat. The work of breathing, combined with hot weather and exercise, often precipitates decompensation in dogs with laryngeal paralysis, causing severe hyperthermia in some cases.

Brachycephalic airway disease is described in detail elsewhere; however, the pathophysiology of the associated upper airway obstruction warrants discussion here. Brachycephalic animals have substantial resistance to airflow because of their stenotic nares,[8] overlong soft palates,[9] and often hypoplastic tracheas.[10] In addition, bulldogs (and presumably other brachycephalic breeds) have excessive pharyngeal tissue that narrows the upper airway. When awake, bulldogs recruit the sternohyoideus muscles to dilate the pharynx with every breath. The activity in these muscles is greater than that seen in the same muscles in nonbrachycephalic breeds. During rapid eye movement sleep in bulldogs, apnea is associated with decreased activity of the pharyngeal dilator muscles. Apnea is terminated by massive bursts of pharyngeal dilator muscle activity. These massive bursts of activity are associated with edema and fibrosis of the dilator muscles.[11-13] Over time, this muscle fibrosis may mean that bulldogs are less capable of dilating their airways during inspiration. In some brachycephalic dogs, prolonged partial upper airway obstruction leads to eversion of the mucosa of the lateral ventricles (everted laryngeal saccules).[14] The increased negative pressure in the airway, generated to overcome resistance to flow, pulls the mucosa lining the lateral ventricles into the laryngeal lumen. The turbulent airflow over the mucosa causes edema and swelling. This bulging mucosa can obstruct more than 50% of the glottis. Over time, the laryngeal cartilage frame can weaken in brachycephalic dogs and the larynx can progressively collapse.[15,16]

Animals with severe, acute upper airway obstruction are at risk of developing noncardiogenic pulmonary edema.[17] This syndrome of pulmonary edema secondary to upper airway obstruction also occurs in humans and is incompletely understood.[18-21] Proposed mechanisms for edema formation include:

1. The markedly decreased intrathoracic pressure caused by inspiration against an obstruction.[18] The extreme negative pressure may increase venous return to the heart, increasing pulmonary arterial pressure. At the same time, the negative intrathoracic pressure creates a pressure gradient across the alveolar-capillary membrane that favors flux of fluid from the pulmonary capillaries into the pulmonary interstitium and alveoli. Although logical, this proposed mechanism does not explain why the edema most often develops after relief of the airway obstruction rather than during the obstructive episode.[20]

2. Increased permeability of the pulmonary capillaries due to the mechanical disruption of the capillary walls.[21] Recently, frank pulmonary hemorrhage has been reported secondary to upper airway obstruction.[21] Presumably, the pulmonary hemorrhage described in the human patient of this report represents a more severe manifestation of the same disorders that cause pulmonary edema. Disruption of the pulmonary capillaries secondary to increased capillary wall stress was implicated. Wall stress is defined as:

$$\text{Wall stress} = \frac{\text{Transmural capillary pressure}}{} \times \frac{\text{Radius of vessel}}{\text{Vessel wall thickness}}$$

In an experimental canine model, stress failure of the pulmonary capillary wall occurred at a transmural capillary pressure of 70 mm Hg.[22]

3. Increased capillary permeability may occur secondary to severe hypoxia.[20]

Some animals with upper airway obstruction have concurrent problems including gagging/retching, regurgitation, or vomiting. In some instances these problems are directly associated with the upper airway obstruction (e.g., foreign body penetration of the caudal pharynx can cause gagging, and the associated swelling can cause partial upper airway obstruction). In other cases, pharyngeal or laryngeal stimulation is presumed to cause the gagging or retching episodes. This is reported in approximately 10% of brachycephalic dogs prior to corrective upper airway surgery.[9] In severe cases, animals may suffer respiratory and cardiac arrest after gagging or vomiting; this is likely caused by massive vagal discharge.

In some dyspneic animals, regurgitation is associated with evidence of an air-filled esophagus or a hiatal hernia on thoracic radiographs. Although hiatal hernia has been described in association with laryngeal paralysis,[23] the hiatus itself is often anatomically normal. Presumably the profound negative pressure generated in the intrapleural space pulls the cardia and part of the fundus of the stomach into the thorax. Once the caudal esophageal sphincter has been displaced cranially into the thorax, its function is compromised and gastroesophageal reflux can occur. Gastroesophageal reflux has been seen in dogs with both clinical[24] and experimental[25] hiatal hernia, and the associated reflux esophagitis can decrease esophageal motility.[26] The hiatal hernia usually resolves with successful treatment of the upper airway obstruction, but some animals may need symptomatic treatment of residual esophagitis.

Animals with upper airway obstruction and concurrent vomiting or regurgitation are at risk of aspiration, which is most commonly described in dogs with laryngeal paralysis.[27-29] These animals cannot adduct the larynx during swallowing and vomiting because recurrent laryngeal nerve degeneration affects both the laryngeal adductor and abductor muscles. In humans with respiratory muscle fatigue, the cough mechanism is adversely affected.[6] Diminished cough reflexes may also occur in animals with upper airway obstruction and increased respiratory effort. Human patients with respiratory muscle weakness can have decreased mucociliary clearance[30] and are prone to develop atelectasis,[31] both of which predispose to pneumonia.

Differential Diagnosis

A wide range of diseases affect different sections of the upper respiratory tract, and can cause stertor or stridor and partial upper airway obstruction. Some diseases occur commonly in certain breeds (e.g., laryngeal paralysis in older, large-breed dogs). It is tempting to make a diagnosis based on the signalment and clinical signs alone; however, many upper airway diseases can cause similar if not identical clinical signs. The clinician is encouraged to keep an open mind, perform a thorough examination, and have an extensive list of possible causes in mind when evaluating an animal with upper airway obstruction.

Stertorous respiration is associated with diseases affecting the nasal passages, choanae, and nasopharynx. Nasal diseases that may affect dogs severely enough to cause stertor include neoplasia, fungal infection (most commonly aspergillosis), trauma, and occasionally rhinitis secondary to severe dental disease or inhaled foreign bodies.[32] In cats, severe viral rhinitis secondary to herpes or calicivirus infection, neoplasia, *Cryptococcus* infection, and severe chronic bacterial rhinitis may be associated with stertorous respiration.[33]

Choanal diseases are not described often in the veterinary literature; however, conditions affecting this region almost invariably produce signs of upper airway obstruction. In dogs, nasal neoplasms can extend into the choanae. Congenital atresia,[34] foreign bodies,[35] and scarring secondary to trauma can also occlude this area. Membranous obstruction of the choanae has been described in several cats and termed nasopharyngeal stenosis.[36-38]

Nasopharyngeal and pharyngeal diseases potentially associated with airway obstruction in dogs include neoplasms, foreign body penetrations[39] and secondary abscesses, and mucoceles.[40] In cats, nasopharyngeal polyps[41] and grass foreign bodies[42] have been associated with stertorous respiration. Occasionally, primary oral tumors will grow large enough in dogs and cats to create respiratory distress. In the majority of these cases, however, the primary signs of oral neoplasia are dysphagia, drooling, halitosis, and a bloody oral discharge. Tonsillar squamous cell carcinoma warrants specific mention as a diagnostic possibility because of its unusual behavior. In many cases, the primary tonsillar tumor is small, but the metastatic lesions in the local lymph nodes can be large[43] and compress the pharynx, larynx, and trachea.

Brachycephalic airway syndrome can cause stertor and stridor in bulldogs, Boston terriers, and pugs. Acquired laryngeal paralysis should be suspected in older, large-breed dogs with worsening stridor. In young Bouviers, huskies, rottweillers, and dalmatians, marked inspiratory dyspnea can be associated with congenital laryngeal paralysis. Congenital subglottic stenosis has been reported in one dog.[44] Foreign body or insect inhalation, laryngeal trauma, and abscesses should all be considered. Laryngeal obstruction as an unusual manifestation of anticoagulant intoxication has also been described.[44] Neoplasms or abscesses in the cranial mediastinum or cervical region can affect recurrent laryngeal nerve function. Neoplasia of the larynx,[46] and especially of the thyroid,[47] can cause clinical signs compatible with laryngeal paralysis. Thyroid carcinomas can invade the cervical musculature, esophagus, trachea, and larynx, causing inspiratory stridor.[47]

In cats, laryngeal paralysis, inflammatory or granulomatous laryngeal disease, and laryngeal and tracheal lymphosarcoma should be considered as possible causes of the clinical signs. Other tracheal neoplasms, foreign bodies, and tracheal avulsions can cause signs similar to laryngeal paralysis. In cats, tracheal perforation associated with intubation can cause signs of upper airway obstruction. In these cases, the diagnosis should be suspected because of the association of the dyspnea with recovery from anesthesia and the development of subcutaneous emphysema.[48,49]

Tracheal or bronchial foreign bodies[50] or tumors,[51] eosinophilic tracheal granuloma,[52] parasitic infestation of the trachea,[53,54] anticoagulant rodenticide intoxication,[55] tracheal polyps,[56] and tracheal cuterebriasis[57] can all cause signs of upper airway obstruction. Intrathoracic tracheal compression by esophageal foreign bodies or mediastinal tumors, abscesses, or hematomas also cause similar signs. The animal with a collapsing trachea usually has a history of intermittent, chronic, honking cough, which may not be evident on physical examination in cases with acute decompensation and respiratory obstruction.

Complications that often occur in conjunction with upper airway obstruction, including noncardiogenic pulmonary edema and aspiration pneumonia, should also be considered. Animals with laryngeal paralysis should be examined for evidence of central and peripheral nerve disease.

Diagnostic Testing and Initial Management

In animals with upper airway obstruction, diagnostic testing and initial management must be considered together. Many of these animals have used up their physiologic reserves and are not stable. Routine diagnostic procedures that involve restraint, including jugular venipuncture and thoracic radiography, can cause acute worsening of respiratory signs. Animals with respiratory distress must therefore be carefully assessed and diagnostic tests performed in a stepwise manner.

Animals with mild to moderate stertor or stridor can generally be examined without sedation or supplemental oxygen. While collecting a detailed history, the clinician can observe the animal's respiratory rate, pattern, and effort. In cases with stertor, the external nares should be examined carefully. In dogs with a history of stertor and mucopurulent or hemorrhagic nasal discharge, depigmentation of the nasal planum is highly suggestive of nasal fungal infection. Facial symmetry is evaluated because nasal and frontal sinus neoplasia often causes facial distortion in dogs. In cats, facial distortion is associated with neoplasia or with *Cryptococcus* infection. The animal's mouth is gently opened, and the hard and soft palate, pharynx, and tonsils are evaluated. Oral examinations are performed with caution: extensive manipulation and palpation in the mouth can cause massive vagal discharge in some animals. In tractable cats, the presence of a nasopharyngeal polyp can be detected by quickly passing an index finger caudally over the hard and soft palates. In normal cats, the finger will slip dorsally at the caudal edge of the hard palate. In cats with nasopharyngeal polyps, the polyp pushes the soft palate ventrally and this will often be easily palpable. The salivary glands, lymph nodes, pharynx, larynx, and trachea are gently palpated. The larynx, trachea, and lungs are auscultated. The heart is auscultated and pulse quality is assessed. The abdomen and peripheral lymph nodes are palpated. A neurological examination is performed to evaluate animals with laryngeal paralysis for evidence of central or peripheral neuropathies. Based on the findings from the history and physical examination, further diagnostic tests including blood work, and thoracic and cervical radiographs can be planned. Some diagnostic tests, including nasal and skull radiographs or computerized axial tomography (CAT scan), laryngoscopy, and pharyngoscopy, require general anesthesia.

It is often difficult to perform anything more than a cursory examination on animals with severe stridor and airway obstruction. The stress of an unfamiliar environment and handling can cause these animals to decompensate and respiratory arrest. The initial goal of managing such cases should be stabilization to allow the animal to tolerate further diagnostic procedures. Intravenous access is mandatory in a severely dyspneic animal. An intravenous catheter should be placed and secured with minimal restraint. Oxygen supplementation can be provided with a tent, mask, or an oxygen cage. In some animals with severe respiratory obstruction, oxygen supplementation may not relieve the dyspnea. In hyperthermic animals with no evidence of heart disease or pulmonary involvement, a bolus (10 ml/kg) of cool intravenous fluids is administered to reduce core temperature. External cooling should also be considered using ice packs, fans, and wetting the animal as needed.

Some animals respond well to intravenous acetylpromazine maleate (0.01 to 0.05 mg/kg), indicating that a substantial amount of the respiratory distress might be due to the perception of dyspnea and associated panic. Increased inspiratory effort and increased negative intrathoracic pressure associated with panic results in worsening airway collapse. Pulse oximetry may be useful to assess hemoglobin saturation with oxygen if animals will tolerate placement of the probe. Some severely dyspneic animals will stabilize enough to allow a rapid but complete physical examination. In others, the physical examination and further diagnostic testing can only be performed once the animal has been anesthetized and intubated.

The method of anesthetic induction and intubation depends somewhat on the urgency of obtaining control over the airway. All animals should be premedicated with an anticholinergic to prevent vagally mediated asystole. Animals with mild to moderate stridor can be induced with boluses of injectable anesthetic agents titrated to allow examination of laryngeal function (see Chapters 15 and 41). In severely stridorous, dyspneic animals, the main priority is to rapidly secure a patent airway. In these animals, the ventral neck should be clipped before induction of anesthesia, provided this does not increase respiratory distress. A designated surgeon and a tracheostomy kit should be available in case intubation per os is not possible. A variety of types and sizes of endotracheal tubes is available. In some instances, medium to large red rubber catheters can be threaded through a partially obstructed larynx or trachea and allow effective ventilation and oxygenation until a tracheostomy is performed. Intubation should only be attempted with an appropriately sized laryngoscope that has a functioning light source.

Once an effective, fully functional airway is secured, further diagnostic tests can proceed in a logical order. At the same time, appropriate monitoring can be instituted to allow accurate assessment of ventilation and gas exchange. An arterial catheter should be placed to allow sampling for blood gas analysis and direct blood pressure monitoring. A pulse oximeter probe is placed on the tongue. End tidal carbon dioxide is measured. Thoracic radiographs are made to evaluate the lungs for evidence of pneumonia or edema. Radiographic changes compatible with aspiration pneumonia include an alveolar pattern with air bronchograms in the ventral and cranial lung fields. Animals with noncardiogenic pulmonary edema secondary to upper airway obstruction tend to have dorsocaudal interstitial or alveolar infiltrates.[17] When aspiration pneumonia is suspected, a transtracheal wash is performed through a sterile endotracheal tube.

In cases presenting primarily for stertor, diagnostic tests include nasal radiographs and rhinoscopy. Visualization of the choanae and nasopharynx with a flexible endoscope may be indicated. The nasopharynx can also be partially visualized by retracting the soft palate rostrally using a spay hook. Obvious lesions are biopsied either through the endoscope biopsy port, or blindly using cup forceps inserted into the nose to a depth measured from radiographs. In some cases, diagnostic biopsy samples can be obtained by placing a bulb syringe in one nostril, occluding the opposite nostril, and flushing forcefully with saline. Samples are retrieved from the caudal pharynx. In cases with stridor in which the diagnosis cannot be made from the physical examination, laryngoscopy, pharyngoscopy, or thoracic radiographs, tracheoscopy and bronchoscopy are performed.

In most instances, it is important to definitively treat the underlying cause of the airway obstruction at the time of diagnosis. For example, in brachycephalic dogs, the stenotic nares should be widened and the soft palate shortened immediately after anesthetic induction and visual inspection. In cats diagnosed with nasopharyngeal polyps, the polyp is removed and a ventral bulla osteotomy is performed. In some cases (e.g., dogs with laryngeal paralysis), immediate treatment will depend on the experience of the surgeon. If immediate correction is not possible, placement of a temporary tracheostomy tube will ensure a patent airway during anesthetic recovery. In a dog with collapsing trachea, the diagnosis can often be obtained or at least strongly suspected prior to anesthesia. If deemed necessary, surgery or stent placement can be planned appropriately, but tracheostomy should be avoided in dogs with a collapsing trachea.

Tracheotomy is best performed under controlled circumstances. The animal should be intubated, the ventral neck clipped and prepared for aseptic surgery, and the animal positioned in dorsal recumbency (Figure 5-1). A skin incision is made on the ventral midline extending caudally from the cricoid cartilage for 4 to 10 cm, depending on the size of the animal. The sternohyoid muscles are split and retracted. Monofilament sutures are placed around a tracheal cartilage immediately cranial

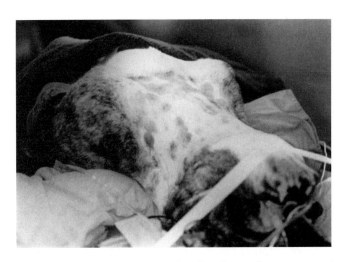

Figure 5-1. A bulldog positioned in dorsal recumbency prepared for a tracheostomy. (Courtesy of Dr. Daniel Brockman.)

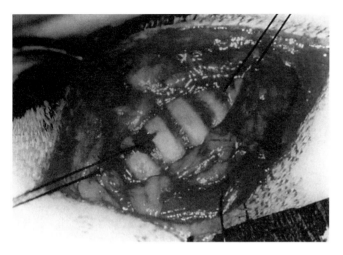

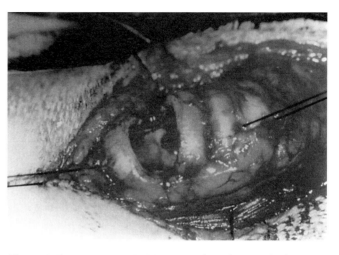

Figure 5-2. *Monofilament sutures placed around a tracheal cartilage immediately cranial and caudal to the proposed tracheotomy. The suture ends are tied and left long. These sutures allow the tracheostomy to be raised into the incision to facilitate replacement of the tracheostomy tube if necessary.*

Figure 5-3. *A transverse incision is made in the annular ligament between two tracheal rings, at least three rings caudal to the cricoid cartilage.*

and caudal to the proposed tracheotomy, and the suture ends are tied and left long. These sutures allow the tracheostomy to be raised into the incision to facilitate replacement of the tracheostomy tube if necessary (Figure 5-2). The cuff on the oral endotracheal tube is deflated and a transverse incision is made in the annular ligament between two tracheal rings, at least three rings caudal to the cricoid cartilage (Figure 5-3). Experimentally, tracheostomies made one-third of the circumference of the trachea healed with less than 5% reduction of tracheal lumen diameter.[58] Clinically, tracheostomy incisions that are half the size of the tracheal circumference appear to be without clinical complications.

The tracheostomy tube should be no larger than 75% of the tracheal diameter, ideally allowing manual occlusion of the tube to assess whether the primary upper airway problem (e.g., swollen, overlong soft palate) has resolved sufficiently to allow the animal to breathe around and therefore without the tracheostomy tube. The tube should be cuffed if positive pressure ventilation is required, and should have an inner cannula to facilitate cleaning (Figure 5-4). The trachea is suctioned free of blood and secretions and the tracheostomy tube inserted. The tube is secured with sutures to the skin of the neck, and with an umbilical tape encircling the neck. In some brachycephalic dogs, it is necessary to loosely suture the tube to the trachea to prevent displacement. Vertical and transverse flap tracheostomies have also been described in dogs, but do not appear to offer substantial advantages over the transverse tracheostomy technique described here.[59,60]

Air passing through the tracheostomy tube bypasses the upper airway and is not warmed, humidified, or filtered. Inspiration of dry, cool gas can cause increased production of thick viscous respiratory secretions and decreased mucociliary activity, resulting in decreased clearance of mucus and debris.[61] Mucus that is moved by the mucociliary apparatus is deposited on the end of the tracheostomy tube and can obstruct the tube within 2 to

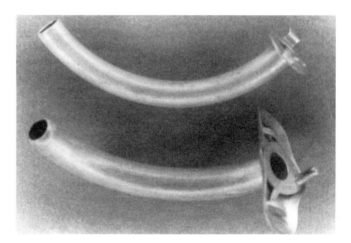

Figure 5-4. *An older metal tracheostomy tube with the inner cannula removed and shown. Intermittent removal of the inner cannula allows mucus to be cleaned from the end of the tube and prevents tube obstruction.*

6 hours. Postoperative care of a patient with a tracheostomy tube should include intravenous fluids to ensure adequate hydration, and either nebulization at the tracheostomy site or the use of a disposable humidifier on the tracheostomy tube.[62] Humidification should provide air that has 100% saturation with water vapor.[61] Intermittent nebulization with water droplets is commonly used to moisten airway secretions. Experimental studies in rabbits ventilated and nebulized for 6 hours have raised concerns about excessive duration of nebulization, which can cause pulmonary changes including increased artery wall thickness, and interstitial and alveolar edema.[63] Mucus accumulating on the distal end of the tracheostomy tube is eliminated by removing and cleaning the inner cannula of the double lumen tube every 2 to 6 hours. When an emergency tracheostomy is performed and double lumen tracheostomy tubes are not available, the tracheostomy tube

should be removed and replaced with a new tube as frequently as every 4 to 6 hours if needed. Replacement is facilitated by pulling up on the stay suture placed in the tracheal ring caudal to the tracheostomy.

Suctioning of the trachea should be avoided if possible, because both the passage of the catheter[64] and the applied negative pressure[65] can cause tracheobronchial trauma. Other adverse effects of suction include marked hypoxia, which can persist for up to 15 minutes after catheter insertion in dogs.[66] Cardiac arrhythmias[67] and pneumothorax[68] are other significant reported complications of suction. If suction is deemed necessary, the animal should be preoxygenated, a soft catheter less than half the size of the trachea should be used, and ideally a controlled vacuum pressure of 70 to 100 mm Hg is used.[69]

Once the upper airway obstruction is successfully treated and the swelling has resolved, airway patency can be tested by covering the end of the tracheostomy tube. The animal should be able to breathe comfortably around the tube if the tube is less than 75% of the tracheal diameter. Occasionally, mucus accumulation between the exterior of the tube and the tracheal mucosa causes inability to breathe when the tube is occluded. If other clinical indications suggest that the upper airway obstruction has been resolved, a test removal of the tracheostomy tube may be indicated. When the tube is removed, the tracheostomy site is left to heal as an open wound. The skin should not be debrided and closed, because leakage of air from the tracheostomy site on exhalation would cause severe subcutaneous emphysema.

The author wishes to acknowledge the advice of Dr. R.O. Davies and the assistance of Ms. Sharon Ward.

REFERENCES

1. Ohnishi T, Ogura JH: Partitioning of pulmonary resistance in the dog, *Laryngoscope* 79:1847, 1969.
2. Grandage J, Richardson K: Functional anatomy. In Slatter DH, editor: *Textbook of small animal surgery*, ed 2, vol I. Philadelphia, 1993, WB Saunders.
3. Guyton AC, Hall JE: *Textbook of medical physiology*, ed 9, Philadelphia, 1996, WB Saunders.
4. Milic-Emili J, Zin WA: Breathing responses to imposed mechanical loads. In Fishman AP, section editor; Cherniack AP, Widdicombe JG, volume editors: *Handbook of physiology, the respiratory system*, vol 2, ed 2, Baltimore, 1986, Williams and Wilkins.
5. Younes M: Mechanisms of respiratory load compensation. In Dempsey JA, Pack AI, editors: *Regulation of breathing*, ed 2, New York, 1995, Marcel Dekker Inc.
6. Rochester DF, Truwit JD: Respiratory muscle failure in critical illness. In Shoemaker WC, editor: *Textbook of critical care*, ed 3, Philadelphia, 1995, WB Saunders.
7. Love S, Waterman AE, Lane JG: The assessment of corrective surgery for canine laryngeal paralysis by blood gas analysis: A review of 35 cases, *J Small Anim Pract* 28:597, 1987.
8. Harvey CE: Upper airway obstruction surgery I: Stenotic nares surgery in brachycephalic dogs, *J Am Anim Hosp Assoc* 18:535, 1982.
9. Harvey CE: Upper airway obstruction surgery II: Soft palate resection in brachycephalic dogs, *J Am Anim Hosp Assoc* 18:538, 1982.
10. Coyne BE, Fingland RB: Hypoplasia of the trachea in dogs: 103 cases (1974-1990), *J Am Vet Med Assoc* 201:768, 1992.
11. Petrof BJ et al: Pharyngeal myopathy of loaded upper airway in dogs with sleep apnea, *J Appl Physiol* 76:1746, 1994.
12. Hendricks JC, Petrof BJ, Panckeri K et al: Upper airway dilating muscle hyperactivity during non-rapid eye movement sleep in English bulldogs, *Am Rev Resp Dis* 148:185, 1993.
13. Schotland HM, Insko EK, Panckeri KA et al: Quantitative magnetic resonance imaging of upper airway musculature in an animal model of sleep apnea, *J Appl Physiol* 81:1339, 1996.
14. Harvey CE: Everted laryngeal saccule surgery in brachycephalic dogs, *J Am Anim Hosp Assoc* 18:545, 1982.
15. Leonard HC: Collapse of the larynx and adjacent structures in the dog, *J Am Vet Med Assoc* 137:360, 1960.
16. Harvey CE: Upper airway obstruction surgery IV: Partial laryngectomy in brachycephalic dogs, *J Am Anim Hosp Assoc* 18:548, 1982.
17. Kerr L: Pulmonary edema secondary to upper airway obstruction in dogs: A review of nine cases, *J Am Anim Hosp Assoc* 25:207, 1989.
18. Lee KWT, Downes JJ: Pulmonary edema secondary to laryngospasm in children, *Anesthesiology* 59:349, 1983.
19. Kamal RS, Agha S: Acute pulmonary oedema: A complication of upper airway obstruction, *Anesthesia* 39:464, 1984.
20. Weissman C, Damask MC, Yang J: Noncardiogenic pulmonary edema following laryngeal obstruction, *Anesthesiology* 60:163, 1984.
21. Schwartz DR, Maroo A, Malhotra A et al: Negative pressure pulmonary hemorrhage, *Chest* 115:1194, 1999.
22. Mathieu-Costello O, Willford DC, Fu Z et al: Pulmonary capillaries are more resistant to stress failure in dogs than in rabbits, *J Appl Physiol* 79:908, 1995.
23. Burnie AG, Simpson JW, Corcoran BM: Gastro-esophageal reflux and hiatus hernia associated with laryngeal paralysis in a dog, *J Small Anim Pract* 30:414, 1989.
24. Prymak C, Saunders HM, Washabau RJ: Hiatal hernia repair by restoration and stabilization of normal anatomy: An evaluation in four dogs and one cat, *Vet Surg* 18:386, 1989.
25. Baue AE, Hoffer RE: The effects of experimental hiatal hernia and histamine stimulation on the intrinsic esophageal sphincter, *Surg Gynecol Obstet* 125:791, 1967.
26. Henderson RD, Mugahe F, Jeejeebhoy KN et al: The motor defects of esophagitis, *Can J Surg* 17:112, 1974.
27. Ross JT, Matthiesen DT, Noone K et al: Complications and long-term results after partial laryngectomy for the treatment of idiopathic laryngeal paralysis in 45 dogs, *Vet Surg* 20:169, 1991.
28. Holt DE, Harvey CE: Idiopathic laryngeal paralysis: Results of treatment by bilateral vocal fold resection in 40 dogs, *J Am Anim Hosp Assoc* 30:389, 1994.
29. Trout NJ, Harpster NK, Berg J et al: Long-term results of unilateral ventriculocordectomy and partial arytenoidectomy for the treatment of laryngeal paralysis in 60 dogs, *J Am Anim Hosp Assoc* 30:401, 1994.
30. Mier A, Laroche C, Agnew JE et al: Tracheobronchial clearance in patients with bilateral diaphragmatic weakness, *Am Rev Resp Dis* 142:545, 1990.
31. Schmidt-Nowara WW, Altman AR: Atelectasis and neuromuscular respiratory failure, *Chest* 85:792, 1984.
32. Van Pelt DR, McKiernan BC: Pathogenesis and treatment of canine rhinitis, *Vet Clin North Am Small Anim Pract* 24:789, 1994.
33. Van Pelt DR, Lappin MR: Pathogenesis and treatment of feline rhinitis. *Vet Clin North Am Small Anim Pract* 24:807, 1994.
34. Coolman BR, Marretta SM, McKiernan BC et al: Choanal atresia and secondary nasopharyngeal stenosis in a dog, *J Am Anim Hosp Assoc* 34:497, 1998.
35. Wells MJ, Coyne JA, Prince JL: What is your diagnosis? *J Am Vet Med Assoc* 180:83, 1982.
36. Mitten RW: Nasopharyngeal stenosis in four cats, *J Small Anim Pract* 29:341, 1988.
37. Novo RE, Kramek B: Surgical repair of nasopharyngeal stenosis in a cat using a stent, *J Am Anim Hosp Assoc* 35:251, 1999.
38. Griffon DJ, Tasker S: Use of a mucosal advancement flap for the treatment of nasopharyngeal stenosis in a cat, *J Small Anim Pract* 41:71, 2000.
39. White RAS, Lane JG: Pharyngeal stick penetration injuries in the dog, *J Small Anim Pract* 29:13, 1988.
40. Weber WJ, Hobson HP, Wilson SR: Pharyngeal mucoceles in dogs, *Vet Surg* 15:5, 1986.
41. Kapatkin AS, Matthiesen DT, Noone KE et al: Results of surgery and long-term follow-up in 31 cats with nasopharyngeal polyps, *J Am Anim Hosp Assoc* 26:387, 1990.
42. Riley P: Nasopharyngeal grass foreign body in eight cats, *J Am Vet Med Assoc* 202:299, 1993.
43. Withrow SJ: Tumors of the gastrointestinal system: A, Cancer of the oral cavity. In Withrow SJ, MacEwan EG, editors: *Small animal clinical oncology*, ed 2, Philadelphia, 1996, WB Saunders.

44. Venker-van Haagen AJ, Engelse EJJ, van den Ingh TSGAM: Congenital subglottic stenosis in a dog. *J Am Anim Hosp Assoc* 17:223, 1981.
45. Peterson J, Streeter V: Laryngeal obstruction secondary to brodifacoum toxicosis in a dog, *J Am Vet Med Assoc* 208:352, 1996.
46. Saik JE, Toll SL, Diters RW et al: Canine and feline laryngeal neoplasia: A 10-year survey, *J Am Anim Hosp Assoc* 22:359, 1986.
47. Ogilvie GK: Tumors of the endocrine system. In Withrow SJ, MacEwan EG, editors: *Small animal clinical oncology*, ed 2, Philadelphia, 1996, WB Saunders.
48. Hardie EM, Spodnick GJ, Gilson SD et al: Tracheal rupture in cats: 16 cases, *J Am Vet Med Assoc* 214:508, 1999.
49. Mitchell SL, McCarthy R, Rudloff E et al: Tracheal rupture associated with intubation in cats: 20 cases (1996-1998), *J Am Vet Med Assoc* 216:1592, 2000.
50. Lotti U, Niebauer GW: Tracheobronchial foreign bodies of plant origin in 153 hunting dogs, *Comp Cont Ed Pract Vet* 14:7, 1992.
51. Carlisle CH, Biery DN, Thrall DE: Tracheal and laryngeal tumors of the dog and cat: Literature review and 13 additional patients, *Vet Radiol* 32:229, 1991.
52. Brovida C, Castagnaro M: Tracheal obstruction due to an eosinophilic granuloma in a dog: Surgical treatment and clinicopathological observations, *J Am Anim Hosp Assoc* 28:8, 1992.
53. Metcalfe SS: Filaroides osleri in a dog, *Aust Vet Pract* 27:65, 1997.
54. Cobb MA, Fischer MA: Crenosoma vulpis infection in a dog, *Vet Rec* 130:452, 1992.
55. Blocker TL, Roberts BK: Acute tracheal obstruction associated with anticoagulant rodenticide intoxication in a dog, *J Small Anim Pract* 40:577, 1999.
56. Sheaffer KA, Dillon AR: Obstructive tracheal mass due to an inflammatory polyp in a cat, *J Am Anim Hosp Assoc* 32:431, 1996.
57. Fitzgerald SD, Johnson CA, Peck EJ: A fatal case of intrathoracic cuterebriasis in a cat, *J Am Anim Hosp Assoc* 32:353, 1996.
58. Harvey CE, Goldschmidt MH: Healing following short duration transverse incision tracheotomy in the dog, *Vet Surg* 11:77, 1982.
59. Smith MM, Saunders GK, Leib MS et al: Evaluation of horizontal and vertical tracheotomy healing following short duration tracheostomy in dogs, *Vet Surg* 23:416, 1994.
60. Macintire DK, Henderson RA, Wilson ER et al: Transverse flap tracheostomy: A technique for temporary tracheostomy of intermediate duration, *J Vet Emerg Crit Care* 5:25, 1995.
61. Tsuda T, Noguchi H, Takumi Y et al: Optimum humidification of air administered to a tracheostomy in dogs: Scanning electron microscopy and surfactant studies, *J Anaesth* 49:965, 1977.
62. Mebius C: A comparative evaluation of disposable humidifiers, *Acta Anaesthesiol Scand* 27:403, 1983.
63. John E, Ermocilla R, Golden J et al: Effects of gas temperature and particulate water on rabbit lungs during ventilation, *Pediatr Res* 14:1186, 1980.
64. Sackner MA, Lander J, Greenletch N et al: Pathogenesis and prevention of tracheobronchial damage with suction procedures, *Chest* 64:284, 1973.
65. Plum F, Dunning MF: Techniques for minimizing trauma to the tracheobronchial tree after tracheotomy, *N Eng J Med* 254:193, 1956.
66. Naigow D, Powaser MM: The effect of different endotracheal suction procedures on arterial blood gases in a controlled experimental model, *Heart Lung* 6:808, 1977.
67. Shim C, Fernandez R, Fine N et al: Cardiac arrhythmias resulting from tracheal suctioning, *Am International Med* 71:1149, 1969.
68. Vaughan RS, Menke JA, Giacoia GP: Pneumothorax: A complication of endotracheal tube suctioning, *J Pediatr* 92:633, 1978.
69. Young CS: Recommended guidelines for suction, *Physiotherapy* 70:106, 1984.

CHAPTER 6

Acute and Chronic Cough

Elizabeth A. Rozanski • John E. Rush

Cough is a common presenting complaint for dogs and, to a lesser extent, cats. Cough is a sign of an underlying disorder, not a disease in itself. Therefore, the cause of the cough should be identified and the underlying disease, not just the cough, should be treated. The cause of cough may be simple to identify and easy to correct in many cases. In other animals, the etiology can be obscure, diagnostic testing unrewarding, and the cough may remain unresponsive to therapeutic manipulation. It is therefore important to have a strong grasp of the underlying pathophysiology and as well as the common and uncommon causes of cough.

Definition and Clinical Signs

Cough is defined as a sudden expiratory effort, initially against a closed glottis, producing a noisy expulsion of air from the lungs. A cough usually signals an effort to clear the lungs or upper airway of real or perceived foreign material. Cough is therefore not a final diagnosis, but rather a clinical sign noted with a variety of underlying causes. A cough can be classified as acute or chronic. Coughing is considered chronic if it persists for 2 months or longer.

Historical information and a description of the cough may help to pinpoint the etiology. Cough may also be described as moist, dry, productive, or honking. A moist cough suggests the presence of airway secretions. Animals may be observed to either swallow or produce sputum after a bout of coughing, and in these cases the cough is considered productive. Cough may also be classified regarding the time of day that it occurs (e.g., night or morning) or coupled with an event such as drinking, eating, running, or pulling on a leash. In cats, cough may be confused with retching or attempts to vomit

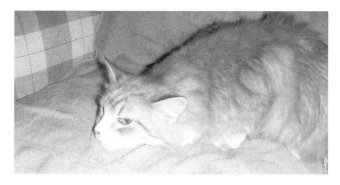

Figure 6-1. *A cat demonstrating the characteristic posture of cough. Note the extended head and neck.*

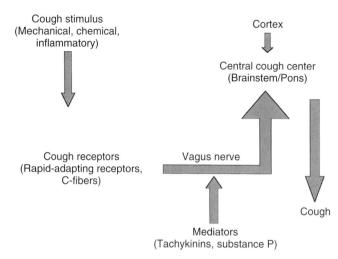

Figure 6-2. *Flow chart demonstrating the cough pathway. Note the involvement of the stimulus, cough receptors, mediators, and efferent pathways.*

(Figure 6-1). In a variety of diseases, cough is often the primary presenting complaint, particularly when cough is a new clinical sign. However, in some dogs with chronic or multisystemic signs, cough may not be specifically identified as a complaint unless the client is precisely questioned.

Pathophysiology

Coughing can be both a voluntary and an involuntary act, although in animals it is difficult to determine the immediate trigger. Most coughing in animals is presumed to be an involuntary response. Stimuli to cough include pressure on the outside of the airway or the presence of foreign material, excessive secretions, or noxious gases in the airway. Cough serves as an important function both by aiding in the clearance of foreign debris and by enhancing the actions of the mucociliary escalator.[1] The cough reflex is the primary defense mechanism of the pulmonary system.[1,2]

The cough pathway has been extensively investigated in animals.[3-7] It includes the cough receptors and sensory nerves in the airway, the vagus nerve, the central cough center (brainstem, pons) and the effectors including the glottis and expiratory muscles (Figure 6-2).[1,3] Innervation for these receptors and the sites for triggering cough is supplied exclusively by the vagus nerve.[1,3,8] Therefore, some structures that are not usually considered to be part of the respiratory tract (e.g., the external auditory meatus and the tympanic membrane) may also be involved in the cough reflex.[8]

The first step in creation of a cough is stimulation of the cough receptors, which are made up of sensory nerves. Species differences exist in sensory nerves; however, much of the research on cough receptors has been performed in animals.[1,3-7,9,10] At least three different receptors are involved in stimulation of a cough response: the rapidly adapting stretch receptors, the pulmonary C-fibers and the bronchial C-fibers.[2,3] The rapidly adapting stretch receptors (or "irritant" receptors) are located within the mucosa of the tracheobronchial tree. During normal breathing, these myelinated receptors discharge sporadically, and they respond to light mechanical stimulus.[2,3] These are the receptors that are most likely to be stimulated by foreign debris.

C-fibers are unmyelinated receptors located close to blood vessels. They respond to lung hyperinflation as well as to endogenous and exogenous stimulants. The pulmonary C-fibers are located within peripheral airways and are supplied by blood from the pulmonary circulation. The bronchial C-fibers are located within larger airways and are supplied by the bronchial circulation. Both of these C-fiber receptors are more sensitive to chemical stimulation than mechanical stimulus.[11,12] Not all C-fibers are involved in the generation of cough, and substantial species differences exist. C-fibers are also important in bronchoconstriction and in the neural control of respiration.

The cough pathway may be stimulated by mechanical or chemical factors.[2,3] Endogenous triggers of coughing include the presence of airway secretions and airway inflammation. Exogenous agents include smoke and aspirated foreign materials such as food or water. Certain diseases can magnify the response to a specific agent, resulting in increased cough. For example, dogs with experimentally induced *Bordetella bronchiseptica* infection have a marked increase in the response of the rapidly adapting stretch receptor.[7] Anatomical differences also affect the resulting cough response because airways differ in their reactions to various stimuli. The more proximal airways (i.e., larynx and trachea) are very sensitive to mechanical stimuli, but are less sensitive to chemical stimulation. The more distal airways (e.g., the bronchi and bronchioles) are more sensitive to chemical stimulus and less responsive to mechanical stimulation. This is largely a reflection of the type of receptors present in each location. Direct stimulation of the larynx results in the *expiratory reflex*, which is a cough without prior inspiration. This reflex may be appreciated in the initial cough triggered during attempts at endotracheal intubation in cats. Stimulation of receptors from distal airways typically results in an inspiratory phase prior to the cough. The prior inspiration serves to maximize the subsequent expiratory airflow rate.

Chemical mediators, released by receptors in response to stimulation, serve to modulate the cough response. These mediators include substance P, calcitonin gene-related peptide (CGRP), neurokinin A (NKA), and other tachykinins.[9] The relative roles of these neuropeptides in modification or stimulation of cough is still under investigation. Substance P (SP) has been extensively investigated. It is a potent proinflammatory agent in the airways that causes increased vascular permeability, vasodilation, and submucosal gland secretion.[9] Research to date suggests that the neuropeptides (including SP) are the final mediators of many abnormalities in the inflamed airways, including cough. Neuropeptides are degraded by neutral endopeptidase (NEP), angiotensin converting enzyme (ACE), and other enzymes. Modification of neuropeptide degradation may ultimately be useful in management of cough. Practically, in human medicine, cough that is linked to ACE inhibitor use (e.g., benazepril or enalapril) is thought to reflect either delayed degradation of SP or local increases in bradykinin that stimulate the C-fibers. ACE inhibitor–associated cough has rarely been reported in veterinary medicine and, in fact, most studies show substantial improvement in cough following the addition of an ACE-inhibitor due to better control of congestive heart failure.[13]

Sensory and neuropeptide activity is altered in human asthmatics when compared to healthy controls. Whereas cough and bronchoconstriction are triggered by closely related stimuli, these phenomena are clinical signs actually initiated by separate sensory pathways.[11] For example, cough suppressants such as codeine have no effect on bronchoconstriction. The mast cell stabilizer cromoglycate blocks bronchoconstriction but has no effect on cough.[1,11] This concept appears to be significant in understanding the pathophysiology of cough and bronchoconstriction. This distinction has not been described in spontaneously-occurring animal disease such as feline asthma, although laboratory evidence with experimental animal models suggests that similar physiology may exist in many species.[1,3-5]

The cough reflex has been objectively tested in people and experimental animals. In this test, an agent known to trigger cough (e.g., capsaicin, a red pepper extract) is nebulized at increasing concentrations until two or more coughs occur.[14] Individuals who cough at lower concentrations are regarded as having an increased cough reflex. This test is thought to be useful to provide more objective data about the symptom of cough, but it has not found clinical utility in clinical veterinary medicine.

Differential Diagnosis

Many underlying diseases are recognized to cause cough (Box 6-1). Cough can be seen in animals with disease in the nasal passages, larynx, trachea, bronchi, alveoli, pleural space; and in animals with cardiac disease. Broad categories or etiologic agents include allergic/inflammatory, cardiac, infectious, neoplastic, parasitic, trauma, and physical factors. Multiple causes of cough exist in some animals (e.g., the aged dog with heart disease and collapsing trachea), and in these cases the cough may be triggered by more than one disease. It is usually helpful to consider species, age, breed or body conformation, history, and physical examination findings when considering differential diagnoses, in order to develop a diagnostic plan.

BOX 6-1
Causes of Cough in Small Animals

Allergic/Inflammatory

Feline asthma
Chronic bronchitis
Chronic obstructive pulmonary disease (COPD)
Pulmonary infiltrates with eosinophilia (PIE)
Eosinophilic pneumonitis

Cardiovascular

Pulmonary edema
Left atrial enlargement
Pulmonary embolism (uncommon)

Infectious

Tracheobronchitis
Pneumonia
　Bacterial
　Viral
　Fungal
　Protozoal

Neoplastic

Primary
　Lung

Primary, cont'd
　Trachea
　Larynx
Metastatic
Heart-base tumor
Compression due to enlarged lymph nodes

Parasites

Filaroides
Aelurostrongylus
Paragonimus
Capillaria
Dirofilaria
Others

Trauma and Physical Abnormalities

Foreign body
Collapsing trachea
Tracheal hypoplasia
Tracheal stenosis
Smoke inhalation

Diagnostic Testing

Diagnostic testing for acute and chronic cough is usually based, at least in part, on the signalment, history, and physical examination findings. In some cases (e.g., mild infectious tracheobronchitis with typical historical and physical examination findings) no further testing may be required. However, in almost all pets with cough, a thoracic radiograph is an essential initial diagnostic test. Thoracic radiography provides useful information about the lung parenchyma, the pleural space, and the cardiovascular system. Further diagnostic testing is often based upon the result of the thoracic radiographs. For example, if pleural effusion is evident, then thoracocentesis is appropriate; whereas if alveolar infiltrates are noted in a cranioventral location, then tracheal aspiration with cytology and culture should be performed.

Routine laboratory testing such as a complete blood count, chemistry profile, urinalysis, and fecal examination are helpful to complete the minimum database and to exclude some systemic and parasitic causes of cough. Fluoroscopy may be indicated if dynamic airway obstruction is suspected, and direct visualization of the airways (i.e., laryngoscopy and bronchoscopy) with subsequent sample collection for cytology and bacterial culture may be useful in infectious or inflammatory causes of cough. Echocardiography and electrocardiography are very useful in evaluating the patient with suspected left-sided heart failure or the patient with cor pulmonale due to chronic bronchitis. Ultrasonographic evaluation of noncardiac structures is often useful for suspected mass lesions and pleural effusion of unknown etiology. Heartworm (serology) and lungworm (Baermann fecal) testing is recommended in animals from endemic areas.

Pulmonary function tests may or may not be abnormal in animals with cough. Arterial blood gases may document hypoxemia or hypercarbia but do not provide information about the underlying etiology. More specialized pulmonary function testing (e.g., plethysomography) may help to clarify the type of impairment present and can also be used as a tool to judge the response to therapy.

Initial Management Pending Results of Diagnostic Testing

The most successful management of cough involves treatment and resolution of the underlying cause. Specific disease-oriented therapy often results in near complete resolution of coughing. When cough is accompanied by dyspnea or respiratory distress, oxygen therapy is indicated while diagnostic testing is proceeding. In most cases, cough does not require immediate treatment prior to completion of a complete history, physical examination, and thoracic radiograph.

If cough is associated with bronchoconstriction, bronchodilator therapy can result in partial resolution of the cough. For animals with infectious etiologies and productive cough, nebulization and coupage can improve clearance of airway secretions and debris and thereby improve the effectiveness of the cough reflex.

Unfortunately, in some animals coughing persists despite therapy for the underlying etiology. This is especially true for animals with chronic nonproductive cough. In these cases, cough suppressants may be indicated. Excessive or frequent coughing, to the point of exhaustion for the patient or insomnia on the part of the patient or the client, is often the reason for use of cough suppressant therapy. Some dogs experience syncopal episodes precipitated by paroxysms of coughing, and in many cases cough suppression can reduce the frequency of syncope. Even in these cases, it is important to identify the underlying disease and the reason(s) to suppress coughing. Cough suppression is contraindicated (or relatively contraindicated) in dogs with infectious disease and productive cough.

Medications that suppress cough include drugs that directly inhibit the cough receptors including the narcotics (e.g., butorphanol, hydrocodone), antiinflammatory agents (specifically glucocorticoids), and bronchodilators (e.g., the methylxanthines and β_2-agonists). The most appropriate choice of cough suppressant depends upon the underlying disease.

In most small animals with cough, a specific disease or disorder can be identified as the etiology. Airway inflammation is a common denominator for many diseases causing cough, and modulating the inflammatory response may be appropriate in many cases. Treatment of the primary process, when possible, will result in the most effective long-term control of clinical signs.

REFERENCES

1. Chang AB: Cough, cough receptors, and asthma in children, *Pediatric Pulmonology* 8:59-70, 1999.
2. Fuller RW, Jackson DM: Physiology and treatment of cough, *Thorax* 45:425-430, 1990.
3. Widdicombe JG: Neurophysiology of the cough reflex, *Eur Respir J* 8:1193-1202, 1995.
4. Dixon M, Jackson DM, Richards IM: A study of the afferent and efferent nerve distribution to the lungs of dogs, *Respiration* 39:144-149, 1980.
5. Davies A, Dixon M, Callahan D et al: Lung reflexes in rabbits during pulmonary stretch receptor block by sulphur dioxide, *Respir Physiol* 34:83-101, 1978.
6. Widdicombe JG: Afferent receptors in the airways and cough, *Respir Physiol* 114:5-15, 1998.
7. Dixon M, Jackson DM, Richards IM: The effect of respiratory tract infection on histamine-induced changes in lung mechanics and irritant receptor discharge in dogs, *Am Rev Respir Dis* 120: 843-848, 1979.
8. Karlsson J, Sant'Ambrogio G, Widdicombe J: Afferent neural pathways in cough and reflex bronchoconstriction, *J Appl Physiol* 65:1007-1023,1988.
9. Sekizawa K, Jia YX, Ebihara T et al: Role of substance P in cough, *Pulmonary Pharmacology* 9: 323-328, 1996.
10. Ujiie Y, Sekizawa K, Aikawa T et al: Evidence for substance P as an endogenous substance causing cough in guinea pigs, *Am Rev Respir Dis* 148:1628-1632, 1993.
11. Choudry NB, Fuller RW, Anderson N et al: Separation of cough and reflex bronchoconstriction by inhaled local anaesthetics, *Eur Resp J* 3:579-583, 1990.

12. Coleridge HM, Coleridge JCG, Baker DG et al: Comparison of the effects of histamine and prostaglandin on afferent C-fibre endings and irritant receptors in intrapulmonary airways, *Adv in Exp Med Biol* 99:291-305, 1978.
13. Kitagawa H, Wakamiya H, Kitoh K et al: Efficacy of monotherapy with benazepril, an angiotensin converting enzyme inhibitor, in dogs with naturally acquired chronic mitral insufficiency, *J Vet Med Sci* 59:513-520, 1997.
14. Fuller RW, Karlsson J, Choudry NB et al: Effect of inhaled and systemic opiates on responses to inhaled capsaicin in humans, *J Appl Physiol* 65:1125-1130, 1988.

CHAPTER 7

Panting

Susan G. Hackner

Panting is defined as rapid, shallow respiration, with a respiratory frequency of 200 to 400 breaths per minute and a decreased tidal volume, such that alveolar ventilation remains relatively unchanged.[1-4] It is a normal thermoregulatory mechanism in many species, including the dog and cat.[2,4,5] Panting is seldom a primary complaint but is commonly observed on presentation or during hospitalization. Because of the usually innocuous causes of panting, it is often overlooked. It may, however, be an indicator of more serious underlying disease or drug therapy.

Physiology

Panting is the major method of thermoregulation in small animals exposed to heat or exercise.[2,4,6] By rapidly replacing moist air over the evaporative surfaces of the nasal passages and the mouth with fresh, dry air, panting increases evaporative heat loss.[2,5,7] During panting, the mechanical capabilities of the respiratory system are devoted to efficient air flow through the upper airway to maximize evaporative cooling.[5,8] Evaporative loss is enhanced by a concurrent rise in lingual and nasal blood flow (up to sevenfold).[7,9,10] Secretions from the lateral nasal glands increase up to fortyfold,[2,11] and it has been suggested that the role of these glands is analogous to that of sweat glands in humans.

Additional heat generated by muscular work is avoided by panting with a rhythmic motion that approaches the resonant frequency of the respiratory system[5,8]: that is, the elastic properties of the lungs and thorax allow expansion and contraction at this rate with a minimum of external work.[8] The oxygen consumption of respiratory muscles during thermal panting is minimally increased, and is less than that observed for a comparable level of ventilation produced by hypercapnia.[8,12]

Panting is characterized by a high respiratory frequency and a low tidal volume.[3,4,13] Dead space ventilation is proportionally increased relative to alveolar ventilation and minute ventilation.[14,15] Although the magnitude of tidal volume is decreased, it remains slightly greater than dead space such that, over a wide range of heat stress and relative humidity, gas exchange is adequate and arterial blood gases and intracellular pH are well defended.[8,16] This pattern of ventilation and gas exchange is analogous to contemporary methods of high frequency positive pressure ventilation.[14] Only after prolonged exposure to extreme heat stress do some animals exhibit deterioration of their blood gases, and heat exhaustion is finally associated with severe respiratory alkalosis.[1,8,16]

Panting is controlled by the thermoregulatory centers of the brain.[1,13] When the blood becomes overheated, the hypothalamus initiates neurogenic signals to decrease the body temperature, resulting in vasodilation and panting. The actual panting process is controlled by the panting center, associated with the pneumotaxic respiratory center located in the pons.[13]

Temperature detection occurs both centrally and peripherally. The anterior hypothalamic-preoptic area contains large numbers of heat-sensitive neurons.[13] These function as heat sensors, the neurons increasing their firing rate twofold to tenfold in response to an increase in body temperature of 1° C.[13] Peripheral temperature receptors are found in the skin, the spinal cord, the abdominal viscera, and around the great veins of the cranial abdomen and thorax. These receptors, however, mainly detect cold rather than heat, and play a lesser role in protection from overheating than do the central receptors.[13] Sensory signals from both central and peripheral receptors are transmitted to the posterior hypothalamus, where temperature-controlling effector mechanisms are initiated.[13] The effector pathways appear to be primarily autonomic.[7,17]

The integrated responses of the hypothalamus function to maintain the body temperature within a narrow, crucial range, known as the *set point* of the temperature control system. The feedback gain of the temperature control system is extremely high; that is, profound changes in ambient temperature result in minimal changes in body temperature.[13] Due to the oxygen cost of panting, however, thermoregulation is possible only within limits. Limitations depend on the energy requirements of the respiratory muscles, on the temperature set point, and on the feedback gain.[18]

It has been shown that ambient temperature leads to marked panting only above 30° C, and that panting is increased when the relative humidity of the air increases.[18] Panting can be stimulated by increases in cellular metabolism that result in heat production. This is known as chemical thermogenesis and is caused by increased concentrations of epinephrine, norepinephrine, and thyroxine.[13]

Dehydrated and hypovolemic dogs show a delayed panting threshold[19,20] that has been ascribed to the presence of brain receptors sensitive to extracellular solute concentration.[19]

Clinical Signs

Panting is seen as rapid, shallow breathing, without evidence of respiratory distress. The respiratory rate is generally between 200 and 400 breaths per minute. Three patterns of panting have been demonstrated as the demand for respiratory evaporation increases: (1) nasal inhalation and exhalation; (2) nasal inhalation, with exhalation through the nasal passages and mouth; and (3) inhalation and exhalation through the nasal passages and mouth.[6] Pattern 1 occurs with mildly elevated ambient temperatures (below 26° C) and with mild exercise in cold weather. Patterns 2 and 3 occur at rest in ambient temperatures above 30° C and during exercise. These latter patterns rarely occur independently; instead, there is normally continual oscillation between the two, with proportionally greater pattern 3 respiration as temperature and/or exercise speed increase. Pattern 3 is associated with greater alveolar ventilation requirements.

Differential Diagnosis

Panting is a normal physiological response to increased ambient temperature, exercise, hyperthermia, or fever. It is also commonly seen with anxiety, pain, or nervousness (due, at least in part, to chemical thermogenesis).[13] As such, panting is a common, nonspecific finding in both healthy and diseased animals. It is, however, also associated with a number of specific diseases and drugs (Box 7-1).

Hyperadrenocorticism and corticosteroid therapy often result in panting. Proposed pathophysiological mechanisms include abdominal fat deposition, muscle wasting, and respiratory muscle weakness.[21] Panting has

---

BOX 7–1
Causes of Panting

Elevated ambient temperature
Fever, hyperthermia
Anxiety, nervousness
Pain
Hyperadrenocorticism
Glucocorticosteroid therapy
Pheochromocytoma
Hyperthyroidism
Hypocalcemia
Narcotic administration
Cardiac disease/tachyarrhythmias
Brain disease

---

been reported in 25% of dogs with pheochromocytoma.[22] It is likely that the pathophysiology involves epinephrine-induced chemical thermogenesis. Thyrotoxicosis rarely produces panting at rest but often results in panting with even mild stress.[23] Abnormalities in respiratory function in humans with hyperthyroidism include decreased vital capacity, decreased pulmonary compliance, and increased minute ventilation.[24] These findings have been ascribed to respiratory muscle weakness and increased CO_2 production, but chemical thermogenesis is likely contributory. Approximately 50% of hypocalcemic dogs pant.[25] The pathophysiology is unclear, but it is likely related to anxiety and pain associated with tetany.[25]

Panting has been reported as a clinical sign in patients with cardiac disease, particularly feline cardiomyopathy.[26] A mechanism has not been proposed, but either anxiety or angina is feasible. It is the author's opinion that patients with tachyarrhythmias commonly pant.

Narcotics commonly result in panting, which appears to be dose-related, independent of the route of administration, and higher with pure agonist opioids (e.g., morphine, oxymorphone, or hydromorphone) compared with mixed agonist-antagonists (e.g., butorphanol).[27-29]

Patients with brain disorders occasionally pant. This may be due to a direct effect on the thermoregulatory system of the hypothalamus or to anxiety.

Diagnostic Testing

The first step in the approach to a panting animal is to determine whether panting is merely a response to elevated ambient temperature or to anxiety associated with a visit to the veterinarian, or whether it is an indicator of underlying disease. The latter is suggested by a history of increased panting at home. Careful history taking should include a drug history (e.g., administration of corticosteroids or narcotics) as well as any evidence of underlying disease. Polyuria and polydipsia may suggest hyperadrenocorticism, hyperthyroidism, or pheochromocytoma. Weight gain or hair loss may indicate hyperadrenocorticism. Muscle twitching or facial rubbing are compatible with hypocalcemia. Abnormal behavior or seizures should raise suspicion for brain disease.

The physical examination should distinguish panting from tachypnea or dyspnea. Panting is seen as more rapid, shallow respiration without evidence of distress. In the panting patient, evidence of underlying disease may include an elevated body temperature, tachycardia or tachyarrhythmia, an enlarged thyroid gland, muscle twitching, altered mentation, or changes compatible with hyperadrenocorticism (e.g., pot-bellied appearance, alopecia, or calcinosis cutis).

History and physical examination findings should guide an appropriate diagnostic workup, which may include a complete blood count, biochemical profile, thyroxine concentration, endocrine testing, electrocardiogram, and/or abdominal ultrasonography. Arterial blood gas analysis in the panting animal is generally normal but may show some degree of respiratory alkalosis.

Initial Management

No specific therapy is indicated for panting. Attempts should be made to reduce ambient temperature, if elevated, and to minimize anxiety. If the patient is febrile or hyperthermic, adequate hydration should be ensured to allow efficient thermoregulation. Therapy should be directed to the underlying condition.

REFERENCES

1. Andersson BE, Jonasson H: Temperature regulation and environmental physiology. In Swenson MJ, Reece WO, editors: *Duke's physiology of domestic animals*, ed 11, Ithaca, 1993, Cornell University Press.
2. Reece WO: Respiration in mammals. In Swenson MJ, Reece WO, editors: *Duke's physiology of domestic animals*, ed 11, Ithaca, 1993, Cornell University Press.
3. Cunningham JG: Overview of respiratory function: Ventilation of the lung. In Cunningham JG, editor: *Textbook of veterinary physiology*, Philadelphia, 1992, WB Saunders.
4. Erickson HH: Exercise physiology. In Swenson MJ, Reece WO, editors: *Duke's physiology of domestic animals*, ed 11, Ithaca, 1993, Cornell University Press.
5. Ruckebusch Y, Phaneuf L-P, Dunlop R: Mechanics of respiration. In Ruckebusch Y, Phaneuf L-P, Dunlop R, editors: *Physiology of large and small animals*, Philadelphia, 1991, BC Decker.
6. Goldberg MB, Langman VA, Taylor CR: Panting in dogs: Paths of air flow in response to heat and exercise, *Respir Physiol* 43(3):327, 1981.
7. Ronert H, Pleschka K: Lingual blood flow and its hypothalamic control in the dog during panting, *Pflugers Arch* 367(1):25, 1976.
8. Easton PA, Abe T, Young RN et al: Costal and crural diaphragm function during panting in awake canines, *J Appl Physiol* 77(4):1983, 1994.
9. Thomson EM, Pleschka K: Vasodilatory mechanisms in the tongue and nose of the dog under heat load, *Pflugers Arch* 387(2):161, 1980.
10. Baile EM, Guillemi S, Pare PD: Tracheobronchial and upper airway blood flow in dogs during thermally induced panting, *J Appl Physiol* 63(6):2240, 1987.
11. Blatt CM, Taylor CR, Habal MB: Thermal panting in dogs: The lateral nasal gland, a source of water for evaporative cooling, *Science* 177(51):804, 1972.
12. Hales JRS, Findlay JD: The oxygen cost of thermally-induced and CO_2-induced hyperventilation in the ox, *Respir Physiol* 4(3):353, 1968.
13. Guyton AC, Hall JE: Body temperature, temperature regulation, and fever. In Guyton AC, Hall JE, editors: *Textbook of medical physiology*, ed 10, Philadelphia, 2000, WB Saunders.
14. Meyer M, Hahn G, Piiper J: Pulmonary gas exchange in panting dogs: A model for high frequency ventilation, *Acta Anaesthesiol Scand Suppl* 90:22, 1989.
15. Meyer M, Hahn G, Buess C et al: Pulmonary gas exchange in panting dogs, *J Appl Physiol* 66(3):1258, 1989.
16. Albers C, Usinger W, Scholand C: Intracellular pH in unanesthetized dogs during panting. *Respir Physiol* 23(1):59, 1975.
17. Saxena R, Kumar S, Tandon S et al:, Role of vagus during exercise in thermal panting, *Indian J Physiol Pharmacol* 24(3):190, 1980.
18. Albers C: Respiratory control of body temperature: A theoretical model, *Respir Physiol* 30(1-2):137, 1977.
19. Baker MA, Turlejska E: Thermal panting in dehydrated dogs: Affects of plasma volume expansion and drinking, *Pflugers Arch* 413(5):511, 1989.
20. Horowitz M, Nadel ER: Effect of plasma volume on thermoregulation in the dog, *Pflugers Arch* 400(2):211, 1984.
21. Feldman EC, Nelson RW: Hyperadrenocorticism (Cushing's syndrome). In Feldman EC, Nelson RW editors: *Canine and feline endocrinology and reproduction*, ed 2, Philadelphia, 1996, WB Saunders.
22. Feldman EC, Nelson RW: Pheochromocytoma and multiple endocrine neoplasia. In Feldman EC, Nelson RW editors: *Canine and feline endocrinology and reproduction*, ed 2, Philadelphia, 1996, WB Saunders.
23. Feldman EC, Nelson RW: Feline hyperthyroidism (thyrotoxicosis). In Feldman EC, Nelson RW editors: *Canine and feline endocrinology and reproduction*, ed 2, Philadelphia, 1996, WB Saunders.
24. Ingbar DH: The respiratory system in thyrotoxicosis. In Braverman LE, Utiger RD, editors: *The thyroid: A fundamental and clinical text*, ed 6, Philadelphia, 1991, JB Lippincott.
25. Feldman EC, Nelson RW: Hypocalcemia and primary hypoparathyroidism. In Feldman EC, Nelson RW editors: *Canine and feline endocrinology and reproduction*, ed 2, Philadelphia, 1996, WB Saunders.
26. Nelson RW, Couto CG: Myocardial diaseases of the cat. In Nelson RW, Couto CG, editors: *Small animal internal medicine*, St Louis, 1998, Mosby.
27. Cullen LK, Raffe MR, Randall DA et al: Assessment of the respiratory effects of intramuscular morphine in conscious dogs, *Res Vet Sci* 67(2):141, 1999.
28. Lucas AN, Firth AM, Anderson GA et al: Comparison of the effects of morphine administered by constant-rate intravenous infusion or intermittent intramuscular injection in dogs, *J Am Vet Med Assoc* 218(6):884, 2001.
29. Dyson DH, Atilola M: A clinical comparison of oxymorphone-acepromazine and butorphanol-acepromazine sedation in dogs, *Vet Surg* 21(5):418, 1992.

CHAPTER 8

Pleural Space Disease

Deborah C. Silverstein

Definitions and Clinical Signs

Pleural space disease is defined as an accumulation of air, fluid, and/or soft tissue within the pleural cavity. The etiology, quantity, and rate of development of the pleural space–filling defect determine the severity of clinical signs. Most animals do not exhibit obvious respiratory embarrassment until there is a significant impairment of the ability to expand the lungs. The observed respiratory signs occur secondary to a decrease in lung vital capacity, caused by the reduction in maximum tidal volume that can be achieved at peak inspiration. Thus, the inspiratory reserve volume is diminished. The lung volume at end-expiration (functional residual capacity) is also decreased, reducing the expiratory reserve volume. The lungs are subsequently predisposed to atelectasis, and impairment of ventilation and oxygenation occurs.

Dyspnea, tachypnea, shallow breathing, open mouth breathing, cyanosis, reluctance to lie down, orthopnea, +/− coughing, fever, depression, weight loss, anorexia, jugular pulses, arrhythmias, cardiac murmurs, ascites, and/or pericardial effusion may be present in animals with pleural space disease.

Pleural space disease is often suspected based on the clinical signs and auscultation abnormalities. Muffled or absent heart or breath sounds over large areas of the thorax may occur unilaterally or bilaterally, ventrally or dorsally, all depending on the nature and magnitude of the disorder. If a pleural filling defect is suspected, percussion of the chest wall may help characterize the nature of the abnormality. To percuss the chest, a finger is placed on an intercostal space and tapped with a finger of the opposite hand while listening for an increase or decrease in the sonic resonance of the sounds. This procedure is repeated over several areas of the chest bilaterally. A high-pitched, long-duration, tympanic sound suggests an air-filling abnormality, whereas a low-pitched, short-duration, dull sound may indicate fluid-filling disorders. Chest compression should also be performed in cats; a significant decrease in compressibility of the cranial thorax is often associated with a cranial mediastinal mass and pleural effusion.

Pathophysiology

The pleural cavity is a potential space between the lungs and the chest wall; it typically contains 1 to 5 ml of fluid, which lubricates the lungs during respiratory movements.[1,2] The pleura is a serosal surface that consists of a single layer of flattened endothelial cells with an underlying connective–tissue layer containing blood vessels and lymphatics.[3] The parietal pleura lines the thoracic walls, the mediastinum, and diaphragm; is rich in lymphatics; and receives its blood supply from the systemic circulation. The visceral pleura covers the serosal surface of the lungs, and its blood supply is provided by the pulmonary circulation.[3] Normally, there is continuous production of pleural fluid from the capillaries of the parietal pleura into the pleural space: this is absorbed by the visceral pleural capillaries and parietal lymphatic network.[2]

Starling's forces and lymphatic function control the dynamics of pleural fluid formation and absorption. The hydrostatic pressure in the systemic capillaries that provide blood to the parietal pleura is approximately 30 cm H_2O; whereas the hydrostatic pressure of the pleural fluid is −5 cm H_2O because of the opposing elastic recoil of the thoracic wall and lungs. Thus, there is a net hydrostatic pressure of 35 cm H_2O in favor of fluid movement from the parietal pleura into the pleural space. In addition, the colloid osmotic pressure (COP) of the pleural fluid is approximately 3 cm H_2O, compared to the COP of the capillaries, which is about 34 cm H_2O.[4] Therefore, there is a net COP of 31 cm H_2O in favor of fluid movement from the pleural space into the parietal pleura. However, the hydrostatic pressure of the pulmonary capillaries supplying the visceral pleura is 11 cm H_2O, creating a net hydrostatic pressure gradient of only 16 cm H_2O between the visceral pleura and the pleural space. The net colloid osmotic pressure that encourages fluid absorption from the pleural space remains at 31 cm H_2O, resulting in a net pressure of 15 cm H_2O favoring fluid absorption from the pleural space by the visceral pleura.[2]

The permeability of the capillary wall is the final determinant of Starling's forces, resulting in the final filtration volume, as described in the following formula:

$$\text{Fluid movement} = K \times ([[(HP_{c\,parietal} - HP_{c\,visceral}) - HP_{if}] - [COP_c - COP_{if}])$$

Where K = Filtration coefficient (in ml/sec/cm^2/cm H_2O); HP_c = mean capillary hydrostatic pressure (cm H_2O); HP_{if} = mean intrapleural fluid hydrostatic pressure (cm H_2O); COP_c = colloid osmotic pressure of the capillaries (cm H_2O); and COP_{if} = colloid osmotic pressure of fluid in the intrapleural space (cm H_2O).

The parietal pleural lymphatics also absorb pleural fluid and protein from the pleural space. This is increasingly important in disease states that result in a high protein pleural effusion because an increase in the COP of the pleural fluid decreases the absorption of fluid by the pulmonary capillaries. Lymphatic flow is stimulated by normal respiratory movements, and movement of the diaphragmatic and thoracic musculature.

Transudative pleural effusion results when there is increased pleural fluid formation or decreased fluid absorption. Potential causes of increased pleural fluid formation include an increase in capillary hydrostatic pressure (e.g., right-sided heart failure in dogs, left or right-sided heart failure in cats, pericardial effusion, diaphragmatic hernia, or neoplasia); decreased intravascular colloid osmotic pressure (e.g., hypoalbuminemia); or an increase in vascular endothelial permeability (e.g., systemic inflammatory response syndrome, chronic chylothorax, or cisplatin therapy in cats[5]). Decreased pleural fluid absorption occurs secondary to inflammation of the pleura, to neoplastic or embolic obstructions of the thoracic duct or lymph nodes, or lymphatic hypertension (see Chapter 78).

Additional causes of pleural effusion include hemothorax (see Chapter 81), pyothorax (see Chapter 80), and chylothorax (see Chapter 79). Hemothorax may occur secondary to trauma, neoplasia, coagulopathy, pulmonary thrombosis, thymic rupture, lung lobe torsion, infection, or postoperative complications. Pyothorax is often caused by migrating foreign bodies, puncture wounds of the chest wall, hematogenous spread of infectious agents, tracheal or esophageal perforation, pulmonary abscess or tumor rupture. Chylothorax occurs when chyle from the cisterna chylothoracic duct leaks into the pleural space. This may be idiopathic, secondary to an increase in systemic venous pressures (e.g., right heart failure, heartworm disease, mediastinal neoplasia, cranial vena cava thrombi, or fungal granulomas), thoracic duct rupture or obstruction, lung lobe torsion, lymphangiectasia, or trauma. The effusive form of feline infectious peritonitis may cause a high-protein, low– to moderate–cell count pleural and/or abdominal effusion in cats.

Air commonly enters the pleural space via thoracic wall injuries, esophageal perforations (e.g., extension from a pneumomediastinum), or rupture of the trachea or lung lesions (e.g., infection, bullae, or neoplasia). As air accumulates and the intrapleural pressure increases, the parietal and visceral pleurae separate and the lungs collapse. A tension pneumothorax occurs when the intrapleural pressure exceeds atmospheric pressure during inspiration and expiration. This is due to a one-way valve leak, typically in the lung, which allows air to enter the pleural space during inspiration and traps the air in the pleural space as the tissues around the perforation collapse, thus preventing the air from returning to the airways for exhalation. More air is added to the pleural space with each breath until the lungs collapse to their minimum volume and cause potentially fatal respiratory impairment.

The most common causes of space-occupying soft tissue disease in the pleural space include diaphragmatic hernia and mediastinal or pleural masses (see Chapters 83 and 84). Diaphragmatic hernias may be congenital or secondary to abdominal trauma. Cats may be predisposed to right-sided herniation.[6]

Differential Diagnosis

The differential diagnoses for an animal with pleural space disease include other causes of respiratory distress, such as primary pulmonary parenchymal disease, lower airway disease, upper airway obstruction, chest wall disease, abdominal enlargement, or pulmonary thromboembolism.

Diagnostics

Animals with pleural space disease may have severe respiratory compromise that prevents a full diagnostic workup. Close monitoring of the patient's respiratory rate and effort, mucous membrane color and capillary refill time, heart rate and pulse quality, Pao_2, hemoglobin saturation, blood pressure, and electrocardiogram should be performed in compromised patients. If a pleural space–filling defect is suspected, immediate diagnostic and therapeutic thoracocentesis is indicated (see Chapter 20).

In animals with pleural effusion, fluid analysis using biochemical, cytological, and physical characteristics will provide valuable diagnostic information. Fluid samples should be placed in a tube containing EDTA for cytologic examination and cell counts, and a clot tube for physical and biochemical analysis (e.g., specific gravity, total protein, clotting characteristics, and triglyceride concentrations). Fluid should be saved for aerobic and anaerobic cultures if cytology and appearance suggest a septic process. Fibronectin concentrations have been shown to help differentiate malignant from cardiogenic pleural effusions in dogs and cats.[7]

Confirmation of pleural space–filling disorders is made with thoracic radiographs, but only if the patient is not severely dyspneic. As little as 100 ml of pleural fluid is detectable in a medium-sized dog using standard radiographic views of the thorax.[8] Removal of fluid or air prior to taking radiographs will not only help to stabilize the animal but also improve the radiographic visualization of the lung fields, heart, and mediastinum. Radiographic changes associated with pleural effusion include blurring of the cardiac silhouette, interlobar fissure lines, rounding of the lung margins at the costophrenic angles, widening of the mediastinum, separation of the lung borders from the thoracic wall, and scalloping of the lung margins at the sternal border (Figure 8-1).[9,10] Collapse of lung lobes associated with pleural effusion tends to be uniform, leading to retention of the original shape of the partially collapsed lung and referred to as "form elasticity." If fibrinous or fibrous peel has accumulated on the visceral pleura, there is a subsequent loss of form elasticity and the lungs assume a more rounded appearance, often suggestive of a

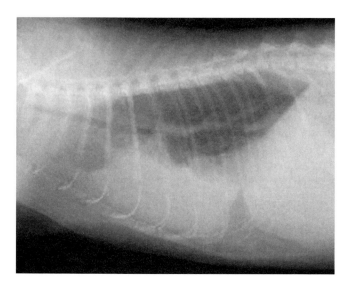

Figure 8-1. *Lateral thoracic radiograph showing pleural effusion. Radiographic findings characteristic of pleural effusion include blurring of the cardiac silhouette, interlobar fissure lines, rounding of the lung margins, widening of the mediastinum on ventrodorsal or dorsoventral views, separation of the lung borders from the thoracic wall, and scalloping of lung margins at the sternal border.*

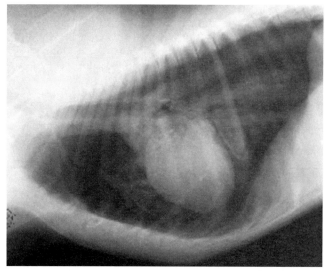

Figure 8-2. *Lateral thoracic radiograph showing pneumothorax. Radiographic findings characteristic of pneumothorax include dorsal displacement of the heart on lateral views of the thorax, retraction of the lung from the chest wall, and increased density of the collapsed lung lobes.*

chronic inflammatory process. Horizontal beam radiographs facilitate the differentiation of free versus encapsulated fluid and allow better visualization of the thoracic structures. Lateral and erect ventrodorsal views enable the detection of as little as 50 ml of fluid in a 15-kilogram animal.[8]

Radiographic changes associated with pneumothorax include dorsal displacement of the heart on the lateral view, retraction of the lung from the chest wall, and an increased density of the collapsed lung lobes (Figure 8-2).

Radiographic changes in animals with a diaphragmatic hernia include loss of visualization of the diaphragmatic line, loss of the cardiac silhouette, displacement of the lung fields dorsally or laterally, the presence of a gas- or ingesta-filled luminal structure within the thoracic cavity, and pleural effusion (Figure 8-3). Positive contrast celiography (using a water-soluble contrast agent dosed at 1.1 ml/kg) may be indicated in more difficult cases, although omental and fibrous adhesions might seal the diaphragmatic rent and lead to a false-negative diagnosis.

Ultrasonography is another useful diagnostic aid in animals with abnormal soft tissue or fluid accumulation within the pleural space. Because sound waves do not propagate through air, an extensive ultrasound examination of the thorax and noncardiac structures is not possible when the lungs are fully inflated or if a pneumothorax is present. Ultrasound is used to better visualize fluid or soft tissue abnormalities of the thoracic wall, and pleural, mediastinal, pulmonary, pericardial, and diaphragmatic structures.[11] Echocardiography is used to evaluate cardiac structure and function. Fluid within the pleural space enhances the propagation of sound and facilitates visualization of soft tissue abnormalities within the thorax. Ultrasound often enables percutaneous aspi-

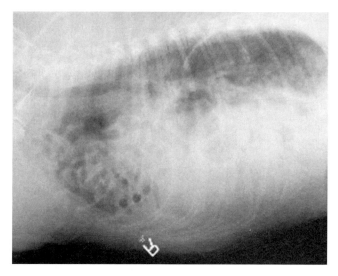

Figure 8-3. *Lateral thoracic radiograph showing a diaphragmatic hernia. Radiographic findings characteristic of diaphragmatic hernia include loss of diaphragmatic visualization, loss of the cardiac silhouette, displacement of the lung fields dorsally or laterally, evidence of a gas or ingesta-filled luminal structure within the thoracic cavity, and pleural effusion.*

ration or core biopsy of abnormal structures in order to obtain a cytological or histopathological diagnosis.

Thoracoscopy can assist in the diagnosis and treatment of pleural, mediastinal, pulmonary, and pericardial disease. It has been used experimentally and clinically in dogs.[12-20] Thoracoscopy can be performed in dogs with pleural effusion to visualize intrathoracic structures and obtain diagnostic biopsy samples with minimal complications.[21-23]

Magnetic resonance imaging (MRI) and computed tomographic (CT) scanning of the thorax are additional diagnostic tools that might aid in the diagnosis of pleural space disease, although general anesthesia is often necessary. CT-guided percutaneous aspiration or core biopsy is also possible.

Diagnostic and/or therapeutic exploratory thoracotomy may be necessary, and the surgical approach to the thorax is often guided by CT or MRI findings.

Initial Management Pending Results of Diagnostic Tests

The initial management of the patient with suspected or confirmed pleural space disease includes minimal handling, oxygen supplementation, and thoracocentesis (see Chapter 20). Any fluid collected should be saved for diagnostic evaluation. It is important that enough air or fluid is removed to make the animal more comfortable, but it is not necessary to remove all of the air or fluid. If the fluid or air returns rapidly and requires repeated chest drainage, an indwelling chest tube should be placed. Ongoing pleural space hemorrhage in patients with normal coagulation may require an exploratory thoracotomy.

In animals with severe respiratory impairment, intubation and positive pressure ventilation with 100% oxygen may be necessary. An attempt should be made to evacuate the pleural space as soon as possible. Reexpansion pulmonary edema may occur if the lungs have been chronically collapsed. It is important to remember that positive pressure ventilation of animals with a tension pneumothorax is contraindicated until a drainage site has been created from the pleural space to the atmosphere (e.g., a chest tube or lateral thoracotomy in severe situations).

REFERENCES

1. Burgen ASV, Steward PB: A method for measuring the turnover of fluid in the pleural and other serous cavities, *J Lab Clin Med* 52:118-124, 1958.
2. Agostoni E: Mechanics of the pleural space, *Physiol Rev* 52(1):57-128, 1972.
3. Evans HE: The respiratory system. In Evans HE, editor: *Miller's anatomy of the dog*, Philadelphia, 1993, WB Saunders.
4. Miserochi G, Agostoni E: Contents of the pleural space, *J Appl Physiol* 30:208-213, 1971.
5. Knapp DW, Richardson RC, DeNicola DB et al: Cisplatin toxicity in cats, *J Vet Intern Med* 1:29-35, 1987.
6. Padrid P: Canine and feline pleural disease, *Vet Clin North Am Small Anim Pract* 30(6):1295-1307, 2000.
7. Hirschberger J, Pusch S: Fibronectin concentration in pleural and abdominal effusions in dogs and cats, *J Vet Intern Med* 10(5): 321-325, 1996.
8. Lord PF, Suter PF, Chan KF et al: Pleural, extrapleural, and pulmonary lesions in small animals: A radiographic approach to differential diagnosis, *J Am Vet Radiol Soc* 13:4-17, 1972.
9. Thrall DE: The pleural space. In Thrall DE, editor: *Textbook of veterinary diagnostic radiology*, Philadelphia, 2002, WB Saunders.
10. Myer W: Radiography review: Pleural effusion, *J Am Vet Radiol Soc* 19:75-79, 1978.
11. Tidwell AS: Ultrasonography of the thorax (excluding the heart), *Vet Clin North Am Small Anim Pract* 28(4):993-1015, 1998.
12. Faunt KK, Jones BD, Turk JR et al: Evaluation of biopsy specimens obtained during thoracoscopy from lungs of clinically normal dogs, *Am J Vet Res* 59:1499-1502, 1998.
13. Garcia F, Prandi D, Pena T et al: Examination of the thoracic cavity and lung lobectomy by means of thoracoscopy in dogs, *Can Vet J* 39:285-291, 1998.
14. Zhang DH, Chen YN, Li HD: Thoracoscopy using flexible fiberoptic bronchoscopy: A preliminary report of experimental and clinical studies, *Zhonghua Nei Ke Za Zhi* 28(1):3-6, 60, 1989.
15. Watanabe G, Misaki T, Nakajima K et al: Thoracoscopic radiofrequency ablation of the myocardium, *Pacing Clin Electrophysiol* 21(3):553-558, 1998.
16. Walton RS: Video-assisted thoracoscopy, *Vet Clin North Am Small Anim Pract* 31(4):729-759, 2001.
17. Walsh PJ, Remedios AM, Ferguson JF et al: Thoracoscopic versus open partial pericardectomy in dogs: Comparison of postoperative pain and morbidity, *Vet Surg* 28(6):472-479, 1999.
18. Radlinsky MG, Mason DE, Biller DS et al: Thoracoscopic visualization and ligation of the thoracic duct in dogs, *Vet Surg* 31(2): 138-146, 2002.
19. MacPhail CM, Monnet E, Twedt DC: Thoracoscopic correction of persistent right aortic arch in a dog, *J Am Anim Hosp Assoc* 37(6): 577-581, 2001.
20. Jackson J, Richter KP, Launer DP: Thoracoscopic partial pericardiectomy in 13 dogs, *J Vet Intern Med* 13(6):529-533, 1999.
21. Kovak JR, Ludwig LL, Bergman PJ et al: Use of thoracoscopy to determine the etiology of pleural effusion in dogs and cats: 18 cases (1998-2001), *J Am Vet Med Assoc* 221(7):990-994, 2002.
22. Ben Isaac FE, Simmons DH: Flexible fiberoptic pleuroscopy: Pleural and lung biopsy, *Chest* 67(5):573-576, 1975.
23. Dupre GP, Corlouer JP, Bouvy B: Thoracoscopic pericardectomy performed without pulmonary exclusion in 9 dogs, *Vet Surg* 30(1): 21-27, 2001.

CHAPTER 9

Hypoventilation

Vicki L. Campbell • Sandra Z. Perkowski

Carbon dioxide (CO_2) is a by-product of aerobic metabolism and is removed from the body through the lungs via a process called ventilation.[1,2] Arterial carbon dioxide tension (Pa_{CO_2}) may be used clinically to determine the ventilatory status of the patient. Elevated Pa_{CO_2}, known as hypercarbia, is most commonly caused by alveolar hypoventilation due to decreased minute ventilation, increased dead space ventilation with a fixed tidal volume, or increased CO_2 production with a fixed tidal volume. In addition, an increased inspired concentration of CO_2 may also lead to hypercarbia. Decreased minute ventilation is the most common cause of hypercarbia and is therefore the main focus of this chapter.[1]

Definition

Ventilation is defined as the tidal exchange of air between the lungs and the atmosphere that occurs during breathing.[3] The amount of tidal exchange that occurs in 1 minute is defined as the respiratory minute volume (RMV). RMV is the product of the tidal volume and the respiratory rate[4]; however, RMV does not accurately reflect ventilation at the level of the alveolus because anatomical and physiological dead space exist. Dead space is defined as the portion of gas during a breath that does not reach the region of the lung where gas exchange occurs. Alveolar ventilation is the portion of gas during a breath that reaches the region of the lung where gas exchange occurs.[2]

Alveolar ventilation is defined as the RMV minus the dead space ventilation.[1] Alveolar ventilation can be determined by two methods. The first consists of measuring the anatomic dead space, calculating the dead space ventilation, and subtracting this value from the total ventilation.[4] The second method is more practical and determines alveolar ventilation in the healthy animal by measuring the concentration of CO_2 in the end-expiratory gas. The measured end-expiratory concentration of CO_2 reflects CO_2 production. It is almost completely alveolar in origin in the healthy patient because the CO_2 concentration in the atmosphere, and therefore in dead space gas at the end of inspiration, is negligible.[1,4] The alveolar ventilation is then calculated by taking the volume of CO_2 exhaled over time ($\dot{V}_{CO_2}$) divided by the alveolar fractional concentration of the CO_2 (F_{CO_2}). The partial pressure of CO_2 in the alveolus (PA_{CO_2}) is proportional to the fractional concentration of gas in the alveoli:

$$PA_{CO_2} = F_{CO_2} \times K$$

where $K = 0.863$. The PA_{CO_2} can therefore be used to determine alveolar ventilation ($\dot{V}$). K is a constant that equates dissimilar units for $\dot{V}_{CO_2}$ (ml CO_2/min) and $\dot{V}_A$ (L/min) to Pa_{CO_2} pressure units (mm Hg).[5] This leads to the equation:

$$Alveolar\ ventilation\ (\dot{V}_A) = \frac{\dot{V}_{CO_2}}{PA_{CO_2}} \times 0.863$$

Due to the highly diffusible nature of CO_2, the PA_{CO_2} is essentially equal to the Pa_{CO_2}, which allows Pa_{CO_2} to be used to determine alveolar ventilation. Rearranging the equation and substituting the easily measured Pa_{CO_2} for PA_{CO_2}, the following equation is derived:[2,5]

$$Pa_{CO_2} = \frac{\dot{V}_{CO_2}}{\dot{V}_A} \times 0.863$$

Thus, the relationship of arterial carbon dioxide tension, CO_2 production, and alveolar ventilation is established.

The above equation allows hypoventilation to be defined as alveolar ventilation that is lower than that required to maintain a normal arterial carbon dioxide tension, based on the level of CO_2 production.[1,2,4,5] Arterial carbon dioxide tension can therefore be utilized to determine the ventilatory status of patient. Based on the equation, there is a very important relationship between alveolar ventilation and arterial and alveolar partial pressure of CO_2. For example, if the alveolar ventilation is halved, then arterial and alveolar P_{CO_2} will double as long as CO_2 production is kept constant.[4]

Clinically, hypoventilation is defined as a Pa_{CO_2} greater than 45 mm Hg in the dog and greater than 40 mm Hg in the cat. Normal Pa_{CO_2} values vary depending on the individual analyzer, but in general they range from 35 to 45 mm Hg in the dog and 30 to 40 mm Hg in the cat.[6-8]

Clinical Signs

The clinical signs associated with hypoventilation are related to the systemic effects of hypercarbia, to uncompensated respiratory acidosis, or to the manifestations of the condition that is causing hypoventilation.

Hypoventilation can present clinically as shallow breathing. This type of breathing pattern is represented by a small tidal volume, and is commonly associated with a rapid respiratory rate in an effort to maintain normal alveolar minute volume.[2,9] When the tidal volume is small, inadequate ventilation of the alveoli occurs and hypercapnia ensues. In contrast, a slow or erratic respiratory rate despite adequate tidal volumes may also cause alveolar hypoventilation. For example, if an animal is only breathing once a minute, the alveoli are not being effectively ventilated and the animal becomes hypercarbic due to CO_2 retention.

A decreased tidal volume or very slow respiratory rate are two clinical signs commonly observed in patients that are hypoventilating due to decreased RMV, with rapid, shallow breathing being the most common manifestation.[2,9] However, certain conditions can cause hypoventilation even though the RMV is increased. For example, pulmonary thromboembolism causes an increase in physiologic dead space. Many animals compensate for the increased dead space by increasing the minute ventilation, which clinically is revealed as tachypnea or hyperpnea. However, the pulmonary thromboembolism may be so massive that despite increased respiratory minute volume, CO_2 retention occurs. In this situation, the animal is hypoventilating by definition because it cannot adequately remove carbon dioxide from the body due to inadequate alveolar ventilation, even though the RMV is actually increased.[2,10]

Hypercarbia has also been shown to increase the magnitude of naturally occurring sighs; this is known as the inspiratory-augmenting reflex. This phenomenon is thought to be due to central stimulation of the reflex by elevated $Paco_2$.[11]

Hypercarbia secondary to hypoventilation causes a primary respiratory acidosis. In the acutely hypercarbic animal, acidosis tends to be more severe because there has not been time for metabolic compensation to occur. Hypercarbia directly causes myocardial depression and peripheral vasodilation.[12-14] However, respiratory acidosis increases sympathetic tone in vivo by stimulating catecholamine release, resulting in increased cardiac output and blood pressure despite reduced total peripheral resistance.[12-15] Hypercarbia also increases coronary perfusion, but myocardial oxygen consumption remains unchanged despite the increase in coronary perfusion.[15] Sympathetic nervous system stimulation secondary to hypercarbia may cause tachycardia, hypertension, or arrhythmias.[12] Hypercarbia also causes cerebral vasodilation and can lead to increased intracranial pressure.[16] This is especially true under anesthesia because many inhalant anesthetics blunt the normal relationship between CO_2, cerebral blood flow, and increased sympathetic tone.[16,17] Mental dullness, narcosis, coma, and muscle weakness are also seen with severe respiratory acidosis.

Additional clinical signs depend on the cause of the hypoventilation (e.g., neuromuscular disease, muscle wasting, peripheral or central neurological disease, respiratory depressant drugs, toxins, neuromuscular blockers, or chronic lung disease with associated hypoxemia).

Pathophysiology of Control of Breathing

In the healthy animal, CO_2 is very tightly controlled through several mechanisms in order to maintain a normal $Paco_2$ (eucapnia). Factors that control alveolar ventilation, and thus control arterial CO_2 concentrations, include central and peripheral neuronal control, central and peripheral chemoreceptors, and respiratory mechanics and muscles (Figure 9-1). When these mechanisms begin to fail, CO_2 control becomes altered and the $Paco_2$ deviates from the eucapnic range.

Numerous steps occur during a normal breath, any one of which can be adversely affected by disease or drugs and result in hypoventilation. An understanding of the control of breathing and the feedback mechanisms involved is necessary to fully comprehend the pathophysiology of hypoventilation. In addition, a thorough understanding of the pathophysiology of the causes and effects of hypercarbia is crucial in understanding how and why to treat the hypercarbic patient.

NEURONAL CONTROL OF THE RESPIRATORY CENTER

A breath is generated in the medullary neurons. The medulla contains several types of neurons for control of the respiratory rhythm, and these neurons are responsible for timing the breath in respect to inspiration and expiration.[1,2,18,19] The pons contains the pneumotactic center and the apneustic center, which are responsible for fine motor control of the breath, especially prevention of overfilling of the lungs and control of the rhythm between breaths.[1,18,19] The cortex is involved in the control of respiration and allows the respiratory pattern to be altered during activities such as sniffing, coughing, or vocalizing.[2,19] The suprapontine reflexes aid in controlling the respiratory pattern during events such as sneezing or swallowing.[19]

The upper motor neurons that arise from the medulla and spinal cord synapse onto the lower motor neurons

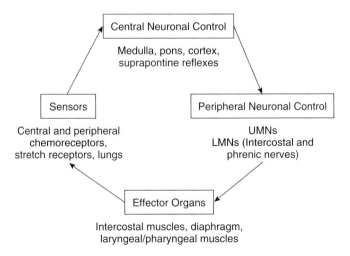

Figure 9-1. Components of the control of breathing (UMN, Upper motor neuron; LMN, lower motor neuron).

of the respiratory muscles to allow involuntary rhythmic breathing, voluntary control of breathing (e.g., vocalizing), and involuntary nonrhythmic control of the respiratory system (e.g., swallowing).[19] The lower motor neurons that innervate the intercostal muscles, and the phrenic nerve that controls the diaphragm, are important to maintain adequate movement of the chest wall and diaphragm and thereby allow an appropriate tidal volume for each breath. The phrenic nerve normally arises from cervical vertebral segments C5, C6, and C7; runs in the fascia adjacent to the external jugular vein; and then converges to form the phrenic nerve cranial to the thoracic inlet. The phrenic nerve unites with a branch from the caudal cervical ganglion or the sympathetic trunk adjacent to the ganglion, courses through the mediastinum, and then branches to innervate the diaphragm as its only motor nerve. The intercostal nerves are the ventral branch of their respective thoracic nerves and generally come off thoracic vertebrae T2 through T12.[20]

The most detrimental disruption of the central neuronal control of breathing leading to an abnormal or inadequate ventilatory drive occurs when there is disruption of the medullary neurons, the site where the breath is generated.[1] Numerous causes are possible, but the most likely are trauma, neoplasia, hemorrhage, cerebral edema, or respiratory depressant drugs. All anesthetics, opioids, and barbiturates lead to depression of the medullary neurons.[10]

The integrity of the pons combined with the medulla is necessary to maintain a normal respiratory rhythm.[18] Disruption of the pons may lead to an apneustic breathing pattern, in which inspiration is no longer halted due to feedback into the pons but rather is stopped due to reaching maximum lung capacity.[1] Injury to the pons can also lead to an erratic breathing pattern, which may cause an inadequate RMV. Cortical depression or suprapontine reflex disruption is unlikely to be a significant cause of hypoventilation because these regions do not have significant roles in the generation of the breath.

Upper motor neuron, lower motor neuron, or neuromuscular junction disease can lead to significant hypoventilation.[10] If there is disruption of the upper motor neurons from the medulla or the lower motor neurons of the phrenic and intercostal nerves, the tidal volume will become inadequate. This is commonly seen in dogs with cervical vertebral lesions at C2 through C4.[21] Disruption of the phrenic nerve may lead to hypoventilation due to diaphragm paralysis or paresis. A C5 through C7 lesion may cause hypoventilation due to disruption of the branches of the phrenic nerve.[20] In addition, lower motor neuron disease or neuromuscular junction disease affecting the intercostal muscles causes decreased tidal volume and leads to hypoventilation.

Stretch receptors in the muscles and airways are also involved in neuronal control of the breath. They respond to increases in transmural pressure with each breath and negatively feed back onto the central neuronal controls to inhibit respiration at peak inspiration. The opposite occurs with the deflation reflex during exhalation. This reflex is known as the Hering-Breuer reflex and is controlled by the vagus nerve. These stretch receptors be-

come more sensitized after microembolism and can stimulate the afferents associated with the vagus resulting in rapid, shallow breathing.[19] Studies have indicated that tonic vagal influences may also be involved in control of the respiratory pattern and frequency, independent of the vagal influence of phasic lung inflation.[22] However, these vagal influences are not required for the normal response to hypercapnia, hypoxia, or exercise.[23]

CENTRAL AND PERIPHERAL CHEMORECEPTORS

The central chemoreceptors control about 85% of the response to carbon dioxide,[19] although some studies indicate a lower contribution.[24] These chemoreceptors are located in close proximity to the medullary neurons that are responsible for generation of the breath. They respond to changes in the pH of the cerebral spinal fluid (CSF). Because carbon dioxide diffuses freely across the blood-brain barrier, a rise in Pa_{CO_2} causes a roughly equal rise in the CO_2 of the CSF. On average, the CO_2 level is normally about 10 mm Hg higher in the CSF, cerebral tissue, and jugular veins than it is in arterial blood.[19] Over a period of 24 hours of hypercarbia, sodium bicarbonate ($NaHCO_3$) passively distributes into the CSF to offset the rise in CO_2.[25] An acute rise in CO_2 of the CSF stimulates ventilation due to the decrease in the CSF pH.[25] Acidosis as a result of the breakdown products from intracranial hemorrhage will cause hyperventilation. Metabolic acidosis also stimulates the central chemoreceptors and increases ventilation.[26]

The central chemoreceptors also respond to low oxygen tensions. At mild to moderately low arterial oxygen tensions (Pa_{O_2} <60 mm Hg) the central chemoreceptors are stimulated to increase ventilation. However, these receptors eventually become depressed when arterial oxygen tension becomes severely low (Pa_{O_2} <13 mm Hg).[19] The mechanism of central ventilatory depression during periods of severe hypoxia is not fully understood, but is possibly due to increased levels of inhibitory neurotransmitters such as γ-aminobutyric acid (GABA) or endogenous opioids. The end result is stimulation of the "gasping center," which results in an agonal breathing pattern.[19]

The peripheral chemoreceptors are made up of both the carotid bodies and the aortic bodies. Of these two, the carotid bodies play a much more significant role in controlling ventilation than the aortic bodies, which are more involved with altering the cardiovascular system. These chemoreceptors respond to low Pa_{O_2}, high Pa_{CO_2}, increased hydrogen ion, and decreased perfusion rate.[19]

The carotid bodies consist of large sinusoids that have a high perfusion relative to their metabolic rate. Thus the difference between the arterial and venous P_{O_2} is very small, allowing high sensitivity to changes in P_{O_2} and a very rapid response to changes (approximately 1 to 3 seconds). The carotid body contains the glomus, or type I cells. These cells secrete multiple neurotransmitters (most importantly, dopamine) that alter the chemoreceptor sensitivity of the carotid body. When neurotransmitter release is stimulated, the respiratory pattern is altered to improve ventilation.[19] Low arterial oxygen tension is thought to decrease adenosine triphosphate (ATP) in the carotid bodies, resulting in increased glucose uptake and a subsequent increase in type I cell neurotransmitter release.

The respiratory pattern is altered when there is a decrease in dissolved plasma oxygen tensions. It is important to note that the PaO_2 must typically be less than 60 mm Hg before it causes significant changes in the breathing pattern. However, the response to hypoxemia is enhanced in the presence of hypercarbia.[19,27] Arterial hypercarbia or acidosis stimulates the type I cells by stimulating the carbonic anhydrase system in the cells; this results in increased ventilation. However, this response to either carbonic or nonrespiratory acidosis is only about one sixth of the change that occurs due to central chemoreceptor stimulation.[19]

The carotid and aortic bodies also contain baroreceptors, which respond to changes in blood pressure. Elevated blood pressure causes respiratory depression via the baroreceptors. Consequently, massive catecholamine release can lead to hypoventilation or apnea.[19] All of the chemoreceptors are affected by anesthetic agents and do not respond as effectively to changes in $PaCO_2$, pH, or PaO_2 in the anesthetized animal. Hypoventilation is a common complication in spontaneously breathing anesthetized dogs and cats.[28-37]

RESPIRATORY MECHANICS AND MUSCLES

The effector organs involved in respiration include the muscles of respiration, the lung parenchyma, the chest wall, and any elements that might affect these mechanical components of respiration. Because the respiratory mechanical components are the effector organs on which the neuronal pathways terminate, they are crucial in generating an appropriate tidal volume for each breath.

The muscles involved in the production of a normal breath include the diaphragm and the intercostal muscles, with the diaphragm being the major muscle of respiration. In addition, the muscles of the upper airway must function normally for proper inspiration.[2] Carotid body stimulation causes recruitment of inspiratory and expiratory muscle activity.[38] If the muscles are working improperly or are impeded, then ineffective ventilation can occur due to inadequate tidal flow in and out of the alveoli. The muscles may be affected by neuromuscular disease or blockade, as well as by fatigue or weakness from prolonged periods of increased work of breathing. Increased work of breathing can occur when there is upper airway obstruction or severe hypoxemia, loss of lung compliance (e.g., as in pulmonary fibrosis), or loss of chest wall compliance (e.g., as occurs when there is restriction of chest expansion due to a tight bandage or abdominal distention).[10] In the case of neuromuscular disease, a combination of muscle weakness and increased elastic load is responsible for rapid, shallow breathing that leads to hypercapnia.[9]

Hypoventilation can occur if the lung parenchyma is prevented from inflating fully.[10] Full inflation of the lungs may be inhibited if there is restriction of the intratho-

racic space by pleural space disease (e.g., pleural effusion, pneumothorax, or neoplasia). Primary lung disease, in which the lung parenchyma has decreased compliance and areas of atelectasis, may lead to hypoventilation. Anesthetic agents, as well as patient positioning, will reduce the functional residual capacity of the lungs; this can decrease the RMV. Increased airway resistance, such as with upper airway obstruction, may also prevent adequate tidal flow to the alveoli and lead to hypoventilation. Upper airway obstruction is a common cause of hypercarbia in veterinary medicine.

If the chest wall loses its integrity (e.g., during flail chest or a thoracic wall puncture), loss of negative pressure in the thoracic cavity results in lung collapse due to normal pulmonary elastic recoil. The resulting atelectasis causes hypoventilation of the collapsed lung lobes.

Respiratory mechanics can be affected by pain, resulting in hypoventilation due to a decrease in RMV. This is especially true in animals with thoracic pain, such as the postoperative thoracotomy or thoracic trauma patient. Adequate pain management in these cases is extremely important in ensuring adequate tidal volumes, but requires careful consideration. Because most pure opioid agonists tend to cause respiratory depression,[39-41] they should be used with careful monitoring in thoracotomy or thoracic trauma cases. Despite reports of intramuscular morphine causing a dose dependent increase in RMV in awake dogs,[42] other studies have shown that intravenous morphine administration in awake dogs is a respiratory depressant[40] and panting caused by intramuscular morphine or oxymorphone administration in postthoracotomy dogs reduces RMV and leads to hypercarbia.[41] Alternate techniques, including the use of local analgesics, may be preferred in some cases. In the dog it has been demonstrated that intercostal nerve blockade may be an effective means of providing analgesia while maintaining normoventilation in the thoracotomy case.[41] Another study demonstrated that intrapleural bupivacaine decreased pain scores and hypoxemia compared to intravenous buprenorphine, although hypoventilation did not occur with either drug in that study.[43] If local analgesics are not sufficient to control the pain, and opioid administration may be harmful to the animal, assisted ventilation should be considered to enable simultaneous treatment of both the pain and the hypoventilation.

Pathophysiology of Additional Causes of Hypercarbia

In addition to hypercarbia due to decreased RMV, CO_2 retention can occur with increased dead space ventilation, increased metabolic CO_2 production with a fixed respiratory minute volume, or increased inspired CO_2.

Increased alveolar dead space, or physiological dead space, is a type of ventilation-perfusion $(\dot{V}/\dot{Q})$ mismatching in which ventilation is in excess of perfusion. In this case, the animal has the ability to maintain normal tidal gas flow to the alveoli and commonly has a normal to increased respiratory minute volume. However, decreased perfusion to many of the alveoli results in inability of the lungs to appropriately remove CO_2 from the body. High ventilation/low perfusion states are seen with pulmonary thromboembolism, or extremely low cardiac output in which pulmonary capillary perfusion is significantly decreased. Hypercarbia also occurs when excessive anatomic dead space is present. This commonly occurs in small patients when an endotracheal tube is excessively long or a large volume Y-piece is utilized within a breathing circuit.[1] By definition, animals that are hypercarbic secondary to excessive dead space and are breathing with a fixed tidal volume are hypoventilating.

Increased metabolic CO_2 production with a fixed respiratory minute volume (e.g., during malignant hyperthermia, iatrogenic hyperthermia, or fever) also causes hypercarbia. In anesthetized animals, the normal response to CO_2 is blunted due to central nervous system depression and the animal cannot compensate appropriately by increasing its RMV.[1] In addition, if the animal is on a ventilator with a fixed RMV, hypercarbia may occur if there is increased metabolic CO_2 production (e.g., during excessive nutritional support). By definition these animals are hypoventilating.

The most common cause of increased inspired CO_2 is rebreathing of CO_2 secondary to expired or saturated soda lime in an anesthetic circuit.[1] This is considered to be an iatrogenic cause of hypercarbia.

Differential Diagnosis

There are many differential diagnoses for hypoventilation (Box 9-1). The basic categories are logical if the mechanism of the normal breath and the feedback mechanisms are considered. General categories include central neurological, lower motor neuron disease, neuromuscular disease, abnormal function of either peripheral or central chemoreceptors, abnormal respiratory mechanics, and increased airway resistance. Other causes of hypercarbia (e.g., increased dead space relative to perfusion, increased dead space from an anesthesia or ventilator circuit, increased CO_2 production with a fixed respiratory minute volume, or increased inspired CO_2) should also be considered.

Diagnostic Testing

The best way to diagnose hypoventilation is measurement of arterial P_{CO_2}. In the dog, the sample is most commonly obtained from the dorsal metatarsal, dorsal pedal, cranial tibial, femoral, auricular, or radial artery. In the cat, the sample is most commonly obtained from the femoral artery.

Venous carbon dioxide tension (Pv_{CO_2}) may be cautiously utilized to help rule out hypoventilation. Venous CO_2 tends to be about 5 to 10 mm Hg higher than arterial in the normal animal.[7,8,44] Also in the normal animal, peripheral capillary blood (e.g., from the pinna of the ear) has a similar P_{CO_2} to arterial samples due to minimal CO_2 production from tissues in these areas.[44] Cardiovascularly normal dogs under anesthesia have lingual venous blood gases comparable to arterial blood gases due to extensive arterial-venous fistulae in the tongue.[45] In cats, Pv_{CO_2} has limited correlation to Pa_{CO_2}.[7]

Many variables may cause elevation of venous carbon dioxide tension independent of alveolar ventilation. Therefore, venous CO_2 must be used with caution during hypovolemic, cardiac, or distributive shock because the blood may become stagnant in the periphery and the CO_2 may be locally, but not systemically, elevated.[44,45] If the Pv_{CO_2} is normal, hypoventilation almost certainly can be ruled out. However, elevated Pv_{CO_2} values should not be utilized to confirm hypoventilation.

End tidal CO_2 (ET_{CO_2}) monitoring can be an extremely useful tool for monitoring ventilation, typically in intubated animals either under anesthesia or on a ventilator but also in unintubated animals.[46] Mainstream or sidestream ET_{CO_2} monitors display a capnograph with a measured ET_{CO_2} value. The ET_{CO_2} has a strong correlation to Pa_{CO_2} in spontaneously and mechanically ventilated normal dogs under inhalant anesthesia,[47,48] with the ET_{CO_2} typically 2 to 6 mm Hg lower than the Pa_{CO_2} in normal dogs.[47] These monitors should be used with caution, however, because they can give the clinician a false sense of security. An ET_{CO_2} value greater than 45 mm Hg has a strong correlation with hypoventilation.[46] Numerous factors can lower ET_{CO_2}; however, including high physiological dead space (high $\dot{V}/\dot{Q}$) secondary to poor pulmonary capillary perfusion, a large amount of anatomic dead space, high respiration rates, or a leak in the anesthetic or ventilator circuit.[47] In addition, the ET_{CO_2} tends to more severely underestimate the Pa_{CO_2} at ET_{CO_2} values greater than 55 or 60 mm Hg.[37,48] Therefore, end-tidal capnography should be used as an aid to watch trends, in conjunction with arterial blood gas monitoring. Sidestream monitors can be used to measure ET_{CO_2} in an unintubated animal by placing the tubing 1 to 2 cm into a nostril, but leakage of room air around the tubing may give artificially low numbers.[46]

A spirometer is a useful tool under anesthesia or during mechanical ventilation to determine whether the animal is producing an adequate tidal volume. Pulmonary function machines can be utilized in intubated animals to determine lung compliance, tidal volume, lung resistance, CO_2 production, O_2 consumption, and chest wall compliance.[2] These monitors are expensive and commonly require anesthesia but can give insight into an animal's ability to produce an adequate respiratory minute volume. Pneumotachography has been used for measurement of tidal breathing flow-volume loops in awake dogs with airway obstruction and may be a useful diagnostic test of pulmonary function.[49-51]

Transcutaneous carbon dioxide can be measured using heated electrodes attached to the skin. However, these are expensive, need frequent calibration, and the results are difficult to interpret in the poorly perfused patient.[52] Normal cats under isoflurane anesthesia have shown good correlation between transcutaneous CO_2, ET_{CO_2}, and Pa_{CO_2}; however, a correct conversion formula

BOX 9-1
Differential Diagnosis of Hypoventilation/Hypercarbia

Decreased Respiratory Minute Ventilation

I. **Central Neurological Disease**
   1. Medulla, cerebrum, pons
      a. Drugs
         i. Opioids
         ii. General anesthetics
      b. Trauma
      c. Neoplasia
      d. Intracranial hemorrhage
      e. Cerebral edema
      f. Severe metabolic disturbances
      g. Severe hypothermia <80° (F)
   2. Cervical disease
      a. Trauma
         i. Spinal cord hemorrhage
         ii. Cervical fracture
      b. Tumor
      c. Surgery
      d. Infectious
      e. Intervertebral disk disease
      f. Inflammatory
      g. High epidural
      h. Anterior horn cell disease

II. **Lower Motor Neuron Disease/ Neuromuscular Disease**
   1. Myasthenia gravis
   2. Neuromuscular blockers
   3. Botulism
   4. Tick paralysis
   5. Demyelination
   6. Polyradiculoneuritis
   7. Toxoplasmosis

III. **Chemoreceptor Abnormalities**
   1. Drugs
      a. Anesthetic agents
   2. Peripheral acidosis
      a. Metabolic derangements
   3. CSF acidosis
      a. Intracranial hemorrhage
      b. Metabolic derangements

IV. **Abnormal Respiratory Mechanics**
   1. Pulmonary fibrosis
   2. Respiratory fatigue from increased work of breathing
   3. Pickwickian syndrome
   4. Pleural space disease
      a. Pneumothorax
      b. Hemothorax
      c. Chylothorax
      d. Hydrothorax
      e. Malignant effusion
      f. Space-occupying mass
      g. Diaphragmatic hernia
   5. Loss of elasticity of chest wall/lungs
      a. Extrathoracic compression
      b. Fibrosis
   6. Loss of structural integrity of chest wall
      a. Flail chest
      b. Chest wound
   7. Decreased functional residual capacity
      a. Anesthetic agents
      b. Patient positioning (especially dorsal recumbency)

V. **Increased Airway Resistance**
   1. Upper airway obstruction
      a. Mucus plugs
      b. Neoplasia
      c. Foreign body
      d. Recurrent laryngeal nerve damage
      e. Laryngeal edema
      f. Inflammatory laryngitis
      g. Polyps
   2. Increased circuit resistance under anesthesia
   3. Tracheal or mainstem bronchus collapse
   4. Brachycephalic syndrome
   5. Bronchoconstriction
      a. Asthma
      b. Chronic bronchitis

Increased Dead Space Ventilation

I. **Increased Physiological Dead Space** *(High $\dot{V}/\dot{Q}$)*
   1. Poor cardiac output
   2. Shock
   3. Pulmonary emboli
   4. Pulmonary hypotension
   5. Pulmonary bulla

II. **Increased Anatomical Dead Space**
   1. Excessive dead space in ventilator/anesthesia breathing circuit
   2. Excessively long endotracheal tube

Increased Carbon Dioxide Production with a Fixed Tidal Volume

I. **Malignant hyperthermia**

II. **Reperfusion injury**

III. **Excessive nutritional support in a ventilated patient**

IV. **Fever**

V. **Iatrogenic hyperthermia**

Increased Inspired Carbon Dioxide

I. **Expired or old soda lime**

for transcutaneous CO_2 to $Paco_2$ has not been established.[53] More clinical studies are needed to understand the usefulness of this technique in veterinary medicine.

Numerous tests can be performed to look for the underlying cause of hypoventilation. Every evaluation should start with a thorough history, physical examination, complete blood count, serum chemistry analysis, and urinalysis.[2] In addition to lung function testing and arterial blood gas analysis, chest radiographs, abdominal radiographs, abdominal ultrasound, cervical radiographs, coagulation profile, titers for neuromuscular disease and infectious diseases, toxin screen, electromyelogram, CT or MRI scanning, CSF fluid analysis, endocrine function testing, nerve conduction velocities, electroencephalograms, and nerve and muscle biopsies may be indicated depending on the clinical signs of the animal.[2]

Initial Management Pending Results of Diagnostic Tests

It is important to recognize and treat hypercarbia because it may result in acidosis and risk of elevated intracranial pressure. During hypoventilation, as with any respiratory emergency, the most important initial priority is to ensure that the patient has a patent airway and is breathing. If the airway is obstructed, then oxygen should be administered. Attempts to relieve the obstruction or an emergency tracheotomy should be performed immediately. The animal should be intubated if it is not breathing. Next, the cardiovascular system should be assessed and cardiopulmonary resuscitation performed if necessary. Management of hypovolemic, cardiac, or distributive shock should ensue to help alleviate hypercarbia due to increased physiological dead space secondary to low pulmonary capillary perfusion.

Controversy often arises when determining whether or not to give oxygen to an animal that is hypoventilating and simultaneously hypoxemic. Giving oxygen to a hypoventilating and severely hypoxemic animal may result in an increased $Paco_2$, especially in animals with end-stage parenchymal lung disease. It has been reasoned that this phenomenon is due to a decrease in the hypoxic stimulus to breathe; however, new studies have shown that worsened hypercarbia secondary to oxygen administration may be due to alterations in ventilation/perfusion matching caused by relief of hypoxic pulmonary vasoconstriction.[2] If the Pao_2 is less than 60 mm Hg and the animal is severely dyspneic or cyanotic, supplemental oxygen is recommended in order to maintain oxygen delivery to the tissues. If there is serious concern about further increases in $Paco_2$, the animal should be intubated and mechanically ventilated so that RMV can be controlled and oxygen administered simultaneously.

Readily treatable causes of hypoventilation should be addressed immediately. Any opioids, sedatives, anesthetics, or neuromuscular blockers should be reversed or the animal intubated and ventilated until the agents have been metabolized. If a diagnosis of hypoventilation is determined and the underlying cause is not immedi-

ately reversible, several treatment options are available. The most effective means of treating hypoventilation is to mechanically ventilate the animal. This can be a very labor intensive and expensive process requiring highly specialized staff and equipment, and does not necessarily treat the underlying disease process. Since increased sympathetic tone is associated with hypercarbia, mechanical ventilation may decrease blood pressure both by producing normocapnia and by decreasing venous return.[12] However, positive pressure ventilation may be life saving and allow time for additional diagnostics to be performed.

Bronchodilators such as aminophylline and theophylline have been advocated to treat hypoventilation. These xanthine derivatives inhibit phosphodiesterase, thereby increasing cyclic adenosine monophosphate (cAMP). As a result, they relax smooth muscle in the bronchi and pulmonary vasculature but also have weak inotropic effects, chronotropic effects, mild centrally mediated CNS stimulation, and central ventilatory stimulation.[54] Their benefit in treating hypoventilation remains controversial.

Numerous respiratory stimulants have been used to treat hypoventilation but care must be exercised in their use because they may lead to respiratory fatigue by increasing the work of breathing. Caffeine may be used intravenously to stimulate the respiratory center and increase tidal volume, and in the authors' experience this drug is especially effective in puppies with bronchopneumonia. Doxapram has been used in newborn puppies and kittens to stimulate respiration: the mechanism of respiratory stimulation is thought to be predominantly due to stimulation of the medullary respiratory neurons and through reflex action on the peripheral chemoreceptors. Unfortunately, doxapram has many additional side effects including generalized central nervous system stimulation. In addition, it increases the work of breathing and hence causes increases in oxygen consumption and carbon dioxide production.[54]

Progesterone has been used as a treatment for hypoventilation in human medicine[2,55] but is not commonly used to treat hypoventilation in veterinary medicine. Progesterone probably increases the sensitivity of the central respiratory center to CO_2, thus increasing RMV and lowering alveolar CO_2.[55,56] In human medicine, almitrine bismesylate acts on the carotid body to stimulate ventilation in response to hypoxia and also affects the pulmonary vasculature to enhance hypoxic pulmonary vasoconstriction. However, this drug causes pulmonary hypertension if used long term.[2] Fluoxetine, a 5-hydroxytryptamine (5-HT or serotonin) reuptake inhibitor has been utilized in human patients as a possible treatment for obese subjects with sleep-related hypoventilation.[57] The tricyclic antidepressant protriptyline has also been utilized in sleep-related apnea.[2] It has not been determined if these drugs are beneficial in veterinary medicine. Acetazolamide is a carbonic anhydrase inhibitor that induces metabolic acidosis. It has been proposed for treatment of hypoventilation in anticipation that the metabolic acidosis will stimulate ventilation. This is extremely dangerous, however, and is not advocated.[2] In human medicine, phrenic nerve pacing has been utilized to help with central or primary alveolar hypoventilation or high cervical cord injuries.[2]

Sodium bicarbonate is contraindicated in patients that are acidotic due to hypoventilation. Hypercapnia usually worsens after sodium bicarbonate administration, leading to deterioration of the acid-base status.[58] The acid-base status of the animal should be assessed prior to administration of NaHCO$_3$. If it is necessary to administer NaHCO$_3$ to a hypercarbic animal, then ventilatory support should be available and provided if needed.

Once initial management of hypoventilation has begun, then further diagnostics can be performed and other treatment options will depend on the underlying disease process.

REFERENCES

1. Nunn JF: Carbon dioxide. In Nunn JF, editor: *Nunn's applied respiratory physiology,* ed 4, Oxford, 1993, Butterworth-Heinemann.
2. Robinson RW, Zwillich CW: Hypoventilation, central apnea, and disordered breathing patterns. In Bone RC, editor: *Pulmonary and critical care medicine,* St Louis, 1998, Mosby.
3. Stedman TL: *Stedman's medical dictionary,* ed 25, Baltimore, MD, 1990, Williams & Wilkins.
4. West JB: Ventilation. In West JB, editor: *Respiratory physiology—the essentials,* ed 5, Baltimore, MD, 1995, Williams & Wilkins.
5. Martin L: *All you really need to know to interpret arterial blood gases,* Malvern, PA, 1992, Lea & Febiger.
6. Haskins SC: Blood gases and acid-base balance: Clinical interpretation and therapeutic implications. In Kirk RW, editor: *Current veterinary therapy VIII,* Philadelphia, 1983, WB Saunders.
7. Middleton DJ, Ilkiw JE, Watson AD: Arterial and venous blood gas tensions in clinically healthy cats, *Am J Vet Res* 42(9):1609-1611, 1981.
8. Wingfield WE, Van Pelt DR, Hackett T et al: Usefulness of venous blood in estimating acid-base status of the seriously ill dog, *J Vet Emerg Crit Care* 4(1):23-27, 1994.
9. Misuri G, Lanini B, Gigliotti F et al: Mechanism of CO$_2$ retention in patients with neuromuscular disease, *Chest* 117(2):447-453, 2000.
10. Nunn JF: Ventilatory failure. In Nunn JF, editor: *Nunn's applied respiratory physiology,* ed 4, Oxford, 1993, Butterworth-Heinemann.
11. Nishino T, Honda Y: Effects of PaCO$_2$ and PaO$_2$ on threshold for the inspiratory-augmenting reflex in cats, *J Appl Physiol* 53(5):1152-1157, 1982.
12. Cullen DJ, Eger EI: Cardiovascular effects of carbon dioxide in man, *Anesthesiology* 41(4):345-349, 1974.
13. Kontos HA, Richardson DW, Paterson JL: Vasodilator effect of hypercapnic acidosis on human forearm blood vessels, *Am J Physiol* 215(6):1403-1405, 1968.
14. Kontos HA, Thames MD, Lombana A et al: Vasodilator effects of local hypercapnic acidosis in dog skeletal muscle, *Am J Physiol* 220(6):1569-1572, 1971.
15. Vance JP, Smith G, Brown DM et al: Response of mean and phasic coronary arterial blood flow to graded hypercapnia in dogs, *Br J Anaesth* 51:523-529, 1979.
16. Ponte J, Purves MJ: The role of the carotid body chemoreceptors and carotid sinus baroreceptors in the control of cerebral blood vessels, *J Physiol* 237:315-340, 1974.
17. Skovsted P, Price ML, Price JL: The effects of carbon dioxide on preganglionic sympathetic activity during halothane, methoxyflurane, and cyclopropane anesthesia, *Anesthesiology* 37(1):70-75, 1972.
18. Cohen MI, Piercey MF, Gootman PM et al: Respiratory rhythmicity in the cat, *Fed Proc* 35(9):1967-1974, 1976.
19. Nunn JF: Control of breathing. In Nunn JF, editor: *Nunn's applied respiratory physiology,* ed 4, Oxford, 1993, Butterworth-Heinemann.
20. Kitchell RL, Evans HE: The spinal nerves. In Evans HE, editor: *Miller's anatomy of the dog,* ed 3, Philadelphia, 1993, WB Saunders.
21. Beal MW, Paglia DT, Griffin GM et al: Ventilatory failure, ventilator management, and outcome in dogs with cervical spinal disorders: 14 cases (1991-1999), *JAVMA* 218(10):1598-1602, 2001.
22. Phillipson EA: Vagal control of breathing pattern independent of lung inflation in conscious dogs, *J Appl Physiol* 37(2):183-189, 1974.
23. Favier R, Kepenekian G, Desplanches D et al: Effects of chronic lung denervation on breathing pattern and respiratory gas exchanges during hypoxia, hypercapnia and exercise, *Resp Physiol* 47:107-119, 1982.
24. Heeringa J, Berkenbosch A, de Goede J et al: Relative contribution of central and peripheral chemoreceptors to the ventilatory response to CO$_2$ during hyperoxia, *Resp Physiol* 37:365-379, 1979.
25. Bleich HL, Berkman PM, Schwartz WB et al: The response of cerebrospinal fluid composition to sustained hypercapnia, *J Clin Invest* 43(1):11-16, 1964.
26. Kaehny WD, Jackson JT: Respiratory response to HCl acidosis in dogs after carotid body denervation, *J Appl Physiol: Resp, Env & Exercise Physiol* 44(1):28-35, 1978.
27. Fitzgerald RS, Parks DC: Effect of hypoxia on carotid chemoreceptor response to carbon dioxide in cats, *Resp Physiol* 12:218-229, 1971.
28. White GA, Matthews NS: Frequency of hypoventilation during general anesthesia for routine elective surgery, *Vet Med* 94(3):247-251, 1999.
29. Hodgson DS, Dunlop CI, Chapman PL et al: Cardiopulmonary effects of anesthesia induced and maintained with isoflurane in cats, *Am J Vet Res* 59(2):182-185, 1998.
30. McMurphy RM, Hodgson DS: Cardiopulmonary effects of desflurane in cats, *Am J Vet Res* 57(3):367-370, 1996.
31. Grandy JL, Hodgson DS, Dunlop CI et al: Cardiopulmonary effects of halothane anesthesia in cats, *Am J Vet Res* 50(10):1729-1732, 1989.
32. Hikasa Y, Ohe N, Takase K et al: Cardiopulmonary effects of sevoflurane in cats: Comparison with isoflurane, halothane, and enflurane, *Res Vet Sci* 63(3):205-210, 1997.
33. Hikasa Y, Kawanabe H, Takase K et al: Comparisons of sevoflurane, isoflurane, and halothane anesthesia in spontaneously breathing cats, *Vet Surg* 25(3):234-243, 1996.
34. Steffey EP, Gillespie JR, Berry JD et al: Circulatory effects of halothane and halothane-nitrous oxide anesthesia in the dog: Spontaneous ventilation, *Am J Vet Res* 36(2):197-200, 1975.
35. Jaspar N, Mazzarelli M, Tessier C et al: Effect of ketamine on control of breathing in cats, *J Appl Physiol* 55(3):851-859, 1983.
36. Siafakas NM, Bonora M, Duron B et al: Dose effect of pentobarbital sodium on control of breathing in cats, *J Appl Physiol* 55(5):1582-1592, 1983.
37. Klide AM: Cardiopulmonary effects of enflurane and isoflurane in the dog, *Am J Vet Res* 37(2):127-131, 1976.
38. Smith CA, Ainsworth DM, Henderson KL et al: Differential responses of expiratory muscles to chemical stimuli in awake dogs, *J Appl Physiol* 66(1):384-391, 1989.
39. Jacobson JD, McGrath CJ, Smith EP: Cardiorespiratory effects of four opioid-tranquilizer combinations in dogs, *Vet Surg* 23:299-306, 1994.
40. Pelligrino AO, Riegler FX, Albrecht RF: The comparative ventilatory effects of morphine, morphine-3- and morphine-6-glucuronide in the awake dog, *Anesthesiology* 69:A812, 1988.
41. Berg RJ, Orton EC: Pulmonary function in dogs after intercostal thoracotomy: Comparison of morphine, oxymorphone, and selective intercostal nerve block, *Am J Vet Res* 47(2):471-474, 1986.
42. Cullen LK, Raffe MR, Randall DA et al: Assessment of the respiratory actions of intramuscular morphine in conscious dogs, *Res Vet Sci* 67:141-148, 1999.
43. Conzemius MG, Brockman DJ, King LG et al: Analgesia in dogs after intercostal thoracotomy: A clinical trial comparing intravenous buprenorphine and interpleural bupivacaine, *Vet Surg* 23:291-298, 1994.
44. Rodkey WG, Hannon JP, Dramise JG et al: Arterialized capillary blood used to determine acid-base and blood gas status of dogs, *Am J Vet Res* 39(3):459-464, 1978.
45. Wagner AE, Muir WW, Bednarski RM: A comparison of arterial and lingual venous blood gases in anesthetized dogs, *J Vet Emerg Crit Care* 1(1):14-18, 1991.
46. Hendricks JC, King LG: Practicality, usefulness, and limits of end-tidal carbon dioxide monitoring in critical small animal patients, *J Vet Emerg Crit Care* 4(1):29-39, 1994.

47. Hightower CE, Kiorpes AL, Butler HC et al: End tidal partial pressure of CO_2 as an estimate of arterial partial pressure of CO_2 during various ventilatory regimens in halothane-anesthetized dogs, *Am J Vet Res* 41:610-612, 1980.
48. Grosenbaugh DA, Muir WW: Accuracy of noninvasive oxyhemoglobin saturation, end-tidal carbon dioxide concentration, and blood pressure monitoring during experimentally induced hypoxemia, hypotension, or hypertension in anesthetized dogs, *Am J Vet Res* 59(2):205-212, 1998.
49. Amis TC, Kurpershoek C: Tidal breathing flow-volume loop analysis for clinical assessment of airway obstruction in conscious dogs, *Am J Vet Res* 47(5):1002-1006, 1986.
50. Amis TC, Smith MM, Gaber CC et al: Upper airway obstruction in canine laryngeal paralysis, *Am J Vet Res* 47(5):1007-1010, 1986.
51. Amis TC, Kurpershoek C: Patterns of breathing in brachycephalic dogs, *Am J Vet Res* 47(10):2200-2204, 1986.
52. Schweiger JW, Rasanen J: Monitoring during ventilatory support. In Stock MC, Perel M, editors: *Handbook of mechanical ventilatory support*, ed 2, Baltimore, MD, 1997, Williams & Wilkins.
53. Mann FA, Wagner-Mann CC, Branson KR: Transcutaneous oxygen and carbon dioxide monitoring in normal cats, *J Vet Emerg Crit Care* 7(2):99-109, 1997.
54. Plumb DC: *Veterinary drug handbook*, ed 2, Ames, IA, 1995, Iowa State University Press.
55. Orenstein DM, Boat TF, Stern RC et al: Progesterone treatment of the obesity hypoventilation syndrome in a child, *J Pediatr* 90(3):477-479, 1977.
56. Goodland RL, Reynolds JG, McCoorde AB et al: Respiratory and electrolyte effects induced by estrogen and progesterone, *Fertility & Sterility* 4(4):300-317, 1953.
57. Kopelman PG, Elliot MW, Simonds A et al: Short term use of fluoxetine in asymptomatic obese subjects with sleep-related hypoventilation, *Int J Obes Relat Metab Disord* 16:825-830, 1992.
58. Moon PF, Gabor L, Gleed RD et al: Acid-base, metabolic, and hemodynamic effects of sodium bicarbonate or tromethamine administration in anesthetized dogs with experimentally induced metabolic acidosis, *Am J Vet Res* 58(7):771-776, 1997.

CHAPTER 10

Respiratory Muscle Fatigue and Failure

Joan C. Hendricks

Definition and Utility

Respiratory muscle fatigue is a concept rather than a clearly and objectively defined pathological entity. The utility of the concept is that increased effort and the recruitment of additional muscles to aid respiration can serve as the earliest indication of abnormal loading of the respiratory system. Long before arterial blood gas measurements provide objective evidence of respiratory failure (i.e., the increase in $Paco_2$ that signals that the respiratory system's efforts have been exhausted), the assessment of clinical signs related to changes in respiratory mechanics aids in diagnosing the degree of respiratory effort and discomfort.

When the work of breathing increases, respiratory muscle patterns change and muscles that are not ordinarily used for respiration are recruited. In addition, the animal makes postural and other behavioral adaptations to reduce the workload. Generally, these changes are readily noted on physical examination and may even be quantifiable. Although it is unfortunate that there are no objective measures that change linearly as the animal loses respiratory reserve (e.g., no pulmonary equivalent to the creatinine clearance) it is most fortunate that as-

sessment of respiratory muscle fatigue can be accomplished through the quick, noninvasive, and inexpensive method of observing the patient.

Interpreting Changes in Breathing

Most causes of respiratory problems in dogs and cats occur with a normal respiratory control system (afferent nerves, central nervous system) and normal effector organs (efferent nerves, muscles, ribcage cartilage and bones, and an intact body wall). That is, the pump system itself is initially normal, but the pulmonary system or other organs that affect breathing are providing signals to the control system that lead to changes in the breathing pattern in an attempt to normalize the blood gases. If unrelieved, the additional workload can lead to respiratory muscle fatigue and eventual failure.

The less common situation occurs when either the central respiratory control system in the brain, the peripheral nerves that innervate respiratory muscles, or the respiratory muscles themselves is the primary cause of the pathology leading to hypoventilation (see Chapter 9). Such an aberration of the control system may lead to profound changes in respiratory pattern, including reduced tidal volume, very slow or irregular respiration, or bizarre patterns such as apneustic or agonal breathing. In this case, the impact on the respiratory muscles depends on the specific abnormality. These conditions will not lead to respiratory muscle fatigue if they simply reduce respiratory effort. If, however, partial paralysis affects some muscles, the remaining muscles may be susceptible to fatigue.

Although respiratory pattern changes may indicate profound abnormalities of the respiratory system and can herald impending respiratory failure, it is worth mentioning that respiratory patterns also change in response to nonrespiratory inputs. Because the respiratory center integrates inputs from higher centers, changes in breathing occur in response to excitement, pain, anxiety, or any change in level of consciousness such as sleep or sedation. Because of its role in pH homeostasis, the respiratory system assists in correction of changes in pH, leading to hyperventilation and respiratory alkalosis in response to metabolic acidosis and to slowed respiratory frequency in response to metabolic alkalosis. Of course, thermal polypnea (panting) results from increased ambient temperature. Some endocrine conditions (e.g., endogenous or exogenous hyperadrenocorticism and feline hyperthyroidism) can alter respiration. Irritation of the respiratory system between the larynx and lower bronchi can result in cough or increased expiratory effort that can be mistaken for a response to loading.

A thorough historical and clinical assessment of the animal will generally reveal such conditions. They are mentioned here because the most prominent sign is sometimes the change in respiratory pattern; however, focusing on the respiratory system may waste time and prove to be fruitless. Conversely, if the animal is predisposed to respiratory difficulty by an underlying condition, such additional stresses may lead to overt manifestation of respiratory abnormalities. The algorithm in Figure 10-1 provides a decision tree that may be useful in considering how to pursue the causes of respiratory changes, especially when

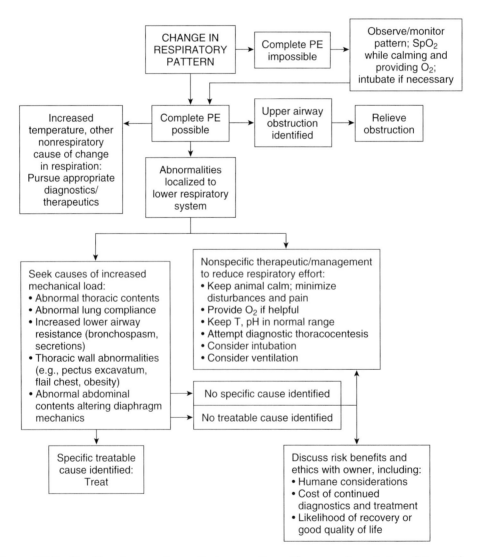

Figure 10-1. *Algorithm for assessing patients presenting with apparent respiratory distress (change in respiratory pattern).*

the degree of apparent respiratory distress delays or precludes definitive diagnostic testing.

CHANGES IN RESPIRATORY PATTERN RESULTING FROM INCREASED RESPIRATORY LOAD

The term "dyspnea" actually means "sensation of breathlessness" and, strictly speaking, cannot be used to describe objective signs of respiratory difficulty. The precise origin of the sensation, studied in humans, has been difficult to define. The possibilities include the vagal afferents from the lung; stretch receptors in muscles or joints of the chest wall; or sensors of inflammation or stretch in the airway mucosa. Changes in pH, Pao_2, or $Paco_2$ that are integrated in the brainstem could also somehow provide signals that are consciously perceived. Whatever the source of the conscious perception of respiratory discomfort, adjustments of breathing pattern and of muscle recruitment are readily observed. Changes in breathing pattern may not always be accompanied by conscious awareness of a change in respiratory loading.

The normal respiratory pump mechanism in small quadrupeds relies almost entirely on effort from the diaphragm alone, aided during inspiration by a small additional number of muscles that stiffen the intercostal spaces and rotate the ribs cranially and laterally (the intercostals and the cervical strap muscles such as the sternohyoid and scalenes; Figure 10-2, *A*). Because of the position of the diaphragmatic central tendon rostral to the caudal costal margin, diaphragmatic contraction pulls the ribs cranially and slightly inward. The inward vector of the contraction is counteracted by contraction of the extrinsic chest wall muscles, so that the ribs normally rotate cranially and laterally during inspiration, increasing the volume of the chest cavity, reducing intrathoracic pressure compared to atmospheric pressure, and leading to an inrush of air. The animal with a normal-sized, patent airway can allow the trachea and pharynx to be somewhat compressed or twisted as it performs normal behaviors, and can alter respiration during eating, vocalization, or exercise. When the chest wall, thoracic contents, and abdominal contents are normal, respiratory movements are nearly effortless, and are unnoticeable to the untrained observer. Even close observation or palpation of the chest wall and cervical respiratory muscles reveals only minimal contractions. Expiration occurs without any muscular effort (see Figure 10-2, *A*).

Increased respiratory loading can occur due to narrowing of the airway lumen at any level (e.g., nares, pharynx, larynx, trachea, or bronchi); decreased compliance of the thoracic contents; increased volume of thoracic contents; or abnormal abdominal contents that change the position and mechanics of the diaphragm (Figure 10-2, *B*). Changes in the shape or function of the chest wall associated with rib fractures, obesity, or chest wall tumors, for example, can also lead to reduced mechanical efficiency and therefore increase the work of breathing. When any component of this system is thus altered, adjustments are made to reduce the work of breathing *before* actual muscle fatigue or frank respiratory failure occurs.

Respiratory muscle fatigue is a concept that is distinct from the muscle fatigue that occurs when tetanic muscle contractions lead to failure of a muscle to contract despite continued electrical stimulation, as can be produced in vitro in an isolated muscle. Rather, respiratory muscle fatigue is best conceptualized as a coordinated response to increased loading that threatens to overwhelm the ability to maintain blood gas homeostasis. This "central fatigue" leads to effort-reducing adjustments that reduce wear and tear on muscles long before the isolated muscles would begin to fail, and consists of postural and behavioral changes, changes in respiratory muscle recruitment, and changes in respiratory pattern.

POSTURAL AND BEHAVIORAL CHANGES

Early adjustments include attempts to decrease airway resistance by increasing the cross-sectional area of the airways; this is done by straightening the head and neck to reduce flexion of the pharynx and larynx and by avoiding behaviors that narrow the airways (e.g., swallowing). Opening the mouth greatly increases the oropharyngeal airway diameter. This adjustment is made readily by dogs, but much less readily by cats, in whom the effort to breathe through the nose despite nasal obstruction will sometimes continue even to the point of frank hypoventilation and failure. Most animals will also become quiet, an appropriate adjustment to muscle exertion that would increase the need for oxygen and the production of carbon dioxide. However, some young or excitable animals will continue to be active and even playful despite the added load on their respiratory systems.

Later postural adjustments can include adopting a sitting position with forelimbs abducted. The sitting position compresses the abdominal contents against the diaphragm and allows the abdominal contents to serve as a fulcrum to hold the central tendon of the diaphragm in its rostral position. This optimizes the mechanical advantage of the diaphragm by optimizing the position of the fibers on the length:tension curve. It also maintains the rostral position of the origin of the fibers from the central tendon. This tends to counteract the effects of abnormal chest contents (e.g., pleural effusions) that would otherwise tend to move the diaphragm caudally. The abducted forelimbs apparently allow the ribs to swing cranially and laterally without hindrance. Perhaps for the same reason, animals with respiratory distress will generally avoid lying down in any position and will forcefully fight restraint that compresses the ribcage.

RESPIRATORY MUSCLE RECRUITMENT

The laryngeal abductors, intercostal muscles, and cervical respiratory muscles such as the scalenes and sternohyoid may be recruited when inspiratory effort increases, but these are difficult or impossible to appreciate in the awake patient. The abduction of the alae nasi, therefore, is often the first indication beyond postural adjustments that respiratory workload has increased. Additional orofacial

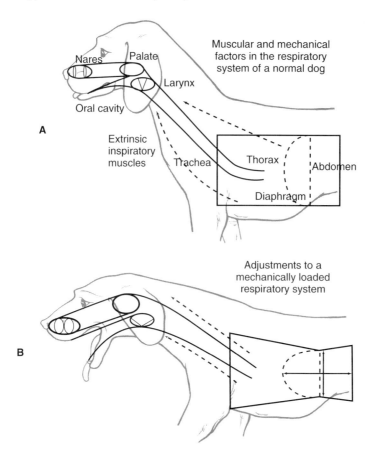

Figure 10-2. *Schematic of respiratory muscles and narrow point of the airways in animals with A, normal and B, increased respiratory workloads. Airway and body cavity boundaries are depicted with solid lines. Vectors or respiratory muscle influences are indicated with broken lines.*

muscles may also be observed to contract with each inspiration so that the tongue is protruded, mandible depressed, and the lips retracted rhythmically. If the work of expiration has increased, recruitment of abdominal musculature to provide active expiration may also be noted. This latter may be most easily appreciated in overweight or longhaired animals through palpation rather than visual observation. This expiratory effort may also serve the function of shortening expiration as part of increasing the frequency of breathing, as occurs in normal exercise. This complex of changes when workload increases is depicted schematically in Figure 10-2, *B.*

CHANGES IN THE MECHANICS OF THE CHEST WALL: "PARADOXICAL BREATHING"

When the central tendon of the diaphragm moves caudally due to abnormal thoracic contents, and the degree of contraction of the diaphragmatic fibers has increased due to increasing workload, the normal mechanical results of diaphragmatic contractions change. The normal direction of the force resulting from diaphragmatic fiber contractions pulls the ribs cranially and slightly inward; the inward vector is counteracted by the laterally located

extrinsic chest wall muscles (e.g., the scalenes) that arise in the neck. However, when the central tendon is more caudal, the diaphragm is then oriented so that contraction of the fibers that insert along the costal margin tends to pull the caudal ribs inward. When the diaphragm is contracting forcefully because of increased drive, this contraction is no longer fully counteracted by the external chest wall muscles. Thus the caudal ribcage actually collapses inward with each inspiratory effort, reducing rather than increasing the volume of the thorax at this level. The abdominal contents are displaced caudally by the shortening of the diaphragm's fibers and the contraction of the caudal ribs, and the abdomen may be seen to increase in volume during inspiration. These grossly abnormal mechanics are highly inefficient because increased work by other respiratory muscles is necessary to increase the thoracic volume in the more cranial regions. When paradoxical breathing movements are observed, it is reasonable to expect that the workload on the respiratory system is so greatly increased that it cannot be sustained indefinitely. Either the cause of the increased workload must be treated (e.g., by surgery to remove an upper airway obstruction) or the work of breathing must be taken over by artificial means (i.e., by mechanical ventilation).

CHANGES IN RESPIRATORY PATTERN

Depending on the exact nature of the mechanical change, the respiratory pattern may change by increasing or decreasing frequency and by changing the inspiratory to expiratory ratio. Changes in tidal volume may also occur. Of all of these, the change in respiratory frequency is the most straightforward to quantify and can serve as a very simple objective monitoring tool for the patient. When the system is near failure, marked irregularities may be noted, with periods of respiratory effort alternating with periods of apnea.

Consequences of Respiratory Distress and Failure

In the effort to increase inspiration, animals commonly swallow air. This aerophagia can lead to gross distention of the esophagus and stomach with air, sometimes producing obvious abdominal dilation. In some animals this result of respiratory distress may be more apparent to the owners than the primary respiratory cause. Failure to have a high index of suspicion for respiratory causes of esophageal, gastric, and even intestinal dilation can have profound consequences if expensive, time-wasting, and possibly dangerous diagnostic and therapeutic procedures are undertaken to pursue esophageal and gastric dilation. We have seen animals undergo barium swallows and even gastropexy when the primary disease was actually brachycephalic airway obstruction, laryngeal paralysis, or nasopharyngeal polyp.

At the terminal stages, when oxygenation is not maintained or CO_2 accumulates, respiratory failure leads to changes in the animal's mentation. Hypoxic animals do not show interest in their environment, and hypercapnia leads to sedation. Profound hypoxia leads to agonal or gasping respiration because the normal respiratory center ceases to function and a different brainstem center that is resistant to hypoxia takes over. Usually, little can be done to reverse the situation at this point.

Clinical Implications of Diagnosing Respiratory Muscle Fatigue

The fact that early signs of increased respiratory workload can generally be appreciated and monitored by physical examination allows appropriate direction of diagnostic and therapeutic efforts. The algorithm in Figure 10-1 is intended to provide a guide when respiratory muscle fatigue is initially noted. Because frank respiratory failure (increased CO_2) occurs when the animal has decompensated, at that point reversal can occur only if muscles are rested (by taking over ventilation) and/or the cause of load is dramatically decreased (e.g., by removing pleural fluid or air or by removing an upper airway obstruction). Thus it is far preferable to be aware that the animal may be at risk for decompensation and to be able to undertake appropriate testing before frank respiratory failure occurs. It is also important to provide the owners with appropriate information so that they are prepared to make decisions about the expensive and labor-intensive prospect of providing mechanical ventilation if the need arises. Of course, depending on the overall situation, it may be more appropriate for humane, ethical, and financial reasons to consider euthanasia in cases of respiratory failure.

A final note, which may seem obvious but is often overlooked, is that respiratory failure is a pump failure. Oxygen supplementation may prolong life, but obviously will not lower carbon dioxide or reverse mechanical problems that are overloading respiratory muscles.

PART TWO

Respiratory Tract Diagnostics

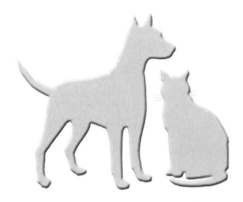

CHAPTER 11

Physical Examination of the Respiratory Tract

Neil K. Harpster

Evaluation of the cat or dog with respiratory disease begins in the examination room with the veterinarian in the position of historical investigator and the patient, ideally, in a calm and cooperative mood. The first order of business is to obtain a thorough and detailed history regarding the patient's clinical signs and patterns observed in its normal environment. This is preferably taken from a person who has had significant exposure and opportunity to observe the patient. When the pet is presented by a friend or uninvolved family member, the reported history may be less than adequate, and direct communication with the primary caretaker at home should be pursued.

In addition to obtaining an accurate description of the patient's abnormal clinical signs at home, questions pertaining to any changes in activity level or other daily routines should be raised. In particular, in elderly patients where the possibility of multiple organ disease is in-

creased, specific questions should be directed at changes in eating and drinking patterns, fluctuations in body weight, alterations in urination or defecation habits, and modifications of personality or behavioral traits.

When a complete and accurate patient history is combined with a thorough physical examination, total knowledge of respiratory tract anatomy, and good clinical experience, the ideal situation has been secured for optimal diagnosis and management of a patient. However, this only holds true if appropriate diagnostic equipment and tests are available and are pursued.

Anatomy of the Respiratory Tract

The respiratory system is composed of the lungs and the passageways for air that lead to the specific locations for gas exchange within the lungs. Although air may enter via either the nasal or the oral cavity, only the nasal cavity is considered a component of the respiratory tract. The nasal cavity is the most cranial (or the facial) portion of the respiratory passageway. It extends from the external nares to the choanae and is divided into right and left sides by the nasal septum. The nasal cavity and nasal turbinates mainly serve the function of warming and moistening inspired air, but also function to remove foreign materials from it. In addition the nasal glands, notably the lateral nasal glands along with the laryngeal glands, serve as major sources of moisture. This enhances heat dissipation in warm environments and during panting in the dog.[1] Based on airflow studies, the lateral nasal gland has been shown to play a significant role in the thermoregulatory system in the dog. A second study subsequently confirmed its importance based on the correlation between the volume of secretion and both heat load and panting.[2]

The nasopharynx or nasal portion of the pharynx extends from the choanae to the intrapharyngeal ostium. The intrapharyngeal ostium lies cranial to the larynx and is formed by the coalescence of the oral pharynx and nasal pharynx. The nasal portion of the nasopharynx is bounded ventrally by the hard palate, dorsally by the vomer bone, and laterally by the palatine bones. More caudally, the boundaries of the nasopharynx include the base of the skull and its muscular attachments dorsally and the soft palate ventrally.

The larynx is a complex musculocartilaginous organ that guards the entrance to the trachea. It extends from the intrapharyngeal ostium to the trachea. The major functions of the larynx encompass its roles as a portion of the air passageway; in prevention of aspiration of food, water and other substances; and in vocalization. The cavity of the larynx is divided into three transverse portions: (1) the antechamber or the laryngeal vestibule, which extends from the laryngeal opening (i.e., aditus laryngis) to the ventricular folds; (2) a central, narrow portion termed the glottis, composed dorsally of the paired arytenoid cartilages and ventrally by the paired vocal cords, which form a narrow passageway within the larynx termed the rima glottidus; and (3) the infraglottic cavity, which lies caudal to the glottis extending from the rima glottis to the trachea. The infraglottic cavity is wide dorsally, where it comprises the cricoid cartilage lamina, and is more narrow ventrally.

The trachea is normally a noncollapsible, tubelike structure that extends from the cricoid cartilage of the larynx to its bifurcation into the right and left main stem bronchi dorsal to the cranial portion of the heart base. Its proximal boundary lies on a plane approximately through the disk between the fourth and fifth thoracic vertebrae. The trachea is composed of a consecutive series of C-shaped hyaline cartilages, numbering approximately 35 in the dog.[3] The space remaining dorsally by the failure of the incomplete tracheal cartilage rings to meet or overlap is bridged by smooth fibers of the transversely oriented trachealis muscle and by associated connective tissue. The tracheal rings are united in a longitudinal plane by bands of fibroelastic tissue, termed tracheal annular ligaments. These annu-

lar ligaments are approximately one quarter the width of the tracheal rings.[4]

The bronchi or bronchial tree are responsible for conduction of air from the trachea to the respiratory bronchioles. At the tracheal bifurcation the bronchi originate as a right and left principal or main stem bronchus. The right main stem bronchus gives rise to the right upper lobe bronchus, then the intermediate or accessory lobe bronchus, and then divides into bronchi supplying the middle and caudal right lung lobes. Meanwhile, the left main stem bronchus divides into two bronchi, one giving rise to the cranial and caudal portions of the left cranial lung lobes and the other supplying the left caudal lung lobe. The major bronchus to each individual lung lobe is termed a lobar bronchus. Then within each lobe the lobar bronchi divide into segmental or tertiary bronchi. Each segmental bronchus, and the lung tissue it ventilates, is termed a bronchopulmonary segment. The segmental bronchi undergo dichotomous branching until the respiratory bronchioles are formed. The respiratory bronchioles in turn give rise to alveolar ducts, alveolar sacs, and pulmonary alveoli. All three of these respiratory compartments serve in the transfer of oxygen from the inspired gas into the alveolar capillaries, and in the removal of carbon dioxide.

Observation in the Examination Room

While in the examination room questioning the owner, it is beneficial to have the pet in full display so it may be observed. This can provide an opportunity to see behaviors that concern the owner or that have been observed at home (e.g., coughing, wheezing, snorting, or choking). This direct observation experience can be expanded by having the owner walk the dog outside on a leash, or by allowing the pet free movement about the examination room.

Important clues can often be obtained as to the anatomical position and nature of the respiratory tract disorder when attention is paid to the patient's respiratory patterns. Color and capillary refill time of visible mucous membranes are additional clues concerning cardiac and respiratory tract function. These observations should be carried over and continued during the actual physical examination.

Observation of the patient's respiratory or breathing patterns may not be helpful on casual inspection in the examination room environment, depending upon the severity of the respiratory disorder and the level of excitement of the patient. The pertinent features are the rate, regularity, depth, and apparent effort being expended in breathing.[5] In both dogs and cats an increased respiratory rate is the anticipated normal finding in the examination room, and panting is an equally common finding in the dog. Open-mouth breathing is another common observation in the nervous, panting dog; however, it may also be an expected pathophysiological response in the patient with bilateral nasal obstruction, and is not uncommon in the presence of inspiratory dyspnea.

As mentioned previously, abnormal patterns of respiration are often characteristic of certain pathophysiological alterations in lung performance. For example, in obstructive upper airway disease the characteristic breathing pattern at rest is a slow respiratory rate and an exaggerated inspiratory effort in an attempt to develop a large tidal or inspiratory volume. This respiratory pattern increases the volume of air delivered to the alveoli by increasing the duration of inspiration. On the other hand, in restrictive lung disease (e.g., pneumothorax, pleural effusion, or pulmonary fibrosis) the common breathing pattern is distinguished by small tidal volumes (shallow inspiration) and an increased respiratory rate.

Patients with multiple rib fractures and an unstable segment of chest wall, termed *flail chest,* may exhibit localized paradoxical chest wall movement characterized by inward movement of the unstable fractured rib segment during inspiration and outward movement during expiration. Although this abnormal chest wall motion may have some impact on overall lung performance, significant abnormalities in measured respiratory parameters in this setting are more likely the result of hypoventilation secondary to painful respiration and the presence of underlying lung contusion.

In contrast, paradoxical respiration associated with respiratory muscle fatigue is characterized by opposing movements of the chest and abdominal wall during inspiration and expiration. That is, during inspiration the caudal ribcage collapses inward, reducing rather than increasing the volume of the thorax. The abdominal contents are displaced caudally, and the abdomen may appear to increase in volume during inspiration. Paradoxical respiration can occur in animals with a variety of respiratory disorders and represents a significant increase in the work of breathing and the imminent risk of onset of respiratory muscle fatigue and failure.

In certain respiratory disorders, specific postural adaptations are assumed by the patient to enhance ventilation. Orthopnea, or dyspnea in any but the erect sitting or standing position, is usually the result of bilateral pulmonary edema (as seen in left heart failure or electrical shock) or bilateral diaphragmatic paralysis.[6] Trepopnea, or dyspnea in one lateral recumbent position but not the other, may be the result of unilateral lung disease, unilateral pleural effusion, or unilateral airway obstruction. In contrast platypnea, or dyspnea in the upright position, is usually secondary to intracardiac shunts or vascular shunts in the lungs.[7]

Examination of the Nasal Cavity

Major limitations are imposed upon physical examination of the nasal cavity by the bony structures that surrounded it. The examination is begun by observing for symmetry over the facial region, which is made up predominantly of the incisive, nasal, and maxillary bones dorsally and the incisive, maxillary, and palatine bones ventrally. This includes careful examination of the nasal plane and facial areas with the patient's mouth closed; and then, after opening the mouth, inspection of the roof of the mouth for the presence of any swelling, ulceration, or defects.

Further examination of the nasal cavity should include visual inspection of the nostrils for discharge that is most commonly purulent or bloody, and examination of each nasal cavity for airflow or patency. This latter examination can be accomplished by holding a small strand of cotton over first one nostril and then the other to observe for movement during expiration. Improved sensitivity to abnormalities of airflow is achieved by placing the dog's or cat's nostril adjacent to the examiner's ear and listening to the individual inspiratory and expiratory passage of air through the right and left nostrils while the opposite nostril is digitally occluded. This nostril airflow evaluation is very useful in establishing the presence of complete or partial occlusion of the nasal cavity.

One last area that should be examined in any patient with a concern of nasal disease is the upper dental arch, including both the teeth and associated gums. The upper canine teeth, when infected or abscessed, are particularly prone to result in extension of the infection into the nasal cavity, resulting in a purulent nasal discharge on the affected side.

Examination of the Pharynx and Associated Cervical Region

The pharynx serves as a common passageway for both the respiratory and the digestive systems. This anatomical arrangement unquestionably increases the risk of aspiration because of the proximity of ingested food and water to the lower respiratory tract during their passage into the cervical esophagus.

Disorders affecting the pharynx are quite varied and can include tumors; foreign bodies; nasal, sinus, or tonsillar infections; and anatomical malformations involving the soft palate (e.g., cleft palate or elongated soft palate in brachycephalic breeds). Clinical signs vary considerably and can encompass heat intolerance, noisy breathing, coughing, choking, retching, occasional vomiting, and even a nasal discharge. There can be considerable overlap of clinical signs arising from pharyngeal disorders and those arising from other upper respiratory anatomic sites, as well as from the gastrointestinal system.

Examination of the pharynx is limited in the fully conscious patient because of its anatomical positioning. The best that one might expect to obtain in the most cooperative patient is a limited inspection of the soft palate and adjacent structures, including the base of the tongue and palatine tonsils. With sedation a more comfortable and complete examination can be accomplished, and should include digital palpation of the hard and soft palate, as well as inspection behind the soft palate. Investigation of any disease process affecting the pharynx or nasopharynx should include palpation of the submandibular lymph nodes and the adjacent salivary glands.

Examination of the Larynx

Diseases affecting the larynx are more common in the dog and cat than those affecting the pharynx, although the clinical signs may be quite similar. It may also prove equally difficult to do a thorough examination of the larynx in the fully awake dog or cat.

Poor exercise and heat tolerance and noisy respiratory sounds are the common and expected observations when laryngeal disease is present. In the examination room, noisy respiration and an inspiratory stridor are anticipated. Occasionally, when these are not apparent, an inspiratory stridor can be heard on thoracic auscultation and when the stethoscope is placed over the larynx. One additional useful examination tool is applying digital pressure over the larynx while closely observing the inspiratory airflow. In normal large and giant breeds of dogs, even severe digital pressure applied to the larynx results in little effect on airflow. However, when the larynx is narrowed by laryngeal paralysis or the presence of an intraluminal mass, mild to moderate digital pressure over the larynx results in a significant and readily detectable reduction in airflow. Unfortunately, this examination tool is not useful in smaller dogs or cats because of less intrinsic rigidity of the larynx.

To accurately assess the cause and severity of laryngeal disease, an intraoral examination is required, utilizing either sedative(s) or general anesthesia. Whereas examination of the larynx under full general anesthesia is appropriate for dogs and cats with inflammatory or neoplastic processes involving the larynx, many anesthetics interfere with laryngeal function. For evaluation of the patient with suspected laryngeal dysfunction due to laryngeal paralysis, light sedation with acepromazine (0.1 to 0.2 mg/kg IM) may prove helpful.

Examination of the Cervical Trachea

Physical examination of the trachea is confined to the cervical portion. Normally, the trachea is a round, rigid, tubelike structure that is minimally compressible and insensitive with mild to moderate palpation. Any deviation from this pattern should be considered abnormal. Examination should include digital palpation along the course of the cervical trachea from the larynx to the thoracic inlet. Abnormalities on examination may include a trachea that is smaller than the expected diameter (so-called hypoplastic trachea); a widened, dorsoventrally flattened trachea that is easily compressed with mild digital pressure (tracheomalacia or tracheal collapse); and increased tracheal sensitivity manifested by easily induced coughing in the absence of distinct anatomic abnormalities.

When increased tracheal sensitivity is present in the absence of tracheal deformities, more generalized respiratory tract conditions should be considered. Specific causes may include infections involving bacterial, viral,

or fungal agents; aspiration pneumonia or aspiration of foreign materials; and respiratory tract allergic disorders. Under these circumstances further diagnostic studies are warranted to establish a definitive cause.

Examination of the Thorax

As mentioned previously, examination of the thorax should begin by careful observation of the patient's respiration and respiratory patterns in the examination room while obtaining the pet's history and listening to the owner's observations at home.

The actual physical examination should begin with thoracic palpation to define the position of the maximal cardiac impulse, determine the presence of any respiratory rhonchi, and to evaluate for chest wall masses or deformities. A rhonchus is a prominent or loud rale that arises in the trachea or one of the larger bronchi. It is characterized not only by its prominence on auscultation, but also by being referred to the chest wall as a palpable vibration or fremitus. Palpation is followed by thorough auscultation of the chest, which should include the thoracic inlet. Increased inspiratory sounds may arise within the intrathoracic trachea or bronchi; or be referred from the upper respiratory tract, which may include the pharynx, larynx, or extrathoracic trachea. When the increased inspiratory sounds are louder over the thorax their origin is more likely to be intrathoracic, whereas their origin is expected to be extrathoracic when the increased inspiratory sounds are loudest over the thoracic inlet or cervical trachea.

Thoracic auscultation should be initiated by a complete examination of the heart, bilaterally, followed by a thorough examination of all lung fields. Poor patient cooperation and noisy respiration due to panting, hyperventilation, purring, growling, or vocalization are the main obstacles to good thoracic auscultation. In dogs, thoracic auscultation may be enhanced by holding the mouth closed with or without digital occlusion of one nostril. The nostril occlusion approach seems to work best with puppies and young adolescents, and is less well tolerated in aggressive, strong-willed, adult dogs, especially those with ventilation abnormalities. Purring in feline patients can usually be overcome by placing mild digital pressure just cranial to the larynx.

Optimal thoracic auscultation requires a cooperative patient and complete examination of all lung fields. In the normal dog or cat the anticipated inspiratory sounds on auscultation are characteristically soft, low-pitched flow or airway sounds whereas the expiratory sounds are softer and lower-pitched, and may even be absent. These are termed normal bronchovesicular sounds. However, in patients with respiratory disease abnormal lung sounds are usually present and generally are fairly characteristic of the underlying disorder. These abnormal lung sounds are usually referred to as rales, rhonchi, or wheezes and may or may not be associated with alterations in the duration and effort of inspiration or expiration. Rales are defined as small rhonchi, and are further identified as either moist or dry. Moist rales are characterized by low-pitched, fine, popping inspiratory sounds, usually heard best in a perihilar distribution and typically found in patients with pulmonary edema, hemorrhage, or pneumonia. These animals commonly have some degree of respiratory distress, although expiration and the expiratory sounds tend to be unremarkable. In pulmonary edema secondary to left-sided congestive heart failure, moist rales tend to occur earliest and resolve last in a right hilar position. With severe cardiogenic pulmonary edema, moist rales may also be present in a left hilar position or diffusely distributed in all lung fields.

Dry rales, on the other hand, are characterized by higher-pitched inspiratory popping or "inspiratory crackles." Dry rales are the anticipated finding in patients with acute or chronic airway disease (e.g., bronchitis or asthma) and may be accompanied by increased expiratory effort. In animals with chronic bronchitis, dry, crepitant rales tend to be fairly evenly distributed over all lung fields, whereas with other respiratory conditions varying distributions of abnormal lung sounds may be observed and tend to lack any consistent pattern. Both moist and dry rales are considered to be discontinuous or interrupted sounds, whereas rhonchi and wheezes are continuous sounds longer than 250 ms.[5]

Characteristically, wheezes and rhonchi are abnormal airway sounds that occur secondary to narrowing of the tracheobronchial airway, usually a bronchus. The bronchial pathology responsible for the abnormal sounds may be secondary to increased secretion or other fluid development, an inflammatory or other structural change, or dynamic compression of the airway. Wheezes are high-pitched sounds with a dominant frequency of 400+ Hz, whereas rhonchi are lower-pitched airway sounds having a dominant frequency of around 200+ Hz. Although wheezes and rhonchi may be present during either inspiration or expiration, they are more commonly observed during expiration due to normal bronchial narrowing during expiration.

Thoracic percussion is another substantial aid in the examination of patients with diseases involving the thoracic cavity. Percussion is defined as a diagnostic procedure designed to determine the density of a part by means of tapping the surface with the finger or a plessor.[8] Although percussion may be performed on any patient, its greatest benefits are likely to be gained in larger dogs and cats, and increase with clinical experience. Percussion is ideally performed with the patient standing. If the examiner is right-handed, the middle finger of the left hand is placed over the right thorax just above the sternum at the costochondral junction and just behind the right shoulder blade. This finger is tapped firmly with the middle finger of the right hand as the left hand is moved dorsally toward the thoracic vertebrae. The hands should be reversed if the examiner is left-handed. This process is repeated at two to four consecutive distances caudally to the first position until the entire right chest has been percussed; then the left chest should be similarly percussed.

The purpose of thoracic percussion is to determine whether the tympanic sounds created by thoracic wall percussion are normal, increased, or decreased. Bilateral pleural effusion is a classic cause of bilaterally reduced tympanic sounds in a ventral position. Dorsal to the fluid line the tympanic sounds tend to be normal. Other potential causes of decreased tympanic sounds in which the findings are not bilaterally symmetrical include diaphragmatic hernia, intrathoracic masses, consolidation of lung lobes, and unilateral pleural effusion. Causes of increased tympanic sounds on thoracic percussion include pneumothorax, emphysema, and asthma.

Despite the characteristic patterns described above, some variations in the consistency of these patterns do occur. Lateral and ventrodorsal thoracic radiographs should always be taken to support the working diagnosis when abnormal respiratory patterns are present, when lung sounds are abnormal on auscultation, and whenever thoracic percussion is deemed abnormal.[9]

Abdominal Evaluation in the Patient with Respiratory Disease

Although the abdomen is not considered a portion of the respiratory system, it can reflect alterations in function of the respiratory system. Similarly, abnormalities involving the abdominal cavity may on occasion inhibit or interfere with respiratory system functions, primarily by its proximity to the thoracic cavity. Diaphragm movement, in particular, is the common mediator that can be called upon to enhance ventilation when abnormalities of respiratory function exist, although the muscles of the abdominal wall may also play a minor, less significant role.[10]

Abdominal abnormalities such as large masses (especially those arising in the liver), as well as large peritoneal effusions, can significantly interfere with diaphragm movement. A similar situation may occur with paralysis of the diaphragm. Although these abnormalities in themselves are unlikely to result in clinically significant hypoxemia, polypnea, or dyspnea, they may be responsible for reduced exercise tolerance or may contribute significantly to respiratory dysfunction when other, primary respiratory abnormalities coexist.[11]

One other circumstance in which the abdomen appears to play an active role in a respiratory disorder is in patients with small airway (small bronchi or bronchiole) disease (e.g., in feline patients with asthma or in canine patients with chronic bronchitis). Clinically, this respiratory pattern is characterized by a mild expiratory tensing of the abdominal muscles or by an active abdominal expiratory push and is normally accompanied by a prolongation of the expiratory phase of respiration.

Conclusions

The respiratory system is a complex, extensive airway that stretches from the external nares to the alveoli. It is responsible for the transport of oxygen from the atmosphere to all the living cells of the body and, in turn, the transport of carbon dioxide from the cells back to the atmosphere.[3] Alterations in the normal function of the respiratory tract usually lead to a reduction in oxygen transfer into arterial blood resulting in hypoxemia and, subsequently, difficult or labored respiration, termed dyspnea.

Physical examination of the respiratory tract is extremely helpful in establishing the anatomical location of a particular problem and in formulating a list of potential causes. The respiratory tract presents major barriers to the examiner, however, by its encasement within bony and cartilaginous enclosures. Some of these problems may be circumvented by clinical experience and exposure, but even then, rarely can an absolutely unequivocal definitive diagnosis be established. Additional imaging or interventional diagnostic procedures are usually required in order to confirm a suspected working diagnosis or to establish a definitive diagnosis.

REFERENCES

1. Schmidt-Nielson K, Bretz WL, Taylor CR: Panting in dogs: Unidirectional air flow over evaporative surfaces, *Science* 169:1102-1104, 1970.
2. Blatt CM, Taylor CR, Habel M: Thermal panting in dogs: The lateral nasal gland a source of water for evaporate cooling, *Science* 177:804-805, 1972.
3. Evans HE, Christenson GC: *Miller's anatomy of the dog,* ed 2, Philadelphia, 1979, WB Saunders.
4. Guyton AC: *Textbook of medical physiology,* Philadelphia, 1961, WB Saunders.
5. Snider GL: History and physical examination. In Baum GL, Wolinsky E, editors: *Textbook of pulmonary disease,* ed 5, Philadelphia, 1993, WB Saunders.
6. Ries AL, Mahler DA: Chronic dyspnea. In Mahler DA, editor: *Dyspnea,* Mount Kisca, NY, 1990, Futura.
7. Mahler DA: Positional dyspnea. In Mahler DA, editor: *Dyspnea,* Mount Kisca, NY, 1990, Futura.
8. *Stedman's Medical Dictionary,* Baltimore, MD, 1961, Williams & Wilkins.
9. Prueter JC, Hamilton TA: Pulmonary parenchymal disorders. In Morgan RV, editor: *Handbook of small animal practice,* Philadelphia, 1997, WB Saunders.
10. Wilkins RL, Hodgkin JE: History and physical examination of the respiratory patient. In Burton GG, Hodgkin JE, Ward JJ, editors: *Respiratory care: A guide to clinical practice,* ed 3, Philadelphia, 1991, J.B. Lippincott.
11. Crossman W, Braunwald E: Pulmonary hypertension. In Braunwald E, editor: *Heart disease: A textbook of cardiovascular medicine,* Philadelphia, 1992, WB Saunders.

CHAPTER 12

Thoracic Imaging

H. Mark Saunders • Dennis Keith

The investigation of suspected thoracic disease relies heavily on diagnostic imaging, particularly radiography. Thoracic radiographs are used to verify suspected disease, identify the extent and location of the lesion, detect additional complicating abnormalities, plot the course of the disease, and select further alternative imaging procedures. However, thoracic radiographs have limitations. Diagnostic information may be limited by poor radiographic quality, an uncooperative patient, reader inexperience, and improper assimilation of the radiographic findings with the clinical picture. Furthermore, radiographic findings are rarely disease specific. Although the final radiographic diagnosis may be equivocal, a working list of potential differential diagnoses can often be established from the radiographs. The primary clinical diagnosis is rarely based on the radiographic findings; radiographic abnormalities must be integrated with clinical history, physical examination results, and laboratory data.

Radiographs often supply early, critical diagnostic information, and because of financial limitations, may be the only imaging study performed. The goal is to optimize the diagnostic value of thoracic radiographs: that is, to obtain the most information while reducing interpretive errors. This information must be gathered and analyzed in a timely and accurate fashion. Complete elimination of error is impossible, but by understanding the influence of technical factors and human perceptual and cognitive factors, errors can be reduced.

Alternative imaging modalities, principally ultrasonography and computed tomography, are now available to supplement information provided by thoracic radiographs. The radiographic findings and specifics of the additional information needed are used to select the most appropriate alternative imaging modalities. The ability of fluoroscopy, ultrasonography, and computed tomography to answer further diagnostic questions requires an understanding of each modality's indications and limitations.

Thoracic radiographic imaging abnormalities are typically organized in the literature using a structure-by-structure approach. Effective use of this presentation method in other textbooks obviates the need to repeat the format. The aims of this chapter are to convey the methods used to maximize the gathering of thoracic radiographic information and to minimize interpretive error by understanding the sources of diagnostic error. Finally the indications, limitations, and findings of thoracic fluoroscopy, ultrasonography, and computed tomography will be addressed.

Optimizing Thoracic Radiographic Information

OPTIMIZING RADIOGRAPHIC QUALITY

High quality thoracic radiographs are necessary for lesion detection and accurate diagnoses. Because many factors influence the quality of individual radiographic projections, it is important to develop criteria to determine whether particular images are of sufficient quality to provide a diagnosis. When radiographic quality is substandard, the radiographic views should be repeated. The inconvenience and cost associated with retaking radiographs will be compensated for by improved diagnostic quality. The major factors directly influencing diagnostic quality are exposure, detail, contrast, and patient positioning.

Radiographic Exposure

The optimal degree of film blackness on a thoracic radiograph can be measured objectively, but subjectively varies widely among observers. Objectively, there is a useful range of "optical density" (i.e., 0.25 to 2.0 OD with optimum around 1.0 OD) for ideal viewing on a standard radiographic illuminator.[1] Subjectively, it is more important to achieve a consistent and therefore familiar appearance of the thoracic structures. This allows for more accurate comparisons over time and helps minimize the tendency for false positives or negatives because of inability to perceive lesions.

The wide range of tissue densities in the thorax makes it difficult to choose a single radiographic technique that optimizes visualization of all structures. Adequate exposure of all areas of the thorax in some patients may require two identical views using different radiographic techniques. For a routine thoracic radiograph, adequate x-ray penetration and subsequent film exposure should be sufficient to reveal structures in the most tissue-dense portions of the thorax using a standard illuminator (viewbox). On the lateral views, this typically means being able to see the thoracic vertebral dorsal spinous processes superimposed on the scapulae (Figure 12-1), and on the VD/DV view, being able to see the vertebral bodies superimposed on the heart base. Unfortunately, adequate film density in these regions results in a relative overexposure of the peripheral lung fields, necessitating the use of a bright light for evaluation. Some exposure balance in these areas of disparate thoracic tissue density (e.g., heart base versus peripheral lung field) can be achieved by using a higher kVp (relative to mAs) radiographic technique.[2] The resultant radiograph will have the longer gray-scale (lower contrast) needed for viewbox evaluation. The cranial abdomen is included on thoracic radiographs, but the relative underexposure of this region will hamper evaluation.

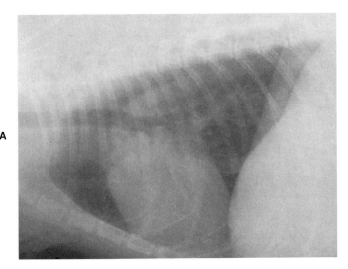 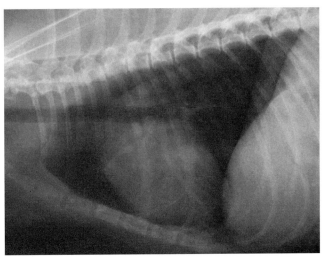

A   B

Figure 12-1. *Two left lateral recumbent thoracic radiographs of the same dog obtained using different exposure settings. **A,** Underexposed view obtained at 2.5 mAs and 72 kVp. The dorsal spinous processes of the cranial thoracic vertebra are not visible because of inadequate x-ray penetration of the thicker shoulder region. The pulmonary parenchyma appears more radiopaque than normal because of the relative underexposure. **B,** Properly exposed view obtained at 6.0 mAs and 76 kVp. The cranial thoracic vertebral dorsal spinous processes are visible. The pulmonary parenchyma is normal with the pulmonary vessels clearly visible contrasting with the radiolucent pulmonary parenchyma. Complete evaluation of the pulmonary parenchyma, especially the cranioventral lung field, requires using a bright light or device to limit extraneous viewbox light.*

Radiographic Detail

Thoracic radiographs with high detail greatly enhance diagnostic accuracy. High detail thoracic radiographs typically would require using slow speed film-screen systems. These high detail film-screen systems require longer exposure times for adequate film density, and the resultant detail may be compromised by respiratory motion. Hence, thoracic radiographic detail is a compromise: obtain a radiograph of adequate detail required for a diagnosis while eliminating motion unsharpness. Respiratory motion during the radiographic exposure is unavoidable, but shortening the exposure time and slowing or pausing the patient's respiratory motion during the exposure can minimize motion.

Exposure time determines the duration of x-ray production. The total quantity of x-ray photons produced is proportional to the product of x-ray tube current (milliamperes or mA) and time (seconds).[3] The product, milliampere-seconds (mAs), represents the quantity or number of x-ray photons produced during a radiographic exposure. Therefore, the easiest way to decrease exposure time while maintaining optimal film blackness is to proportionally increase the current. If the exposure time is halved, the current must be doubled to maintain the same mAs. Because of this inverse relationship, the highest current setting available (mA) is usually used during small animal thoracic radiography.

Milliampere-seconds, and therefore exposure time, can be further reduced if there is a comparable increase in kilovoltage peak (kVp). If the energy of the x-ray photons (kVp) is increased, each photon has a greater chance of passing through the patient and contributing to the radiographic density. Relatively small changes in kVp can reduce the mAs required to produce an optimal image. The "16% to 20% rule" is a helpful radiographic principle used to further reduce exposure time when motion unsharpness results from patients that are panting or have rapid respiratory rates.[4] If the exposure time is cut by 50%, the resulting loss of radiographic density by the 50% reduction in mAs can be compensated for by a 16% to 20% increase in kVp. The radiograph will have the same optical density at half the original exposure time.

Several techniques can be used to pause or slow a patient's breathing. Positive pressure ventilation (end inspiration) is preferred in anesthetized patients, but should be of short duration to prevent interference with cardiac return. Narcotics or sedatives that produce panting should be avoided before thoracic radiography. In conscious patients, simply startling them by blowing on the face or calling their name is sometimes sufficient to produce respiratory pauses long enough for an exposure.

Radiographic Contrast

Lesion conspicuity is defined as a ratio between the lesion contrast and the surround complexity in the image.[5] Because the surround complexity includes factors such as the patient's anatomy, the location of a lesion, and the presence of pathology, these factors are inherently constant during a radiographic procedure. Improving lesion conspicuity, especially for lesions in complex regions, therefore relies on enhancing lesion contrast. Image contrast can be improved by choosing the appropriate film-screen combination and radiographic technique, but it can be adversely affected by unwanted film exposure (fog).

The ability of a particular radiographic film to enhance image contrast is defined by its characteristic curve (also known as the "H&D curve").[3] When the slope of this curve is greater than one, image contrast is enhanced. However, there is a practical limit to this feature because very high contrast film tends to have a limited dynamic range and less exposure latitude (i.e., small changes in exposure setting result in over- or underexposure). In general, film should be selected based on balancing the reciprocal relationship between improved contrast and limited latitude or dynamic range. This balance varies depending on patient type, the training and skill of the radiographic technician, the x-ray machine used, and the preferences of the image interpreters.

Radiographic techniques using relatively high mAs and low kVp settings accentuate subject contrast (Figure 12-2). However, in human medicine, studies have shown that high kVp techniques tend to increase diagnostic accuracy.[2] The authors hypothesized that diagnostic improvements from the high kVp technique occurred when lower structural complexity outweighed the reduction in lesion contrast. The added advantage of higher thoracic kVp techniques is greater exposure latitude, so thoracic radiographs are typically obtained using medium to high kVp techniques.

Unintended film density, or fog, significantly reduces the image contrast by causing the "white" parts of the image to appear gray. Fog can result from film exposure to light, heat, pressure, or humidity. Maintaining image contrast and minimizing fog requires attention to proper film handling, storage, and processing. Film boxes should be stored side-by-side like books rather than stacked flat. If stacked flat, film in the bottom boxes of a stack will be fogged due to prolonged pressure by the weight of the rest of the film. Darkroom safelights using excessive bulb wattage or mounted too near the work surface will cause light fog as the films are handled. To minimize chemical fog, automatic film processors or manual wet tanks must be properly maintained to ensure proper chemical strength, temperature, and film transport.

Film fog and reduced image contrast are also caused by scatter radiation. Scatter radiation results from redirection of the x-ray energy in the patient. If the redirected x-ray photon strikes the image receptor, the information from that photon does not represent the attenuation characteristics of the patient.[1] These photons contribute to an almost constant background fog level on the film images. The two main defenses against scatter radiation are x-ray beam collimation (discussed later) and use of a grid. The grid is placed between the patient and the cassette to eliminate photons that are not traveling parallel with the primary beam. It consists of a series of lead strips and spacers that allow only photons traveling in a straight line between the focal spot and the film to pass through. Scattered photons are absorbed by the lead. Using grids during thoracic radi-

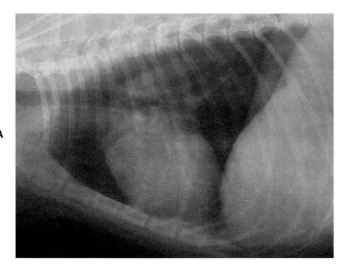

A

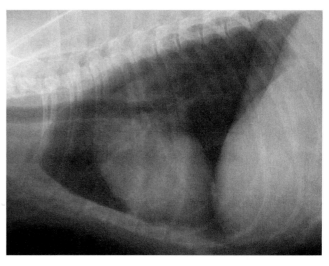

B

*Figure 12-2. Left lateral recumbent thoracic radiographs of the same dog obtained using different exposure settings to alter radiographic contrast. **A,** Higher mAs (4.0) and lower kVp (76) technique enhances subject contrast resulting in a radiograph with higher, or short-scale, contrast. The spine, ribs, and pulmonary vessels stand out against the pulmonary parenchyma causing the radiograph to appear more crisp and sharp. **B,** Lower mAs (2.0) and higher kVp (95) technique results in a radiograph with lower, or long-scale, contrast. The pulmonary vessels are still visible, but the pulmonary parenchyma appears slightly more radiopaque. The ribs are not as apparent superimposed on the pulmonary parenchyma.*

ography of most veterinary patients reduces the adverse effects of scatter radiation on image quality. Grid ratio is the height of the lead strips in the device to the space between them.[6] Typical grid ratios are 8:1 or 10:1. Grids with very high ratios (i.e., greater than 12:1) require greatly increased mAs during the radiographic exposure, which increases motion unsharpness; therefore their use may be counterproductive.

Patient Positioning

The diagnostic value of the thoracic radiograph is highly dependent on proper positioning of the patient during the radiographic procedure. Patient rotation adversely affects the radiographic appearance of normal thoracic structures, and thoracic limb superimposition hampers evaluation of the cranial mediastinum and lung lobes. An appreciation of normal anatomic variation is only gained by routinely reviewing thoracic views of symmetrically positioned patients. However, when the patient is rotated, the radiographic appearance of structures varies from normal and presents an interpretation dilemma for the inexperienced reader: Does the abnormal appearance represent a true abnormality or an artifact of malpositioning? For example, patient rotation on the lateral recumbent radiograph result in apparent tracheal elevation and splitting of the mainstem bronchi. The reader may erroneously conclude that cardiomegaly, particularly of the left atrium, is present. Patient rotation on either the VD or DV view often alters the appearance of the cardiac silhouette leading to the false impression of cardiomegaly.[7,8]

Symmetrically positioning the patient with the thoracic limbs pulled cranially reduces superimposition of soft tissue on the cranial mediastinum and cranial lung lobes. Superimposition of the limbs increases the overall opacity and reduces lesion contrast in this region, resulting in possible missed pulmonary nodules or overinterpretation of pulmonary parenchymal disease. The head should also be held in a neutral position to straighten the fixed tracheal length. If the head and neck are positioned ventrally, the trachea may deviate dorsally in the cranial mediastinum during expiration, creating the illusion of a cranial mediastinal mass.

Lesions in areas excluded from the radiograph cannot be detected. Readers must make an effort to note whether the entire thorax is included on the radiograph. Positioning and collimation errors typically result in exclusion of the thoracic inlet region or lumbophrenic angles on the lateral thoracic view, and costophrenic angles and lung apices on the ventrodorsal/dorsoventral view. On the other hand, unnecessary scatter radiation can be produced from extraneous structures that are included in the primary beam. Because this reduces image contrast, every effort should be made to limit the image to only the thorax.

Collimation

Image quality is adversely affected by lack of primary x-ray beam collimation. In all radiographic projections, the primary beam should be limited to the body part of interest. Collimating the primary beam reduces scatter (secondary) radiation by preventing photon interaction with structures beyond the region of interest.[1] The volume of tissue irradiated by the primary beam largely determines the amount of scatter radiation. Because the patient cannot be made thinner, limiting the primary beam area is the only realistic measure used to reduce scatter radiation. Scatter radiation contributes to overall film density and reduces image contrast.[1] In digital imaging, scatter radiation increases image noise. Using a grid in conjunction with a properly collimated primary beam can further reduce the adverse effects of scatter radiation on image quality.

Respiratory Phase

The phase of the respiratory cycle during which the radiograph is obtained directly influences radiographic quality. To prevent interpretive errors associated with an inappropriate respiratory phase, the reader must be able to differentiate inspiration from expiration on radiographs (Figure 12-3). Some useful characteristics of inspiration on the lateral projection are that the cranial borders of the lung lobes are even with, or cranial to, the first rib, and the lumbophrenic angles are caudal to T12. On an inspiratory VD projection, the diaphragmatic cupola is usually caudal to the eighth thoracic vertebra and the costophrenic angles are caudal to the tenth rib.[9]

Standard thoracic radiographs are made with the patient in full inspiration so that the lungs are inflated and radiolucent. Full inspiratory phase views will maximize the contrast between normal radiolucent lung parenchyma and any suspected radiopaque pulmonary abnormalities (e.g., bronchopneumonia, pulmonary nodules). In an expiratory phase view, the pulmonary parenchyma will appear slightly radiopaque and pulmonary vascular detail will decrease. By failing to recognize an expiratory phase

radiograph, the reader may conclude that an interstitial pattern representing pulmonary pathology is present.[9] Expiratory phase radiographs also may result in the false interpretation of cardiomegaly. The cardiothoracic ratio is a subjective radiographic measure of the portion of the thoracic cavity area occupied by the cardiac silhouette area. After becoming accustomed to evaluating inspiratory phase radiographs, the smaller thoracic cavity volume characteristic of an expiratory phase radiograph may cause the cardiac silhouette to falsely appear larger than normal.

On occasion, an expiratory phase radiograph is indicated when contrast between radiopaque, partially inflated lung parenchyma and a suspected radiolucent abnormality (e.g., a pulmonary bulla) is desired. Expiratory phase thoracic views are also more sensitive for detecting the presence of a pneumothorax.[10]

OPTIMIZING RADIOGRAPHIC INTERPRETATION

Once high quality thoracic radiographs are obtained, diagnostic interpretation can proceed. The viewing environment, access to important clinical history, lesion conspicuity, reader experience, and reader frame of mind all affect radiographic interpretation and account for most missed diagnoses. The greatest sources of interpretation error arise from human perceptual and cognitive limits. Perceptual error accounts for approximately 40% of total error; of this, 10% is caused by sampling errors (i.e., improper search methods) and 30% is caused by recognition errors.[11,12] The remaining 60% of errors are caused by cognitive limitations, otherwise classified as decision error.[11] Although total error elimination is impossible, understanding error sources and adhering to accepted tenets of radiographic interpretation can reduce error to an acceptable level.

A
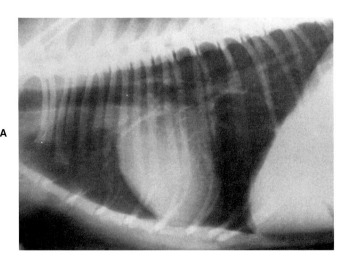

B
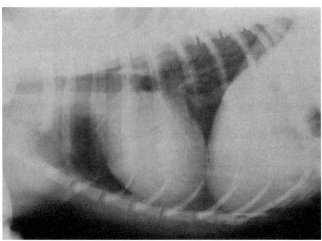

Figure 12-3. Left lateral recumbent thoracic radiographs obtained at maximum inspiratory and expiratory phases of the respiratory cycle. **A,** Separation between the caudal heart and diaphragmatic border, caudally located lumbophrenic angles, cranial lung borders extending beyond the first rib, normal cardiothoracic ratio, and normal radiolucent lungs are seen in an inspiratory phase view. **B,** In an expiratory phase view, the caudal heart and diaphragmatic border overlap, the lumbophrenic angles are cranially located, the heart appears large in relation to the thorax, and the lungs appear more radiopaque.

The inherent complexity of thoracic radiographs and viewing conditions directly impact the reader's ability to recognize abnormalities. Research has shown that optical scattering from background illumination through low density areas of a thoracic radiograph (e.g., cardiac silhouette), light from adjacent unused illuminated view panels, light leakage around films, and ambient room light all decrease the reader's ability to detect small, low contrast objects on the radiograph.[13] The decrease in contrast sensitivity occurs because retinal photoreceptor cells are desensitized by optical scattering from the extraneous light.[14] Procedures to enhance viewing conditions and thereby contribute to reduced reader error will be discussed in the next section.

Sources of Interpretive Error

Radiographic reading can be divided into three phases: search, recognition, and decision. Sources of error arise from all three phases. Factors that influence the amount of total error include reader experience, available clinical history, presence of native abnormalities, lesion conspicuity (e.g., contrast, size, and structural complexity), knowledge of disease prevalence in the population, consequences of an incorrect decision, and timing of the radiographic procedure.

Search. Studies of human thoracic radiographic search error indicate that 10% to 20% of the lung fields are not covered by the reader's high-resolution vision.[12] The high-resolution portion of the visual field consists of the central retina, called the fovea, and an area immediately adjacent to the fovea extending out about 6 degrees.[11] The fovea measures about the size of the thumb nail at arms length; visual acuity beyond the fovea is approximately 60% of that of the central fovea.[11] Because the entire radiographic image is not searched with high-resolution vision, peripheral visual input and rapid eye movements are two mechanisms compensating for the steep decline in visual acuity beyond the central region. Although important in the overall scheme of the search, detection of abnormalities from peripheral input is far less accurate. Detection accuracy of pulmonary nodules was one half when the nodule was 5 degrees from the axis of gaze.[15] Other studies have shown that one third of missed pulmonary nodules are not included within a useful field of view sufficient to detect the nodule 90% of the time (considered scanning errors).[11] Problems with rapid eye movements will be discussed later, but despite these compensatory mechanisms, search errors still account for 10% of perceptual and cognitive errors.[12]

The radiographic search process has been shown to prematurely end with the detection of native, or unrelated, abnormalities.[16] Satisfaction of search (SOS) describes a phenomenon in which the detection of one abnormality interferes with the detection of other abnormalities on the same radiograph. SOS can be caused by both early termination of search and by inappropriate allocation of visual attention and is dependent on the number and nature of the native abnormalities in the image. Decreased vigilance has been shown to cause SOS and supports the hypothesis that premature halt of search causes SOS.[16] Premature halt of search has been concluded not to be a sampling problem. Ninety percent of missed nodules on human thoracic radiographs containing a native abnormality were fixated and received prolonged visual attention but were not reported and therefore represented a decision error.[16] SOS can work in both directions: pulmonary nodules can be detected at the expense of finding native abnormalities, and vice versa.[16]

Controversy exists whether knowledge of the clinical history affects SOS. Although some studies have found no substantial SOS effect in the presence of an appropriate clinical history, others have shown that knowledge of the clinical history had an important effect on the detection of unexpected abnormalities, which seemed to nullify the SOS phenomenon.[16,17]

Recognition. The radiograph is searched with the high-resolution visual region, modified with peripheral inputs and rapid eye movements. The reader's eye quickly darts over the radiograph, fixating on structures for 300 milliseconds or less. Recognition errors arise when a lesion is fixated on by the reader's eye, but the lesion is not recognized and reported. For example, in a study exploring pulmonary nodule detection on human chest radiographs, approximately one-third of nodules were fixated by the reader but not recognized.[11] The probability of nodule detection during a single fixation is determined by the fundamental nodule-surrounding relationship and a covert decision-making function.[11] The fundamental nodule-surrounding relationship is also referred to as lesion conspicuity, which can be quantified as the lesion contrast/surrounding complexity.[5] Lesion contrast is the joint property of the lesion and surrounding tissue; normal background anatomic structures contribute to surrounding complexity. It is often unclear whether the failure to report a lesion is a covert decision not to perceive (recognition error), or the lesion is perceived and there is an overt decision not to report. This uncertainty blurs the boundary between perception and cognition.[11]

Decision. Roughly one task-related decision is made during each second of radiograph scanning.[18] Decision error accounts for the most prevalent type of error (as much as 60%) in reviewing a radiograph.[12] For example, a pulmonary nodule may receive prolonged fixations for several seconds, even comparison fixations on the contralateral lung field, indicating increased visual scrutiny, but the nodule is not reported. In this case the nodule is perceived but the outcome is an overt decision not to report.[11] Each fixation cluster is considered a decision, but the viewer is not aware of the decision made during the scanning—the lingering eye movements provide evidence of perception and indirect evidence of a covert decision.[12] In these instances, the viewer is deciding whether the camouflaged object is a true lesion or a normal anatomical variant. In eye motion studies of radiographic viewing, visual dwelling indicated the location of false-positive and false-negative decisions.[19] Ninety percent of false-positive decisions were caused by some perturbation in the image that aroused the suspicion of the viewer. Most false-negative nodules also received prolonged visual attention, implying an active decision not to report the nodule.

Methods to Overcome Interpretive Errors

These perceptual and cognitive errors in part explain why at least 30% of all pulmonary nodules on human chest radiographs are missed on the initial reading by competent radiologists.[20] To reduce reader error, either the lesion must be made more apparent on the radiograph, or the reader must become better at lesion perception and decision-making. Technical methods of enhancing lesion conspicuity are dealt with in other sections of this chapter. Methods to overcome perceptual and cognitive deficits concentrate on efforts to enhance the reading environment and altering viewing search methods to mitigate reader inexperience.

Viewing Conditions. First, several simple recommendations can be made concerning viewing conditions. All views taken in the study should be hung on viewing panels at the same time; this requires a sufficient number of panels in the viewer. A bright light or hot light with adjustable illumination levels should be available. Because of the wide range of film density on a thorax radiograph, overexposed areas are inevitable and are effectively examined only with a bright light. Extraneous light in the viewing area should be reduced. Ambient room lights should be dimmed or turned off. Adjacent, unused viewer panels should be turned off, and light escaping around films should be masked. Improved reader performance has been documented when only the radiograph was illuminated and adjacent viewing areas were masked.[21] Performance slightly decreased when adjacent viewing panel lights were off and covered with chest radiographs or illuminated and covered with chest radiographs. Convenient viewing masking tools can be made to block extraneous light. A darkened sheet of exposed, processed x-ray film with a 15-cm hole cut in the middle, or simply a black film rolled into a tube through which the radiologist views the film are effective.[21] The radiographic reading area should be quiet, allowing the reader to concentrate on interpretation with minimal distractions.

Search Methods. The experience level of the reader determines the manner in which the radiograph is searched and interpreted. As previously mentioned, only portions of the radiograph are searched using the high-resolution visual region. Experimental evidence suggests that experienced radiologists perceive abnormalities using a global approach in which perception results from rapid parallel processing of the entire retinal image.[22] Studies have shown that radiologists' eye movements fixate on abnormal regions on thoracic radiographs within the first few seconds of viewing, indicating that they perceive most abnormalities directly without first identifying distinctive features.[23] Feature analysis is reserved for difficult cases, but is also used extensively in teaching radiographic pattern recognition. Successful global analysis of the radiograph relies heavily on the reader satisfying a visual concept. This theory describes the relations between the visual data derived from the retina and remembered generalizations about the meaning of similar data.[24] In other words, it may be necessary to have seen similar abnormalities in the past, so as to form an appropriate vi-

sual concept for the current abnormality.[25] Incorrect diagnoses may therefore arise from lack of experience. Experienced radiologists follow global analysis with discovery scanning. The latter phase occurs by efficient scanning of the remaining image and is controlled by vigilance for unexpected abnormalities.[16]

In a study measuring interobserver performance in reading chest radiographs, board-certified radiologists as a group demonstrated a higher level of diagnostic accuracy than either radiology residents or nonradiologist physicians.[26] Even among experienced radiologists, however, there was substantial performance variability in interpreting a standardized set of chest radiographs. The highest performing radiologists demonstrated less variability in the interpretation of normal radiographs relative to abnormal radiographs than did their counterparts. Furthermore, the top-performing radiologists were more confident in their interpretations than were their peers. Although it is commonly assumed that radiologists are better visual analyzers than a majority of their colleagues, studies have shown that radiologists do not possess superior visual and analysis skills compared with lay people when it comes to searching art pictures for hidden targets.[27]

For the inexperienced reader, the thoracic radiograph represents an assortment of incomprehensible gray shadows and borders, which are often incorrectly assimilated into phantom structures. Only after familiarity with the thoracic radiographic appearance is the reader able to comprehend the visual cues of size, shape, opacity, location, and distortion. To overcome inexperience, novices must rely on a more analytical, systematic, and focused search pattern rather than the quicker, global visual search employed by experienced radiologists. Inexperienced readers should thoroughly examine the thoracic radiograph by dividing the thorax into five structural categories: extrathoracic, mediastinum, pleura, cardiac, and pulmonary. This search method promotes a systematic review of important thoracic structural categories in hopes of reducing sampling error. The systematic, analytic search pattern will break down without discipline, but it also should gradually disappear with experience.

Because studies of the effect of clinical history on search patterns have produced conflicting results, it is difficult to make concrete recommendations. It is probably advisable to initially view the thoracic radiographs without knowledge of the clinical history. Unbiased review should result in a more thorough search of the entire radiograph and a more complete differential diagnosis list for the found abnormality. A review of the radiograph following assimilation of the clinical history may then result in a more focused search, similar to the discovery scanning phase, with increased vigilance for the suspected abnormality. Detection of multiple abnormalities should not result in satisfaction of search (SOS). Override the tendency to halt the search once an abnormality is detected, and do not permit one abnormality to capture all the visual attention.

An effective strategy aimed at decreasing reader search error is dual, or multiple readings of the same image.[11] The radiographic study is viewed twice at different times. The dual reading is best performed by two different readers; it is less effective if the radiograph is read by the same reader at two different times. Multiple readings increase personnel costs, and the method only works if a system has been devised to deal with reader disagreement. The simplest, least expensive, but least effective method if disagreement occurs is to either "believe the positive" or "believe the negative." The most effective method for optimizing multiple reading performance is arbitration, where a third party resolves the difference between the two primary readers.

INCREASING DIAGNOSTIC ACCURACY

Proper viewing conditions and search patterns improve recognition of radiographic abnormalities. Making correct diagnostic decisions relies on recognizing common radiographic signs and realizing the value of additional positional views.

Conspicuity

Despite the best intentions to improve radiographic quality and minimize sources of reader error, thoracic radiographic lesions may escape detection because of lack of lesion visibility. Lesion invisibility may be caused by insufficient lesion size (e.g., the lesion falls below the detection threshold of the film-screen system), insufficient lesion contrast with the surrounding tissue, or superimposition of the lesion on complex normal structures. For instance, the visibility of a nodule on a chest film depends not only on the physical properties of the lesion such as size, shape, and density, but also on the properties of the surrounding tissue. The quantitative measure, conspicuity, was developed to explore the relationship between the probability of nodule detection on thoracic radiographs and the complexity of normal structures that surround the nodule.[5] The concept of conspicuity was originally devised to describe the effect of random and structural noise on the detection of targets by peripheral vision; this measure was found to correlate well with the probability of detecting faint nodules on thoracic radiographs.[5] Conspicuity is defined as the ratio of lesion contrast and surrounding tissue complexity. This mathematical formula is valid only for circumscribed lesions, in which the border is either definitely identified or extrapolated with a high level of confidence. The term conspicuity is now commonly used in a broad sense to describe abnormalities that become visible when their size, shape, or density becomes sufficient to overwhelm the complexity of the surrounding structures.

For example, metastatic pulmonary nodules only become apparent when their size and density is sufficient for detection. The visibility limit of soft tissue nodules in human lungs is generally regarded to be about 3 mm because the resolution of the film-screen system is insufficient to detect smaller nodules.[11] Yet many lung cancers in humans are rarely detected until nodules are 8 to 10 mm in diameter because there are many "noise" nodules between 3 and 10 mm in diameter.[11,28] Two factors

probably influence the reader's decision not to report smaller (less than 10 mm) nodules: the prevalence of cancer in the population and the consequences of a false positive decision.[28] The reader is believed to perceive these nodular-like structures but is unwilling to report a nodule for fear of making too many false-positive reports. When strict decision criteria are applied, the toll of false-negative results is accepted. For example, given a disease prevalence of 5%, a size threshold criterion of at least 8 mm must be used to achieve a predictive value of 90% (i.e., to be correct 90% of the time in calling a nodule positive).[28] Although the precise prevalence of disease may not be known, the reader actually takes into account the signalment, history, and clinical signs when examining the radiographs.

Many other lesions in the thorax do not become visible until they reach sufficient size, radiopacity, or volume to become conspicuous. The ability to perceive these lesions may be enhanced by certain radiographic positional views. For example, small volumes of pleural effusion remain radiographically undetected until a threshold volume has been exceeded. Results from studies using experimental hydrothorax indicated that in both the VD and lateral recumbent views, the presence of 100 ml of fluid was visible in a medium-sized dog.[29] In the lateral recumbent view, fluid accumulated dorsal to the sternum, forming a scalloped border as the lung lobes retracted from the thoracic wall. Rounding of the costophrenic angles and widening of the interlobar fissures, particularly along the caudoventral mediastinal reflection, occurred on the VD view. As little as 50 ml of pleural fluid in a 15-kg dog was detected on the erect, VD horizontal beam view; widening of the caudoventral mediastinal reflection and rounding of the costophrenic angles occurred.

Similar to experimental induction of hydrothorax, experimental injection of air into the pleural space caused a radiographically apparent pneumothorax when 5 mls/kg was injected.[10] Although the study was not designed to determine the threshold limit for detecting pneumothorax, certain radiographic views were better for detecting pneumothorax. The left lateral recumbent view and horizontal beam VD view made during expiration were the most sensitive views for detecting pneumothorax; of these two views, the expiratory, horizontal beam VD was better. In general, expiratory views were superior to inspiratory views for detecting pneumothorax because the lungs became more opaque and contrasted with the free pleural air on the expiratory views.[10]

RECOGNIZING COMMON RADIOGRAPHIC SIGNS

Air Bronchograms

Air bronchograms are one of the characteristics of an alveolar pulmonary pattern and occur when the alveoli are either filled with fluid or collapse. The more rigid bronchi remain air-filled against the soft tissue opacity of the lung (Figure 12-4). It is important to recognize arborization of the bronchi to confirm a true air bron-

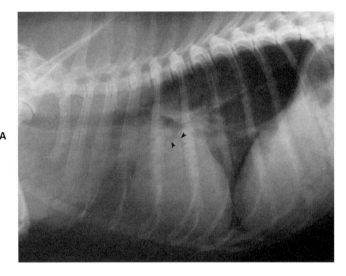

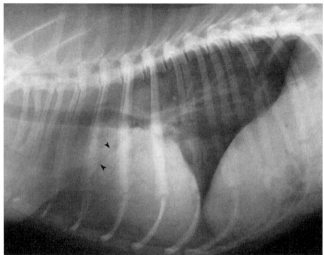

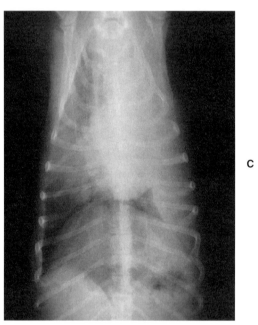

Figure 12-4. *Three thoracic radiographic views of a Jack Russell Terrier with pulmonary hemorrhage caused by rodenticide poisoning. **A,** On the right lateral recumbent view there is an alveolar pulmonary pattern involving the left cranial lung lobe with a visible air bronchogram (arrowheads). There is a silhouette sign of the cranial heart border caused in part by the left cranial lobe consolidation. **B,** The air bronchogram (arrowheads) on the left lateral recumbent view is compatible with an alveolar pattern involving the right cranial lung lobe that is contributing to the silhouette sign of the cranial heart border. **C,** On the ventrodorsal view, there is a uniform soft tissue radiopacity of the left cranial and caudal lung lobes and a silhouette sign of the left heart border. Both radiographic signs are compatible with an alveolar pulmonary pattern. The alveolar pattern of the right cranial and middle lung lobes is less severe than that involving the left lung lobes.*

chogram. Because air bronchograms are caused by air-filled bronchi, they are unique to the pulmonary parenchyma and can be used to establish pulmonary involvement in a soft tissue opacity.[29,30] Atelectasis, pneumonia, severe pulmonary hemorrhage, and severe pulmonary edema can all result in an alveolar pulmonary pattern and air bronchograms.

Silhouette Sign

The silhouette sign is a traditional but confusing term used to describe effacement of the border of an object by an adjacent structure of similar radiographic opacity, such as would occur with alveolar pulmonary consolidation or a pulmonary mass (see Figure 12-4).[31] A true silhouette sign only occurs when the organs or structures creating the opacity are in contact with each other. For instance, the right cranial lung lobe contacts the cranial border of the heart more than does the left cranial lobe. Therefore, alveolar consolidation of the right cra-

nial lobe is more likely to result in a silhouette sign of the heart. Conversely, if there is cranioventral alveolar consolidation and no silhouette of the cranial heart border, the consolidation is more likely in the left cranial lobe. Similarly, a thoracic wall mass may be superimposed on the heart in the lateral view, but if the mass is not large enough to contact the heart, the heart borders will remain visible.

A silhouette sign in the thorax may result from soft tissue opacities other than pulmonary masses or alveolar consolidation. Pleural fluid will produce a silhouette sign when it is in contact with the heart or diaphragm; this is particularly evident on the DV view, where fluid will accumulate along the sternum and heart. Abdominal organs herniating through the diaphragm can also cause a silhouette sign with either the heart or the diaphragm. Pleural effusion often accompanies a diaphragmatic rupture, and this fluid will cause a silhouette sign with the herniated abdominal organs, heart, and diaphragm.

Tracheal Stripe

The tracheal stripe sign becomes evident when an air-filled megaesophagus is present. Also called an esophageal stripe sign, the tracheal stripe refers to a thick soft tissue band produced by the summation of the ventral esophageal wall with the dorsal tracheal wall.[32] The ventral esophageal wall becomes evident when the esophageal lumen fills with air. Although the tracheal stripe sign is most evident with an air-filled megaesophagus, short segments of a tracheal stripe can be seen if the cranial thoracic esophagus is partially filled with air because of aerophagia.

Extrapleural Sign

Extrapleural lesions arise from structures outside the parietal or mediastinal pleura and therefore include masses originating from the thoracic wall, diaphragm, and mediastinum. Radiographically, the extrapleural sign, denoting an extrapleural mass, is characterized by a uniform convex radiopacity protruding into the thorax.[29] The broad base of the opacity is oriented towards the parietal pleura; the protruding edge of the radiopacity is typically well delineated and tapers evenly on either side with the normal parietal pleura. Although appearing similar to an extrapleural mass, the edge of a peripheral pulmonary soft tissue mass fails to taper evenly with the parietal pleura. Pulmonary masses and consolidations can be further differentiated from pleural masses by the presence of air bronchograms in areas of pulmonary consolidation.[29]

POSITIONAL RADIOGRAPHY

Manipulating the position of the patient and the radiographic beam to improve visualization of lesions and abnormalities may maximize the diagnostic information provided by a radiographic study. The standard patient positions used in thoracic radiography include right lateral, left lateral, dorsal, and ventral recumbency. In addition to changing the position of the patient, the vertical x-ray beam can be reoriented in a horizontal direction to further exploit the physiologic response of the patient.

One general rule-of-thumb for selecting the position of the patient for a radiographic procedure is that the lesion should be placed as close as possible to the cassette. This minimizes the lesion-to-film distance and the geometric unsharpness caused by magnification.[33] However, the opposite rule applies if the lesion is in the lungs. It has been shown that lesions in the lungs of dogs are more difficult to detect when the affected lung is placed in a dependent position (i.e., closer to the cassette).[34]

Selecting Right Versus Left Lateral Recumbency

Selecting the appropriate patient position for the lateral radiographic view depends on the location of the expected lesion. Because an effort should be made to position the patient with the lesion in the nondependent lung, a careful physical examination before the radiographic procedure is important. If auscultation reveals abnormalities in particular lung lobes or thoracic quadrants, the patient should be positioned so that the more normal side is down on the x-ray machine table. If no abnormalities are detected on the physical examination to indicate the location of pulmonary abnormalities, then it is often appropriate to obtain both lateral radiographs to ensure greater diagnostic sensitivity. It has been shown in dogs that the most sensitive projection for detecting pulmonary metastasis is the right lateral recumbent position.[35] Furthermore, both the right and left lateral recumbent position radiographs were more sensitive than the ventrodorsal radiograph.[35]

Selecting Dorsal Versus Ventral Recumbency

It has become commonplace to obtain both right and left lateral radiographs in thoracic studies, and the ventrodorsal radiograph is also a staple. Realizing the advantages and disadvantages of the ventrodorsal and dorsoventral views may help the clinician more carefully select the appropriate projections for a given situation.

Dorsoventral radiographs result in easier identification and evaluation of the caudal pulmonary arteries in dogs; this can be especially useful in cases of cardiopulmonary disease. However, compared with the ventrodorsal projection, the craniocaudal axis of the heart appears shorter, the relationship between the spine and the cardiac silhouette is more variable, and less of the accessory lung lobe is visible on the dorsoventral view.[36] In cats, differences between ventrodorsal or dorsoventral radiographs are much less dramatic.[37]

When pleural fluid is present, patient position influences the location of the fluid within the thorax. A loss of radiographically detectable borders (silhouette sign) is seen when the heart, mediastinal structures, and pulmonary lesions are submersed in fluid (Figure 12-5). In this situation, placing the patient in dorsal recumbency (for a ventrodorsal radiograph) improves visualization of the heart and mediastinum. Therefore, when a pleural effusion is suspected, and the temperament and clinical status of the patient permits positioning in dorsal recumbency, a ventrodorsal projection is usually preferable.[38]

The Effects of Rotation on Radiographic Appearance

Patient rotation introduces significant additional variability to the appearance of normal structures on thoracic radiographs, and can confound even experienced observers. The effects of malpositioning are most evident during evaluation of the cardiac silhouette; greater than 5 degrees of rotation results in alteration of the size of the cardiac silhouette.[8] Patient rotation on the VD view of dogs can be assessed by evaluating the vertebral dorsal spinous processes; the processes should not project beyond the silhouette of the vertebral body.[7]

Tangential Versus En Face Lesion Evaluation

Some lesions may be more appropriately evaluated if the radiographic beam passes tangentially through the lesion, rather than en face through it. This technique is commonly used to detect rib proliferation or lysis

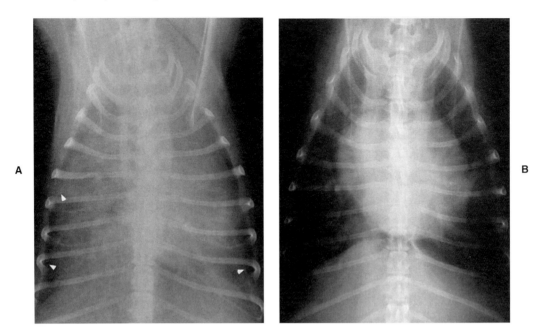

Figure 12-5. *Two thoracic radiographic views of a Shih Tzu with pleural effusion.* **A,** *Positioning the dog for a dorsoventral view causes the pleural effusion to accumulate in the ventral portion of the thorax. A silhouette sign of the cardiac border occurs as the pleural effusion surrounds the heart. Pleural effusion is also accumulating in the pleural fissures and separates the lung lobes (white arrowheads).* **B,** *Ventrodorsal view obtained following the dorsoventral view. The pleural effusion now gravitates to the dependent dorsal portion of the thorax, away from the heart, so that the cardiac silhouette becomes visible.*

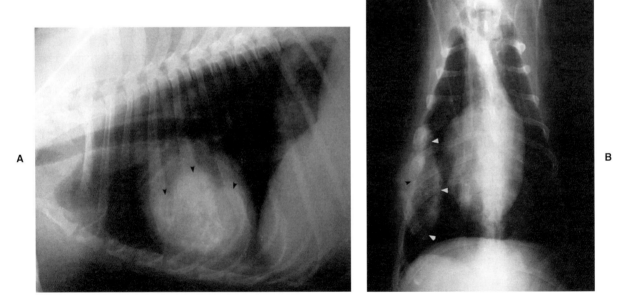

Figure 12-6. *Two thoracic radiographs of a golden retriever with osteosarcoma arising from the right fifth rib.* **A,** *A lobulated, mineralized mass (black arrowheads), superimposed on the cardiac silhouette, is seen on the left lateral recumbent view.* **B,** *The thoracic wall mass (white arrowheads) has caused an extrapleural sign, which is characterized by a broad-base along the thoracic wall, convex protrusion into the thoracic cavity, and evenly tapered edges with the normal thoracic wall. There is lysis of the right fifth rib associated with the mass (black arrowhead) and periosteal proliferation on the right fourth and sixth ribs.*

associated with an overlying thoracic wall soft tissue mass, or when evaluating the extent of trauma-associated rib fractures (Figure 12-6). Additional radiographs made at nonstandard intervals of rotation may be required to image certain lesions in tangent. The x-ray beam should also be collimated to reduce scatter and to maximize detail in the area of interest.

Horizontal Beam Techniques

On most x-ray machines, the x-ray beam can be oriented in a horizontal direction (parallel with the ground) instead of the typical vertical orientation used for radiographing small animals. Horizontal beam techniques take advantage of gravity to move organs, fluid, or air towards or away from the region of interest. Combination of a horizontal x-ray beam with atypical patient positions is used to detect fluid or air in the pleural space, or to move pleural fluid away from suspected masses. For example, a horizontal beam with the patient held vertical for a VD view can be used to move pleural effusion away from a suspected cranial mediastinal mass. If a pulmonary bulla is partially filled with fluid, a standing lateral, horizontal beam view will demonstrate a flat fluid-gas linear interface in the bulla. Thoracic wall lesions and pulmonary or pleural masses may be better viewed using the horizontal beam technique.

If a separate cassette holder with grid is not available for the horizontal beam view, the radiographic technique should be adjusted to account for the absence of a grid. In general, the focal-film distance used for horizontal beam radiography should remain the same as for vertical beam techniques (typically around 40 inches). Because many veterinary patients may not tolerate lengthy restraint (to allow fluid movement) in unusual positions, positional radiography has given way to other diagnostic modalities (e.g., ultrasound) to provide similar information.

Expiratory Views

Thoracic radiographs of small animals are typically made during inspiration. Because awake animals will not breath-hold, the degree of inspiration and thoracic inflation can vary. In certain abnormalities, however, intentional expiratory phase radiographs may actually improve lesion detection. The applicable concept is that lesion detection is markedly influenced by the contrast between the lesion and the background structures. Typically, lesions of interest within the lung are of soft tissue opacity; by reducing the opacity of the lung (inspiration), contrast between the pulmonary parenchyma and the lesion is increased. However, when the lesion of interest in the lung is a bulla or other relatively lucent lesion, increasing the opacity of the adjacent lungs theoretically increases lesion detectability. Therefore lesion density influences decisions on whether inspiratory or expiratory views should be obtained.

The physiological effect of the respiratory phase on the lesion of interest should also be considered. In cases of collapsing trachea, the width of the affected portion of the trachea may vary with respiratory phase. In these cases it may be appropriate to obtain both inspiratory and expiratory phase radiographs for comparison. In many cases where dynamic changes are seen in the appearance of structures based on physiologic processes, fluoroscopy is a more efficient modality to completely evaluate the entire respiratory cycle.

Fluoroscopy

Primarily because of equipment expense, the availability of fluoroscopy is essentially limited to large veterinary specialty and academic hospitals. The prime advantage of fluoroscopy is the added dimension of dynamic, real-time imaging that permits an assessment of function. Fluoroscopy is required for functional assessments of swallowing, esophageal motility, diaphragmatic excursions, respiratory motion, cardiac motion, and tracheal collapse.

Fluoroscopy can be used to help differentiate the origin of lesions (e.g., pleural, pulmonary, or mediastinal) and types of diaphragmatic hernias or ruptures. Interventional procedures (e.g., cardiac catheterization and aspiration or biopsy of thoracic masses) require fluoroscopy. Because of limited availability and greater use of alternative imaging modalities (i.e., ultrasound and CT), fluoroscopy is less often used to guide aspiration and biopsy procedures and to differentiate mass lesions of pleural, pulmonary, or mediastinal origin.

Cardiac catheterization procedures and evaluation of the tracheal diameter to detect evidence of tracheal collapse still require fluoroscopy. Although tracheal collapse may be suspected using expiratory and inspiratory phase lateral radiographs, confirmation of dynamic tracheal narrowing is best diagnosed with fluoroscopy (Figure 12-7). Tracheal lumen collapse often occurs at the thoracic inlet during inspiration, and the intrathoracic portion, immediately cranial to the carina, often collapses during expiration. If tracheal collapse is not obvious during normal breathing, dynamic collapse may become evident during active coughing.

Noncardiac Thoracic Ultrasonography

Thoracic imaging using ultrasonography was initially disregarded because it was widely believed that most thoracic structures would be inaccessible to ultrasound wave propagation. With greater operator experience, the important complementary role of ultrasonography with radiography in thoracic imaging is now realized. Ultrasonography will never replace the need for thoracic radiographs. First, the abnormality prompting the need for the ultrasound examination must be identified on the radiograph. The location of the abnormality is then used to focus the ultrasound examination to a specific area of the thorax. In order for thoracic ultrasonography to be effective, the normally aerated lung lobes must become

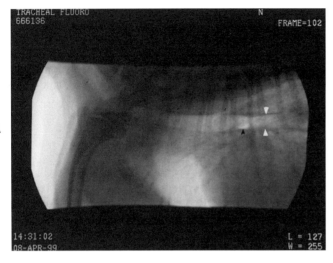 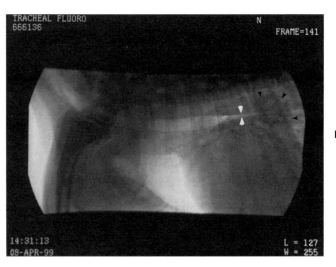

Figure 12-7. Lateral digital fluoroscopic images obtained of a miniature poodle presented for coughing. *A,* On the inspiratory phase image, the tracheal diameter is normal and the mainstem bronchus (white arrowheads), *caudal to the carina* (black arrowhead), *is open. B,* On the expiratory phase view, obtained during a slight cough, there is collapse of the mainstem bronchus (white arrowheads) *caused by left atrial enlargement* (black arrowheads) *secondary to chronic valvular disease.*

consolidated, collapsed, or displaced by a pleural effusion or mass. The lesion location determines whether the patient must be repositioned to take advantage of gravity's effect on a pleural effusion or a collapsed lung lobe. Imaging from the dependent portion of the thorax is occasionally required to create an acoustic window and visualize the lesion. Even with a mass or pleural effusion present, a majority of the thorax remains obscured by partially aerated lung. Thoracic scanning is usually done through the intercostal spaces, and transducers with a small contact area minimize artifacts created by the ribs. The highest frequency transducer allowing adequate depth penetration should be used. Although routine thoracic ultrasonography can be performed in the unsedated patient, aspiration/biopsy procedures are best done with general anesthesia.

Thoracic ultrasonography is particularly useful to clarify the following abnormalities seen on radiographs: (1) pleural effusion presence, amount and character; (2) possible mediastinal mass; (3) differentiating thoracic wall from pulmonary masses; and (4) differentiating pulmonary consolidation from mass. Finally, ultrasound is particularly effective to guide aspiration or biopsy procedures of pleural effusion and thoracic masses.

PLEURAL EFFUSION

Ultrasonography is an excellent modality for determining the presence of small volumes of pleural effusion, providing gross estimations of effusion volume and assessing effusion characteristics based on echogenicity. Unlike radiography, where pleural effusion silhouettes intrathoracic structures such as the mediastinum, pleural fluid acts as an excellent acoustic medium, reduces lung volume, and thereby allows ultrasound imag-

ing of normally inaccessible, deeper structures. The pleural effusion should not be removed from stable patients before the ultrasound examination.

When scanning the normal thorax through the intercostal spaces, the hyperechoic reflective pleuropulmonary interface is seen sliding intimately against the costal pleura lining the thoracic wall. Pleural effusion separates the costal from pulmonary pleura, and the resultant space fills with fluid of varying echogenicity. A transudate-type effusion appears anechoic; cells, fibrin, or protein in the fluid will cause it to become more echogenic.[39] Chronic pleural effusions may contain fibrin tags.

The medical literature reports that ultrasonographic differentiation between benign and malignant pleural effusion is possible if nodular pleural structures are visible.[40] Pleural nodules must be greater than 5 mm in diameter on the parietal or pulmonary pleura in order to be detected. Visible nodules appear as round or oval, broad-based hyperechoic structures that are well-delineated against the pleural effusion. Pleural metastasis without effusion is difficult to visualize.[40] Although not substantiated in the veterinary literature, conceptually, similar imaging circumstances would have to be present in veterinary patients.

MEDIASTINAL MASSES

The mediastinum is best evaluated on thoracic radiographs. The normal mediastinum cannot be imaged with ultrasound because of adjacent aerated lung. Ultrasonography is indicated when radiographs indicate mediastinal widening caused by a possible mass, or when a mediastinal abnormality is suspected but obscured by pleural effusion. Mediastinal structures become accessible when aerated lungs are displaced by either a mediastinal mass large enough to contact the thoracic wall, or by a pleural effusion. Usually only the ventral portion of the mediastinum can be evaluated; even under ideal conditions of a large pleural effusion, the dorsal portion remains obscured by aerated lung lobes.[40] The location of the radiographically identified mediastinal abnormality determines whether the ultrasound transducer is positioned for a parasternal, suprasternal, or substernal approach. In the case of a mediastinal mass, the transducer must be positioned where the mass contacts the thoracic wall or diaphragm. Greater flexibility in transducer location and improved visibility of the ventral mediastinum occurs when a concurrent pleural effusion is present. Imaging small mediastinal masses may require scanning from the dependent side to take advantage of the physical displacement of fluid or lung lobe collapse.[41]

Mediastinal masses vary in their appearance between and within diseases.[39] In a survey of noncardiac thoracic abnormalities in dogs and cats, mediastinal masses were most often caused by lymphadenopathy and therefore appeared multiple or multilobular. Fluid-containing masses only occurred in cats.[39] Incidental, idiopathic mediastinal cysts were singular structures with large amounts of anechoic fluid contained by a thin wall. A cystic thymoma was characterized by a thick, irregular wall and filled with echogenic fluid. The appearance of these cystic structures differed from reported branchial cysts of thymic origin in that the latter had multiple cysts containing proteinaceous, cellular fluid and a concurrent pleural effusion.[42]

THORACIC WALL VERSUS PULMONARY MASS

Ultrasonography is indicated to differentiate thoracic wall masses from pulmonary masses and to differentiate focal thoracic mass lesions (e.g., neoplasia, abscess, granuloma, or hematoma) from diffuse lesions (e.g., cellulitis or hemorrhage).[43] A mass arising from the thoracic wall can be identified ultrasonographically based on location, rib involvement, shape, and respiratory movement. Thoracic wall masses are superficially located; aggressive masses arising from or secondarily involving the ribs will create either an irregular rib border because of a periosteal reaction or an absent deep acoustic shadow where the rib has been totally destroyed. Thoracic wall masses may appear ultrasonographically similar to the extrapleural sign seen radiographically. The mass may have a convex border extending from the wall into the thoracic cavity, tapered borders at the periphery, and a smooth border between the mass and the lung surface.[43,44] Thoracic wall masses move synchronously with the thoracic wall, and the pulmonary pleural interface slides deep to the mass. The ultrasonographic appearance of masses varies with tissue composition (e.g., solid or cavitated). Thoracic wall cellulitis or hemorrhage is characterized by the absence of a well-defined mass and the presence of fluid in the subcutaneous tissue.

A suitable acoustic window must be present to image pulmonary masses using ultrasound. The mass must be peripherally located in the lung and in contact with either the chest wall or a concurrent pleural effusion. Alternatively, a mass more centrally located in the lung must have an acoustic window created by superficial collapsed or consolidated lung. Pulmonary masses are differentiated from thoracic wall masses by synchronous movement with respiration, and sliding of the mass against the thoracic wall. This movement, referred to as the gliding sign, was present in 92% of pulmonary masses in humans.[45] Unlike thoracic wall masses, the edges of pulmonary masses cannot be delineated ultrasonographically; their edges are obscured by superficial aerated lung.[45]

The acoustic appearance of pulmonary masses also varies depending on the mass structure. In one retrospective study, the majority of pulmonary masses were neoplastic and appeared homogenous and hypoechoic compared to the adjacent lung (Figure 12-8).[39] Smooth borders between the mass and adjacent lung were more commonly seen with neoplastic masses.[39] Pulmonary masses may have a complex echogenic appearance; cavities filled with variably echogenic fluid or air may represent necrotic areas. Masses may be avascular or contain abnormal vessels.[41]

PULMONARY CONSOLIDATION VERSUS MASS

Ultrasound is also used to differentiate areas of pulmonary consolidation or collapse from pulmonary masses. Ultrasonography cannot be used to image the normal aerated pulmonary parenchyma deep to the pulmonary pleura. However, when peripheral alveoli collapse or become filled with fluid, ultrasound waves can then penetrate these consolidated or collapsed areas of the pulmonary parenchyma.[46] Pulmonary consolidation is typically associated with inflammatory disease (e.g., pneumonia), severe pulmonary edema, or severe pulmonary hemorrhage. Lung lobe collapse occurs secondary to a large volume pleural effusion, bronchial obstruction, prolonged lateral recumbency, or lung lobe torsion.

Areas of pulmonary consolidation or collapse are differentiated from pulmonary masses by shape, border delineation, and echotexture characteristics. Pulmonary consolidation often maintains the shape and triangular architecture of normal lung lobes. Consolidation may involve the entire lung lobe or gradually blend in with normal lung; the distinct delineation seen between pulmonary masses and aerated lung is absent. Although some pulmonary masses may appear homogenous, consolidated lung appears more uniform than a pulmonary mass and may resemble hepatic echotexture.[41] Unlike masses, regions of pulmonary consolidation should not contain fluid- or air-filled cavities.

Additional ultrasonographic characteristics of pulmonary consolidation and inflammatory lung disease in humans are air bronchograms, fluid bronchograms, and scattered echogenic foci caused by residual air in the consolidated lung parenchyma.[47] Air bronchograms, analogous to those seen radiographically, appear ultrasonographically as linear, hyperechoic branching structures with deep acoustic reverberation.[46] Fluid bronchograms, which cannot be detected radiographically, appear as branching, nonpulsatile, anechoic tubular structures.[46] Fluid bronchograms can be differentiated from pulmonary vessels using color Doppler.[48] Fluid bronchograms are a

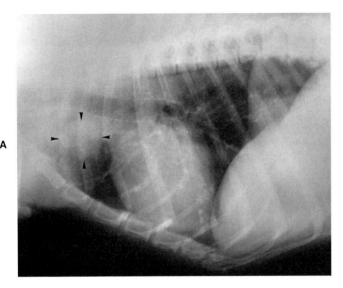

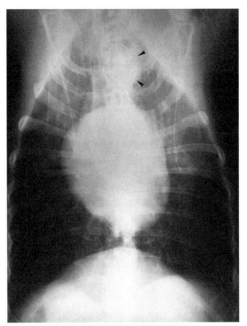

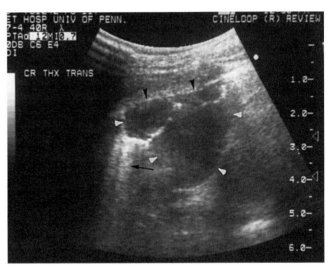

Figure 12-8. *Left lateral recumbent, ventrodorsal radiographs of the thorax and a thoracic ultrasonographic image obtained of a 10-year old boxer.* **A,** *On the left lateral recumbent view, there is a 4-cm diameter soft tissue mass in the cranial thorax* (black arrowheads). *The mass is more likely of pulmonary rather than mediastinal origin because of the well-defined dorsal border.* **B,** *On the ventrodorsal view, the mass is superimposed on the C7 to T1 vertebrae and cranial mediastinum. Only the left, abaxial, convex border of the mass is visible* (black arrowheads). **C,** *Transverse ultrasonographic image obtained with a 4-7 MHz curvilinear array transducer placed between the right first and second ribs. The patient was heavily sedated, placed in a right lateral recumbent position, and imaging was performed from the dependent side. Right pulmonary atelectasis brought the mass in contact with the thoracic wall. The 3-cm deep, lobulated, hypoechoic mass* (white arrowheads) *is bordered superficially by the thoracic wall* (black arrowheads) *and deep by aerated lung with reverberation artifacts* (black arrow). *Ultrasound-guided aspirates were performed of the mass. Pulmonary carcinoma was suspected based on examination of the aspirated material.*

sign of pneumonia in humans and arouse suspicion of bronchial obstruction.[48] Small pockets of gas trapped in the consolidated or collapsed lung create hyperechoic foci with distal reverberation artifacts.[41]

DIAPHRAGMATIC HERNIA AND RUPTURE

Ultrasonography can be used to confirm a radiographically suspected diaphragmatic hernia or traumatic rupture. On the thoracic radiographs, a pleural effusion may obscure the diaphragmatic/hepatic silhouette and herniated abdominal viscera. The ultrasound study may be quick and rewarding or difficult and demanding depending on the extent of diaphragmatic disruption, the volume of herniated viscera, and the presence of pleural effusion. The ultrasound study can proceed using two approaches: attempt to identify either the loss of di-

aphragmatic integrity or the presence of abdominal viscera in the thorax.

The normal hyperechoic interface cranial to the liver seen on an abdominal ultrasound study is commonly called the diaphragm but is actually the pleuropulmonary surface. The diaphragm is not ultrasonographically seen as a distinct structure unless fluid is present cranial (pleural) or caudal (peritoneal) to the diaphragm.[39] It is difficult to examine the diaphragm for potential disruption unless adjacent fluid is present. Examination of diaphragm integrity is further complicated by the mirror-image artifact that incorrectly places the liver cranial to the diaphragm on the ultrasound image.[49] Imaging the diaphragm through the intercostal spaces is difficult, and loss of diaphragm integrity may be more easily determined from the transhepatic approach with the transducer at the xiphoid. This approach places the ultrasound beam perpendicular to the diaphragm and minimizes the mirror-image artifact.[41] Small diaphragmatic tears are difficult to identify ultrasonographically if the hyperechoic interface of the aerated caudal lung lobes lies adjacent to the tear.[43]

Ultrasound can also be used to identify abdominal viscera in the pleural or pericardial space. This approach may be more rewarding than searching for diaphragmatic disruptions. Traumatic diaphragmatic ruptures often have a concurrent pleural effusion that aids ultrasonographic examination of the pleural space. Abdominal viscera must be differentiated from consolidated lung lobes; the liver can be identified by following caudally oriented portal veins and the absence of fluid or air bronchograms.[43] For a congenital peritoneopericardial diaphragmatic hernia, the appearance of abdominal viscera adjacent to the heart within the pericardial sac, and loss of the diaphragm contour near midline are considered diagnostic.[39,43] The ultrasonographic diagnosis of diaphragmatic hernia or traumatic rupture still relies heavily on a high index of suspicion derived from the thoracic radiographs.

ASPIRATION/BIOPSY PROCEDURES AND COMPLICATIONS

Ultrasound is indicated to guide diagnostic aspiration or therapeutic drainage of pleural effusion; aspiration of pulmonary consolidation; and aspiration/biopsy of mediastinal, pulmonary, and thoracic wall masses. These procedures can be successfully performed once acoustic windows are identified, permitting appropriate access to the abnormality. Some abnormalities may only be accessible from the dependent side when accumulated pleural effusion or lung lobe collapse creates acoustic windows. Aspiration of pleural effusion is often performed with little to no sedation, but thoracic mass aspiration/biopsy procedures, especially those of pulmonary masses, should be performed under general anesthesia. General anesthesia permits intermittent cessation of respiratory motion during needle insertion into the pulmonary mass and reduces the possibility of pulmonary laceration.

Needle guidance can be performed by either of two methods: transducer needle guides or freehand. Transducer needle guides are designed to fix the needle path in the ultrasound beam plane, thereby making needle visualization easier and simplifying the procedure. Unfortunately, needle guides limit the flexibility required to aspirate and biopsy small or marginally accessible lesions. The freehand technique relies on the operator to coordinate and maintain the needle path in the ultrasound beam plane. This technique is more technically demanding, and experience is required to coordinate the scan plane and needle approach. The primary advantage of the freehand technique is increased flexibility of the needle approach.

Successful aspiration or therapeutic drainage of pleural effusion depends on the fluid type and amount of fibrin septa. Anechoic fluid generally represents a transudate-type fluid and can be easily aspirated using a 22-gauge needle. Highly echogenic, and therefore more cellular, inspissated fluid may represent hemorrhagic effusion, empyema,

or chylothorax and require larger-gauge needles to obtain a sample. Fibrin strands and pleural adhesions, commonly seen with chronic effusions, often obstruct the needle during aspiration. Successful aspiration of a small volume pleural effusion may require scanning and access from the dependent side of the thorax.

Ultrasound is commonly used to guide aspiration or biopsy procedures of thoracic wall, pulmonary, and mediastinal masses. Fine-needle aspiration of thoracic masses is easy to perform and associated with few complications. Most aspirations are performed using 22-gauge needles of various lengths. In human medicine, fine-needle aspiration is generally considered less diagnostic compared with large-bore cutting needle biopsy.[48] However, in a retrospective survey of veterinary thoracic ultrasound-guided aspiration procedures, cytology was considered diagnostic in 51 of 56 patients (91%), with no reported complications.[39]

Large-bore biopsy procedures are generally performed using 14-, 16-, or 18-gauge cutting-type biopsy needles. Semiautomatic and automatic biopsy devices are now routinely used rather than the original manual cutting needles. These spring-loaded devices have simplified the biopsy procedure so that one person can scan, direct the needle, and fire the biopsy gun.[50] The ability to obtain adequate samples with smaller-gauge needles using the spring-load devices has reduced complication rates to approach those rates found with fine needle aspiration procedures.[51,52] Complications secondary to thoracic ultrasound-guided biopsies in humans are reportedly low: pneumothorax (2% to 4%), hemoptysis (1% to 2%), and pneumothorax requiring chest tube placement (1% to 2%).[48] Aspiration/biopsy procedures guided by fluoroscopy were associated with higher complication rates.[48] Case selection may influence the complication rate because fluoroscopy is typically used to guide aspirations of deeper masses where the needle must traverse normal lung. Aerated lung and pulmonary vessels can be avoided when ultrasonography is used to guide the needle.

Pneumothorax is a potential complication following mediastinal mass, pulmonary mass, or pulmonary consolidation aspiration or biopsy. Pneumothorax is typically diagnosed on radiographs, but the ultrasonographic recognition of pneumothorax is critical after performing thoracic aspiration/biopsy procedures. The ultrasonographic diagnosis of a pneumothorax is made when the gliding sign (i.e., respiratory-related movement of the pulmonary pleura) disappears, the pulmonary mass or consolidated area suddenly disappears, and the pulmonary pleural line broadens and is accompanied by reverberation artifacts.[40,53] Small pockets of pleural air may produce comet tail artifacts. The degree of lung lobe collapse and volume of pneumothorax is more accurately assessed radiographically.

Thoracic Computed Tomography

Computed tomography (CT) is becoming more available for alternative imaging of veterinary patients. The benefits of CT for imaging a variety of thoracic disorders in human medicine are well documented; many of the same indications apply in veterinary medicine.[54,55] Similar to radiography, CT uses x-rays, but the cross-sectional nature of CT scanning eliminates problems created on radiographs when lesions can be hidden by superimposed structures. Compared with conventional radiography, CT has significantly poorer spatial resolution but significantly better contrast resolution.[56] The improved contrast resolution is a major advantage of CT compared with radiography because subtle differences between a soft tissue tumor and adjacent normal tissue can be distinguished on a CT scan. Because CT scans represent digital data, the brightness and contrast of the images can be manipulated to highlight soft tissue (e.g., mediastinal tissue) or lung parenchyma. The air in the lungs provides an excellent background against which to evaluate pulmonary vasculature, pulmonary parenchyma, and airways. Spiral or helical CT scanners, especially those with multi-slice capability, can scan through an entire thorax in a matter of seconds rather than minutes. Despite the speed of modern CT scanners, thoracic CT studies of veterinary patients usually require general anesthesia to momentarily suspend respiratory motion during scanning.

THORACIC CT TECHNIQUES

CT of the thorax is best performed using spiral (also known as helical) CT. Conventional slice-by-slice CT, with the required interscan delay of several seconds, can produce slice misregistration because of respiratory motion. When slice misregistration occurs, small lesions can be missed and multiplanar or 3-D reconstructions are degraded. With spiral CT the table and patient move continuously while the x-ray tube rotates such that the x-ray tube essentially traces a spiral or helical path around the patient. A volumetric set of data is obtained because data acquisition is synchronous with patient movement. Volume data acquisition occurs during a single breath hold, eliminates slice misregistration, and results in superior multiplanar and 3-D reconstructions.[57]

Despite the inherent speed of early spiral CT scanners, faster multi-row detector units are now commercially available. The early spiral CT scanners have a single row of x-ray beam detectors opposite the x-ray tube such that only a single finite volume of tissue several millimeters thick can be sampled per x-ray tube rotation. Although single-row detector spiral CT units are considerably faster than conventional CT scanners, imaging large volumes of the thorax along the length of the patient (i.e., z-axis) requires either a long patient breath hold or fast patient translation, the latter resulting in lower z-axis resolution. New multi-detector row spiral CT scanners (i.e., multi-slice) can acquire information from 4 to 16 individual sections of tissue with a single x-ray tube rotation, thereby allowing rapid scanning of large volumes of tissue while preserving z-axis resolution.[58] Faster volumetric data acquisition and improved 3-D reconstructions with multi-detector spiral CT units are particularly crucial for CT angiographic studies.

There is no one optimal set of acquisition parameters for thoracic CT. Similar to radiography, kVp, mAs, and slice acquisition time are adjusted with the patient's size. Slice thickness, slice interval, slice reconstruction overlap, and table travel speed are set based on the distance covered in the thorax, desired image resolution, patient's respiratory status, and need for multiplanar or 3-D reconstructions. With spiral CT, the term *pitch* is used to describe the relationship between patient table travel per one 360-degree tube revolution and the slice thickness. Pitch is equal to table travel speed/slice thickness. A pitch of 1 to 1.5 or 1.7 is generally used for the thorax; the higher pitches are required to cover larger thoracic volumes in a single breath hold.

The raw data is obtained and further processed by various reconstruction algorithms to ultimately create the CT image. The image is composed of a matrix of pixels representing a volume, or voxel, of tissue in the patient. Each pixel is assigned a CT number that is ultimately derived from the density of tissue represented by that pixel.[56] CT numbers, also known as Hounsfield units (HV), are quantitative; the tissue's CT number can be used in an attempt to determine the nature of the tissue. CT numbers normally range from −1000 to +3000. Water is centered at 0, air at −1000, soft tissue ranges from −300 to −100, and dense bone or iodinated contrast agent can extend from +300 to 3000.

Once the image of the patient is reconstructed from the raw data, the reader can perform postprocessing of the displayed image by adjusting the window and leveling.[56] CT images typically possess 12 bits of gray scale (for a total of 4096 shades of gray), but most computer monitors display only 8 bits (256 shades of gray). The 12-bit CT image must be reduced to 8-bit by postprocessing (i.e., adjusting the window and level of the CT image). The window width defines the range of displayed grays; the CT number centered in the window is the window level. In other words, if a display is set to a window width of 1024 and a window level of 0, the 256 shades of gray represent the CT numbers −512 to +512. But if the window level is raised to 100, then the values represented are −412 to +612. CT images with narrow window widths have greater contrast; high window levels result in brighter images. By adjusting the window width and level, the reader essentially adjusts the image contrast and brightness, respectively, depending on the tissue of interest. For example, mediastinal tissue can be examined by adjusting the window width and level to around 350 and 40, respectively, and then changed to a window width of 1000 and level of −700 to examine lung parenchyma (Figure 12-9). Digital image processing allows adequate evaluation of bone, soft tissue, and lung on a single CT study without the need to rescan the patient at different exposure settings.

THORACIC CT INDICATIONS

In veterinary medicine, thoracic CT is typically performed when abnormalities are seen or suspected on thoracic radiographs and additional information is needed about the extent and exact location of a lesion.

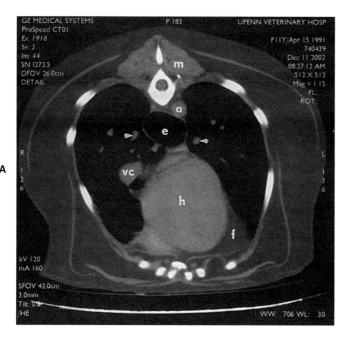
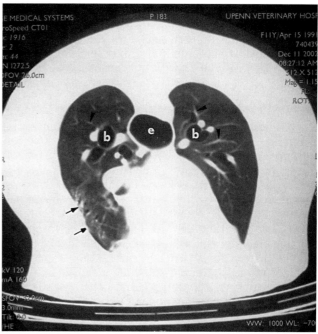

Figure 12-9. *Two noncontrast transverse CT scans of the canine thorax displayed using different window width and level settings.* **A,** *The dog was positioned in ventral recumbency, the CT slice was obtained through the caudal region of the heart, and the image has been postprocessed to display soft tissue (window width = 706, window level = 30), The aorta (a), caudal vena cava (vc), heart (h), pericardial fat (f), air-dilated esophagus (e), epaxial musculature (m), and pulmonary vessels (white arrowheads) are seen.* **B,** *Identical CT slice postprocessed to display the bronchi, pulmonary parenchyma, and vessels (window width = 1000, window level = −700). The soft tissue can no longer be distinguished because of increased image brightness and decreased contrast. The pulmonary parenchyma, smaller pulmonary vessels (black arrowheads) and bronchi (b) are seen. An area of mild pulmonary consolidation (black arrows) is now seen in the right ventral pulmonary region. This was caused by residual atelectasis from the patient having been placed in right lateral recumbency before positioning for the CT study.*

There are, however, rare instances when a thoracic CT may be performed because the thoracic radiographs are unexpectedly normal. Abnormalities of the thoracic wall, pleura, mediastinum, pulmonary parenchyma, major mediastinal vessels, and pulmonary vasculature can be further assessed with CT. CT can also be used to guide aspiration and/or biopsy procedures. A CT study is often needed for planning and dosimetry with patients receiving high-energy radiation therapy.

Thoracic CT typically involves obtaining a separate series of scans preintravenous and postintravenous administration of an iodinated contrast agent. Major mediastinal vessels and contrast enhancement of suspected masses might be identified on the post-contrast series. If more specific information pertaining to the major mediastinal or pulmonary vessels is required, the vascular administration of contrast agent can be carefully timed with scan acquisition to produce a CT angiographic study.

THORACIC WALL AND PLEURA

Thoracic wall lesions are typically seen radiographically; however, the true extent and origin of the lesion may not be readily apparent. CT is indicated to differentiate a par-

ticularly large thoracic wall mass from a pulmonary mass. Additional small thoracic wall lesions may be seen on the CT study that are not seen on thoracic radiographs. If rib destruction is questioned radiographically, results of the CT study can help determine the presence and extent of rib lysis and can be used to plan surgical resection.

Pleural effusion causes a silhouette sign of intrathoracic soft tissue structures on thoracic radiographs. If a majority of the effusion cannot be removed, and additional information about intrathoracic structures is needed, the inherently better contrast resolution of CT allows the reader to distinguish soft tissue from pleural effusion. Furthermore, pleural effusion will not enhance post-contrast administration. The patient should be positioned for the CT study so that the pleural effusion does not surround the area of interest; similar to radiographic principles, a soft tissue mass becomes more evident on CT if surrounded by aerated lung.[54] CT may also be indicated in a patient with suspected traumatic diaphragmatic rupture in which it is difficult to assess diaphragmatic integrity because of silhouetting of the diaphragmatic border by accompanying pleural effusion.

In veterinary patients with spontaneous pneumothorax, a CT study may be indicated to identify suspected pulmonary bullae or rupture of a cavitated neoplasm. On radiographs, large pulmonary bullae may be seen, but small bullae and ruptured bulla are difficult to identify. CT may also reveal large bullae, but small bullae (less than 0.3 cm) may be difficult to detect.[54]

PULMONARY PARENCHYMA

Further description of pulmonary masses, parenchymal infiltration, airway disease, or suspected lung lobe torsion are all indications for performing thoracic CT. Larger pulmonary masses are usually seen on radiographs; however, a mass located on the midline may be partially obscured by the spine on radiographs and better defined on CT. Pulmonary masses seen on radiographs can be further described with CT. The size, internal composition (e.g., solid versus cystic), involved lung lobe, and detection of smaller masses not seen radiographically may influence subsequent therapeutic decisions. In humans, the presence and pattern of calcification in solitary pulmonary nodules is used to differentiate benign from malignant nodules.[59] Thin section (2- to 3-mm slice thickness) CT is 10 to 20 times more sensitive than is standard radiography for detecting intranodular calcification. Furthermore, CT numbers (Hounsfield units, HU) of the nodule allow objective, quantitative assessment of calcification. The vascularity of benign and malignant pulmonary nodules differs, and the degree of contrast enhancement is a characteristic used to make this important distinction in humans. Absence of significant lung nodule enhancement (less than 15 HU) on CT has been shown to be strongly predictive of benignity with a 98% sensitivity but only 58% specificity.[60] Thoracic spiral CT is also used for lung cancer screening in humans. In populations at high risk for developing lung cancer, preliminary results have shown that spiral CT is potentially a more useful screening method for detecting early peripheral lung cancers than is chest radiography.[61] Similar results could be expected in veterinary medicine, but pulmonary metastatic screening is less likely to be performed because of limitations of CT availability, cost, and need for anesthesia of veterinary patients.

Other potential indications for thoracic CT in veterinary patients with pulmonary lesions are suspected lung lobe torsion, bronchial disease, alveolar or interstitial disease, and pulmonary bulla. CT can be used to help differentiate alveolar pulmonary consolidation from pulmonary masses and further characterize bronchial disease.[62] In human medicine, thin-section thoracic CT is used to assess pulmonary parenchymal changes in patients with acute respiratory distress syndrome and idiopathic interstitial pneumonia.[63,64]

MEDIASTINUM

Thoracic CT is an excellent modality for ruling out mediastinal masses, heart base masses, lymphadenopathy, esophageal masses, and major vessel infiltration or deviation by a mass. Many of these abnormalities are likely to have been identified on thoracic radiographs and contrast studies (e.g., esophogram) but confirmation of the suspected lesion, the extent of involvement, and surgical or radiation therapy planning information can be obtained from the CT study. CT is particularly useful for identifying tracheobronchial lymphadenopathy and caudal mediastinal masses not associated with the esophagus. The post-IV contrast series is used to identify major mediastinal vessels that may be deviated or invaded by mediastinal masses.

PULMONARY VASCULATURE

The most common indication for CT examination of the pulmonary vasculature is when pulmonary thromboembolism (PTE) is suspected. Although radiographic abnormalities may be present in dogs with PTE, the changes are usually nonspecific.[65] Conventional pulmonary angiography, digital subtraction angiography, and ventilation-perfusion (V/Q) scintigraphy have been traditional special studies performed in dogs to diagnose PTE.[66] Before the advent of spiral CT, V/Q scintigraphy was recommended as the best available method to screen dogs with suspected PTE.[66] In humans, however, V/Q scintigraphy has poor diagnostic sensitivity and sensitivity as a screening test.[67] Conventional pulmonary angiography is considered the gold standard in humans but is invasive and risky and therefore underutilized. Although thoracic CT requires anesthesia, the CT study is minimally invasive and involves no residual radioactivity. Therefore spiral CT angiography has progressively replaced pulmonary angiography and V/Q scintigraphy in human patients.[68]

Examining the pulmonary arteries with CT requires a fast spiral CT scanner and careful coordination between IV contrast injection and scan acquisition that essentially results in a CT angiogram. In experimentally-induced PTE in dogs, readers of spiral CT angiograms identified 64% to 76% of gelfoam pulmonary emboli in the lobar, segmental, and subsegmental arteries.[67] Emboli were seen as complete or partial intraluminal filling defects on transverse and 3-D reconstructed images (Figure 12-10). Reader detection sensitivity was 96% for vessels greater than 4 mm and 80% for vessels less than 3 mm; specificity was 98.8%. Similar high sensitivity and specificity are reported in studies using spiral CT for detecting PTE in humans. Faster CT scanners have allowed thinner collimated beams (2 to 3 mm); the improvement in spatial resolution has meant that reconstruction of contiguous rather than overlapping sections is now recommended, and that emboli can be detected in the subsegmental arteries.[68] Additional cited benefits of spiral CT angiography for PTE detection in humans are the lower percentage of nondiagnostic studies (because the lung parenchyma, mediastinum, and thoracic wall structures are also evaluated) and a greater agreement among readers of CT scans compared with V/Q scintigraphy.[69-71]

Spiral CT angiography has become the initial imaging modality for people with suspected PTE. Conventional pulmonary angiography is reserved for patients where the

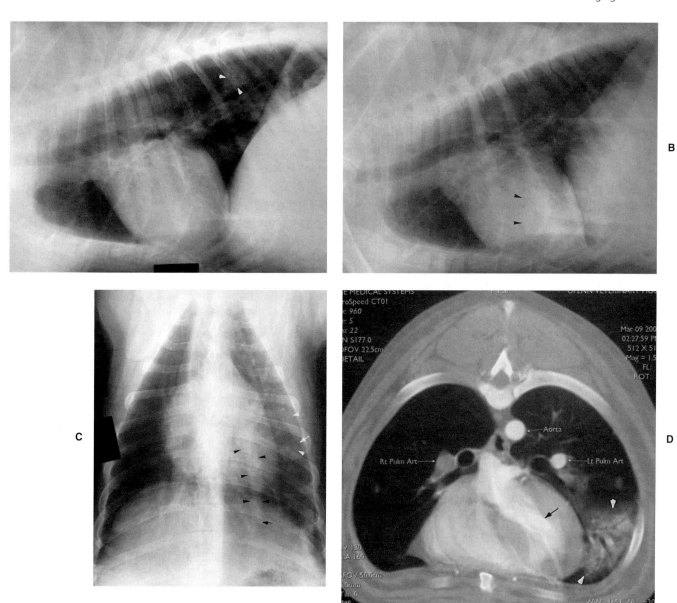

Figure 12-10. Three thoracic radiographic views and a CT scan of an 8-year-old rottweiler with multiple pulmonary thromboemboli. **A,** Left lateral recumbent thoracic radiograph on which right-sided cardiac enlargement and a caudodorsal focal region of interstitial pulmonary opacity (white arrowheads) are seen. **B,** Right lateral recumbent thoracic radiograph with a subtle region of ventral alveolar pulmonary consolidation superimposed on the heart (black arrowheads). Compare the increased radiopacity of this region on the right lateral versus the left lateral recumbent view. **C,** Dorsoventral view on which there is enlargement (black arrowheads) and peripheral blunting (black arrow) of the left caudal pulmonary artery. There is increased radiopacity of the cranial and caudal segments of the left cranial lung lobe (white arrowheads). The pleural fissure is visible (white arrow) between these two segments because of either a small pleural effusion or pleural edema. **D,** A transverse CT pulmonary angiogram scan obtained through the eighth thoracic vertebra. Iodinated contrast material is present in the left ventricle (black arrow). Contrast material is absent in the right pulmonary artery (compared with the left pulmonary artery). Intraluminal hyperdense material, similar to soft tissue, in the right pulmonary artery represents the thrombus. Additional thrombi were seen in smaller branches of the left pulmonary artery (images not shown). Alveolar consolidation of the caudoventral region of the left cranial lung lobe (white arrowheads) is more clearly seen on the CT study compared with the radiographs.

clinical suspicion for PTE remains high despite normal CT results, especially if the technical conditions of the CT examination (e.g., respiratory motion) limit the depiction of acute PTE to the central pulmonary arteries.[68]

REFERENCES

1. Bushberg JT, Seibert JA, Leidholdt EM et al: Screen-film radiography. In Bushberg JT, editor: *The essential physics of medical imaging*, ed 2, Philadelphia, 2002, Lippincott Williams & Wilkins.
2. Revesz G, Shea FL, Revesz G: The effects of kilovoltage on diagnostic accuracy in chest radiography, *Radiology* 142:673-676, 1982.
3. Bushberg JT, Seibert JA, Leidholdt EM et al: X-ray production, x-ray tubes, and generators. In Bushberg JT, editor: *The essential physics of medical imaging*, ed 2, Philadelphia, 2002, Lippincott Williams & Wilkins.
4. Han CM: Exposure variables. In Han CM, Hurd CD, editors: *Practical diagnostic imaging for the veterinary technician*, ed 2, St Louis, 2000, Mosby.
5. Kundel HL, Revesz G: Lesion conspicuity, structured noise, and film reader error, *Am J Roentgenol* 126:1233-1238, 1976.
6. Han CM: Achieving radiographic quality. In Han CM, Hurd CD, editors: *Practical diagnostic imaging for the veterinary technician*, ed 2, St Louis, 2000, Mosby.
7. Holmes RA, Smith FG, Lewis RE et al: The effects of rotation on the radiographic appearance of the canine cardiac silhouette in dorsal recumbency, *Vet Radiol* 26:98-101, 1985.
8. Perkins R: Effects of radiographic positioning on the heart shadow in dogs, *Mod Vet Pract* 60:801-805, 1979.
9. Silverman S, Suter PF: Influence of inspiration and expiration on canine thoracic radiographs, *JAVMA* 166:502-510, 1975.
10. Kern DA, Carrig CB, Martin RA: Radiographic evaluation of induced pneumothorax in the dog, *Vet Radiol & Ultrasound* 35:411-417, 1994.
11. Kundel HL: Perception errors in chest radiography, *Sem Resp Therapy* 10:203-210, 1989.
12. Nodine CF, Kundel HL: Using eye movements to study visual search and to improve tumor detection, *RadioGraphics* 7:1241-1250, 1987.
13. Baxter B, Ravindra H, Normann RA: Changes in lesion detectability caused by light adaptation in retinal photoreceptors, *Invest Radiol* 17:394-401, 1982.
14. Ravindra H, Normann RA, Baxter B: Changes in visual sensitivity explained with references to light adaptation of cone-type photoreceptors in the retina, *Invest Radiol* 18:105-106, 1983.
15. Carmody DP, Nodine CF, Kundel HL: An analysis of perceptual and cognitive factors in radiographic interpretation, *Perception* 9:339-344, 1980.
16. Samuel S, Kundel HL, Nodine CF et al: Mechanism of satisfaction of search: Eye position recordings in the reading of chest radiographs, *Radiology* 194:895-902, 1995.
17. Berbaum KS, Franken EA, Anderson KL: The influence of clinical history on visual search with single and multiple abnormalities, *Invest Radiol* 28:191-201, 1993.
18. Kundel HL, Nodine CF, Thickman D et al: Searching for lung nodules: A comparison of human performance with random and systemic scanning models, *Invest Radiol* 22:417-422, 1987.
19. Kundel HL, Nodine CF, Krupinski EA: Searching for lung nodules: Visual dwell indicates location of false-positive and false-negative decisions, *Invest Radiol* 24:472-478, 1989.
20. Guiss LW, Kuenstler P: A retrospective view of survey photofluorograms of persons with lung cancer, *Cancer* 13:91-95, 1960.
21. Alter AJ, Kargas GA, Kargas SA et al: The influence of ambient and viewbox light upon visual detection of low-contrast targets in a radiograph, *Invest Radiol* 17:402-406, 1982.
22. Kundel HL, Nodine CF: Interpreting chest radiographs without visual search, *Radiology* 116:527-532, 1975.
23. Kundel HL, La Follette PS: Visual search patterns and experience with radiological images, *Radiology* 103:523-528, 1972.
24. Arnheim R: *Visual thinking*, Berkeley, 1969, University of California Press.
25. Kundel HL, Nodine CF: A visual concept shapes image perception, *Radiology* 146:363-368, 1983.
26. Potchen EJ, Cooper TG, Sierra AE et al: Measuring performance in chest radiography, *Radiology* 217:456-459, 2000.
27. Nodine CF, Krupinski EA: Perceptual skill, radiology expertise, and visual test performance with NINA and WALDO, *Acad Radiol* 5:603-612, 1998.
28. Kundel HL: Predictive value and threshold detectability of lung tumors, *Radiology* 139:25-29, 1981.
29. Lord PF, Suter PF, Chan KF et al: Pleural, extrapleural and pulmonary lesions in small animals: A radiographic approach to differential diagnosis, *J Am Vet Radiol Soc* 13:4-17, 1972.
30. Myer W: Radiographic review: The alveolar pattern of pulmonary disease, *J Am Vet Radiol Soc* 20:10-14, 1979.
31. Longuet R, Phelan J, Tanous H et al: Criteria of the silhouette sign, *Radiology* 122:581-585, 1977.
32. Watrous BJ: The esophagus. In Thrall DE, editor: *Textbook of veterinary diagnostic radiology*, ed 4, Philadelphia, 2002, WB Saunders.
33. Bushberg JT, Seibert JA, Leidholdt EM et al: Image quality: The essential physics of medical imaging, Philadelphia, 2002, Lippincott Williams & Wilkins.
34. Pechman RD: Effect of dependency versus nondependency on lung lesion visualization, *Vet Radiol* 28:185-190, 1987.
35. Lang J, Wortman JA, Glickman LT et al: Sensitivity of radiographic detection of lung metastasis in the dog, *Vet Radiol* 27:74-78, 1986.
36. Ruehl WW, Thrall DE: The effect of dorsal versus ventral recumbancy on the radiographic appearance of the canine thorax, *Vet Radiol* 22:10-16, 1981.
37. Carlisle CH, Thrall DE: A comparison of normal feline thoracic radiographs made in dorsal versus ventral recumbency, *Vet Radiol* 23:3-9, 1982.
38. Groves TF, Ticer JW: Pleural fluid movement: its effect on the appearance of ventrodorsal and dorsoventral radiographic projections, *Vet Radiol* 24:99-105, 1983.
39. Reichle JK, Wisner ER: Noncardiac thoracic ultrasound in 75 feline and canine patients, *Vet Radiol & Ultrasound* 41:154-162, 2000.
40. Mathis G: Thoraxsonography: part I: Chest wall and pleura, *Ultrasound in Med & Biol* 23:1131-1139, 1997.
41. Stowater JL, Lamb CR: Ultrasonography of noncardiac thoracic disease in small animals, *JAVMA* 195:514-520, 1989.
42. Lui S, Patnaik AK, Burk RL: Thymic branchial cysts in the dog and cat, *JAVMA* 182:1095-1098, 1983.
43. Tidwell AS: Ultrasonography of the thorax (excluding the heart), *Vet Clin North Am Small Anim Pract* 28:993-1015, 1998.
44. Saito T, Kobayashi H, Kitamura S: Ultrasonographic approach to diagnosing chest wall tumors, *Chest* 94:1271-1275, 1988.
45. Targhetta R, Bourgeois JM, Marty-Double C et al: Peripheral pulmonary lesions: Ultrasonic features and ultrasonically guided fine needle aspiration biopsy, *J Ultrasound Med* 12:369-374, 1993.
46. Targhetta R, Chavagneux R, Bourgeois JM et al: Sonographic approach to diagnosing pulmonary consolidation, *J Ultrasound Med* 11:667-672, 1992.
47. Acunas B, Celik L, Acunas A: Chest sonography: Differentiation of pulmonary consolidation from pleural disease, *Acta Radiologica* 30:273-275, 1989.
48. Mathis G: Thoraxsonography: part II: Peripheral pulmonary consolidation, *Ultrasound in Med & Biol* 23:1141-1153, 1997.
49. Kremkau FW, Taylor KJ: Artifacts in ultrasound imaging, *J Ultrasound Med* 5:227-237, 1986.
50. Hoppe FE, Hager DA, Poulos PW et al: A comparison of manual and automatic ultrasound-guided biopsy techniques, *Vet Radiol* 27:99-101, 1986.
51. Tikkakoski T, Päivänsalo M, Siniluoto T et al: Percutaneous ultrasound-guided biopsy: Fine needle biopsy, cutting needle, or both? *Acta Radiologica* 34:30-34, 1993.
52. Yang PC, Lee YC, Yu CJ et al: Ultrasonographically guided biopsy of thoracic tumors: A comparison of large-bore cutting biopsy with fine-needle aspiration, *Cancer* 69:2553-2560, 1992.
53. Targhetta R, Bourgeois JM, Chavagneux R et al: Diagnosis of pneumothorax by ultrasound immediately after ultrasonically guided aspiration biopsy, *Chest* 101:855-856, 1992.
54. Burk RL: Computed tomography of thoracic disease in dogs, *JAVMA* 199:617-621, 1991.
55. Garland MR, Lawler LP, Whitaker BR et al: Modern CT applications in veterinary medicine, *RadioGraphics* 22:55-62, 2002.

56. Bushberg JT, Seibert JA, Leidholdt EM et al: *Computed tomography: The essential physics of medical imaging*, ed 2, Philadelphia, 2002, Lippincott Williams & Wilkins.
57. Volk P, Soucek M, Daepp M et al: Lung: Spiral volumetric CT with single-breath-hold technique, *Radiology* 176:864-867, 1990.
58. Mahesh M: Search for isotropic resolution in CT from conventional through multiple-row detector, *RadioGraphics* 22:949-962, 2002.
59. Erasmus JJ, Connolly JE, McAdams HP et al: Solitary pulmonary nodules: Part I, Morphologic evaluation for differentiation of benign and malignant lesions, *RadioGraphics* 20:43-58, 2000.
60. Swenson SJ, Viggiano RW, Midthun DE et al: Lung nodule enhancement at CT: Multicenter study, *Radiology* 214:73-80, 2000.
61. Kaneko M, Eguchi K, Ohmatsu et al: Peripheral lung cancer: Screening and detection with low-dose spiral CT versus radiography, *Radiology* 201:798-802, 1996.
62. Phillips S, Barr S, Dykes N et al: Bronchiolitis obliterans with organizing pneumonia in a dog, *J Vet Intern Med* 14:204-207, 2000.
63. MacDonald SLS, Rubens MB, Hansell DM et al: Nonspecific interstitial pneumonia and usual interstitial pneumonia: comparative appearances at and diagnostic accuracy of thin-section CT, *Radiology* 221:600-605, 2001.
64. Desai SR, Wells AU, Rubens MB et al: Acute respiratory distress syndrome: CT abnormalities at long-term follow-up, *Radiology* 210:29-35, 1999.
65. Flückiger MA, Gomez JA: Radiographic findings in dogs with spontaneous pulmonary thrombosis or embolism, *Vet Radiol* 25:124-131, 1984.
66. Koblik PD, Hornof WJ, Harnagel SH et al: A comparison of pulmonary angiography, digital subtraction angiography, and 99mTC-DTPA/MAA ventilation-perfusion scintigraphy for detection of experimental pulmonary emboli in the dog, *Vet Radiol* 30:159-168, 1989.
67. Hurst DR, Kazerooni EA, Stafford-Johnson D et al: Diagnosis of pulmonary embolism: Comparison of CT angiography and MR angiography in canines, *JVIR* 10:309-318, 1999.
68. Remy-Jardin M, Remy J: Spiral CT angiography of the pulmonary circulation, *Radiology* 212:615-636, 1999.
69. Kim K, Müller NL, Mayo JR: Clinically suspected pulmonary embolism: Utility of spiral CT, *Radiology* 210:693-697, 1999.
70. Coche EE, Müller NL, Kim K et al: Acute pulmonary embolism: Ancillary findings at spiral CT, *Radiology* 207:753-758, 1998.
71. Mayo JR, Remy-Jardin M, Müller NL et al: Pulmonary embolism: Prospective comparison of spiral CT and ventilation-perfusion scintigraphy, *Radiology* 205:447-452, 1997.

CHAPTER 13

Diagnostic Pulmonary Scintigraphy

A. Reid Tyson • Clifford R. Berry

Nuclear medicine techniques for evaluating lung ventilation and perfusion provide a unique and noninvasive method to obtain functional images of specific physiology. Although these physiological processes are not directly visualized in routine radiology or other alternate imaging techniques, nuclear medicine provides direct physiological information using radiopharmaceutical localization of specific target organs or biochemical reactions. Radiopharmaceuticals can provide early detection of abnormalities that may precede radiographic changes by days to weeks.[1,2]

Nuclear medicine studies consist of labeling a carrier (pharmaceutical) with a radionuclide that by definition is unstable.[1,2] This combination is called a radiopharmaceutical. Often the carrier mimics a physiological process within the body. The radionuclide is used only for external imaging of the location of the carrier within the patient. By attaching a radionuclide to different pharmaceuticals, one can image different physiological processes. For example, when macroaggregated albumin (MAA) is bound to the radionuclide Technetium-99m (^{99m}Tc) and

is injected into a peripheral vein, the particles lodge on the arteriolar side of the first capillary bed encountered, in this case the pulmonary capillary bed.[1,2] The size range of the MAA particles is between 10 and 30 μm.[1,2] The carrier in this case is not tracing a physiological process but provides a framework to define blood flow to the lungs. This concept of first-pass capillary blockade is used in a number of radionuclide experiments. In clinical patients suspected of pulmonary thromboembolism (PTE), this radiopharmaceutical provides a rapid assessment of global pulmonary artery perfusion.

As the radionuclide undergoes radioactive decay (i.e., attempts to achieve nuclear stability), gamma rays (electromagnetic radiation) are emitted from the nucleus. The emitted gamma rays are detected externally by a large sodium iodide crystal within the gamma camera. The detected gamma rays are then counted and positioned according to their origin within the patient by the gamma camera. The count density within a given x,y position on the gamma camera is then transferred to the imaging monitor for display and can be stored for further manipulation or display processing. The localization of the radiopharmaceutical can be imaged in a static acquisition mode (the radiopharmaceutical is assumed to be relatively stable in its biodistribution) or in a dynamic acquisition mode (the accumulation of the radiopharmaceutical is known to change over time).

The most common pulmonary scintigraphic study performed in veterinary medicine is the ^{99m}Tc-macroaggregated albumin (MAA) lung perfusion study, which aids in the detection and diagnosis of PTE and helps to determine the severity and location of the thromboembolic disease. In humans, the nuclear perfusion study is used in combination with a ventilation study in which a radiopharmaceutical is inhaled, resulting in images specific for the distribution of ventilation within the lungs. The static perfusion and ventilation images are then manipulated using a computer that creates a new image called a parametric image. This image is produced by dividing the count density information in the ventilation image by the count density information in the perfusion image. This ventilation/perfusion (V/Q) image is then analyzed for areas of normal ventilation with abnormal (diminished) perfusion, termed *V/Q mismatch.*[1-3]

Although the true incidence of PTE is not known in veterinary medicine, the implications for early recognition and treatment have been well documented in humans.[4] In people, it has been shown that PTE is associated with significant mortality, with a mortality rate approaching 30% in untreated PTE.[1,2,4] This mortality rate is reduced by early recognition and treatment. In veterinary medicine, PTE has been associated with cardiac disease, post adulticide complications with lung lobe infarction from heartworm disease, sepsis, autoimmune hemolytic anemia, hyperadrenocorticism, neoplasia, disseminated intravascular coagulopathy, chronic glomerular disease with associated protein loss, and amyloidosis.[5-13]

The usefulness of pulmonary scintigraphy has been previously reported in animals and humans.* Rapid assessment of pulmonary perfusion using ^{99m}Tc-MAA has been well documented.[1,3,14] In humans, the scintigraphic findings are classified as normal, high probability, intermediate, or low probability scans (Box 13-1). Large clinical trials in humans (PIOPED Investigation) have shown that pulmonary perfusion scintigraphy (compared with selective pulmonary angiography) has a 41% sensitivity and a 97% specificity for patients with high probability lung scans for pulmonary embolism.[4] When evaluating all abnormal scintigraphy scans for the presence of pulmonary embolism, the sensitivity was 98%, while the specificity was only 10%.[4] The conclusions drawn from this large scale study indicated that
- A high-probability scan usually indicates pulmonary embolism, but only a minority of humans with pulmonary embolism have high-probability scans.
- A low-probability scan with a strong clinical impression that pulmonary embolism is not likely makes the possibility of pulmonary embolism remote.

*References 1, 3, 4, 7, 9, 13.

BOX 13-1
PIOPED Classification Scheme for Interpretation of Ventilation Perfusion Abnormalities

High Probability
- ≥2 Large (>75% of a segment) segmental perfusion defects without corresponding ventilation or roentgenographic abnormalities or substantially larger than either matching ventilation or chest roentgenogram abnormalities
- ≥2 Moderate segmental (>25% and <75% of a segment) perfusion defects without corresponding ventilation or roentgenographic abnormalities or substantially larger than either matching ventilation or chest roentgenogram abnormalities
- ≥4 Moderate segmental perfusion defects without ventilation or chest roentgenogram abnormalities

Intermediate Probability
- Not falling into normal, low-, or high-probability categories
- Borderline high or borderline low
- Difficult to categorize as high or low

Low Probability
- Nonsegmental perfusion defects (e.g., very small effusion causing blunting of the costophrenic angle, cardiomegaly, enlarged aorta, hila, and mediastinum and elevated diaphragm)
- Single moderate mismatched segmental perfusion defect with normal chest roentgenogram
- Any perfusion defect with a substantially larger chest roentgenogram abnormality
- Large or moderate segmental perfusion defects involving no more than 4 segments in 1 lung and no more than 3 segments in 1 lung region, with matching ventilation defects either equal to or larger in size and chest roentgenogram either normal or with abnormalities substantially smaller than perfusion defects
- >3 small segmental perfusion defects (<25% of a segment) with a normal chest roentgenogram

Normal
- No perfusion defects present
- Perfusion outlines exactly the shape of the lungs as seen on the chest roentgenogram (hilar and aortic impressions may be seen, chest roentgenogram and/or ventilation study may be abnormal)

- A normal lung scan makes the diagnosis of acute pulmonary embolism very unlikely.[4]

One experimental study in dogs performed a comparison of digital subtraction angiography (DSA), ventilation (^{99m}Tc-DTPA)/perfusion (^{99m}Tc-MAA) scintigraphy, and selective pulmonary angiography.[14] Using selective pulmonary angiography as the "gold standard," the researchers demonstrated an 85% accuracy rate for diagnosis of pulmonary embolism with either digital subtraction angiography or ventilation/perfusion imaging. The sensitivity and specificity for pulmonary ventilation/perfusion imaging in this study were 79% and 95%, respectively. The authors of this study drew a number of important conclusions regarding diagnosis of PTE.[14,15] The incidence of PTE appears to be relatively low in veterinary medicine, hence veterinary clinicians will likely remain relatively inexperienced at interpreting

TABLE 13-1. Veterinary Criteria for Interpretation of Perfusion Imaging Abnormalities Based on ^{99m}Tc-MAA Perfusion Scintigraphy and Thoracic Radiographs[15]

Perfusion Study	Ventilation Study (if available)	Thoracic Radiographs	Diagnosis
Normal	Normal	Normal	No evidence of PTE
Lobar defect (1)	Normal	Normal	PTE probable
Lobar defect (2 or more)	Normal	Normal	PTE highly probable
Lobar defect (1 or more)	Matched abnormality	Matched areas of pulmonary consolidation, atelectasis, or infiltrate	Indeterminate—requires selective angiography or DSA study for confirmation of PTE
Normal	Lobar defect (reverse mismatch)	Matched abnormality, typically area of atelectasis	Reverse mismatches are usually due to recumbent atelectasis

TABLE 13-2. Common Radionuclides Used in Pulmonary Scintigraphy and Decay Characteristics

Radionuclide	Mode of Radioactive Decay	Photon Energy (keV)	Physical Half-Life	Study
Technetium-99m	Isomeric transition	140	6.01 hours	^{99m}Tc-MAA—pulmonary perfusion ^{99m}Tc-DTPA—pulmonary ventilation
Xenon-133	Beta minus decay	81	5.3 days	Pulmonary ventilation study
Gallium-67	Electron capture	93, 185, 300	78.1 hours	Inflammation
Indium-111	Electron capture	172, 247	2.82 days	Inflammation
Iodine-123	Electron capture	159	13.1 hours	Label specific (e.g., ^{123}I-iodoamphetamine— macrophage imaging)
Oxygen-15	Positron (beta plus) decay	511	2 minutes	Water distribution, perfusion studies
Fluorine-18	Positron (beta plus) decay	511	109 minutes	Label specific, (^{18}FDG—glucose metabolism studies)

any of the imaging techniques (i.e., DSA, $\dot{V}/\dot{Q}$ scintigraphy, and selective angiography). The optimal imaging procedure for diagnosing PTE should therefore have high lesion-to-normal tissue contrast that enhances the rate and degree of lesion identification. It should also have a high diagnostic specificity because many of the animals may not have PTE. Radiographic findings in dogs with PTE, although often suggestive of a pulmonary vascular abnormality, rarely provide a definitive diagnosis. In addition, PTE rarely results in a single vascular lesion and there is a continuum of pulmonary pathological responses to thromboemboli in a given animal. Therefore, it is likely that the V/Q scan will remain useful in dogs with PTE despite the presence of pulmonary opacities on thoracic radiographs. Chronic obstructive lung disease, the primary disease process that limits the specificity of V/Q scintigraphy in humans, is relatively uncommon in dogs. Based on these considerations, V/Q scintigraphy represents the test of choice to evaluate dogs with suspected pulmonary thromboembolism.[14,15]

The ^{99m}Tc-MAA perfusion study is relatively easy to perform compared with the difficulty of performing the aerosolized ^{99m}Tc-DTPA study, which has complicating radiation safety factors when administering the aerosol to the animal via a mask without a muzzle seal. Revised criteria have been published for evaluation of pulmonary perfusion scans in animals without a concurrent ventilation study (Table 13-1).[15] With these criteria in mind, a normal set of thoracic radiographs along with an abnormal perfusion study should be considered diagnostic for pulmonary embolism.

Other scintigraphic studies can be employed for diagnosis of different pulmonary abnormalities. These include mucociliary studies to test for ciliary dyskinesia, evaluation of radiopharmaceutical uptake by primary or metastatic tumors, and detection of infection or inflammatory disorders such as *Pneumocystis carinii*.

Radiopharmaceuticals

Unbound Technetium-99m (^{99m}Tc) has a natural affinity for the thyroid gland, salivary gland, and gastric mucosa, and is primarily excreted via the kidneys. The chemistry of ^{99m}Tc allows it to bind to many different ligands when reduced to ^{99m}TcO$_2$, enabling it to target specific organs or biological functions. With a half-life of 6.01 hours and a gamma ray energy of 140 KeV (within the ideal energy range of gamma camera imaging), ^{99m}Tc-pertechnetate has many favorable characteristics. Commonly used radionuclides and the studies for which they are used are listed in Table 13-2.

Pulmonary Perfusion Scintigraphy

In typical pulmonary perfusion scintigraphy, macroaggregated albumin is bound to ^{99m}Tc and injected intravenously.[1,2,15] The particles are approximately 10 to 90 μm in size, with 60% of the MAA particles in the 20 to 40 μm range.[1,2] These become lodged in the pulmonary capillaries, which are 6 to 8 μm in diameter. If the ^{99m}Tc-MAA particles are evenly mixed in the venous blood, their distribution approximates pulmonary blood flow. During a typical pulmonary perfusion scan only 1% to 5% of the capillaries in the lung become occluded.[1,2] Histological examination of the lungs postinjection show that the occlusions are only temporary. Pulmonary macrophages remove the MAA particles, with the biological half-life of MAA being 2 to 10 hours, depending on the particle size. In areas of absent or reduced perfusion, photopenic or "cold" spots are produced on the images.[15] Normal images reveal equal distribution to each lung lobe, with relative areas of photopenia in the mediastinum, hilum, and diaphragmatic margins where soft tissue structures cause depressions within the adjacent lung lobes (Figure 13-1). If a ventilation/perfusion scintigraphic study is planned, the ventilation images should be acquired first because they are count-density deprived relative to the perfusion images.[1,2,15]

Administration of ^{99m}Tc-MAA should be undertaken with caution in dogs with extensive pulmonary thromboemboli. Although deaths have been anecdotally reported in severely affected dogs following ^{99m}Tc-MAA injection, the authors have used ^{99m}Tc-MAA in several hundred patients without incident. In humans, it is conjectured that patients with severe PTE are potentially in a gray area, where they are compromised but compensating. Any further insult could result in patient death.[2] If severe pulmonary embolism (i.e., more than two lobes

affected) is suspected, a decrease in the number of injected particles (less than 60,000 particles per animal) should be considered. This is also recommended in humans with pulmonary hypertension.[1,2] Although complications attributable to ^{99m}Tc-MAA have not been seen by the authors, there is always the possibility of an anaphylactic reaction to the human albumin ligand, particularly if repeat studies are done over time.

^{99m}Tc-MAA is made up immediately prior to injection from a human lyophilized kit. The intravenous injection is made with the animal in sternal recumbency to ensure even distribution of the ^{99m}Tc-MAA throughout the pulmonary parenchyma. Images may begin within several minutes of injection, and are acquired for 300,000 to 500,000 counts per image. A routine study would include right lateral, left lateral, dorsal right oblique, dorsal left oblique, dorsal, and ventral. Images are acquired in a 256 × 256 × 16 static frame mode (see Figure 13-1).

Interpretation of the pulmonary perfusion study should be made with regard to current thoracic radiographs. High quality diagnostic radiographs should be made just prior to the perfusion scintigraphic study. Typically, a normal ^{99m}Tc-MAA study demonstrates even distribution of the radiopharmaceutical throughout all lung fields (see Figure 13-1). Ventrally on the lateral projections there are photopenic oval areas in the middle half of the thorax consistent with the position of the cardiac structures. The photopenic cardiac structures are visualized in the middle of the ventral image. The cardiac structures are less apparent on the dorsal image, particularly if the image is obtained with the dog in sternal recumbency and the camera placed over the animal's back in a true dorsal orientation. Oblique lateral projections of the caudodorsal lung fields are helpful for detecting peripheral perfusion abnormalities in the caudodorsal lung margins. The majority of the ^{99m}Tc-MAA distributes to the caudal lung fields, which receive the highest proportion of blood flow in dogs and cats. It may therefore be difficult to identify photopenic areas in the peripheral lung fields when both lungs are superimposed as seen

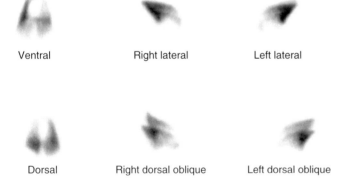

Ventral   Right lateral   Left lateral

Dorsal   Right dorsal oblique   Left dorsal oblique

Figure 13-1. Normal pulmonary perfusion images obtained from a 7-year-old neutered female mixed-breed dog. The static images were obtained 5 minutes after injection of 111 MBq (3 mCi) of ^{99m}Tc-MAA. Note the homogeneous distribution of the radiopharmaceutical throughout all lung fields. (Images courtesy of Dr. Gregory B. Daniel, College of Veterinary Medicine, University of Tennessee, Knoxville, Tenn.)

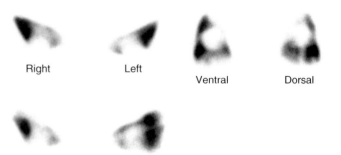

Right   Left   Ventral   Dorsal

Figure 13-2. Pulmonary perfusion static images obtained from a 6-year-old, intact male Walker hound with a clinical history of acute onset of dyspnea. The perfusion study is abnormal because there are large photopenic areas noted in the left cranial and caudal lung lobes and the caudal aspect of the right caudal lung lobe, best seen on the dorsal image. Pulmonary emboli in the corresponding pulmonary arteries were confirmed at necropsy. (Images courtesy of Dr. Gregory B. Daniel, College of Veterinary Medicine, University of Tennessee, Knoxville, Tenn.)

on the right and left lateral images. The biological half-life of ^{99m}Tc-MAA is 2 to 10 hours, with phagocytosis by monocytes and alveolar macrophages being the primary method of clearance.[1,2,15]

Interpretation of abnormal images is based on unequal distribution of the radiopharmaceutical in the lung fields. Pulmonary perfusion abnormalities due to emboli are usually defined as triangular defects with the tip of the photopenic triangle pointing toward the pulmonary hilus (Figure 13-2).[1,2,15] For a diagnosis of pulmonary embolism, the perfusion defect should be pleural based and not central in position. Patchy areas of inhomogeneous pulmonary perfusion that are not pleural based but more central in distribution (Figure 13-3) may be caused by bronchopneumonia, chronic obstructive lung disease, emphysema, pulmonary bulla, pulmonary masses, disseminated neoplasia or other space occupying lesions, asthma, smoke inhalation, mucous plugging of airways with secondary atelectasis, or pulmonary edema.[1,2,15] These differentials can clearly be best worked through and prioritized based on thoracic radiographs and other pertinent physical examination and laboratory findings.

Other considerations regarding perfusion scintigraphy include the presence of right to left intracardiac or extracardiac shunts or animals with diaphragmatic or pleural disease. In the case of right to left shunts, part of the ^{99m}Tc-MAA will pass through the shunt to enter the systemic circulation. The albumin particles will block the first systemic capillary bed encountered and result in an abnormal distribution of the radiopharmaceutical, something easily recognized in the brain and kidneys. Other causes of pleural or diaphragmatic abnormalities (e.g., pleural effusion, pleural masses, diaphragmatic hernia, or diaphragmatic paralysis) may also result in uneven distribution of the ^{99m}Tc-MAA. These changes, however, are ruled out as true perfusion abnormalities based on thoracic radiographic findings.

Ventilation Scintigraphy

Ventilation scintigraphy in small animals is more labor intensive and requires more extreme precautions during administration of the radioaerosol. Most awake dogs and cats resist placement of a face mask for delivery of the radiopharmaceutical. Anesthesia, with nebulization of liquid ^{99m}Tc-diamine-triamino-penta-acetic acid (DTPA) directly into the endotracheal tube, is the easiest way to ensure direct homogeneous delivery of the radiopharmaceutical without the risk of muzzle or local environmental contamination. Clearly, this is not the ideal situation in dogs or cats with respiratory compromise. A closed circuit rebreathing system is required, with a filter that traps any exhaled radioaerosol. Typical oxygen delivery rates of 10 to 12 L/min are used, and the patient is allowed to breathe the radioaerosol for 3 to 5 minutes.

The lung fields should be evaluated with the patient on the gamma camera, so that the persistence scope can be used to determine an end point. Typical inhaled doses are in the range of 3.7 MBq for cats (0.1 mCi) to 9.25 MBq for dogs (0.25 mCi). A suitable radioaerosol particle diameter for even alveolar distribution (range 0.5 to 0.8 μm) is required to ensure that the ^{99m}Tc-DTPA particles are deposited in the terminal bronchioles and alveoli.

Once enough counts are present within the lung field, the patient is imaged in the standard positions for pulmonary perfusion scintigraphy for at least 60 seconds each (50,000 to 100,000 counts per image). As stated earlier, because the ventilation images are going to be significantly count-density limited compared with the perfusion images, this study should be acquired first. The final image should be the dorsal image. After the dorsal image is acquired, if a ^{99m}Tc-MAA study is going to be performed, the patient should be left in the same position in sternal recumbency with the gamma camera centered over the thorax dorsally. The ^{99m}Tc-MAA is then injected and after several minutes, the dorsal image of the perfusion study acquired. It is important to maintain the same position of the patient to allow postimage processing of the dorsal ventilation and perfusion images (e.g., calculation of a parametric image, in which the count density information and relative distribution of the ventilation and perfusion images are divided by each other). In a normal study, the relative distribution of the ventilated radioaerosol should be similar to the distribution of the perfusion radiopharmaceutical.

Normal ventilation images should show an even distribution of the radioaerosol throughout the lung fields. Ventilation abnormalities should be correlated with any abnormalities noted on the radiographs, such as areas of pulmonary disease (interstitial, bronchial, or alveolar) or complete lobar consolidation.

Ventilation clearance studies have also been used. After the initial ventilation images are acquired, serial static dorsal or ventral images are acquired over the next 60 to 90

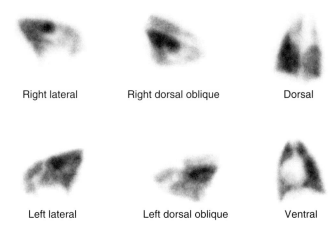

| Right lateral | Right dorsal oblique | Dorsal |
| Left lateral | Left dorsal oblique | Ventral |

Figure 13-3. *Pulmonary perfusion images obtained from a 13-year-old female collie with a clinical history of coughing for several weeks. Numerous perfusion defects are seen within the ventral right and left cranial lung lobes. Corresponding radiographic abnormalities consistent with bronchopneumonia were identified.* (Images courtesy of Dr. Gregory B. Daniel, College of Veterinary Medicine, University of Tennessee, Knoxville, Tenn.)

minutes at 10-minute intervals.[16] Pulmonary clearance half-times can then be calculated. The mean (± standard deviation) clearance half-time in dogs is 48 (±12) minutes.[16] Clearance half-times are calculated from decay corrected time activity curves using a least squares monoexponential fit. Clearance of the ^{99m}Tc-DTPA from the lungs is based on local absorption into the blood stream across the pulmonary capillary bed and renal excretion. This clearance is dependent on normal alveolar-capillary membrane permeability, and pulmonary clearance half-times of ^{99m}Tc-DTPA can be altered secondary to certain disease states. In one experimental study using a pulmonary artery occlusion model the ^{99m}Tc-DTPA clearance half-times were increased in the occluded lung (54 ± 19 minutes) compared to the preoccluded clearance half-time (45 ± 7 minutes) and the mirror lung at the time of the occlusion (43 ± 11 minutes).[16] Other pulmonary disease states in humans (e.g., interstitial lung disease, chronic obstructive pulmonary disease, and smoking) can lead to increased or accelerated ^{99m}Tc-DTPA clearance half-times.[18-20]

Ventilation/perfusion (V/Q) parametric imaging is based on acquisition of dorsal images of the patient using a ventilation (^{99m}Tc-DTPA) technique and a separate perfusion (^{99m}Tc-MAA) imaging study. Once these images are acquired, the two can then be divided (perfusion into ventilation) and a parametric image calculated. Evaluation of each lung field or lung lobe allows determination of the presence of V/Q mismatch. If the V/Q in an area exceeds the mean value elsewhere in the lung (typically around 0.75 to 1.25), this indicates that ventilation is normal but perfusion is limited.[1,3] High V/Q is considered the "classic" mismatch in dogs and cats with pulmonary emboli.[14,15] Matched ventilation and perfusion abnormalities (e.g., photopenic anatomical areas on both the ventilation and the perfusion images) can be seen with chronic obstructive pulmonary disease, bronchitis and bronchiectasis, pulmonary blebs or bulla, congestive heart failure, asthma, bronchogenic carcinoma, inhalation injury, and pulmonary trauma or hemorrhage.[1,2,15,19,20]

Mucociliary Scintigraphy

Normal mucociliary clearance moves particulate debris out of the major airways (principal bronchi and trachea) and into the larynx. The debris is either coughed out or swallowed and excreted by the gastrointestinal tract. Mucociliary clearance can be evaluated by depositing radioactive particulate matter on the airway mucosa and following it over time using the external gamma camera.[21] The mucociliary droplet test has been used as a screening test for ciliary dyskinesia, in which the cilia are characterized by abnormal structure and function (amotile or dysmotile).[21-23] Radiopharmaceuticals used include ^{99m}Tc-MAA or ^{99m}Tc-sulfur colloid.

General anesthesia and intubation are required.[21] A single droplet (30 μl) of the radiopharmaceutical is preloaded into the tip of a long 5 Fr polyethylene catheter, which is placed in the lumen of a shorter 10 Fr catheter that serves as the outer sleeve. After disconnecting the patient from the anesthesia machine, the catheter is advanced to the caudal thoracic trachea, just before the level of the carina. The distance for catheter advancement is premeasured on the outside of the patient, or measured using a lateral thoracic radiograph. The inner catheter is then advanced 1 cm beyond the outer sleeve. The radiopharmaceutical is deposited into the tracheal lumen using air injected into the inner sleeve catheter. The inner catheter is retracted into the outer catheter, both catheters are pulled back out of the endotracheal tube and the anesthesia machine is reconnected. A series of static images is obtained over the next 15 minutes (1 minute each, acquired every 3 to 4 minutes). External markers are used to determine the original position of the radiopharmaceutical droplet and the thoracic inlet. The velocity is calculated by computing the distance traveled by the radiopharmaceutical relative to the elapsed time.

Evaluation of the static images should show the beginning of clearance almost immediately. Typically the radiopharmaceutical droplet breaks up over time, with multiple clearance waves of radioactivity moving away from the site of deposition toward the head and larynx. Lack of droplet movement is considered diagnostic for ciliary dyskinesia. Absolute particle clearance velocities can be calculated but have been shown to increase from puppyhood to maturity and then decrease with age (immature dogs = 4 mm/min; young dogs = 9 mm/min, middle-age dogs = 7 mm/min; and older dogs = 3 mm/min).[23]

Scintigraphic Imaging in Pulmonary Infection and Inflammation

Scintigraphic imaging of inflammatory changes has been established in human medicine since the 1970s, but has not been utilized extensively in veterinary medicine. Gallium-67 citrate infection imaging is used to test for generalized pulmonary inflammatory or infectious conditions in humans.[2] Gallium-67 citrate (^{67}Ga) has an affinity for ferric ion binding sites, which are present on plasma proteins such as transferrin as well as on inflammatory proteins associated with degranulating white blood cells (e.g., lactoferrin, ferritin, and siderophores). An adequate blood supply to the area and a change in vascular permeability are requisites for localization to the site of inflammation. Because of its high affinity for iron, normal organs of distribution for ^{67}Ga include the liver, spleen, and bone marrow. It has a 78-hour physical half-life and is typically imaged at 6, 24, and 48 hours postintravenous injection. Gallium-67 citrate has been shown in people to accumulate in areas of pulmonary infection, granulomatous diseases, pneumonia, lung abscess, acute respiratory distress syndrome, and potential sites of neoplasia.[2] Gallium-67 citrate lung uptake has also been shown to occur in association with adverse reactions to drugs such as cyclophosphamide, bleomycin, and amiodarone.[2] Gallium-67 citrate will also localize in certain tumors, although the mechanism is poorly understood. It appears that some tumor cells have numerous transferrin receptors on their cell surfaces that transport ^{67}Ga into the cells where it binds to other iron-binding proteins such as ferritin and lactoferrin.[2] Gallium-67 citrate uptake in lymphoma, mesothelioma, and other lung cancers has been shown to have a diagnostic sensitivity of 85% to 90% in humans.[2,19,20] The clinical utility of ^{67}Ga for inflammatory or neoplastic imaging in veterinary patients has yet to be explored.

Conclusion

Pulmonary scintigraphy in veterinary medicine is primarily used to evaluate for the presence of pulmonary thromboemboli. Due to the lack of sensitivity of intermediate and low probability perfusion studies in humans, newer techniques using non-selective pulmonary angiography and spiral computed tomography have been developed.[24-27] Ventilation imaging may provide additional information, particularly if coupled with ventilation clearance times, although these techniques have not yet been shown to be beneficial in the veterinary clinical setting. Mucociliary clearance and inflammatory imaging of the pulmonary parenchyma are alternate relatively sensitive and specific scintigraphic techniques now available for veterinary patients.

REFERENCES

1. Palmer EL, Scott JA, Strauss HW: *Practical nuclear medicine,* Philadelphia, 1992, WB Saunders.
2. Thrall JH, Ziessman HA: *Nuclear medicine: The requisites,* St. Louis, 1995, Mosby.
3. West JB: *Respiratory physiology: The essentials,* ed 5, Philadelphia, 1995, Williams & Wilkins.
4. The PIOPED Investigators: Value of the ventilation/perfusion scan in acute pulmonary embolism, *J Am Med Assoc* 263(20):2753-2759, 1990.
5. LaRue MJ, Murtaugh RJ: Pulmonary thromboembolism in dogs: 47 cases (1986-1987), *J Am Vet Med Assoc* 197(10):1368-1372, 1990.
6. Klein MK, Dow SW, Rosychuk RA: Pulmonary thromboembolism associated with immune-mediated hemolytic anemia in dogs: Ten cases (1982-1987), *JAVMA* 195(2):246-249, 1989.
7. Pouchelon J-L, Chetboul V, Devauchelle P et al: Diagnosis of pulmonary thomboembolism in a cat using ultrasonography and pulmonary scintigraphy, *J Sm Anim Pract* 38:306-310, 1997.
8. Sottiaux J, Franck M: Pulmonary embolism and cor pulmonale in a cat, *J Sm Anim Pract* 40:88-91, 1999.
9. Johnson LR, Lappin MR, Baker DC: Pulmonary thromboembolism in 29 dogs: 1985-1995, *J Vet Intern Med* 13:338-345, 1999.
10. Venco L, Calzolari D, Morini S: Pulmonary thromboembolism in a dog with renal amyloidosis, *Vet Radiol Ultrasound* 39:564-565, 1998.
11. Dennis JS: Clinical features of canine pulmonary thromboembolism, *Comp Cont Ed* 15:1595-1603, 1993.
12. Slauson DO, Grible DH: Thrombosis complicating renal amyloidosis in dogs, *Vet Pathol* 8:352-363, 1971.
13. Bunch SE, Metcalf MR, Crane SW et al: Idiopathic pleural effusion and pulmonary thromboembolism in a dog with autoimmune hemolytic anemia, *J Am Vet Med Assoc* 195:1748-1753, 1989.
14. Koblik PD, Hornof WJ, Harnagel SH: A comparison of pulmonary angiography, digital subtraction angiography and 99mTc-DTPA/MAA ventilation-perfusion scintigraphy for detection of experimental pulmonary emboli in the dog, *Vet Radiol* 8:159-168, 1989.
15. Berry CR, Daniel GB, O'Callahan M: Pulmonary scintigraphy. In Berry CR, Daniel GB, editors: *Handbook of veterinary nuclear medicine,* Raleigh, 1996, North Carolina State University.
16. Harnagel SH, Hornof WJ, Koblik PD et al: The use of 99mTc radioaerosol ventilation and macroaggregated albumin perfusion imaging for the detection of pulmonary emboli in dogs, *Vet Radiol* 30:22-27, 1989.
17. Clercx C, van den Brom WE, Stokhof AA et al: Pulmonary scintigraphy in canine lobar and sub lobar airway obstruction, *Lung* 167:213-224, 1989.
18. Clercx C, van den Brom WE, van den Ingh TSGAM et al: Scintigraphic analysis as a diagnostic tool in canine experimental lung embolism, *Lung* 167:225-236, 1989.
19. DeNardo BL: Lung imaging. In Martin P, editor: Clinical nuclear medical imaging, Hyde Park, NY, 1981, Medical Examination Publishing.
20. Spies WG, Spies SM, Mintzer RA: Radionuclide imaging in diseases of the chest (Parts I & II), *Chest* 83(1):122-127; 83(2):250-255, 1983.
21. Toal RL, Edwards DF: Mucociliary scintigraphy. In Berry CR, Daniel GB, editors: *Handbook of veterinary nuclear medicine,* Raleigh, 1996, North Carolina State University.
22. Edwards DF, Patton CS, Kennedy JR: Primary ciliary dyskinesia in the dog, *Prob Vet Med* 4(2):291-319, 1992.
23. Whaley SL, Muggenburg BA, Seller FA et al: Effect of aging on tracheal mucociliary clearance in beagle dogs, *J Appl Physiol* 62(3):1331-1334, 1987.
24. Karabulut N, Goodman LR: The role of helical CT in the diagnostic work-up for pulmonary embolism, *Emerg Radiol* 6:10-16, 1999.
25. Remy-Jardin M, Remy J, Artaud D et al: Spiral CT of pulmonary embolism: Technical considerations and interpretive pitfalls, *J Thorac Imaging* 12:103-117, 1997.
26. Remy-Jardin M, Remy J, Artuad D et al: Peripheral pulmonary arteries: Optimization of the spiral CT acquisition protocol, *Radiology* 204:157-163, 1997.
27. Flückiger MA, Gomez JA: Radiographic findings in dogs with spontaneous pulmonary thrombosis or embolism, *Vet Radiol* 25(3):124-131, 1984.

CHAPTER 14

Rhinoscopy and Sampling from the Nasal Cavity

Ross Doust • Martin Sullivan

Rhinoscopy and sample collection from the nasal cavity form an important part of a thorough evaluation of nasal cavity disease. Both procedures should follow diagnostic imaging (e.g., radiography, computed tomography, or magnetic resonance imaging) to avoid artefactual change from hemorrhage.[1-7]

All patients having rhinoscopy and nasal sampling must be anesthetized and have an endotracheal tube with an inflated cuff. Where possible the pharynx should be packed with gauze or sponge to reduce the risk of aspiration of blood, nasal exudate, or lavage fluids.[2,8]

Rhinoscopy

BACKGROUND AND DEFINITION

Rhinoscopy is the nonsurgical visualization of the nasal cavities and nasopharynx. A variety of instruments (detailed below) can be used. The procedure provides information that may not be otherwise available. The nasal and nasopharyngeal anatomies require that separate rostral and caudal rhinoscopic procedures be performed. Rostral rhinoscopy allows evaluation of the nasal cavity through the external nares, whereas caudal rhinoscopy facilitates evaluation of the nasopharynx, caudal choanae, and caudal nasal cavities via the oropharynx.[9-12]

INDICATIONS

Rhinoscopy should be performed as part of a complete diagnostic nasal investigation in any case that demonstrates evidence of nasal, paranasal sinus, or nasopharyngeal disease. Clinical signs associated with nasal, nasopharyngeal, or sinus diseases include sneezing, reverse sneezing, nasal discharge, epistaxis, stertor (snoring or snorting sounds), stridor (inspiratory noise and wheezing), facial swelling or deformity, and mouth breathing.[3,9,13,14]

Rhinoscopy may help to define the type, location, and extent of disease before treatment is initiated. Biopsy for histopathological, cytological, or microbiological examinations is facilitated by rhinoscopy. In cases with acute clinical signs, rhinoscopy may be the diagnostic and therapeutic procedure of choice. These procedures should be considered early in animals with sudden onset of sneezing, snorting, or gagging because these signs may suggest foreign body inhalation.[9,10,12]

CONTRAINDICATIONS

Rhinoscopy may be contraindicated in cases with a coagulopathy. In animals with epistaxis, a clotting profile should be performed prior to rhinoscopy because hemorrhage can result from mucosal trauma by either the rhinoscope or the biopsy. Even if the clotting profile is normal, provision should be made for intravascular volume support (e.g., intravenous fluids, cross match for blood transfusion) and for local hemorrhage control in case it might be needed.[8,15]

General anesthesia is necessary for rhinoscopy because the procedure can elicit a forceful sneeze or reverse sneeze reflex even in animals in a deep plane of anesthesia. Rhinoscopy is therefore contraindicated in animals in which there is a possibility of raised intracranial pressure. In patients with head trauma, it is preferable whenever possible to delay anesthesia until normal intracranial pressure is confirmed.[12]

INSTRUMENTATION

A variety of instruments can be used for rhinoscopy. The rostral nasal cavities can be assessed with an otoscope. In cases of suspected nasal aspergillosis, an otoscope will often provide sufficient access to the affected areas to allow visualization of eroded turbinates and fungal plaques, and biopsy for cytology and fungal culture. The appropriate size of the otoscopic speculum varies with the size of the patient.[10]

An extremely limited view of the caudal nasopharynx in medium to large dogs can be gained with the use of a dental mirror.[12,14,16]

Small arthroscopes offer good visualization of the nasal cavities by rostral rhinoscopy. It is also possible to perform caudal rhinoscopy with a rigid endoscope via a pharyngotomy approach. Arthroscopes are usually 2 to 3 millimeters in diameter and can be used with an appropriately sized sheath that has a flushing or biopsy channel. Arthroscopes are available with a variety of viewing angles. The viewing angle is defined by the angle of the tip of the arthroscope, with a larger angle giving a more side-on view. This may allow better visualization of a lesion, although it does require some practice to navigate through the nose. The disadvantages of arthroscopes are their reduced maneuverability compared with flexible endoscopes and the sharp edges at the tip of the arthroscope that can damage the nasal mucosa (especially diseased, friable areas). Arthroscopic sheaths are usually blunt and should improve protection, although they increase the outside diameter of the rhinoscope.[12,16,17]

Flexible endoscopes are available in 2.5 to 5.0 mm external diameter sizes. Flexible endoscopes are more expensive but are preferred when available because of their increased maneuverability and softer exterior, which allow them to be used for rostral and caudal rhinoscopy (especially in larger patients). With all types of rhinoscopy it is essential that the size of the endoscope is appropriate for the patient, being aware that with smaller scopes the size of the biopsy channel may limit rhinoscopically guided biopsies.[12,16,17]

TECHNIQUE

Preparation

General anesthesia is essential for rhinoscopic examination. There is a strong sneeze reflex in dogs and cats that may persist even under general anesthesia, making conscious rhinoscopy and sample collection impossible. A complete preanesthetic evaluation should be performed with laboratory tests as indicated by the patient's status. Routine testing should include hematology, a biochemistry profile, and a urinalysis. Coagulation profiles, buccal mucosal bleeding time (BMBT), platelet count, and fibrin degradation products should be assessed prior to further nasal disease investigation in animals with epistaxis. It is possible for frank hemorrhage to pass from the nasal cavity and nasopharynx into the pharynx and be swallowed rather than appear at the external nares. BMBT testing provides simple, rapid, and inexpensive indication of the presence of a coagulopathy caused by a platelet function defect. Fibrin degradation products (FDPs) are elevated in circumstances of extensive coagulation because fibrinolysis is also increased.[8,11,15,17]

Ehrlichiosis serology should be performed in endemic areas or for at-risk patients. Blood pressure measurement should be considered in cases of epistaxis, particularly in cats.

Routine precautions should be taken to minimize the risk of aspiration of fluids or blood during rhinoscopy or biopsy. An appropriately sized endotracheal tube, correctly placed with the cuff inflated, is essential. After intubation the pharynx should be packed with an absorbent sponge or gauze swabs to absorb excess fluid. Prior to extubation the pack is removed and the pharynx evaluated for blood or fluid, which can be removed with the aid of suction. The endotracheal tube should be removed as late as possible. Some anesthesiologists advocate leaving the cuff partially inflated during withdrawal to help remove blood or fluid from the trachea.[8,17]

After induction of anesthesia, diagnostic imaging procedures (e.g., radiography, computed tomography, and magnetic resonance imaging) should be carried out prior to rhinoscopy to avoid imaging artifacts created by iatrogenic epistaxis. Biopsy, including rhinoscopically guided biopsy, should be performed following a complete rhinoscopic examination to reduce the risk of iatrogenic hemorrhage obscuring rhinoscopic evaluation.[8,10]

Prior to rhinoscopy the oral cavity should be examined carefully, visually and by palpation, to detect mucosal and anatomic changes. Examination should include visual assessment of the oropharynx, tonsils, tongue, soft and hard palates, teeth, and lips. A thorough dental examination must be performed, including probe examination of each dental sulcus. The soft and hard palates should be digitally examined.[8,9,11,13,18]

For rostral rhinoscopy the patient should be placed in sternal recumbency with the muzzle supported in a horizontal position, facilitating access to the nasal cavity via the external nares. Placing the patient with the nose extending over the edge of the table aids manipulation of the rhinoscope (particularly rigid endoscopes). For caudal rhinoscopy the patient may be placed in sternal or dorsal recumbency. It is essential that a mouth gag be in place to prevent the patient from biting down on the flexible endoscope. Nasopharyngoscopy requires a deep plane of anesthesia because the gag reflex is pronounced.[14,17]

Rhinoscopic viewing may be improved in a darkened room. The mucosa may be viewed through a fluid or air interface. Nasal secretions and hemorrhage will obscure the view, and a constant flow of saline or air, or repeated cycles of saline lavage and aspiration, may be necessary to adequately visualize the cavity. Light source intensity can influence interpretation of mucosal color, and mucosal capillary blanching may occur with a constant airflow.[14,17]

Rostral Rhinoscopy

Entry to the nasal cavities via the external nares and the channel provided by the large alar cartilages can be difficult. The endoscope is inserted ventromedially, then straightened and the nasal planum elevated to allow advancement into the common meatus. Once the alar cartilage is passed, the endoscope is oriented so that the nearly flat surface of the medial septum is vertical. From here the nasal conchae (three primary scrolls of bone rising laterally) and the nasal meatus (major air passages) can be appreciated.

Caudal Rhinoscopy

A variable view is obtained depending on the equipment available. A dental mirror and rostral retraction of the caudal edge of the soft palate will allow some visualization of the nasopharynx in medium to large breed dogs. Warming the mirror to body temperature and endotracheal intubation can reduce fogging of the mirror. The soft palate may be retracted rostrally using a spay hook, stay sutures, Babcock (lung-holding) forceps, or swab forceps. In cats almost all of the nasopharynx to the level of the caudal prominences of the pterygoid bone can be visualized with this method, although lesions on the ventral nasopharynx (dorsal surface of the soft palate) may be obscured.[8,11,13,14,19]

A retroflexed (180-degree) flexible endoscope provides the best view of the nasopharynx and caudal choanae. The endoscope can be flexed prior to insertion with the tip dorsally and passed beyond the caudal edge of the soft palate, which should drop over the tip, allowing it to be retracted rostrally. Care should be taken to avoid damage to the larynx by directing the endoscope laterally during insertion. The view of the nasopharynx and caudal choanae will be inverted. If a biopsy is required, the biopsy forceps must be placed in the channel prior to flexing the endoscope because passing biopsy forceps through a flexed endoscope can cause serious (and expensive) damage. The length of the endoscope tip and the elasticity of the soft palate limit the view.[14,15,17]

An alternative approach is to pass a flexible or rigid endoscope over the soft palate from a pharyngotomy incision. Place the patient in lateral recumbency, then clip and aseptically prepare the area immediately caudal to the vertical ramus of the mandible. Place a finger into the pharynx and identify the larynx and hyoid apparatus. Select a site in the dorsal-lateral pharynx caudal to the epihyoid bone. Tent the site with curved forceps of an appropriate size for the patient. Sharply incise the skin, platysma, and sphincter colli muscles and the pharyngeal mucosa over the forceps. Direct the endoscope between the open jaws of the forceps. Once the endoscope is in the pharynx, withdraw the forceps.

Complications

Mild to moderate hemorrhage may occur after rhinoscopy or biopsy. This usually subsides within a few minutes.[1,8]

INTERPRETATION OF RESULTS

Oral Examination

Masses dorsal to the soft palate can be detected by digital palpation of the soft palate in most cases, particularly nasopharyngeal polyps in cats. Nasal tumors may erode through the palatine or pterygoid bones or may develop on the ventral aspect of these bones, resulting in protrusion or a softening of the hard palate area.[13]

Draining tracts or oronasal fistulae may be detected, either as a congenital abnormality in young animals or secondary to dental disease, trauma, or neoplasia in older animals. Probe examination of the dental sulcus of the teeth may demonstrate a deep pocket of erosion or infection that may result in an oronasal fistula that is not obvious on visual examination.

The palatine tonsil normally sits mostly within the tonsillar fossa. Excessive protrusion of the tonsil may result from inflammation, infection, or neoplasia or may result from excessive inspiratory pressure, particularly in brachycephalic animals or other patients in which the nasal cavity is partly occluded.

Rostral Rhinoscopy

The normal meatus are narrow, convoluted, and limit the depth of penetration possible with a rhinoscope. Severe mucosal edema or congestion may narrow the apparent size of the meatus. An increase in the size of the meatus (cavitated appearance) indicates turbinate destruction consistent with fungal or erosive rhinitis. The convoluted structure of the ethmoturbinates and the root of the maxilloturbinates usually hinder caudal passage of the rhinoscope. Visualization of the nasopharynx by rostral rhinoscopy, except in large dogs or when using a fine endoscope (2 to 3 mm outside diameter), indicates some degree of turbinate destruction. Considerable turbinate erosion is necessary before the nasofrontal duct or frontal sinus ostia can be appreciated.[14,17]

The normal nasal mucosa should appear pink and smooth with a fine network of submucosal capillaries. These may be made less visible by mucosal edema or hyperemia, nasal discharge or hemorrhage, too bright a light source, or by constant flushing with air or cold saline.

Hemorrhage, although a common sequel to rhinoscopy, can be easier to induce or increased if there is an increase in mucosal inflammation and tissue friability. Mucosal hyperemia or surface irregularities such as erosions and ulcers may also be seen.[14,17]

Whitish mucoid or fluffy masses on the mucosal surface, particularly with turbinate erosion, indicate fungal infection. Although in some cases there is a similar appearance to mucopurulent discharge material, the reflective surface tends to be shiny. The color of fungal colonies may vary from whitish to green tinged, and they may be seen in the nasal cavity and maxillary or frontal sinuses (Figure 14-1). A mixture of mucoid, purulent, or sanguineous discharges can accompany fungal infections, obscuring visualization of fungal plaques. When suspected fungal plaques are seen they should be biopsied for cytology and culture to confirm the diagnosis.[10,14,17]

Mucoid discharge and mucosal hypertrophy or hyperemia are consistent with hypertrophic (idiopathic) rhini-

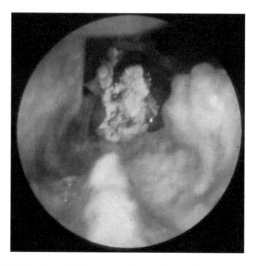

Figure 14-1. *Rostral rhinoscopy. Extensive turbinate destruction is present and a large fungal plaque is evident resting on the mucosa.*

tis. This is largely a diagnosis based on signalment (common in whippets and rough collies), clinical signs (e.g., chronic mucoid to mucopurulent nasal discharge not or only partly responsive to antibacterial therapy, recurring immediately on cessation), and exclusion (no other primary lesions found). For this reason it may be advisable to periodically reevaluate these cases to determine if another cause has been missed.

Tissue in the meatus may be neoplastic or inflammatory and should always be examined histopathologically for a definitive diagnosis. Inflammatory tissue may be a fungal granuloma (e.g., feline cryptococcosis, sporothricosis, or canine rhinosporidiosis) or idiopathic (e.g., nasal polyps). Tumors most commonly occur in the caudal area of the nasal cavity and may be difficult to access if there is limited destruction of the rostral conchae. The exception to this is squamous cell carcinoma, which can be found within the external nares. Because mucopurulent or sanguineous discharge may also make visualization of nasal tumors difficult, unguided biopsy is often necessary.[8,17,20,21]

Nasal discharge may also make identification and retrieval of foreign bodies difficult. The presence, location (unilateral or bilateral), and type of discharge should be noted. The location should be referred back to radiographs and periodontal examination results. In some cases a profuse discharge may be found on rhinoscopy that has not been noted by owners. This can occur either because the patient is removing the discharge (by licking) before it is seen, or because the majority of the discharge is draining caudally.[12,22]

Caudal Rhinoscopy

Healthy nasopharyngeal mucosa is usually pink and smooth. Irritated mucosa appears hyperemic and friable and may have hyperplastic lymphoid follicles. These follicles have a miliary appearance as small whitish lumps protruding from the mucosal surface and, seen in chronic reverse sneezing, are associated with long-term antigenic stimulation of the nasopharyngeal mucosa.

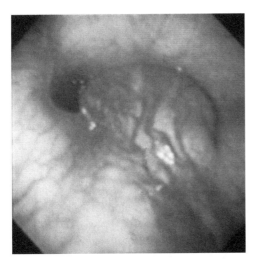

Figure 14-2. *Caudal rhinoscopy. A large mass is present in the nasopharynx occluding the caudal choanae.*

Anatomical landmarks include the eustachian tube orifices, soft palate, juncture of hard and soft palates, vomer bone and its rostral continuation as the nasal septum, pituitary gland area/projection, and the caudal aspects of the left and right nasal choanae. The juncture of the hard and soft palates may be identified by digital pressure in the oral cavity.[17]

Abnormalities that can be detected range from benign conditions (e.g., nasopharyngeal stenosis or nasopharyngeal polyps in cats, foreign bodies, and nasal mites) to malignancies (Figure 14-2). Malignant tumors are less commonly identified in the nasopharynx than in the nasal cavity itself.[11]

Sample Collection

BIOPSY

Biopsy is the collection of tissue samples for histopathology, cytology, culture, virus isolation, or other tests. Samples range from fine needle aspirate biopsies to excisional biopsies through a rhinotomy approach, and each has its own specific indications, advantages, and disadvantages. Excisional biopsies include grab, wedge, suction, and punch biopsies. Excisional biopsies are preferable to flushing techniques for the collection of suitable samples.[2,5,23]

Indications and Contraindications

Nasal mucosal abnormalities, tissue growths, and fungal plaques should all be sampled. Biopsies can be used for culture (microbial and fungal), cytological, or histopathological evaluation. Tissue biopsy may be the only way to positively differentiate different disease processes. Although there is always some degree of hemorrhage, in most biopsies the risk of major hemorrhage is small. Reported cases of severe hemorrhage following nasal biopsy have had an underlying coagulopathic etiology identified. Coagulopathies may be considered a specific contraindication for biopsy techniques other than fine needle aspirate biopsy.[1,8,10,12]

INSTRUMENTATION

The instrumentation required depends on the technique chosen. Rhinotomy requires a standard surgical kit and periosteal elevator, Gelpi retractor, oscillating saw (preferred) or osteotome and mallet, air drill or Jacob's chuck, and pins. Trephination may be performed with a trephine or a large-diameter Steinmann pin. Flexible endoscopes often have a specific flexible biopsy forceps that can be passed through a channel in the endoscope. These forceps usually collect very small tissue fragments (i.e., less than 2 mm), although the sample can be taken under direct visualization, allowing accurate collection.[20,23]

Unguided or blind biopsies may be gathered with a variety of instruments. The two most common techniques are grab and suction biopsies. Grab biopsies use athroscopic biopsy instruments (Figure 14-3) or, in larger dogs,

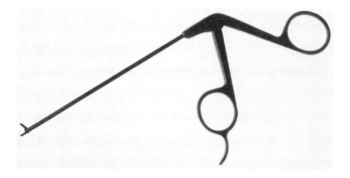

Figure 14-3. *Arthroscopic forceps for nasal biopsy. These are suitable for animals ranging from cats to giant dogs.*

mare endometrial cup biopsy forceps. Suction biopsies use a stiff urinary catheter or other tubing, with the end cut at 45 degrees; and a 50-ml syringe to provide suction.[2]

Punch biopsy has also been described using a tissue biopsy needle (e.g., tru-cut needle).[2,4]

Technique

Rhinotomy is usually reserved for cases in which there is a focal lesion or when other techniques have not been successful. Rhinotomy is an invasive biopsy method performed using a dorsal or ventral approach, depending on the location and extent of the disease process previously identified by diagnostic imaging or rhinoscopy. Complications of rhinotomy include severe hemorrhage, entry to the calvarium, pain, emphysema, airway obstruction, and nasal discharge. Intraoperative hemorrhage can be minimized by lavage with semi-frozen sterile saline, or by temporary occlusion of the external carotid arteries, although the latter should be unnecessary for a biopsy. Packing of the nasal cavity following surgery should be avoided because it promotes hyperventilation and subcutaneous emphysema, and can be painful to remove. Blood transfusions may be necessary if there is excessive hemorrhage during or after surgery.[12,16,23-25]

Trephination involves a limited approach to a specific area of the nasal cavity or paranasal sinuses. It is particularly useful for disease limited or extending to the frontal sinus. Grab biopsies can then be taken, and the skin incision closed. Trephine holes in the frontal sinuses may also be used to place drains for the treatment of fungal rhinitis.[12]

Nasal biopsies are most commonly collected by closed techniques, either rhinoscopically guided, or blind. Rhinoscopy and diagnostic imaging (e.g., radiography, computed tomography, or magnetic resonance imaging) are used to identify target areas for closed biopsy. Several biopsies should be taken to reduce the random effect. In cases where the lesions are accessible, arthroscopic biopsy forceps can be placed parallel to the rhinoscope and the biopsy site visualized during collection. When the lesion cannot be directly visualized rhinoscopically, or there is insufficient space to allow both the rhinoscope and the biopsy forceps, biopsies can be taken blind. When closed biopsies are performed

blind, the medial canthus of the eye is used as a landmark for the maximum depth of insertion to avoid penetrating the cribriform plate. Biopsy forceps are measured from the nasal planum to the medial canthus and premarked to indicate the maximum depth of penetration. The cribriform plate, which is already more friable than normal bone due to the large number of fenestrations, may be excessively so due to destructive disease processes such as neoplasia or fungal rhinitis.[2,8]

Suction biopsies are obtained by introducing a catheter/tube to approximately the level of the lesion and applying suction while moving the catheter in and out. Gentle suction is applied while the syringe is withdrawn.[2,4]

Punch biopsies have been described using a Tru-cut biopsy needle. The needle is inserted into the nasal cavity. If stiff resistance is felt, the needle is withdrawn slightly and redirected. There is usually some increase in resistance if entering a soft tissue mass. Several samples are taken at different angles. This technique may not be as efficient for sampling nasal cavities where there is not a soft tissue proliferative disease process.[2]

Touch preparations can be made from biopsy samples for cytological examination prior to formalin fixation for histopathology. Small specimens should be placed on a premoistened piece of lens or filter paper in the formalin to prevent loss.[2]

Complications

Mild to moderate hemorrhage will usually occur after nasal biopsy. If it is severe or persistent, the nasal cavity and nasopharynx may be packed with cotton buds soaked in dilute (1:100,000) epinephrine or 0.5% phenylephrine, and a moist sponge inserted into the nasopharynx to prevent flow of the blood caudally. Care should be taken not to exceed a safe dose of either drug. In extremely rare instances a transfusion is required and if the hemorrhage is severe and persistent, carotid ligation or embolization on the affected side may be considered. Suction should always be used gently to minimize bleeding that could interfere with the procedure.[26]

CYTOLOGY

Cytology is the microscopic examination of cells collected from the body. There are four broad categories of cell collection: fine needle aspirate biopsy (FNAB), brush cytology, exfoliative cytology, and touch cytology. Fine needle aspirate biopsy involves the use of a 21- to 23-G needle placed into a mass or organ, and the application of suction to gather cells into the body of the needle. FNAB is not commonly used in nasal disease unless the lesion is directly visible. Brush cytology uses a brush to collect cells from a lesion or mucosal surface. Exfoliative cytology is the collection of cells that have been shed from a lesion or mucosal surface. The most common collection method for exfoliative cytology is to flush the organ or area with sterile saline. Touch preparations are made from tissue samples (e.g., from a biopsy prior to fixation). Nasal flush techniques are not diagnostic as often as other biopsy techniques.[2,4,5]

Care should be taken to avoid over-interpretation of cytology because some metaplastic cells may appear neoplastic. Findings must be interpreted in conjunction with history, physical examination, rhinoscopy, and clinical and laboratory findings. Negative or nonspecific findings on cytology do not rule out serious disease processes such as neoplasia or fungal rhinitis, which often have an inflammatory cell population. Rhinoscopy and radiography should always be performed prior to any cell collection techniques.[3,24,28]

Indications and Contraindications

Cytological evaluation is indicated in all cases of nasal disease. Aggressive collection techniques such as suction biopsies should be avoided in cases of coagulopathy, where fine needle aspirate biopsy and gentle retrograde flushing techniques are appropriate.

Instrumentation

Cytology samples can be collected by a variety of simple techniques. Flushing of the nasal cavity may be performed with either a normal urinary catheter or a Foley catheter with a balloon of sufficient size to occlude the nasopharynx (e.g., 10 ml in cats and small dogs, 30 ml in most medium to large dogs [Figure 14-4]). Flushing is performed with sterile, nonbacteriostatic physiological saline.[4,28,29]

Touch or squash preparations may be made using biopsy samples collected as above. All samples are prepared on glass slides. Slides should be wiped with a clean dry tissue prior to use to remove particulate debris that may impede a smooth, even spread.[4,28]

Technique

Nasal flushing is always performed in anesthetized animals with endotracheal intubation. The pharynx is packed with gauze swabs to reduce the risk of aspiration and for collection of large fragments that may be dislodged. The nasal cavity can then be flushed using 5- to 10-ml aliquots of sterile saline. Fluid is collected by aspiration after flushing and by catching it in sample containers at the external nares and on gauze swabs at the external nares and pharynx.[29]

Alternatively, a Foley catheter is inserted in a retrograde fashion into the nasopharynx; the pharynx is packed with gauze swabs to collect leakage; and the nasal cavity is flushed through the Foley catheter. Samples may be collected by free catch at the external nares, either into sample pots or onto gauze swabs, or by inserting a rubber tube into the nasal cavity and aspirating.[4,29]

Touch imprints or squash preparations are made of collected tissue fragments. Touch imprints (impression smears) are made by removing excess fluid and blood from the surface of the sample by dabbing it gently onto gauze swabs or blotting paper. The sample is then gently pressed onto the surface of a glass slide. Several impressions should be made sequentially on the same slide from the same cut surface to reduce the blood contami-

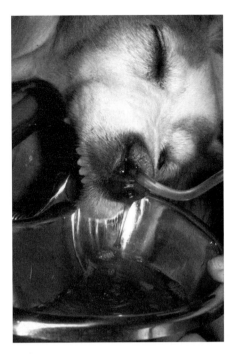

Figure 14-4. *Nasal flushing carried out in an attempt to retrieve diagnostic samples.*

nation on the later smears. Squash preparations are preferred when the tissue fragment is too small to handle and there is sufficient sample to preserve some for histopathology. The smear is made by placing a small fragment onto a glass slide and placing a second slide over the sample at right angles to the first slide. The top slide is dragged lengthways over the first to smear the sample. The second slide is examined.[4]

Nasal flush samples may be smeared directly or centrifuged, and the sediment smeared onto glass slides using a standard blood smear technique. All slides are air-dried, stained, and examined by routine methods. Romanovsky-type stains are preferred for examination of cytology. There are Romanovsky stains available that are simple to use in the practice situation (e.g., Diff-Quick), along with a variety of stains that are used in the laboratory or in practices where a large number of cytology and peripheral blood smears are examined. An advantage of the Romanovsky stain is that cell morphology will be familiar to most operators from peripheral blood smears, and published cytology pictures will mostly use a variation of this stain. Operators should become familiar with the techniques and interpretation of a particular stain. New methylene blue staining can be used to highlight the granules of mast cells if they do not stain well with Romanovsky stains. Periodic acid-Schiff (PAS) stains are used to highlight fungal hyphae.[4,29]

Submitting samples to laboratories for cytological examination has the advantage of allowing an expert opinion and higher quality staining techniques than are available in most practices. The obvious disadvantage is that it removes the immediate diagnostic value. Fluid samples for submission should be sent in EDTA tubes and be accompanied by an air-dried or methanol-fixed smear. Samples should not be packed with formalin samples because formalin fumes can significantly change the staining characteristics of cytology samples.[4]

INTERPRETATION OF BIOPSY AND CYTOLOGY RESULTS

As is the case with all ancillary diagnostic aids, histopathology and cytology should be interpreted in the context of the clinical presentation. It is important to distinguish between normal and pathological cell and bacterial populations. Epithelial cell morphology varies with the site and depth of the sample. Nonkeratinized squamous epithelial cells, with or without adherent bacteria, are found in the external nares and oropharynx, whereas the nasal turbinates are lined with ciliated pseudostratified columnar epithelial cells. Hemorrhage is a common finding in nasal samples because the nasal epithelium is easily traumatized by collection techniques.[3,4]

Exudates associated with bacterial, viral, and fungal infections usually have a predominance of neutrophils, along with variable numbers of macrophages, lymphocytes, and plasma cells. The same cell population can be seen with any inflammatory condition of the nasal cavity. A pathogenic bacterial infection may be suspected when there is a monomorphic bacterial population with some bacteria seen within neutrophils, rather than the normal pleomorphic population of bacteria that colonize epithelial cells with minimal neutrophil involvement. Bacterial infections of the nasal cavity are usually secondary to mucosal injury, often due to foreign bodies, trauma, fungal infection, or neoplasia.

Chronic hyperplastic rhinitis biopsies have hyperplasia of the mucosa and a mixed inflammatory cell population, whereas in lymphocytic-plasmacytic rhinitis there is an infiltration of lymphocytes and plasma cells within the nasal mucosa. Lymphocytic-plasmacytic rhinitis may reflect a chronic allergic stimulus. Cytologically, an abundance of lymphocytes and plasma cells may reflect a reactive hyperplasia of submucosal lymphoid aggregates.[3,8,30]

Viral inclusions are occasionally seen in nasal samples, and herpesvirus infection in cats may produce intranuclear inclusions in epithelial cells.

Fungal hyphae may not stain well and can usually be seen as clear, filamentous structures within dense accumulations of cells and debris. Specialized stains (e.g., periodic acid-Schiff or Gomori's methanamine silver) may improve the visualization of fungal hyphae. Fungal morphology is not a reliable method for identifying the species involved; culture is necessary. *Aspergillus* spp. and *Penicillium* spp. are the most common causes of fungal rhinitis in the dog. Fungal rhinitis in the dog is usually localized rather than a manifestation of a systemic mycosis. These appear as 2.0 to 4.5 μm wide, septate branching hyphae, often found enmeshed in clumps of necrotic debris (Figure 14-5). *Rhinosporidia seeberi* causes polypoid nasal growths in the dog; it appears as round to oval 7-μm spores in nasal exudates or tissue imprints and stains bright pink. The spores contain eosinophilic globules and have thin, bilaminar walls. The

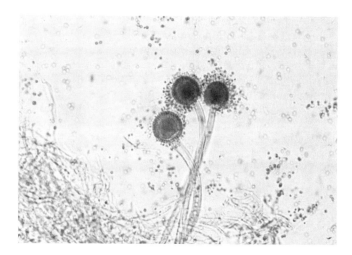

Figure 14-5. Aspergillus fumigatus *obtained from a nasal swab and smeared.*

presence of large sporangia containing numerous endospores is supportive but not often seen.[3,21,28,31,32]

Cryptococcus neoformans is a saprophytic yeast causing rhinitis and sinusitis, most commonly in cats. The significant subspecies are *Cryptococcus neoformans var neoformans* and *var. gatii*. It may be diagnosed from touch imprints or aspirates of nasal lesions without flushing or biopsy techniques. *C. neoformans* is basophilic, round to oval, 3.5 to 7.0 μm in diameter, with a thick polysaccharide capsule. It stains poorly with Wright's or Diff-Quick. India ink is not taken up by *Cryptococcus*, so it remains silhouetted on the stain, but air bubbles and fat globules may confuse inexperienced operators. *C. neoformans* infection can be confirmed with a latex capsule agglutination test (LCAT) performed on serum, which can also be used to monitor response to treatment. Other mycoses seen in the cat include *Aspergillus* spp., *Histoplasma capsulatum*, and *Blastomyces dermatitidis*.[*]

Pneumonyssoides caninum and *Linguatula serrata* have been reported in dogs. Adult or larval *P. caninum* may be found on the nasal mucosa. It may be an incidental finding or cause mucosal irritation, sneezing, or reverse sneezing. *L. serrata* attaches to the nasal mucosa and may induce sneezing, coughing, and epistaxis. Adults may be viewed rhinoscopically, and larvated eggs may be found in nasal exudates. *Capillaria aerophila* is usually found in the lower respiratory tract but has been found in the nasal sinuses. The eggs are characteristically barrel-shaped with bipolar end plugs. Sedimentation of nasal flush samples may be useful to recover ova. Exudates with parasites usually contain an increased number of eosinophils with neutrophils and other white cells.[16,28,35]

Nasal foreign bodies are typically inhaled plant material. The cytology samples should be examined for signs of foreign material, usually in the form of variable sized and shaped particles. Persistent foreign bodies result in chronic rhinitis secondary to mucosal damage.

*References 3, 13, 16, 26-28, 33, 34.

Exudates with a predominance of eosinophils may indicate environmental antigen stimulation, although eosinophils may also be present with parasites, fungi, bacteria, and neoplasia; all need to be ruled out before inhalant allergic rhinitis can be diagnosed.[3,16]

Neoplasia is usually seen in older animals, but may occasionally be seen in very young animals. Eighty to ninety percent of nasal tumors are malignant; however, metastasis is uncommon, or occurs late in the course of the disease. Histopathology is necessary for the definitive diagnosis of tumor type and grade of malignancy, but cytology can provide a useful screening test. Cytology samples from nasal cavities with neoplasia typically contain erythrocytes, inflammatory cells, bacteria, and necrotic debris. Neoplastic cells may or may not be present, depending on the sample collection technique and the exfoliative nature of the tumor. Hemorrhage, which may be prominent with well-vascularized tumors, or concomitant discharge may obscure diagnostic cells. The absence of neoplastic cells does not rule out nasal neoplasia. Fine needle aspirate biopsy, catheter biopsy, and touch preparations of biopsy samples are more likely to yield neoplastic cells than are nasal flush samples.[2-5,8,24,29]

Tumors of epithelial origin are most common. Adenocarcinoma is the most common, followed by squamous cell carcinoma and undifferentiated carcinomas. Carcinomas consist of clusters of round to oval cells with a variable nucleus:cytoplasm ratio, which is less pronounced in well-differentiated carcinomas. Cytologically, they may be difficult to differentiate from hyperplastic epithelial cells. Adenocarcinomas are often associated with production of mucus, apparent as an amorphous to fibrillar deeply pink–staining material. Squamous cell carcinomas usually have a variety of developmental stages, from small hypochromatic cells to large round or angular cells with pale basophilic cytoplasm and large nuclei. Perinuclear clearing, if apparent, strongly suggests squamous cell origin.[3,8,24,36,37]

Mesenchymal tumors include fibrosarcoma, chondrosarcoma, osteosarcoma, hemangiosarcoma, and undifferentiated sarcomas. Mesenchymal tumors exfoliate poorly or may be covered with normal or hyperplastic epithelium until advanced. Aspiration or catheter biopsy preparations produce a more cellular sample than nasal flush. Sarcoma cells are plump oval to fusiform or spindle shaped, with the cytoplasm streaming away from the nucleus. Sarcomas tend to exfoliate individually or in small clumps, unlike carcinomas, which exfoliate in large sheets. Osteosarcoma and chondrosarcoma cells may have abundant basophilic cytoplasm and pink granules. Malignant melanoma is not a common nasal tumor but is a common tumor of the palate and may invade the nasal cavity.[3,28,29,36-40]

Round cell tumors of the nasal cavity include lymphosarcoma, mast cell tumors, and transmissible venereal tumors. Round cell tumors usually exfoliate readily as a homogenous population of individual round cells with distinct cell margins. Lymphosarcoma is usually a monomorphic population of large immature lymphocytes. Small mature lymphocytes predominate in nonneoplastic conditions with submucosal lymphoid hyperplasia. Mast cell tumors usually have bloody aspirates with numerous mast cells and few eosinophils, whereas allergic rhinitis tends to have more eosinophils and few mast cells. Transmissible venereal tumor is more commonly associated with the genital regions, but due to the social habits of dogs it may be transmitted to the nasal area. The tumor cells have round nuclei, a variable chromatin pattern, and a single prominent nucleolus. There is a moderate amount of cytoplasm that is lightly basophilic, usually containing clear vacuoles. Mitoses may be numerous, and inflammatory cells of a mixed type may be present.[3,28,41-43]

Benign growths occur more commonly in the feline nasal passages. Fungal granulomas may occur with cryptococcal infection. Benign inflammatory polyps occur in the nasal cavity and nasopharynx. These are separate entities, for which the etiopathogenesis is obscure. Nasal polyps originate in the nasal cavity, and histopathologically there is polypoid inflammatory tissue with prominent vasculature and osseous metaplasia. Osseous metaplasia and prominent vasculature are not found in nasopharyngeal polyps, which probably arise in the auditory canal. Cats with nasopharyngeal polyps should have an otic examination.[20,44]

MICROBIOLOGICAL SAMPLING

Samples are collected from the nasal cavity for culture of bacteria and mycoses and for antibiotic sensitivity profiles. The normal nasal cavity has a rich population of commensal bacteria, although these may become opportunistic pathogens secondary to other nasal diseases (e.g., neoplasia, fungal rhinitis, and idiopathic hyperplastic rhinitis). Samples may be collected from the conjunctiva, nasal cavity, or oropharynx in cats for isolation of viral and chlamydial causes of feline upper respiratory tract diseases.

Indications and Contraindications

Any nasal discharge should be cultured. Purulent or mucopurulent discharges are more likely to contain bacteria. There are no contraindications to bacterial culture and sensitivity testing. Cases of feline upper respiratory tract disease should be sampled as early in the disease process as possible. Fungal culture should be performed in cases where there is a suspicion of fungal rhinitis.

Instrumentation

A bacteriology swab and bacterial transport media are all that is required for bacterial or fungal culture. Guarded bacteriology swabs reduce the risk of contamination from the external nares. Biopsy samples are superior for culture, particularly fungal culture. Feline swabs should be placed into virus transport media immediately following collection for transport.

Technique

Bacterial culture may be performed on a variety of samples. Tissue biopsies are the ideal samples. When taking

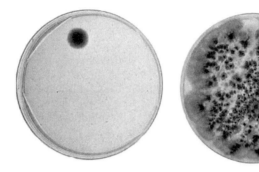

Figure 14-6. *Culture plates. The impact of obtaining a guided swab is evident from the sparse growth obtained on the left plate from a blind swab compared to the right plate from a guided swab.*

a swab from the nasal cavity it is important to avoid contamination from the external nares and where possible in guided fashion (Figure 14-6). Where available, a guarded swab is superior. As with nasal biopsies, the maximum depth of insertion is based on the medial canthus of the eye.

For conjunctival, nasal, or oropharyngeal swabs for feline upper respiratory tract disease, take a sterile swab, moisten with tears or saliva, and firmly scrape the surface (conjunctiva or mucosa) being sampled. Immediately place the swab into the transport medium, and freeze for transport.[32]

Interpretation of Results

Overinterpretation of bacteriological cultures should be avoided. A positive culture should not be immediately identified as the primary etiopathogenic agent. When a secondary nasal infection exists, culture and sensitivity testing is useful to identify the organism(s) and define effective treatment.

Positive culture of fungal disease should be interpreted as such and treatment instituted, unless there is evidence of gross contamination. *Aspergillus* spp. and *Penicillium* spp. infection may occur secondary to, or concomitant with, nasal tumors.

The major causes of chronic feline upper respiratory tract disease are feline herpesvirus-1 (FHV-1), feline calicivirus (FCV), and *Chlamydia psittaci*. Other pathogens, such as *Bordetella bronchiseptica*, *Mycoplasma felis* or feline reovirus, should be considered significant.[33,45]

Feline herpesvirus may not be isolated in chronic cases of feline upper respiratory tract disease, where it has been the primary pathogen. Feline herpesvirus can destroy the nasal turbinates, allowing secondary bacterial and fungal infection. FHV-1 in cats develops a true latent carrier state and is usually only shed under conditions of stress or prolonged corticosteroid use, making recovery difficult. Feline calicivirus is shed continuously from carrier cats and is therefore more reliably isolated. Coinfection with viral diseases such as feline leukemia virus (FeLV) or feline immunodeficiency virus (FIV) should be considered in all cases.[16,33,45-47]

REFERENCES

1. Forbes Lent SE, Hawkins EC: Evaluation of rhinoscopy and rhinoscopy assisted mucosal biopsy in diagnosis of nasal disease in dogs: 119 cases (1985-1989), *JAVMA* 201:1425-1429, 1992.
2. Withrow SJ, Susaneck SJ, Macy DW et al: Aspiration and punch biopsy techniques for nasal tumors, *J Am Anim Hosp Assoc* 21:551-554, 1985.
3. French TW: The use of cytology in the diagnosis of chronic nasal disorders, *Compendium on Continuing Education for the Practicing Veterinarian* 9:115-120, 1987.
4. Meyer DJ: The management of cytology specimens, *Compendium on Continuing Education for the Practicing Veterinarian* 9:10-16, 1987.
5. Withrow SJ: Diagnostic and therapeutic nasal flush in small animals, *J Am Anim Hosp Assoc* 13:704-707, 1977.
6. Gartrell CL, O'Handley PA, Perry RL: Canine nasal disease – part I, *Compendium on Continuing Education for the Practicing Veterinarian* 17:323-328, 1995.
7. Clercx C, Wallon J, Gilbert S et al: Imprint and brush cytology in the diagnosis of canine intranasal tumours, *J Small Anim Pract* 37:423-427, 1996.
8. Tasker S, Knottenbelt CM, Munro EAC et al: Aetiology and diagnosis of persistent nasal disease in the dog: A retrospective study of 42 cases, *J Small Anim Pract* 40:473-478, 1999.
9. Gabor L, Price JE, Laurendet HM et al: Paroxysmal sneezing in a 7-year-old cat, *Aust Vet J* 75:320, 328, 335, 1997.
10. Sullivan M: Nasal discharge in the dog. In Gorman NT, editor: *Canine medicine and therapeutics*, ed 4, Oxford, 1998, Blackwell Science.
11. Tyler JW: Endoscopic retrieval of a large, nasopharyngeal foreign body, *J Am Anim Hosp Assoc* 33:513-516, 1997.
12. McKiernan BC: Sneezing and nasal discharge. In Ettinger SJ, Feldman SC, editors: *Textbook of veterinary internal medicine*, ed 4, Philadelphia, 2000, WB Saunders.
13. Allen HS, Broussard J, Noone K: Nasopharyngeal diseases in cats: A retrospective study of 53 cases (1991-1998), *J Am Anim Hosp Assoc* 35:457-461, 1999.
14. Sullivan M: Rhinoscopy. In Brearley MJ, Cooper JE, Sullivan M, editors: *A color atlas of small animal endoscopy*, London, 1991, Wolf Publications.
15. Littlewood JD: A practical approach to bleeding disorders in the dog, *J Small Anim Pract* 27:397-409, 1986.
16. Norsworthy GD: Finding the cause of chronic nasal discharge in cats, *Vet Med* 90:1038-1046, 1995.
17. Padrid PA, McKiernan BC: Endoscopy of the upper respiratory tract of the dog and cat. In Tams TR, editor: *Small animal endoscopy*, ed 2, London, 1999, Mosby.
18. Bellows J: A misdiagnosed cause of chronic sneezing in a dog, *Vet Med* 96:103-104, 2001.
19. Rudd RG, Richardson DC: A diagnostic and therapeutic approach to nasal disease in dogs, *Compendium on Continuing Education for the Practicing Veterinarian* 78:103-113, 1985.
20. Galloway PE, Kyles A, Henderson JP: Nasal polyps in a cat, *J Small Anim Pract* 38:78-80, 1997.
21. Caniatti M, Roccabiance P, Scanziani E et al: Nasal rhinosporidiosis in dogs: Four cases from Europe and a review of the literature, *Vet Rec* 142:334-338, 1998.
22. Davidson AP, Mathews KG, Koblik PD et al: Diseases of the nose and nasal sinuses. In Ettinger SJ, Feldman SC, editors: *Textbook of veterinary internal medicine*, ed 4, Philadelphia, 2000, WB Saunders.
23. Hedlund CS: Rhinotomy techniques. In Bojrab MJ, Ellison GW, Slocum B, editors: *Current techniques in small animal surgery*, ed 4, Baltimore, 1997, Williams & Wilkins.
24. Thiesen SK, Hosgood G, Lewis DD: Intranasal tumors in dogs: Diagnosis and treatment, *Compendium on Continuing Education for the Practicing Veterinarian* 18:131-138, 1996.
25. Beck ER, Withrow SJ: Tumors of the canine nasal cavity, *Vet Clin North Am Small Anim Pract* 15:531-532, 1985.
26. Hedlund CS, Tangner CH, Elkins AD et al: Temporary bilateral carotid artery occlusion during surgical exploration of the nasal cavity of the dog, *Vet Surg* 12:83-85, 1983.
27. Taboada J: Cryptococcosis. In Ettinger SJ, Feldman SC, editors: *Textbook of veterinary internal medicine*, ed 4, Philadelphia, 2000, WB Saunders.

28. Andreason CB, Rakich PM, Latimer KS: Nasal exudates and masses. In Cowell RL, Tyler RD, Meinkoth JM, editors: *Diagnostic cytology and hematology of the dog and cat,* ed 2, St Louis, 1999, Mosby.
29. MacEwen EG, Withrow SJ, Patnaik AK: Nasal tumors in the dog: Retrospective evaluation of diagnosis, prognosis, and treatment, *JAVMA* 170:45-48, 1977.
30. Burgener DC, Slocombe RF, Zerbe CA: Lymphoplasmacytic rhinitis in five dogs, *J Am Anim Hosp Assoc* 23:565-568, 1987.
31. Easley JR, Merton DJ, Levy MG et al: Nasal rhinosporidiosis in the dog, *Vet Pathol* 23:50-56, 1986.
32. Ford RB: Viral upper respiratory infection in cats, *Compendium on Continuing Education for the Practicing Veterinarian* 13:593-602, 1991.
33. Cape L: Feline idiopathic chronic rhinosinusitis: A retrospective study of 30 cases, *J Am Anim Hosp Assoc* 28:149-155, 1992.
34. Evinger JV, Kazacos KR, Cantwell HD: Ivermectin for treatment of nasal capillariasis in a dog, *JAVMA* 186:174-175, 1985.
35. Norris AM: Intranasal neoplasms in the dog, *J Am Anim Hosp Assoc* 15:231-236, 1970.
36. Madewell BR, Priester GA, Gillette EL et al: Neoplasms of the nasal passages and paranasal sinuses in domesticated animals as reported by 13 veterinary colleges, *Am J Vet Res* 37:851-856, 1976.
37. Confer AW, DePaoli A: Primary neoplasms of the nasal cavity, paranasal sinuses and nasopharynx in the dog, *Vet Pathol* 15:18-30, 1978.
38. Todoroff RJ, Brodey RS: Oral and pharyngeal neoplasia in the dog: A retrospective survey of 361 cases, *JAVMA* 175:567-571, 1979.
39. Dorn CR, Priester WA: Epidemiologic analysis of oral and pharyngeal cancer in dogs, cats, horses and cattle, *JAVMA* 169:1202-1206, 1976.
40. Duncan JR, Prasse KW: Cytologic examination of the skin and subcutis, *Vet Clin North Am Small Anim Pract* 6:637-645, 1976.
41. Weir EC, Pond MJ, Duncan JR et al: Extragenital occurrence of transmissible venereal tumor in the dog: Literature review and case reports, *J Am Anim Hosp Assoc* 14:532-536, 1978.
42. Bright RM, Gorman NT, Probst CW et al: Transmissible venereal tumor of the soft palate in a dog, *JAVMA* 183:893-895, 1983.
43. Anderson DM, Robinson RK, White RAS: Management of inflammatory polyps in 37 cats, *Vet Rec* 147:684-687, 2000.
44. Sykes JE, Anderson GA, Studdert VP et al: Prevalence of feline *Chlamydia psittaci* and feline herpesvirus-1 in cats with upper respiratory tract disease, *J Vet Intern Med* 13:153-162, 1999.
45. August JR: Feline viral respiratory disease, *Vet Clin North Am Small Anim Pract* 14:1159-1171, 1984.
46. Pederson NC, Ho EN, Brown ML et al: Isolation of a T-lymphotropic virus from domestic cats with an immunodeficiency-like syndrome, *Science* 235:790-793, 1987.
47. Knowles JO, Gaskell RM, Gaskell CJ et al: Prevalence of feline calicivirus, feline leukaemia virus, and antibodies to FIV in cats with chronic stomatitis, *Vet Rec* 124:336-338, 1989.

CHAPTER 15

Laryngoscopy and Pharyngoscopy

David E. Holt

Direct examination of the larynx and pharynx is an important diagnostic procedure in animals presenting with signs of upper airway disease. Examination of the pharynx is also important in animals presenting for gagging or difficulty prehending or swallowing food. Animals with pharyngeal disorders such as foreign bodies, perforation, or nasopharyngeal polyps can present with respiratory distress, gagging, and difficulty swallowing of varying severity. Laryngoscopy is the examination of the larynx, generally under light general anesthesia, to determine patency and function. Pharyngoscopy is the examination of the oropharynx and nasopharynx and associated structures, including the choana, soft palate, tonsils, palatine arches, and epiglottis. This chapter will focus on laryngoscopy and pharyngoscopy in the context of upper airway disease.

Indications

In many instances a diagnosis, or at least the anatomical location of the animal's disease, is suggested by the history, clinical signs, and physical examination findings. Laryngoscopy and pharyngoscopy are used to confirm the tentative diagnosis, evaluate the disease, and plan appropriate treatment. In cases of severe upper airway obstruction, laryngoscopy is indicated simply as a means of assisting intubation and rapidly obtaining a functional airway to stabilize the animal before further evaluation.

Pharyngoscopy is indicated as part of the diagnostic work-up of chronic nasal disease. Chronic nasal discharge and inability to move air through the nasal passages can be associated with obstructions of the choana or nasopharynx that may be congenital due to nasopharyngeal polyps, secondary to trauma or due to neoplasia. Obstruction of the cranial nasopharynx by a membrane of tissue has been described in young cats.[1-3] These lesions can be visualized using a retroflexed endoscope. Nasopharyngeal polyps should be suspected in young cats with stertorous respiration, nasal discharge, and difficulty swallowing. Rapid oral palpation in the conscious animal with the index finger often reveals ventral displacement of the soft palate by the polyp. Pharyngoscopy under general anesthesia allows the veterinarian to make a definitive diagnosis and rule out other diseases affecting the nasopharynx.[4]

In dogs with brachycephalic airway syndrome, laryngoscopy and pharyngoscopy allow evaluation of the length of the soft palate and examination of the larynx for eversion of the mucosa of the lateral ventricles (everted laryngeal saccules) and laryngeal collapse. In bite wound and choke chain crushing injuries involving the larynx, laryngoscopy is vital to evaluate laryngeal integrity and function and to assess the possibility of laryngeal repair. In pharyngeal foreign body perforations, pharyngoscopy is often required to remove the foreign body safely and treat the resulting wound appropriately.[5]

Many older, large breed dogs present with upper airway stridor and other signs suggestive of laryngeal paralysis. A thorough physical examination and diagnostic work-up is performed to rule out other possible causes of the clinical signs (e.g., thyroid carcinoma and tracheal neoplasia) and other associated problems (e.g., polyneuropathy, megaesophagus, and aspiration pneumonia). Laryngoscopy under light anesthesia then allows confirmation of laryngeal paralysis and exclusion of other laryngeal or pharyngeal diseases that might cause similar clinical signs. Laryngoscopy is also imperative postoperatively to assess the results of arytenoid abduction.

Laryngoscopy and pharyngoscopy are necessary to obtain biopsy specimens for definitive diagnosis of oral, pharyngeal, or laryngeal neoplasms. Direct examination, in addition to routine staging and advanced imaging of the primary neoplasm if necessary, allows the clinician to decide the feasibility of primary tumor resection.

Laryngoscopy and pharyngoscopy are also indicated in animals that have difficulty breathing after extubation, particularly after nasal, oral, pharyngeal, laryngeal, or tracheal surgery. The veterinarian must rapidly evaluate airway patency and laryngeal function, especially following procedures with the potential for recurrent laryngeal nerve damage (e.g., tracheal ring prosthesis placement).

In some instances, animals with respiratory distress and clinical signs of partial upper airway obstruction can present with a nonspecific history and physical examination findings that fail to point towards a specific diagnosis. In these cases, laryngoscopy and pharyngoscopy are indicated as part of a complete investigation to identify the underlying cause of the respiratory distress.

Contraindications

There are few absolute contraindications to laryngoscopy and pharyngoscopy. The opportunity to evaluate laryngeal function may be extremely brief in animals with severe upper airway obstruction. These animals may require immediate intubation to secure a patent airway and allow for effective ventilation. Stimulation of the larynx and pharynx can occasionally result in massive vagal discharge and severe bradycardia or cardiac arrest; therefore all animals undergoing laryngoscopy and pharyngoscopy should be premedicated with an anticholinergic drug. Ideally, all animals requiring laryngoscopy and pharyngoscopy should be fasted for 12 hours prior to anesthesia to minimize the risk of regurgitation or vomiting, but this is not possible in animals with moderate to severe respiratory compromise. In this situation, a secure seal must be confirmed between the endotracheal tube cuff and the trachea, and the animal is extubated only after the gag response has returned to minimize the possibility of aspiration.

Some animals with laryngeal paralysis have concurrent megaesophagus. True abnormalities of esophageal function may be difficult to diagnose preoperatively because a normal esophagus may appear air-filled and dilated on thoracic radiographs due to aerophagia. A barium swallow to document esophageal function is contraindicated in animals with respiratory distress. Nevertheless, esophageal dysfunction should be suspected in any animal with laryngeal dysfunction. If present, megaesophagus greatly increases the risk of postoperative aspiration pneumonia.

Many animals presenting with severe upper airway obstruction have concurrent problems (e.g., hyperthermia and respiratory muscle fatigue). Older bulldogs often have scarring of the pharyngeal dilator muscles.[6] Dogs with laryngeal paralysis may have an associated generalized polyneuropathy[7,8] and concurrent aspiration pneumonia. These conditions are not direct contraindications to laryngoscopy and pharyngoscopy per se, but they must be carefully considered because they all decrease the likelihood of a straightforward anesthetic recovery and normal respiration in the immediate postoperative period.

Instrumentation

Endotracheal tubes of varying sizes and stiffness must be available to facilitate intubation. In some animals with severe airway obstruction, the only tube that will pass the obstruction may be a narrow, red rubber catheter, through which oxygen can be continuously insufflated. In spite of the small lumen size, animals can often be adequately oxygenated through a red rubber catheter until a tracheostomy can be performed to bypass the upper airway obstruction. The use of stylets to stiffen endotracheal tubes and thereby facilitate intubation is somewhat controversial. Some clinicians feel that there is an increased risk of perforating the dorsal tracheal membrane if a stylet is used improperly. At least two laryngoscopes with blades of appropriate length and functioning lights may be required. One laryngoscope depresses the epiglottis ventrally; the second is often necessary to move the soft palate dorsally, especially in brachycephalic dogs, to allow an unobstructed view of the larynx.

Flexible endoscopes give the veterinarian an excellent view of the nasopharynx when the endoscope is retroflexed. Flexible fiberoptic endoscopes contain glass fiber bundles to transmit and receive light. Disruption of the bundles' arrangement, water leakage, and breakage of the glass fibers are all detrimental to image quality. Video endoscopes use a microelectronic chip on the distal tip of the scope to transmit images to a video processor, which in turn displays the image on a television screen. In cats the nasopharynx can be visualized endoscopically using either a retroflexed cystoscope or a small bronchoscope. Alternatively, a small spay hook is used to retract the soft palate cranially and expose the nasopharynx. This technique works particularly well in cats with nasopharyngeal polyps.

A surgical instrument pack for an emergency tracheostomy should be open at the time of anesthetic induction in severely dyspneic animals or in cases in which the likelihood of easy intubation is in doubt. Surgical instruments for biopsy of oral, pharyngeal, or laryngeal lesions are also necessary. Laryngeal biopsy is often facilitated by long-handled laryngeal cup forceps.

In dyspneic animals in which a tentative diagnosis cannot be made before anesthesia, the veterinarian must be prepared to perform the entire diagnostic investigation, and perhaps surgical correction of the condition, during the anesthetic episode for laryngoscopy and pharyngoscopy. This may include cervical and thoracic imaging, tracheoscopy and bronchoscopy, and an endotracheal wash or bronchoalveolar lavage. Facilities for these procedures should be available.

Technique

In stable animals, a thorough physical examination and diagnostic work-up is performed prior to laryngoscopy. Although a partial upper airway obstruction may be suspected, other potential causes of respiratory distress should be carefully considered. Diseases affecting the trachea, bronchi, lungs, chest wall, pleural space, diaphragm, and heart can sometimes cause clinical signs similar to those of upper airway disease. Concerns about concurrent megaesophagus, neuromuscular disease, and aspiration pneumonia have already been mentioned. Animals in respiratory distress must be examined with caution because any struggling or stress will increase oxygen consumption and may precipitate decompensation. An oral examination is desirable but can cause vagally mediated bradycardia. Evidence of mucous membrane cyanosis raises concern about the severity of the animal's respiratory compromise and should also prompt consideration of congenital heart diseases (associated with cyanosis in young animals), methemoglobinemia, hypoventilation, and primary lung disease. External palpation of larynx, pharynx, and the cervical area may reveal masses such as thyroid carcinoma, lymphosarcoma, or a mucocoele responsible for the airway compromise. Thoracic auscultation and thoracic wall palpation helps define potential cardiac, pleural, chest wall, or diaphragmatic diseases that may contribute to the animal's respiratory distress. Thoracic radiographs should be obtained prior to anesthesia in stable animals; in unstable animals, radiographs should be made once a reliable airway is secured with an endotracheal or tracheostomy tube.

One, or preferably two secure, reliable intravenous catheters are required before proceeding with laryngoscopy. An anticholinergic premedication is administered and the animal is given flow-by or face-mask oxygen supplementation prior to and during anesthesia induction. Many different anesthetic protocols have been used in dogs and cats for laryngoscopy and pharyngoscopy (see Chapter 33). The plane of anesthesia must be extremely light for laryngeal function to be accurately assessed. Most clinicians currently use small boluses of propofol or thiobarbiturates for this purpose. Unpublished information indicates that phenothiazines may decrease arytenoid movement in normal dogs. This decrease can be reversed by administering doxapram.[9] During laryngoscopy, respiratory effort, mucous membrane color, and pulse quality are carefully monitored. Ideally, indirect oscillometric or Doppler blood pressure monitoring and pulse oximetry are also used. Oxygen supplementation is provided at the nares or mouth until the animal is intubated.

Once the anesthetic has taken effect, a length of gauze is placed behind the upper canine teeth to hold the mouth open, the tongue is gently grasped with a gauze sponge and pulled forward out of the mouth, and the laryngoscope is used to depress the epiglottis and visualize the larynx. Movement of the corniculate processes of the arytenoid cartilages is observed while an assistant describes the phase of respiration. Normally during inspiration, the arytenoid cartilages should abduct then return to a paramedian position during expiration. In animals with laryngeal paralysis, the arytenoid cartilages either do not move or move paraxodically to the phase of respiration (i.e., during inspiration, the lower pressure within the airway draws the arytenoids together; during expiration, the arytenoids are pushed apart). This paradoxical movement can superficially mimic normal movement; therefore attention must be paid to the phase of respiration during movement of the larynx. Failure of adequate arytenoid abduction indicates either laryngeal paralysis or an animal that is in too deep a plane of anesthesia. As a general rule, the animal should be in a plane light enough to be attempting to gag before lack of arytenoid movement is interpreted as paralysis.

The initial examination of the oropharynx is performed at the same time as laryngoscopy. The oropharynx is examined using the laryngoscope blade and light source. In brachycephalic dogs, the length of the soft palate is assessed and the larynx examined for eversion of the mucosa of the lateral ventricles and evidence of collapse. Once these examinations have been performed, the animal is intubated.

Examination of the nasopharynx or manipulation of a pharyngeal foreign body generally requires a deeper plane of anesthesia. The nasopharynx should initially be viewed directly by retracting the soft palate rostrally with either a spay hook or a stay suture placed at the caudal edge of the soft palate. In cats with nasopharyngeal polyps, rostral retraction of the palate often causes the polyp to protrude into the oropharyx where it can be grasped and removed. Rarely, the soft palate may need to be incised to gain access to small nasopharyngeal polyps.

The rostral nasopharynx can be further examined with an endoscope. The endoscope is inserted into the caudal oropharynx, then retroflexed into the nasopharynx. The rostral nasopharynx and choanal openings are then examined. A small endoscope can also be useful in examining wounds in the pharynx caused by foreign body penetration. The magnified view provided by the endoscope can be used to determine if any pieces of foreign material remain in the pharyngeal wound.

Interpretation of Results

The difficulties in interpreting failure of arytenoid abduction during laryngoscopy have already been mentioned. The results of laryngoscopy must be interpreted in light of the phase of respiration and the plane of anesthesia. In general, if the animal is light enough to gag when the epiglottis is depressed by the laryngoscope blade, failure of arytenoid abduction indicates paralysis. Although not as common as bilateral paralysis, unilateral paralysis can occur in dogs and cats. It is also important to remember that laryngeal paralysis is not an "all or nothing" disease, and results of laryngoscopy can depend on the timing of the examination relative to the course of the disease.

Laryngeal electromyography (EMG) can be performed if the diagnosis is in doubt. EMG needles do not have to be inserted into the dorsal cricoarytenoid muscle specifically because the caudal laryngeal nerves innervate all of the intrinsic muscles of the larynx except the cricothyroideus muscles. Fibrillation potentials, positive sharp waves, and "dive bomber" electrical activity in the muscles of the larynx support a diagnosis of denervation and paralysis. Ultrasonographic examination of the larynx has been described in awake dogs[10] and following further study this technique may allow diagnosis of laryngeal paralysis in the awake animal.

REFERENCES

1. Mitten RW: Nasopharyngeal stenosis in four cats. *J Small Anim Pract* 29:341, 1988.
2. Novo RE, Kramek B: Surgical repair of nasopharyngeal stenosis in a cat using a stent, *J Am Anim Hosp Assoc* 35:251, 1999.
3. Griffon DJ, Tasker S: Use of a mucosal advancement flap for the treatment of nasopharyngeal stenosis in a cat, *J Small Anim Pract* 41:71, 2000.
4. Allen HS, Broussard J, Noone K: Nasopharyngeal disease in cats: A retrospective study of 53 cases (1991-1998), *J Am Anim Hosp Assoc* 35:457, 1999.
5. White RAS, Lane JG: Pharyngeal stick penetration injuries in the dog, *J Small Anim Pract* 29:13, 1988.
6. Petrof, BJ, Pack AI, Kelly AM et al: Pharyngeal myopathy of loaded upper airway in dogs with sleep apnea, *J Appl Physiol* 76:1746, 1994.
7. Gaber CE, Amis TX, LeCouteur RA: Laryngeal paralysis in dogs: A review of 23 cases, *J Am Vet Med Assoc* 186:377, 1985.
8. Braund KG, Steinberg S, Shores A et al: Laryngeal paralysis in immature and mature dogs as one more sign of a more diffuse polyneuropathy, *J Am Vet Med Assoc* 194:1735, 1989.
9. Tobias KM: Personal communication, 2000.
10. Bray JP, Lipscombe VJ, White RAS et al: Ultrasonographic examination of the pharynx and larynx of the normal dog, *Vet Radiol Ultrasound* 39:566, 1998.

CHAPTER 16

Bronchoscopy

Ned F. Kuehn • Rebecka S. Hess

Background and Definition

Bronchoscopy or tracheobronchoscopy is a reliable procedure for the diagnosis, and occasionally for the treatment, of respiratory tract diseases. Bronchoscopy is indicated in patients with chronic or acute respiratory disease considered to be due to airway compromise. Animals with diffuse small airway disease (<2-mm diameter) or interstitial lung disease are less likely to benefit from direct visualization of the airways; however, diagnostic samples may be obtained via bronchoalveolar lavage. Although rigid scopes can be utilized, flexible fiberoptic bronchoscopes are superior for visualization and procurement of diagnostic samples deeper into the airway system. Bronchoscopy allows the clinician to visually evaluate the lumen and walls of the trachea; carina; principal bronchi (right and left mainstem bronchi); and, to a variable extent, the secondary and tertiary segmental bronchi. Bronchoscopy also makes possible the procurement of diagnostic samples (e.g., biopsy specimens, bronchoalveolar lavage fluid, and samples for culture), as well as retrieval of aspirated foreign objects or particulate matter within the airway system.

Anatomy and Nomenclature

Lung lobe names are based on bronchial division and not on the presence of external fissures or relation of lobes to surrounding structures in the dog and cat.[1] Each lung has a cranial lobe, ventilated by the cranial bronchus, and a caudal lobe, ventilated by the caudal bronchus. In addition, the right lung has a middle lobe ventilated by the middle bronchus and an accessory lobe ventilated by the accessory bronchus. The left cranial lobe is divided into cranial and caudal sections because there is no left middle lobe.

Endobronchial nomenclature for the systematic evaluation of the canine airway system has been proposed (Figure 16-1).[2] The nomenclature enables the bronchoscopist to relocate lesion sites, associate bronchoscopic findings with diagnostic imaging studies, and convey bronchoscopic findings, as well as specific location to other clinicians. A similar scheme has not been established for cats.

Airway branching in the dog is strongly monopodial.[3] Lobar bronchi are identified by the side of the bronchial tree from which they stem and by the order in which they originate from the principal bronchus.[2] The lobar bronchus to the left cranial lung lobe is therefore designated as LB1 (left bronchus 1) and that to the left caudal lung lobe as LB2. The lobar bronchus to the right cranial lung lobe is designated RB1; the right middle

lung lobe, RB2; the right accessory lung lobe, RB3; and finally, the right caudal lung lobe, RB4.

Segmental bronchi are identified by their orientation and sequence of origination from the lobar bronchus. Except for the right middle lung lobe, the segmental bronchi in all of the other lung lobes arise in either a dorsal or ventral direction. The dorsal series of segmental bronchi are designated by the capital letter D and those of the ventral series by the capital letter V. Therefore, the segmental bronchus designated as RB3D1 is the first dorsal segmental bronchus (D1) arising from the lobar bronchus of the accessory lung lobe (RB3).

Unlike the segmental bronchi of the other lung lobes, those of the right middle lung lobe are directed in a cranial and caudal orientation. The segmental bronchi of the right middle lung lobe directed cranially are designated by the capital letter R (rostral), and those directed caudally are designated by the capital letter C. Hence, the segmental bronchus identified as RB2R1 refers to the first rostrally directed segmental bronchus (R1) arising from the lobar bronchus of the right middle lung lobe (RB2). Likewise, the segmental bronchus identified as RB2C1 is the first caudally directed segmental bronchus (C1) arising from the lobar bronchus of the right middle lung lobe (RB2).

In medium and large breeds of dogs, some subsegmental bronchi can be visualized with flexible fiberoptic bronchoscopes. These can be identified by order of origin (but not anatomical direction) using sequential lower-case letters. Although anatomical origin might conceivably be identified by using a series of six lower-case letter designations (d-dorsal, v-ventral, m-medial, l-lateral, c-caudal, r-rostral), this proves to be difficult and confusing. Instead, for simplicity, the first subsegmental bronchus

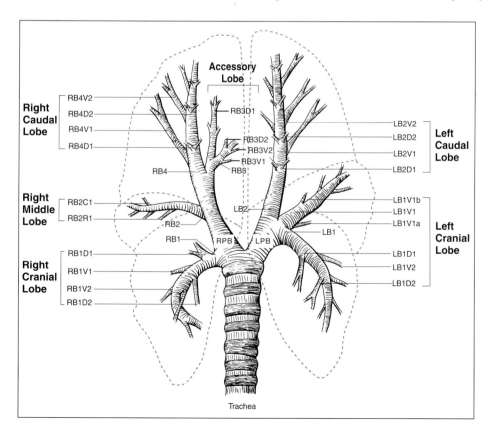

Figure 16-1. Diagrammatic representation of the canine endobronchial tree. The principal, lobar, segmental, and subsegmental bronchi are identified using the endobronchial nomenclature for the canine airway system described in the text. (From Amis TC, McKiernan BD: Systematic identification of endobronchial anatomy during bronchoscopy in the dog, Am J Vet Res 12:2649, 1986.)

encountered is designated by the letter a, the second by the letter b, and so on. Therefore, RB1V1b is the second subsegmental bronchus (b) originating from the first ventral segmental bronchus (V1) arising from the right cranial bronchus (RB1) to the right cranial lung lobe.

Indications

Diagnostic indications for the use of tracheobronchoscopy vary (Box 16-1).[1,4] Generally, the procedure is performed when physical examination; thoracic radiographs; blood or serological studies; and, possibly, therapeutic trials have failed to identify an underlying cause for lower respiratory tract disease. Small animal patients with chronic cough, hemoptysis, and chronic or acute respiratory distress may benefit most from the procedure when other studies have failed to establish a cause for the respiratory disease. Animals with disease determined to be affecting the pulmonary vasculature alone, or those with isolated discrete pulmonary lesions, are unlikely to benefit from bronchoscopy.

Therapeutic indications for bronchoscopy are less common and include removal of foreign material; suction of aspirated materials; removal of viscous secretions or mucous plugs; and, occasionally, to aid in difficult intubation.

Contraindications

Bronchoscopy is generally a safe procedure when performed by an experienced endoscopist. The decision to perform bronchoscopy must balance the risks and benefits to the patient. Careful assessment of the patient prior to

---

BOX 16-1
Diagnostic Indications for Bronchoscopy

Procurement of diagnostic samples
• Obtain material for microbiologic studies
• Bronchoalveolar lavage
• Bronchial brushing
• Transbronchial biopsy of lung tissue
• Transbronchial lymph node aspiration
Investigation of unexplained clinical signs
• Hemoptysis
• Cough (or change in nature of cough)
• Wheezes or stridor
Evaluation of radiographic lung lesions of unexplained etiology
• Pulmonary densities or infiltrates
• Atelectasis or localized hyperlucency
Assessment of airway integrity
• Airway patency (extramural, endomural, or intramural obstruction lesions)
• Tracheal or bronchial tears
• Tracheobronchial or bronchoesophageal fistula
• Lung lobe torsion
• Tracheal or bronchial collapse
Assessment of extent of airway injury
• Inhalation of noxious gases
• Aspiration of gastric contents or caustic substances

---

and after the procedure is important. The category of patients often at high risk are those with unstable cardiac failure or arrhythmias or those with respiratory insufficiency associated with moderate to severe hypoxemia or hypercarbia.[1,4] The procedure must be approached cautiously in patients suspected to have partial tracheal obstruction due to stenosis or an aspirated foreign body. Hemorrhage may be a complication following biopsy in patients with uremia, pulmonary hypertension, or coagulopathies.[5] Immunocompromised individuals may be at increased risk for infection following bronchoscopy. Finally, in patients with lung abscessation, there is increased risk of flooding the airways with purulent material.

Instrumentation

Rigid or flexible fiberoptic endoscopes may be utilized for examination of the airway system. Flexible fiberoptic endoscopes are preferred because they allow a more complete examination of the bronchial tree (Figures 16-2 and 16-3). Either type of scope will allow visualization of the trachea, carina, and principal and lobar bronchi. Flexible fiberoptic endoscopes permit further detailed evaluation of the segmental and subsegmental bronchi.

Rigid fiberoptic endoscopes are available in varying lengths and diameters. Two or three rigid scopes would be required to evaluate animals of various sizes.[1] For animals under 7 to 10 kg, a 3.5-mm diameter by 30-cm length rigid scope would be suitable. A rigid scope with an 8.0-mm diameter by 45-cm length will be required for animals between 10- and 23-kg body weight. For animals of greater than 23-kg body weight, a rigid esophagoscope may be used as a bronchoscope. Flexible fiberoptic endoscopes that can be used for bronchoscopy consist of bronchofiberscopes and, for larger animals, pediatric gastroduodenoscopes.[1] Pediatric and adult flexible bronchoscopes with diameters ranging from 3.6 mm to 5 mm are suitable for cats and most dogs. The work-

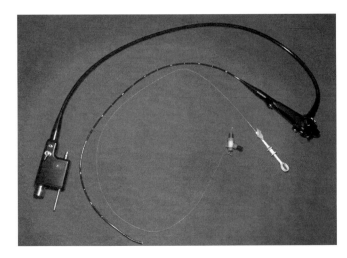

Figure 16-2. Flexible bronchoscope (6.0-mm diameter) used for bronchoscopy in dogs, along with brush forceps. Also photographed is a double swivel elbow with a 7.6-mm port used to connect the anesthesia machine, oxygen, and endoscope to the tracheal tube.

ing length of most human bronchoscopes is limited to 57 cm, which limits passage of the scope only as far as the distal trachea or carina in large or giant breed dogs. A pediatric gastroduodenoscope with a 5-mm to 8-mm outer diameter and a 1-m or longer working length is often required in these dogs.

Fiberoptic instrument technology has been well reviewed.[6] Flexible fiberoptic scopes utilized for bronchoscopy should have an instrument port and channel, suction, bidirectional tip deflection capability, bending capability of not less than 100 degrees in at least one direction, and an external light source. Essential additional equipment includes Y- or T-shaped endotracheal tube adapters, sterile endotracheal tubes, brush catheters, biopsy and retrieval forceps, microbiology specimen brushes, and specimen traps for bronchoalveolar lavage. Appropriate photographic equipment might be considered if slides or other visual or digital images are to be obtained.

Technique

The bronchoscope should be sterilized according to manufacturer's recommendations prior to each procedure. Meticulous cleaning of the outside of the scope with a sponge or soft brush, then cleaning the channels using brushes supplied by the manufacturer, is mandatory to remove dirt and organic debris prior to sterilization. Immersion of the scope in a liquid disinfecting solution recommended by the manufacturer (usually glutaraldehydes or iodophors) is the most common method of sterilization. Ethylene oxide gas may also be used, but strict adherence to the manufacturer's guidelines regarding venting of the scope must be followed to prevent damage to the instrument's bending section sheath. After exposure to ethylene oxide gas, the instrument requires aeration in an OSHA approved vented chamber for approximately 10 hours to dispel absorbed ethylene oxide gas. Endoscopic

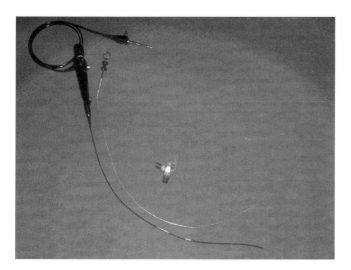

Figure 16-3. *Flexible bronchoscope (3.0-mm diameter) used for bronchoscopy in cats and small dogs along with biopsy forceps. Also photographed is a double swivel elbow with a 7.6-mm port used to connect the anesthesia machine, oxygen, and endoscope to the tracheal tube.*

accessories such as biopsy forceps, grasping forceps, snares, cytology brushes, and water bottles are in most cases autoclavable (follow manufacturer's guidelines).

Fiberoptic scopes are delicate and should be handled with the utmost care. Rough handling of the scope (e.g., sharply bending the light cord or insertion tube, dropping the scope, or closing the instrument in the hinges of the carrying case) may result in costly repairs. Instruments passed down through the biopsy channel should not have kinks or rough edges. Meticulous cleaning, followed by lubrication of the air and water suction valves, is essential for proper operation of the scope. Finally, the equipment should be stored in a safe and secure location such as either the original carrying case or hung in a closet specifically dedicated for endoscopic instruments.

General anesthesia is required to perform bronchoscopy. The animal is placed in sternal recumbency with the head elevated on a headrest such as a rolled towel so that the nose is parallel to the table. An oral speculum should be used to prevent the animal from accidentally biting and damaging the scope. The animal should be intubated with the largest possible sterile endotracheal tube to facilitate passage of the scope. The endotracheal tube may be shortened to allow as complete visualization of the trachea as possible. A sterile Y- or T-shaped swivel adapter is then attached to the end of the endotracheal tube to allow the passage of oxygen and anesthetic gas during the procedure. The adapter has a self-sealing port for passage of the bronchoscope.

The scope should be lubricated with a sterile, water-soluble lubricant before passage. It is then passed through the self-sealing port, down the endotracheal tube, and advanced carefully towards the carina and bronchi. In order to avoid laceration and subsequent pneumomediastinum or tension pneumothorax, the scope should never be forced into secondary or tertiary airways.

Adequate ventilation is critically important but may be difficult to maintain during bronchoscopy. Intermittent cessation of the procedure may be required to allow adequate ventilation and oxygenation of the patient. High flow rates of anesthetic gas may be required during bronchoalveolar lavage due to the concomitant suctioning of anesthetic gases with lavage fluid during the collection phase of the procedure. High-frequency jet ventilation may be utilized to overcome the hypoventilation associated with bronchoscopy during standard mechanical ventilation.[7] Oxygen may be delivered to the patient directly through the hollow center of a rigid scope or through the biopsy channel of a flexible fiberoptic endoscope if prolonged examination is required. Indirect respiratory monitoring using pulse oximetry and end-tidal capnography may be used to provide valuable information about the status of the patient during the procedure.

Tracheobronchoscopy is more difficult in the cat and in very small dogs. With very small animals, the endoscope will likely need to be passed directly through the larynx and into the trachea. Care must be given to avoid trauma to the arytenoid cartilages or vocal folds during passage of the scope through the glottis. A sterile, water-soluble lubricant should be applied to the scope to reduce the risk of laryngeal injury as the scope is moved forwards and backwards. If resistance is encountered during passage of the scope, the procedure should be discontinued until the cause can be determined. Due to the tendency for cats to develop severe laryngospasm, the arytenoid cartilages should be swabbed with a local anesthetic such as proparacaine or lidocaine using a cotton-tipped applicator stick prior to bronchoscopy. Short-acting intravenous anesthetics are best in very small dogs and cats. In these animals, intubation and preoxygenation for 30 to 45 seconds, followed by extubation and insertion of the scope, is advised. A small diameter rigid or flexible scope is passed directly through the larynx to examine the trachea and carina. Extensive evaluation of the lobar bronchi, however, is difficult.

Canine tracheobronchial anatomy encountered during bronchoscopy has been thoroughly reviewed.[2,8] The first lobar bronchus encountered upon entry of the right principal bronchus is that of the right cranial lung lobe. The second lobar bronchus, encountered just past that of the right cranial lung lobe, is that to the right middle lung lobe. The lobar bronchus to the right accessory lobe arises from the ventromedial to medial aspect of the right principal bronchus just caudal to the entry into the right middle lung lobe. The right principal bronchus becomes the entrance to the right caudal lung lobe immediately caudal to the lobar bronchus of the right accessory lung lobe. On the left side, the first lobar bronchus encountered is that of the left cranial lung lobe. The left principal bronchus becomes the left caudal lobar bronchus just past the left cranial lobar bronchus.

The bronchoscope should be gently directed through the airway system. Aggressive manipulation or forced passage of the scope may cause hemorrhage or tearing of the tracheobronchial wall. Following systematic evaluation of the tracheobronchial tree and subsegmental airways, specimens may be collected for cytology, bacterial or fungal culture, biopsy, and bronchoalveolar lavage.[1,4]

Cytologic specimens obtained through the endoscope by brushing the tracheal or bronchial mucosa are superior to those obtained via tracheal wash and aspiration. Specially designed brushes contained within a plastic sheath are advanced through the lumen of a rigid endoscope or through the biopsy channel of a fiberoptic endoscope and directed to the site of interest, where the brush is advanced through the plastic sheath. The brush is then reintroduced into the plastic sheath and the entire assembly is removed from the scope. Cytological preparations are made by gently rolling the brush with the sample on a clean glass slide.

Transbronchial needle aspiration of paratracheal, carinal, hilar, and peripheral lung lesions may be performed using specially designed aspiration needles, which are passed through the biopsy channel of a flexible fiberoptic bronchoscope. Fluoroscopy is often required to place the scope in the correct location. The needle is advanced through the catheter sheath and passed through the bronchial wall into the lesion. Suction is applied using a syringe while moving the needle in and out of the lesion. The sample is then prepared in the same way as other fine needle aspirates.

Sterile bacterial cultures of deep airway specimens can also be obtained with a specially designed system consist-

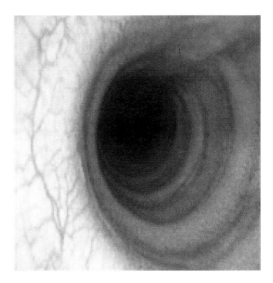

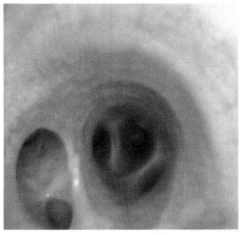

Figure 16-4. *Normal trachea and lower airways in a 4-year-old female Afghan hound.*

ing of a sterile brush contained within a telescoping double catheter occluded by a polyethylene glycol plug. The plugged telescoping double catheter system is passed through the endoscope and the brush is extended into the secretions that are to be cultured. The brush is then retracted into the inner catheter and the assembly is removed from the scope. The brush can then be advanced out of the catheter, the wire is cut with sterile scissors, and the brush is placed in transport media for bacterial culture.

Transbronchial lung biopsy is possible using specially designed biopsy forceps that pass through the endoscope. This technique may be attempted to determine the cause of diffuse interstitial, alveolar, or nodular lung diseases. The biopsy forceps are passed through the instrumentation channel of the endoscope and pushed through the bronchial wall to obtain lung tissue. Major complications such as hemorrhage or pneumothorax are possible with this technique.

Bronchoalveolar lavage is indicated for lobar and diffuse lower airway or interstitial lung diseases. The procedure is relatively safe and can be quickly performed. In patients with lobar disease, the procedure is performed by

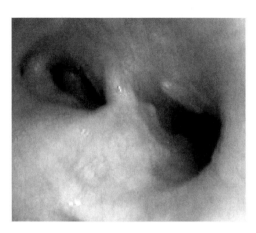

Figure 16-5. *Edematous lower airway observed in a 14-year-old male castrated mixed-breed dog diagnosed with allergic tracheobronchitis based on bronchoalveolar lavage cytology (eosinophilic [47%] and suppurative inflammation).*

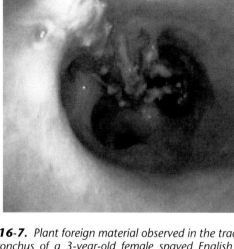

Figure 16-7. *Plant foreign material observed in the trachea and right bronchus of a 3-year-old female spayed English springer spaniel. Partial removal of the foreign material during bronchoscopy and treatment with antibiotics were curative.*

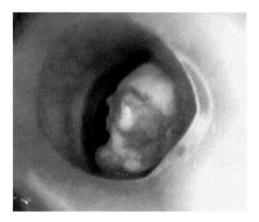

Figure 16-6. *Tracheal chondrosarcoma in an 11-year-old male castrated Labrador retriever. The tumor was diagnosed with surgically obtained biopsy.*

BOX 16-2
Abnormal Bronchoscopic Findings

Tracheal or bronchial wall
- Redness or pallor
- Absence of mucosal surface luster
- Edema
- Vascular engorgement
- Irregular mucosal surface
- Indistinct cartilage rings
- Protrusion of cartilage
- Mucosal ulceration or necrosis
- Mucosal atrophy or thickening
- Pendulous dorsal tracheal membrane
- Tumor

Tracheal or bronchial lumen
- Abnormal secretions (mucus, hemorrhage)
- Stenosis
- Obstruction or foreign body
- Compression
- Torsion
- Shape anomalies (widening, flattening, constriction, sacculation)
- Abnormal branching
- Abnormal movement during respiration or on coughing

---

insertion of the tip of the bronchoscope into the secondary bronchus leading to the affected lobe. With diffuse lung diseases, the scope is inserted randomly in selected secondary bronchi in the right and left lungs. Bronchoalveolar lavage is discussed in detail in Chapter 17.

Interpretation of Results

The normal tracheal and bronchial mucosa is a uniform, light pink color and appears moist with only a minimal amount of mucous secretions (Figure 16-4).[1,4] A network of fine submucosal blood vessels is present. The tracheal cartilage rings are readily visualized, and the dorsal tracheal membrane should be narrow and taut. The carina appears as a sharp wedge dividing the trachea into the two principal bronchi. The right principal bronchus usually appears as a near direct continuation of the trachea,

whereas the left principal bronchus forms a more acute angle with the trachea. The entrances into the principal and various subsegmental bronchi should appear round with crisp, sharply defined edges and should remain open during respiration. A systematic evaluation of all accessible parts of the bronchial tree should be undertaken in a consistent manner. Abnormalities in size, shape, or color of the airways, as well as the presence or absence of abnormal secretions such as mucus or blood, should be recorded (Figures 16-5, 16-6, and 16-7; Box 16-2).[9]

REFERENCES

1. Roudebush P: Tracheobronchoscopy, *Vet Clin North Amer* 20:1297, 1990.
2. Amis TC, McKiernan BD: Systematic identification of endobronchial anatomy during bronchoscopy in the dog, *Am J Vet Res* 12:2649, 1986.
3. Phalen RF, Oldham MJ: Tracheobronchial airway structure as revealed by casting techniques, *Am Rev Respir Dis* 128:S1, 1983.
4. Ford RB: Endoscopy of the lower respiratory tract of the dog and cat. In Tams TR, editor: *Small animal endoscopy*, Philadelphia, 1990, Mosby.
5. Fulkerson WJ: Current concepts: Fiberoptic bronchoscopy, *New Eng J Med* 311:511, 1984.
6. Barlow DE: Fiberoptic instrument technology. In Tams TR, editor: *Small animal endoscopy*, Philadelphia, 1990, Mosby.
7. Bjorling DE, Lappin MR, Whitfield JB: High-frequency jet ventilation during bronchoscopy in a dog, *J Am Vet Med Assoc* 187:1373, 1985.
8. Venker-van Haagen AJ: Bronchoscopy of the normal and abnormal canine, *J Am Anim Hosp Assoc* 15:397, 1979.
9. Venker-van Haagen AJ, Vroom MW, Heijn A et al: Bronchoscopy in small animal clinics: An analysis of the results of 228 bronchoscopies, *J Am Anim Hosp Assoc* 21:521, 1985.

CHAPTER 17

Bronchoalveolar Lavage

Eleanor C. Hawkins

Background and Definition

Bronchoalveolar lavage (BAL) is a diagnostic technique for sampling from the alveoli and small airways. It is also helpful in the diagnostic evaluation of some interstitial diseases.[1-3] Sterile isotonic saline is instilled into a bronchus in a volume large enough to reach the alveoli communicating with the airway. The saline is then retrieved for analysis, along with cells and other compounds lining the airways and alveoli. Bronchoalveolar lavage is most commonly performed during bronchoscopy. Fortunately, simple, inexpensive techniques that can be performed in any practice have recently been described for nonbronchoscopic BAL.

Bronchoalveolar lavage is distinct from tracheal or bronchial washes. Airway washes collect material from the surface of large airways only. Bronchoalveolar lavage collects material from deep within the lung, with only minor contribution from the large airways except in cases of bronchitis. The retrieval of material from the deep lung by BAL is identifiable by a grossly visible layer of foam on top of the fluid indicating the presence of surfactant and cytologically (in health) by large numbers of alveolar macrophages within the fluid.

Many veterinarians and veterinary students are initially dismayed by the relatively large volumes of saline instilled into the lungs to perform BAL; therefore the technique is still not used routinely in nonreferral settings. However, BAL has been used widely for many years in people and animals of all sizes, and the effects of BAL have been studied and reported in detail. In the 1970s, using healthy dogs to study the possibility of therapeutic whole lung lavage with saline, effects were transient even using volumes of saline as high as 4 liters/dog.[4-7] Bronchoalveolar lavage is considered a routine diagnostic technique in human medicine and should be employed routinely in the diagnosis of certain lung diseases in veterinary medicine as well. The ability to perform BAL sequentially in the same individual also makes it a powerful tool in the investigation of disease progression or therapeutic response.

A sufficient volume of BAL fluid can be recovered for most types of analysis. Routine analysis of fluid in the veterinary clinical setting consists of cytology, bacterial culture, and sometimes fungal or mycoplasmal culture. Other diagnostic assays that are used in the clinical analysis of BAL fluid from human patients include viral cultures, antigen tests for cryptococcosis, polymerase chain reaction tests for specific organisms, and the application of monoclonal markers for specific tumors.

Bronchoalveolar lavage fluid analysis has also been used extensively in research settings to study local immune responses, cellular damage, and drug disposition in people and laboratory animals. Numerous papers have been published using dogs and cats as subjects. For instance, immune responses have been investigated through cell counts, measurement of inflammatory mediators, cellular function assays, and maintenance and testing of macrophages in cell culture.[8-17] Phenotypic subtyping of lymphocytes in BAL fluid from healthy dogs and dogs undergoing treatment for pulmonary neoplasia has been reported.[8,18,19] Biochemical markers such as alkaline phosphatase and lactate dehydrogenase can be used as indicators of cellular damage.[20,21] In addition, studies of various drugs have used BAL as a means to estimate concentrations within the epithelial lining fluid (ELF) or phagocytes.[22-24]

There is one major technical difficulty in measuring components of BAL fluid. The degree of dilution imposed on the ELF is variable, depending on factors such as the volume of saline instilled, the volume of fluid recovered, and the dwell time of saline within the lung. This problem is rarely significant in the clinical situation because relative cell counts and the presence of pathogenic organisms or neoplastic cells are generally unaffected by the degree of dilution. Nevertheless, consistency in technique is helpful in the clinical setting and essential in research. Markers of dilution are often used in research to estimate the dilution of ELF. Urea and albumin are most commonly used, with urea being preferable in diseased populations.[25] Urea is freely diffusible and should be present in ELF at the same concentration as in plasma. If lavage is performed quickly, so that minimal additional urea can diffuse into the instilled saline, the volume of ELF in the BAL fluid can be calculated by the following formula[26]:

$$Volume_{ELF} = Volume_{BAL} \times \frac{Urea_{BAL}}{Urea_{Plasma}}$$

This method is known to overestimate ELF volume, but with dwell times of less than 2 minutes the error is less than twofold.[27,28] No technique is entirely accurate in determining the volume of ELF in BAL fluid, and differences between study groups must be several-fold in order to be significant.

Indications

Bronchoalveolar lavage is a valuable diagnostic technique for patients that are not in respiratory distress with lung disease involving the small airways, alveoli, or interstitium. Bronchoalveolar lavage should be performed routinely in patients undergoing diagnostic bronchoscopy because the additional risk is minimal. A large volume of lung is sampled by BAL, especially compared with lung aspiration. Large volumes of fluid are retrieved, providing abundant material for analysis. Note that tracheal wash usually provides an adequate specimen from patients with historic and radiographic findings suggestive of overt bacterial bronchopneumonia or aspiration pneumonia, and does not require the patient to undergo general anesthesia.

Bronchoalveolar lavage performed during bronchoscopy (B-BAL) can be directed to specific areas of the lung that are identified as abnormal by thoracic radiography or gross examination of the airways. B-BAL is therefore indicated in the investigation of localized disease or where gross examination of the airways or other bronchoscopic collection techniques will be useful. Nonbronchoscopic BAL (NB-BAL) does not allow for directed sampling, although likely collection sites can be presumed. NB-BAL is indicated in the investigation of diffuse lung disease when the equipment or expertise needed for bronchoscopy is not available, or when the owner's finances preclude bronchoscopy.

Bronchoalveolar lavage is used as a therapeutic modality in people with alveolar proteinosis, an uncommon condition in which surfactant accumulates within the alveoli and interferes with ventilation. Lavage with many liters of saline is required for each treatment. A recent report describes treatment of a dog with aleolar proteinosis using lung lavage.[29] To the author's knowledge only one other dog and no cats have been reported to have this disease.[30] Bronchoalveolar lavage is not indicated in the treatment of aspiration pneumonia because it probably exacerbates airway obstruction by pushing particles deeper into the lung. At this time, BAL is considered primarily a diagnostic procedure in veterinary medicine.

Diagnostic Yield

Techniques for collection of pulmonary specimens for cytological analysis, including BAL, offer the clear advantages of lower risk and less expense compared with lung biopsy, which is the gold standard for diagnosis of pulmonary disease. For any cytological specimen to provide an accurate diagnosis, the disease process must involve the specific area sampled; the diseased area must release organisms or abnormal cells into the collected material; and secondary infection, inflammation, or hemorrhage must not mask an underlying disease. Therefore, the diagnostic yield of any pulmonary specimen collection technique depends on patient selection and final diagnosis. As examples, tracheal wash has a high yield in the diagnosis of *Bordetella*-induced bronchitis but a low yield in the diagnosis of interstitial lung disease, and lung aspiration has a high yield in the diagnosis of neoplasia when the needle can be placed directly into a mass lesion.

The large volume of fluid retrieved for analysis by BAL increases its potential for providing a diagnosis, particularly compared with lung aspirates. Sufficient material is obtained for making multiple slides for special staining, for aerobic and anaerobic bacterial culture, for fungal or mycoplasmal culture, or for other specific tests (e.g., antigen assays or polymerase chain reaction [PCR]) in the investigation of infectious disease. The high quality cytological preparations that can be produced and large numbers of cells available for examination facilitate the diagnosis of neoplasia.

Several reports are available in the literature describing the diagnostic yield of BAL in dogs and cats. Unfortunately, total case numbers are low. A study of dogs with overt fungal pneumonia showed that organisms were detected cytologically in BAL fluid from 6 of 9 dogs (67%).[31] Tracheal wash of the same dogs resulted in diagnostic organisms in half of the dogs. *Cryptococcosis* was identified in BAL fluid from a cat with normal thoracic radiographs.[32] A study of dogs with multicentric lymphoma determined that identification of lung involvement by BAL exceeded the sensitivity of thoracic radiographs and was equal to that of histopathology based on previous reports.[33] Lymphoma was identified in 31 of 47 dogs (66%) by BAL and in only 16 dogs (34%) by radiography.[33] Tracheal wash was successful in identifying lymphoma in only 4 of 41 dogs (10%).[33] *Toxoplasma gondii* tachyzoites were found in BAL fluid from cats with experimentally induced infection in all cats with clinical signs and in many without.[34] Lavage was more sensitive than histopathology in detecting organisms. Tachyzoites have also been found in BAL fluid from a client-owned cat with pneumonia due to toxoplasmosis.[35]

A retrospective study of dogs that underwent BAL at teaching hospitals found that BAL fluid cytology provided a definitive diagnosis in 17 of 68 cases (25%) and was supportive of the diagnosis in 34 cases (50%).[36] As with any cytological specimen, a definitive diagnosis was only possible when cells showed clear criteria of malignancy in the absence of inflammation or when intracellular bacteria or extracellular pathogens were seen. These numbers may underestimate the yield of BAL in routine practice because of the referral nature of the population. Referred cases may have failed diagnosis by other means and may have failed to respond to therapeutic trials for common diseases. On the other hand, only cases with a definitive clinical diagnosis were included in the analysis, which excluded cases in which BAL also failed to provide a diagnosis.

Information from the above studies regarding the diagnosis of neoplasia is useful.[33,36] Lymphoma of the lung is readily diagnosed by BAL. The technique should be considered for clinical trials where accurate staging of disease is needed and for treating patients that develop clinical or radiographic signs of lung disease to differentiate recurrence of neoplasia from infection. Carcinoma is much more likely to be identified than sarcoma. Carcinoma was definitively identified by BAL in 8 of 14 dogs (57%) and cells suspicious for malignancy were identified in an additional 4 dogs (29%), whereas sarcoma was identified in none of 7 dogs (0%).[36]

The value of BAL, as with all other pulmonary specimen collection techniques, is in positive findings. Identification of infectious agents or neoplastic cells can provide a definitive diagnosis. Characterization of the inflammatory response can be supportive of certain diagnoses, but failure to identify infectious agents or abnormal cells cannot be used to rule out specific diagnoses. The safety and low cost of BAL relative to lung biopsy makes attempts to obtain a positive result with this technique worthwhile.

Side Effects

The physiological effects of BAL have been studied in detail in healthy subjects of many species. In humans, BAL is considered a safe procedure with minor side effects.[3] Effects on lung function include a transient decrease of forced expiratory volume in 1 second (FEV_1), vital capacity (VC), peak expiratory flow (PEF), and arterial oxygen tension (Pao_2). Bronchospasm is rare except in patients with hyperreactive airways. Fever is seen in 10% to 30% of patients and usually responds to antipyretics.

In dogs the effects of whole lung lavage using much larger volumes of saline than those used for diagnostic purposes have been described.[4-6] These studies were performed to investigate the feasibility of repeated, large volume, whole lung lavages to remove inhaled radioactive particles accumulating in the lungs following a nuclear accident. Early alterations include decreased arterial oxygen tension; increased respiratory rate; and smaller tidal volumes, which appear to be the result of ventilation/perfusion abnormalities due to retention of saline and loss of surfactant. Some fluid is retained within the lungs following lavage, but within 48 hours there were minimal histologic changes or pulmonary function abnormalities. No cumulative or long-term effects were reported. Further, diagnostic lavage can be repeated at 48-hour intervals without affecting the cytological findings within the fluid.[7] Body temperatures over 39.5° C were found following BAL in some experimental dogs, with temperatures returning to normal within 48 hours.[6] Persistence of fever has not been noticed clinically in dogs or cats.

Healthy dogs (n = 9) were monitored by pulse oximetry for 20 minutes following NB-BAL.[37] Supplementation with 100% oxygen through an endotracheal tube was maintained during the first 10 minutes. Oxygen saturation decreased below 90% in only one dog at a single time point (Sao_2 = 87%). No clinical signs of complications were noted, and thoracic radiographs were unremarkable 48 hours post-BAL.

Healthy cats (n = 4) were monitored by measuring arterial blood gases for 2 hours following NB-BAL.[38] While the cats were breathing room air, partial pressures of oxygen dropped from a mean of 81 mm Hg prior to BAL to 58 mm Hg 3 minutes post-BAL. Values steadily increased to a mean of 62 mm Hg at 10 minutes and 70 mm Hg at 20 minutes. The mean value had returned to baseline (83 mm Hg) at 1 hour postlavage. The decrease in oxygen tension was prevented with supplementation with 100% oxygen through an endotracheal tube, as evidenced by a mean oxygen pressure of 263 mm Hg 3 minutes post-BAL.

In the clinical situation, however, patients undergoing BAL have some degree of pulmonary compromise and may be susceptible to more severe decreases in lung function. Nevertheless, BAL is generally considered a safe procedure in humans with lung disease and is routinely done on an outpatient basis. Supplemental oxygen and monitoring by pulse oximetry and ECG are recommended.[3] Human patients with a history of asthma are premedicated with bronchodilators.[3] Complications of BAL in dogs and cats with lung disease without dyspnea are rare. In a retrospective study, 2 of 101 dogs (2%) undergoing BAL at a referral hospital died.[36] Both dogs were overtly dyspneic prior to BAL, and in one dog, additional invasive diagnostic procedures were also performed at the time of BAL. At necropsy both dogs had extensive multisystemic disease. During the same period, an additional 47 dogs with lymphoma (66% with lung involvement) were lavaged with no complications.[33]

Tracheal tear due to overinflation of the endotracheal tube cuff is a potential complication of NB-BAL in cats.[39] An endotracheal tube of sufficient size should be used, and care should be taken while inflating the cuff to create an airtight seal. Excessive inflation of the cuff must be avoided.

It is theoretically possible to rupture a cavitary lesion during BAL, although to the author's knowledge this has not been seen as a complication in dogs or cats. It is prudent to decrease the volume of saline infused per bolus in patients with suspected cavitary lesions.

Contraindications

Ideally, BAL is performed in patients that show no evidence of respiratory distress while breathing room air. Although the hypoxemia that occurs with BAL is transient and responsive to oxygen supplementation, patients must be able to tolerate general anesthesia and additional respiratory compromise. Bronchoalveolar lavage should not be performed in animals that have overt respiratory distress in spite of supplementation with oxygen. Relative risks and benefits of the procedure must be considered carefully in patients that fall between these extremes. Before any clinical patient undergoes BAL, the veterinarian should be prepared to provide supplemental oxygen for up to 2 hours following the procedure if necessary.

Technique

Collection of high-quality BAL fluid requires that a sufficient volume of saline is instilled into an airway to reach the alveoli connected to that airway. In addition, a snug fit between the airway and the bronchoscope or lavage catheter must be achieved so that fluid from the deep lung is retrieved. A variety of techniques are available to achieve these goals. For consistency in results, standard protocols should be followed as much as possible. The techniques described below are protocols that are used by the author and for which cytological values from healthy dogs and cats have been published.

Monitoring of clinical patients during BAL should include continuous assessment of respiration, heart rate (via electrocardiography), and mucous membrane color. Whenever possible, pulse oximetry should be utilized to assess oxygen saturation, and arterial blood pressure should be monitored. Cats with historical or suspected airway disease should be treated prior to BAL with a bronchodilator to avoid bronchospasm associated with airway manipulation. Aminophylline (not sustained release; cats, 5 mg/kg; dogs, 11 mg/kg) can be given orally 1 or 2 hours prior to anesthesia, or terbutaline can be administered subcutaneously (cats, 0.01 mg/kg; can be repeated) 30 minutes prior to BAL.

BRONCHOSCOPIC BAL

Bronchoalveolar lavage performed through a flexible bronchoscope allows sampling of specific lung lobes. The bronchoscope, including the channel, must be sterilized. Routine bronchoscopic examination of the airways is performed first to assist in the selection of grossly abnormal lobes for BAL, and because saline remaining in the airways following BAL will interfere with visualization. In every case, it is recommended that several lobes be lavaged to increase the diagnostic yield.[31,36] In compromised patients, preoxygenation with 100% oxygen is suggested for several minutes prior to BAL.

For each lobe that is to be lavaged, the bronchoscope is passed into successively smaller airways until a snug fit is achieved between the scope and the airway. It may be necessary to reposition the scope into an adjacent airway, still within the desired lobe, to find a good fit. The author routinely uses a 4.8-mm outer diameter pediatric bronchoscope, which generally lodges in a mainstem or lobar bronchus of cats, and 2 or 3 generations lower in most dogs.

Sterile, nonbacteriostatic, 0.9% sodium chloride (saline) solution is instilled through the biopsy channel of the bronchoscope into the airway by preloaded syringe. Immediately on completion of instillation, suction is applied to the same syringe to recover BAL fluid. If negative pressure is obtained rather than a return of fluid, less suction is applied to the syringe to minimize airway collapse. If negative pressure remains a problem, the scope is withdrawn a few millimeters. Airway collapse is most often a problem in dogs with chronic airway inflammation (bronchitis). If the scope is withdrawn too far, it will no longer be snug within the airway into which the fluid was instilled and subsequent suction attempts will produce mostly air. Vacuum suction and a specimen trap can be used instead of a syringe for fluid recovery, but it is more difficult to control the degree of suction and cells are more likely to become damaged in the process. After retrieval of as much fluid as possible from the first bolus of saline, the process is repeated for one or more additional boluses. Additional lobes are then lavaged using the same procedure. Following completion of BAL, 100% oxygen is provided through the endotracheal tube.

The volume of saline instilled has not been standardized in either people or animals. In humans, saline is instilled until a sufficient volume of fluid has been retrieved to perform indicated tests. Common total volumes are 100 to 300 ml/lobe.[3] The volume per bolus is limited by the volume of lung below the obstructed airway to avoid barotrauma. The number of boluses used is not critical as long as more than one bolus is used and consistent technique is followed. Fluid retrieved from the first bolus has the largest contribution of material from the large airways. It generally has a lower total cell count, increased neutrophils, and increased epithelial cells compared with fluid from subsequent boluses.[7,37,40-42]

In dogs, using a 4.8-mm outer diameter scope, the author routinely uses two boluses of 25 ml (50 ml total) in each lung lobe lavaged. In dogs less than 8 kg and cats or if using a smaller diameter scope that lodges more deeply within the lung (therefore leaving fewer alveoli to be filled), the author decreases the volume of fluid to 10 ml/bolus and instills four or five boluses per site. Regardless of the volume per bolus, preloaded syringes are used.

Indications of an excellent quality specimen include the presence of foam rising to the top of the fluid and a recovered volume of fluid exceeding 50% of the volume instilled (Figure 17-1). In cases with severe airway collapse, it may be impossible to achieve good fluid recovery. Additional boluses may increase the chances of ob-

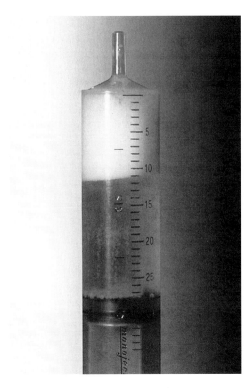

Figure 17-1. Foam floating on top of the specimen is one indication of successful sampling of material from the alveoli.

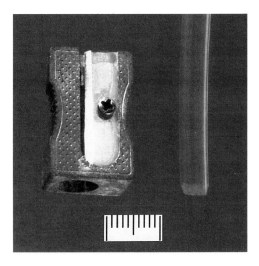

Figure 17-2. Preparation of the catheter for performing nonbronchoscopic bronchoalveolar lavage in dogs. The metal, hand-held pencil sharpener has been autoclaved. The fenestrated end of the 16 French stomach tube has been cut off. The pencil sharpener is used to make a slight taper on the end of the tube to facilitate the tube fitting snugly within an airway lumen. Sterile technique is maintained.

taining a representative specimen from the deep lung. In a retrospective study of BAL in clinical canine patients using two boluses of 25 ml each per lobe, the mean return volume was 24 ml (48%).[36]

NONBRONCHOSCOPIC BAL IN DOGS

Nonbronchoscopic BAL in dogs can be performed using an inexpensive (approximately $1) feeding tube.[37] The NB-BAL catheter is prepared as follows, maintaining sterile technique throughout. A 122-cm, 16 Fr Levin-type polyvinyl chloride stomach tube (Argyle stomach tube, Sherwood Medical Co, St. Louis, MO) is shortened by cutting off both ends. The distal end is cut off to eliminate the side openings. The proximal end is cut off to remove the flanged end and to decrease the total length of the tube. The final length should be approximately, but no shorter than, the distance from the open end of the dog's endotracheal tube to the last rib. Recovered fluid volume can be improved by slightly tapering the distal end of the tube using a simple, metal, single-blade, hand-held pencil sharpener that has been autoclaved and is used only for this purpose (Figure 17-2). A standard syringe adapter is attached to the proximal end of the NB-BAL catheter for attaching the syringes of saline.

The dog is anesthetized using a short-acting protocol that will allow intubation. Short-acting barbiturates, propofol, or the combination of medetomidine and butorphanol can be used following premedication with glycopyrrolate or atropine. The dog is intubated using a sterile endotracheal tube. Intubation is carried out as cleanly as possible to minimize oral contamination of the specimen. The dog is positioned in dorsal recumbency. 100% oxygen is provided for several minutes through the endotracheal tube.

The NB-BAL catheter is passed through the endotracheal tube. In compromised patients, continued oxygen delivery can be achieved by passing the NB-BAL catheter through a bronchoscope swivel port. The NB-BAL catheter is passed into the airways until resistance is felt. The tube is withdrawn a few centimeters, then passed again until resistance is felt consistently at the deepest level to achieve a snug fit within an airway. Rotating the tube slightly on its axis may also facilitate lodging within an airway rather than abutting an airway division.

With the tube held in place, boluses of 25 ml of saline are instilled through the catheter immediately followed by 5 ml of air to minimize dilution of the specimen by the relatively large volume of the catheter relative to a bronchoscope channel. This process is greatly facilitated by prefilling 35-ml syringes with 25 ml of saline and 5 ml of air. The syringe is held upright during instillation so that the air follows the saline into the catheter (Figure 17-3). Immediately after instillation, suction is applied by the same syringe. If negative pressure is obtained, suction pressure is decreased. If negative pressure persists, the catheter is slowly withdrawn until fluid begins to appear in the syringe. If the catheter is withdrawn too far, it will no longer be snug within the airway into which the fluid was instilled and subsequent suction attempts will produce mostly air. The procedure is repeated for at least one more bolus of saline (50 to 75 ml total). Following BAL the dog is administered 100% oxygen through the endotracheal tube.

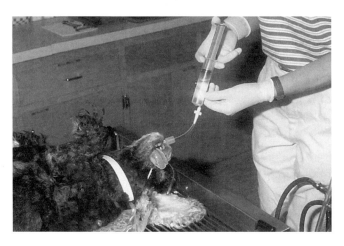

Figure 17-3. Performing nonbronchoscopic bronchoalveolar lavage in a dog. The dog is in dorsal recumbency. The lavage catheter has been passed until it is wedged within an airway. The syringe contains saline and air and is held upright so that the saline is infused first, followed by the air.

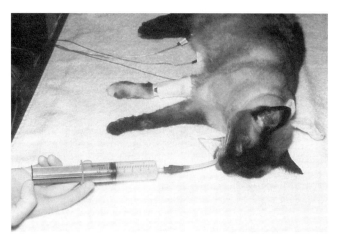

Figure 17-4. Performing nonbronchoscopic bronchoalveolar lavage in a cat. The cuff of the endotracheal tube is carefully inflated to create a seal. The saline is infused into the tube using a standard syringe adapter. The procedure must be performed without delay once the syringe adapter is in place.

Based on mean recovery volumes from 9 healthy dogs, expected return from the first bolus is 44%, from the second bolus is 60%, and from a third bolus is 68%.[37] Decreased return can be anticipated in dogs with airway collapse.

Although this method of NB-BAL does not allow for directed specimen collection, the technique resulted in lavage of the right caudal lung lobe in 7 of 9 dogs and of the left caudal lung lobe in 2 dogs, based on the catheter position identified by thoracic radiographs prior to BAL. Therefore this technique is likely of most value for dogs with disease involving the caudal lobes. If disease is apparently localized to a specific caudal lobe, radiographic identification of catheter position and random attempts at replacement would likely allow for specimen collection from that lobe.

The specific feeding tube described was selected because it is readily available, of minimal expense, is sufficiently stiff to prevent folding or kinking within the endotracheal tube or airways and for the operator to feel resistance, and is sufficiently pliable to travel within the airways to lodge snugly in an airway lumen. In addition, the 5.3-mm diameter of the feeding tube is comparable to the outer diameter of bronchoscopes used in studies reporting BAL fluid cytology in dogs and should lodge in a similar generation of airways.[8,36,43,44] The NB-BAL catheter can be passed through an endotracheal tube as small as size 6, and the technique is therefore applicable to most dogs.

For dogs that are too small for this technique, the NB-BAL catheter can be passed directly through the larynx. Increased oral contamination is expected, but care can be taken to minimize contamination during passage. Where results of bacterial culture are critical, guarded bronchoscopic culture swabs can be passed blindly for specimen collection. Alternatively, a smaller diameter tube can be used to perform lavage.

NONBRONCHOSCOPIC BAL IN CATS

Nonbronchoscopic BAL in cats is easily performed through a sterile endotracheal tube. The cat is premedicated with glycopyrrolate or atropine. Short-acting anesthesia that will allow intubation is induced using standard protocols such as with ketamine and diazepam. Intubation is performed carefully to minimize oropharyngeal contamination. To ensure a clean intubation, lidocaine should be applied topically to the larynx and a laryngoscope used in every case. The cuff of the endotracheal tube is expanded to ensure an airtight seal, but overinflation of the cuff must be avoided to prevent tracheal tear.[39] In general, less than 3 ml of air should be needed for an appropriately sized tube.[39] The cat is placed in lateral recumbency. If the disease process is asymmetrical, than the most affected side should be placed against the table. Using this technique the majority of the lavage fluid is probably obtained from the cranial/middle lung lobes on the dependent side.

Following preoxygenation for a few minutes with 100% oxygen, the anesthetic adapter is removed from the endotracheal tube and replaced with a standard syringe adapter. At this point BAL must be performed quickly because the cat cannot ventilate adequately through the narrow syringe adapter lumen. Lavage is performed using three boluses of sterile saline, each of a volume of 5 ml/kg body weight. For a 4-kg cat, each bolus is 20 ml for a total lavage volume of 60 ml. The bolus is instilled through the endotracheal tube and immediately retrieved by suction (Figure 17-4). The procedure is rapidly repeated for each bolus. Cats generally take one or two breaths between each bolus.

Immediately after the procedure, the syringe adapter is removed and the cat's hindquarters are elevated for a few moments to allow additional fluid to drain from the endotracheal tube. Then the anesthetic adapter is replaced on the tube and 100% oxygen is provided.

Based on mean retrieved volumes from healthy cats, approximate expected return volumes from this method of NB-BAL are 32% from the first bolus, 57% from the second, and 80% from the third.[45] A technique for NB-BAL in cats using a feeding tube has also been described.[46,47]

POST-BAL PATIENT CARE

Immediately after BAL all patients are administered 100% oxygen by endotracheal tube for 5 to 10 minutes. Gentle positive pressure ventilation using the anesthesia reservoir bag may facilitate the opening of collapsed alveoli, as may positioning the patient in sternal recumbency. The patient is observed carefully for several minutes following discontinuation of oxygen supplementation. If pallor of mucous membranes is observed or measured oxygen saturation decreases, oxygen administration is reinstated. Attempts are made to discontinue the oxygen every 5 minutes. If the patient begins to recover from anesthesia before it is possible to discontinue oxygen administration through the endotracheal tube, a decision must be made whether or not to use gas anesthesia to allow continued control of the airway. In all but severely compromised patients, the patient can be allowed to recover and the endotracheal tube removed. In most of these cases, oxygen supplementation via face mask or oxygen cage is sufficient to maintain adequate oxygenation. It is rare for previously stable patients to require more than 5 to 10 minutes of oxygen supplementation following BAL.

If a patient fails to respond to oxygen supplementation, the potential for bronchospasm or pneumothorax should be considered. Bronchospasm is most likely to occur in cats with reactive airway disease. Wheezes may be auscultated and increased expiratory efforts observed. Bronchodilators should be administered. Pneumothorax could occur secondary to rupture of a cavitary lesion or, rarely, from a tracheal tear related to intubation and cuff overinflation. The latter generally causes subcutaneous emphysema. If decreased lung sounds are auscultated, therapeutic thoracocentesis should be performed. Pneumothorax as a result of BAL has not been observed by the author.

Retained fluid is isotonic and is absorbed from the alveoli; however, it is normal to auscult crackles for up to 24 hours after BAL.[6] Radiographic evidence of fluid and atelectasis should resolve within 2 days.[6,37]

Specimen Processing

Fluid should be kept in plastic or silicone-treated syringes or tubes pending analysis because phagocytes adhere readily to glass. Fluid for culture should be placed promptly in appropriate transport media. Fluid for cytological analysis should be processed within 1 hour for optimal results.[48] Specimens that cannot be processed soon after collection should be refrigerated and processed within 12 hours.[3]

WHEN TO COMBINE BAL FLUID FOR ANALYSIS

It is advisable to process BAL fluid from different lobes separately for cytological evaluation. In a retrospective study of BAL in dogs, additional cytological information was obtained by evaluating multiple lobes in about one third of cases even though diffuse disease was indicated radiographically.[36] A study of BAL cytology from dogs with fungal pneumonia showed organisms were not visible in every lobe lavaged in 3 out of 6 dogs in which organisms were identified cytologically.[31] In addition, the author has found that fungal and protozoan infections may only manifest one visible organism on an entire slide.[31,34] Preparing slides from multiple lobes results in examination of increased numbers of slides for organisms in low concentrations. It is acceptable to combine fluid from all lobes sampled for culturing unless the disease appears to be localized to a specific lobe. In this instance, unnecessary dilution would occur.

It is generally appropriate to combine BAL fluid from separate boluses from the same lung lobe. In human medicine, some pulmonologists advocate discarding return from the first bolus because of its relatively greater representation from the larger airways.[2,3] Others believe that this practice is unnecessary.[49] In dogs and cats, it is unlikely that the minor contribution of the large airways to a BAL specimen would be clinically relevant. However, if the underlying disease process primarily affects the large airways and not the deep lung, then the dilution of material from the large airways by material from the deep lung might affect results. For instance, in one dog with chronic bronchopneumonia, only *Bordetella* was recovered from a tracheal wash, whereas only *Pseudomonas* was recovered from a BAL specimen. If large airway disease is suspected, either the fluid returned from the first bolus of BAL should be processed separately or a specifically directed airway specimen (e.g., bronchial wash, tracheal wash, bronchial brushing, or bronchial biopsy) should be submitted in addition to the BAL specimen.

CYTOLOGICAL EXAMINATION

Total nucleated cell counts are performed on undiluted BAL fluid using a hemocytometer. The cell sizes prevent accurate results using automated counters. The concentration of cells in BAL fluid is often too dilute for evaluation of direct smears. Instead, concentrated preparations must be made using techniques such as cytocentrifugation, which provides high quality slides. Volumes of 100 to 200 μl/slide are generally required. Wright-Giemsa or quick Romanowsky stains are used routinely. Special stains to further characterize abnormal cell populations or to facilitate the identification of organisms may be useful in some cases. Fluid should not be strained through gauze prior to processing to remove mucus strands because certain cells or organisms may be selectively retained.

Cytological characterization includes the performance of differential cell counts. A minimum of 200 cells should be counted, and qualitative changes are noted. Macrophages are examined for evidence of activation and for phagocytized organisms, debris, red blood cells, or hemosiderin. Neutrophils are examined for degenerative changes and intracellular organisms. All cells are examined for criteria of malignancy. As with any cytological specimen, care must be taken in interpreting criteria of malignancy in the face of inflammation. The entire slide should be carefully scrutinized for the presence of infectious agents. Only one organism may be present on the slides of a patient with fungal, protozoal, or parasitic disease.

BACTERIAL CULTURE

Ideally, quantitative or semiquantitative culturing methods should be employed for BAL fluid. The large airways are not completely sterile in health, and some oral contamination can occur during the procedure. The determination of the significance of cultured bacteria is further complicated by the presence of increased numbers of organisms within the airways of patients with reduced airway clearance (particularly chronic bronchitis) relative to healthy patients. The significance of these organisms is not known, but overt inflammation and clinical signs are not always present. On the other hand, BAL dilutes the concentration of any pathogens that are present.

To minimize costs it is common in veterinary medicine to employ routine culturing techniques. If quantitative cultures are not performed, lavage fluid should be inoculated directly onto culture plates, as well as inoculated into enrichment media to identify slow-growing organisms and organisms present in low numbers.

MYCOPLASMA CULTURE

The role of *Mycoplasma* in respiratory disease of the dog and cat is still not well characterized. A role for the organisms as a cause for lung disease in cats has been proposed, and the organisms have been cultured from BAL fluid of cats with pneumonia.[50,51] As mucosal inhabitants, bronchial brushings or washings may provide a superior specimen to BAL. Specific handling and culturing techniques are necessary.

FUNGAL CULTURE

Culture of BAL fluid for fungal organisms improves the sensitivity of the technique for diagnosing fungal pneu-

monia.[52] Cultures should only be performed in laboratories equipped to handle these organisms.

Interpretation of Results

CYTOLOGY

A great deal of variability is present among healthy dogs and cats with regard to BAL fluid cell counts (Table 17-1). Slight deviations compared with normal values should not be overinterpreted. Increased variability is added by inconsistency in collection techniques and specimen processing. Regardless, the predominant cell type in health is the alveolar macrophage (Figure 17-5). Lymphocytes can be difficult to distinguish cytologically from small macrophages, and variability in expected numbers has been reported.[53] Immunofluorescent, immunocytochemical, and flow cytometric techniques can be used for accurate differentiation of mononuclear cells. Neutrophils are present in slightly greater numbers in fluid returned from the first bolus in dogs and people.[7,37, 40-42]

Eosinophil counts can be high in clinically healthy cats and dogs.[44,54] Eosinophil counts from the same cats lavaged eight times at intervals of 1 or more weeks varied by 1% to 52% compared with values from their first lavage.[55] Therefore, the finding of relative eosinophilia

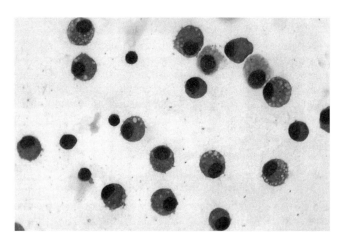

Figure 17-5. *Bronchoalveolar lavage fluid from a healthy dog. The predominant cell type is the alveolar macrophage. (Wright-Giemsa, 250×)*

	Canine B-BAL[58] (Mean ± SD)	Canine NB-BAL[37] (Mean ± SD)	Feline B-BAL[63] (Mean ± SE)	Feline NB-BAL[45] (Mean ± SD)
TNCC (/μl)	200 ± 86	352 ± 115	241 ± 101	337 ± 194
Macrophages (%)	70 ± 11	81 ± 11	71 ± 10	78 ± 15
Neutrophils (%)	5 ± 5	15 ± 12	7 ± 4	5 ± 5
Eosinophils (%)	6 ± 5	2 ± 3	16 ± 7	16 ± 14
Lymphocytes (%)	7 ± 5	2 ± 5	5 ± 3	0 ± 1

TABLE 17-1. **Reported Cell Counts of BAL Fluid From Healthy Dogs and Cats Using the Described Collection Techniques**

TNCC, Total nucleated cell count; *SD,* standard deviation; *SE,* standard error.

should be interpreted with careful consideration also given to the total nucleated cell count, patient history, and other clinical data. Mast cells are usually less than 1% to 2% of white blood cells in normal dogs.[56,57]

Epithelial cells are usually less than 5% of nucleated cells, and greater numbers suggest a large contribution to the fluid from the large airways.[3] An exception is fluid collected using the NB-BAL technique described for dogs. As many as 2 to 5 clumps of epithelial cells/hpf were noted in fluid from the first boluses, presumably from disruption of cells during efforts to blindly lodge the lavage catheter within the airways.[37]

Most emphasis is placed on the relative cell counts when identifying an inflammatory response of the lungs. The relative counts are independent of the variability in dilution inherent in BAL specimens. It is not possible to accurately assign specific numbers to distinguish normal from abnormal relative cell counts because of the variability seen in health. Criteria used to identify abnormal inflammatory responses in dogs reported in the previously mentioned retrospective study were based on the 90th percentile values of relative cell counts from BAL fluid collected using the bronchoscopic method from 30 histologically normal lung lobes from five healthy dogs.[36,58] Based on these criteria, relative neutrophil counts greater than 12% are considered to indicate neutrophilic inflammation, eosinophil counts greater than 14% are considered to indicate eosinophilic inflammation, and lymphocyte counts greater than 16% are used to indicate lymphocytic inflammation.

In clinical practice, total nucleated cell counts are also used to temper the interpretation of increases in relative counts. Very low total nucleated cell counts may indicate that the fluid collected is more likely a bronchial wash than BAL fluid. Marginally increased relative cell counts in combination with a low total nucleated cell count are not as likely to be clinically significant as those associated with an increased total nucleated cell count.

Because macrophages normally make up the majority of cells in BAL fluid, an increase in these cells is only identifiable by increased cell numbers. However, clinically relevant pulmonary inflammation can be expected to result in a concurrent increase in relative neutrophil, eosinophil, or (occasionally) lymphocyte counts. Macrophagic inflammation is better assessed by cytological criteria of differentiation (e.g., increased size, less basophilic cytoplasm, vacuolization, and phagocytized debris).[59] Macrophage activation can be seen in clinically normal dogs and cats, particularly if they are exposed to smoke, smog, or other particulates. As with eosinophilia, this finding must be interpreted with consideration of other available information.

Neutrophils are scrutinized for evidence of degenerative change (e.g., pyknotic, karyorrhectic, or karyolytic nuclei). The presence of these changes is supportive of a septic process; however, it is not uncommon for the neutrophils to appear normal in the face of infection.[59]

Macrophages and neutrophils are scrutinized for the presence of intracellular organisms. Intracellular bacteria indicate active infection. Intra- or extracellular pathogenic fungal organisms, parasite larvae or ova, or protozoal organisms are diagnostic for active infection.

Slides are scanned for abnormal cell populations. As with other cytological specimens, criteria of malignancy may represent hyperplasia and metaplasia rather than neoplasia if an inflammatory response is present.

BACTERIAL CULTURES

Large airways can be inhabited by bacteria in health, and increased numbers can be expected in patients with reduced airway clearance (a complication of diseases such as chronic bronchitis, bronchiectasis, and ciliary dyskinesia). Therefore, growth of bacteria from BAL fluid does not necessarily indicate infection. In people, growth of greater than 10^5 colonies/ml of fluid is associated with pneumonia. Growth of greater than 10^3 colonies/ml may represent infection, particularly in patients that have recently received antibiotics.[60] A study involving 47 dogs determined that bacterial growth of 1.7×10^3 colonies/ml was associated with airway infection.[61] Results of BAL fluid cultures correlate well with results from specimens collected with guarded catheter swabs, although slightly lower thresholds are used to diagnose pneumonia when swabs are used.[60]

Quantitative cultures are rarely performed in veterinary medicine. Infection is confirmed if intracellular bacteria are identified cytologically. The growth of organisms on agar plates inoculated directly with BAL fluid has also been considered to represent infection.[62] Infection is unlikely in the absence of neutrophilic inflammation. The cases that pose a diagnostic problem are those with neutrophilic inflammation, no intracellular bacteria, and growth of organisms only following incubation of BAL fluid in enrichment media. These cases may have true infection but have relatively low numbers of organisms because of the dilution of the specimen or because of recent treatment with antibiotics. Alternatively, these cases may not have true infection.

Unfortunately, in veterinary medicine BAL is often not recommended until after antibiotics fail to resolve the clinical signs. Antibiotics within the lung may persist in sufficient concentrations to interfere with culturing efforts for as long as 1 week (and probably longer with some of the newer, longer-lasting antibiotics) even when these antibiotics have been clinically ineffective. The clinical condition of the patient may not allow a delay before BAL is performed. Therefore, BAL fluid should also be placed in enrichment broth to promote the growth of bacteria present in low numbers. The significance of positive cultures must then be interpreted with caution. This diagnostic dilemma can often be avoided by performing BAL prior to initiation of antibiotics and by collecting high-quality specimens using careful techniques to minimize contamination.

Conclusion

Bronchoalveolar lavage is a clinically useful technique for obtaining specimens from the lung. Its diagnostic value for dogs and cats with pulmonary disease will continue to grow as we obtain increased experience with the technique and as sensitive and specific laboratory methods applicable to the collected fluid continue to be developed.

REFERENCES

1. Yohn SE, Hawkins EC, Morrison WB et al: Confirmation of a pulmonary component of multicentric lymphosarcoma with bronchoalveolar lavage in two dogs, J Am Vet Med Assoc 204:97-101, 1994.
2. Goldstein RA, Rohatgi PK, Bergofsky EH et al: Clinical role of bronchoalveolar lavage in adults with pulmonary disease, Am Rev Respir Dis 142:481-486, 1990.
3. Klech H, Pohl W: Technical recommendations and guidelines for bronchoalveolar lavage (BAL), Eur Respir J 2:561-585, 1989.
4. Muggenburg BA, Mauderly JL, Pickrell JA et al: Pathophysiologic sequelae of bronchopulmonary lavage in the dog, Am Rev Respir Dis 106:219-232, 1972.
5. Muggenburg BA, Mauderly JL: Lung lavage using a single-lumen endotracheal tube, J Appl Physiol 38:922-926, 1975.
6. Muggenburg BA, Mauderly JL, Halliwell WH et al: Cardiopulmonary function and morphologic changes in beagle dogs after multiple lung lavages, Arch Environ Health 35:85-91, 1980.
7. Pinsker KL, Norin AJ, Kamholz SL et al: Cell content in repetitive canine bronchoalveolar lavage, Acta Cytol 24:558-563, 1980.
8. Vail DM, Mahler PA, Soergel SA : Differential cell analysis and phenotypic subtyping of lymphocytes in bronchoalveolar lavage fluid from clinically normal dogs, Am J Vet Res 56:282-285, 1995.
9. Jones SE, Davila DR, Haley PJ et al: The effects of age on immune responses in the antigen-instilled dog lung: Antibody responses in the lung and lymphoid tissues following primary and secondary antigen instillation, Mechanisms of Ageing and Development 68:191-207, 1993.
10. Collie DDS, DeBoer DJ, Muggenburg BA et al: Evaluation of association of blood and bronchoalveolar eosinophil numbers and serum total immunoglobulin E concentration with the expression of nonspecific airway reactivity in dogs, Am J Vet Res 58:34-39, 1997.
11. Chang SC, Hsu HK, Lin CY: Usefulness of bronchoalveolar cell profile in early detection of canine lung allograft rejection, Immunology Letters 29:265-270, 1991.
12. Dambro NN, Grad R, Witten ML et al: Bronchoalveolar lavage fluid cytology reflects airway inflammation in beagle puppies with acute bronchiolitis, Ped Pul 12:213-220, 1992.
13. Gillette SM, Powers BE, Orton EC et al: Early radiation response of the canine heart and lung, Radiat Res 125:34-40, 1991.
14. Padrid P, Snook S, Finucane T et al: Persistent airway hyperresponsiveness and histologic alterations after chronic antigen challenge in cats, Am J Respir Crit Care Med 151:184-193, 1995.
15. Padrid P, Snook S, Mitchell R et al: Data derived from an experimental model of feline asthma. In Proceedings of the eleventh annual forum, Washington, DC, 1993, American College of Veterinary Internal Medicine.
16. Hawkins EC, Kennedy-Stoskopf S, Levy JK et al: Effect of FIV infection on lung inflammatory cell populations recovered by bronchoalveolar lavage, Vet Immunol Immunopathol 51:21-28, 1996.
17. Weissman DN, Bice DE, Muggenburg BA et al: Primary immunization in the canine lung, Am Rev Respir Dis 145:6-12, 1992.
18. Dirscherl P, Beisker W, Kremmer E et al: Immunophenotyping of canine bronchoalveolar and peripheral blood lymphocytes, Vet Immunol Immunopathol 48:1-10, 1995.
19. Khanna C, Anderson PM, Hasz DE et al: Interleukin-2 liposome inhalation therapy is safe and effective for dogs with spontaneous pulmonary metastases, Cancer 79:1409-1421, 1997.
20. Hampson ECGM, Eyles DW, Pond SM: Effects of paraquat on canine bronchoalveolar lavage fluid, Toxicol Appl Pharmacol 98:206-215, 1989.
21. Henderson RF: Use of bronchoalveolar lavage to detect lung damage, Environ Health Perspect 56:115-129, 1984.
22. Hawkins EC, Boothe DM, Guinn A et al: Concentration of enrofloxacin and its active metabolite in alveolar macrophages and pulmonary epithelial lining fluid of dogs, J Vet Pharmacol Therap 21:18-23, 1998.
23. Vaden SL, Heit MC, Hawkins EC et al: Fluconazole in cats: Pharmacokinetics following intravenous and oral administration and penetration into cerebrospinal fluid, aqueous humour and pulmonary epithelial lining fluid, J Vet Pharmacol Therap 20:181-186, 1997.
24. Jones SA, Boothe HW, Boothe DM et al: Concentration of marbofloxacin in canine alveolar macrophages (abstract), J Vet Intern Med 14:355, 2000.
25. Jones KP, Edwards JH, Reynolds SP et al: A comparison of albumin and urea as reference markers in bronchoalveolar lavage fluid from patients with interstitial lung disease, Eur Respir J 3:152-156, 1990.
26. Rennard SI, Basset G, Lecossier D et al: Estimation of volume of epithelial lining fluid recovered by lavage using urea as a marker of dilution, J Appl Physiol 60:532-538, 1986.
27. Marcy TW, Rankin JA, Reynolds HY: Limitations of using urea to quantify epithelial lining fluid recovered by bronchoalveolar lavage, Am Rev Respir Dis 135:1276-1280, 1987.
28. Thompson AB, Spurzem JR, Rennard SI: Bronchoalveolar lavage in interstitial lung disease. In Schwarz MI, King TE, editors: Interstitial lung disease, St Louis, 1993, Mosby.
29. Silverstein D, Greene C, Gregory C et al: Pulmonary alveolar proteinosis in a dog, J Vet Intern Med 14:546-551, 2000.
30. Jefferies AR, Dunn JK, Dennis R: Pulmonary alveolar proteinosis (phopholipoproteinosis) in a dog, J Small Anim Pract 28:203-214, 1987.
31. Hawkins EC, DeNicola DB: Cytologic analysis of tracheal wash specimens and bronchoalveolar lavage fluid in the diagnosis of mycotic infections in dogs, J Am Vet Med Assoc 197:79-83, 1990.
32. Hamilton TA, Hawkins EC, DeNicola DB : Bronchoalveolar lavage and tracheal wash to determine lung involvement in a cat with cryptococcosis, J Am Vet Med Assoc 198:655-656, 1991.
33. Hawkins EC, Morrison WB, DeNicola DB et al: Cytologic analysis of bronchoalveolar lavage fluid from 47 dogs with multicentric malignant lymphoma, J Am Vet Med Assoc 203:1418-1425, 1993.
34. Hawkins EC, Davidson MG, Meuten DJ et al: Cytologic identification of Toxoplasma gondii in bronchoalveolar lavage fluid of experimentally infected cats, J Am Vet Med Assoc 210:648-650, 1997.
35. Brownlee L, Sellon RK: Diagnosis of naturally occurring toxoplasmosis by bronchoalveolar lavage in a cat, J Am anim Hosp Assoc 37:251-255, 2001.
36. Hawkins EC, DeNicola DB, Plier ML: Cytological analysis of bronchoalveolar lavage fluid in the diagnosis of spontaneous respiratory tract disease in dogs: A retrospective study, J Vet Intern Med 9:386-392, 1995.
37. Hawkins EC, Berry CR: Use of a modified stomach tube for bronchoalveolar lavage in dogs, J Am Vet Med Assoc 215:1635-1639, 1999.
38. Hawkins EC, DeNicola DB: Collection of bronchoalveolar lavage fluid in cats using an endotracheal tube, Am J Vet Res 50:855-859, 1989.
39. Hardie EM, Spodnick GJ, Gilson SD et al: Tracheal rupture in cats: 16 cases (1983-1998), J Am Vet Med Assoc 214:508-512, 1999.
40. Kelly CA, Kotre CJ, Ward C et al: Anatomical distribution of bronchoalveolar lavage fluid as assessed by digital subtraction radiography, Thorax 42:624-628, 1987.
41. Martin TR, Raghu G, Maunder RJ et al: The effects of chronic bronchitis and chronic airflow obstruction on lung cell populations recovered by bronchoalveolar lavage, Am Rev Respir Dis 132:254-260, 1985.
42. Rennard SI, Ghafouri M, Thompson AB et al: Fractional processing of sequential bronchoalveolar lavage to separate bronchial and alveolar samples, Am Rev Respir Dis 141:208-217, 1990.
43. Rebar AH, DeNicola DB, Muggenburg BA: Bronchopulmonary lavage cytology in the dog: Normal findings, Vet Pathol 17:294-304, 1980.
44. Baudendistel LJ, Vogler GA, Frank PA et al: Bronchoalveolar eosinophilia in random-source versus purpose-bred dogs, Lab Anim Sci 42:491-496, 1992.
45. Hawkins EC, Kennedy-Stoskopf S, Levy JK et al: Cytologic characterization of bronchoalveolar lavage fluid collected through an endotracheal tube in cats, Am J Vet Res 55:795-802, 1994.
46. McCarthy G, Quinn PJ: The development of lavage procedures for the upper and lower respiratory tract of the cat, Irish Vet J 40:6-9, 1986.
47. McCarthy GM, Quinn PJ: Bronchoalveolar lavage in the cat: Cytologic findings, Can J Vet Res 53:259-263, 1989.
48. McCullough S, Brinson J: Collection and interpretation of respiratory cytology, Clin Tech Sm Anim Prac 14:220-226, 1999.
49. Baughman RP, Golden JA, Keith FM: Bronchoscopy, lung biopsy, and other diagnostic procedures. In Murray JF, Nadel JA, editors: Textbook of respiratory medicine, Philadelphia, 2000, WB Saunders.
50. Randolph JF, Moise NS, Scarlett JM et al: Prevalence of mycoplasmal and ureaplasmal recovery from tracheobronchial lavages and of mycoplasmal recovery from pharyngeal swab specimens in cats with or without pulmonary disease, Am J Vet Res 54:897-900, 1993.

51. Foster SF, Barrs VR, Martin P et al: Pneumonia associated with Mycoplasma spp in three cats, *Aust Vet J* 76:460-464, 1998.

52. Baughman RP, Dohn MN, Loudon RG et al: Bronchoscopy with bronchoalveolar lavage in tuberculosis and fungal infections, *Chest* 99:92-97, 1991.

53. Mayer P, Laber G, Walzl H: Bronchoalveolar lavage in dogs: Analysis of proteins and respiratory cells, *J Vet Med A* 37:392-399, 1990.

54. Padrid PA, Feldman BF, Funk K et al: Cytologic, microbiologic, and biochemical analysis of bronchoalveolar lavage fluid obtained from 24 healthy cats, *Am J Vet Res* 52:1300-1307, 1991.

55. King RR, Fox LE: Eosinophil fluctuation in bronchoalveolar lavage fluid from normal cats (abstract), *J Vet Intern* 7:119, 1993.

56. Sommerhoff CP, Osborne ML, Gold WM et al: Functional and morphologic characterization of mast cells recovered by bronchoalveolar lavage from Basenji greyhound and mongrel dogs, *J Allergy Clin Immunol* 83:441-449, 1989.

57. Baldwin F, Becker AB: Bronchoalveolar eosinophilic cells in a canine model of asthma: Two distinctive populations, *Vet Pathol* 30:97-103, 1993.

58. Kuehn NF: Canine bronchoalveolar lavage profile. Thesis for Masters of Science Degree, Purdue University, 1987.

59. Rebar AH, Hawkins EC, DeNicola DB: Cytologic evaluation of the respiratory tract, *Vet Clinics N Am Sm Anim Prac* 22:1065-1084, 1992.

60. Souweine B, Veber B, Bedos JP et al: Diagnostic accuracy of protected specimen brush and bronchoalveolar lavage in nosocomial pneumonia: Impact of previous antimicrobial treatments, *Crit Care Med* 26:236-244, 1998.

61. Peeters DE, McKiernan BC, Weisiger RM et al: Quantitative bacterial cultures and cytological examination of bronchoalveolar lavage specimens in dogs, *J Vet Intern Med* 14:534-541, 2000.

62. Padrid P: Chronic lower airway disease in the dog and cat, *Prob Vet Med* 4:320-344, 1992.

63. King RR et al: Bronchoalveolar lavage cell populations in dogs and cats with eosinophilic pneumonitis. In *Proceedings of the seventh veterinary respiratory symposium*, Chicago, 1988, The Comparative Respiratory Society.

CHAPTER 18

Tracheal Washes

Rebecca S. Syring

Background and Definition

The tracheal wash is a minimally invasive diagnostic technique used to sample the respiratory tract of dogs and cats. Tracheal washes are used primarily to obtain samples from the large airways (trachea and primary bronchi) and are considered less helpful in the diagnosis of interstitial or alveolar lung disease. Specimens obtained from tracheal washes can be evaluated cytologically to identify and characterize the inflammatory response and to identify any infectious agents or neoplastic cells. Bacterial or fungal cultures can be performed on these specimens to confirm an infectious etiology.

Tracheal washes can be performed by either a transtracheal or endotracheal route. It has been suggested that the transtracheal wash (TTW) may be superior to an endotracheal wash (ETW) for sampling smaller airways and alveoli. Because sedation is usually not required for a TTW, the patient's cough reflex remains intact during the procedure, therefore potentially providing a sample from the smaller airways and alveoli. To the author's knowledge, no studies have been published comparing the diagnostic yield of TTW to ETW.

A few clinical studies have compared the diagnostic yield of endotracheal washes with bronchoalveolar lavage (BAL), in which ETW immediately preceded BAL.[1-3] In dogs with multicentric lymphoma, pulmonary involvement was detected in 4 of 41 dogs via ETW.[3] Although lymphoma was also detected via BAL in all 4 of these dogs, pulmonary involvement was documented in 23 additional dogs using BAL.[3] Similarly, in 9 dogs that had systemic fungal infections with suspected pulmonary involvement, ETW was successful in identifying *Blastomyces* in 3 dogs. However, in this same population, BAL isolated *Blastomyces* in 5 dogs and *Histoplasma* in 1 dog.[2] A case report of a cat with pulmonary *Cryptococcus* stated that infectious agents were detected in both the ETW and BAL, however the ETW contained fewer organisms.[1] These studies suggest that although tracheal washes may provide useful diagnostic information, they are less sensitive than BAL.

Only one clinical study investigates TTW compared with BAL; however, this study includes both TTW and ETW into a general category of tracheal washes and does not report results individually.[4] In this study, both a tracheal wash (TTW or ETW) and a BAL were performed in 66 dogs. The cytological interpretation of the samples retrieved differed between procedures in 68% of dogs. In this study, BAL more often detected hemorrhage, infectious agents, and neoplasia compared with tracheal washes. In addition, the cytological pattern of inflammation differed in 41% of animals between the two procedures.[4] Because the type of tracheal wash performed was not reported in this study, it is not possible to determine if one type of tracheal wash might more closely correspond to results from BAL. In addition, because the primary disease process in these dogs was not always confirmed histopathologically, it is not possible to discern which of these techniques was more accurate.

Compared with BAL, the tracheal wash is a simple, noninvasive, diagnostic technique that can be performed without special training or expensive equipment. As such, it may be used as an initial screening test for the diagnosis of respiratory diseases. When a tracheal wash either fails to provide a diagnosis or the results do not fit with the clinical picture, then BAL should be considered.

Indications

Tracheal washes are most helpful in diagnosing large airway disease. The procedure can be performed in patients with lower airway, alveolar, and interstitial lung disease; however, diagnostic yield is reportedly inferior to that of BAL.[2,3] This procedure is indicated in animals with persistent coughing, wheezing, or radiographic evidence of respiratory disease, particularly when other noninvasive diagnostics have failed to provide a diagnosis. Cytological characterization of the tracheal wash will help to narrow the differential list when inflammatory cells are found. For example, tracheal wash with primarily eosinophilic inflammation increases suspicion for an allergic or parasitic etiology. Identification of parasitic larvae or eggs within the tracheal wash specimen may provide a definitive diagnosis.

Although it is stated that tracheal washes mainly sample the large airways, it appears that the TTW is a suitable diagnostic tool for bacterial pneumonia. An experimental study in dogs found TTW to be an equally sensitive technique for isolating known *Streptococcus pneumoniae* infections compared with transbronchial biopsy, lung aspirates, and bronchoscopic cultures.[5] However, the TTW was less specific (i.e., fewer pure cultures) than transbronchial biopsy, lung aspirates, or bronchoscopic brush culture.[5] A more recent study in human patients found transtracheal aspiration to be a sensitive (77%) and specific (95%) technique for diagnosing bacterial pneumonia.[6] Positive bacterial cultures have been reported in 44% to 57% of animals with suspected lower respiratory tract disease when samples were obtained via TTW.[7-9]

There is little information about the efficacy of tracheal washes to diagnose pulmonary neoplasia. As previously mentioned, the tracheal wash can determine pulmonary infiltration with malignant lymphoma; however, it is less sensitive than BAL.[3] Primary lung tumors originating from the airway (e.g., bronchogenic carcinoma) may be more likely to exfoliate into tracheal wash specimens than metastatic neoplasia, which is more likely to reside in the interstitium. However, in a recent retrospective study of dogs with primary lung tumors, the TTW failed to identify neoplastic cells in all 6 dogs that had this procedure performed.[10]

The ETW is recommended for smaller patients (cats and small dogs), those patients who cannot be adequately restrained for a TTW, or patients who are scheduled to undergo general anesthesia for other reasons. Whereas this procedure causes less tracheal injury and is technically less difficult, diagnostic sampling of the small airways may not occur because the patient is unlikely to cough while anesthetized. In addition, ETW is associated with a higher risk of oropharyngeal contamination.

Contraindications

Although a TTW is minimally invasive and generally does not require sedation, respiratory distress may be exacerbated in dyspneic patients. This procedure is contraindicated in fractious or uncooperative patients because undue stress to the patient and tracheal injury (e.g., laceration) can result. Although light sedation may make TTW feasible in a fractious patient, ETW with anesthesia may be more appropriate.

TTW should not be performed in animals with abnormalities in primary (thrombocytopenia or thrombocytopathia) or secondary (hypocoagulability) hemostasis because uncontrollable bleeding at the site of tracheal puncture may occur. In addition, TTW should be avoided in patients with severe skin disease on the ventral neck because it may result in contamination of the tracheal wash and inoculation of debris into the airway. TTW may be more difficult in patients with megaesophagus and could result in tracheal wash contamination if the esophagus cannot be moved out of the way. The TTW may exacerbate airway irritation in dogs with severe tracheal collapse and could result in precipitation of a respiratory crisis.

ETW may be a more suitable diagnostic tool in any of the above listed situations. The ETW is contraindicated in patients too unstable for general anesthesia or patients in severe respiratory distress where extubation may not be possible following the procedure, particularly if mechanical ventilation is not an option.

Side Effects

In general, tracheal washes are associated with minimal side effects or complications. Transient worsening of respiratory status and exacerbation of coughing may occur following either TTW or ETW. This is rarely clinically significant unless the patient's respiratory status is already markedly compromised. These procedures can cause airway irritation and bronchoconstriction, particularly in patients with chronic airway disease (e.g., cats with feline asthma). Treatment with a bronchodilating agent (theophylline or terbutaline) prior to the procedure may help to minimize this side effect.

Subcutaneous emphysema and pneumomediastinum can occur following TTW; however, this rarely causes clinical consequence. If a significant leak from the trachea develops, pneumomediastinum could potentially progress to a pneumothorax and result in respiratory distress. Other uncommon complications of TTW include tracheal laceration, esophageal perforation, endotracheal hemorrhage, cardiac arrhythmias, and inoculation of infection into the needle tract.[11] In addition, it is possible that a portion of the catheter could be severed during the procedure, resulting in a bronchial foreign body.

If mechanical suction is employed for ETW, it is important to limit the extent and duration of negative pressure used during suctioning. Pressures exceeding the recommended 100 to 170 mm Hg of negative pressure [12] can cause untoward effects such as tracheal mucosal injury, regional pulmonary atelectasis, cardiovascular instability, and hypoxia.[13]

Instrumentation

Clippers, gauze sponges, and antiseptic scrub (e.g., 4% chlorhexidine gluconate) are needed to prepare a sterile field on the ventral neck for a TTW, and 2% lidocaine should be used to provide local anesthesia. Sterile gloves should be worn during both TTW and ETW to prevent contamination of the sample, and syringes (10 and 20 ml) should be prefilled with a sterile lavage fluid using aseptic technique.

Transtracheal washes can be performed with a through-the-needle, long intravenous catheter* (19- to 22-gauge, 8-inch catheter for cats and small dogs; 19-gauge, 12- or 24-inch catheter for large dogs). This type of catheter is optimal because the needle can be withdrawn from the trachea and covered following catheter placement to minimize tracheal injury or catheter damage during the procedure. If this catheter is not available, a 16-gauge needle or a 14-gauge over-the-needle catheter can be inserted into the trachea, and a sterile 3.5 Fr red rubber catheter can be fed through the needle and down the trachea.

To perform an endotracheal wash, a sterile laryngoscope should be used to facilitate rapid intubation and to minimize oropharyngeal contamination. A sterile endotracheal tube should be used for this procedure. A red rubber catheter will be needed to deliver the lavage fluid into the trachea. In addition, mechanical suction, a suction catheter,† and a sterile suction trap‡ (Figure 18-1) may be needed to collect the sample.

Sterile saline (0.9%) should be used for the tracheal wash, avoiding bacteriostatic preparations, which would inhibit bacteria growth. The use of 0.9% saline provides an isotonic solution that will preserve cellular and bacterial integrity for cytological evaluation and culture. Hypotonic solutions (sterile water, 0.45% saline) should be avoided because cell lysis will occur and preclude cytological evaluation.

Technique for Transtracheal Wash

Transtracheal washes should be performed without sedation in cooperative animals, thereby allowing the patient to cough when saline is infused into the trachea,

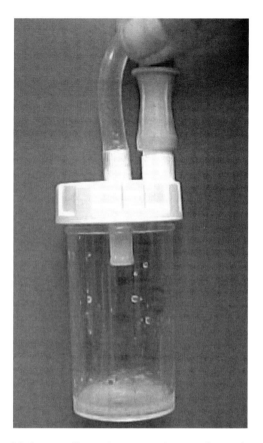

Figure 18-1. *A sterile specimen container can be used to collect the endotracheal lavage sample. This container has two ports, one that can be attached to a mechanical suction device and the other that can be attached to a suction catheter placed into the patient's airway. Following collection of the sample, the two ports can be connected to provide a closed container for transport to the laboratory.*

improving sampling from the lower airways, and improving diagnostic yield. If sedation is required to facilitate catheter placement in uncooperative or fractious animals, pure opioids (e.g., oxymorphone 0.05 to 0.2 mg/kg IV) or a combination of ketamine and diazepam are recommended. Pure opioids can be fully reversed with an opioid antagonist (e.g., naloxone 0.022 mg/kg IV) once the catheter has been placed into the airway so that the patient can cough during the procedure. Ketamine, on the other hand, does not inhibit the cough reflex.

The patient should be positioned in sternal recumbency with the neck dorsiflexed. If the patient has unilateral lung disease, the procedure can also be performed in lateral recumbency with the affected lungs positioned on the dependent side. A full surgical preparation with wide margins should be performed on the ventral neck of the animal, including the larynx and proximal cervical trachea (Figure 18-2, *A*). Lidocaine (2 to 5 mg/kg in dogs) can be infused intradermally and into the subcutaneous tissue to provide local anesthesia during the procedure. The onset of action for lidocaine is 10 to 15 minutes.[14] Strict asepsis should be adhered to throughout the procedure.

*Intracath®, Becton Dickinson Vascular Access, Sandy, Utah.
†Safe T Vac® Suction Catheter, Kendall Co., Mansfield, Mass.
‡Bard® Mucous Specimen Trap, CR Bard Inc., Covington, Ga.

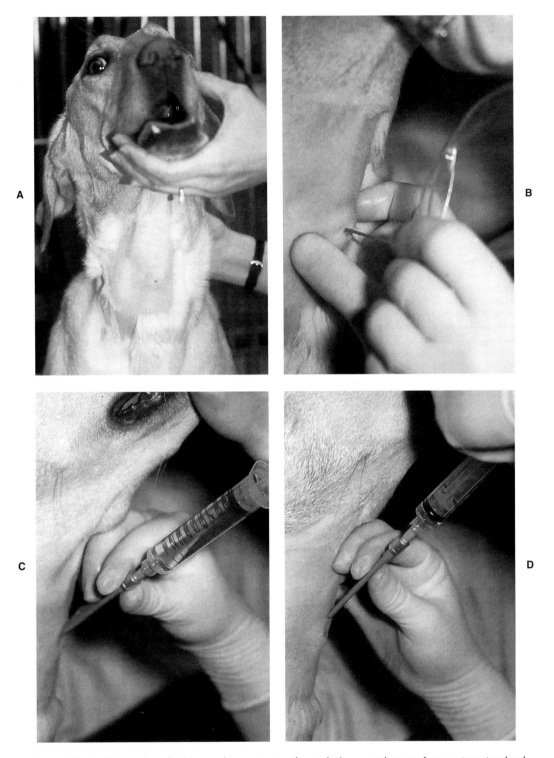

Figure 18-2. *This series of pictures demonstrates the technique used to perform a transtracheal wash.* (From King LG: *Bacterial infections of the respiratory tract in dogs and cats,* Trenton, NJ, 1997, Veterinary Learning Systems.)

The catheter can be inserted into the trachea either through the cricothyroid ligament or just distal to the larynx on the midline between two tracheal rings (Figure 18-3). The cricothyroid ligament has been recommended for small dogs and cats, whereas either method is ac-ceptable for large dogs. When palpating the larynx, the cricothyroid ligament can be felt as a wide, triangular depression located between the prominent thyroid carti-lage orally and the cricoid cartilage aborally. Personal ex-perience with the cricothyroid approach is that patients

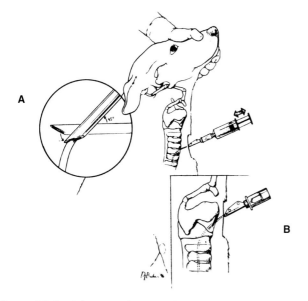

Figure 18-3. *Schematic drawing of two accepted techniques for transtracheal washing.* **A,** *Insertion of the catheter between two tracheal rings (used most commonly in large breed dogs).* **B,** *Insertion of the catheter through the cricothyroid ligament. The needle should be inserted with the bevel down; once the trachea has been entered, the needle is raised to a 45-degree angle to allow the catheter to be fed down into the trachea.* (From King LG: *Bacterial infections of the respiratory tract in dogs and cats,* Trenton, NJ, 1997, Veterinary Learning Systems.)

often retch or swallow after catheter placement, making the procedure more difficult.

A small stab incision can be made in the skin to facilitate needle placement, although this is not always necessary. After the needle has been inserted through the skin, the larynx or trachea is stabilized with one hand. The needle is then inserted, with the bevel down, into the trachea using steady pressure (see Figure 18-2, *B*). When the needle has entered the airway, the tip of needle should be lowered and the catheter should be fed its entire length into the airway. The patient may start coughing at any point after penetrating the tracheal lumen. If resistance is noted, the needle should be backed out a small distance and the catheter fed again because the needle may have been abutting the opposite wall of the trachea. Once the catheter has been fed into the airway, the needle can be withdrawn from the trachea and covered with a needle guard. The stylet should be removed at this time.

A syringe prefilled with sterile saline (3 to 5 ml for cats and small dogs, 10 to 20 ml for larger dogs) can be attached to the catheter and flushed into the catheter (see Figure 18-2, *C*). The syringe should then be aspirated slowly to retrieve lavage fluid. At this time, the patient should be gently coupaged to encourage coughing, which will improve the quality of the sample. If the syringe fills with air, it can be detached to evacuate the air and reattached for additional aspiration. This procedure should continue with additional saline-filled syringes until an adequate sample is obtained. Only a small por-

tion of the fluid instilled into the airway may be retrieved (about 0.5 to 2 ml) following TTW, and the remaining fluid is quickly absorbed by the bronchopulmonary tree (see Figure 18-2, *D*). It has been reported that up to 1 ml/kg of saline can be injected into the airway at one time without causing signs of respiratory distress[15]; however, no study has been published validating this recommendation. After a sufficient sample has been obtained, the catheter should be removed from the trachea and gentle pressure and a bandage applied to limit bleeding and air leakage from the site.

Technique for Endotracheal Wash

Endotracheal washes require the patient to be at an adequate plane of anesthesia to facilitate intubation. Short-acting anesthetic agents (e.g., propofol or thiopental) are recommended to allow quick induction and recovery following the procedure. Ketamine and diazepam can also be used; however, these agents are associated with a slower anesthetic recovery.

The patient is usually positioned in sternal recumbency for the procedure. Alternatively, the patient can be placed in lateral recumbency with the affected side down, which may aid in obtaining a diagnostic sample from patients with focal disease. Topical lidocaine can be sprayed into the pharynx of cats to decrease laryngospasm and facilitate intubation. A laryngoscope should be used to assist intubation to minimize oropharyngeal contamination of the endotracheal tube. A sterile endotracheal tube is required, and if possible the patient's endotracheal tube should not be connected to the anesthetic circuit until after the procedure has been completed (Figure 18-4, *A*).

As soon as the patient has been intubated, a sterile red rubber catheter is introduced into the airway through the endotracheal tube and fed as far as possible beyond the tip of the endotracheal tube. A syringe prefilled with sterile saline (3- to 5-ml aliquots for cats and small dogs, 10- to 20-ml aliquots for larger dogs) is attached to the catheter and flushed into the airway (see Figure 18-4, *B*). A catheter adapter* may be required to secure the syringe to the catheter. Care should be taken to hold onto the catheter while flushing to prevent the catheter from becoming detached and lodging within the trachea.

Endotracheal wash fluid can be retrieved by a variety of techniques. The syringe used to flush the saline into the airway can be flushed with air then manually aspirated to retrieve the sample. Mechanical suction can also be used, which may result in a higher yield. A mechanical suction device that can provide regulated low-pressure suction (100 to 170 mm Hg)[12] can be attached to a suction catheter† and sterile specimen container‡ (see Figure 18-1). Using this technique, the red rubber catheter is removed from the airway and the suction catheter is quickly fed into the trachea beyond the en-

---

*Catheter Adapter, Becton Dickinson Co., Franklin Lakes, N.J.
†Safe-T-Vac Suction Catheter, Kendall Co., Mansfield, Mass.
‡Bard Mucous Specimen Trap, CR Bard Inc., Covington, Ga.

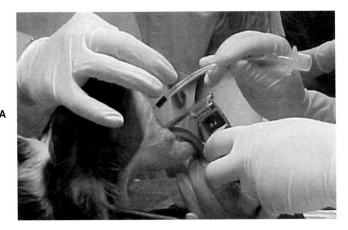
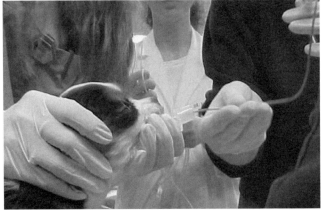

Figure 18-4. *This series of pictures demonstrates the technique used to perform an endotracheal lavage.*

dotracheal tube. Gentle intermittent suction is applied to retrieve a fluid sample. Saline flushes can be repeated until an adequate sample has been obtained.

Sample Handling

The tracheal wash sample should immediately be allocated for cytological evaluation and saved for microbiologic culture. Samples can be submitted in a variety of containers (e.g., capped syringe or vial) for cytological evaluation, depending on the preference of the diagnostic laboratory. Highly cellular samples should be placed in an EDTA tube to prevent clot formation and clumping of cells.[16] If cytological evaluation cannot be performed immediately, slides should be prepared to preserve cellular integrity or the sample should be refrigerated. Labeling the sample with the method by which it was obtained and providing a medical history including any microbial concerns are extremely important measures to facilitate appropriate testing because microorganisms such as *Mycoplasma* spp. and fungal agents require special culture techniques.

Most microbiology laboratories prefer to receive the actual fluid rather than a swab of the sample, if possible because a larger sample size increases the possibility of isolating microorganisms. However, if the sample cannot be plated within 3 hours, it should be placed in a vial containing transport media to prolong the viability of microorganisms and to prevent bacterial overgrowth. Samples placed in transport media can remain at room temperature for up to 4 hours for isolation of aerobic bacteria but should be refrigerated if they are stored beyond that time. By refrigerating samples and placing them in transport media, aerobic cultures can be performed on the sample for about 2 to 3 days. Optimally, culture for anaerobic bacteria should be performed within 10 minutes of collection if the sample is kept under anaerobic conditions (e.g., in a syringe with all air expelled and capped with a rubber stopper) without transport media. Special transport media are available

---

BOX 18-1
Bacteria Isolated From the Lower Respiratory Tracts of Healthy Dogs[19,20]

Acinetobacter spp.
Corynebacterium spp.
Enterobacter aerogenes
Klebsiella pneumoniae
Moraxella spp.
Pasteurella multocida
Staphylococcus (coagulase positive and negative)
Streptococcus (alpha and nonhemolytic)

BOX 18-2
Bacteria Isolated From the Lower Respiratory Tracts of Healthy Cats[18,21]

Acinetobacter	*Klebsiella*
Bordetella	*Micrococcus*
Corynebacterium	*Pasteurella multocida*
Enterbacter	*Pseudomonas*
Escherichia coli	*Staphylococcus*
Flavobacterium	*Streptococcus*

---

for anaerobic cultures, which may sustain the viability of microorganisms for up to 2 days when refrigerated.[17]

Interpretation of Results

The tracheobronchial tree and lungs are not sterile in healthy dogs and cats. In fact, several studies have isolated a variety of bacteria from the trachea and lower respiratory tract in 40% to 50% of healthy dogs and cats (Boxes 18-1 and 18-2).[18-21] These bacteria are usually present in low numbers (less than 10^3 CFU/ml)[19] and are not associated with clinical signs of illness, radiographic abnormalities, or cytological evidence of inflammation. Positive bacterial cultures from tracheal washes must therefore be interpreted in light of clinical signs and other diagnostic test results.

Quantitative or semiquantitative cultures can be used to determine whether a cultured organism represents a true infection or is a contaminant or part of the normal airway flora. Microbial quantitation has not been routinely performed in veterinary medicine but is becoming more routine. In humans, bacterial isolation at concentrations less than 10^4 CFU/ml is considered to be either a contaminant or insignificant. Isolation of greater than 10^5 CFU/ml of bacteria is supportive of infection, with most significant bacterial infections being present in concentrations greater than 10^6 to 10^8 CFU/ml.[22] Culture results should be interpreted with caution in patients receiving antibiotics prior to tracheal wash because these cultures may yield false negative results or less than 10^3 CFU/ml of bacteria.

Because tracheal washes are performed by instilling saline into the airway, any bacteria isolated will be diluted, making quantitation inaccurate. Protocols can be developed in collaboration with the diagnostic laboratory to standardize the volume of fluid used during the procedure and culture to more accurately quantitate the results.

Tracheal wash samples can vary in the degree of cellularity. Direct smears can be evaluated in highly cellular samples; however, cytocentrifugation is often required to concentrate cells for evaluation. Cytological evaluation should include an estimate of cellularity, differential cell counts, characterization of cell morphology, and identification of any neoplastic cells or infectious agents. Tracheal wash samples from normal airways may contain respiratory epithelial cells, occasional inactive macrophages, small amounts of mucus, and rare neutrophils or lymphocytes.[16]

Identification of intracellular bacteria is specific for bacterial infection but not particularly sensitive because microorganisms may be detected cytologically in only one third to one half of patients with bacterial pneumonia.[11,23-24] Culture and sensitivity testing is warranted if neutrophilic inflammation is present or if there is clinical evidence suggestive of pneumonia, even if bacteria are not seen cytologically. When possible, antibiotics should be discontinued for at least 1 week prior to testing to limit the possibility of false negative cultures.[11]

Conclusion

Tracheal washes can provide useful information for a variety of airway and lung disorders of dogs and cats. They can be performed quickly and inexpensively in most patients and should be used as an initial diagnostic test in patients with respiratory disease. Cytological evaluation should be performed routinely on tracheal wash fluid, and microbial culture should be routine in those patients with suspected infections or evidence of neutrophilic inflammation.

REFERENCES

1. Hamilton TA, Hawkins EC, DeNicola DB: Bronchoalveolar lavage and tracheal wash to determine lung involvement in a cat with cryptococcosis, J Am Vet Med Assoc 198:655-666, 1991.
2. Hawkins EC, DeNicola DB: Cytologic analysis of tracheal wash specimens and bronchoalveolar lavage fluid in the diagnosis of mycotic infections in dogs, J Am Vet Med Assoc 197:79-83, 1990.
3. Hawkins EC, Morrison WB, DeNicola DB et al: Cytologic analysis of bronchoalveolar lavage fluid from 47 dogs with multicentric malignant lymphoma, J Am Vet Med Assoc 203:1418-1425, 1993.
4. Hawkins EC, DeNicola DB, Plier ML: Cytological analysis of bronchoalveolar lavage fluid in the diagnosis of spontaneous respiratory tract disease in dogs: A retrospective study, J Vet Intern Med 9:386-392, 1995.
5. Moser KM, Maurer J, Jassy L et al: Sensitivity, specificity, and risk of diagnostic procedures in a canine model of Streptococcus pneumoniae pneumonia, Am Rev Resp Dis 125:436-442, 1982.
6. Sanchez-Mejorada G, Calva JJ, Ponce de Leon S et al: Usefulness and risks of transtracheal aspiration in the diagnosis of pulmonary infections, Rev Invest Clin 43:285-292, 1991.
7. Angus JC, Jang SS, Hirsch DC: Microbiological study of transtracheal aspirates from dogs with suspected lower respiratory tract disease: 264 cases (1989-1995), J Am Vet Med Assoc 210: 55-58, 1997.
8. Harpster NK: The effectiveness of the cephalosporins in the treatment of bacterial pneumonias in the dog, J Am Anim Hosp Assoc 17:766-771, 1981.
9. Creighton SR, Wilkins RJ: Bacteriologic and cytologic evaluation of animals with lower respiratory tract disease using transtracheal aspiration biopsy, J Am Anim Hosp Assoc 10:227-232, 1974.
10. McNiel EA, Ogilvie GK, Powers BF et al: Evaluation of prognostic factors for dogs with primary lung tumors: 67 cases (1985-1992), J Am Vet Med Assoc 211:1422-1427, 1997.
11. Greene CE: Respiratory infections. In Greene CE, editor: Infectious diseases of the dog and cat, ed 2, Philadelphia, 1990, WB Saunders.
12. Young CS: Recommended guidelines for suction, Physiotherapy 70:106-108, 1984.
13. Young CS: A review of the adverse effects of suction, Physiotherapy 70:104-106, 1984.
14. Skarda RT: Local and regional anesthetic and analgesic techniques: Dogs. In Thurman JC, Tranquilli WJ, Benson GJ, editors: Lumb and Jones' veterinary anesthesia, Baltimore, 1996, Williams & Wilkins.
15. Thayer GW: Infections of the respiratory system. In Greene CE, editor: Clinical microbiology and infectious diseases of the dog and cat, Philadelphia, 1984, WB Saunders.
16. Cowell RL, Tyler RD, Baldwin CJ: Transtracheal and bronchial washes. In Cowell RL, Tyler RD, editors: Diagnostic Cytology of the Dog and Cat, Goleta, Calif, 1989, American Veterinary Publications.
17. Lappin MR, Turnwald GH: Microbiology and infectious diseases. In Willard MD, Tvedten H, Turnwald GH, editors: Small animal clinical diagnosis by laboratory methods, Philadelphia, 1994, WB Saunders.
18. Dye JA, McKiernan BC, Rozanski EA et al: Bronchopulmonary disease in the cat: Historical, physical, radiographic, clinicopathologic, and pulmonary functional evaluation of 24 affected and 15 healthy cats, J Vet Intern Med 10:385-400, 1996.
19. Lindsey JO, Pierce AK: An examination of the microbiologic flora of normal lung of the dog, Am Rev Resp Dis 117:501-505, 1978.
20. McKiernan BC, Smith AR, Kissil M: Bacterial isolates from the lower trachea of clinically healthy dogs, J Am Anim Hosp Assoc 20:139-142, 1984.
21. Padrid PA, Feldman BF, Funk K et al: Cytologic, microbiologic, and biochemical analysis of bronchoalveolar lavage fluid obtained from 24 healthy cats, Am J Vet Res 52:1300-1307, 1991.
22. Fagon JY, Chastre J, Hance AJ et al: Detection of nosocomial lung infection in ventilated patients: Use of a protected specimen brush and quantitative culture techniques in 147 patients, Am Rev Resp Dis 138:110-116, 1988.
23. Hirsch DC: Bacteriology of the lower respiratory tract. In Kirk RW, editor: Current veterinary therapy IX, Philadelphia, 1986, WB Saunders.
24. Thayer GW, Robinson SK: Bacterial bronchopneumonia in the dog: A review of 42 cases, J Am Anim Hosp Assoc 20:731-735, 1984.

CHAPTER 19

Fine Needle Aspirates

Steven G. Cole

Fine needle aspiration (FNA) is an extremely useful technique that is easily performed in the clinical setting. FNA provides samples for both cytological analysis and microbiological culture and is a valuable tool in the diagnosis of many intrathoracic disease processes. Although the procedure is commonly used to obtain samples from discrete thoracic wall and mediastinal masses, FNA is also indicated to characterize pulmonary nodules and mass lesions, as well as diffuse diseases of the pulmonary interstitium.

Fine needle aspiration is usually performed after prior diagnostic tests (generally thoracic radiographs or ultrasound) have identified intrathoracic disease. The yield of FNA is high, with published reports in the veterinary literature documenting that a diagnostic sample is obtained in approximately 90% of cases with intrathoracic disease.[1-4] These results are consistent regardless of the type of lesion or the method used in performing the procedure. Because it is relatively noninvasive, FNA may be performed in lieu of (or in conjunction with) needle core biopsy or surgical biopsy of mass lesions. In addition, the procedure may also supplement transtracheal, endotracheal, or bronchoalveolar lavage in animals with regional, diffuse, or disseminated pulmonary interstitial disease.

In addition to excellent diagnostic yield, the diagnostic accuracy of fine needle aspiration is also high in animals with intrathoracic disease. In a study of ultrasound guided aspiration of focal pulmonary parenchymal lesions, sensitivities of 88% for carcinoma and 83% for blastomycosis were documented.[4] The specificity and positive predictive value of FNA for both disease processes was 100%.[4] Similar results have also been reported with fluoroscopically guided aspirates and with blind aspiration of animals with diffuse interstitial disease.[1,3]

Indications

Fine needle aspiration is indicated for characterization of mediastinal and thoracic wall masses, solitary or multiple discrete pulmonary nodules or masses, and regional or diffuse interstitial disease of the pulmonary parenchyma. FNA may be used to obtain valuable diagnostic and prognostic information, especially in patients that may not tolerate more invasive diagnostic tests.

Contraindications

The most important contraindications to performing fine needle aspiration are coagulopathy (especially in cases of thrombocytopenia or thrombocytopathia), pulmonary hypertension, and the presence of pulmonary bullae.[1,4,5] Other contraindications to FNA include the inability to adequately visualize discrete lesions, inadequate sedation or analgesia, and the inability to manage postprocedure complications. Significant respiratory distress and poor clinical condition have been correlated with higher complication rates and unfavorable outcomes and thus are also relative contraindications to FNA for patients in this category.[3]

Choice of Site for FNA

The specific approach and procedure chosen for FNA depends on the type of lesion (mass lesion versus diffuse disease), location of the lesion (central versus peripheral), and unique characteristics (tractable versus fractious, stable versus compromised) of a given patient. For animals with discrete masses or lung consolidation, ultrasonography, fluoroscopy, or computed tomography may be used to visualize the lesion while performing the procedure. Ultrasonography, in particular, is an extremely valuable tool in performing fine needle aspiration. Ultrasound guidance allows for precise localization of the needle and for the identification and avoidance of vascular structures. In addition, a practiced ultrasonographer can perform FNA rapidly and with a minimal amount of patient manipulation or discomfort.

When the use of ultrasound is limited (e.g., the presence of aerated lung tissue or air in the pleural cavity between the lesion and the ultrasound transducer), alternate techniques are indicated. Fluoroscopy is simple to perform and allows visualization of the entire thoracic cavity. Computed tomography (CT) also allows precise visualization of the entire thorax and the needle path, although CT-guided aspiration is generally more expensive and technically difficult to perform.

Finally, in animals with regional, diffuse or disseminated pulmonary parenchymal disease, a blind aspiration technique may be employed to acquire a representative sample for analysis. The site of aspiration depends on the regions affected, with care taken to avoid cardiac and vascular structures. In animals with diffuse disease, the caudal lung lobes may be aspirated by introducing the needle in the seventh to ninth intercostal space at a level two thirds of the distance from the costochondral junction to the vertebral bodies.[3,5]

Instrumentation and Technique

Fine needle aspiration is performed with 20- to 25-gauge needles of varying lengths, although 22-gauge, $1\frac{1}{2}$-inch needles are most often used. Deeper lesions may be sampled using a 22-gauge $2\frac{1}{2}$-inch, $3\frac{1}{2}$-inch, or 5-inch spinal needle without a stylet. Other materials necessary for FNA include 6-ml or 12-ml syringes, extension tubing, and glass slides to prepare specimens for cytology. Transport media for fungal or bacterial culture should also be available when appropriate.

A variety of techniques for ultrasound-guided fine needle aspiration have been described in the recent veterinary literature.[2,4,6] Other reports document techniques for fluoroscopic and CT guidance, as well as blind techniques used in aspirating intrathoracic lesions.[1,3,5,7] In practice, the technique used for fine needle aspiration is similar regardless of the type of lesion or method used for visualization.

After the lesion to be aspirated has been identified, the least traumatic needle approach is determined, facilitated if possible by real-time ultrasound, fluoroscopy, or computed tomography. Sedation or general anesthesia is administered, depending on the technique and the temperament and clinical status of the patient. The patient is placed in sternal or lateral recumbency and the skin overlying the lesion is clipped and aseptically prepared. The needle, attached either directly or via a short extension set to a 6- to 12–ml syringe, is introduced through the skin and is advanced into the lesion. Imaging techniques allow precise localization of the needle within the lesion to be aspirated. If general anesthesia is employed, ventilation may be briefly suspended to minimize motion during the procedure. Once within the lesion, negative pressure is applied two to five times as a sample is obtained. Following release of negative pressure, the needle is withdrawn. The syringe is removed from the needle or extension set, filled with air, and then reattached. The sample is expelled onto a glass slide, and smears are made as quickly as possible. Alternatively, the sample may be prepared and submitted for microbiological culture.

One or two aspirates are performed for each lesion, although the quality of the samples obtained may dictate the number of aspirates performed. One of the drawbacks of the negative pressure aspiration technique is excessive sample hemodilution. An alternate technique has been described to prevent this occurrence.[6] With this technique, the attached syringe is prefilled with air. Once the needle is introduced, no negative pressure is applied. Rather, the needle is rapidly moved back and forth within the lesion five to ten times and then withdrawn. The sample, which has collected within the needle lumen, is then expelled onto a glass slide or microbiological culturette.

Complications and Postprocedure Management

Reported complications resulting from intrathoracic fine needle aspiration in veterinary patients include pneumothorax, hemothorax, intrapulmonary hemorrhage, and hemoptysis. In general, however, significant complications are unusual. This is especially true for ultrasound-guided aspiration, with two studies reporting clinically recognizable complication rates of 0%.[2,4] Complication rates of 17% for fluoroscopic-guided aspiration and 43% for blind aspiration were noted in two separate studies, and these tended to be seen in animals with diffuse or disseminated disease processes.[1,3]

Potential complications from fine needle aspiration may be minimized by careful screening for conditions that place patients at additional risk (e.g., pulmonary bullae, coagulopathy, or pulmonary hypertension). A ruptured pulmonary bulla, for example, may lead to the development of tension pneumothorax. Coagulopathy and pulmonary hypertension both predispose patients to bleeding complications. Although fine needle aspiration may generally be performed with minimal physical or chemical restraint, excessive patient motion may lead to inadvertent damage to intrathoracic structures. Therefore judicious use of sedation, analgesia, or anesthesia should be considered to maximize patient comfort and safety during the procedure. In addition, general anesthesia and assisted ventilation may be required in animals with significant respiratory distress. This is also the case if fluoroscopic or CT visualization is necessary to aspirate nonperipheral lesions. In these situations, control of ventilation is essential to ensure adequate targeting of the lesion and to minimize the potential for damage to normal structures.

Patient management following FNA depends on the presence and magnitude of complications stemming from the procedure. Certainly, all animals should be closely monitored for tachypnea, dyspnea, cough, hemoptysis, or deterioration of hemodynamic status following FNA. In addition, packed cell volume and total solids should be rechecked immediately postprocedure and 2 hours later. Pulse oximetry or, ideally, arterial blood gas analysis are indicated to assess pulmonary function. Ideally, chest radiographs could be obtained immediately after the procedure and repeated several hours later, but the decision to perform radiography may be based on changes in physical examination or clinical parameters.

Once identified, appropriate management of any problems following fine needle aspiration is essential. Although many instances of pneumothorax following FNA are subclinical and self-limiting, thoracocentesis is indicated if significant pneumothorax is identified. Rare cases require repeat thoracocentesis or the placement of a chest tube for continuous evacuation of the pleural space. Similarly, animals with bleeding complications may require transfusion of blood products or pleural drainage in severe cases. Patients with compromised pulmonary function should receive supplemental oxygen, and mechanical ventilation must be considered in cases of ventilatory or respiratory failure. Although these potential complications may be serious or even life threatening, it should be noted that the large majority of patients have no clinically significant complications following FNA of intrathoracic lesions.

Conclusion

Samples obtained by fine needle aspiration are ideal for cytopathological evaluation, as well as for microbiological culture. In this way, FNA is extremely useful in the characterization of mediastinal, thoracic wall, and pulmonary parenchymal disease processes of various etiologies.[1,2,4,5,8] Because of its low cost, high yield, and relative simplicity, FNA should be considered a first-line procedure that provides valuable diagnostic and prognostic information that can then be used to guide further diagnostic and therapeutic strategies for patients with intrathoracic disease.

REFERENCES

1 McMillan MC, Kleine LJ, Carpenter JL: Fluoroscopically guided percutaneous fine-needle aspiration biopsy of thoracic lesions in dogs and cats, *Vet Radiol* 29:194-197, 1988.
2. Reichle JK, Wisner ER: Non-cardiac ultrasound in 75 feline and canine patients, *Vet Radiol Ultrasound* 41:154-162, 2000.
3. Teske E, Stokhof AA, van den Ingh TSGAM et al: Transthoracic needle aspiration biopsy of the lung in dogs with pulmonic diseases, *J Am Anim Hosp Assoc* 27:289-294, 1991.
4. Wood EF, O'Brien RT, Young KM: Ultrasound-guided fine-needle aspiration of focal parenchymal lesions of the lung in dogs and cats, *J Vet Intern Med* 12:338-342, 1998.
5. Roudebush P, Green RA, Digilio KM: Percutaneous fine-needle aspiration biopsy of the lung in disseminated pulmonary disease, *J Am Anim Hosp Assoc* 17:109-116, 1981.
6. Menard M, Papageorges M: Technique for ultrasound-guided fine needle biopsies, *Vet Radiol Ultrasound* 36:137-138, 1995.
7. Finn-Bodner ST, Hathcock JT: Image-guided percutaneous needle biopsy: Ultrasound, computed tomography, and magnetic resonance imaging, *Seminars in Vet Med and Surg (Sm Anim)*, 8:258-278, 1993.
8. Ogilvie GK, Haschek WM, Withrow SJ et al: Classification of primary lung tumors in dogs: 210 cases (1975-1985), *J Am Vet Med Assoc* 195:106-108, 1989.

CHAPTER 20

Thoracocentesis

Valérie Sauvé

Background and Definition

Greek word elements define thoracocentesis, or thoracentesis, as the act of *puncture and aspiration of the thorax*. The pleural space is a potential space, which in the normal animal contains a few milliliters of serous fluid and has a negative pressure.

In different disease states, fluid can accumulate in the pleural space and the retrieval of this fluid can be of great diagnostic and therapeutic aid. Early identification of the disease process and adequate therapy can improve outcome; drainage of large amounts of pleural fluid can improve dyspnea, pulmonary mechanics, and in some instances hemodynamics. Air retrieval from a significant pneumothorax can have the same benefits.

Indications

In the guidelines published by the American Thoracic Society in 1988, indications to perform thoracocentesis include (1) the presence of any undiagnosed pleural effusion and (2) therapeutic thoracocentesis to relieve respiratory signs caused by a large effusion.[1] When the etiology of the effusion can be reasonably deduced by the clinical presentation and the patient is not dyspneic, the procedure may be postponed and the response to therapy followed.[1]

Analysis of fluid collected by thoracocentesis can be of great benefit to a patient whose diagnosis is not confirmed. In a study of 82 human patients with pleural effusions undergoing diagnostic thoracocentesis, the procedure yielded improvement in the diagnosis and/or treatment in 56% and a change in the presumptive prethoracocentesis diagnosis in 45% of patients.[2] In another human study of 78 thoracocentesis procedures, pleural fluid analysis was judged to be clinically useful in 92% of the cases, but a definitive diagnosis was achieved in only 18%.[3] In most cases, pleural fluid analysis finds its utility in supporting a presumptive diagnosis.[1]

In a dyspneic animal, respiratory compromise can arise from the upper airways, lower airways, pleural space, pulmonary parenchyma, chest wall, or from neurological or metabolic causes. Historical findings (e.g., previous heart disease, trauma, bite wounds, or neoplasia) and auscultation and physical examination will often identify patients with pleural disease. Animals with a large pleural effusion or significant pneumothorax often have a short, shallow respiratory pattern. The chest wall excursions may be minimal considering the degree of respiratory effort. Dull heart and lung sounds can be appreciated unilaterally or bilaterally; ventrally, with fluid accumulation; and caudodorsally, in the presence of a pneumothorax. Percussion may be dull ventrally if fluid is present, or hyperresonant where air has accumulated. A diagnostic thoracocentesis should be performed if there is any suspicion that pleural space disease could be contributing to the dyspnea. Thoracocentesis should be performed before radiographs if the animal is severely dyspneic. Thoracic ultrasonography, if available, may be a rapid means of confirming the presence of fluid.

A small pneumothorax may not be clinically significant and may not require any therapy unless concurrent pulmonary pathology (e.g., pulmonary contusion) is present. However, a moderate to severe or tension pneumothorax will be demonstrated by tachypnea or dyspnea, may be rapidly life threatening, and should be relieved promptly by thoracocentesis. Both sides of the chest should be aspirated because the mediastinum may not be permeable to air and asymmetrical air accumulation is common.

Animals with hemothorax often present for circulatory collapse rather than dyspnea because significant ventilation impairment does not occur until 30 to 60 ml/kg (dogs) or 20 ml/kg (cats) of fluid is present in the pleural space.[4,5] If possible, hemorrhagic effusions should not be removed because the effused red blood cells will be absorbed back into the circulation. Furthermore, patients with nontraumatic hemothorax may be coagulopathic, and thoracocentesis may only contribute to further bleeding. However, if the patient's respiratory function is compromised by the effusion, sufficient blood should be removed from the pleural space to allow comfortable breathing. Autotransfusion may be considered if the hemorrhagic effusion is secondary to trauma and more than 10 ml/kg of blood is present.[4]

If thoracocentesis is required more then twice to relieve a patient's dyspnea, if no improvement occurs following thoracocentesis, if a significant amount of air or blood is aspirated, or if negative pressure cannot be reached within the pleural space, a thoracostomy tube with continuous or intermittent suction is probably indicated for ongoing management of the patient.[6]

Finally, pleural fluid may mask intrathoracic structures; therefore, performing thoracocentesis before thoracic radiography may be indicated. Radiographs then allow quantitation of the fluid remaining in the chest as a baseline to follow reaccumulation.[7] The diagnostic value of thoracic radiographs after thoracocentesis has been questioned in human medicine; in one study (excluding the finding of a pneumothorax), only four new findings were found in 105 films evaluated postthoracocentesis.[8]

Contraindications and Complications

If significant dyspnea is present because of either pleural effusion or pneumothorax, the relative contraindications

and potential complications should be considered in a risk-benefit evaluation and the thoracocentesis should be performed in the safest way possible.

In the human literature, contraindications to performing thoracocentesis include severe alterations in hemostasis, hemodynamic instability, severe respiratory insufficiency, a very small effusion, and uncooperative patients.[1-2] In addition, human intensivists have been reluctant to perform thoracocentesis in ventilated patients with small effusions, or when positive end-expiratory pressure (PEEP) is in use because of an increased risk of iatrogenic pneumothorax. In one study of 29 ventilated human patients, blind thoracocentesis resulted in pneumothorax in 6% of cases.[9] In another human study using ultrasound guidance, no pneumothorax was caused in 45 procedures.[10] Therefore it appears that mechanical ventilatory support should not be considered a contraindication, especially if ultrasound guidance is used.

Various studies in humans have had inconsistent results in showing the different risk factors for complications following thoracocentesis. These risk factors include coagulopathy, chest wall infection, very small effusion, inability of the patient to cooperate, removal of large amounts of fluid (greater than 1.5 L), therapeutic as opposed to diagnostic tap, performance by inexperienced persons without direct supervision, unstable medical condition, use of a large needle, the need for multiple needle passes, the presence of loculation, underlying neoplastic or chronic obstructive lung disease, radiation therapy, and repeated thoracocenteses in the same patient.[1,11]

Potential complications are numerous and have been reported in humans to include pneumothorax, hemothorax, pneumohemothorax, organ laceration, subcapsular splenic hematoma, hemoabdomen, acute death, shearing of the catheter tip requiring thoracotomy, pain, persistent cough, dyspnea, negative tap, subcutaneous hematoma, seroma, vasovagal reaction, reexpansion pulmonary edema, hypovolemia, air embolism, tumor seeding through the needle track, and pleural infection.[1,3,12]

Iatrogenic pneumothorax caused by laceration of lung tissue at the time of needle insertion, or at the end of the tap when the lung is reexpanding, is certainly one of the greater risks. Other proposed mechanisms of pneumothorax include air being drawn into the chest during manipulation of the collecting system, or along the needle track, if high negative intrapleural pressures are present.[13] Treatment of an iatrogenic pneumothorax may require no intervention; a thoracocentesis; or, in some instances, a thoracostomy tube with continuous suction.

The frequency of iatrogenic pneumothorax postthoracocentesis in human medicine has been stated to be between 3% and 20%, with approximately 20% of those patients requiring a chest drain.[1] Three large retrospective studies in people documented a frequency of postthoracocentesis pneumothorax of 7.6% in 679 taps, and chest tubes were needed in 48% of the patients that developed pneumothorax.[14-16] In another 7 prospective studies of 612 thoracocentesis attempts in 463 patients, the incidence of pneumothorax was 8.6%, and chest tubes were required in 30.1% of patients that developed a pneumothorax.[3,12,17-21] In a more recent study of 205 human patients, in whom 255 thoracocentesis procedures were performed, a pneumothorax was reported in 5.4%, and chest tube placement was required in only 0.78% of all cases.[11]

The prevalence of the other major and minor complications has been reported, but has been less studied because the other complications occur rarely, are anecdotal, or are associated with little morbidity.[8,12,19]

Routine immediate postthoracocentesis thoracic radiographs used to be recommended for identification of potential complications (mostly pneumothorax). Other complications (e.g., hemothorax, reexpansion pulmonary edema, and organ laceration) are typically detected by clinical deterioration in the postprocedure period. The recommendation to routinely radiograph patients after thoracocentesis has been challenged in recent years, and current guidelines suggest that it is not necessary to radiograph the vast majority of stable patients after the procedure in the absence of suspicion, clinical indications, or risk factors.[8,19] Air aspiration during the tap may indicate the need for thoracic radiographs because a high percentage of these patients will have a pneumothorax.[8,19]

Instrumentation

Different techniques have been described, using different instrumentation. The size and body condition of the patient, the nature and quantity of the pleural pathology, and the preference of the user will dictate appropriate instrumentation. Clipping and surgical preparation will be required; ideally, sterile gloves should be worn.

In cats, a butterfly catheter is usually used mounted on a three-way stopcock and a 10- to 20-ml syringe. Butterfly catheter needles 19 to 23G in size are appropriate, with the larger-bore needles used if thicker fluid (e.g., pyothorax or hemothorax) is present or suspected. In small dogs in good or thin body condition, a butterfly catheter can also be used. In large or obese dogs, an 18- to 22G 1½- to 2-inch needle, or an over-the-needle 14- to 18G 2- to 5¼-inch catheter may be used, attached to an extension set, with a three-way stopcock and a 20- or 60-ml syringe (Figure 20-1). In some instances, it may be helpful to add holes near the tip of larger-bore catheters with a sterile surgical blade. The use of a through-the-needle 14G, 8- to 24-inch catheter without a stylet has also been described.[22,23]

Advantages stated for the use of catheters rather than needles include stability and decreased risk of lung laceration, with patient cooperation and immobility being less imperative.[22] However, in a prospective study of 52 human patients undergoing thoracocentesis, no significant difference in the rate of complications was found between needle and needle-catheter procedures, but there was a significant decrease in the rate of complications when ultrasound guidance was used to introduce a needle.[20] The special catheter kit used in that study is not used in veterinary medicine and has been reported to be rigid and traumatic compared with other catheter systems.[13] Other evidence shows that the use of ultrasonog-

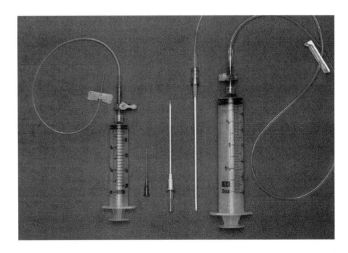

Figure 20-1. *Instrumentation for thoracocentesis. The size and body condition of the patient, the nature and quantity of the pleural pathology, and the preference of the user will dictate appropriate instrumentation. A butterfly catheter mounted on a three-way stopcock and a 10- to 20-ml syringe, 18- to 22G 1½- to 2-inch needle, or an over-the-needle 14- to 18G 2- to 5¼-inch catheter may be used, attached to an extension set, with a three-way stopcock and a 20- or 60-ml syringe.*

raphy to guide thoracocentesis may not decrease the incidence of complications.[24]

Several specific devices or prepackaged trays are available for use in human patients but have not been used in clinical veterinary medicine. In both the human and veterinary literature, small pleural catheters have been described to be left in place for repetitive drainage, replacing conventional thoracostomy tubes.[21,25] The use of a vacuum bottle has been associated in human medicine with an increased rate and severity of iatrogenic pneumothorax and has been strongly discouraged.[8]

Technique

The animal is routinely placed in sternal recumbency or standing to perform a thoracocentesis. However, when a pneumothorax is present, lateral recumbency is also appropriate. Most animals tolerate this procedure well, but adequate sedation is important when required. Medications that could cause respiratory or cardiac depression should be avoided. In a depressed or cooperative patient, minimal handling while administering flow-by oxygen may be ideal. Local anesthesia may be used (e.g., 1 to 2 ml of 2% lidocaine), and will be necessary when a large bore catheter is used. Infiltration of the subcutaneous tissue and muscle layers should be performed after skin preparation.

The tap is performed at the 7th or 8th intercostal space. The chest can be divided into thirds, the costochondral junction separating the ventral and midsection. According to the predicted pleural pathology, the tap should be performed at the costochondral junction if fluid is suspected or at the junction between the mid and dorsal third if air is suspected. If the animal is in lateral recumbency for air retrieval, the highest point or mid-thorax should be used. Long catheters are inserted in the mid-thorax area to retrieve pleural fluid. When very small amounts of fluid are present, or when there is difficulty obtaining a sample, ultrasound guidance may be required.

An area of the chest several inches in diameter should be clipped and surgically prepared. Ideally, sterile gloves should be worn, and strict asepsis should be followed. A tap may require two or three people, with one person who is sterile handling the needle or catheter; ideally, with another handling the syringe and three-way stopcock; and with a third person restraining the animal. The needle or catheter should be introduced into the thorax just cranial to the rib to avoid the costal vessels and nerve. The hand holding the needle or catheter should be resting on the chest wall to prevent excessive motion.

NEEDLE THORACOCENTESIS

The needle can be introduced slowly at a 45- or 90-degree angle, bevel facing the thoracic cavity, while a small negative pressure is maintained on the syringe to detect penetration of the pleural cavity by aspiration of air or fluid. The syringe can also be intermittently suctioned as the needle is gradually introduced through the thoracic wall. If reorientation is required, the needle should be partially removed, redirected, and then reintroduced into the chest cavity. Once in the chest and freely obtaining air or fluid, the needle may be reoriented ventrally, parallel to the chest wall, to prevent laceration of the lungs. Clamping a hemostat on the needle at the skin surface may prevent excessive movement in discordance with the patient.

A splash of frothy blood and negative pressure during aspiration is probably consistent with penetration of the lung parenchyma, and the needle should be removed. Similarly, the needle should be removed if the patient moves excessively or experiences violent coughing.

After collection of specimens for laboratory analysis, as much fluid or air as possible should be retrieved using the three-way stopcock, with the exception of patients with hemothorax, in whom blood may be left in the chest for reabsorption. Thoracocentesis should be performed on both sides of the thoracic cavity whenever possible.

CATHETER THORACOCENTESIS

An over-the-needle catheter can be used for removal of pleural fluid. The catheter is advanced through the chest wall very gradually. Once a flash of fluid is obtained in the hub of the catheter, the catheter is advanced slightly over the stylet to cover its tip, and then the two directed ventrally. The catheter should then feed easily over the stylet, which is then removed and the extension set with three-way stopcock and syringe is attached to allow complete evacuation of the chest contents. As long as the catheter tip is below the fluid line, air should not be introduced in the thorax while the stylet is being removed; however, the catheter can be clamped with a sterile hemostat while connecting it to the suction device. When fluid stops flowing, the catheter can be slowly pulled out (Figure 20-2).

The through-the-needle technique is similar. The needle is pulled out of the chest wall after completely feeding the soft catheter in the chest. The needle is then covered by the needle protector to prevent injury to the operator, patient, or catheter.

When larger catheters are used, a larger area of skin should be surgically prepared. By pulling the skin forward, the skin can be penetrated two intercostal spaces caudal to the site of penetration of the chest cavity, thereby preventing leaks through the needle track after the procedure, and possible development of pneumothorax. A small skin stab incision with a surgical blade will facilitate insertion of large catheters.

ULTRASOUND-GUIDED THORACOCENTESIS

Indications to use ultrasound guidance include the presence of a small effusion, dry taps in the presence of a large effusion, inability to properly position a debilitated patient, failure of fluid to layer out on radiographs, and coagulopathy.[12] Ultrasonography allows identification of the most appropriate site for puncture and measurement of the depth of the fluid, avoiding the lung parenchyma. The needle track can be visualized and confirmation of sufficient fluid removal can be made.[26]

Interpretation of Results

Retrieval of air from the pleural space, assuming that there is no leak in the collection system, is consistent with an open or closed pneumothorax, either acquired or spontaneous. If fluid is retrieved from the pleural cavity, samples should be collected in an EDTA tube (lavender top) for total nucleated cell count, total protein, and cytology; in a serum tube (red top) for biochemical analysis; and in a culture-transport medium. Total protein measurement and total nucleated cell counts will differentiate transudates, modified transudates, and exudates. Cytology and biochemical analysis (e.g., triglycerides, pH, glucose, bilirubin, and lactate) may be performed to further characterize the effusion and further orient diagnostic and therapeutic procedures.[27,28]

Iatrogenic blood contamination may present as a small amount of frothy blood, consistent with lung parenchyma puncture. Alternatively, aspiration of blood at the beginning or the end of the tap, especially with patient movement, is consistent with vessel injury or damage to viscera such as the liver if the needle has been incorrectly positioned or if there is a diaphragmatic hernia. True hemorrhagic effusions are uniform throughout the tap. If blood or bloody fluid is obtained, clotting of the sample should be assessed. Blood in the pleural space should be defibrinated rapidly by lung motion and should not clot unless massive peracute bleeding is present.

Inability to retrieve confirmed pleural fluid from the pleural cavity may result from pocketing or loculation of

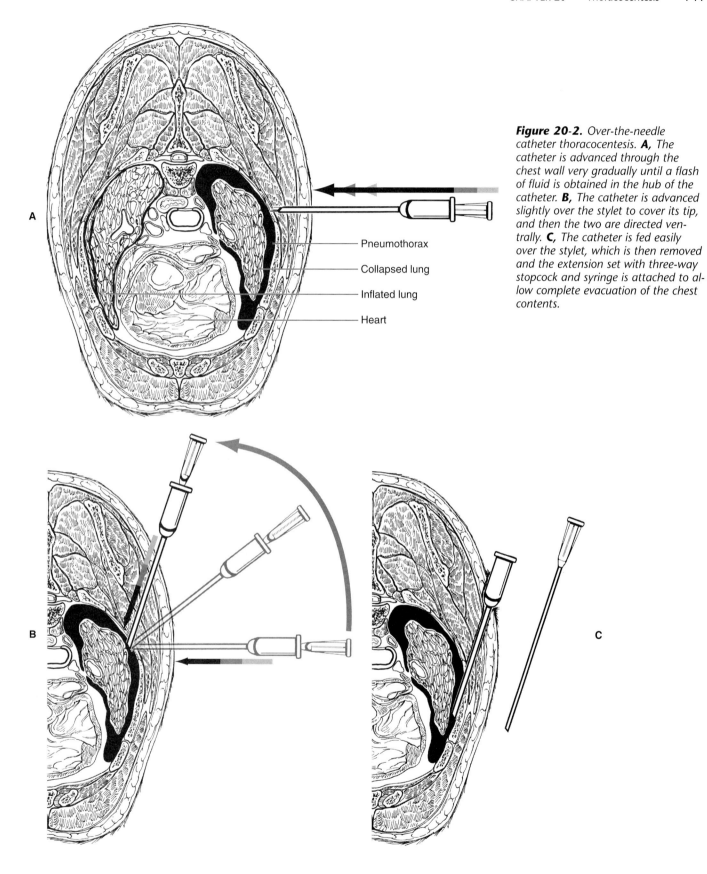

A

Pneumothorax

Collapsed lung

Inflated lung

Heart

B

C

Figure 20-2. *Over-the-needle catheter thoracocentesis.* **A,** *The catheter is advanced through the chest wall very gradually until a flash of fluid is obtained in the hub of the catheter.* **B,** *The catheter is advanced slightly over the stylet to cover its tip, and then the two are directed ventrally.* **C,** *The catheter is fed easily over the stylet, which is then removed and the extension set with three-way stopcock and syringe is attached to allow complete evacuation of the chest contents.*

the fluid, obstruction of the needle, inappropriate needle length, or chronic pleural effusion with fibrous adhesions. Aspiration at different sites, use of ultrasound guidance, and changing the position of the patient may help facilitate fluid retrieval.

REFERENCES

1. American Thoracic Society: Guidelines for thoracentesis and needle biopsy of the pleura, *Am Rev Respir Dis* 140:257-258, 1989.
2. Fartoukh M, Azoulay E, Galliot R et al: Clinically documented pleural effusions in medical ICU patients: How useful is routine thoracocentesis? *Chest* 121(1):178-184, 2002.
3. Collins TR, Sahn SA: Thoracentesis: Clinical value, complications, technical problems, and patient experience, *Chest* 91(6): 817-822, 1987.
4. Ludwig LL: Surgical emergencies of the respiratory system, *Vet Clin North Am Small Anim Pract* 30(3):531-553, 2000.
5. Cockshutt JR: Management of fracture-associated thoracic trauma, *Vet Clin North Am Small Anim Pract* 25(5):1031-1046, 1995.
6. Raffe MR: Respiratory care. In Raffe MR, Wingfield WE, editors: *The Veterinary ICU book*, Jackson, WY, 2002, Teton New Media.
7. Blair GP: Routine chest radiography after thoracocentesis, *Ann Intern Med* 126(6):491, 1997.
8. Peterson WG, Zimmerman R: Limited utility of chest radiographs after thoracocentesis, *Chest* 117(4):1038-1042, 2000.
9. Godwin JE, Sahn SA: Thoracentesis: A safe procedure in mechanically ventilated patients, *Ann Intern Med* 113:800-802, 1990.
10. Lichtenstein D, Hulot J-S, Rabiller A et al: Feasibility and safety of ultrasound-aided thoracocentesis in mechanically ventilated patients, *Intensive Care Medicine* 25:955-958, 1999.
11. Colt HG, Brewer N, Barbur E: Evaluation of patient-related and procedure-related factors contributing to pneumothorax following thoracocentesis, *Chest* 116(1):134-138, 1999.
12. Seneff MG, Corwin RW, Gold LH et al: Complications associated with thoracocentesis, *Chest* 90(1):97-100, 1986.
13. Swinburne AJ, Bixby K, Fedullo AJ et al: Pneumothorax after thoracocentesis, *Arch Intern Med* 151:2095-2096, 1991.
14. Jenkins DW Jr, McKinney MK, Szpak MW et al: Veres needle in the pleural space, *South Med J* 76:1383-1385, 1983.
15. Raptopoulos V, Davis LM, Lee G et al: Factors affecting the development of pneumothorax associated with thoracocentesis, *AJR Am J Roentgenol* 156:917-920, 1991.
16. Moore PV, Mueller PR, Simeone JF et al: Sonographic guidance in diagnostic and therapeutic interventions in the pleural space, *AJR Am J Roentgenol* 149:1-5, 1987.
17. Bartter T, Mayo PD, Pratter MR et al: Lower risk and higher yield for thoracocentesis when performed by experienced operators, *Chest* 91:817-822, 1993.
18. Yu CJ, Yang PC, Chang DB et al: Diagnostic and therapeutic use of chest sonography: Value in critically ill patients, *AJR Am J Roentgenol* 159:695-701, 1992.
19. Doyle JJ, Hnatiuk OW, Torrington KG et al: Necessity of routine chest roentgenography after thoracocentesis, *Ann Intern Med* 124(9): 816-820, 1996.
20. Grogan DR, Irwin RS, Channick R et al: Complications associated with thoracocentesis, *Arch Intern Med* 150:873-877, 1990.
21. Grodzin CJ, Balk RA: Indwelling small pleural catheter needle thoracentesis in the management of large pleural effusion, *Chest* 111(4):981-988, 1997.
22. Schall WD: Thoracocentesis, *Vet Clin North Am* 4(2):395-401, 1974.
23. Gott PH: A simplified method for thoracentesis and pleural drainage, *Am Rev Respir Dis* 92:295-296, 1965.
24. Kohan JM, Poe RH, Israel RH et al: Value of chest ultrasonography versus decubitus roentgenography for thoracocentesis, *Am Rev Respir Dis* 133:1124-1126, 1986.
25. Frendin J, Obel N: Catheter drainage of pleural fluid collections and pneumothorax, *J Small Anim Pract* 38:237-242, 1997.
26. Matsumata T, Kanematsu T, Sugimachi K: Ultrasound guided pleural tap, *Int Surg* 76:172-173, 1991.
27. Light RW: Pleural effusion, *N Engl J Med* 346(25):1971-1977, 2002.
28. Cowell RL, Tyler RD, Meinkoth JH: Abdominal and thoracic fluid. In Cowell RL, Tyler RD, Meinkoth JH, editors: *Diagnostic cytology and hematology of the dog and cat*, ed 2, St Louis, 1999, Mosby.

CHAPTER 21

Respiratory Tract Cytopathology

Patricia M. McManus

Introduction to Cytopathology

Diagnosis of respiratory disorders commonly requires cytological evaluation of tissues collected from the upper or lower respiratory tract or the pleural space. Although cytological evaluation is usually done by clinical pathologists in large referral diagnostic laboratories or academic institutions, time constraints often mandate that clinicians examine slides and act on their own observations prior to receiving the pathologist's report. Cytopathology has the potential to provide useful information regarding inflammation, infectious agents, and neoplasia, but knowledge of what to expect in normal tissue is a prerequisite for evaluation of the abnormal. In addition, an understanding of the techniques used in preparation and staining of smears is imperative to avoid misidentification and misinterpretation. This chapter addresses some of these issues.

Techniques

Detailed discussion of smear and staining techniques is best found in texts specifically addressing this subject,[1,2] but a few general points are worth clarifying. Successful microscopic examination of cells in a cytological preparation depends on creation of an artifact, in that spherical cells must be flattened in order to visualize interior cytoplasmic and nuclear structures. Identification of cells and infectious agents is difficult to impossible if cells are not flattened adequately (Figure 21-1). The quality of spreading within any one smear tends to be highly variable; therefore, skill in recognition of adequately spread cells must be developed.

Solid tissues can be sampled by direct impression, fine needle aspiration, nonaspiration fine needle biopsy, surface scrapings, swabs, or brushings. Of these, direct impressions tend to be the least helpful, in that generally only easily exfoliated cells (e.g., blood and inflammatory cells) are found. Tissue cells (e.g., spindle and epithelial cells) are more efficiently obtained using slightly more aggressive techniques.

Pleural fluids are processed according to their cellularity. Fluids with greater than 30,000 cells/μl can be handled without concentration by preparing direct smears. Concentration techniques are advised when nucleated cell counts are less than 30,000 cells/μl. In fluids that have between 2000 and 30,000 cells/μl, simple centrifugation and smearing of the sediment is generally adequate. Cytocentrifugation is advised when cell counts are less than 2000/μl. Buffy coat preparations are recommended for very bloody fluids in which the packed cell volume (PCV) is greater than 5% to 10%.

Slides should always be labeled as they are being prepared to prevent confusion later. Labeling should include the name of the owner, case number, date, and site. Labeling tools can include lead pencils, diamond pencils, or fine-tip black permanent markers. Green, blue, and red permanent markers are not really very permanent and should be avoided.

The next step in preparation is fixation and staining. Quick staining methods should be applied to effect rather than according to the manufacturer's timing suggestions, which only apply to thin blood smears. There is no danger of overstaining, but understaining can result in nondiagnostic preparations. The preferred method of staining is a more complex Romanowsky hematological stain (e.g., Wright-Giemsa). The processing is longer (approximately 12 minutes) but results in greater cytological detail (Box 21-1).

Generally it is best to dedicate a very good microscope for evaluation of blood and cytology smears and use a separate microscope for urine and fecal analysis. Recommended objectives for cytological evaluation include 4×, 10×, 20×, 50× oil, and 100× oil. Using a 50×-oil lens simplifies processing of slides because a coverslip is not necessary to examine cells and there is no fear of getting oil on a 40× dry lens.

Storage of slides after examination is just as important as storage of radiographs. Slides used as part of medical decision making are part of the medical record and should not be discarded. Oil can be removed by simply wiping it off using a tissue (e.g., Kleenex). Kimwipes and lens paper will scratch the smears. Using tissues that are impregnated with lotions or aloe vera is not recommended because they leave a film on the slide that is incompatible with immersion oil. Slides should then be stored, either in empty, cardboard slide boxes or slide file cabinets (Figure 21-2). Labeling of boxes or drawers by date is generally adequate, although a system using accession numbers can also be implemented. Coverslipping is not necessary prior to storing. Smears stored back to front will not be dam-

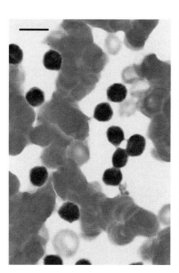 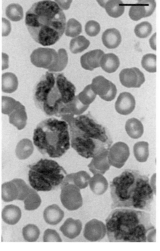

A   B

Figure 21-1. *Two sites within the same blood smear demonstrating the effect of smear thickness on cell identification.* **A,** *The nucleated cells are too thick to identify as monocytes.* **B,** *Improved smear technique allows easy identification of the cells. Bars = 10 μm. Wright-Giemsa stain.*

BOX 21-1
Protocol for Wright-Giemsa Stain* (Harleco®)

- Place dried smears on staining rack
- Cover entire smear with methanol using Pasteur pipette; leave on 1 minute
- Decant methanol
- Cover entire smear with filtered Wright-Giemsa stain; leave on 3 minutes
- Pipette an equal amount of deionized (or distilled) water on top of Wright-Giemsa stain; leave on 6 minutes
- Wash smears with deionized (or distilled) water and let dry

*Stain should be filtered using No. 42 Whatman filter; prepare a moderately large amount as a stock for staining.

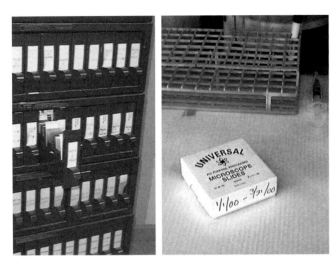

Figure 21-2. *Slides can be stored in either file cabinets designed for slides or in empty slide boxes. Labeling can be by accession number or date.*

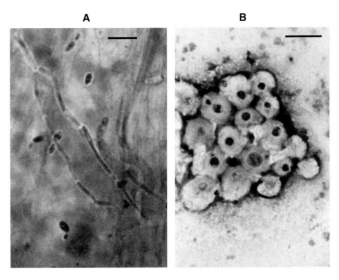

Figure 21-3. A, *Fungal hyphae and spores, typical for opportunistic fungal infections (bar = 10 μm).* **B,** *Yeast forms* (Cryptococcus neoformans) *from the nose of a cat (bar = 25 μm). Wright-Giemsa stain.*

aged when reasonable care is practiced during filing and retrieval.

Nasal Cytology

PURPOSE/SAMPLING

Evaluation of nasal specimens can result in determination of an inflammatory profile, identification of a specific infectious agent, and/or the diagnosis of neoplasia. Sampling of nasal passages is best done via lavage, aspirates, swabs, brushings, or scrapings.[3-5] Direct impressions of almost any lesion, regardless of the underlying cause, generally result in collection of superficial mucosal cells, inflammatory cells, and secondary bacterial agents. This type of profile may not reflect the primary disease process.

NORMAL

Normal elements detected in a nasal sample include nonkeratinized squamous epithelial cells or ciliated columnar cells, normal oropharyngeal flora such as *Simonsiella* spp., and a small amount of light pink–stained mucus. With traumatic procedures there may also be blood and nucleated cells appropriate to blood.

COMMON PROFILES

Common inflammatory profiles include acute (neutrophilic), chronic active or subacute (mixed neutrophils and macrophages), chronic (macrophages), lymphocytic-plasmacytic, and occasionally eosinophilic. Lymphocytic-plasmacytic inflammation is commonly mixed with acute inflammation and a secondary bacterial infection.

A bacterial infection should be suspected with acute inflammation, although bacteria are rarely the primary pathogen. Bacteria stain dark blue in Romanowsky-stained smears, regardless of Gram-staining characteristics. A monomorphic population of intracellular and extracellular organisms suggests a bacterial infection. Extracellular or squame-associated bacteria, which are mixed in type, suggest oropharyngeal contamination.

Fungal infections common to the upper respiratory tract include hyphal forms of *Aspergillus* spp. and *Penicillium* spp., which are both branching, septate, and 2 to 4.5 μm wide (Figure 21-3, *A*). Common yeast forms include *Cryptococcus neoformans* (Figure 21-3, *B*), primarily in cats, and *Rhinosporidium seeberi* in dogs.

Neoplasms of the upper respiratory tract likely to be encountered in cytological evaluations include adenocarcinoma, squamous cell carcinoma, lymphosarcoma (LSA), fibrosarcoma, chondrosarcoma, and osteosarcoma. Nasal adenocarcinomas, the most common tumor type,[6] can be either highly anaplastic, with marked pleomorphism, or consist of small uniform cells, with high nuclear to cytoplasmic ratios. The latter form can be difficult to distinguish from LSA (Figure 21-4). Chondrosarcomas are often distinguished by the presence of a bright purple- to magenta-stained extracellular matrix. The staining intensity of this matrix can result in poor staining of the chondroblasts themselves. This same material can be present in aspirates of osteosarcomas but is generally less abundant.

CONFUSION

Dysplastic and hyperplastic epithelial tissue should not be confused with neoplasia. Furthermore, squamous metaplasia can occasionally be observed in association with long-standing severe inflammation. In cases of lymphocytic-plasmacytic inflammation, lymphocytes can be

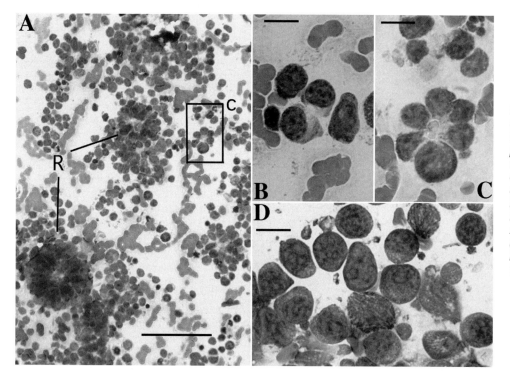

Figure 21-4. Nasal carcinomas can be difficult to distinguish from lymphosarcomas in cytological preparations. **A, B, C,** Cells taken from a cat with nasal carcinoma confirmed by biopsy. **D,** Cells from a dog with lymphosarcoma. The key to identification of carcinomas is demonstration of cell:cell adhesion and rosetting of clustered cells (R and **C**). **A,** Bar = 75 μm; **B, C,** and **D,** bars = 10 μm. Wright-Giemsa stain.

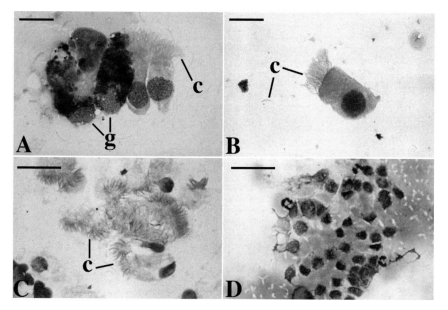

Figure 21-5. Tracheal wash with ciliated columnar epithelial cells. **A, B,** Extremely well-preserved cells, something unusual in a TW. Goblet cells (g) contain dark purple mucus granules that may be mistaken for large cocci following rupture of these cells. Intact goblet cells that become isolated from other columnar cells are sometimes mistaken for mast cells. Columnar cells are usually more difficult to identify, as in **C** and **D**. Free cilia (c) should not be misidentified as thin, rod-shaped bacteria. Bacteria generally stain dark blue in Romanowsky stained smears, whereas mucin granules are purple and cilia are light pink. Bars = 10 μm. Wright-Giemsa stain.

numerous; therefore, criteria for a diagnosis of lymphosarcoma must be strictly applied (i.e., a homogeneous population of immature lymphocytes).

Trachea

PURPOSE/SAMPLING

Tracheal washes (TW) are used to delineate the type of inflammatory profile present in the trachea and bronchi (and possibly, bronchioles and alveoli) and potentially identify a specific infectious agent. TW are rarely helpful in the diagnosis of neoplasia. Typically, the trachea is sampled either by transtracheal or endotracheal techniques.[3]

NORMAL

Normal wash cytology contains low to moderate numbers of ciliated columnar epithelial cells, occasional goblet cells and macrophages, and a small amount of mucus (Figure 21-5). It can be difficult to distinguish a normal wash from missampling. If a normal TW interpretation conflicts with clinical findings, a second wash should be considered.

COMMON PROFILES

Inflammatory profiles common to tracheal washes include acute, chronic active or subacute, chronic or granulomatous (epithelioid macrophages and multinucleate giant cells), and eosinophilic. The cytologist cannot assume that the location of the inflammation is alveolar, in that inflammation limited to the trachea or even the oropharynx may result in an inflammatory TW. For this reason interpretations generated by a clinical pathologist are not anatomically specific (e.g., acute bronchopneumonia). This diagnosis is best reserved for histopathology, where the inflammation is seen in the context of anatomic structures. When histopathology is not available, a diagnosis of pneumonia is based on a combination of the cytological and radiographical interpretations, coupled with the physical examination.

Acute inflammation is typically associated with a bacterial infection. As with nasal specimens, a monomorphic population of intracellular and extracellular organisms suggests a bacterial infection, which may be primary or secondary. Mixed types of bacteria may indicate contamination, perforating wounds, or aspiration.

Chronic inflammation can be seen in animals with neoplasia; parasitic, fungal and protozoal infections; chronic congestive processes; lung lobe torsion; and pulmonary embolism. Although fungal infections are included in this list, many fungal infections of the lung are opportunistic and are likely to be seen in association with acute inflammation and bacterial infections. Opportunistic infections include the same hyphal forms that can be seen in nasal infections. Their presence should be anticipated in animals with aspiration pneumonia. On the other hand, the systemic mycoses (e.g., *Blastomyces dermatitidis*, *Cryptococcus neoformans*, *Coccidioides immitis*, and *Histoplasma capsulatum*), detected as yeasts, are more likely to result in chronic or granulomatous inflammation, which is characterized by epithelioid and multinucleate macrophages.

Eosinophilic inflammation is associated with hypersensitivity, parasitism, neoplasia (e.g., bronchogenic carcinoma), idiopathic eosinophilic infiltrative disorders, and occasionally fungal infections. Likely parasites include

lungworms such as *Filaroides* spp., *Aelurostrongylus abstrusus*, *Crenosoma vulpis*,[7] and heartworms *(Dirofilaria immitis)*. Fortunately, distinguishing the two broad groups of worms is simple. Lungworm infections are generally diagnosed by detection of tightly coiled larvae that usually stain turquoise blue (Figure 21-6, *A*). Heartworms are seen as thin, straight to slightly curvy microfilaria approximately 200 to 300 μm in length (Figure 21-6, *B*). Very small, dark blue nuclei may be evident (Figure 21-6, *C*). Lungworm larvae are almost twice as long as heartworm microfilaria and are much thicker. Parasitic infections may or may not be associated with a strong eosinophilic response, but if eosinophils are consistently noted, especially within a pyogranulomatous setting, a careful low-power scan of all areas of several slides is advised. In addition, fecal analysis for nematode larvae, using the Baermann technique, is recommended.[7]

Other cells occasionally seen in TW include lymphocytes, mast cells, basophils, and plasma cells. These cell types are always low in frequency, and a high proportion of any of these cells would be a very abnormal profile. For example, many lymphocytes within a tracheal wash are suggestive of lymphosarcoma.

Mucus production increases with almost any type of inflammation or chronic irritation; therefore, pink- to purple-stained mucus is a common constituent of TW. Fine to thick spirals of mucus, termed Curschmann's spirals, may represent mucus from small airways although they do not add specificity to the interpretation (Figure 21-7, *A*).

Oropharyngeal squames with associated oral flora (Figure 21-7, *B*) usually indicate oral contamination of the sample, which can either be procedural or pathological. Appropriate interpretation requires inspection for a neutrophilic response targeting the bacteria. The presence of inflammation, with mixed intracellular bacteria and squamous cells, is supportive of the clinical diagnosis of aspiration pneumonia, although the inflammation

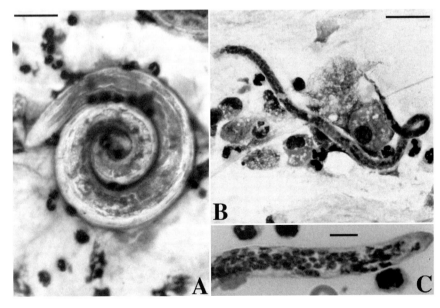

Figure 21-6. Lung nematodes in a tracheal wash. *A* is a larval form of Aelurostrongylus abstrusus *from a cat.* *B* and *C* are Dirofilaria immitis microfilariae *from a dog.* *A* and *B* are taken at the same magnification, but notice the size difference between the two larval forms. *C* is a close-up of the small nuclei visible in stained D. immitis microfilariae. Nuclei are not as distinct in A. abstrusus larvae. Morphology of canine lungworm larvae is similar. *A* and *B* bars = 25 μm. *C* bar = 5 μm. Wright-Giemsa stain.

could also be within the oropharynx. Again, findings should be interpreted in the context of other diagnostic clues such as clinical signs and radiographs.

Hemorrhagic or congestive processes can result in the presence of erythrophagocytosis or hemosiderosis. Hemosiderin is classically golden-brown, refractile granular material; however, in TW macrophages it can be gray-blue and non-refractile. If unsure, a Prussian blue stain for iron can help identify hemosiderin within macrophages. Associations include trauma, neoplasia, congestive heart failure, foreign bodies, pulmonary embolism, coagulopathies, lung lobe torsion, eosinophilic inflammation, and chronic infection. Significance should be considered in context of other changes found. Blood, without evidence of erythrophagocytosis and hemosiderin, suggests procedure-related contamination, which is more likely to be a complication of transtracheal collection than endotracheal sampling.

CONFUSION

Columnar epithelial cells are often numerous in inflammatory TW, but they are usually poorly preserved and difficult to identify (see Figure 21-5, *D*). Smudged epithelial cells and free cilia should not be mistaken for lymphocytes and bacteria, respectively. Cilia stain light pink, whereas bacteria are more consistently dark blue. Smudged cells are represented by only bare nuclei. Nuclei of the epithelial cells approximate the size of lymphocyte nuclei, but the chromatin tends to be less coarse and more homogeneous and the nucleoli are very tiny. As a general precautionary strategy, it is wise not to infer an identity to any cell represented by only the nucleus.

Small to moderately large clusters of hyperplastic epithelial cells, displaying increased anisocytosis and cytoplasmic basophilia, may occasionally be observed in association with inflammation. These hyperplastic cells may be cuboidal to low columnar with moderately large and prominent nucleoli. Detection of carcinoma cells in TW is extremely rare; therefore, low to moderate numbers of mildly to moderately atypical epithelial cells, in the context of severe inflammation, should be interpreted as reactive. A definitive diagnosis of carcinoma should be reserved for profiles featuring markedly pleomorphic epithelial cells with a minor inflammatory component.

Eosinophilic infiltrates can occasionally create confusion. First, regional variations within lavage samples are possible, so that some areas may be predominantly eosinophilic, whereas other areas contain mostly neutrophils or macrophages. Finding collections of eosinophils, even with many neutrophils and bacteria, suggests that eosinophilic inflammation is concurrent or possibly the primary cause for the animal's clinical signs. Secondly, eosinophil granules in sight-hound breeds such as greyhounds and whippets often do not stain pink, and appear more like vacuoles (Figure 21-8, *A*). This is problem enough in blood smear evaluations but could potentially completely misdirect a differential diagnosis if the cells in a TW are misidentified as degenerate neutrophils or macrophages. Finally, eosinophil granules from cats are rod shaped, resembling pink- to red-stained, rod-shaped bacteria; however, bacteria stain dark blue (Figure 21-8, *B*). Context and staining characteristics will help the examiner distinguish the structures.

Layering of inflammatory cells and infectious agents, especially lungworm larvae, can occur in wash fluids. This layering can result in all the larvae being on only one of several slides prepared from sediment or zones of

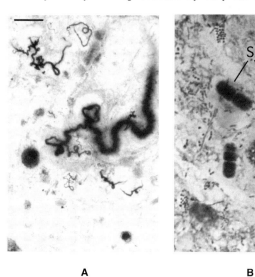

A   B

Figure 21-7. Tracheal wash. Curschmann's spirals **(A)** may represent mucus from small airways but they do not add specificity to a cytological interpretation (bar = 25 μm). The large rod-shaped bacteria in **B** are Simonsiella organisms, which are normal oropharyngeal flora. The organisms adhere to each other side to side, which results in their appearance as giant bacteria. Bar = 10 μm. Wright-Giemsa stain.

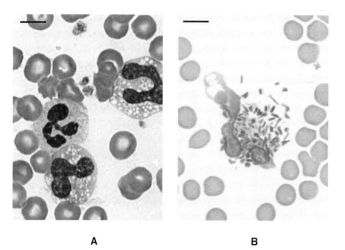

A   B

Figure 21-8. Canine and feline eosinophils. The two vacuolated cells in **A** are eosinophils from a greyhound. Their granules fail to pick up the eosin stain, so they appear vacuolated. These cells can be difficult to distinguish from macrophages or degenerate neutrophils in cytological preparations. **B,** A partially ruptured feline eosinophil. Cat eosinophilic granules are rod-shaped and can be misidentified as bacteria; however, bacteria generally stain dark blue, whereas the eosinophil's granules stain pink. Bars = 10 μm. Wright-Giemsa stain.

inflammation, which contain differing cell distributions. This tendency toward layering can be compensated for by evaluation of several areas of a few slides.

Finally, it seems likely that the tracheal wash profile does not always represent alveolar patterns. A review of bronchopneumonia in 42 dogs reported that in 11 of these dogs the TW was not inflammatory.[8] A retrospective study of over 100 cats infected with *Toxoplasma gondii* found that the alveolar infiltrate seen in these cats is primarily histiocytic.[9] However, the few *Toxoplasma gondii* infections detected in tracheal washes by the author have been associated with acute inflammation accompanied by a large amount of necrotic cellular debris and moderate numbers of macrophages.

Bronchi

PURPOSE/SAMPLING

Sampling of the bronchi, similar to that of the trachea, can provide information regarding the type of inflammation and possibly the etiological agent. Sampling is done via either bronchoalveolar lavage or bronchial brushings. Bronchoalveolar lavage (BAL), compared with TW, may be more predictive of alveolar histological patterns.[10] There is also a slightly greater likelihood that sampling could aid in the diagnosis of neoplasia, although it is still a poor choice for this purpose.[11,12] Bronchial brushings are used for selective sampling of bronchial lesions.

NORMAL

Bronchoalveolar lavage results in a semiquantitative evaluation of the contents of airways below the trachea.[13-15] Aliquots from the left bronchus are generally distinguished from the right and submitted as separate samples. A consistent dosage of lavage fluid should be instilled so that comparisons regarding nucleated cells per microliter are possible. Usually counts are low, necessitating the use of a cytocentrifuge to prepare smears.[16] In addition to the routine cytological description, a BAL report includes nucleated cells/μl, red blood cells (RBC)/μl, and the cell differential. Quantitative analysis yields normal cell counts of about 200 to 500 nucleated cells/μl. Normal findings include mostly mononuclear cells and columnar epithelial cells, and occasional goblet cells, mast cells, neutrophils, and eosinophils.[17] Mucus is scant.

Bronchial brushings from healthy animals contain moderate to many low to moderately high columnar epithelial cells, rare small clusters of mature lymphocytes, and a very small amount of mucus.

COMMON PROFILES

The types of inflammation and disease associations are the same as for TW, but BAL findings do not always duplicate TW findings, with up to 68% discordance reported.[10] In staging lymphosarcoma, studies show a greater sensitivity in detection of neoplasia using BAL compared with TW.[11,12]

Bronchial brushings can be cytologically unremarkable even in the face of inflammatory TW and BAL. Bronchial brushings are most useful if carefully applied to visible lesions.

CONFUSION

Clinically healthy cats are reported to have high percentages of eosinophils in quantitatively normal BAL fluids.[18] In this study, the mean nucleated cell count for 24 cats, after instillation of 50 ml of fluid, was 301 $\pm$ 126 cells/μl (80 to 665/μl), with a mean eosinophil count of 25% $\pm$ 21% (2% to 83%) in the differential. High nucleated cell counts should be used to confirm the potential for a true eosinophilic inflammatory response.

Romanowsky-stained goblet cells contain many dark purple granules, creating the potential for misidentification as distorted mast cells in a cytocentrifuged BAL smear. In addition, if there is a large amount of mucus in a BAL sample, quantitative analysis is likely to be inaccurate.

Bronchial brushing may result in the collection of aggregates of lymphocytes. These represent bronchus-associated lymphoid tissue and must be distinguished from lymphosarcoma. The presence of predominantly small lymphocytes supports an interpretation of normal or possibly hyperplastic lymphoid tissue.

Lungs

PURPOSE/SAMPLING

Direct aspiration of lung tissue is generally performed when other procedures have failed to provide a specific diagnosis. The most common type of lesion to aspirate is a mass suspicious for neoplasia that is detected by diagnostic imaging.[19] Compared with the above procedures, this technique is the most likely to yield specific information regarding neoplasia.

NORMAL

The term "normal profile" does not apply for this procedure because it is highly unlikely that a lung viewed as normal radiographically would be aspirated. Nondiagnostic smears, consisting of mostly blood, a few macrophages, and a small amount of mucus, are common. Mechanically exfoliated mesothelial cells are occasionally detected due to inadvertent sampling of the pleura (Figure 21-9).

COMMON PROFILES

The same inflammatory profiles previously described for tracheal washes are possible in samples obtained by direct aspiration of the lung. Typically, lung aspirates are performed when neoplasia is suspected; therefore, acute inflammation and bacterial infections are usually not diagnosed in this manner.

The most common tumor type to be diagnosed via direct aspiration is carcinoma (Figure 21-10).[19] Bronchogenic carcinomas can be well differentiated, consisting of colum-

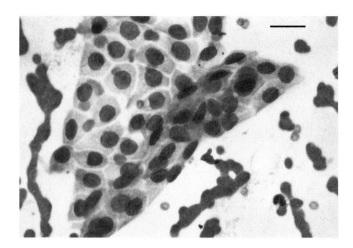

Figure 21-9. *Lung aspirate: Mechanically exfoliated, nonreactive mesothelial cells appear as sheets of flat, uniform, squamous cells. Bar = 25 μm. Wright-Giemsa stain.*

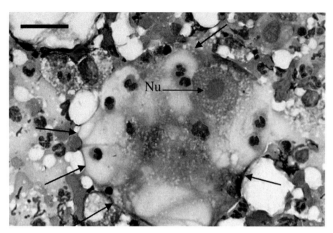

Figure 21-10. *Lung aspirate showing feline metastatic mammary gland adenocarcinoma. The arrows point to the cell boundaries of a single, giant carcinoma cell. Inside the cell are neutrophils displaying the phenomenon known as* emperipolesis, *where inflammatory cells migrate into or through another cell. Nu = nucleolus. Bar = 25 μm. Wright-Giemsa stain.*

nar epithelial cells, making them difficult to distinguish from hyperplastic tissue. Malignant histiocytosis is another neoplasm that exfoliates readily with direct aspiration. The neoplastic histiocytes must clearly display marked pleomorphism beyond that expected for reactive macrophages in order for a cytological diagnosis to be made; otherwise, histological evaluation is needed to confirm this diagnosis. Most spindle cell tumors do not exfoliate readily and are difficult to diagnose using direct aspiration methods.[20] Hemangiosarcomas, in particular, are almost never represented in smears, although evidence of chronic inflammation, hemosiderosis, and hemorrhage are common in these tumors. Regardless of the specific diagnosis, neoplasia is typically accompanied by a mix of inflammatory cells (e.g., macrophages and neutrophils), as well as evidence of hemorrhage, necrosis, and possibly epithelial cell hyperplasia.

CONFUSION

Tissue reacting to the presence of severe inflammation can be mistaken for neoplasia. Hyperplastic cells that are most often mistakenly interpreted as neoplastic include epithelial cells and fibroblasts. Macrophages can also be misleading when they become large, foamy, and multinucleate.

Inadvertent sampling of liver tissue via the diaphragm occasionally occurs. Hepatocytes are generally easily identified as contaminants because they have a specific uniform cuboidal morphology; however, if the liver is abnormal, missampling may not be obvious.

Pleural Effusions

PURPOSE/SAMPLING

Sampling and analysis of pleural fluid is always indicated when an effusion is perceived to exist clinically or radiographically.[21] Fluid analysis potentially offers diagnosis of

a specific cause of the effusion (e.g., neoplasia or infection). Contradictory reports in the human literature question whether cytological evaluation is necessary if the quantitative analysis indicates a transudative process.[22-24] This controversy has not been debated in the veterinary literature, but based on the author's experience, cytological evaluation of most fluids, regardless of quantitative analysis, is advised. Smear inspection often offers insight that the quantitative analysis misses. Clumping of cells can spuriously decrease nucleated cell counts and result in counts typical of transudates. This is fairly common in carcinoma-induced malignant effusions where large clusters of pleomorphic adherent cells can result in inaccurate cell counts. On the other hand, the need for cytological evaluation of acute hemorrhagic effusions is questionable. When the quantitative analysis is basically consistent with blood, with a nucleated cell count proportionate to that of the peripheral blood, cytological evaluation rarely allows determination of a specific cause.

NORMAL

Fluid analysis includes gross characteristics, total protein (TP), nucleated and red blood cell counts, a cell differential, a description of potentially neoplastic cells, and a search for infectious agents. Total protein is traditionally measured by refractometry rather than using a chemical analyzer; therefore, values of less than 2.5 gm/dl are not further quantified. Normal pleural fluid is scant and difficult to collect from healthy dogs and cats; it is transudative with a protein less than 2.5 gm/dl and a nucleated cell count less than 500 cells/μl.

COMMON PROFILES

Transudative effusions are characterized by low nucleated cell counts and few red blood cells. The most numerous nucleated cells present are non-phagocytic macrophages and non-degenerate neutrophils, in approximately equal numbers. In addition, occasional mast cells, eosinophils, lymphocytes and mesothelial cells are detected, usually at frequencies less than 5%.

Pure transudates are characterized by a TP less than 2.5 gm/dl and a nucleated cell count less than 1500/μl.[2] Pure transudates generally reflect increased hydrostatic pressure or decreased oncotic pressure. Modified transudates, with protein greater than 2.5 gm/dl and nucleated cells between 3000/μl[25] and 7000/μl[2], are most likely to be seen secondary to liver or heart failure and neoplasia.[26] Feline infectious peritonitis-induced effusions may be characterized quantitatively as modified transudates, but the globulin content of the fluid is higher than with heart failure and neoplasia, and neutrophils predominate.[27]

Inflammatory exudates are characterized by elevations in both the nucleated cell count and the TP, although exceptions occur. Potential causes include bacterial, fungal, protozoal, and parasitic infections; neoplasia; lung lobe torsion; and immune-mediated pleuritis. Neutrophils usually predominate in exudative processes, although there are occasions when macrophages can almost match neutrophils in number. The most striking examples of high numbers of macrophages in an exudate seen by the author have been in association with lung lobe torsion. One patient with a lung lobe torsion seen at the Veterinary Hospital of the University of Pennsylvania had 45,500 nucleated cells/microliter, with 44% macrophages, 54% neutrophils, 1% lymphocytes, and 1% reactive mesothelial cells. Generally, a relative increase in macrophages suggests chronicity to the effusion (e.g., chronic bacterial or fungal infections) and neoplasia.

Chylous effusions are characterized by a triglyceride concentration greater than 100 mg/dl[28] but with highly variable nucleated cell counts.[29] Evaluation of serum triglyceride, serum cholesterol, and fluid cholesterol is not necessary to confirm this interpretation. Usually, small lymphocytes predominate (Figure 21-11), but with chronicity, neutrophils and macrophages may eventually exceed lymphocytes.[30] Chylous effusions most commonly reflect partial or complete obstruction of the thoracic duct, which then results in back-up of chyle within the lymphatic system and subsequent lymph seepage from intact lymphatics.[29] The obstruction can be either physical or functional. Potential causes include cardiomyopathy in cats,[31-33] constrictive pericarditis in dogs,[34] lung torsion in dogs,[35] granulomatous disease,[36] and neoplasia.[37] Occasionally the cause remains unknown. Traumatic rupture of the thoracic duct is an uncommon cause of chylous effusions.[29,30,38,39]

Occasionally lymphocytic effusions are observed that cytologically resemble chylous effusions. They contain mostly small, mature, morphologically unremarkable lymphocytes but have triglyceride concentrations less than 100 mg/dl. Despite the low triglyceride content, this type of effusion is still thought to result from lymphatic obstruction. The triglyceride content of the lymph arising from the gastrointestinal tract is diet related; therefore, a chronically anorexic animal may have peritoneal lymph with a low triglyceride concentration.[28] It is also possible that either lymphangiectasia or obstruc-

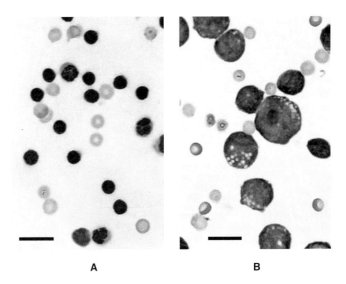

Figure 21-11. Pleural effusions. **A,** Feline chylous effusion consisting of mostly small lymphocytes with very dense chromatin, no visible nucleoli, and a narrow rim of cytoplasm. Bar = 10 μm. Wright-Giemsa stain. **B,** Malignant effusion from an FeLV-infected cat with mediastinal lymphosarcoma. The neoplastic cells are moderately large to very large lymphoblasts with round or clefted nuclei, moderately coarse to fine chromatin, large nucleoli, and a small amount of variably vacuolated cytoplasm. Bar = 10 μm. Wright-Giemsa stain.

tion of pleural lymphatics is not impinging on or involving the thoracic duct; therefore, peritoneal chyle is not contributing to the effusion. Finally, nonchylous lymphocytic effusions can be seen with thymomas and well-differentiated lymphosarcomas, although the latter diagnosis is uncommon in the chest.

Pseudochylous effusions are extremely rare in small animal medicine, although the term has been inappropriately applied to chylous effusions arising for reasons other than traumatic thoracic duct rupture. Pseudochylous effusions are milky and opaque, as are chylous effusions; however, they are characterized by high cholesterol content.[29] The cholesterol is derived from cell breakdown in a setting of severe chronic inflammation. Cytologically these effusions contain cholesterol crystals, necrotic cellular debris, and inflammatory cells (Figure 21-12). The most common causes reported in the human literature are tuberculosis and rheumatoid pleuritis.

Malignant effusions can have variable nucleated cell counts, red blood cell counts, and TP. Inflammation and hemorrhage are common complications. Based on a recent study, between 30% and 40% of effusions secondary to neoplasia contain no detectable neoplastic cells and are classed by other features such as modified transudates, inflammatory exudates, and hemorrhage.[40] Malignant effusions secondary to carcinoma and lymphosarcoma are the most likely to contain neoplastic cells (see Figure 21-11). Hemangiosarcoma-induced hemorrhagic effusions virtually never contain identifiable malignant cells. Mesotheliomas stimulate effusions, but the malignant mesothelial cells may not display enough atypia to warrant a cytological interpretation of

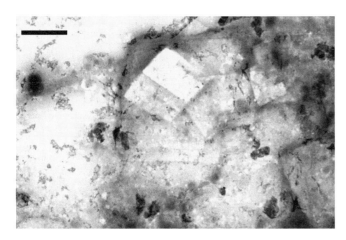

Figure 21-12. *Pseudochylous effusion. The relatively clear, angular structures are cholesterol crystals. The slightly smudged, poorly defined small dark structures are nuclei from disintegrating neutrophils. Bar = 25 μm. Wright-Giemsa stain.*

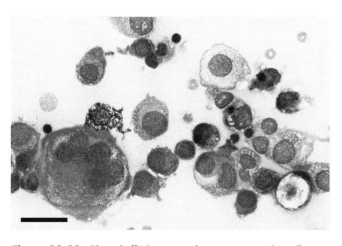

Figure 21-13. *Pleural effusion secondary to metastatic malignant melanoma in a dog. The primary tumor was located on an eyelid. Although the neoplastic cells are essentially amelanotic, there is a suggestion of very fine pigment granules in some cells (e.g., the multinucleate cell, bottom left). Cells containing large dense granules are melanophages. Bar = 25 μm. Wright-Giemsa stain.*

neoplasia, although occasional exceptions occur. Malignant melanoma is a rare cause for pleural effusions (Figure 21-13). Pigmentation of the neoplastic cells may or may not be apparent, although melanophages can occasionally be detected. Morphology of malignant melanoma cells is unpredictable, with the potential for spindle, epithelioid, and/or round cells.

Hemorrhagic effusions have packed cell volumes greater than 5%, with evidence of erythrophagocytosis or hemosiderosis. Causes include trauma, coagulopathies, and bleeding neoplasia. They are often complicated by an inflammatory component, which is detected by comparing the nucleated cell count with the peripheral blood count. A significant difference, favoring the fluid, indicates an inflammatory component to the hemorrhage.

Eosinophilic effusions contain greater than 10% eosinophils. They can be transudative or exudative. They are seen in association with the same disorders listed for nasal and tracheal specimens (i.e., hypersensitivities, parasitism, neoplasia, and idiopathic eosinophilic infiltrative disorders such as eosinophilic granulomatous disease or hypereosinophilia). Neoplasms reported to incite eosinophilic effusion in dogs and cats include carcinoma, lymphosarcoma, and hemangiosarcoma.[41] In dogs mast cell neoplasia should also be considered,[41] but mast cell neoplasia in cats seldom incites an eosinophilic response.

Pleural effusions are often multifactorial. For example, an animal can have a transudate with an inflammatory component, where the TP is low but the cell differential indicates a preponderance of neutrophils that cannot be explained by blood contamination. Both exudates and transudates can be complicated by a mild to moderate hemorrhagic component. The PCV may not be remarkably elevated, but erythrophages and hemosiderophages are found in the fluid.

CONFUSION

Reactive mesothelial cells can become numerous or pleomorphic in the presence of inflammation or chronic hemorrhage in canine pleural effusions. They can be difficult to distinguish from a neoplastic population. Reactive mesothelial cells are less evident in feline fluids. Adherent macrophages in both cats and dogs may be misinterpreted as carcinoma, especially if they are proliferative and multinucleate. Nucleated cell counts can be spuriously decreased by clumping or adhesion of cells (e.g., mesothelial cells and malignant epithelial cells).

Measuring TP by refractometry is subject to the same interferences as seen in the determination of plasma TP. Lipids, bilirubin, and hemolysis can all spuriously elevate TP. Lipid interference is particularly common with chylous effusions. Furthermore, if a sample is collected in an EDTA tube, but the quantity is very small, the EDTA can spuriously elevate the TP to extreme levels, even greater than 10 gm/dl. Interferences should be considered whenever receiving TP results that seem disproportionately high compared with plasma or serum levels.

Conclusion

Cytopathology of the respiratory tract can augment other diagnostic tools used in assessment of respiratory disorders. Sample collection tends to be easy, fast, and relatively noninvasive, although anesthesia is often required. Nasal tissue sampling can offer clues as to the type of inflammation and the potential cause, including neoplasia. Tracheal and bronchial sampling is useful for inflammatory patterns and infectious agents. Both direct lung aspiration and pleural fluid evaluation have the potential for diagnosis of neoplasia, in addition to inflammatory patterns and infectious agents. Quantitative and qualitative analysis of pleural fluids offers evidence regarding the mechanism for the effusion. On the other hand, cytological evaluation cannot determine invasiveness of a tumor within normal tissues or determine tissue distribution by inflammatory cell infiltrates. The lack of architectural relationships between cells and tissue result in a less definitive diagnosis as to the specific tumor identity compared with histopathology. Lastly, negative cytological findings must always be viewed as inconclusive because inability to detect an etiological agent or neoplastic cells does not rule them out.

REFERENCES

1. Baker R, Lumsden JH: *Color atlas of cytology of the dog and cat,* ed 1, St Louis, 1999, Mosby.
2. Cowell RL, Tyler RD, Meinkoth JH: *Diagnostic cytology and hematology of the dog and cat,* ed 2, St Louis, 1999, Mosby.
3. Baker R, Lumsden JH: The respiratory tract: Nasal, bronchial and tracheal wash. In Baker R, Lumsden JH, editors: *Color atlas of cytology of the dog and cat,* ed 1, St Louis, 1999, Mosby.
4. Forbes Lent SE, Hawkins EC: Evaluation of rhinoscopy and rhinoscopy-assisted mucosal biopsy in diagnosis of nasal disease in dogs: 119 cases (1985-1989), *J Am Vet Med Assoc* 201:1425-1429, 1992.
5. Caniatti M, Roccabianca P, Ghisleni G et al: Evaluation of brush cytology in the diagnosis of chronic intranasal disease in cats, *J Small Anim Pract* 39:73-77, 1998.
6. Tasker S, Knottenbelt CM, Munro EA et al: Aetiology and diagnosis of persistent nasal disease in the dog: A retrospective study of 42 cases, *J Small Anim Pract* 40:473-478, 1999.
7. Georgi AU Jr: Parasites of the respiratory tract, *Vet Clin North Am Small Anim Pract* 17:1421-1442, 1987.
8. Thayer GW, Robinson SK: Bacterial bronchopneumonia in the dog: A review of 42 cases, *J Am Anim Hosp Assoc* 20:731-736, 1984.
9. Dubey JP, Carpenter JL: Histologically confirmed clinical toxoplasmosis in cats: 100 cases (1952-1990), *J Am Vet Med Assoc* 203:1556-1566, 1993.
10. Hawkins EC, DeNicola DB, Plier ML: Cytological analysis of bronchoalveolar lavage fluid in the diagnosis of spontaneous respiratory tract disease in dogs: A retrospective study, *J Vet Int Med* 9:386-392, 1995.
11. Yohn SE, Hawkins EC, Morrison WB et al: Confirmation of a pulmonary component of multicentric lymphosarcoma with bronchoalveolar lavage in two dogs, *J Am Vet Med Assoc* 204:97-101, 1994.
12. Hawkins EC, Morrison WB, DeNicola DB et al: Cytologic analysis of bronchoalveolar lavage fluid from 47 dogs with multicentric malignant lymphoma, *J Am Vet Med Assoc* 203:1418-1425, 1993.
13. Hawkins EC, DeNicola DB, Kuehn NF: Bronchoalveolar lavage in the evaluation of pulmonary disease in the dog and cat, *J Vet Int Med* 4:267-274, 1990.
14. Hawkins EC, DeNicola DB: Collection of bronchoalveolar lavage fluid in cats, using an endotracheal tube, *Am J Vet Res* 50:855-859, 1989.
15. Smith BP: Pleuritis and pleural effusion in the horse: A study of 37 cases, *J Am Vet Med Assoc* 170:208-211, 1977.
16. Schumann GB, Linker G: Cytopreparatory techniques for bronchoalveolar lavage specimens, *Lab Med* 23:115-119, 1992.
17. Rebar AH, DeNicola DB, Muggenburg BA: Bronchopulmonary lavage cytology in the dog: Normal findings, *Vet Pathol* 17:294-304, 1980.
18. Padrid PA, Feldman BF, Funk K et al: Cytologic, microbiologic, and biochemical analysis of bronchoalveolar lavage fluid obtained from 24 healthy cats, *Am J Vet Rec* 52:1300-1307, 1991.
19. Wood EF, O'Brien RT, Young KM: Ultrasound-guided fine-needle aspiration of focal parenchymal lesions of the lung in dogs and cats, *J Vet Int Med* 12:338-342, 2000.
20. Logrono R, Filipowicz EA, Eyzaguirre EJ et al: Diagnosis of primary fibrosarcoma of the lung by fine-needle aspiration and core biopsy, *Arch Pathol Lab Med* 123:731-735, 1999.
21. Gookin JL, Atkins CE: Evaluation of the effect of pleural effusion on central venous pressure in cats, *J Vet Int Med* 13:561-563, 1999.
22. Zakaria A, Caruso JL, Herndon J et al: Cytologically proved malignant pleural effusions: Distribution of transudates and exudates, *Chest* 113:1302-1304, 1998.
23. Valeriano F, Scolari N, Villa A: Positivity of pleural fluid cytologic examination in transudate pleural effusions, *Chest* 114:1798-1799, 1998.
24. Teklu B: Cytology on transudative pleural effusions, *Chest* 116:846, 1999.
25. Baker R, Lumsden JH: Pleural and peritoneal fluids. In Baker R, Lumsden JH, editors:. *Color atlas of cytology of the dog and cat,* ed 1, St Louis, 1999, Mosby.
26. Bunch SE, Metcalf MR, Crane SW et al: Idiopathic pleural effusion and pulmonary thromboembolism in a dog with autoimmune hemolytic anemia, *J Am Vet Med Assoc* 195:1748-1753, 1989.
27. Shelly SM, Scarlett-Krantz J, Blue JT: Protein electrophoresis on effusions from cats as a diagnostic test for feline infectious peritonitis, *J Am Anim Hosp Assoc* 24:495-500, 1988.
28. Waddle JW, Giger U: Lipoprotein electrophoresis differentiation of chylous and nonchylous pleural effusions in dogs and cats and its correlation with pleural effusion triglyceride concentration, *Vet Clin Pathol* 19:80-85, 1990.
29. Meadows RL, MacWilliams PS: Chylous effusions revisited, *Vet Clin Pathol* 23:54-62, 1994.
30. Fossum TW, Birchard SJ, Jacobs RM: Chylothorax in 34 dogs, *J Am Vet Med Assoc* 188:1315-1318, 1986.
31. Birchard SJ, Ware WA, Fossum TW et al: Chylothorax associated with congestive cardiomyopathy in a cat, *J Am Vet Med Assoc* 189:1462-1464, 1986.
32. Davies C, Forrester SD: Pleural effusion in cats: 82 cases (1987 to 1995), *J Small Anim Pract* 37:217-224, 1996.
33. Fossum TW, Miller MW, Rogers KS et al: Chylothorax associated with right-sided heart failure in five cats, *J Am Vet Med Assoc* 204:84-89, 1994.
34. Campbell SL, Forrester SD, Johnston SA et al: Chylothorax associated with constrictive pericarditis in a dog, *J Am Vet Med Assoc* 206:1561-1564, 1995.
35. Gelzer AR, Downs MO, Newell SM et al: Accessory lung lobe torsion and chylothorax in an Afghan hound, *J Am Anim Hosp Assoc* 33:171-176, 1997.
36. Howard J, Arceneaux KA, Paugh-Partington B et al: Blastomycosis granuloma involving the cranial vena cava associated with chylothorax and cranial vena caval syndrome in a dog, *J Am Anim Hosp Assoc* 36:159-161, 2000.
37. Peaston AE, Church DB, Allen GS et al: Combined chylothorax, chylopericardium, and cranial vena cava syndrome in a dog with thymoma, *J Am Vet Med Assoc* 197:1354-1356, 1990.
38. Fossum TW, Forrester SD, Swenson CL et al: Chylothorax in cats: 37 cases (1969-1989), *J Am Vet Med Assoc* 198:672-678, 1991.
39. Birchard SJ, Fossum TW: Chylothorax in the dog and cat, *Vet Clin North Am Small Anim Pract* 17:271-283, 1987.
40. Hirschberger J, DeNicola DB, Hermanns W et al: Sensitivity and specificity of cytologic evaluation in the diagnosis of neoplasia in body fluids from dogs and cats, *Vet Clin Pathol* 28:142-146, 1999.
41. Fossum TW, Wellman M, Relford RL et al: Eosinophilic pleural or peritoneal effusions in dogs and cats: 14 cases (1986-1992), *J Am Vet Med Assoc* 202:1873-1876, 1993.

CHAPTER 22

Lung Biopsy and Thoracoscopy

Greg M. Griffin

Introduction

In many patients with lung disease it is difficult, if not impossible, to achieve a definitive diagnosis without first obtaining a biopsy. In many instances, however, the invasiveness and risk associated with the procedure to obtain the biopsy cannot be justified. The ideal technique for obtaining biopsies of the lung and other intrathoracic structures should be minimally invasive, have a low complication rate, and have a high diagnostic yield. Unfortunately, in pulmonary disease few procedures fulfill all of these criteria. In this chapter we will review indications for lung biopsy; discuss the various techniques for obtaining the biopsy; and discuss in some depth the option of thoracoscopic lung biopsy, a procedure that is commonplace in human medicine.

Indications, Contraindications, and Complications of Lung Biopsy

For the most appropriate treatment and prognosis of any respiratory condition,[1] we must base our decisions on the most accurate morphological and etiological diagnosis that can be obtained without imposing an unacceptable risk to the patient. Definitive diagnosis of infectious, inflammatory, or neoplastic conditions that result in diffuse interstitial or focal nodular pulmonary lesions may require lung biopsy. Lung biopsy can be performed in any patient, but we must think carefully before performing it.[2] Could a diagnosis be achieved through less invasive techniques? If a diagnosis can be obtained by use of bronchoalveolar lavage or fine needle aspirate cytology or culture, for example, then invasive procedures to obtain tissue biopsies of the lung should not be performed.

Lung biopsy is contraindicated in patients with pulmonary hypertension, uncorrectable coagulopathies, and pulmonary bullae.[1,3] The major complication of lung biopsy is pneumothorax,[1,3-8] which has been variably reported to occur in 6% to 44% of human patients. In many cases, pneumothorax is persistent and requires the placement of thoracostomy tubes. Other complications include hemorrhage, both intrathoracic and intrapulmonary (rarely resulting in hemoptysis); empyema; inadvertent damage to other intrathoracic structures; and tumor seeding in neoplastic conditions.[4,7,8]

Because pneumothorax is the most common complication of lung biopsy, serial postbiopsy chest radiographs are recommended.[1] In light of the severe life-threatening complications that can occur after lung biopsy, it is recommended that these procedures only be performed at a facility that has capabilities for critical care and emergency thoracic surgery, should these become necessary in the postbiopsy patient.

Techniques for Lung Biopsy

Several techniques of varying invasiveness—and correspondingly varying diagnostic yield—are available to obtain samples from the lung. As expected, the higher the chance of a definitive diagnosis, the higher the risk of complications. Techniques that carry less risk and thus lower yield include transtracheal aspirates, endotracheal or bronchoalveolar lavage, thoracocentesis, and bronchoscopy.[1] Unfortunately, misinterpretation and nondiagnostic samples are always a concern with cytological diagnostics.[8] Procedures that obtain larger samples of lung tissue include transbronchial aspirates and biopsies, transthoracic aspirates and biopsies, thoracoscopic biopsy (Figure 22-1), and open surgical lung biopsy.[1,3,4,6,7] The technique chosen depends on the location and type of lesion. For diagnosis of focal lesions, a more specifically targeted technique is needed than for diagnosis of a diffuse condition. If an abscess is suspected, an endobronchial technique may be tried first because of the risk of empyema.[1] If multiple nodules are suspected to be metastatic in origin, a primary tumor can often be located outside the chest, thereby avoiding a lung biopsy. If fungal disease is suspected, serology may be of some benefit.

TRANSBRONCHIAL ASPIRATES AND BIOPSIES

Transbronchial aspirates and biopsies are performed under fluoroscopic or bronchoscopic guidance using specially designed needles, catheters, and biopsy instru-

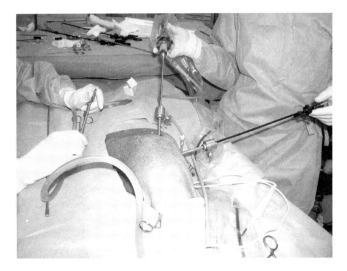

Figure 22-1. *Thoracoscopy in progress.*

ments. These techniques are most appropriate for sampling lymph nodes or masses near the airways but are not useful for lesions in peripheral lung tissue.[1] For aspirates, the needle is passed between the cartilage rings of the bronchus and negative pressure is applied. The major risks are bleeding and pneumothorax; the bigger the needle, the more likely it is that complications will occur.[1] To perform transbronchial biopsies, the biopsy instrument is passed into the bronchus under fluoroscopic or bronchoscopic guidance. The instrument is wedged into a peripheral bronchus, the jaws are opened, and tissue is grasped and pulled out. One advantage of using a bronchoscope is that it can be pushed into the bronchus after the biopsy to help slow the bleeding. Complications are similar to transbronchial aspirates. These procedures can be performed relatively easily on the caudal lung lobes, but it is almost impossible to gain access to the distal bronchi of the cranial or middle lobes. Another limitation is the small sample size and the crush artifact, which results in little information being obtained about the lung architecture, something that is especially important in interstitial diseases.

TRANSTHORACIC ASPIRATES AND NEEDLE BIOPSIES

Transthoracic aspirates and needle biopsies allow samples to be taken from the chest wall, lung, and mediastinal tissues. These procedures are much easier to perform if the lesion to be sampled is large. Local anesthesia can be used with or without sedation, and general anesthesia can be used if necessary. The procedure is usually performed under fluoroscopic, computed tomography, or ultrasound guidance. Ultrasound often provides good visualization of chest wall and peripheral lung lesions. Great care must be taken when sampling lesions in the dorsal thoracic cavity because of the proximity of the major vessels.[1] Infectious or neoplastic conditions can often be as readily diagnosed with fine needle aspirates as with needle biopsies, but aspirates may be of little help in nonin-

fectious or nonneoplastic conditions. However, needle biopsies are associated with less crush artifact than transbronchial biopsies, thus possibly giving a definitive diagnosis in cases of interstitial disease. Complications of transthoracic sampling include pneumothorax, hemorrhage, pericardial tamponade, and tumor seeding. In one veterinary study of 41 dogs and 2 cats having transthoracic needle aspirates, 31% developed pneumothorax post aspirate and 6.2% required the placement of thoracostomy tubes.[8] Five patients died. An accurate diagnosis was made in 83% of cases.[8]

OPEN SURGICAL LUNG BIOPSY

Although open surgical lung biopsy is the most invasive of all the techniques, it allows the greatest and most definitive yield.[1] Open surgical biopsy can be performed via a median sternotomy, if the entire thoracic cavity is to be examined, or through a lateral thoracotomy, if only one side of the thoracic cavity is involved. Mini-thoracotomies to obtain a small sample of lung tissue can also be performed.[9] In certain cases, open lung biopsy may be the procedure of choice. Such cases would include single focal lesions, whether neoplastic, infectious, or foreign body related. In these cases with a single lesion, the procedure could be both diagnostic and curative.

THORACOSCOPY

Thoracoscopy has become a widely used technique in human surgery, and minimally invasive techniques (Figures 22-2 and 22-3) are becoming more commonplace in veterinary medicine.[3,6,10-13] Thoracoscopic lung biopsy offers several advantages over open thoracotomy.[3-7] Most important, it is less painful,[11] has lower wound healing complications, allows excellent visualization with magnification (Figure 22-4), and should allow a similar sample to be obtained.[10,14-16] A recent veterinary study has shown thoracoscopy to be very useful in cases with pleural effusion, the cause of which could not be diagnosed by less invasive means.[17] In veterinary medicine, no study has compared the complication rates and diagnostic yield of open thoracotomy versus thoracoscopy. In human medicine, several studies have shown that thoracoscopy provides similar diagnostic samples with less discomfort, shorter hospital stays, and no difference in complication rate.[18,19] One paper reported the complication rates as 15% and 17% for thoracoscopy and open thoracotomy, respectively.[19] The mortality rate was higher in the open thoracotomy patients. In general, open thoracotomy was selected for the more critical patients because they could not tolerate the one-lung ventilation required for thoracoscopy.[19] In all deaths in both groups, the patients were in respiratory failure preoperatively. Thoracoscopy, or video assisted thoracic surgery (VATS) as it is also called, provided better visualization than when a mini–open thoracotomy was performed.[19] Although biopsies obtained thoracoscopically had slightly more artifact because of tissue manipulation, this was not sufficient to affect the ability to make a diagnosis.[18] Disadvantages of thoracoscopy in-

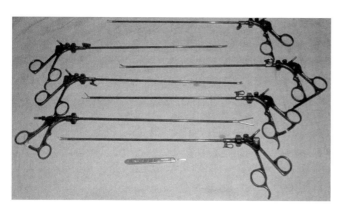

Figure 22-2. *Instruments routinely used for thoracoscopic procedures.*

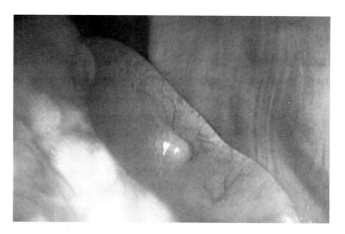

Figure 22-4. *Thoracoscopic appearance of normal lung.*

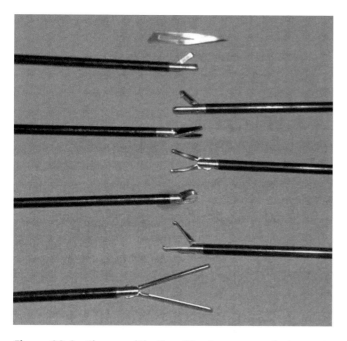

Figure 22-3. *Close up of the tips of the thoracoscopy instruments.*

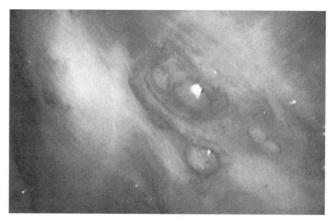

Figure 22-5. *Thoracoscopic view of small pleural lesions.*

clude the cost of all the specialized equipment needed and the expertise needed to perform the procedure.[3,4,7] Thoracoscopy or VATS requires a suitably sized, rigid thoracoscope (usually 5- to 10-mm diameter); a light source; a camera and monitor; operating ports for instruments and scope; and special instruments required for the procedures. In humans, lung biopsy has been performed thoracoscopically safely and effectively using endoscopic staplers,[20,21] Nd:YAG lasers,[22] and endoscopic loop ligatures.[23] Thoracoscopy can be performed with the patient in dorsal or lateral recumbency.[3-5,7] Careful anesthetic monitoring (including heart rate; blood pressure; oxygen saturation; end tidal carbon dioxide; and, if possible, blood gas analysis) is essential because these patients will have some degree of pulmonary compromise as a result of the procedure.[15,16]

Several methods are used to achieve adequate visualization during thoracoscopy, including thoracic insufflation, bilateral controlled pneumothorax, and single lung ventilation (Figure 22-5).[4,14-16] Bilateral pneumothorax is the easiest to use and is adequate for most procedures. A semi-open pneumothorax is established when the scope is introduced through a non-airtight cannula. Bilateral controlled pneumothorax has been shown to be well tolerated in dogs, with only minor decreases in blood oxygen tension and mild increases in arterial carbon dioxide and mean arterial pressure.[14]

Alternatively, one-lung ventilation allows the greatest visualization and working space within the thoracic cavity. To achieve one-lung ventilation, a double lumen endotracheal tube, endobronchial tube, or bronchial blocker must be used. Bronchoscopic guidance is often needed to place these tubes appropriately. Care should be taken to ensure that the tube is in the correct location because the location of the bronchus of the right cranial lung lobe can make placement difficult. One-lung ventilation causes significant decreases in oxygen tension, but it can be performed in dogs that are closely monitored and breathing 100% oxygen.[15]

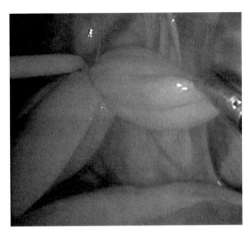

Figure 22-6. *Thoracoscopic lung biopsy using the loop ligature method.* (Photograph courtesy of Dr Lori Ludwig, Animal Medical Center, New York.)

Thoracic insufflation with carbon dioxide or nitrous oxide can be performed without major cardiopulmonary effects. The pressure within the thoracic cavity must be continually monitored and should be kept at 5 to 8 mm Hg.[14] To use this technique, an airtight camera and airtight operating cannulas are required. For one-lung ventilation and bilateral pneumothorax, an airtight seal is not a priority.

Once the patient is positioned and ready for thoracoscopy, the first cannula and then the camera are introduced into the chest, and a complete exploration is performed. When the area to be biopsied has been identified, two additional cannulas are placed through the chest wall, through which the instruments will be passed.[3-5,7] The biopsy is taken using either an endoscopic stapler or loop ligature (Figure 22-6).[20,21,23] Once the sample is retrieved from the chest, the area is inspected for bleeding. A thoracostomy tube is placed postoperatively; this is later removed once any air leak, if present, has sealed.

In the author's experience, most patients recover very well and rapidly from thoracoscopic procedures. Complications of thoracoscopic lung biopsy include pneumothorax, hemorrhage, and wound healing problems.[3,4,10] There is no veterinary study comparing the complication rate of thoracoscopy with open thoracotomy, but thoracoscopy appears to offer us a safe, minimally invasive way to obtain high quality lung biopsy samples without putting the patient through untoward risk and with the added benefit of avoiding the pain of open thoracotomy.[11]

REFERENCES

1. Bauer TG: Lung biopsy, *Vet Clin North Am Small Anim Pract* 30(6):1207-1225, 2000.
2. Temes RT, Joste NE, Qualls CR et al: Lung biopsy: Is it necessary? *J Thorac Cardiovasc Surg* 118:1097-1100, 1999.
3. McCarthy TC, McDermaid SL: Thoracoscopy, *Vet Clin North Am Small Anim Pract* 20(5):1341-1352, 1990.
4. Remedios AM, Ferguson J: Minimally invasive surgery: Laparoscopy and thoracoscopy in small animals, *Compend Contin Educ Pract Small Anim* 18(11):1191-1199, 1996.
5. McCarthy TC: Diagnostic thoracoscopy, *Clin Tech Small Anim Pract* 14:213-219, 1999.
6. Garcia F, Prandi D, Pena T et al: Examination of the thoracic cavity and lung lobectomy by means of thoracoscopy in dogs, *Can Vet J* 39:285-291, 1998.
7. Potter L: Video-assisted thoracic surgery. In *Veterinary endosurgery*, St Louis, 1999, Mosby Year Book Inc.
8. Teske E, Stokhof AA, van den Ingh TSGAM et al: Transthoracic needle aspiration biopsy of the lung in dogs with pulmonic diseases, *J Am Anim Hosp Assoc* 27:289-294, 1991.
9. Kirby TJ, Mack MJ, Landreneau RJ et al: Lobectomy-Video-assisted thoracic surgery versus muscle sparing thoracotomy: A randomized trial, *J Thorac Cardiovasc Surg* 109:997-1002, 1995.
10. Faunt KK, Jones BD, Turk JR: Evaluation of biopsy specimens obtained during thoracoscopy from lungs of clinically normal dogs, *Am J Vet Res* 59:1499-1502, 1998.
11. Walsh PJ, Remedios AM, Ferguson JF et al: Thoracoscopic versus open partial pericardectomy in dogs: Comparison of postoperative pain and morbidity, *Vet Surg* 28:472-479, 1999.
12. Jackson J, Richter KP, Launer DP: Thoracoscopic partial pericardectomy in 13 dogs, *J Vet Intern Med* 13:529-533, 1999.
13. Isakow K, Fowler D, Walsh P: Video-assisted thoracoscopic division of the ligamentum arteriosum in two dogs with persistent right aortic arch, *J Am Vet Med Assoc* 217:1333-1336, 2000.
14. Faunt KK, Cohn LA, Jones BD et al: Cardiopulmonary effects of bilateral hemithorax ventilation and diagnostic thoracoscopy in dogs, *Am J Vet Res* 59:1494-1498, 1998.
15. Cantwell SL, Duke T, Walsh PJ et al: One-lung versus two-lung ventilation in the closed chest anesthetized dog: A comparison of cardiopulmonary parameters, *Vet Surg* 29:365-373, 2000.
16. Bennett RA, Orton EC, Tucker A et al: Cardiopulmonary changes in conscious dogs with induced progressive pneumothorax, *Am J Vet Res* 50:280-284, 1989.
17. Kovak JR, Ludwig LL, Bergman PJ et al: Use of thoracoscopy to determine the etiology of pleural effusion in dogs and cats: 18 cases (1998-2001), *J Am Vet Med Assoc* 221:990-994, 2002.
18. Kadokura M, Colby TV, Myers JL et al: Pathologic comparison of video-assisted thoracic surgical lung biopsy with traditional open lung biopsy, *J Thorac Cardiovasc Surg* 109:494-498, 1995.
19. Ferson PF, Landreneau RJ, Dowling RD et al: Comparison of open versus thoracoscopic lung biopsy for diffuse infiltrative pulmonary disease, *J Thorac Cardiovasc Surg* 106:194-199, 1993.
20. Lewis RJ: Simultaneously stapled lobectomy: A safe technique for video-assisted thoracic surgery, *J Thorac Cardiovasc Surg* 109: 619-625, 1995.
21. Hazelrigg SR, Landreneau RJ, Mack M et al: Thoracoscopic stapled resection for spontaneous pneumothorax, *J Thorac Cardiovasc Surg* 105:389-393, 1993.
22. Keenan RJ, Landreneau RJ, Hazelrigg et al: Video-assisted thoracic surgical resection with the neodymium:yttrium-aluminum-garnet laser, *J Thorac Cardiovasc Surg* 110:363-367, 1995.
23. Liu HP, Chang CH, Lin PJ et al: Thoracoscopic loop ligation of parenchymal blebs and bullae: Is it effective and safe? *J Thorac Cardiovasc Surg* 113:50-54, 1997.

PART THREE

Pulmonary Function Testing

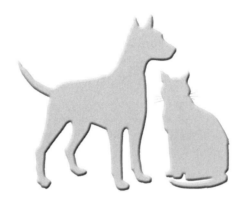

CHAPTER 23

Pulmonary Mechanics

Janice A. Dye • Daniel L. Costa

Introduction

Pulmonary function testing is routinely used in human medicine to objectively characterize functional deficits in patients with respiratory disease. In veterinary medicine, although respiratory diseases are a common problem, diagnostic testing is largely limited to localizing disease to and within the respiratory system and to identifying underlying infectious or neoplastic processes. With the exception of blood gas analysis, testing methods to identify specific pathophysiological processes or to define disease severity and progression on a functional basis are not routinely available. Yet this is precisely the information needed to advance our

knowledge of some of the more challenging respiratory disease syndromes in small animals (e.g., canine chronic bronchitis,[1] feline bronchopulmonary disease,[2] and chronic interstitial or fibrotic lung disease[3-6]). Just imagine how difficult it would be to manage a patient with diabetes mellitus, renal disease, or hepatic disease without the ability to monitor changes in blood glucose, urea nitrogen, or bile acids, respectively. Analogously, if pulmonary function tests (PFTs) were more widely available, we could objectively evaluate the small animal respiratory patient. In turn, we could better define clinical spectrums of disease and characterize the underlying etiologies and disease mechanisms. Most important, we could monitor natural disease progression (or resolution) and better assess the efficacy of specific treatment protocols.

Part of the difficulty in using PFTs in veterinary clinical medicine is that companion animals are by nature uncooperative and therefore difficult to study using standard spirometric approaches that were developed for adult human beings. Although spirometric testing is noninvasive, rapid, and easy to perform on awake hu-

Disclaimer: The information described in this article has been reviewed by the National Health and Environmental Effects Research Laboratory, U.S. Environmental Protection Agency, and approved for publication. Approval does not signify that the contents necessarily reflect the view and policy of the agency, nor does mention of trade names or commercial products constitute endorsement or recommendation for use.

man subjects, procedures such as maximal expiratory maneuvers require a level of conscious cooperation that is simply not possible in animals.

Nevertheless, a wealth of information exists on the lung mechanical properties of cats and dogs. Nearly 100 articles have been published assessing pulmonary function in the cat, and an equivalent database exists in the dog. In physiology studies, for example, cats have been used extensively to define key reflexes involved in the control of breathing and to determine lung and airway smooth muscle responses to bioactive mediators and pharmaceutical agents.[7,8] In toxicology studies, cats and dogs exposed to inhaled substances (e.g., environmental tobacco smoke, sulfur dioxide,[9] ozone,[10] and diesel exhaust[11]) have undergone pulmonary function testing to establish the toxicity of these agents. As animal models of human lung disease, cats and dogs with experimentally induced pathology (e.g., allergic pneumonitis or bronchitis,[12-15] viral-mediated bronchiolitis,[16-18] or surfactant deficiency[19,20]) have undergone functional assessments to establish the efficacy of new drugs or ventilatory support techniques. With few exceptions, however, it has not been possible to incorporate these experimental testing procedures into veterinary clinical medicine because they include the use of nonrecoverable anesthetics (such as urethane) or unacceptably invasive procedures such as tracheostomy placement or pleural space cannulization.[21]

A few individuals have sought to modify these techniques such that meaningful, albeit somewhat more limited, functional information can be obtained from companion animals. In this chapter we will present some of these approaches, focusing on those that are most applicable for routine clinical use: tidal breathing flow-volume loop assessments; and measures of upper airway resistance, lung resistance, and static or dynamic lung compliance.

Knowledge of basic respiratory physiology is essential in order to understand how PFTs can aid in the diagnosis and management of respiratory disease in small animals. To begin, we will review the basic processes related to movement of air in and out of the respiratory tract under normal conditions. We will then discuss how these processes are disrupted by disease, emphasizing relationships between structural pathological changes and corresponding functional deficits. Brief descriptions of the methods and instrumentation required, advantages and disadvantages of certain procedures, and limitations of data interpretation are included. We will use case examples and, where available, information from clinical studies in cats and dogs to emphasize the utility of these assessments in veterinary medicine. Lastly, we will discuss obstacles that must be overcome as we look towards more routine use of PFTs in the future, in particular the need to standardize testing procedures and to establish appropriate reference ranges. Recent advances in lung function testing in human infants will be explored because pediatric patients, not unlike cats and dogs, are often uncooperative and difficult to study. Therefore some of the same approaches may prove useful for evaluation of the small animal patient.

Respiratory Physiology

The simple act of taking a breath is an amazingly coordinated process. The purpose of breathing is to provide adequate gas exchange for the animal's current metabolic demand, no more and no less. In health, this is accomplished very efficiently. In fact, the average small animal patient takes 10,000 to 30,000 breaths every day without any real effort or thought as to how this is happening. But as disease develops, the respiratory system becomes less efficient and the respiratory muscles must work harder to compensate for this inefficiency. The ability to appreciate or detect respiratory disease in small animals depends on the extent of disease, as well as the activity level of the patient. Incipient disease is often unappreciated by the owner because the animal either minimizes its activity or compensates by subtly altering its breathing pattern and frequency when necessary. As disease progresses, respiratory inefficiency becomes more apparent, especially during periods of increased metabolic demand, and the patient may be presented for exercise intolerance. By the time an animal is presented at rest but with excessively labored respiration, it is clearly in overt respiratory distress. It may be unclear whether the patient has developed acute, fulminant disease, or whether it is experiencing an acute exacerbation of long standing but heretofore occult disease. Many animals effectively hide their illness until critically low levels of lung reserve remain. More routine use of PFTs in veterinary medicine may permit earlier recognition of disease, allowing therapeutic intervention prior to the establishment of chronic, likely irreversible changes.

How does air flow in and out of the lungs of healthy animals with such efficiency? Normally, the elastic and resilient lung is tethered within the thoracic cavity by a thin layer of pleural fluid. The lung's size and shape readily conforms to that of the more rigid chest wall and diaphragm. During resting or tidal breathing, inspiration is initiated as the diaphragm flattens and the chest wall expands outward. In so doing, the lung parenchyma is expanded, and with it the alveolar spaces and small conducting airways become somewhat distended both in length and diameter. Conversely, as the lung collapses during expiration, there is a dynamic narrowing of the small airways. By contrast, the diameter of the nasal passageways, trachea, and larger airways (bronchi) remains relatively unchanged under normal conditions.

The total amount of air moving in and out of the lung during tidal breathing is referred to as the tidal volume (TV or V_T). The breathing frequency (f; breaths/minute or bpm) multiplied by the TV (ml/breath) is equal to the minute volume (MV; ml/minute). At rest, dogs and cats normally breathe nasally. Hence during a typical ventilatory cycle, air must first pass through the nares, then through the nasal passageways and nasopharynx, through the laryngeal opening, continuing into the tracheobronchial tree where it traverses a series of ever-narrowing tubes until at last it reaches the alveolar space, the site of gas exchange. The flow of air is, of course, reversed during expiration. In all mammalian lungs, the O_2-rich inspired air must traverse through the same series of tubes as the CO_2-enriched expired air, and there is continual mixing of new and spent air in the process. Nevertheless, in health, an animal is able to effectively transport sufficient quantities of air to and from the alveolar units to maintain relatively constant O_2 and CO_2 partial pressures within arterial blood. Blood gas analysis allows assessment of the efficiency of gas exchange, considering the lung as one large ventilatory unit. Decreases in arterial O_2 concentrations (hypoxemia) may be detected with or without concurrent increases in CO_2 retention and are associated with hypoventilation, alveolar diffusion impairment, shunts, or ventilation-perfusion mismatch.[22] Such data are complementary to that obtained by pulmonary functional assessments.

By dividing a breath into its component inspiratory and expiratory phases, each phase can be characterized by changes in three parameters: volume, airflow, and pressure. Figure 23-1 is a schematic depicting the changes occurring over a complete ventilatory cycle in a healthy adult cat. For obvious reasons, on average the volume of inspired air must equal that of the expired air. By definition, lung volume increases during inspiration (becomes positive) and decreases during expiration (Figure 23-1, *A*). Airflow describes the volume of air moving in (or out) of the lung over a specific time (ml/sec) (Figure 23-1, *B*). By convention, inspiratory flow rates are often given negative values, although absolute values may also be used. In cats and dogs, the peak inspiratory flow (PIF) typically occurs in mid- to late inspiration, after which the flow rate rapidly returns to zero, thus marking the end of inspiration. Airflow quickly reverses direction (becomes positive) and the maximal or peak expiratory flow (PEF) occurs in early to midexpiration. The flow rate then gradually decreases until the end of the breath.

The pressure changes depicted represent the differential pressures that develop between the atmosphere and the various regions of the thoracic cavity (e.g., the alveolar space or the pleural space) (see Figure 23-1, *C* and *D*). Note that as the chest wall and lungs expand during inspiration, the alveolar pressure drops below zero due in part to frictional resistance generated as the air flows through the air passageways. Note also that the pleural space pressure remains somewhat negative even at the end of expiration (see Figure 23-1, *D*). The solid symbols depict shifts in the actual pressure curve that occur due to the elasticity of the lung parenchyma.

Owing to cyclic generation of these pressure gradients, air from more proximal regions of the respiratory tract moves deeper and deeper into the lung and back out again, over and over. In health, relatively small pressure gradients are required to effectively transport sufficient quantities of air to and from the alveolar spaces. In fact, normally at the end of expiration, a small volume of air remains in the alveoli due to the slightly negative end-expiratory intrapleural pressure mentioned above (see Figure 23-1, *D*), thereby helping to prevent collapse of the tiny alveolar gas exchange units between breaths. In turn, the alveolar septa are held under a certain de-

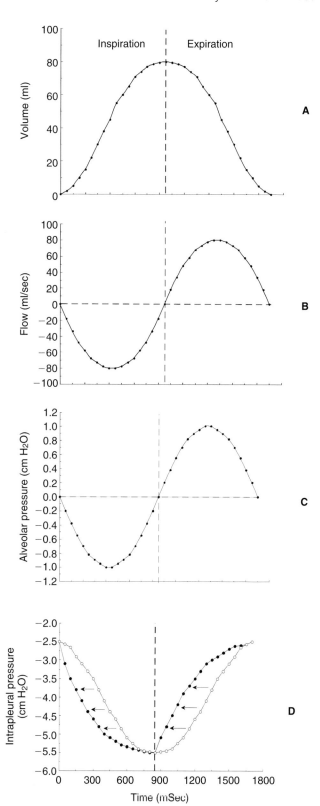

Figure 23-1. *Schematic of a single breathing cycle in a healthy adult cat including changes in **(A)** lung volume; **(B)** airflow; **(C)** alveolar pressure relative to ambient pressure (note that alveolar pressure drops below zero due, in part, to resistance generated as the air flows through the airways); and **(D)** intrapleural pressure. Solid symbols depict the shift in the pressure curve occurring due to elastic recoil of the lung parenchyma.*

gree of constant tension. Furthermore, because the alveolar septa are connected to the walls of the bronchioles, this tension or interdependency serves to provide radial traction around the small airways, in essence maintaining their patency as well. During tidal breathing, the volume of air remaining within the lung at the end of expiration is referred to as the functional residual capacity (FRC). It represents the balance point between the inward elastic recoil of the lungs and the outward elastic recoil of the chest wall.

Although the analogy is somewhat oversimplified, the inflated lung acts in a manner similar to a stretched rubber band. A certain amount of energy is required initially to stretch the rubber band or to expand the lungs (i.e., the energy needed to overcome the elastic and resistive work of breathing). But in so doing, tension is generated within the elastic components of the lung parenchyma. After inspiration ceases, the lung passively recoils because of this tension and returns to its original or end-expiratory size and shape. In the process, an identical volume of air is passively expired.

In small animals, 60% or more of the inspiratory frictional resistance generated during a tidal breath is due to airflow through the nose, pharynx, and larynx.[23] During exercise, when airflow rates increase dramatically, animals often switch to oral breathing in order to bypass this zone of high resistance. In a like manner, when airflow is impeded by localized disease within the nasopharyngeal region (e.g., by space-occupying masses or brachycephalic airway syndrome) animals often resort to oral breathing even at rest. Measurement of flow and volume changes over a single ventilatory cycle in these animals during nasal breathing would reveal alterations in inspiratory flow rates and airflow patterns. Not surprisingly, this approach (i.e., the use of tidal breathing flow-volume loop analysis) was first used clinically to evaluate upper respiratory disease in dogs.

Tidal Breathing Flow-Volume Loop (TBFVL) Analysis for Upper Respiratory Tract Disease

The primary advantage of TBFVL assessment is that one can quantify changes in airflow, volume, and in the temporal aspects of the ventilatory cycle—all in the conscious, nonsedated patient. Specialized equipment is necessary, however (Figure 23-2, A). The patient must be fitted with a sufficiently snug but nonrestrictive face mask to ensure negligible air leakage during the procedure. The mask must conform to the patient's face so that it neither disturbs airflow nor results in excessive dead space. Disproportionate dead space dampens the overall flow signal and allows background noise to become more problematic. The mask is then connected to a pneumotachograph, a device used to measure airflow changes. The pneumotachograph is heated to a constant temperature to avoid wide fluctuations in the inspired versus expired gas temperature. An associated pressure

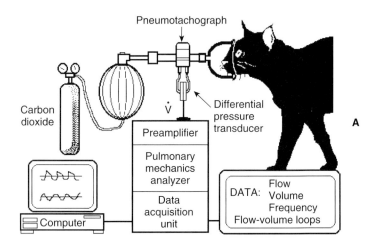

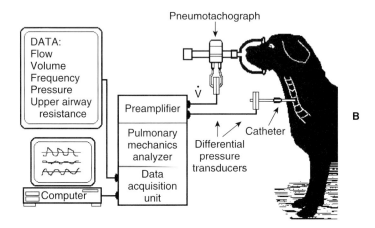

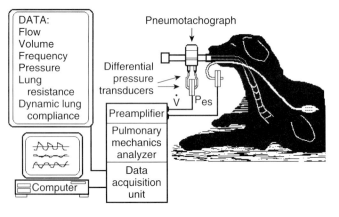

Figure 23-2. *Equipment setup for obtaining respiratory system functional information in small animals, including:* ***(A)*** *TBFVL data acquisition (± breathing increased CO$_2$ concentrations) for use in unanesthetized patients;* ***(B)*** *upper airway pressure (Puaw) and resistance (Ruaw) measurements in unanesthetized large breed dogs; and* ***(C)*** *lung resistance and compliance measurements in anesthetized small animals.*

transducer is required to transmit the electrical signal to a preamplifier and receiver unit. The size (sensitivity) of the pneumotachograph and pressure transducer required is dictated by the size of the patient (i.e., the minimum flow signal generated). For each patient, the system must be calibrated prior to data acquisition.

Using a pulmonary mechanics analyzer (BUXCO Electronics, Sharon, Conn.) and analytical software program (Respiratory Loop Analysis Software, BUXCO Electronics, Sharon, Conn.), the flow signal can be electronically differentiated into its component volume and time measurements, yielding quantitative breath-by-breath or averaged data on airflow rates, volume, and time parameters. For ease of visual inspection of the data, airflow changes are plotted against volume changes to generate the so-called flow-volume or F-V loop. Although the temporal aspects of the breath are not evident in the F-V loop, this information is collected during data acquisition (i.e., frequency [bpm], time [mSec] associated with inspiration [Ti], and expiration [Te]). Information from the flow, volume, and time assessments can be combined to calculate an extensive list of ancillary parameters: time ratios (e.g., Te/Ti); inspiratory to expiratory flow ratios at the same lung volume (e.g., PIF/PEF, IF50/EF50); flow ratios at different lung volumes (e.g., PEF/EF25); or changes in volume over a defined period (e.g., ml exhaled during the first 0.1 second of a breath).[24,25] In theory, a range of normal values can be established for these parameters, allowing quantification of the abnormalities present in affected patients.

Although potentially promising, the primary disadvantage of this approach is its inherent insensitivity due to lack of maximal respiratory effort. As such its usefulness in detecting incipient or mild disease may be limited. During evaluation, it is important that the animal generates sufficiently deep and consistent breaths. Some animals, in particular cats, become apprehensive when the face mask is applied. They may adopt a shallow, rapid breathing pattern that is not indicative of their true tidal breathing capabilities. Alternatively, they may sniff, lick, vocalize, growl, or even purr during many of the breaths acquired. It is necessary therefore to establish a set of criteria by which only acceptable breaths are selected for inclusion in the final TBFVL analysis.

Analogous to the approach used to assess laryngotracheal disease in human infants,[26] Amis and colleagues originally used TBFVL analysis to evaluate dogs with upper respiratory disease.

They first characterized TBFVLs from healthy dogs including breeds with differing nasal anatomy.[24,27] In brief, for each breath a loop is generated as airflow changes are plotted against volume changes. By convention, the loop starts at the 3:00 o'clock position and proceeds in a clockwise direction until closing in on itself (Figure 23-3, *A*). Thus, the lower half of the loop delineates inspiratory changes and the upper half depicts expiration. Amis and colleagues demonstrated that in healthy, large breed, mesaticephalic (Labrador-type) dogs, TBFVLs are quite symmetrical, with the mirror images reflecting along either side of the zero flow axis (see Figure 23-3, *A*). In mesaticephalic dogs the average expiratory time (Te) is slightly longer than the inspiratory time (Ti), resulting in a relatively constant Te/Ti ratio of 1.26 (0.26).[27]

By contrast, Amis and colleagues demonstrated that many dogs with upper respiratory disease have charac-

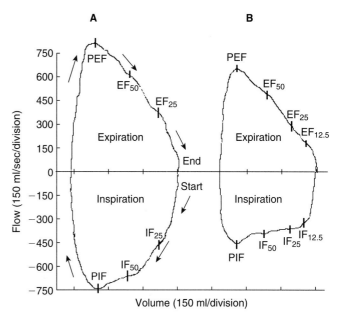

Figure 23-3. *TBFVLs in dogs. Loop* **A** *is a composite loop representing healthy large breed (mesaticephalic) dogs. The mean values as reported by Amis and colleagues[24] are: TV = 460 ml; PEF = 780 ml/sec; PIF = 740 ml/sec; f = 32 bpm; MV = 14.8 L/min; Te = 1170 mS; Ti = 920 mS; Te/Ti = 1.26; PEF/PIF = 1.07; PIF/IF50 = 1.09; PIF/IF25 = 1.26; IF50/IF25 = 1.16. By comparison, loop* **B** *was obtained in a Labrador–mixed breed dog after surgery for bilateral laryngeal paralysis. Indices: TV = 425 ml; PEF = 600 ml/sec; PIF = 415 ml/sec; f = 22 bpm; MV = 9.4 L/min; Te = 1420 mS; Ti = 1300 mS; Te/Ti = 1.09; PEF/PIF = 1.43; PIF/IF50 = 1.11; PIF/IF25 = 1.04; IF50/IF25 = 0.93. Interpretation: mild inspiratory airflow restriction is present.*

teristic TBFVL shape changes and decreased Te/Ti ratios. Dogs with relatively fixed or nonmovable obstruction (e.g., pharyngeal or laryngeal masses) have reductions in both inspiratory and expiratory flow rates, with uniform flattening of the F-V hemicurves.[24] Dogs with dynamic upper airway obstruction, however, have predominantly inspiratory flow restrictions.[28] Furthermore, depending on the severity of disease and ventilatory effort at the time of evaluation, dogs with laryngeal paralysis may produce normal TBFVLs, or loops consistent with fixed (inspiratory/expiratory) obstruction or with nonfixed (inspiratory) obstruction.[28] Amis and colleagues confirmed that many of the TBFVL parameters calculated for healthy brachycephalic dogs are dissimilar from those of mesaticephalic dogs, indicating that functional airflow restrictions are often present in dogs of these breeds.[27]

In the case examples that follow, McKiernan and colleagues[25] demonstrated that TBFVL assessments are also sensitive enough to detect airflow changes in cats with upper respiratory disease. These investigators first established a range of normal values for these parameters in healthy cats (Table 23-1).[25] They observed that, similar to healthy dogs, healthy cats exhibit a very symmetrical TBFVL (Figure 23-4, *A*). In fact, the inspiratory and expiratory times in cats are nearly identical, yielding an average Te/Ti ratio of 1.0 (±0.15).

TABLE 23-1. TBFVL Changes in a 2-Year-Old Himalayan Cat With Bronchopulmonary Disease

Parameter (Units)	Day 0	Day 1	Day 8	2 Months	Cat
CLINICAL STATUS	DYSPNEIC	SLIGHT IMPROVEMENT	MUCH IMPROVED	CLINICAL RELAPSE	NORMAL VALUES[25]
Volume					
TV (ml)	50	38	32	28	58 ± 15
MV (ml)	1550	1292	1380	1036	2500
Time					
RR or *f* (bpm)	31	34	43	37	43 ± 7
Ti (mS)	776	744	642	533	717 ± 140
Te (mS)	1160	1028	735	1080	704 ± 134
Te/Ti	1.49	1.38	1.14	2.03	1.0 ± 0.15
Flow					
PIF (ml/sec)	96	80	73	85	111 ± 27
PEF (ml/sec)	92	58	67	81	114 ± 29
PEF/PIF	0.96	0.73	0.91	0.95	1.04 ± 0.18
EF50/IF50	0.51	0.61	0.85	0.35	1.16 ± 0.22
EF25/IF25	0.47	0.56	0.74	0.39	1.06 ± 0.19
EF12.5/IF12.5	0.49	0.65	0.60	0.41	0.94 ± 0.20
PIF/IF50	1.10	1.10	1.2	1.14	1.23 ± 0.15
IF50/IF25	1.24	1.28	1.2	1.27	1.12 ± 0.08
IF25/IF12.5	1.27	1.32	1.16	1.28	1.11 ± 0.06
PEF/EF50	2.04	1.32	1.29	3.1	1.10 ± 0.06
PEF/EF25	2.8	1.81	1.81	3.5	1.35 + 0.17
PEF/EF12.5	3.4	2.07	2.58	4.26	1.73 ± 0.33

By contrast the non-symmetrical loop (Figure 23-4, *B*) was obtained from a 3-year-old domestic longhair cat presented for making unusual breathing sounds, especially while eating. The cat's breathing pattern was regular but relatively slow (mean *f* = 25 and TV = 77 ml). Visual inspection of the F-V loop revealed severe blunting of maximal expiratory flows and uniform flattening of the expiratory F-V curve. The peak inspiratory flow (PIF) occurred prematurely in inspiration, after which airflow appeared to taper off abnormally. In addition, there was moderate prolongation of the expiratory time relative to inspiratory time (Te/Ti = 1.25). These changes are most consistent with a fixed upper airway obstruction; however, there also appears to be a dynamic component to the obstruction. Oropharyngeal examination of the cat while under anesthesia revealed a nasopharyngeal mass involving the soft palate.

By comparison, the loop in Figure 23-4, *C* was obtained from a 7-year-old domestic shorthair cat. This cat presented for making noisy or unusual sounds when breathing. The cat's breathing pattern was somewhat irregular (mean *f* = 37 and TV = 73 ml). Abnormalities present in the TBFVL included variable flattening and intermittent reversal of inspiratory flow during midinspiration. The Ti was prolonged relative to Te (Te/Ti = 0.73). No expiratory abnormalities were detected. Results were consistent with a dynamic upper airway obstruction. Oral examination of the cat under anesthesia revealed a large, right-sided,

somewhat pedunculated tonsillar mass. Presumably, depending on the angulation of the head while the loops were acquired, the mass was intermittently drawn into the laryngeal opening during inspiration, resulting in profound inspiratory flow restriction. However, when the mass was displaced by reversal of airflow during exhalation, there was no evidence of expiratory airflow obstruction.

By providing a means of quantifying airflow obstruction, several investigators have used TBFVL analysis in dogs to assess the efficacy of different surgical approaches used in correcting laryngeal paralysis or collapse.[29-31] As an illustration, the loop in Figure 23-3, *A* is a composite loop representing healthy mesaticephalic, large breed dogs. By comparison, the loop in 23-3, *B* was obtained from a 14-year-old mixed breed dog 1 week after undergoing a left-sided laryngeal tie-back for bilateral laryngeal paralysis. Of note, the dog also had a generalized decrease in muscle mass and mild rear limb conscious proprioceptive deficits. At rest, its breathing pattern was slow and regular (*f* = 22 bpm, TV = 425 ml, MV = 9400 ml). The inspiratory time was only mildly prolonged compared with expiration (Te/Ti = 1.09; normal 1.26 ± 0.26). The overall loop shape was nearly symmetrical, although mild blunting of the inspiratory flow rates (compared with expiratory flow rates) was still evident (e.g., PEF/PIF = 1.43; normal 1.07 ± 0.13). These measurements were much improved compared with those obtained preoperatively.

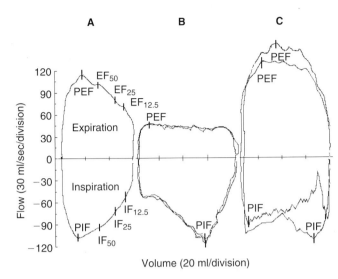

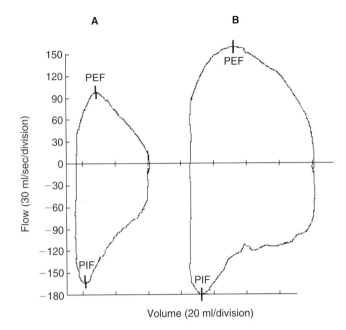

Figure 23-4. *Comparison of TBFVLs from healthy cats and cats with upper respiratory disease. Loop **A** is a composite loop representative of healthy adult cats. Values for select indices obtained in healthy cats are presented in Table 23-1. By comparison, loop **B** was obtained in a 3-year-old DLH cat presented for noisy breathing. Indices: TV = 77 ml; MV = 1925 ml; f = 25 bpm; Ti = 1080 mS; Te = 1350 mS; Te/Ti = 1.25; PIF = 121 ml/sec; PEF = 55 ml/sec; PEF/PIF = 0.45; PIF/IF50 = 1.23; IF50/IF25 = 0.87; IF25/IF12.5 = 1.39. Loop **C** was obtained in a 7-year-old DSH cat presented for making unusual sounds when breathing. Indices: TV = 73 ml; MV = 2700 ml; f = 37 bpm; Ti = 960 mS; Te = 698 mS; Te/Ti = 0.73; PIF = 114 ml/sec; PEF = 158 ml/sec; PEF/PIF = 1.40; PIF/IF50 = 1.71; IF50/IF25 = 0.92; IF25/IF12.5 = 1.05. (See text for loop interpretation.)*

Figure 23-5. *These TBFVLs were obtained in a 14-year-old Persian cat before **(A)** and after **(B)** receiving chemotherapy for a thymoma. (See text for loop interpretation.)*

Tidal Breathing Flow-Volume Loop Analysis for Lower Respiratory Tract Disease

Although the changes are not as visually apparent, TBFVL analysis can also be used to critically evaluate intrathoracic or intrapulmonary disease in dogs and cats. To illustrate, the F-V loops depicted in Figure 23-5 were obtained from a 14-year-old Persian cat. Functionally this cat had restrictive lung disease because it was not able to fully inflate the lungs due to the presence of a large intrathoracic, extrapulmonary mass. The mass had been previously debulked and was diagnosed histologically as a thymoma. After a time the cat represented with signs of respiratory insufficiency. On physical examination the cat was mildly tachypneic and the cranial thorax was noncompressible. As part of the reevaluation, the loop in 23-5, *A* was obtained. Consistent with restrictive lung disease, TBFVL measurements revealed a relatively small TV (45 ml; normal 58 ± 15 ml) with a normal rate (*f* = 46 bpm; normal 43 ± 7) and thus a moderately reduced MV (2070 ml/min; normal around 2500 ml/min). The shape of the inspiratory half of the loop appeared somewhat concave and the PIF was elevated (166 ml/sec; normal 111 ± 27 ml/sec). Although the overall expiratory loop shape and expiratory flow

rates were within normal limits (PEF = 104 ml/sec; normal 114 ± 29 ml/sec), the Te/Ti ratio was notably increased (1.61; normal 1.0 ± 0.15) consistent with the presence of expiratory airflow limitation. Six weeks later, after receiving COAP chemotherapy, the cat was clinically improved and the loop in Figure 23-5, *B* was obtained. TBFVL analysis revealed that with a respiratory rate in the upper normal range (*f* = 50 bpm), and considerable improvement in the TV (71 ml), the MV assessment was notably increased (3550 ml/min). Furthermore, the Te/Ti ratio had normalized (Te/Ti = 0.90). In spite of the fact that the loop shape abnormalities persisted, the flow rates, in particular the maximal expiratory flow rates, were much improved (PEF = 186 ml/sec). It is possible that some of the inspiratory curve shape changes were related to the altered nasal anatomy of the Persian breed.

TBFVL analysis can also be used to detect airflow changes in animals with lower respiratory disorders. For example, in dogs with excessive collapsibility of the large conducting airways, the TBFVL abnormalities observed depends on the region(s) of primary collapse. If the extrathoracic portion of the trachea has inadequate cartilaginous support, it will tend to collapse during inspiration when the pressure within the airway drops below that of the atmosphere. The chondromalacic airways below the thoracic inlet tend to remain open during inspiration because the intraluminal pressure remains greater than that of the pleural space. Consequently, TBFVLs from these patients reveal relative inspiratory flow limitations and prolongation of Ti relative to Te.[32] Conversely, during expiration these same intrathoracic airways tend to collapse because the intrathoracic pressure becomes less negative and may actually exceed that of the airway opening pressure. This is especially problematic during forced expiration or coughing when the intrathoracic pressure becomes markedly increased. Therefore, in dogs with primary intrathoracic tracheal and principal bronchi collapse, expiratory TBFVL abnormalities predominate. And finally, if both the extra- and intrathoracic tracheal regions are involved, or if tracheal collapse occurs in combination with chronic bronchitis, mixed inspiratory/expiratory F-V loop abnormalities are often present.[32,33]

In an earlier report, Amis and colleagues[24] used TBFVL analyses to characterize the airflow restriction occurring in a group of dogs with clinical evidence of chronic bronchitis or tracheal/bronchial collapse. Interestingly, the F-V loops in many of the affected dogs demonstrated concavity or late expiratory phase flattening, consistent with expiratory airflow limitations.[24] Subsequently, Padrid and colleagues[1] used bronchoscopy to identify a group of dogs primarily affected with chronic bronchitis, and demonstrated that in addition to having end-tidal airflow abnormalities, these dogs had decreased Pao_2, and abnormal radioaerosol ventilation scans. Repeated administration of the bronchodilator albuterol was not associated with improvement in the Pao_2 or ventilatory scan assessments. However, in 5 of 7 dogs that had posttreatment TBFVL analysis, bronchodilator therapy was associated with increases in end-tidal airflow that corresponded with the clinical improvement observed in individual animals.[1,32] Although these results are encouraging, the authors caution that larger studies, performed under more stringent conditions, are necessary. Nevertheless, this study demonstrates the utility of PFTs in objectively assessing the efficacy of specific drug therapies.

McKiernan and colleagues[25] used TBFVL analysis to evaluate whether chronically bronchitic cats had evidence of end-tidal airflow restriction. They demonstrated that, compared with healthy adult cats, a group of clinically affected cats had significant (1) increases in the Te/Ti ratios; (2) reductions in expiratory flow rates compared to inspiratory flow rates at the same lung volume; (3) decreases in area-under-the-total and peak-expiratory flow-curve assessments; and (4) decreases in expiratory volume as calculated during the first 0.1 or 0.5 seconds of the tidal breath.[25] These changes are consistent with the presence of bronchial or bronchiolar airflow obstruction.

Because of its ease of use and noninvasiveness, TBFVL analysis can be used repeatedly in the same patient to objectively assess clinical deterioration or response to therapy. By way of example, the loops depicted in Figure 23-6 were obtained from a young adult Himalayan cat presented for chronic but intermittent coughing. During initial presentation (Day 0), the cat was moderately dyspneic and the loop in Figure 23-6, A was obtained. Oral glucocorticoid therapy was initiated and the loop in Figure 23-6, B was obtained the next day (Day 1). Seven days later, after daily glucocorticoid administration, the cat was clinically improved and the loop in Figure 23-6, C was obtained (Day 8). Over the next month, the cat continued to improve and was subsequently tapered off of all glucocorticoid medication.

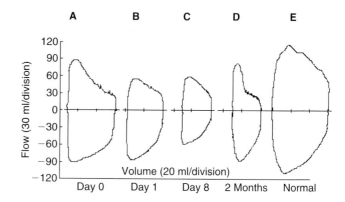

Figure 23-6. *This series of TBFVLs were obtained in a 2-year-old Himalayan cat presented for chronic coughing and intermittent dyspnea (loop **A**). The cat was started on oral glucocorticoid therapy, and follow-up evaluations included loop **B** 1 day later and loop **C** 1 week later. Two months later the cat relapsed clinically and loop **D** was obtained. For comparison, loop **E** is a composite loop representing healthy cats. (See Table 23-1 for changes in the corresponding TBFVL parameters.)*

Shortly thereafter, however, the cat relapsed and the loop in Figure 23-6, D was obtained (2 months). For ease of comparison, a composite loop (Figure 23-6, E) representing healthy cats has been included (see Table 23-1 for comparison of the calculated TBFVL indices).

In this patient, the signs of lower airway obstruction are most evident during expiration, and most of the abnormalities relate to the expiratory phase. As this cat decompensated clinically, the airway obstruction became more severe as evidenced by decrements in the mid- to end-tidal expiratory flow rates, especially in comparison to the peak expiratory flow rates (i.e., the PEF/EF25 and PEF/EF12.5 ratios were markedly elevated). As a result, the cat seemingly modified its breathing pattern to allow relatively more time for expiration (i.e., the Te/Ti ratio increased markedly). Even when the cat appeared to be improved clinically (Figure 23-6, C), the end-tidal airflow and Te/Ti ratios remained abnormal (see Table 23-1). When this cat represented after discontinuation of the glucocorticoid medication, the end-tidal airflow restriction was even greater than during initial presentation. In retrospect, glucocorticoid therapy should probably have been continued until the TBFVL parameters normalized, with more gradual tapering of the dose thereafter.

Enhanced Flow-Volume Loop Analysis

Due to the lack of maximal respiratory effort during TBFVL evaluation, there is a wide range of normal for many of the calculated indices. In an attempt to increase the sensitivity and reproducibility of F-V loop assessments, a variety of approaches have been used to artificially stimulate more maximal ventilatory efforts. The first approach was simply to induce partial rebreathing of the animal's own exhaled CO_2 by increasing the dead space of the tube connected to the pneumotachograph. Although the acute increases in reinspired CO_2 concentrations resulted in increased MV measurements, the results were somewhat variable.

To better define the CO_2 concentration being inhaled, Ambu bags were prefilled with defined gas mixtures containing increasing CO_2 concentrations. Each Ambu bag was then sequentially attached to the nonpatient side of the pneumotachograph (see Figure 23-2, A). This approach was evaluated in healthy cats using 2.5%, 5.0%, 7.5%, 10%, or 12.5% CO_2 with 21% O_2 and the balance N_2.[34] The gas mixtures containing the higher CO_2 concentrations tended to smell like stale air that had escaped from an old inner tube. Most, but not all cats tolerated breathing CO_2 concentrations of 6% to 10%, and occasionally 12.5%, without aversion to placement of the face mask. In healthy cats, the CO_2 increases were linearly associated with commensurate increases in minute ventilation, as well as in many of the standard TBFVL parameters, and TV increased two- to threefold. Notably, breathing frequency was not affected. In healthy cats, CO_2 concentrations of 10% were necessary to achieve statistically significant increases in most end points relative to values obtained on room air.[34] However, breathing of CO_2 concentrations $\geq$10% appeared to induce changes in the overall shape of the F-V loop, possibly due to irritancy or odor, the significance of which is as yet undetermined. On a cautionary note, because hypoxia potentiates the ventilatory response to CO_2, more valid measurements may be obtained if, in addition to increasing the percentage of CO_2, one also increases the O_2 content somewhat to help ensure that hypoxic lung or vascular reflex responses are not inadvertently elicited in the test subject.

As another alternative approach, transient increases in lung volume by stimulation of the medullary respiratory center using doxapram hydrochloride were also evaluated.[35] In healthy cats, increasing doses of doxapram resulted in proportionate increases in many TBFVL indices and area-under-the-curve assessments. Unlike CO_2 stimulation, however, doxapram usage did not appear to affect overall loop shape. Unfortunately, the higher doxapram doses were associated with unacceptable side effects such as excessive salivation, vocalization, nervousness, vomiting, and diarrhea.[35]

Exercise-FVL testing is used in humans to identify subclinical respiratory deficiencies.[36,37] Similarly, horses are exercised on slanted treadmills to increase O_2 consumption and CO_2 production, resulting in MV increases proportionate to the level of exercise. Lumsden and colleagues[38] reported that in horses with upper airway obstruction, the F-V loop shape was more consistent and the coefficients of variation for many of the indices were smaller for breaths acquired during exercise, compared with tidal breathing conditions. Comparable methods are unlikely to be of use in cats, but such an approach has potential for dogs, in particular large breed or working dogs.

Admittedly none of these techniques simulates a true maximal expiratory effort; however, based on one author's experience relative to tidal breathing, breathing

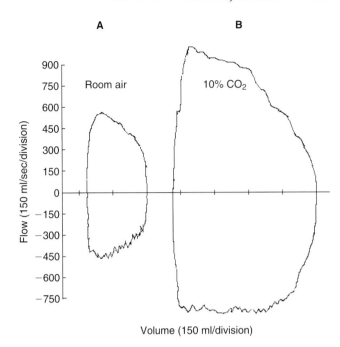

Figure 23-7. These F-V loops were obtained in a 4-year-old bull terrier 6 weeks after corrective surgery for bilateral laryngeal paralysis. In loop **A** the subject was breathing room air; in loop **B** it was breathing 10% CO_2. Note that TV increased (280 to 624 ml), while f decreased (40 to 22 bpm), yielding an increase in MV (11.2 to 20.6 L/min). Peak expiratory flow (PEF) increased (566 to 1050 ml/sec) as did PIF (458 to 836 ml/sec), whereas the Te/Ti ratio was relatively constant.

10% CO_2 approximates half the increases in volume and flow achieved during a maximal expiratory maneuver. Using these or related modifications, it may be possible to effectively increase the sensitivity and reproducibility of the F-V loop assessment but still retain its overall ease and safety. Thus establishment of more narrowly defined reference values for healthy subjects may allow detection of significant differences in mildly affected patients. For example, it appeared that 10% CO_2 levels were necessary to elicit significantly enhanced F-V loop measurements in healthy cats.[34] Diseased patients, however, may require much lower levels to achieve the same enhanced or maximal response.

An example of how breathing 10% CO_2 can unmask flow limitations minimally evident during tidal breathing is shown in Figure 23-7. The F-V loops were acquired from a bull terrier with bilateral laryngeal paralysis that had undergone corrective surgery 6 weeks earlier. The loop shown in Figure 23-7, A was obtained while breathing room air. Although the overall shape is relatively symmetrical, there is evidence of mild blunting of inspiratory flow relative to expiratory flow (i.e., the PEF/PIF ratio was slightly increased at 1.26; normal 1.07 $\pm$ 0.13). In response to breathing 10% CO_2, the lung volume increased 2.2-fold, the PEF rate increased 1.9-fold, and the mid- to end-inspiratory airflow attenuation was more pronounced (Figure 23-7, B).

Another example of how 10% CO_2 can accentuate the patient's ventilatory efforts is shown in Figure 23-8. The

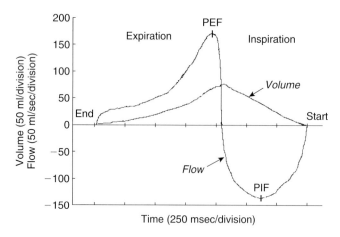

Figure 23-8. *Volume versus time and flow versus time graphs were obtained in a 7-year-old Siamese cat with chronic bronchopulmonary disease while breathing 10% CO_2. Indices: TV = 69 ml; MV = 2340 ml/min; f = 34 bpm; Ti = 720 mS; Te = 972 mS; Te/Ti = 1.35; PIF = 128 ml/sec; PEF = 163 ml/sec; PEF/PIF = 1.28. (See text for interpretation.)*

data were obtained from a 7-year-old Siamese cat with longstanding bronchopulmonary disease. Clinically stable at the time of evaluation, the cat tolerated breathing 10% CO_2. Rather than plotting the typical F-V loop, in Figure 23-8 the changes in lung volume and airflow have been plotted against time. Despite breathing 10% CO_2, the lung volume measurement is only minimally increased over that obtained on room air. This suggests that further increases in lung volume were not possible, likely owing to chronic airway remodeling. In addition, one can readily appreciate the concavity or scooping out of the terminal portion of the expiratory flow-time and expiratory volume-time curves and the disproportionate length of time dedicated to the terminal phase of expiration. As a consequence, this cat seemed to adopt a breathing strategy that allowed more time for the terminal phase of expiration to be more complete. In so doing, on the subsequent breath a proportionately larger volume of inspired air would be able to pass back into the affected alveoli. This case demonstrates that in animals with small airway obstruction, the volume versus time and flow versus time graphs may be more illustrative of end-tidal airflow limitations.

Upper and Lower Airway Resistance and Lung Compliance Assessments

Incorporation of pressure measurements, along with flow and volume assessments, allows for a more in-depth evaluation of breathing mechanics. During examination of the respiratory patient, we attempt to ascertain whether the patient's work of breathing is appropriate—an important but highly subjective clinical assessment. It can be quantified by measuring pressure changes required to generate a breath of known volume or airflow rate, which is the basis of respiratory mechanical as-

sessment, often referred to as function testing. By incorporating pressure changes into ventilatory information, we can calculate direct measures that relate to airflow and tissue mechanics associated with breathing, namely resistance and compliance. These measurements provide clues as to whether the animal has obstructive or restrictive disease.

During inspiration, the alveolar pressure normally becomes slightly negative (see Figure 23-1, *C*), driven by the intrapleural pressure (Ppl) that becomes slightly *more* negative (see Figure 23-1, *D*) relative to ambient pressure. As pressure along the airway drops below atmospheric pressure, air flows inward toward the more negative pressure in the alveolar region. The greater the differential pressure generated, the greater the resultant lung volume. In health, relatively small pressure changes are required to generate a normal tidal breath. The magnitude of the pressure change (P) required is integrally related to several factors, including the tidal volume, the flow rates generated, the ease with which the lung is expanded (lung compliance), and the ease with which air flows through the air passageways (resistance of the upper and lower airways).[39] This is demonstrated mathematically as[23,40]:

$$\Delta P = \frac{\Delta TV}{Compliance} + (\Delta Airflow \times Resistance)$$

Knowing that the diameter of the airways changes with changes in lung volume and with the dynamics of airflow itself, at first glance it may seem impossible to accurately assess all of these parameters simultaneously. On further examination of this equation, however, it becomes apparent that the driving pressure needed to elicit the coincident change in lung volume is closely linked to compliance, whereas that related to airflow is integrally linked to resistance. By imposing certain assumptions on the physiological conditions we use to estimate resistance or compliance, we can define the mechanical behavior of the respiratory system in relatively simple terms. Put another way, if we select two points in the ventilatory cycle where there is no airflow, the corresponding pressure change will primarily be influenced by the elastic properties of the lung. If we select two points where the inspiratory and expiratory volumes are equivalent, the differential pressure will principally reflect resistive effects.

More specifically, resistance can be estimated at a specific point during the inspiratory and expiratory portion of the breath (e.g., at 50% of TV), or it can be computed as a mean of the inspiratory and expiratory phases of the ventilatory cycle. In human experimental physiology laboratories, various methods have been used to make these estimations, many of which require considerable sophistication both in both hardware and software, or involve voluntary participation of the patient (e.g., controlled panting) not readily amenable to veterinary medicine. These methods have been described in practice and in theory elsewhere.[40,41] Fortunately, two methods provide reasonable estimates of resistance and compliance using data collected during tidal breathing. One method, the Mead and Whittenberger[42] approach described nearly 50 years ago, is the more complex but more accurate of the two. With this approach, one first computes compliance from both the inspiratory or expiratory limbs of the breath cycle at a point where there is no airflow. Then, at a given percent of the tidal volume of the next breath, the respective compliant pressure is incorporated into the equation, in essence eliminating the influence of the elastic lung properties from the pressure changes and allowing one to compute resistance. Although straightforward, the algorithms and calculations involved are best left to computer processing. Alternatively, an easier but somewhat less accurate approach uses the isovolume method, sometimes referred to as the poor man's respiratory mechanics.[43] This method uses the same tidal measures of volume, airflow, and pressure, but it computes resistance as an average occurring across inspiration and expiration. The flow and pressure measurements are attained at mid-tidal volumes, ideally at points where airflow is near maximal. With this approach, the volume term on either side of the ventilatory cycle is equivalent. Hence the change in volume is negligible, and the influence of compliance on total pressure is theoretically constant. Thus compliance drops out of the equation and resistance is computed as the quotient of the difference between the pressures and airflows at these two midvolume points. These calculations can be performed by hand by dropping lines across the corresponding points of the volume, flow, and pressure traces (similar to those depicted in Figure 23-1, *A*, *B*, and *D*). Fortunately, pulmonary mechanics software programs exist that make these calculations automatically. In the studies below, the isovolume method was primarily used for estimating resistance and compliance.

Upper Airway Resistance (Ruaw) Assessments

How are ventilatory pressure measurements obtained in small animals? To evaluate upper respiratory airflow disturbances, an over-the-needle catheter may be transcutaneously placed into the lumen of the trachea to assess changes in intratracheal pressure (see Figure 23-2, *B*). This can be accomplished using local anesthesia, similar to the technique used for transtracheal aspiration. The catheter is placed perpendicular to the long axis of the trachea in order to minimize airflow bias at the catheter tip. A pressure transducer connected to the catheter detects pressure changes occurring across the upper airways (Ruaw [i.e., the difference between atmospheric and intratracheal pressure]). Analogous to the TBFVL procedure, a face mask technique can be used to noninvasively obtain measures of volume and airflow. When two transducers are used to measure different aspects of the same functional event, the transducer outputs should be phase-matched to a defined frequency (typically 5 to 10 times the highest *f* encountered) to ensure that any difference in timing is due to the patient and not to the measuring system.[44] Any system-related phasing errors will result in incorrect computations. A pulmonary mechanics analyzer and

software analysis program are used to calculate the overall resistance to airflow, or in this instance, upper airway resistance (Ruaw). Ruaw is a composite of the resistance to airflow through the nares, nasal passages, nasopharynx, larynx, and proximal (upstream) portion of the trachea.

Using this technique, Rozanski and colleagues[45] established normal reference values for Ruaw in mesaticephalic dogs. This minimally invasive approach was well tolerated in untrained, large breed dogs, and the Ruaw values obtained in individual dogs were quite reproducible.[45] Ruaw was calculated using the isovolume method (at 70% of TV) as:

$$R_{uaw} = \frac{\Delta P_{uaw}}{\Delta Flow}$$

The units for Ruaw are cmH$_2$O/L/sec. Hence Ruaw reflects the overall pressure change required to generate a given change in airflow through the upper airways.

A change in the diameter of a single air passageway significantly influences the resistance measurement. Assuming that the length is held constant, if the airway's diameter is progressively reduced, greater and greater pressure changes will be necessary to achieve the same airflow over an equivalent time. Consequently, decrements in airway caliber require generation of greater differential pressure gradients in order to achieve comparable airflow. This, however, is not a linear relationship. In fact, resistance to airflow through the airway is inversely proportional to the radius of the airway taken to the 4th power.[46] Accordingly, if the radius is cut in half, resistance increases sixteenfold. In the respiratory system as a whole, all patent air passageways influence the resistance measurement; however, the upper airways account for ≥60% of the inspiratory frictional resistance occurring during tidal breathing.[23]

Rozanski and colleagues[45] further compared Ruaw values from healthy mesaticephalic dogs with that of healthy dolichocephalic dogs. Despite their elongated nasal profile, collies did not have elevated Ruaw measurements; if anything, there was a trend toward lower absolute Ruaw values in this breed.[45] Conversely, despite their shortened nasal profile, brachycephalic dogs often have increased upper airway resistance due to relatively stenotic nares, elongated soft palates, or hypoplastic tracheas.[47] These examples illustrate the disproportionate influence of decrements in airway caliber (particularly of the upper airways and lower central airways) on the resistance measurement.

Again using the method described in Figure 23-2, *B*, Alsup and colleagues[31] used Ruaw measurements in dogs to validate that the TBFVL improvements noted after corrective surgery for laryngeal paralysis were in fact associated with decreased resistance to airflow through the larynx. Similarly, Greenfield and colleagues[48] used Ruaw measurements in combination with TBFVL analysis to validate an experimental model of canine laryngeal paralysis. Not only did bilateral recurrent laryngeal neurectomy result in analogous clinical signs, the inspiratory airflow impairment was comparable with that of dogs with naturally occurring disease.[48]

Lung Resistance and Compliance Assessments

If assessment of pulmonary function is the priority, the influence of the upper respiratory tract must be excluded, and instead measures of transpulmonary pressure must be obtained. In small animals, alveolar pressure can only be measured indirectly using body plethysmography. Intrapleural pressure (Ppl) can be measured by surgical placement of a cannula into the pleural space. Fortunately, however, pressure changes within the pleural space closely parallel those of the midthoracic esophagus. Thus the least invasive method of obtaining estimates of Ppl is to place a balloon-tipped catheter into the esophagus (just caudal to the heart to avoid movement artifact related to cardiac contractions) and record changes in esophageal pressure (Pes). Although horses commonly tolerate this procedure without general anesthesia, few untrained dogs and presumably no cats would be so tolerant. The esophageal catheter is connected to a pressure transducer (see Figure 23-2, *C*). Volume and airflow measurements could be obtained using a face mask; however, because we are primarily interested in assessing pulmonary disease, and because anesthesia is required for placement of the esophageal catheter, as a rule the animal is intubated and the endotracheal tube is connected directly to the pneumotachograph and associated pressure transducer (see Figure 23-2, *C*).

The main disadvantage of this approach is that it requires a brief period of general anesthesia for placement of the esophageal balloon/endotracheal tube and for data acquisition. Furthermore, because all recoverable anesthetic agents are associated with some degree of respiratory depression, the measurements obtained are likely to be somewhat biased, depending on the agent(s) and the depth of anesthesia. It may be possible to overcome some of the respiratory depression by incorporating methods to partially augment respiratory efforts (e.g., low doses of doxapram or moderate increases in CO_2 during data acquisition). In addition, the endotracheal tube is associated with a certain degree of resistance to airflow. For consistency, when comparing similarly sized healthy and diseased patients, care must be taken to ensure that the endotracheal tubes used are of equivalent length and inner diameter. Alternatively, the airflow resistance of the endotracheal tube may be subtracted from the overall resistance value obtained for the patient. In so doing, however, a portion of the resistance related to the laryngeal/upper tracheal region will also be subtracted.

Analogous to Ruaw, lung resistance (R_L) is calculated by dividing the change in transpulmonary pressure (estimated by Pes) by the change in airflow, again using isovolume conditions. Although all patent airways influence R_L, the large conducting, central airways predominantly influence this measurement.[49] Airway resistance varies inversely with lung volume because the expanding lung parenchyma exerts traction on the walls of the airways. Therefore, lung resistance calculations should always be related to lung volume. The small peripheral airways (defined in humans as 2 mm) normally contribute little to the overall resistance because the airflow per airway is very small and there are so many arranged in parallel, in effect making the combined cross-sectional area of the small airways very large. As such, the R_L measurement is relatively insensitive to small airway changes. It is generally inferred that an increase in R_L is indicative of central airway obstruction with or without concurrent peripheral airway obstruction.

Airway resistance is often increased in humans with chronic inflammatory airway disease (e.g., chronic bronchitis or asthma) due to reductions in airway caliber.[50] Resistance is also influenced by changes in tissues surrounding the airways (e.g., emphysema).[51] During peripheral airway obstruction, lung volume (FRC) is often increased due to air trapping. As the small airways become overly distended, R_L decreases. Unless adjustments are made for the increase in lung volume, the sensitivity of R_L in detecting small airway obstruction is further reduced. In small animals, FRC can be quantified using an open circuit nitrogen washout technique, similar to the method used in human infants.[52] Thus measures of R_L can be used to establish the presence and degree of airway obstruction but cannot discriminate between the conditions that contribute to airway obstruction.

The other commonly used pulmonary mechanical parameter, lung compliance, is used mainly to assess changes in overall lung elasticity or stiffness. As changes in volume, airflow, and pressure are recorded during tidal breathing, if the change in volume is measured at periods when there is no airflow (i.e., at the beginning and end of inspiration), the coincident pressure change related to the resistance term (Δ flow $\times$ resistance) is negated, leaving compliance to be calculated simply as:

$$C = \frac{\Delta TV}{\Delta Ppl}$$

Hence compliance represents the change in lung volume corresponding to a given change in pressure. Compliance determined in this manner is referred to as dynamic lung compliance (C_{dyn}; ml/cm H_2O). Static (or quasistatic) lung compliance is another means of assessing lung distensibility. It can be measured using a number of variations on a theme[40,53,54]; but in each, volume and pressure changes are measured as the lung is incrementally inflated (typically to total lung capacity) and then incrementally deflated. At each step, airflow transiently ceases, thus allowing for computation of compliance with minimal resistive effects. Thoracic static compliance can be likewise estimated; however, with this approach, changes in elasticity may relate not only to lung parenchymal changes but also to changes in the chest wall, and thus pleural space.[51]

A major determinant of dynamic lung compliance is the relaxation state of the smaller airways (i.e., those larger than terminal bronchioles). C_{dyn} is reduced if sufficient numbers of the small airways are constricted or become obstructed.[56] Lung compliance, in particular static compliance,[53] may also be reduced if the lung parenchyma becomes stiffer due to infiltrative processes (e.g., interstitial edema) or fibrotic processes (e.g., cryptogenic fibrosing alveolitis).[57] Conversely, in emphysema and possibly in chronic airway remodeling, as the elastic support structures of the lung parenchyma become weakened or destroyed, Cdyn is abnormally increased.[51] In this situation, R_L also increases due to generalized loss of the radial traction that normally serves to maintain small airway patency.[51]

Few clinical reports in companion animals have used lung mechanical assessments. Conceptually, however, R_L and compliance measurements should prove useful in understanding whether the respiratory disease is obstructive or restrictive and in establishing the extent of the functional impairment. Lung resistance is likely to increase in animals with tracheobronchial collapse or inflammatory airway disease.[1,2,32] Compliance is likely to decrease in patients with diffuse small airway disease. Reductions in compliance are also likely in parenchymal infiltrative diseases (e.g., pulmonary edema related to congestive heart failure,[58] idiopathic pulmonary fibrosis in dogs,[3-5] peribronchiolar fibrosis,[59] and fibrosing alveolitis[6] in cats). Chronic airway wall remodeling—loosely defined as the destructive airway changes occurring as a sequela to persistent airway injury and inflammation[60,61]—may be associated with increased C_{dyn} measurements, because the normal elasticity of the lung is slowly reduced. Bronchiectasis has been reported in dogs[32] and cats,[62] most commonly in association with chronic inflammation. However, the functional abnormalities attributable to bronchiectasis are difficult to distinguish from changes related to the coexisting lung conditions. And finally, although uncommon in small animals, generalized loss/destruction of intraalveolar connections (e.g., emphysema, COPD,[63] chronic pulmonary overinflation states, and bullous emphysema) are likely to be associated with increases in C_{dyn} and small increases in R_L.

By way of specific clinical examples, relatively simple parameters (e.g., TV, MV, and peak inspiratory pressure) are useful objective data in determining whether an animal needs continued mechanical ventilatory support (e.g., after a thoracotomy procedure, with neuromuscular blockade,[64] or for critical patients with primary parenchymal disease[65] or thoracic trauma[66]). Note however, that because ventilated critical patients are under positive pressure ventilation, the Pes measurement is a less reliable indicator of Ppl changes.[67] Thus for human patients receiving mechanical ventilatory support, changes in static compliance are considered a better estimate of whether the pulmonary parenchyma is becoming less distensible. Decrements in total thoracic compliance may be useful, not only in detecting lung parenchymal changes such as edema or pneumonia but also in identifying disorders of the thoracic wall such as pneumothorax or pleural effusion.[55] Because all of these conditions are not uncommon complications in chronically ventilated patients, King and colleagues[55] assessed whether a similar approach could be used to evaluate ventilated small animal patients. These investigators demonstrated that static thoracic compliance could be measured safely and easily in anesthetized, intubated dogs.[55] In addition, when thoracic static compliance was normalized to body weight, values obtained in dogs with respiratory disease were considerably lower than those obtained in healthy dogs.[55] King and colleagues have continued to use similar assessments in animals requiring positive pressure ventilation[65] (e.g., acute respiratory distress syndrome,[68] thoracic trauma with pulmonary contusions,[66] and hypoventilatory states related to spinal cord disorders[69]). Overall, the ability to objectively assess changes in compliance has proven indispensable both for diagnostic and prognostic purposes, as well as for ventilator management in these small animal patients.

As another example, Stobie and colleagues[70] used R_L and C_{dyn} measures in dogs to evaluate the effectiveness of analgesic protocols after a thoracotomy procedure. Results indicated that both anesthesia and thoracotomy were associated with significant changes in lung function, and, moreover, that interpleural administration of the analgesic bupivacaine allowed for an earlier return to normal based on several of the functional assessments evaluated.

Furthermore, Dye and colleagues[2] used R_L and C_{dyn} measures to evaluate airway obstruction in cats with naturally occurring bronchopulmonary disease. Cats were first grouped according to relative disease severity based on scored clinical assessments, then anesthetized using a short-acting barbiturate, and measures of R_L and C_{dyn} were obtained. Data indicated that significant airway obstruction was present in many of the affected cats. Specifically, compared with healthy cats with a mean R_L value of 28.9 cm H_2O/L/sec, the mildly, moderately, and severely affected cats had R_L values of 38.3, 44.8, and 105.2 cm H_2O/L/sec, respectively. Similarly, healthy cats had a mean C_{dyn} value of 19.8 ml/cm H_2O, whereas affected cats had values of 14.7, 17.7, and 13.0 ml/cm H_2O, respectively.[2] Thus despite the fact that most of the cats were not in obvious respiratory distress at the time of evaluation, many cats, in particular those with moderate and severe disease, had considerably abnormal PFT results. The R_L elevations were consistent with obstruction of either the larger airways or with severe, diffuse small airway disease. Cats with decreased C_{dyn} measurements were presumed to have either obstruction of the smaller airways or parenchymal fibrotic/infiltrative disease. Some of the cats had abnormal R_L and C_{dyn} measurements consistent with obstruction/constriction of both the large and small airways. A few cats with particularly longstanding disease had moderate increases in R_L in combination with C_{dyn} increases, possibly due to chronic airway remodeling.

Also in this study, Dye and colleagues[2] administered a test dose of the β_2-agonist terbutaline to assess acute reversibility of the airway obstruction. A few affected cats demonstrated nearly complete reversal, suggesting that the majority of the airway obstruction was caused by excessive smooth muscle constriction. Other cats had only partial reversal, at least acutely (similar to the cat depicted in Figure 23-9, A). Not surprisingly, this cat had particularly longstanding disease. The partial response suggests that other factors in addition to smooth muscle constriction were present (e.g., retention of mucous secretions, intraluminal and submucosal inflammation, or

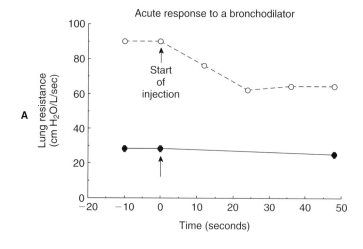

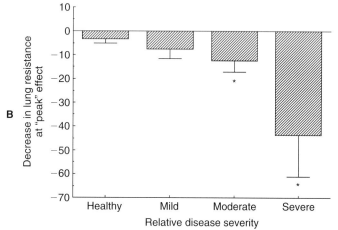

Figure 23-9. A, *Acute response to a test dose of the bronchodilator terbutaline in a cat with chronic bronchopulmonary disease* (open circle) *and a healthy cat* (solid circle). **B,** *Group responses to a test dose of terbutaline in healthy cats and cats with mild, moderate, and severe bronchopulmonary disease. Asterisk* (*) *indicates a significantly greater response than was observed in the healthy cats (p 0.05).*

airway remodeling). Some cats showed negligible improvement following bronchodilator administration. The overall R_L group responses to terbutaline administration are depicted in Figure 23-9, *B.* Compared with healthy control cats, as a group, the moderately and severely affected cats had greater absolute R_L decreases, which was not unexpected remembering that R_L changes inversely with the radius taken to the 4th power. As such, even minor improvements in airflow can be associated with substantial decrements in airflow resistance.

Interestingly, after administration of terbutaline the healthy cats had R_L decrements of approximately 10% and C_{dyn} increases of over 30%. This finding is consistent with the general observation that cats normally have a considerable degree of cholinergic small airway smooth muscle tone.[71] By contrast, resting bronchomotor tone in dogs appears to be minimal.[32] Airway tone is a result of a balance between cholinergic[72] (i.e., acetylcholine-, methacholine-responding receptors), adrenergic (i.e., epi-

nephrine-, β-agonist-responding receptors), and noncholinergic nonadrenergic (NANC) or C-fiber–mediated reflex responses (i.e, tachykinin-, neurokinin-responding receptors).[73] Reflex regulation of airway smooth muscle tone is an area of considerable investigation. A variety of species have been evaluated, no two of which appear to be under identical neurological control. Generally speaking, however, cats appear to be quite similar to humans (and to primates, rabbits, guinea pigs, ferrets, horses, sheep, cattle, and swine), in that the NANC neurons contribute significantly to relaxation of the airway smooth muscle.[7,74-76] In dogs (and rats), virtually all the relaxant innervation to the airway is adrenergically mediated.[76,77]

The cat has been used extensively as a model to investigate the in vivo effects of a variety of bioactive mediators. Some of the bronchoconstrictive mediators evaluated include substance P,[78,79] cold air,[80] cyclooxygenase products and leukotrienes,[8] platelet activating factor (PAF),[81] serotonin (5-HT),[82] oxygen radical species,[83] thromboxanes,[84] and endothelins.[85] Bronchodilatory mediators have included vasoactive intestinal protein (VIP)[86]; PGE_1, 6-keto-PGE_1, and PGI_2[87,88]; and histamine.[78,89] Whether any of these mediators relate to the pathological processes underlying naturally occurring bronchopulmonary disease in cats remains to be determined.

More recent studies suggest that nitric oxide (NO) is involved in the acute NANC-induced airway relaxation in cats[90] and further that NO is an important factor modulating the degree of airway responsiveness (AR) of cats in vivo.[91] This finding is consistent with an earlier report that ozone-induced airway epithelial damage in cats was associated with increased AR to the cholinergic mediator acetylcholine. The authors hypothesized that ozone exposure resulted in decreased production of epithelium-dependent relaxant factor(s).[10] Knowing now that airway epithelial cells are an important source of NO in the lung, one of the relaxant factors alluded to in the previous study was likely to be NO.

In humans, AR is defined as the ease with which airways narrow in response to a nonspecific (nonallergic or nonsensitizing) stimulus.[92] Increased AR is a hallmark feature of asthma[61] and further, the degree of AR may correlate with disease severity and therapy requirements.[93] In the study by Dye and colleagues,[2] a subset of affected cats with relatively normal baseline R_L and C_{dyn} values underwent bronchoprovocation testing to see if they had increased AR analogous to that of human asthmatics during asymptomatic periods. Six (of seven) affected cats had increased AR compared with a group of healthy cats, based on the effective concentration of aerosolized methacholine required to double the baseline R_L measurement ($EC_{200}R_L$).[2] These results suggest (but do not prove) that these cats were predisposed to developing bronchoconstriction and that this may have contributed to their intermittent respiratory signs. On a related note, increased AR has been reported in cats with experimental allergen-induced lung inflammation.[13-15] The AR increases were inhibited by treatment with the potent immunosuppressive drug cyclosporine.[15] Moreover, Miura and colleagues[13] demonstrated that during allergen reexposure, the NANC inhibitory response was diminished in cats, leading to increases in lung resistance. The investigators suggested that protease release during the allergic inflammatory response played a role in dysfunction of airway smooth muscle.

In summary, reflex regulation of airway smooth muscle tone, and thus airway patency, is mediated by multiple, carefully regulated pathways, both inhibitory and excitatory. Although the nature of the regulatory processes varies between species, airway inflammation appears to be a universal disruptor of the balance between constrictor and dilatory input. The ability to define lung function (R_L and C_{dyn}) in small animals is essential not only to document the presence of airway obstruction but also to determine its reversibility. Similarly, lung function assessments can indicate whether the airways are more responsive than normal, thus predisposing the animal to developing obstruction after exposure to irritating or infectious agents.[17,94]

Future Direction and Cautionary Notes

A general limitation of the use of PFTs to assess individual small animal patients is the lack of more specific reference values for comparison. To date, no validated protocols for clinical use are available, and they are unlikely in the foreseeable future. Even in the experimental setting, different investigators use slightly different testing systems, making it difficult to compare results across a number of studies.[40] Until standard protocols are available, investigators should describe the methods and instrumentation used in substantial detail.

Hence one of the goals that must be achieved before PFTs can be used routinely in small animals is the establishment of standard testing protocols. Then, using standard methodologies, longitudinal studies are needed to evaluate sufficient numbers of healthy and affected subjects to define reference values and to generate predictive equations for a variety of clinical syndromes. Reference ranges are likely to need considerable refinement to account for differences in an individual animal's size; age; sex; and, most likely, breed. This reflects the tremendous variability existing especially among dogs, in terms of body size and thoracic shape (from Chihuahuas to Great Danes), and nasal anatomy (from exercise-efficient sight hounds to mouth-breathing bulldogs). Although cats are relatively similar in body size and thoracic shape, differences in nasal anatomy exist (e.g., dolichocephalic Siamese cats, brachycephalic Persians).

Despite these similarities, Dye and colleagues[2] observed that even in healthy cats, C_{dyn} measurements were more variable (coefficient of variance, CV = 37%) than R_L measurements (CV = 22%). Attempts were made to normalize C_{dyn} to some index of the animal's size. There was no clear correlation between C_{dyn} and the animal's body weight, but a significant correlation existed between C_{dyn} and thoracic girth measurements. Clark and colleagues[95] observed that in healthy dogs (ranging in weight from 11.8 to 26.4 kg), C_{dyn} correlated more closely with trunk length than with either body weight or chest circumference. In humans, a number of lung function indices correlate more closely with an individual's height than with weight.[96] Clearly, further work is necessary.

Another major obstacle that must be overcome is the selection of appropriate sedative or anesthetic protocols for PFTs requiring an endotracheal tube, esophageal balloon, or paralysis to achieve total ventilatory control. The anesthetic protocol must allow for safe recovery of the respiratory patient, but it must not unduly influence the underlying pathologic processes. An inhalant anesthetic would seem ideal, however agents such as halothane and isoflurane are considered potent bronchodilators and also appear to induce reflex inhibition of breathing during face mask induction.[97] Likewise, intravenous use of propofol has been shown to have bronchodilatory effects in humans.[98] Use of these or similar agents, or the use of premedicants with anticholinergic activity, is likely to transiently mask the functional deficits we are trying to document. On the other hand, virtually all sedative and anesthetic agents tend to relax the upper airway dilating muscles, further compounding airflow resistance in brachycephalic animals and making any procedure involving sedation or anesthesia in these subjects extremely risky.[42]

Two older agents, α-chloralose and chloral hydrate, have potential for use during PFTs in companion animals. The hypnotic agent α-chloralose preserves vagal and central baroreceptor reflexes, making it a commonly used agent for experimental physiological studies in dogs.[99-101] Lemen and colleages have used it for recovery PFTs in laboratory beagles for over a decade,[17,18,100] reporting that even in puppies, it is safe when administered intravenously up to 8 to 12 times/dog/year, at a cumulative dose of 1.18 gm/kg.[100] Controversy remains whether it is a true anesthetic or simply an immobilizing agent with sedative-hypnotic properties[99]; however, for nonpainful PFT procedures its use seems appropriate. The drug is sparingly soluble,[102] and customized mixing may be necessary, raising possible problems with shelf life and sterility.

Chloral hydrate, a related agent, is another very old sedative hypnotic drug. Despite concerns about its safety, it is currently used extensively in human pediatric patients as an oral agent for non–operating room procedures because it provides an adequate level of sedation without compromising protective reflexes, airway patency, or cardiopulmonary stability.[103,104] Its use in laboratory animals is less common, in part because intraperitoneal administration is not recommended for survival procedures, and oral administration, at least in dogs, is associated with gastric irritation.[101] A recent experimental study in cats used oral chloral hydrate to determine its effect on esophageal smooth muscle tone, in comparison with oral midazolam or an intramuscular cocktail of meperidine, promethazine, and chlorpromazine.[105] Although all sedated cats had some degree of decreased esophageal tone, of the two oral agents, chloral hydrate had the least effect. More definitive studies are needed to determine whether these older agents or whether other newer compounds (possibly in combination), can be used safely in companion dogs and cats and yet effectively preserve pulmonary reflexes and smooth muscle tone. Until standard anesthetic protocols are in place, if sedative/anesthetic agents are used during function testing, one should include a detailed summary of all agents used, including dosages, route(s) of administration, and level of effect. Importantly, these factors influence breathing frequency, lung volume, and bronchomotor tone, and thus may alter PFT assessments.

Although standard end-expiratory lung volume data and tidal F-V curves have provided objective assessment of airway function in pediatric patients, more recent assessments have focused on the latter portion of the expiratory curve in an effort to distinguish maturation changes from those related to airway obstructive disease.[106] For example, in infants with acute bronchiolitis, the ratio of time to reach peak tidal expiratory flow to total expiratory time (tPTEF/Te) allowed demonstration of acute responses to nebulized epinephrine.[107] Still, difficulties arise in interpreting TBFVL data due to dependency on simple differences in measurement conditions[108] and to high inter-subject variability.[109] As such, a variety of approaches have been used in infants in an attempt to simulate the maximal expiratory effort used for FEV$_1$ (forced expiratory volume in 1 second) measurements. In adults, FEV$_1$ is one of the most commonly used and reproducible lung function tests used to assess small airway function.[110] A forced deflation technique, used in pediatric patients with an endotracheal tube in place, can simulate maximal expiratory airflow. Typically the infant is given several manual inflations to establish a consistent volume history. Once total lung capacity is reached on the final inflation, the endotracheal tube is exposed to a constant negative pressure until either expiratory flow ceases or for a maximum of 3 seconds (FEV$_3$).[111] Alternatively, a sedated infant may be fitted with an inflatable jacket designed to apply sudden, but uniform pressure over the thorax and abdomen at the peak of inspiration.[111]

Another approach to assess airway resistance is the use of forced oscillation over a range of frequencies.[36] When used noninvasively for infants (by applying pressure at the mouth), the variable contribution of the upper airways limits the usefulness of the technique for clinical assessment of lung disease.[36] In addition, using a signal processing technique, inductive plethysmography has been used in infants to establish phase relationships between abdominal and thoracic displacement.[112] Despite considerable effort to standardize these approaches for use in very young patients, much work remains.[111]

Similar to the strategies used for function testing in infants, methods to obtain functional assessments less invasively in companion animals have included use of an unrestrained barometric, whole-body plethysmograph[113] or a minimal restraint dual-chamber plethysmograph. Although one cannot discriminate between upper and lower respiratory effects as definitively with this technique, data indicate that this approach is sufficiently sensitive to detect airflow decrements in cats undergoing bronchoprovocation testing[113] or, alternatively, to detect

airflow improvement in asthmatic cats following aerosol administration of a bronchodilator.[114]

Finally, a few miscellaneous precautions are worth mentioning. If an endotracheal tube is used during testing, care must be taken to ensure that the tube is not acting as a critical orifice, creating artifactual flow limitation within the tracheal lumen. If strategies to enhance the ventilatory efforts of the patient are used, one must ensure that the pneumotachograph and pressure transducers are still in range to acquire the augmented signals, and that the system remains appropriately phase-matched. If maneuvers that tend to cause transient hypocapnia are used repeatedly (e.g., rapid lung deflation), changes in CO_2 retention may result in secondary effects on lung vascular and bronchomotor tone. In a similar fashion, alterations in lung volume history as is used during bronchoprovocation testing may recruit additional airspaces, yielding results that underestimate the functional deficits of the steady state diseased condition. And lastly, owing to the potentially labile nature of airway tone and patency, continuous ECG and pulse oximetry monitoring of all animals during and immediately after testing is considered prudent, as is providing general patient support (e.g., supplemental oxygen, anticholinergic or bronchodilating medication) until the animal is stable and fully recovered from the procedure.

As standard protocols are defined and as more complete reference values are available, we hope that PFTs will become more widely used in veterinary clinical medicine. Possibly by combining PFT assessments with other commonly available tests (e.g., blood gas analyses, thoracic radiography, bronchoscopy, and bronchoalveolar cytological/cultural examination), or with newer tests (e.g., pulse oximetry and end-tidal NO or CO_2 concentrations), we can better delineate the clinical spectrums of naturally occurring respiratory disease syndromes. For example, Wiester and colleagues demonstrated that in humans undergoing bronchoprovocation testing, acute decrements in Sao$_2$ measurements were highly correlated with decreases in lung functional endpoints (FEV$_1$ and SR$_{AW}$).[115] Similar innovative approaches may provide noninvasive means for determining AR in companion animals.

With this combined database, we aim to better characterize the etiologies and mechanisms of disease and, most important, to establish the efficacy of specific treatment protocols. Our overall goal is simply to provide a high quality of care for today's pet-owning public. To this end, cooperation between veterinary practitioners; small animal internists and surgeons; and specialists in respiratory physiology, anesthesiology, and critical care medicine will be essential.

ACKNOWLEDGMENTS: No chapter on small animal respiratory disease and function testing would be complete without acknowledging the work of some of the leaders in this field—Drs. Jerry Gillespie, Joan O'Brien, Terry Amis, and N. Ed Robinson, to name but a few. We also wish to thank Drs. Brendan McKiernan, Susan Jones, and Elizabeth Rozanski for their contributions to this field and specifically for their willingness to share the data used in the case examples in this chapter.

REFERENCES

1. Padrid PA, Hornof WJ, Kurpershoek CJ et al: Canine chronic bronchitis: A pathophysiologic evaluation of 18 cases, *J Vet Intern Med* 4(3):172-180, 1990.
2. Dye JA, McKiernan BC, Rozanski EA et al: Bronchopulmonary disease in the cat: Historical, physical, radiographic, clinicopathologic, and pulmonary functional evaluation of 24 affected and 15 healthy cats, *J Vet Intern Med* 10(6):385-400, 1996.
3. Corcoran BM, Cobb M, Martin MWS et al: Chronic pulmonary disease in West Highland white terriers, *Vet Record* 144:611-616, 1999.
4. Corcoran BM, Dukes-McEwan, Rhind S et al: Idiopathic pulmonary fibrosis in a Staffordshire bull terrier with hypothyroidism, *J Small Anim Pract* 40(4):185-188, 1999.
5. Lobetti RG, Milner R, Lane E: Chronic idiopathic fibrosis in five dogs, *J Am Anim Hosp Assoc* 37(2):119-127, 2001.
6. Rhind SM, Gunn-Moore DA: Desquamative form of cryptogenic fibrosing alveolitis in a cat, *J Comp Pathol* 123(2-3):226-229, 2000.
7. Inoue H, Ichinose M, Miura M et al: Sensory receptors and reflex pathways of nonadrenergic inhibitory nervous system in feline airways, *Am Rev Respir Dis* 139(5):1175-1178, 1989.
8. Graybar GB, Harrington JK, Cowen KH et al: Cyclooxygenase mediated airway response to leukotriene D_4 in the cat, *Prostaglandins* 31(1):167-177, 1986.
9. Thompson DC, Szarek JL, Altiere RJ et al: Nonadrenergic bronchodilation induced by high concentrations of sulfur dioxide, *J Appl Physiol* 69(5):1786-1791, 1990.
10. Takata S, Aizawa H, Inoue H et al: Ozone exposure suppresses epithelial-dependent relaxation in feline airway, *Lung* 173(1):47-56, 1995.
11. Pepelko WE, Mattox JK, Yang YY et al: Pulmonary function and pathology in cats exposed 28 days to diesel exhaust, *J Environ Pathol Toxicol* 4(2-3):449-457, 1980.
12. Barch GK, Talbott MW: Allergic bronchoconstriction and its drug-induced reversal in anesthetized ovalbumin-sensitized cats, *Res Commun Chem Pathol Pharmacol* 13(4):623-633, 1976.
13. Miura M, Ichinose M, Kimura K et al: Dysfunction of nonadrenergic noncholinergic inhibitory system after antigen inhalation in actively sensitized cat airways, *Am Rev Respir Dis* 145(1):70-74, 1992.
14. Padrid P, Snook S, Finucane T et al: Persistent airway hyperresponsiveness and histologic alterations after chronic antigen challenge in cats, *Am J Respir Crit Care Med* 151(1):184-193, 1995.
15. Padrid PA, Cozzi P, Leff AR: Cyclosporine inhibits airway reactivity and remodeling after chronic antigen challenge in cats, *Am J Respir Crit Care Med* 154(6 Pt 1):1812-1818, 1996.
16. Cunningham JC, Morgan WJ, Lemen RJ et al: Passive exhalation technique correlates with esophageal balloon measurements of respiratory mechanics in beagle pups, *Am Rev Respir Dis* 136(3):722-726, 1987.
17. Quan SF, Witten ML, Grad R et al: Acute canine adenovirus 2 infection increases histamine airway reactivity in beagle puppies, *Am Rev Respir Dis* 141(2):414-420, 1990.
18. Anderson KA, Lemen RJ, Weger NS et al: Nedocromil sodium inhibits canine adenovirus bronchiolitis in beagle puppies, *Toxicol Pathol* 28(2):317-325, 2000.
19. Mammel MC, Boros SJ, Bing DR et al: Determining optimum inspiratory time during intermittent positive pressure ventilation in surfactant-depleted cats, *Pediatr Pulmonol* 7(4):223-229, 1989.
20. Schulze A, Jonzon A, Sindelar R et al: Assisted mechanical ventilation using combined elastic and resistive unloading in cats with severe respiratory failure: effects on gas exchange and phrenic nerve activity, *Acta Paediatr* 88(6):636-641, 1999.
21. Shardonofsky FR, Skaburskis M, Sato J et al: Effects of volume history and vagotomy on pulmonary and chest wall mechanics in cats, *J Appl Physiol* 71(2):498-508, 1991.
22. Proulx J: Respiratory monitoring: Arterial blood gas analysis, pulse oximetry, and end-tidal carbon dioxide analysis, *Clin Tech Small Anim Pract* 14(4):227-230, 1999.
23. Robinson NE: Airway physiology, *Vet Clin North Am Sm Anim Pract* 22(5):1043-1064, 1992.
24. Amis TC, Kurpershoek C: Tidal breathing flow-volume loop analysis for clinical assessment of airway obstruction in conscious dogs, *Am J Vet Res* 47(5):1002-1006, 1986.
25. McKiernan BC, Dye JA, Rozanski EA: Tidal breathing flow-volume loops in healthy and bronchitic cats, *J Vet Intern Med* 7(6):388-493, 1993.
26. Abramson AL, Goldstein MN, Stenzler A et al: The use of tidal breathing flow volume loops in laryngotracheal disease of neonates and infants, *Laryngoscope* 92:922-926, 1982.
27. Amis TC, Kurpershoek C: Pattern of breathing in brachycephalic dogs, *Am J Vet Res* 47(10):2200-2204, 1986.
28. Amis TC, Smith MM, Gaber CE et al: Upper airway obstruction in canine laryngeal paralysis, *Am J Vet Res* 47(5):1007-1010, 1986.
29. Smith MM, Gourely IM, Kurpershoek CJ et al: Evaluation of a modified castellated laryngofissure for alleviation of upper airway obstruction in dogs with laryngeal paralysis, *J Am Vet Med Assoc* 188(11):1279-1283, 1986.
30. Burbidge HM, Goulden BE, Jones BR: An experimental evaluation of castellated laryngofissure and bilateral arytenoid lateralization for the relief of laryngeal paralysis in dogs, *Aust Vet J* 68:268-272, 1991.
31. Alsup JC, Greenfield CL, Hungerford LL et al: Comparison of unilateral arytenoid lateralization and ventral ventriculocordectomy for the treatment of experimentally induced laryngeal paralysis in dogs, *Can Vet J* 38(5):287-293, 1997.
32. Padrid PA: Chronic tracheobronchial disease in the dog, *Vet Clin North Am Small Anim Pract* 22(5):1203-1229, 1992.
33. Johnson L: Tracheal collapse: Diagnosis and medical and surgical treatment, *Vet Clin North Am Small Anim Pract* 30(6):1253-1266, 2000.
34. McKiernan BC, Rozanski EA, Jones SE et al: The effect of CO_2 on tidal breathing flow volume (TBFVL) loops in conscious cats, *Proceedings of the 8th Comparative Respiratory Symposium,* p. 23, 1989.
35. Marks CK, McKiernan BC: The effect of Dopram®-V on flow-volume loops in conscious cats: *Proceedings of the 14th Comparative Respiratory Symposium,* 48, 1996.
36. Johnson BD, Beck KC, Zeballos RJ et al: Advances in pulmonary laboratory testing, *Chest* 116(5):1377-1387, 1999.
37. Johnson BD, Weisman IM, Zeballos RJ et al: Emerging concepts in the evaluation of ventilatory limitations during exercise: The exercise tidal flow-volume loop, *Chest* 116(2):277-278, 1999.
38. Lumsden JM, Derksen FJ, Stick JA et al: Use of flow-volume loops to evaluate upper airway obstruction in exercising standardbreds, *Am J Vet Res* 54(5):766-775, 1993.
39. Altose MD: Pulmonary mechanics. In Fishman AP, editor: *Fishman's pulmonary diseases and disorders,* ed 3, New York, 1998, McGraw-Hill Health Professions Division.
40. Watson JW: Elastic, resistive, and inertial properties of the lung. In Parent RA, editor: *Treatise on pulmonary toxicology,* ed 1, Boca Raton, 1991, CRC Press.
41. Drazen JM: Physiological basis and interpretation of common indices of respiratory mechanical function, *Environ Health Perspect* 16:11-16, 1976.
42. Mead J, Wittenberger JL: Physical properties of human lungs measured during spontaneous respiration, *J Appl Physiol* 5:779-796, 1953.
43. Amdur MO, Mead J: Mechanics of respiration in unanesthetized guinea pigs, *Am J Physiol* 192:364-368, 1958.
44. Jackson AC, Vinegar A: A technique for measuring frequency response of pressure, volume, and flow transducers, *J Appl Physiol* 47:462-467, 1979.
45. Rozanski EA, Greenfield CL, Alsup JC et al: Measurement of upper airway resistance in awake untrained dolichocephalic and mesaticephalic dogs, *Am J Vet Res* 55(8):1055-1059, 1994.
46. Levitzky MG: Mechanics of breathing. In Levitzky MG, editor: *Pulmonary physiology,* ed 4, New York, 1995, McGraw-Hill.
47. Hendricks JC: Brachycephalic airway syndrome, *Vet Clin North Am Small Anim Pract* 22(5):1145-1153, 1992.
48. Greenfield CL, Alsup JC, Hungerford LL et al: Bilateral recurrent laryngeal neurectomy as a model for the study of idiopathic canine laryngeal paralysis, *Can Vet J* 38(3):163-167, 1997.
49. Drazen JM: Physiologic basis and interpretation of indices of pulmonary mechanics, *Environ Health Perspect* 56:3-9, 1984.
50. West JB: Obstructive diseases. In West JB, editor: *Pulmonary pathophysiology: The essentials,* ed 5, Baltimore 1995, Lippincott Williams & Wilkins.

51. West JB: Other tests. In West JB, editor: *Pulmonary pathophysiology: The essentials,* ed 5, Baltimore 1995, Lippincott Williams & Wilkins.

52. Gernhardt T, Hehre D, Bancalari E et al: A simple method for measuring functional residual capacity by N2 washout in small animals and newborn infants, *Pediatr Res* 19(11):1165-1169, 1985.

53. Gibson GL, Pride NB: Lung distensibility: The static pressure-volume curve of the lungs and its use in clinical assessment, *Br J Dis Chest* 70:143-184, 1976.

54. Costa DL, Lehmann JR, Slatkin EA et al: Chronic airway obstruction and bronchiectasis in the rat after intratracheal bleomycin, *Lung* 161:287-300, 1983.

55. King LG, Drobatz KJ, Hendricks JC: Static thoracic compliance as a measurement of pulmonary function in dogs, *Am J Vet Res* 52(10):1597-1601, 1991.

56. Mitzer W, Blosser B, Yager D: Effect of bronchial smooth muscle contraction on lung compliance, *J Appl Physiol* 72:158-167, 1992.

57. West JB: Restrictive diseases. In West JB, editor: *Pulmonary pathophysiology: The essentials,* ed 5, Baltimore 1995, Lippincott Williams & Wilkins.

58. Miller JE, Eyster G, DeYoung B et al: Pulmonary function in dogs with mitral regurgitation, *Am J Vet Res* 47(12):2498-2503, 1986.

59. Hyde DM, Plopper CG, Weir AJ et al: Peribronchiolar fibrosis in lungs of cats chronically exposed to diesel exhaust, *Lab Invest* 52(2):195-206, 1985.

60. Fernandes DJ, Xu KF, Stewart AG: Anti-remodeling drugs for the treatment of asthma: Requirement for animal models of airway remodeling, *Clin Exp Pharmacol Physiol* 28(8):619-629, 2001.

61. Maddox L, Schwartz DA: The pathophysiology of asthma, *Annu Rev Med* 53:477-498, 2002.

62. Norris CR, Samii VF: Clinical, radiographic, and pathologic features of bronchiectasis in cats: 12 cases (1987-1999), *J Am Vet Med Assoc* 216(4):530-534, 2000.

63. Krotje LJ, McAllister HA, Engwalll MJA: Chronic obstructive pulmonary disease in a dog, *J Am Vet Med Assoc* 191(11):1427-1430, 1987.

64. Haskins SC: Monitoring the anesthetized patient, *Vet Clin North Am Small Anim Pract* 22(2):425-431, 1992.

65. King LG, Hendricks JC: Use of positive-pressure ventilation in dogs and cats: 41 cases (1990-1992), *J Am Vet Med Assoc* 204(7):1045-1052, 1994.

66. Campbell VL, King LG:. Pulmonary function, ventilator management, and outcome of dogs with thoracic trauma and pulmonary contusions: 10 cases (1994-1998), *J Am Vet Med Assoc* 217(10):1505-1509, 2000.

67. Bone RC: Monitoring ventilatory mechanics in acute respiratory failure, *Respir Care* 28:597-604, 1983.

68. Parent C, King LG, Walker LM et al: Clinical and clinicopathologic findings in dogs with acute respiratory distress syndrome: 19 cases (1985-1993), *J Am Vet Med Assoc* 208(9):1419-1427, 1996.

69. Beal MW, Paglia DT, Griffin GM et al: Ventilatory failure, ventilator management, and outcome in dogs with cervical spinal disorders: 14 cases (1991-1999), *J Am Vet Med Assoc* 218(10):1598-1602, 2001.

70. Stobie D, Caywood DD, Rozanski EA et al: Evaluation of pulmonary function and analgesia in dogs after intercostal thoracotomy and use of morphine administered intramuscularly or intrapleurally and bupivacaine administered intrapleurally, *Am J Vet Res* 56(8):1098-1109, 1995.

71. Robinson NE, Sonea I: The adrenergic and cholinergic nervous systems in the lung: Physiology, comparative aspects and therapeutic perspectives, *State-of-the-Art Presentation, Proceedings of the 15th Comparative Respiratory Symposium* 1-5, 1997.

72. Blaber LC, Fryer AD, Maclagan J: Neuronal muscarinic receptors attenuate vagally-induced contraction of feline smooth muscle, *Br J Pharmacol* 86(3):723-728, 1985.

73. Leff AR: State of the art: Endogenous regulation of bronchomotor tone, *Am Rev Respir Dis* 137:1198-1216, 1988.

74. Irwin CG, Boileua R, Tremblay J et al: Bronchodilation: Noncholinergic, nonadrenergic mediation demonstrated in vivo in the cat, *Science* 207(4432):791-792, 1980.

75. Diamond L, O'Donnel M: A nonadrenergic vagal inhibitory pathway to feline airways, *Science* 208(4440):185-188, 1980.

76. Ellis JL, Undem BJ: Pharmacology of non-adrenergic non-cholinergic nerves in airway smooth muscle, *Pulm Pharmacol* 7:205-223, 1994.

77. Russel JA: Responses of isolated canine airways to electrical stimulation and acetylcholine, *J Appl Physiol* 45:690-695, 1978.

78. Andersson P, Persson H: Effect of substance P on pulmonary resistance and dynamic compliance in the anesthetized cat and guinea-pig, *Acta Pharmacol Toxicol (Copenh)* 41(5):444-448, 1997.

79. Diamond L, Szarek JL, Gillespie MN: Substance P fails to mimic vagally mediated nonadrenergic bronchodilation, *Peptides* 3(1):27-29, 1982.

80. Jammes Y, Barthelemy P, Delpierre S: Respiratory effects of cold air breathing in anesthetized cats, *Respir Physiol* 54(1):41-54, 1983.

81. Underwood DC, Kadowitz PJ: Analysis of bronchoconstrictor responses to platelet-activating factor in the cat, *J Appl Physiol* 67(1):377-382, 1989.

82. Skaburskis M, Shardonofsky F, Millic-Emili J: Effect of serotonin on expiratory pulmonary resistance in cats, *J Appl Physiol* 68(6):2419-2425, 1990.

83. Katsumata U, Miura M, Ichinose M et al: Oxygen radicals produce airway constriction and hyperresponsiveness in anesthetized cats, *Am Rev Respir Dis* 141(5 pt 1):1158-1161, 1990.

84. Dyson MC, Kadowitz PJ: Influence of SK&F 96148 on thromboxane-mediated responses in the airways of the cat, *Eur J Pharmacol* 197(1):17-25, 1991.

85. Dyson MC, Kadowitz PJ: Analysis of responses to endothelins 1, 2, and 3 and sarafotoxin 6b in airways of the cat, *J Appl Physiol* 71(1):243-251, 1991.

86. Diamond L, Szarck JL, Gillespie MN et al: In vivo bronchodilator activity of vasoactive intestinal peptide in the cat, *Am Rev Respir Dis* 128(5):827-832, 1983.

87. Chand N, Eyre P: Atypical (relaxant) response to histamine in cat bronchus, *Agents Actions* 7(2):183-190, 1977.

88. Spannake EW, Levin JL, Hyman AI: 6-keto-PGE-1 exhibits more potent bronchodilatory activity in the cat than its precursor, PGI-2, *Prostaglandins* 21(2): 267-275, 1981.

89. Blaber LC, Fryer AD: The response of cat airways to histamine in vivo and in vitro, *Br J Pharmacol* 86(3):309-316, 1985.

90. Aizawa H, Tanaka H, Sakai J et al: L-NAME-sensitive and -insensitive nonadrenergic noncholinergic relaxation of cat airway in vivo and in vitro, *Eur Respir J* 10(2):314-321, 1997.

91. Aizawa H, Takata S, Inoue H et al: Role of nitric oxide released from iNANC neurons in airway responsiveness in cats, *Eur Respir J* 13(4):775-780, 1999.

92. Boushey HA, Holtzman MJ, Seller JR: State of the art: Bronchial hyperreactivity, *Am Rev Respir Dis* 121:389-412, 1980.

93. Juniper EF, Frith PA, Hargreave FE: Airway responsiveness to histamine and methacholine: Relationship of minimum treatment to control symptoms of asthma, *Thorax* 36:575-579, 1981.

94. Holtzman MJ, Morton JD, Shornick LP et al: Immunity, inflammation, and remodeling in the airway epithelial barrier: Epithelial-viral-allergic paradigm, *Physiol Rev* 82(1):19-46, 2002.

95. Clark WT, Jones BR, Clark J: Dynamic pulmonary compliance as a measurement of lung function in dogs, *Vet Record* 101:497-499, 1977.

96. Knudson RJ, Lebowitz MD, Holberg CJ: Changes in the normal maximal expiratory flow-volume curve with growth and aging, *Am Rev Respir Dis* 127:725-734, 1983.

97. Mutoh T, Kanamaru A, Tsubone H et al: Respiratory reflexes in response to nasal administration of halothane to anesthetized, spontaneously breathing dogs, *Am J Vet Res* 61(3):260-267, 2000.

98. Conti G, Dell'Utri D, Vilardi V et al: Propofol induces bronchodilation in mechanically ventilated chronic obstructive pulmonary disease (COPD) patients, *Acta Anaesthesiol Scand* 37(1):105-109, 1993.

99. Holzgrefe HH, Everitt JM, Wright EM:. Alpha-chloralose as a canine anesthetic, *Lab Anim Sci* 37(5):587-595, 1987.

100. Grad R, Witten ML, Quan SF et al: Intravenous choralose is a safe anesthetic for longitudinal use in beagle puppies, *Lab Anim Sci* 38(4):422-425, 1988.

101. Silverman J, Muir WW III: A review of laboratory animal anesthesia with chloral hydrate and chloralose, *Lab Anim Sci* 43(3): 210-216, 1993.

102. Storer RJ, Butler P, Hoskin KL et al: A simple method, using 2-hydroxypropyl-beta-cyclodextran, of administering alpha-chloralose at room temperature, *J Neurosci Methods* 77(1):49-53, 1997.

103. Malis DJ, Burton DM: Safe pediatric outpatient sedation: The chloral hydrate debate revisited, *Otolaryngol Head Neck Surg* 116(1): 53-57, 1997.
104. Malviya S, Voepel-Lewis T, Prochaska G et al: Prolonged recovery and delayed side effects of sedation for diagnostic imaging studies in children, *Pediatrics* 105(3):E42, 2000.
105. Croffie JM, Ellet ML, Lou Q et al: A comparison of the effect of three sedatives on esophageal sphincters in cats, *Dig Dis* 17(2):113-120, 1999.
106. Lodrup Carlsen KC: Tidal breathing at all ages, *Monaldi Arch Chest Dis* 55(5):427-434, 2000.
107. Lodrup Carlsen KC, Carlsen KH: Inhaled nebulized adrenaline improves lung function in infants with acute bronchiolitis, *Respir Med* 94(7):709-714, 2000.
108. Emralino F, Steel AM: Effects of technique and analytic conditions on tidal breathing flow volume loops in term neonates, *Pediatr Pulmonol* 24(2):86-92, 1997.
109. Paetow U, Windstetter D, Schmalisch G: Variability of tidal breathing flow-volume loops in healthy and sick newborns, *Am J Perinatol* 16(10):549-559, 1999.
110. Vollmer WM, McCamant LE, Johnson LR et al: Long-term reproducibility of tests of small airways function: Comparison with spirometry, *Chest* 92(2):303-307, 1990.
111. American Thoracic Society/European Respiratory Society: Respiratory mechanics in infants: Physiologic evaluation in health and disease. A statement of the Committee on Infant Pulmonary Function Testing, *Am Rev Respir Dis* 147:474-496, 1993.
112. Selbie RD, Fletcher M, Arestis N et al: Respiratory function parameters in infants using inductive plethysmography, *Med Eng Phys* 19(6):501-511, 1997.
113. Hoffman AM, Dhupa N, Cimetti L: Airway reactivity measured by barometric whole-body plethysmography in healthy cats, *Am J Vet Res* 60(12):1487-1492, 1999.
114. Rozanski EA, Hoffman AM: Lung function and inhaled albuterol in cats with asthma, *Proceedings 17th ACVIM Forum* 725, 1999.
115. Wiester MJ, Gabriel TT, Steven MA et al: Changes in arterial oxyhemoglobin saturation during histamine-induced bronchoconstriction correlates with changes in SRAW and FEV1 in humans, *Am J Respir Crit Care Med* 151(4):A395, 1995.

CHAPTER 24

Lung Mechanics Using Plethysmography and Spirometry

Elizabeth A. Rozanski • Andrew M. Hoffman

Background Physiology and Definition

The goal of pulmonary function testing (PFT) is to provide an objective evaluation of the efficiency of the respiratory system to move air (ventilate) and exchange gases. Historically, in veterinary medicine, assessment of these two main features of the respiratory system has been subjective, largely based on clinical examination. Recently, arterial blood gas analysis, end-tidal CO_2 analysis, and pulse oximetry have become popular as measures of gas exchange and ventilation, but they do not provide a measure of lung mechanics (i.e., the amount of work required by the animal to maintain those blood gases or saturation). Hence the weakness in veterinary pulmonology is in the area of ventilation and lung mechanics, which constitute half of the picture.

The first lung function tests were described over 150 years ago by Hutchinson, who described a method of measuring vital capacity.[1] Since that time, measurement of lung volume has become routine in both the physiology laboratory and the physician's office. PFT is routinely used in human medicine to provide an objective assessment of pulmonary function and a method for judging response to therapy. In veterinary medicine, PFT is most widely used to assess horses presenting with cough or exercise intolerance.[2] In small animal practice, PFT has been largely used in university settings.[3-6] PFT that has been described in small animal practice includes spirometry and tidal breathing flow-volume loop analysis, plethysmography, and measurement of compliance and resistance.[3-6] This chapter discusses the advantages and limitations of spirometry and plethysmography. Both techniques are currently available and have value for case management, particularly in critical care settings.

Lung Volume Testing

Measurement of lung volumes (Figure 24-1) leads to a better understanding of pathophysiology, especially in the dyspneic patient. There are two major lung volume categories: dynamic lung volumes, including volumes that are displaced with breathing, and static lung volumes, which include gas trapped in the chest.

The dynamic lung volumes include tidal volume (TV), inspiratory reserve volume (IRV), expiratory reserve volume (ERV), and vital capacity (VC). The TV is the amount of air in an average breath at rest, usually 10 to 20 ml/kg in small animals. Functional residual capacity (FRC) is the amount of air remaining in the lungs after tidal expiration. IRV is the amount of air that can be inspired in excess of the normal tidal breath, whereas ERV is the amount of air that can be exhaled in excess of the normal tidal expiration. Residual volume (RV) is the air remaining in the lungs after ERV.

Vital capacity (VC) refers to the sum of ERV, TV, and IRV. Total lung capacity (TLC) is the sum of VC and residual volume (RV) and includes both static (RV) and dynamic (VC) lung volumes. Static volumes include the FRC and the RV. ERV is a dynamic volume that represents the difference between FRC and RV.

Dynamic lung volume measurements are typically measured with a device called a spirometer, a simple instrument that is calibrated to measure volumes. Historically, spirometers have used a water-sealed chamber system, although today many spirometers are electronic. Hand-held spirometers are also available and are used to some extent in evaluating lung volume in dogs and cats. The spirometer is capable of accurately measuring tidal volume and minute ventilation in individual patients (Figure 24-2). It may be attached to an airtight face mask or connected to an endotracheal tube. In addition, a spirometer may be used to accurately measure the volume of air delivered to a patient by a mechanical ventilator. In ventilated patients, large discrepancies may exist between the calculated tidal volume and the actual delivered tidal volume due to the compliance of the ventilatory circuit and its relation to the size of the patient. Whereas the spirometer is not widely used as a pulmonary function tool, it is commonly used in the intensive care unit to better assess ventilated patients and animals with potential hypoventilation.

Static lung volume (FRC and VC) measurement requires a different technique.[1,7] Most commonly, an inert gas dilution method is used; however, plethysmography is considered the gold standard. Gas dilution methodology requires the patient to breathe a known concentration of helium. Helium is relatively insoluble in blood, and over time the concentrations in the lung and the rebreathing device will equilibrate and reach a steady state. Using the equation:

$$C_1 \times V_1 = C_2 \times (V_1 + V_2)$$

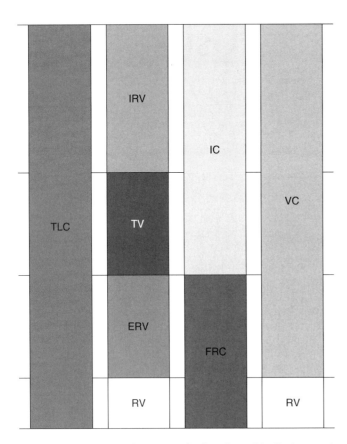

Figure 24-1. Lung volumes are displayed graphically. Lung volumes include tidal volume (TV), inspiratory reserve volume (IRV), expiratory reserve volume (ERV), vital capacity (VC), total lung capacity (TLC), residual volume (RV), and functional residual capacity (FRC).

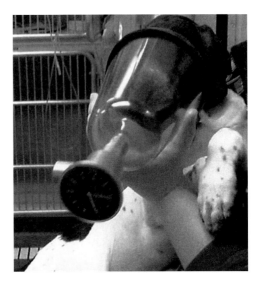

Figure 24-2. A hand-held spirometer may be used to measure tidal volume and minute ventilation in an awake patient using a face mask.

where C equals the concentration of helium and V equals volume, solving for V_2 will result in the determination of FRC:

$$V_2 = V_1 \ (C_1 - C_2)/C_2$$

The starting volume (V_1) and starting concentration of helium (C_1) must be known, and steady state measurements are required for accurate calculations. However, in individuals with air trapping, the FRC measured by plethysmography is greater and more accurate than that measured by helium dilution.

Body plethysmography is a very effective research tool in small animals, but as currently performed requires anesthesia.[8] The technique is based on Boyle's law, which states that there is a constant relationship between pressure (P) and volume (V) at a constant temperature, or mathematically, $P_1 \times V_1 = P_2 \times V_2$. Standard methodology used in plethysmography designed for human use typically includes an airtight box (the plethysmograph) in which the subject sits and breathes through a mouthpiece. The mouthpiece contains a shutter that may be opened and closed electronically. The subject is asked to breathe against the closed shutter at end-expiratory lung volume. Changes in the pressure measured at the mouth (reflecting alveolar pressure) and the changes in pressure in the box (reflecting thoracic gas volume) are recorded. FRC is then calculated as follows:

$$\frac{\Delta V}{\Delta P} \times (P_B - P_{H_2O}) = FRC$$

where ΔV = change in volume, ΔP = change in pressure, P_B = barometeric pressure, and P_{H_2O} = water vapor pressure. In practice, the use of plethysmography requires several assumptions.[7] First, we assume that there is no flow during respiratory efforts against a closed airway, hence FRC is a static lung volume. This assumption is important in validating that the mouth pressure (airway opening pressure, P_{ao}) is equivalent to alveolar pressure (P_{alv}). Theoretically, airflow could occur within the upper airways (shunting) and result in underestimation of alveolar pressure and thus the overestimation of FRC. Practically this has not been a problem except in individuals with significant lower airway obstruction. The second assumption is that changes in pressure are uniform across the lung (i.e., $P_{ao} = P_{alv}$). If pressure changes were not uniform (e.g., in patients with air trapping) this would, in theory, result in measurement of a lower FRC. The final assumption is that air in the gastrointestinal tract is either insignificant or not compressed during occlusion, which is generally true. Despite the need to make these assumptions, there is no question that plethysmographic measurements can be accurately made in small animals under anesthesia in special cases.

In the future, a more user-friendly method will likely employ steady state helium dilution and a computer for rapid results. Finally, FRC can also be computed from CT scans of the chest, but these measurements require 3-D reconstructions and include a tissue component that overestimates FRC.

Barometric Plethysmography for Measurement of Spirometric Indices in Normal Animals

Barometric whole-body plethysmography (BWBP) is a noninvasive method of measuring pulmonary function that has recently been validated in cats.[9] The origin of this method dates back to studies of Neergard (1926– and later, Jaeger (1964), Ingram (1966), and McLead (1971)—that describe marked discrepancies in volume displacement measured at the body surface versus the airway opening at the mouth or nose.[10-13] The difference in volume displacement measured by spirometry (mouth) and plethysmography (body surface) relates to both static and dynamic characteristics of the lung, including lung volume (TV and FRC), resistance to airflow (lung resistance, R_L), the compressibility of thoracic gas, and breathing frequency.[11]

For example, tidal volume measured by plethysmography (volume displacement of the chest and abdomen) is greater than that measured by spirometry (true volume displacement at the mouth) in the presence of:
- Increased lung volume
- Increased R_L as gas behind an obstruction is compressed; as lung resistance increases, the plethysmography and spirometry difference is increased
- Decreased barometric pressure (i.e., high altitude associated with decreased barometric pressure and increased compressibility of gas)
- Increased breathing frequency, which increases the phase lag in the face of gas compression

Barometric whole-body plethysmography (BWBP) is based on the same concept, except that the changes are measured as a net effect during tidal breathing rather than compared as individual signals. In animals, similar phase and magnitude shift was found using double chamber plethysmography.[14] Later this observation was extended to single chamber plethysmography as well.[15,16] BWBP is performed by placing the patient within a single chamber plethysmograph (Figure 24-3).

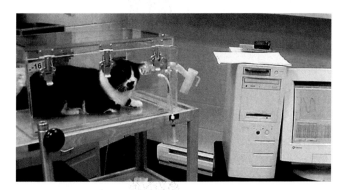

Figure 24-3. *Barometric whole-body plethysmography is performed by placing a cat within a plethysmograph. Note that the cat is free to move about and appears to be resting comfortably.*

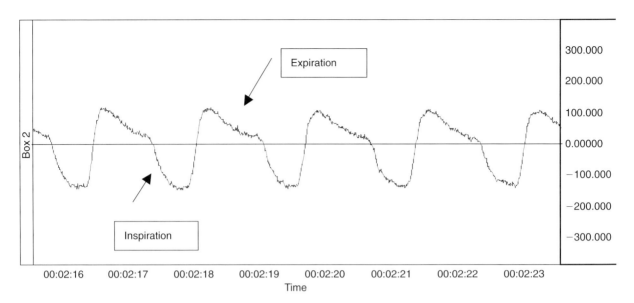

Figure 24-4. *Barometric whole-body plethysmography signal from a normal cat. The inspiratory and expiratory phases are indicated.*

The plethysmograph chamber is airtight, except that it is ventilated with a known bias flow, and a single-screen pneumotachograph with a known resistance is mounted on one wall allowing for a controlled leak of air. A differential pressure transducer sensing changes within the chamber is connected to a preamplifier and a pulmonary function computer. The animal is able to move around the chamber at will.

The breathing pattern is assessed by analysis of the box-pressure signals that vary during breathing. The signals associated with normal unobstructed breathing appear graphically similar to flow signals produced by conventional pneumotachography (Figure 24-4). These signals are produced as the net result of thoracic and nasal airflow causing pressure changes within the plethysmograph. Although these signals are always equal and opposite, warming of the air causes the thoracic volume change to slightly exceed the nasal volume change. Therefore, the net change in chamber pressure is the difference between thoracic and nasal flow. The normal BWBP signal is a measure of the normal difference in lung volume in the chest compared with that at the mouth/nose during a breath. This is in contrast to spirometry with a pneumotachograph that measures flow through the upper airway (nose and mouth).

Baseline values of standard respiratory parameters (e.g., tidal volume and respiratory rate) obtained in healthy cats were similar to those reported in awake, untrained cats during analysis of tidal breathing flow-volume loops acquired with a face mask and an associated pneumotachograph.[5] Cats in particular are very tolerant of BWBP and seem to be very comfortable during testing. In fact, in the distressed cat, 100% oxygen may be used instead of conventional room air bias flow with-

out invalidating the results and with a substantial improvement in patient comfort.

Barometric Whole Body Plethysmography for Measurement of Airway Obstruction

Barometric whole body plethysmography is also an effective method to evaluate patients with airway obstruction. Resistance causes gas expansion during inspiration and compression during expiration, thereby resulting in an increased difference between displacements of volume at the nose (mouth) and body surface. BWBP has been validated in rodents and cats as an alternative noninvasive method of assessing experimental bronchoconstriction.[9,17] During airway obstruction, the signal is created by increased resistance and gas compression in response to increasing airflow limitations and magnified due to discrepancies in thoracic and nasal volumes complicated by a phase lag. The increased pressure changes within the chamber result in the visual appearance of a changed signal (Figure 24-5). In conventional pulmonary function testing, lung resistance (R_L) measurements are thought to reflect narrowing of the larger diameter airways. Using conventional techniques, pause and enhanced pause are two unitless variables that correlate with R_L. In a small group of cats with naturally occurring bronchoconstriction due to asthma, values of pause and enhanced pause were increased when compared with healthy cats; and importantly, these values decreased towards normal following therapy with a bronchodilator.[18] BWBP detects both upper and lower airway diseases be-

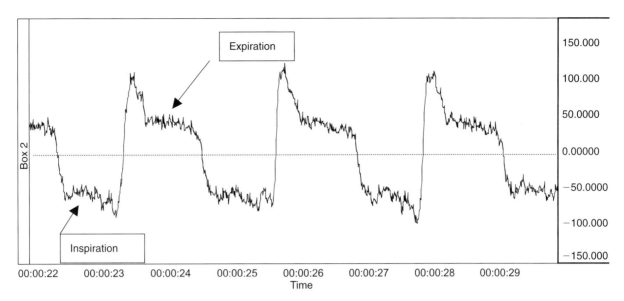

Figure 24-5. *Barometric whole-body plethysmography signal from a cat with bronchoconstriction due to feline asthma. The inspiratory and expiratory phases are marked. Note the difference in signal appearance compared with Figure 24-4.*

cause any site of airway obstruction will result in increased pressure changes associated with breathing.

Barometric Whole Body Plethysmography for Testing Airway Reactivity

Airway reactivity or bronchoprovocation testing is performed in people and in horses in an attempt to detect airway disease (e.g., inflammatory airway disease or chronic obstructive pulmonary disease) earlier in its course. It is also used in individuals with intermittent signs, and to detect response to various treatments. Airway reactivity testing is not performed if bronchoconstriction is already present at initial examination. Classically, bronchoprovocation to test airway reactivity is performed until a set increase occurs from the baseline value of R_L (e.g., a doubling [R_{L200}]) due to narrowing of the airway in response to an agent such as histamine or methacholine. As in naturally occurring bronchoconstriction, pause and enhanced pause have been shown in rodents to correlate with R_L and pleural pressure changes caused by aerosol bronchoprovocation challenges.[19] In cats exposed to the bronchoconstrictive agent carbachol by aerosol, pause and enhanced pause greatly increased during bronchoconstriction.[9] A recent report suggests that airway reactivity diminishes with advancing age in cats.

In small animal patients, airway reactivity has not been widely tested; however, as BWBP becomes more widely available, reactivity testing may become more widespread, particularly in animals with intermittent signs or those in which other diagnostic tests do not elucidate the underlying disease.

Barometric Whole Body Plethysmography for Monitoring Response to Therapy

BWBP is also useful for monitoring patients over time. The test is noninvasive and well tolerated by most small animal patients. Commonly, animals with airway disease require long-term medication and frequent veterinary examinations. BWBP, particularly coupled with reactivity testing, is a useful ancillary method to follow patient progress. BWBP may also be useful to assess the success of airway surgeries (e.g., for brachycephalic airway syndrome or laryngeal paralysis), as well as for immediate assessment of the effect of bronchodilator therapy.[6,17,18]

Indications

Spirometry is indicated to assess tidal volume in patients receiving mechanical ventilation and to assess the adequacy of spontaneous respiratory efforts in animals with lower motor neuron disease, those being weaned from neuromuscular blocking agents, or those recovering from anesthesia.

Barometric whole-body plethysmography is useful to assess a patient with potential airway disease and then to assess the response to therapeutic intervention. Particular indications for cats include (1) asthma or suspected asthma, (2) following therapy for asthma, (3) those animals with intermittent poorly localizing signs of respiratory disease, and (4) suspected fixed airway obstructions. In dogs, specific indications include chronic bronchitis or collapsing trachea. Because some dogs are prone to panting when confined within a plethysmograph, it may be impossible to get adequate measurements. Light sedation may be used, but may result in bronchodilation. BWBP may also be used in exotic pets such as birds, small mammals, and even pot-bellied pigs.

Contraindications

There are no specific patient contraindications to spirometry or plethysmography. Tachypnea or panting at low tidal volumes will invalidate plethysmography results. Animals that are clearly in respiratory distress and appear to have extra-airway sources of disease (e.g., pleural effusion) will not benefit from lung function testing, except if it is needed to exclude concurrent airway obstruction.

Instrumentation and Technique

Hand-held spirometers are available from a number of sources. Pulmonary function computers are less widely available for veterinary use. Buxco Electronics* has marketed the most widely used software and computers designed for pulmonary function testing in clinical small animal medicine, as well as in research settings. A complete discussion of pulmonary function equipment is beyond the scope of this article; however, an understanding of commonly required equipment may be helpful.

In general, pulmonary function equipment and software is designed to calculate pressure, volume, and flow changes. These changes reflect the work the pulmonary system is doing in order to maintain adequate oxygenation and ventilation. For classic pulmonary function testing involving measurement of static or dynamic compliance (C_{stat} or C_{dyn}) and lung resistance (R_L), measurements of flow and pressure are required. Flow (ml/sec) may be measured by a face mask and pneumotachograph and integrated to give volume (ml). Practically, because flow in the healthy patient is sinusoidal, computer-based calculations are much more accurate than hand measurements. Pressure measurements typically require placement of an esophageal balloon in the midthoracic esophagus to approximate transpulmonary pressure. The relationship of pressure to flow and volume during various points in the respiratory cycle is used to calculate the desired values. The units for C_{stat} or C_{dyn} are ml/cm H_2O; and for R_L, cm H_2O/L/sec.

*Buxco Electronics, Sharon, Conn.

In BWBP, different equipment is used. A plethysmograph is an airtight box, constructed of Plexiglas, that is ventilated with a bias flow of room air or 100% oxygen. The bias flow is recommended to prevent over-heating, which will diminish the signal, and also to prevent carbon dioxide retention in the chamber. A single screen pneumotachograph with a known resistance is attached to a corner wall. The pneumotachograph is calibrated before use. To limit the impact of minor barometric pressure changes, a differential pressure transducer is mounted on a neighboring wall with one port open to the chamber and the other port open to a reference chamber. The pressure transducer is connected to a pre-amplifier data acquisition card and then to the computer. The software program recognizes real-time pressure changes and records and stores data for later analysis. Parameters that are recorded by the computer include: peak inspiratory flow (PIF); peak expiratory flow (PEF); tidal volume (TV); end-inspiratory pause (EIP); end-expiratory pause (EEP); frequency (f); expiratory time (Te); inspiratory time (Ti); relaxation time (RT, the time for box pressure to decay to 30% of total box pressure during expiration); pause ([Te/Rt]−1); and enhanced pause (PENH=(Te/[0.3 × RT]−1 × PEF/[PIF × 0.67]).

During BWBP, the patient is placed in the chamber and allowed to relax during data collection. After baseline data collection, further testing may be pursued. Bronchoprovocation (airway reactivity) may be performed if baseline values are not abnormal, and therapeutic interventions (e.g., Beta-2 agonists) may be used if bronchoconstriction is present.

Interpretation

Interpretation of spirometry is based on knowledge of a normal tidal volume for a particular patient and, in general, is defined as either adequate or inadequate. In the awake patient, application of a face mask may influence breathing pattern and possibly result in an increased tidal breath, so appreciation of hyperpnea is limited.

Interpretation of barometric whole-body plethysmography is based on comparison of results with known normal values. In cats, published normal values exist and are listed in Table 24-1, although is likely prudent for the individual laboratory to create its own normal values.[5,9] As previously mentioned, airway reactivity was found to decline with age in healthy cats. No normal values for BWBP have yet been reported in dogs, per-

TABLE 24-1. Selected Barometric Whole Body Plethysmography (BWBP) Values (± SEM) and Values (± SD) Derived From Tidal-Breathing Flow-Volume Loop (TBFVL) Data for Normal Cats[5,9]

	Ti	Te	TV	PEF	PIF	Rate
BWBP	470 ± 40	730 ± 100	35 ± 4	83 ± 12	109 ± 8	58 ± 8
TBFVL	716 ± 139	704 ± 133	58 ± 15	114 ± 29	111 ± 27	43 ± 7

Ti = Inspiratory time in msec; *Te* = expiratory time in msec; *TV* = tidal volume in ml; *PEF* = peak expiratory flow in ml/sec; *PIF* = peak inspiratory flow in ml/sec; *Rate* = respiratory rate in breaths/min. Note (see text) that flow measurements are not representative of the same signal.

haps due to their tendency to pant when confined. In particular, for animals with suspected bronchoconstriction, the values for pause and enhanced pause should be carefully evaluated. Cats with bronchoconstriction have increased values of pause and enhanced pause, as well as changes in signal characteristics (see Figures 24-4, and 24-5). Results may also be interpreted serially following a change in the patient's clinical condition or following a therapeutic intervention. Longitudinal data collection will also allow for long-term follow-up on individual patients, as well as on a variety of patient populations.

Barometric whole-body plethysmography represents an exciting area of pulmonary function testing in small animal patients. In particular, the utility of this form of testing includes its ability to test animals with respiratory distress and its completely noninvasive nature.

REFERENCES

1. Brown RA: Derivation, application and utility of static lung volume measurements, *Resp Care Clin NA* 3(2):183-220, 1997.
2. Hoffman AM, Mazan MR: Programme of lung function testing horses suspected with small airway disease, *Equine Vet Educ* 11:322-328, 1999.
3. Dye J: Feline bronchopulmonary disease, *Vet Clin North Am Small Anim Pract* 22:1187-1201, 1992.
4. McKiernan BC, Johnson LR: Clinical pulmonary function testing in dogs and cats, *Vet Clin North Am Small Anim Pract* 22:1087-1098, 1992.
5. McKiernan BC, Dye JA, Rozanski EA: Tidal breathing flow-volume loops (TBFVL) in healthy and bronchitic cats, *J Vet Int Med* 7:388-393, 1993.
6. Amis TC, Smith MM, Gaber CE et al: Upper airway obstruction in canine laryngeal paralysis, *Am J Vet Res* 47(5):1007-1010, 1986.
7. Coates AL, Peslin R, Rodenstein D et al: Measurements of lung volumes by plethysmography, *Eur Respir J* 10:1415-1427, 1997.
8. Lourenco RV, Chung SY: Calibration of a body plethysmograph for measurement of lung volume, *Am Rev Resp Dis* 95:687-688, 1967.
9. Hoffman AM, Dhupa N, Cimetti L: Airway reactivity measured by barometric whole-body plethysmography in healthy cats, *Am J Vet Res* 60(12):1487-1492, 1999.
10. Neergaard KV, Wirz K: *Messung der stromungswiderstande in den atemwegen des menschen, insbesondere bei asthma und emphysme*, Stachelin R, Berlin, 1926, Med Universitatsklinik Basel.
11. Jaegar MJ, Otis AB: Effects of compressibility of alveolar gas on dynamics and work of breathing, *J Appl Physiol* 19:83-91, 1964.
12. Ingram RH Jr., Schilder DP: Effect of gas compression on pulmonary pressure, flow, and volume relationship, *J Appl Physiol* 21(6):1821-1826, 1966.
13. MacLeod JP, Taylor NWG, Mackelm PT: Phase differences between gas displacement by the thorax and at the airway opening, *Bull Physio-path Resp* 7:433-440, 1971.
14. Pennock BE, Cox CP, Rogers RM et al: A noninvasive technique for measurement of changes in specific airway resistance, *J Applied Physiol* 46(2):399-406, 1979.
15. Dorsch W, Waldherr U, Rosmanith J: Continuous recording of intrapulmonary "compressed air" as a sensitive noninvasive method of measuring bronchial obstruction in guinea pigs, *Euro Journal of Physiol* 391(3):236-241, 1981.
16. Pennock BE: Rib cage and abdominal piezoelectric film belts to measure ventilatory airflow, *J Clin Monit* 6:276-283, 1990.
17. Hamelmann E, Schwarze J, Takeda K et al: Noninvasive measurement of airway responsiveness in allergic mice using barometric plethysmography, *Amer J Resp Crit Care Med* 156:766-775, 1997.
18. Rozanski EA, Hoffman AM: Lung function and inhaled albuterol in cats with asthma, *JVIM* 13:259, 1999.
19. Bergren DR: Chronic tobacco smoke exposure increases airway sensitivity to capsaicin in awake guinea pigs, *J Appl Physiol* 90:695-704, 2001.

CHAPTER 25

Interpretation of Blood Gas Measurements

Steve C. Haskins

Blood gas analysis is the measurement of partial pressures of carbon dioxide and oxygen in the blood. The partial pressure of carbon dioxide in arterial blood defines alveolar minute ventilation. End-tidal and venous blood carbon dioxide measurements, under many circumstances, can be used to estimate arterial carbon dioxide. The partial pressure of oxygen in arterial blood defines the ability of the lungs to oxygenate the blood. Hemoglobin saturation is directly related to the partial pressure of oxygen and, under many circumstances, can be used to approximate the partial pressure of oxygen. The oxygen content of blood is highly dependent on hemoglobin concentration and is important to oxygen delivery. Mixed venous oxygen reflects the balance between oxygen delivery and oxygen consumption; it cannot be used to approximate arterial oxygen and is interpreted with an independent set of rules.

Collection and Storage of Blood Samples Intended for Blood Gas Analysis

Blood should be collected anaerobically. Exposure to air could lower the Pco_2 and change the Po_2 in the sample toward that of room air (0 and 150 mm Hg at sea level, respectively). Small air bubbles that sometimes occur during blood sampling should be avoided; if they occur, they should be immediately expelled from the sample as soon as it is collected. They are not likely to measurably change the analyzed blood gas values because the surface area for gas exchange is small and the exposure time is short. Strong negative pressure when sampling should be avoided because this may pull gases out of solution.[1]

The collector should be sure of the vessel from which the sample is obtained. Arteries and veins are usually adjacent to one another, and the two sample sources generate different measured values, which must be interpreted in the context of their source (Table 25-1).[2]

The sample should be analyzed immediately after collection to minimize *in vitro* metabolic changes to the values of interest. Nucleated white blood cells and platelets consume oxygen and produce carbon dioxide. Red blood cells consume glucose and produce lactic acid that, via carbonic acid, increases carbon dioxide. Important changes in the measured blood gas values may occur with room temperature storage times of as little as 10 minutes.[3] If the analysis cannot be made immediately, the sample should be stored in ice water (ice without water is not sufficient because air pockets prevent efficient cooling). At 4° C, *in vitro* metabolism is slowed to such an extent that samples can be stored for up to 6 hours without important changes in the measured values.[4] The Pco_2 and Po_2 measurements both tend to increase slightly over time with the use of plastic syringes (oxygen diffuses from the plastic into the blood sample faster than it is metabolized by the nucleated blood cells). With glass syringes, the Po_2 tends to decrease over time.[5,6]

Dilution of the blood sample by anticoagulant will also change the measured values. Heparin has a pH of about 5.8, a bicarbonate of about zero, a Pco_2 of about 5 mm Hg, and a Po_2 of about 165 mm Hg. The dead space of a 3-ml syringe and needle is slightly less than 0.1 ml. This represents a 9% dilution of a 1-ml blood sample and a 3% dilution of a 3-ml blood sample. A 9% dilution of a whole blood sample with heparin could decrease the Pco_2 by 11%.[1] It would also tend to change the Po_2, but since oxygen is poorly soluble in water, it may not change the measured value very much. Sample dilution should be minimized and, most importantly, should be consistent between samples.

Measurement and Corrections to Measured Values

Air bubbles are sometimes accidentally injected or aspirated into the analyzer during sample introduction. When they come to rest on the measuring membrane, it will increase the measured Po_2 and decrease the measured Pco_2. The blood sample at the electrode membrane should be visually inspected. Measurements marked with error codes on the analyzer print-out should be repeated. Measurements that seem unbelievable, with respect to the patient, should not be believed. The blood should be re-analyzed, and if there is any doubt about the first sample collection procedure, the patient should be re-sampled.

Blood gases are measured at the temperature of the analyzer water bath, usually 37° C. When the animal's body temperature is different from that of the water bath, *in vitro* changes in the blood gas values occur, associated with the change in temperature of the blood sample (Table 25-2).[3] This difference is caused by changes in the solubility of the gas. An increase in temperature decreases solubility and increases the measured

TABLE 25-2. **The Effect of Temperature on Acid-Base Variables**[3]

°C	°F	pH	Pco_2 (mm Hg)	HCO_3 (mmol/L)	Po_2 (mm Hg)
25	77	7.58	24	22	37
30	86	7.5	30	22.7	51
35	95	7.43	37	23.5	70
37	99	7.40	40	24	80
40	104	7.36	45	24	97

TABLE 25-1. **Mixed, Jugular, and Cephalic Venous Acid-Base Values Compared to Arterial for Normal Dogs**[2]

	Arterial	Mixed Venous	Jugular Vein	Cephalic Vein
pH	7.40 ± 0.03	7.36 ± 0.02	7.35 ± 0.02	7.36 ± 0.02
Pco_2 (mm Hg)	37 ± 3	43 ± 4	42 ± 5	43 ± 3
Base deficit (mmol/L)	−2 ± 2	−1 ± 1	−2 ± 2	−1 ± 1
Bicarbonate (mmol/L)	21 ± 2	23 ± 2	22 ± 2	23 ± 1
Total CO_2 (mmol/L)	22 ± 2	24 ± 2	23 ± 2	24 ± 2
Po_2 (mm Hg)	102 ± 7	53 ± 10	55 ± 10	58 ± 9

vapor pressure of the gas. Correcting for *in vitro* temperature changes more accurately reflects the actual values in the patient at the time the blood sample was taken. It would seem to be a more accurate way to report a series of acid-base values when the body temperature of the subject is fluctuating. It is, however, controversial as to whether to correct for these *in vitro* temperature changes when implementing therapy based upon normothermic reference values.[7] In a piglet model of deep hypothermia, neurological recovery was improved if the measurements were corrected to body temperature.[8] Human adults exhibit improved cognitive function if the measured values are not corrected to body temperature.[9] In human infants, there was no difference in neurological outcome either immediately after surgery[10] or at 1-year follow-up[11] whether or not the measured blood gas values were corrected to body temperature.

Carbon Dioxide

Although blood carbon dioxide level is a balance between production and elimination, the latter is by far the more potent determinant. Chemoreceptors regulate alveolar minute ventilation so as to match carbon dioxide elimination with production, and it is appropriate to consider that arterial carbon dioxide defines alveolar minute ventilation.

An acute change in arterial carbon dioxide causes a near-immediate change in the carbon dioxide levels in the CSF and interstitial tissue. Carbon dioxide is very diffusible across the blood brain barrier. An increase in alveolar minute ventilation and cerebral arteriolar vasodilation occurs within minutes of an acute increase in arterial carbon dioxide, and vice versa.[12,13] The central chemoreceptors and cerebral blood vessels are actually responsive to cerebral spinal fluid (CSF) and cerebral interstitial hydrogen ion concentration, not carbon dioxide, per se.[14,15] A change in CSF and cerebral interstitial carbon dioxide causes a proportional change in hydrogen ion concentration (and an inverse change in pH). After a relatively short time, however, CSF and interstitial bicarbonate concentration adjusts to reverse the change in hydrogen concentration caused by the original change in carbon dioxide. Substantial compensatory changes occur within 4 hours, and the process is virtually complete after approximately 24 hours.[16-19] The original ventilatory and arteriolar vasomotor tone response to the acute change in carbon dioxide subsides because the chemore-

ceptors no longer sense an abnormal CSF or cerebral interstitial hydrogen ion concentration.[12,13,18] A return to normal arterial carbon dioxide at this time again causes an acute change in CSF and cerebral tissue pH, which would have the expected effect on ventilation and cerebral vasomotor tone.[12,18]

ARTERIAL Pco$_2$ (Paco$_2$)

The average Paco$_2$ is about 40 mm Hg in normal humans, slightly lower in the dog (37 mm Hg), and considerably lower in the cat (31 mm Hg) (Table 25-3), with a range of 5 mm Hg. In humans, values below 35 mm Hg represent hypocapnia, whereas values above 45 mm Hg represent hypercapnia. These guidelines have generally been extrapolated to veterinary medicine; however, reported values for normal dogs and cats are somewhat different between the species. A measured Paco$_2$ below 32 mm Hg in the dog and 26 mm Hg in the cat represent hyperventilation and respiratory alkalosis. Paco$_2$ values above 43 mm Hg in the dog and 36 mm Hg in the cat represent hypoventilation and respiratory acidosis. The common causes of hyperventilation and hypoventilation are listed in Tables 25-4 and 25-5, respectively.

A Paco$_2$ in excess of 60 mm Hg may be associated with excessive respiratory acidosis and hypoxemia (when breathing room air) and is usually considered to represent sufficient hypoventilation to warrant definitive therapy. Paco$_2$ values below 20 mm Hg are associated with severe respiratory alkalosis and a decreased cerebral bloodflow, which may impair cerebral oxygenation.

VENOUS Pco$_2$ (Pvco$_2$)

Venous blood is separated from arterial blood by a metabolically active tissue bed, which produces carbon dioxide. Pvco$_2$ is always higher than Paco$_2$, but the difference is usually only about 4 to 6 mm Hg (see Table 25-1) in stable states. Almost 75% of the carbon dioxide produced by tissue metabolism is normally carried to the lungs in the form of bicarbonate.[23] Carbon dioxide that has entered the red blood cell is converted (via carbonic acid equilibration) to H^+ and HCO_3^-; the H^+ is buffered by the hemoglobin and the HCO_3^- diffuses out of the red

TABLE 25-4. **Causes of Hypocapnia**
Hypotension
Fever
Sepsis
Excitement
Exercise
Pain
Pulmonary thromboembolism
Early pulmonary parenchymal disease
Cytokine release in the systemic inflammatory response syndrome
Inappropriate ventilator settings
Compensation for metabolic acidosis

TABLE 25-3. **Arterial Blood Gas Values Reported for Normal Individuals**			
	Human[20]	**Dog**[22]	**Cat**[22]
Pco$_2$ (mm Hg)	40 (35-45)	37 (32-43)	31 (26-36)
Pao$_2$ (mm Hg) (sea level, room air)	95 (80-105)	92 (80-105)	105 (95-115)

TABLE 25-5. **Causes of Hypercapnia**

Hypoventilation
  Neuromuscular disorder
  Medullary dysfunction (excessive depths of anesthesia; intracranial disease)
  Cervical disease or neuromuscular disease
Airway obstruction
  Large airway obstruction (laryngeal paralysis; tracheal collapse)
  Small airway obstruction (chronic airway disease; bronchoconstriction)
Thoracic wall problems
  Open pneumothorax
  Flail chest wall
  Anterior displacement of the diaphragm by abdominal space filling disorders
  Pleural space filling disorder (air; fluid; diaphragmatic hernia)
  Pleural fibrosis
Pulmonary parenchymal disease (late)
Inappropriate ventilator settings
Dead space rebreathing
Recent bicarbonate therapy (in ventilatory compromised patients)
Compensation for metabolic acidosis
Malignant hyperthermia

blood cell in exchange for chloride. Only about 10% of the produced carbon dioxide is carried as dissolved carbon dioxide in the plasma. The arterial/venous gradient is greater when there are problems with carbon dioxide carriage such as during anemia,[24] sluggish peripheral bloodflow,[25] or during carbonic anhydrase inhibitor therapy. The arterial/venous gradient will also be greater during transition states, such as when ventilation is improved after chronic hypercapnia. The ability of hemoglobin to bind H^+ is inversely related to oxygen binding (the Haldane effect), therefore high venous oxygen is also associated with impaired carbon dioxide carriage and an increased arterial/venous Pco_2 gradient.

END-TIDAL Pco_2

A sample of gas taken toward the end of an exhalation represents alveolar gas. The alveolar-arterial Pco_2 gradient is normally very small and therefore the measurement of end-tidal Pco_2 is usually a suitable estimate of $Paco_2$. End-tidal Pco_2 is usually slightly lower than $Paco_2$ (1 to 4 mm Hg in dogs).[26,27]

An increase in alveolar dead space ventilation decreases end-tidal Pco_2 (i.e., it increases the alveolar-arterial Pco_2 gradient). Increased alveolar dead space ventilation occurs in pulmonary thromboembolism[28] and hypovolemia.[29] The alveolar-arterial Pco_2 gradient is also increased in tachypnea, caused by mixing of anatomical dead space and alveolar gas and the inability to obtain a pure alveolar gas sample. End-tidal Pco_2 can still be used as a trend monitor; end-tidal measurements should periodically be correlated to a $Paco_2$ measurement.

End-tidal Pco_2 measurement has been promoted as a way of monitoring the effectiveness of artificial circulation during cardiopulmonary resuscitation.[30] In a cardiac arrested, but ventilated model, alveolar Pco_2 is soon the same as inspired (zero). As the chest or heart compression technique improves cardiac output and tissue bloodflow (and the delivery of venous blood to the lungs), end-tidal Pco_2 should increase proportionately. An end-tidal Pco_2 greater than 18 mm Hg was reported to be associated with better outcomes in humans.[31-33]

Oxygen

The amount of oxygen in the blood can be expressed in three different ways: (1) the partial pressure of oxygen dissolved in the plasma (Po_2; units = mm Hg); (2) the percent saturation of the hemoglobin (So_2; units = %); and (3) the whole blood oxygen content (Content O_2; units = milliliters of oxygen per 100 milliliters of whole blood).

If the measurement is meant to assess pulmonary function, an arterial blood sample is required. The dorsal metatarsal or femoral/medial saphenous arteries are most commonly used; however, the brachial, radial, aural, and lingual arteries may also be accessed. Free-flowing capillary blood has also been used to approximate an arterial blood sample for the purposes of oxygen measurements.[34-37]

The venous blood is separated from arterial blood by a metabolically active tissue bed that consumes oxygen. In contrast to venous carbon dioxide, venous oxygen measurements bear no correlation to arterial oxygen measurements and cannot be used to assess pulmonary function. Venous oxygen measurements are interpreted by an entirely different set of criteria (see below).

Cyanosis is a bluish tissue discoloration caused by the presence of unoxygenated hemoglobin. Arterial blood is normally red because the hemoglobin is well oxygenated, and venous blood is normally blue because the hemoglobin is not well oxygenated. An absolute amount of unoxygenated hemoglobin must be present for cyanosis to be visible, although the amount varies with different lighting conditions and observers. It is commonly cited that it takes 5 grams/deciliter of unoxygenated hemoglobin to manifest cyanosis. Anemic patients may suffer severe hypoxemia without manifesting cyanosis. Although hypoxemia (sometimes called central cyanosis) is the most common cause of cyanosis, it is not the only cause. Sluggish peripheral bloodflow (sometimes called peripheral cyanosis) and methemoglobinemia may also cause cyanosis. Cyanosis should always be considered to be a late and serious sign of pulmonary (usually) or cardiovascular (sometimes) failure. It should invoke a feeling of panic and the institution of aggressive oxygen, ventilation, or fluid therapy. It would not be appropriate to delay therapy of cyanosis for the measurement of blood gases.

ARTERIAL Po_2 (Pao_2)

The Po_2 is the vapor pressure of oxygen dissolved in solution in the plasma. It is independent of hemoglobin and is not affected by anemia. It is measured in a blood

TABLE 25-6. Causes of Hypoxemia

Low inspired oxygen concentration

Inadequate supply of oxygen to the breathing circuit

Dead space rebreathing

Hypoventilation (see Table 25-5)

Venous admixture

Low V/Q

Bronchospasm

Airway narrowing due to fluid/exudate accumulation

Small airway/alveolar collapse

Positional stasis especially with hypoventilation

Increased surface tension due to fluid/exudate accumulation

External compression of lung

Diffusion defect

Inhalation injury

Anatomic shunt

R to L patent ductus arteriosus

R to L ventricular septal defect

Low venous oxygen

Low oxygen delivery

Low cardiac output

Any heart dysfunction

Hypovolemia

Low oxygen content

Anemia

Hypoxemia

High oxygen consumption

Hyperthermia

Muscular activity

gas analyzer with a silver anode/platinum cathode system in an electrolyte solution (polarography) separated from the unknown solution (the blood) by a semipermeable (to oxygen) membrane. The Pao_2, because it is easily and accurately measured, is the usual parameter to define the state of arterial oxygenation. The normal Pao_2 at sea level ranges between 80 and 110 mm Hg. These values vary at altitude because of the decrease in barometric pressure (see below). A Pao_2 greater than 110 mm Hg is labeled hyperoxemia, whereas a Pao_2 less than 80 mm Hg is labeled hypoxemia (Table 25-6). Severe hypoxemia, which requires intervention, is usually defined as a Pao_2 of less than 60 mm Hg.

ARTERIAL HEMOGLOBIN SATURATION (SaO₂)

The percent saturation of the hemoglobin is related to the Pao_2 in a relationship defined by the oxyhemoglobin dissociation curve (Table 25-7). Hemoglobin readily binds oxygen on the steep portion of the oxyhemoglobin dissociation curve. The hemoglobin is near fully saturated at a Pao_2 of 100 mm Hg ($Sao_2 = 97.5\%$); increasing the Pao_2 to 500 mm Hg barely increases the percent saturation ($Sao_2 = 99.9\%$). An Sao_2 of 96% corresponds to a Pao_2 of 80 mm Hg or above. An Sao_2 of 91% corre-

sponds to a Pao_2 of 60 mm Hg, which corresponds to a level of severe hypoxemia below which treatment is warranted. The clinical information derived about the patient from the measurement of hemoglobin saturation (Sao_2) is the same as that obtained from a Pao_2 measurement; they are both a measure of the ability of the lung to deliver oxygen to the blood stream. The numbers of concern are, however, different (Table 25-8).

Sao_2 is often extrapolated from the measured Po_2 via a standard oxyhemoglobin dissociation curve. Accurate derivation of So_2 from Po_2 depends on a normal position of the oxyhemoglobin dissociation curve. Several conditions will shift the curve to the right by increasing the affinity of hemoglobin for oxygen: these include increased temperature, hypercapnia, acidosis, and increased erythrocyte 2,3 DPG or ATP (as occurs in chronic anemia). When the curve is shifted to the right, the So_2 is decreased at any given Po_2. A right-shifted curve facilitates the unloading of oxygen at the tissue level (i.e., for any given Po_2, more oxygen is released from the hemoglobin). A right-shifted curve delays arterialization of blood in the pulmonary capillaries (i.e., it will prolong the time it takes to reach equilibration between alveolar and capillary Po_2), and could eventually reduce peak hemoglobin saturation. Several conditions will shift the curve to the left by decreasing the affinity of hemoglobin for oxygen: these include decreased temperature, hypocapnia, alkalosis, and decreased erythrocyte 2,3 DPG or ATP (as occurs with blood storage). When the curve is shifted to the left, the So_2 is increased at any given Po_2. A left-shifted curve facilitates oxygen loading in the pulmonary capillaries but impedes oxygen unloading to the tissues. P_{50} is a common way to define the position of the oxyhemoglobin dissociation curve and whether it is shifted to the left (a lower P_{50} value) or to the right (a higher P_{50} value).

Table 25-7 is based on calculations for human hemoglobin.[38] The P_{50} for human hemoglobin is between 26 and 27 mm Hg.[14,38-42] The P_{50} for canine hemoglobin is between 28 and 30 mm Hg,[41,43,44] which is close to that of humans; therefore, the values in Table 25-7 are close enough for clinical purposes for the dog. The P_{50} for feline hemoglobin, however, is between 32 and 37 mm Hg,[41-43,45,46] which represents a relative rightward shift of the oxyhemoglobin dissociation curve in the cat. Table 25-7 and blood gas analyzer printouts for Sao_2 (which utilize formulas based on human hemoglobin) are not accurate for the cat.

The percent saturation of hemoglobin (So_2) can also be measured by oximetry. Oximetry is based on the pattern of red to infrared light absorption or reflectance. Each species of hemoglobin (i.e., oxyhemoglobin, reduced hemoglobin, methemoglobin, and carboxyhemoglobin) absorbs light differently. One wavelength of light that maximizes the difference between the hemoglobin species of interest and the others is required to identify each species of hemoglobin.

Sao_2 can be measured with a bench top co-oximeter, which requires an arterial blood sample. This instrument utilizes 4 wavelengths of light and can quantify oxyhemoglobin, carboxyhemoglobin, and methemoglo-

TABLE 25-7. Hemoglobin Saturation (So_2) and Oxygen Content for Various Po_2 Values (Assuming No Shift of the Oxyhemoglobin Dissociation Curve)

Po_2 (mm Hg)	So_2 (%)	Content o_2 (ml/dl)	Po_2 (mm HG)	So_2 (%)	Content o_2 (ml/dl)	Po_2 (mm HG)	So_2 (%)	Content o_2 (ml/dl)
500	99.9	21.6	82	96.1	19.6	46	81.5	16.5
400	99.8	21.3	81	95.9	19.5	45	80.4	16.3
300	99.7	20.9	80	95.8	19.5	44	79.3	16.1
200	99.4	20.6	79	95.7	19.5	43	78.1	15.8
150	98.9	20.3	78	95.5	19.4	42	76.8	15.6
125	98.4	20.2	77	95.4	19.4	41	5.5	15.3
120	98.3	20.1	76	95.2	19.4	40	74.1	15.0
115	98.1	20.1	75	95.1	19.3	39	72.7	14.7
110	98.0	20.0	74	94.9	19.3	38	71.1	14.4
109	97.9	20.0	73	94.7	19.3	37	69.5	14.1
108	97.9	20.0	72	94.5	19.2	36	67.9	13.8
107	97.8	20.0	71	94.3	19.2	35	66.2	13.4
106	97.8	20.0	70	94.1	19.1	34	64.4	13.0
105	97.7	20.0	69	93.9	19.1	33	62.6	12.7
104	97.7	19.9	68	93.6	19.0	32	60.7	12.3
103	97.6	19.9	67	93.4	19.0	31	58.7	11.9
102	97.6	19.9	66	93.1	18.9	30	56.7	11.5
101	97.5	19.9	65	92.8	18.9	29	54.6	11.1
100	97.5	19.9	64	92.5	18.8	28	52.5	10.6
99	97.4	19.9	63	92.2	18.7	27	50.4	10.2
98	97.4	19.9	62	91.8	18.6	26	48.1	9.8
97	97.3	19.9	61	91.5	18.6	25	45.9	9.3
96	97.3	19.8	60	91.1	18.5	24	43.6	8.8
95	97.2	19.8	59	90.6	18.4	23	41.2	8.4
94	97.1	19.8	58	90.2	18.3	22	38.8	7.9
93	97.1	19.8	57	89.7	18.2	21	36.3	7.4
92	97.0	19.8	56	89.2	18.1	20	33.8	6.9
91	96.9	19.8	55	88.6	18.0	19	31.3	6.3
90	96.8	19.7	54	88.0	17.8	18	28.7	5.8
89	96.7	19.7	53	87.3	17.7	17	26.1	5.3
88	96.7	19.7	52	86.7	17.6	16	23.5	4.8
87	96.6	19.7	51	85.9	17.4	15	20.9	4.3
86	96.5	19.6	50	85.1	17.3	14	18.4	3.7
85	96.4	19.6	49	84.3	17.1	13	15.8	3.2
84	96.3	19.6	48	83.4	16.9	12	13.3	2.7
83	96.2	19.6	47	82.5	16.7	11	10.9	2.2

Po_2 = Partial pressure of oxygen (mm Hg); So_2 = oxyhemoglobin saturation (%), calculated from Po_2 using a mathematical model for human hemoglobin[38]; *Content o_2* = oxygen content (ml/dl), calculated by the formula: $(1.34 \times Hb \times So_2) + (0.003 \times Po_2)$.

TABLE 25-8. Correlation Between Pao_2 and Sao_2

Pao_2	Sao_2	Importance
>80	>95	Normal
<60	<90	Serious hypoxemia
<40	<75	Very serious hypoxemia

bin. Oxyhemoglobin is expressed as a fraction of the total amount of hemoglobin, inclusive of dysfunctional hemoglobin molecules such as carboxyhemoglobin and methemoglobin (fractional saturation). Sao_2 can also be approximated with a pulse oximeter, which is an indirect, noninvasive technique. The term "Spo_2" is used to denote Sao_2 measurements derived from a pulse oximeter. Pulse oximeters use two wavelengths of light, and oxyhemoglobin is expressed as a fraction of the hemoglobin capable of binding oxygen, exclusive of dysfunctional hemoglobin molecules such as carboxyhemoglobin and methemoglobin (functional saturation). A co-oximeter and a pulse oximeter express oxyhemoglobin as a different ratio, and to the extent that dysfunctional hemoglobin is present, will display different numbers for oxyhemoglobin.

With a pulse oximeter, a light-emitting diode and the photodetector are attached to a lip, ear, tongue, toe, or tail (thicker appendages generally do not work) and held in place by a light clip. The light from the transmitting diode passes through the tissues to the photodetector. The amount of light absorbed is then calculated by algorithms within the pulse oximeter. There are many tissues between the light-emitting diode and the photodetector that absorb light but are not of interest in this measurement (e.g., skin and other epithelial membranes, interstitial fluids and cellular tissues, and capillary and venous blood). The only tissue of interest is the arterial blood. Hence the "pulse" detector of a pulse oximeter is vitally important to its function. The pulse detector is how the oximeter "becomes informed" as to when the light absorption is caused by the background tissues of no interest (between pulses) and when the light absorption is caused by background tissues plus a flux of arterial blood. The pulse oximeter then simply subtracts the former from the latter to obtain the light absorbance that is caused by hemoglobin in the arterial blood. The oximeter then calculates the percent hemoglobin saturation that would account for the measured light absorbance.

Pulse oximeters represent highly sophisticated technology with a complex series of calculations based on assumptions that may or may not be true for the individual patient. Under ideal circumstances, pulse oximeters are reasonably accurate.[47-51] Under non-ideal circumstances, and in species in which the instruments have not been extensively tested, measurements may be inaccurate. Differences in tissue absorption or light scatter, different thicknesses of tissue, smaller pulsatile flow patterns, small signal-to-noise ratios, and incompletely compensated light emitting diodes may account for some of the inaccuracies associated with pulse oximeters. Inaccuracies may also be generated from baseline read errors (motion), differences in sensor location, and electrical or optical interference (bright room lights). The accuracy of a pulse oximeter is greatest within the range of 80% to 95% and is determined by the accuracy of the empirical formulae that are programmed into the instrument. There are substantial bias and precision variations and response times between products at different levels of saturation.

Two of the most common reasons for poor pulse oximeter performance are poor tissue contact and lack of pulse detection. Hair interferes with good contact between the skin and the light-emitting diode or photodetector. Excessively thick tissues and edema interfere with proper LED-detector alignment. Lack of pulse detection is either caused by poor peripheral perfusion or improper probe placement. Poor peripheral perfusion could be caused by peripheral vasoconstriction (secondary to hypovolemia, heart failure, or hypothermia) or prolonged placement of the probe in one place (clip pres-

sure can cause a decrease in local perfusion, and therefore clips should be moved periodically). Severe anemia[51] can also interfere with the accuracy of pulse oximeter readings.

If the pulse oximeter cannot detect a pulse, it will provide no heart rate or oximetry readings. To some extent, a pulse oximeter is a cardiovascular monitor as well. If the pulse oximeter displays a heart rate and hemoglobin saturation, the operator should check to make sure that the displayed heart rate is the same as the counted heart rate. If the displayed heart rate is wrong, the displayed saturation may also be wrong. Signal displays and signal strength indicators on many pulse oximeters help support the validity of the displayed values. The authors' experience has been that when a pulse oximeter measures inaccurately, it almost always measures inaccurately low. It is therefore recommended to place the pulse oximeter probe at several different locations and take the highest measured value as the one that most closely corresponds to a direct measurement of Sao_2. For most clinical purposes, most pulse oximeters are sufficiently accurate *approximations* of hemoglobin saturation. It is always a good idea to co-measure an arterial blood sample to validate the pulse oximeter measurement, or at least to establish an appropriate off-set for trend monitoring.

The difference between co-oximetry and pulse oximetry is important. Whereas the co-oximeter actually measures and identifies methemoglobin and carboxyhemoglobin, pulse oximeters are just confused by other species of hemoglobin. Pulse oximeters only use two wavelengths of light (i.e., red at 660 nm and infrared at 940 nm) and are designed to measure oxygenated and unoxygenated hemoglobin. If methemoglobin or carboxyhemoglobin is present in elevated concentrations, it will absorb light and will affect the measurement made by the pulse oximeter. Because of the biphasic absorption of methemoglobin at both the 660 nm and 940 nm wavelengths, abnormal accumulations tends to push the pulse oximeter reading toward 80% to 85% (underestimating the measurement when Sao_2 is above 85% and overestimating it when it is below 80%).[52-54] Carboxyhemoglobin absorbs light in a manner similar to oxyhemoglobin at 660 nm but hardly at all at 940 nm; this tends to increase the displayed oxyhemoglobin value.[50,53] Fetal hemoglobin[50] and jaundice[55] have little effect on measured hemoglobin saturation by pulse oximetry. Indocyanine green dye and methylene blue dye absorb light at 660 nm and will generate falsely low saturation measurements.[53]

Sao_2 is not discriminating when an animal is breathing an enriched oxygen mixture. Oximetry can hardly differentiate between a Pao_2 of 100 mm Hg (an Sao_2 of 97.5%) and a Pao_2 of 500 mm Hg (an Sao_2 of 99.9%). This has potential clinical applications. If, for instance, the Pao_2 in a patient breathing 100% oxygen is only 100 mm Hg when it should be at least 500 mm Hg, this provides evidence of very poor lung function and should generate considerable concern about postoperative hypoxemia. If, however, the anesthetist was measuring Spo_2 instead of Pao_2, there would be no warning of any impending problems. The fact that pulse oximetry cannot differentiate between varying degrees of hyperoxemia, however, should not diminish the fact that its claim to fame is the early detection of hypoxemia. In addition, an intraoperative PaO_2 of 500 mm Hg does not, in fact, warrant against postoperative hypoxemia, and so one cannot afford to be lulled into a false sense of security under any circumstances.

Hypoxemia

Hypoxemia is usually defined as a PaO_2 of less than 80 mm Hg. Hypoxemia has only 3 categorical causes: (1) a low inspired oxygen concentration, (2) hypoventilation, and (3) venous admixture. Low inspired oxygen must be considered any time an animal is attached to mechanical apparatus (e.g., face mask, Bain's circuit, anesthetic machine, or ventilator) or is in an enclosed environment (e.g., oxygen cage or anesthetic induction chamber). Hypoventilation has many causes (see Table 25-5) and is defined by an elevated $PaCO_2$. Venous admixture occurs when venous blood can get from the right side of the circulation to the left side of the circulation, without being properly oxygenated.

VENOUS ADMIXTURE

Some venous admixture occurs normally via the bronchial circulation; the thebesian veins, which drain from the myocardium directly into the left ventricle; and via suboptimal arterialization of blood as it traverses regions of the lung with a low ventilation to perfusion ratio (V/Q). Pathological venous admixture can be caused by five physiological mechanisms: (1) an increased number of low V/Q lung units, (2) atelectasis or alveolar filling (not ventilated but perfused lung units), (3) diffusion impairment, (4) anatomical right-to-left shunts, and (5) low venous oxygen content.

Regions of low ventilation/perfusion ratio occur secondary to regional hypoventilaton because of airway narrowing from bronchospasm (reflex or disease-induced), fluid accumulation along the walls of the lower airways, or epithelial edema. The consequence is suboptimal arterialization of the blood flowing through the area, just as global hypoventilation would reduce PaO_2 and increase $PaCO_2$. This is a common mechanism of hypoxemia in mild to moderate pulmonary disease. This mechanism of hypoxemia is typically responsive to oxygen therapy, just as is the hypoxemia of global hypoventilation. Even though the alveoli are hypoventilated, high inspired oxygen concentrations maximize the oxygenation of the blood flowing through the area. PaO_2 values may reach values expected for normal lungs at any given inspired oxygen concentration. Regions of low V/Q could also be attributed to an increase in bloodflow to the region (e.g., because of increased cardiac output or maldistributed cardiac output as may occur in pulmonary thromboembolism). Note that regions of high V/Q do not contribute to hypoxemia; in this case, hyperventilation causes an increase in alveolar and capillary oxygen.

Small airway and alveolar collapse establishes lung regions that are not ventilated but are still perfused. Spontaneous small airway and alveolar collapse can occur in normal lungs in obtunded, recumbent animals because of positional stasis and hypoventilation. Spontaneous small airway and alveolar collapse is a common mechanism of hypoxemia in moderate to severe pulmonary disease. Accumulation of fluids in the airways increases the surface tension of the lining fluid and the tendency for small airway and alveolar collapse. Blood flowing through the area cannot be arterialized. This mechanism of hypoxemia is not responsive to oxygen therapy because oxygen cannot get to the gas exchange area. These lung units must be opened by positive pressure inflation if they are to become functional gas exchange units.

Diffusion impairment, caused by a thickened respiratory membrane, is an uncommon cause of hypoxemia. Fluid leaking into the interstitium of the septal membranes does not accumulate, and there is no thickening of the respiratory membrane. If, however, the type 1 pneumocytes are destroyed by inhalation injury or by inflammatory mediators, they are replaced by thick, cuboidal, type 2 pneumocytes, a process that results in thickening of the respiratory membrane. The diffusion impairment mechanism of hypoxemia is variably responsive to oxygen therapy.

An anatomical shunt occurs when blood flows from the right side of the circulation to the left side without ever passing a functional gas exchange unit. It is caused by abnormal right-to-left extra- or intrapulmonary conduits (e.g., patent ductus arteriosus or ventricular septal defect). This is not a common mechanism of hypoxemia. It is not responsive to oxygen therapy or positive pressure ventilation but requires surgical intervention.

Equilibration between alveolar and capillary PO_2, as the blood flows through the pulmonary capillaries, takes time. Normally equilibration is complete when the blood has traversed approximately one third of the alveolar capillary.[12] Equilibration takes progressively longer when the venous oxygen content becomes progressively lower. Eventually, equilibration cannot occur before the blood reaches the end of the pulmonary capillary. Low venous oxygen is usually attributed to reduced oxygen delivery to the tissues. The continued removal of normal amounts of oxygen from the reduced supply results in decreased systemic capillary and venous oxygen. The subjects of oxygen delivery, oxygen consumption, and venous oxygen will be discussed more extensively at the end of this chapter.

QUANTIFICATION OF VENOUS ADMIXTURE

Quantification of venous admixture provides an assessment of the oxygenating efficiency of the lung. Trends in venous admixture are used to assess the effectiveness of therapy and the progress of the disease. Venous admixture can be assessed by several different methods. If these assessments are made while the patient is breathing room air, all five mechanisms of hypoxemia must be considered. If these assessments are made while the pa-

TABLE 25-9. **Normal Atmospheric and Alveolar Gas Concentrations at Sea Level**

	Air (%) [mm Hg]	Alveolus (%) [mm Hg]
Oxygen	21 [160]	14 [105]
Carbon dioxide	0.03 [0.3]	5 [40]
Nitrogen	78 [593]	74 [565]
Water vapor	1 [8]	7 [50]

TABLE 25-10. **The Effect of Altitude on Barometric Pressure and Inspired Oxygen**[12]

Altitude (ft)	Barometric Pressure Altitude (M)	Inspired P_{O_2} (mm Hg)	% O_2 Required for Sea (mm Hg)	Level P_IO_2
0	0	760	149	20.9
2000	610	707	138	22.6
4000	1220	659	127	24.5
6000	1830	609	118	26.5
8000	2440	564	108	28.8
10,000	3050	523	100	31.3
15,000	4575	429	80	42.8
20,000	6100	349	63	49.3
30,000	9150	226	37	83.2

tient is breathing 100% oxygen, the low V/Q mechanism is excluded.

Alveolar oxygen (PA_{O_2}) is often used in combination with measured arterial oxygen (Pa_{O_2}) as an index of the oxygenating efficiency of the lung. Alveolar oxygen is usually calculated but could also be measured from an end-tidal gas sample. The following discussion explains the calculation of PA_{O_2}.

Atmospheric air primarily contains nitrogen and oxygen, small amounts of water and carbon dioxide, and very small amounts of other gases and pollutants (Table 25-9). The partial pressure of oxygen in atmospheric air at sea level is calculated as barometric pressure (760) × 21% = 160 mm Hg. The inspired P_{O_2} can be calculated for any altitude by inserting the appropriate barometric pressure for that altitude (Table 25-10). The inspired P_{O_2} can be calculated for any oxygen concentration by substituting the appropriate oxygen concentration.

The effective inspired P_{O_2} must account for water vapor because air becomes fully humidified as it is breathed into the alveoli. Since this added water vapor dilutes all of the inspired gases, it is subtracted from the total barometric pressure before multiplying the percent oxygen concentration. The vapor pressure of water is 50 mm Hg at 38° C but varies with body temperature (Table 25-11). The effective partial pressure of inspired oxygen (P_IO_2) at sea level, at 21% atmospheric oxygen, at 38° C body temperature, is calculated as (760 − 50) × 0.21 = 150 mm Hg.

Alveolar oxygen is not, however, equal to inspired oxygen. Venous blood continuously delivers carbon dioxide to the alveoli and removes oxygen from the alveoli as it traverses the capillary bed. For every molecule of

TABLE 25-11. **Water Content and Vapor Pressure of 100% Saturated Air at Various Temperatures**[56]

Temperature (°C)	(°F)	Water Content (mg/L)	Vapor Pressure (mm Hg)	Temperature (°C)	(°F)	Water Content (mg/L)	Vapor Pressure (mm Hg)
0	32	4.8	4.6	25	77	23.1	23.8
2	35.6	5.6	5.3	26	78.8	24.4	25.2
4	39.2	6.4	6.1	27	80.6	25.6	26.7
6	42.8	7.3	7	28	82.4	27.2	28.3
8	46.4	8.3	8	29	84.2	28.8	30
10	50	9.4	9.2	30	86	30.4	31.8
12	53.6	10.7	10.5	31	87.8	32.1	33.7
14	57.2	12.1	12	32	89.6	33.8	35.7
15	59	12.8	12.8	33	91.4	35.7	37.8
16	60.8	13.6	13.6	34	93.2	37.6	39.9
17	62.6	14.8	14.5	35	95	39.6	42.2
18	64.4	15.4	15.5	36	96.8	41.8	44.6
19	66.2	16.2	16.5	37	98.6	44	47
20	68	17.3	17.5	38	100.4	46.3	49.7
21	69.8	18.3	18.7	39	102.2	48.7	52.4
22	71.6	19.4	19.8	40	104	51.2	55.3
23	73.4	20.6	21.1	41	105.8	54.4	58.3
24	75.2	21.8	22.4	42	107.6	57.6	61.5

oxygen that is removed from the alveoli, almost another molecule of carbon dioxide is added to the alveoli, in proportion to the metabolic consumption of oxygen and production of carbon dioxide. The PA_{O_2} can be calculated by subtracting the alveolar P_{CO_2} (PA_{CO_2}) from the $P_{I_{O_2}}$, with two modifications: (1) PA_{CO_2} could be measured (end-tidal P_{CO_2}), but for simplicity and because the alveolar-arterial P_{CO_2} gradient is normally very small, Pa_{CO_2} is usually used to estimate PA_{CO_2} and is substituted for PA_{CO_2} in the calculation of PA_{O_2} and (2) the ratio of carbon dioxide production to oxygen consumption (the respiratory quotient [R/Q]) is not 1.0 but varies between 0.7 and 1.0 in stable states and can exceed this range in unstable states. Respiratory quotient for dogs has been reported to be 0.84[27], 0.90[57], and 0.95 to 1.0.[58] The respiratory quotient in critically ill human beings has been reported to be 0.88[59] and 0.83 to 0.97.[60] This author uses a value of 0.9 for R/Q because it represents a mid-range value of reported values.

The PA_{O_2} is calculated with the formula:

$$([P_b - P_{H_2O}] \times \% \text{ oxygen}) - Pa_{CO_2} (1/RQ)$$

where P_b = barometric pressure; P_{H_2O} = partial pressure of water of saturated air at body temperature; and RQ is the ratio of carbon dioxide production to oxygen consumption. This formula accounts for variations in altitude (P_b), body temperature (P_{H_2O}), oxygen concentration, and respiratory quotient. Under conditions of sea level, 21% oxygen, and normal body temperature, PA_{O_2} can also be calculated with a short formula:

$$150 - Pa_{CO_2} (1.1)$$

where
150 = the $P_{I_{O_2}}$ at sea level, 21% oxygen; and 1.1 = 1/0.9.

Alveolar-Arterial P_{O_2} Gradient ($P[A-a]_{O_2}$)

The alveolar-arterial P_{O_2} gradient ($P[A-a]_{O_2}$) is the difference between the calculated alveolar partial pressure of oxygen (PA_{O_2}) and the measured arterial partial pressure of oxygen (Pa_{O_2}). The $P(A-a)_{O_2}$ is normally less than 10 mm Hg when breathing 21% oxygen[27,58,61,62] and up to 100 mm Hg when breathing 100% oxygen.[26] If the calculated $P(A-a)_{O_2}$ is greater than 15 mm Hg when the animal is breathing room air, or greater that 150 mm Hg when the animal is breathing 100% oxygen, the animal has increased venous admixture. The greater the $P(A-a)_{O_2}$, the greater the venous admixture. The expected $P(A-a)_{O_2}$ at intermediate inspired oxygen concentrations has not been established and must be extrapolated between 10 and 100 mm Hg; values suggestive of venous admixture should be extrapolated between 15 and 150 mm Hg.

The "120" Rule

It has been discussed above that alveolar barometric pressure and the partial pressures of nitrogen and water vapor do not change. The alveolar P_{CO_2} and P_{O_2} are approximately reciprocally related and therefore must total a fixed value of approximately 150 mm Hg at sea level when the animal is breathing 21% oxygen. Assuming a normal $P(A-a)_{O_2}$ of about 10 mm Hg, the added values of Pa_{O_2} + Pa_{CO_2} for arterial blood should be about 140 mm Hg (range 120 to 160 mm Hg). In general, then, an added Pa_{O_2} + Pa_{CO_2} value of less than 120 mm Hg indicates a reduced lung oxygenating efficiency; the further the added value is below 120 mm Hg, the greater is the venous admixture. An added value above 160 is physiologically impossible (there is a measurement error). This "120/160" rule of thumb can only be used when the patient is breathing 21% oxygen at approximately sea level. If the patient is breathing an enriched oxygen mixture or is not at sea level, the original alveolar air equation and the calculation of $P(A-a)_{O_2}$ could be used to estimate venous admixture (or a new "added-value" would need to be calculated).

An "Up/Down Offset" Method

Like alveolar P_{CO_2} and P_{O_2}, Pa_{CO_2} and the Pa_{O_2} are also approximately reciprocally related. The relative change of Pa_{CO_2} and Pa_{O_2} can also be used to assess lung oxygenating efficiency. Assume a central normal Pa_{O_2} of 100 mm Hg and a central normal Pa_{CO_2} of 40 mm Hg. A 20 mm Hg decrease in Pa_{CO_2} (from 40 to 20) would be expected to increase Pa_{O_2} by 22 mm Hg (20 × 1.1) (i.e., from 100 to 122). A 40 mm Hg increase in Pa_{CO_2} (from 40 to 80) would be expected to decrease Pa_{O_2} by 44 mm Hg (40 × 1.1) (i.e., from 100 to 56). If the measured Pa_{O_2} is more than 20 mm Hg below that predicted by this calculation, venous admixture is present. The further the measured Pa_{O_2} is below the predicted value, the greater the venous admixture.

Pa_{O_2}/Fi_{O_2} Ratio

When breathing 21% oxygen, changes in Pa_{CO_2} have an important impact on Pa_{O_2} and must be taken into account when calculating the expected Pa_{O_2} (as in all of the above methods). With progressively higher inspired oxygen concentrations, changes in Pa_{CO_2} have a progressively less important effect on Pa_{O_2} and, for clinical purposes, can legitimately be ignored at inspired oxygen concentrations higher than about 50%. The Pa_{O_2}/Fi_{O_2} ratio (the P/F ratio) is a popular method of expressing lung oxygenating efficiency when the patient is breathing an enriched oxygen mixture. The measured Pa_{O_2} is divided by the fractional inspired oxygen expressed as a decimal: 0.21 to 1.0. In normal lungs the Pa_{O_2}/Fi_{O_2} ratio is greater than 500 mm Hg. Values between 300 and 500 mm Hg represent mild oxygenating inefficiency; values between 200 and 300 mm Hg represent moderate lung inefficiency; and values below 200 mm Hg represent severe venous admixture.

It is also a common convention to divide the Pa_{O_2} by the inspired oxygen expressed as a percent: 21% to 100%. This simply represents a decimal point shift: in normal lungs the Pa_{O_2}/inspired O_2 ratio is greater than 5; values between 3 and 5 represent mild oxygenating inefficiency; values between 2 and 3 represent moderate lung inefficiency; and values below 2 represent severe venous admixture.

The Venous Admixture Formula

This is also called the "shunt" formula; however, the author has avoided this term to reduce confusion because the word "shunt" has been used to mean a specific subset of causes of venous admixture. This formula calculates the percent of cardiac output that would have to flow through the lung as anatomical shunt, assuming that the remaining bloodflow is optimally arterialized, in order to account for the observed difference between the measured venous and arterial oxygen. This formula requires a mixed venous blood sample, preferably from the pulmonary artery, although right atrial and anterior vena cava blood could be substituted. The venous admixture equation is:

$$Q_S/Q_T = (Cco_2 - Cvo_2) / (Cco_2 - Cao_2)$$

where Q_S/Q_T = venous admixture expressed as a percent of cardiac output; Cco_2 = oxygen content of end-capillary blood; Cvo_2 = oxygen content of mixed venous blood; and Cao_2 = oxygen content of arterial blood. Oxygen content (Content o_2; ml/dl) is calculated by the following formula:

$$Content\ o_2 = (1.34 \times So_2) + (0.003 \times Po_2)$$

where 1.34 is the amount of oxygen (milliliters) that each gram of hemoglobin can hold if it is 100% saturated, Hb is the hemoglobin concentration (grams/deciliter), So_2 is the measured or calculated percent hemoglobin saturation with oxygen, and 0.003 is the solubility of oxygen in plasma. PAo_2 is substituted for Pco_2 for the purpose of calculating Cco_2. Venous admixture in normal awake or anesthetized dogs may be up to 10% of the cardiac output.[27,61-63] Values over 10% are considered to be increased and values may exceed 50% in severe, diffuse lung disease.

Whole Blood Oxygen Content and Oxygen Delivery

Whole blood oxygen content (Content o_2) is expressed as milliliters of oxygen per 100 milliliters of whole blood. Content o_2 is an important determinant of oxygen delivery. As can be seen in the formula above for calculating oxygen content, hemoglobin concentration is the predominant determinant of oxygen content. The relationship between oxygen content and Po_2 is also defined by a sigmoid curve, and oxygen content does not increase much when the Po_2 is raised above 100 mm Hg (see Table 25-7); the hemoglobin is mostly fully saturated, and further increases in content are attributed mostly to an increase in dissolved oxygen in the plasma.

Because hemoglobin concentration provides the greatest quantitative contribution to oxygen content, anemia (compared with hypoxemia) is the most potent cause of decreased oxygen content (Table 25-12). At the tissue level, Po_2 is primarily important in that it provides the driving pressure for the flow of oxygen molecules from the plasma to the mitochondria. Content$_a o_2$ is important as a reservoir of oxygen to buffer the decrease in Po_2 that occurs when oxygen molecules diffuse out of the plasma.

Oxygen delivery is the product of oxygen content and cardiac output. Animals can tolerate a decrease in oxygen content if oxygen delivery can be maintained by an increase in cardiac output (Table 25-13). Animals tolerate anemia and poor cardiac output poorly (Table 25-13).

Venous Oxygen

Oxygen delivery needs to be sufficient to meet the oxygen consumption requirements of the patient. Normally, oxygen delivery far exceeds oxygen consumption. Oxygen extraction normally ranges between 20% and 30% of the oxygen delivery. Mixed venous oxygen represents the bal-

TABLE 25-13. **Oxygen Delivery (Do_2) (ml/min/M²) Resulting From Various Combinations of Packed Cell Volume (PCV) and Cardiac Output (Q, ml/kg/min) (Assuming Normal Lung Function and a Pao_2 of 100 mm Hg) (Normal Range for Q is 3.5 to 5.5)***

PCV%	6.5(Q)	5.5(Q)	4.5(Q)	3.5(Q)	2.5(Q)
40	1155	977	799	621	444
30	873	739	604	470	336
25	731	618	506	394	281
20	588	498	407	317	226
15	446	378	309	240	172
10	304	257	210	164	117

*It has been recommended to maintain Do_2 above 550-600 ml/min/M².

TABLE 25-12. **Effect of Anemia, Hypoxemia, and Hyperoxemia on Pao_2, Sao_2, and Content$_a o_2$**

Condition	Fio_2	Pao_2 (mm Hg)	Sao_2 (%)	Hemoglobin (gm/dl)	Content$_a o_2$ (ml/dl)
Normal	0.21	100	98	15	19.9
Anemia	0.21	100	98	5	6.9
Low Pao_2	0.21	50	85	15	17.3
High Pao_2	1.0	500	99.9	15	21.6
Anemia & High Pao_2	1.0	500	99.9	5	8.2
Anemia & Low Pao_2	0.21	50	85	5	5.8

TABLE 25-14. Interpretation of Central Venous Po₂ Measurements

Central or Mixed Venous Po_2 (mm Hg)	Interpretation/Action
>60	Very high Do_2/Vo_2 ratio; determine cause
50-60	High Do_2/Vo_2 ratio; no action required
40-50	Normal
30-40	Low Do_2/Vo_2 ratio; no action required
25-30	Low Do_2/Vo_2 ratio; determine cause; consider corrective action
20-25	Very low Do_2/Vo_2 ratio; corrective action required
<20	Extremely low Do_2/Vo_2 ratio; demands immediate action

ance between whole body oxygen delivery and oxygen consumption. Mixed or central venous Po_2 ranges between 40 and 50 mm Hg in normal dogs (Table 25-14).[61] When oxygen delivery is decreased (e.g., because of low cardiac output, anemia, hypoxemia, or vasoconstriction), the tissues continue to "draw" their normal amount of oxygen and therefore oxygen extraction (expressed as a percent of oxygen delivery) increases, and Content co_2 and venous oxygen decreases. Venous Po_2 values below 30 mm Hg are usually attributed to excessively low oxygen delivery but could be caused by high oxygen consumption (see Table 25-14). Values below 20 mm Hg should be considered life-threatening.

REFERENCES

1. Siggaard-Andersen O: Sampling and storing of blood for determination of acid-base status, Scand J Clin Lab Invest 13:196-204, 1961.
2. Ilkiw JE, Rose RJ, Martin ICE: A comparison of simultaneously collected arterial, mixed venous, jugular venous, and cephalic venous blood samples in the assessment of blood gas and acid-base status in dogs, J Vet Int Med 5:294, 1991.
3. Kelman GR, Nunn JF: Nomograms for correction of blood Po₂, Pco₂, pH, and base excess for time and temperature, J Appl Physiol 21:1484-1490, 1966.
4. Haskins SC: Sampling and storage of blood for pH and blood gas analysis, J Am Vet Med Assoc 170:429-433, 1977.
5. Evers W, Racz GB, Levy AA: A comparative study of plastic (polypropylene) and glass syringes in blood gas analysis, Anesth Analg 51:92-97, 1972.
6. Winkler JB, Huntington CG, Wells DE et al: Influence of syringe material on arterial blood gas determinations, Chest 66:518-521, 1974.
7. Laussen PC: Optimal blood gas management during deep hypothermic paediatric cardiac surgery: Alpha-stat is easy, but pH-stat may be preferable, Paediatric Anaesthesia 12:199-204, 2002.
8. Priestly MA, Golden JA, O'Hara IB et al: Comparison of neurologic outcome after deep hypothermic circulatory arrest with alpha-stat and pH-stat cardiopulmonary bypass in newborn pigs, J Thorac Cardiovasc Surg 12:204-205, 2001.
9. Murkin JM, Martzke JS, Buchan AM et al: A randomized study of the influence of perfusion technique and pH management strategy in 316 patients undergoing coronary artery bypass surgery. II: Neurologic and cognitive outcomes, J Thorac Cardiovasc Surg 110:349-362, 1995.
10. duPlessis AJ, Jonas RA, Wypij D et al: Perioperative effects of alpha-stat versus pH-stat strategies for deep hypothermic cardiopulmonary bypass in infants, J Thorac Cardiovasc Surg 114:991-1001, 1997.
11. Bellinger DC, Wypij D, duPlessis AJ et al: Developmental and neurologic effects of alpha-stat and pH-stat strategies for deep hypothermic cardiopulmonary bypass in infants, J Thorac Cardiovasc Surg 121:374-383, 2001.
12. Lumb AB: Changes in carbon dioxide tension. In Nunn JF, editor: Nunn's applied respiratory physiology, ed 5, Oxford; Boston; 2000, Butterworth Heineman.
13. Raichle ME, Posner JB, Plum F: Cerebral blood flow during and after hyperventilation, Arch Neurol 23:394-403, 1970.
14. Fencl V, Miller TB, Pappenheimer JR: Studies on the respiratory response to disturbances of acid-base balance, with deductions concerning the ionic composition of cerebral interstitial fluid, Am J Physiol 210:459-472, 1966.
15. Kontos HA, Wei EP, Raper AJ et al: Local mechanism of CO₂ action on cat pial arterioles, Stroke 8:226-229, 1977.
16. Pavlin EG, Hornbein TF: Distribution of H+ and HCO₃− between CSF and blood during respiratory acidosis in dogs, Am J Physiol 228:1145-1148, 1975.
17. Hornbein TF, Pavlin EG: Distribution of H+ and HCO₃− between CSF and blood during respiratory alkalosis in dogs, Am J Physiol 228:1149-1154, 1975.
18. Muizelaar JP, van der Poel HG: Cerebral vasoconstriction is not maintained with prolonged hyperventilation, in Hoff JT, Betz AL, editors: Intracranial pressure VII, Berlin, 1989, Springer-Verlag.
19. Christensen MS: Acid-base changes in cerebrospinal fluid and blood, and blood volume changes following prolonged hyperventilation in man, Br J Anaesth 46:348-357, 1974.
20. Martin L: All you really need to know to interpret arterial blood gases, ed 2, Philadelphia, 1999, Lippincott, Williams & Wilkins.
21. Shapiro BA, Peruzzi WT, Templin R: Clinical application of blood gases, ed 5, Chicago, 1994, Mosby-Yearbook.
22. DiBartola SP: Fluid therapy in small animal practice, ed 2, Philadelphia, 2000, WB Saunders.
23. Baggot J: Gas transport and pH regulation. In Devlin TM, editor: Textbook of biochemistry, ed 3, New York, 1992, Wiley-Liss.
24. Kawashima Y, Yamamoto Z, Manabe H: Safe limits of hemodilution in cardiopulmonary bypass, Surgery 76:391-397, 1974.
25. Weil MH, Rackow EC, Trevino R et al: Difference in acid-base state between venous and arterial blood during cardiopulmonary resuscitation, N Eng J Med 315:153-156, 1986.
26. Schuurmans Stekhoven JH, Kreuzer F: Alveolar-arterial O₂ and CO₂ pressure differences in the anesthetized, artificially ventilated dog, Respir Physiol 3:177-191, 1967.
27. Muggenburg BA, Mauderly JL: Cardiopulmonary function of awake, sedated, and anesthetized beagle dogs, J Appl Physiol 37:152-157, 1974.
28. Eriksson L, Wollmer P, Olsson CG et al: Diagnosis of pulmonary embolism based upon alveolar dead space analysis, Chest 96:357-362, 1989.
29. Shibutani K, Muraoka M, Shitasaki S: Do changes in end-tidal PCO₂ quantitatively reflect changes in cardiac output? Anesth Analg 79:829-833, 1994.
30. Gudipati CV, Weil MH, Bisera J: Expired carbon dioxide: a noninvasive monitor of cardiopulmonary resuscitation, Circulation 77:324-329, 1988.
31. Callaham M, Barton C: Prediction of outcome of cardiopulmonary resuscitation from end-tidal carbon dioxide concentration, Crit Care Med 18:358-362, 1990.
32. Ward KR, Sullivan RJ, Zelenak RR et al: A comparison of interposed abdominal compression CPR and standard CPR by monitoring end-tidal PCO₂, Ann Emerg Med 18:831-837, 1989.
33. Levine RL, Wayne MA, Miller CC: End-tidal carbon dioxide and outcome of out-of-hospital cardiac arrest, New Eng J Med 337:301-306, 1997.
34. Sharpe JJ, Nelson AW, Lumb WV: Estimation of arterial acid-base values from toenail blood of the anesthetized dog, Am J Vet Res 29:2365-2369, 1968.
35. Rodkey WG, Hannon JP, Dramise JG et al: Arterialized capillary blood used to determine the acid-base and blood gas status of dogs, Am J Vet Res 39:459-464, 1978.
36. Solter PF, Haskins SC, Patz JD: Comparison of Po₂, Pco₂, pH in blood collected from the femoral artery and a cut claw of cats, Am J Vet Res 49:1882-1883, 1988.
37. Quandt JE, Raffe MC, Polzin D et al: Evaluation of toenail blood samples for blood gas analysis in the dog, Vet Surg 20:357-361, 1991.

38. Kelman GR: Digital computer subroutine for the conversion of oxygen tension into saturation, *J Appl Physiol* 21:1375-1376, 1966.
39. Yoder RD, Seidenfeld BM, Suwa K: Normal hemoglobin-oxygen affinity, *Anesthesiology* 42:741-744, 1975.
40. Canizaro PC, Nelson JL, Hennessy JL et al: A technique for estimating the position of the oxygen-hemoglobin dissociation curve, *Ann Surg* 180:364-367, 1974.
41. Spector WS, editor: *Handbook of biological data,* Philadelphia, 1956, WB Saunders.
42. Baumann R, Bartels H, Bauer C: Blood oxygen transport. In Geiger SR, Farhi LE, Tenney SM et al, editors: *Handbook of physiology: The respiratory system,* vol 4, Bethesda, 1987, American Physiologic Society.
43. Bartels H, Harms H: Sauerstoffdissoziationskurven des blutes von saugetieren, *Pflugers Archiv* 268:334-365, 1959.
44. Ou D, Mahaffey E, Smith JE: Effect of storage on oxygen dissociation of canine blood, *J Am Vet Med Assoc* 167:56-58, 1975.
45. Mauk AG, Huang YP, Skogen FW et al: The effect of hemoglobin phenotype on whole blood oxygen saturation and erythrocyte organic phosphate concentration in the domestic cat (felis catus), *Comp Biochem Physiol* 51:487-489, 1975.
46. Taketa F: Organic phosphates and hemoglobin structure-function relationships in the feline, *Ann NY Acad Sci* 241:524-537, 1974.
47. Jacobson JD, Miller MW, Matthews NS et al: Evaluation of accuracy of pulse oximetry in dogs, *Am J Vet Res* 53:537-540, 1992.
48. Fairman NB: Evaluation of pulse oximetry as a continuous monitoring technique in critically ill dogs in the small animal intensive care unit, *J Vet Emerg Crit Care* 2:50-56, 1993.
49. Hendricks JC, King LG: Practicality, usefulness, and limits of pulse oximetry in critical small animal patients, *J Vet Emerg Crit Care* 3:5-12, 1994.
50. Kelleher JF: Pulse oximetry, *J Clin Monitoring* 5:37-62, 1989.
51. Lee S, Tremper K, Barker SJ: Effects of anemia on pulse oximetry and continuous mixed venous hemoglobin saturation monitoring in dogs, *Anesthesiology* 75:118-122, 1991.
52. Eisenkraft JB: Pulse oximeter desaturation due to methemoglobinemia, *Anesthesiology* 68:279-282, 1988.
53. Alexander CM, Teller LE, Gross JB: Principles of pulse oximetry, *Anesth Analg* 68:368-376, 1989.
54. Barker SJ, Tremper KK, Hyatt J: Effects of methemoglobinemia on pulse oximetry and mixed venous oximetry, *Anesthesiology* 70:112-117, 1989.
55. Veyckermans F, Baele P, Guillaume JE et al: Hyperbilirubinemia does not interfere with hemoglobin saturation measured by pulse oximetry, *Anesthesiology* 70:118-122, 1989.
56. Weast RC, Astle MJ: Weight of saturated aqueous vapor. In Chemical Rubber Company: *Handbook of chemistry & physics,* ed 60, Boca Raton, 1979, Author.
57. Tsukimoto K, Arcos JP, Schaffartzik W et al: Effect of common dead space on V_A/Q distribution in the dog, *J Appl Physiol* 68: 2488-2493, 1990.
58. Mauderly JL, Pickrell JA: Pulmonary function testing of unanesthetized beagle dogs, *Res Anim Med* 665-675, 1973.
59. Brandi LS, Bertolini R, Santini L: Effects of ventilator resetting on indirect calorimetry measurement in the critically ill surgical patient, *Crit Care Med* 27:531-539, 1999.
60. Moriyama S, Okamoto K, Tabira Y et al: Evaluation of oxygen consumption and resting energy expenditure in critically ill patients with systemic inflammatory response syndrome, *Crit Care Med* 27:2133-2136, 1999.
61. Haskins SC, Farver TB, Patz JD: Ketamine in dogs, *Am J Vet Res* 446:1855-1860, 1985.
62. Haskins SC, Patz JD: Effects of small and large face masks and translaryngeal and tracheostomy intubation on ventilation, upper-airway dead space, and arterial blood gases, *Am J Vet Res* 47:945-948, 1986.
63. Finley TN, Lenfant C, Haab P et al: Venous admixture in the pulmonary circulation of anesthetized dogs, *J Appl Physiol* 15:418-424, 1960.

CHAPTER 26

Pulse Oximetry

Joan C. Hendricks

Pulse oximetry is a noninvasive method of assessing the oxyhemoglobin content of perfused tissues. The reading can be obtained within seconds. Therefore within certain limits this technology can provide information about tissue oxygen delivery long before tissue hypoxia leads to signs such as syncope and at far higher saturations than the point at which cyanosis becomes detectable as a clinical sign. Figure 26-1 shows the oxyhemoglobin saturation curve that describes the underlying physiology of the relationship between oxygen saturation of hemoglobin and arterial partial pressure of oxygen (Pao_2). Because the pulse oximeter makes a beeping noise at whatever alarm settings are chosen, it also provides an auditory signal to complement visual observation.

The instrument can be used in a number of practical situations in which a continuous monitor of oxygenation is desirable (e.g., in anesthetized or hypoxic patients). Perhaps one undervalued contribution is its use in cases where the respiratory system appears to be compromised and certain diagnostic tests are thought to be risky. In these patients, monitoring oxygenation by oximetry may provide reassurance that the animal is actually not in danger of desaturating, allowing the tests to proceed.

The use of oximetry has become standard (even required) for anesthesia in humans, for monitoring pediatric ICU cases, and in a variety of adult ICU conditions. As its use has been validated and reported in veterinary medicine, the utility of the device has become apparent for similar purposes. At the same time, models have been developed and marketed specifically for veterinary use. The probes, the sturdiness, and the cost have been adapted to veterinary patients. Unfortunately, the accuracy and reliability have not always been fully tested in units marketed for veterinarians, so that judicious use and critical interpretation are advisable.

Pulse oximetry is currently a widely used method to estimate the oxygenation of veterinary patients. The technology is safe, easy to use, and provides information for most patients that could not be obtained (or at least not obtained as quickly and as often) by other means. However, the technology has both theoretical and practical limits and even under ideal conditions cannot provide complete information about pulmonary function.

Background Physiology and Definition

Pulse oximetry relies on the detection of light absorption when light is transmitted through tissues. Although it was developed based on the absorption spectrum of human oxyhemoglobin, pulse oximetry was recently determined to be valid as an estimate of directly measured hemoglobin saturation (Sao_2), in dogs and cats, as well as large animal species.[1] It is important that the values are interpreted with the understanding that, although the normal values for Sao_2 (96% to 98%) are similar to the normal range of Pao_2 (approximately 80 to 100 mm Hg), the numbers actually reflect different physiological measures, and their relationship is described by a sigmoid curve. The Pao_2 that correlates with a particular Sao_2 varies, depending on 2,3 diphosphoglycerate (DPG) concentrations, blood pH, and temperature.[2] Thus an Sao_2 of 90% may reflect a range of actual Pao_2 values (Figure 26-1).

Pulse oximetry estimates the percent oxygenation of hemoglobin (Spo_2) by sensing the difference between light absorption during pulsations (presumed to be arterial) and the background absorption between pulsations (presumed to be due to venous blood, tissue, and bone). The shift toward red that occurs when most of the hemoglobin is oxygenated, compared with the background of venous blood, provides the waveform. The instrument sends a light signal through the tissue, and the difference in light absorbance in the range of oxygenated blood is measured by a detector.

The signal depends on two cardiopulmonary factors: (1) the degree of difference between the pulsatile oxyhemoglobin and background hemoglobin (the oxygen saturation) and (2) the amplitude of the pulse (perfusion).[3] If pulmonary function is normal, the signal varies only with perfusion; if perfusion is normal, it varies only with oxygenation. However, in many clinical situations both the cardiovascular and the pulmonary systems are affected. At least initially, the contribution of abnormalities in the two systems is usually not known with certainty. Thus, the signal may be influenced by changes in both the cardiovascular and the pulmonary system, and it may not be clear which is more important unless additional tests can

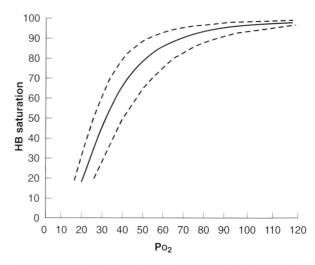

Figure 26-1. *Calculated dissociation curve for T = 37°C, pH = 7.4, together with lines representing calculated values + 95% confidence intervals. (Reproduced with permission from Rossing RG, Cain SM: A nomogram relating Po_2, pH, temperature and hemoglobin saturation in the dog, J Appl Physiol 21:195-201,1966.)*

be performed. Many instruments include signals to assist in distinguishing the pulse amplitude from the oxygenation, but these readouts must be interpreted carefully to avoid making ill-informed decisions.

Whereas the information detected by the pulse oximeter is derived largely from changes in cardiopulmonary function, the signal can also be influenced by local changes in the tissue (e.g., if it is compressed or desiccated, or if the patient moves). Similarly, changes in color of the blood (e.g., conditions leading to jaundice or methemoglobinemia) or variability in ambient light might theoretically alter the signal. Practically speaking, the fact that the signal arises from the difference between the color of pulsatile and venous background levels appears to eliminate problems arising from constant environmental light. The author has not found problems arising from icterus and has limited experience with methemoglobin. Patient movement, however, can seriously interfere with the ability to obtain a reading. Difficulty may be experienced obtaining readings in very darkly pigmented dogs (e.g., Newfoundlands and black Labrador retrievers). In addition, when probes are placed in one spot for a prolonged time, pressure on the underlying tissue may result in a gradual decrease in the Spo_2 reading that returns to normal after repositioning the probe. When the probe is placed on the tongue, gradual drying of the tissues may also lead to erroneous results that can be corrected by moistening.

Indications

Because there are other tests that can provide more reliable information about cardiovascular and pulmonary function, what is the utility of pulse oximetry? With regard to pulmonary function, arterial blood gases remain the most complete and reliable measure; however, arterial puncture may be impossible or dangerous in some patients. Although cageside blood gas machines have now been developed, providing much more prompt and widespread access to these measurements, even the quickest determination takes more than the few seconds required to obtain a pulse oximetry reading. Also, even though newer instruments can make determinations on very small blood volumes, very frequent determinations are still impractical. Thus, constant monitoring of oxygenation is an appropriate use of pulse oximetry even when other tests are readily available.[4]

Therefore we use pulse oximetry in anesthetized patients that are at risk for hypoxia, in ventilated patients between blood gas determinations, and for monitoring the patient's response to procedures that may put it at risk of hypoxia. The instrument is commonly used for patients in respiratory distress to determine whether oxygenation improves with oxygen supplementation, or, conversely, whether the patient's saturation falls when supplemental oxygen is removed. Similarly, pulse oximetry can allow the clinician a measure of reassurance that oxygenation remains adequate during necessary diagnostic testing such as physical examination, radiography, arterial blood sampling, or transtracheal wash. Pulse oximetry during anesthetic induction and recovery provides continuous and nearly real-time information that cannot be obtained by any other means.

Contraindications and Limits

Pulse oximetry carries essentially no direct risk to the patient. The instrument is very easy to use but may provide a reading that is somewhat or even grossly inaccurate. The risk inherent in its use is the possibility of overreliance on the SpO_2 without realizing the limits of the measurement. For a variety of reasons, pulse oximetry cannot replace classical blood gas measurements. First, of course, it provides no information about acid-base status or CO_2 values. Secondly, it may provide no reliable information in particular animals (e.g., those with dark pigment). In addition, there are both theoretical limits and practical limits to the ability of the pulse oximeter to accurately reflect oxyhemoglobin saturation.

THEORETICAL LIMITS

The pulse oximeter cannot assess oxyhemoglobin saturation when there is absent or inadequate pulsatile blood flow between the transmitter and the sensor. This means that poorly perfused tissues may yield no values or, worse, may yield values that are misleading. All machines include some indicator of poor pulse quality and provide a measure of detected pulse rate. Therefore a value obtained when the pulse quality is poor, or when the detected pulse rate is at variance with the actual pulse rate, should be rejected. The best machines display a graphic representation of the shape of the detected pulse wave and sometimes also a quantified measure of the quality of the pulse. These additional features can aid the identification of SpO_2 values that are most likely to be valid.

A second important limit is that calibration curves using a number of different machines in healthy animals have shown that the SpO_2 is linear only above 70%. The SpO_2 result is generally lower than the actual measured SaO_2 at very high values (>96% to 97%), and SpO_2 results tend to overestimate the actual SaO_2 at low values.[5,6] Validation of one model on critically ill small animal patients yielded a confidence interval of 4.4%.[7] Referring to the oxyhemoglobin saturation curve in Figure 26-1, it is obvious that this ±4.4% range in SpO_2 spans a broad range of PaO_2 values. Thus an SpO_2 value of 91% could reflect an actual SaO_2 of 87% to 95%. The patient's actual PaO_2 may be lower than 70 mm Hg or well within the normal range of 80 to 100 mm Hg. In practice, in a given location on a well-perfused animal, the readings generally seem to reflect trends accurately. In order to determine how the readings relate to the individual's actual PaO_2, there is no substitute for comparing SpO_2 with PaO_2 measured directly from arterial blood. When the patient's status is changing, intermittent arterial blood gas determinations should be obtained, with pulse oximetry used for monitoring between arterial blood samples.

PRACTICAL LIMITS

The size and shape of the available probes are not appropriate for some small animals, and particular problems can be encountered in applying probes to cats. In addition, if the patient is aggressive, application to the lips (which commonly give the best reading in a conscious patient) cannot be achieved. The expensive probes cannot be left in place without observation in patients that are likely to chew them. The very slight heat and pressure produced by the probe can lead eventually to necrosis of the tissue if left in place for days (e.g., in ventilated patients). This injury is easily prevented by moving the probe every 2 to 4 hours as part of routine ventilator management.[8]

Instrumentation and Technique

Probes include clips and cylinders, designed for light transmission through soft tissue, and flat devices that are intended to detect a reflected signal bounced off a bony surface. These were developed for the human ear or finger and forehead, respectively. In addition, rectal probes are available for use in veterinary patients. In practice, the author has found the clip to be the most useful applied to the lip, ear pinna, tail, mucosal surfaces, skinfolds, and unpigmented footpads (the latter in cats only).

To obtain a reliable reading, the transmitter and detecting surface must both be in close apposition to the skin or mucosa. The skin must be close-shaven and, ideally, cleaned and degreased with an alcohol swab. The animal's temperature must be high enough so that the tissue is being perfused. Thus in hypothermic or vasoconstricted animals the ears, distal tail, or paws may not provide any readings. Generally, the very best readings are obtained from well-perfused mucosal surfaces such as the lip, penis or prepuce, vulvar folds, or tongue. All of these are readily accessible in an anesthetized patient; but in an aggressive, painful, or even just normally conscious animal, the choices may be limited to the lip or to other skinfolds (e.g., the axilla, gastrocnemius tendon region, or the footpads in the cat). The more distal skinfolds typically provide underestimates of the actual Sao_2, which could lead to an erroneous diagnosis of hypoxia and thus the performance of unnecessary diagnostics or the provision of supplemental oxygen when it is actually not warranted.[7] If at all possible, verification of hypoxia by arterial blood gas analysis is recommended.

Although virtually all animals will tolerate the placement of the oximetry probe, the occasional very aggressive or extremely dyspneic animal will not allow the probe to remain in place long enough to obtain a reading. A higher proportion of conscious animals will not allow the probe to remain in place continuously for more than a few minutes. Because the probes are costly, removal between readings in an active or uncooperative patient is routine. This means that each reading in such patients is from a slightly different location, rather than a perfectly identical reading, and that the great value for continuously monitoring trends may be lost. If the probe is moved to different locations on an individual animal, Spo_2 readings can vary by as much as 12%.[7] Finally, if more than one type of oximeter is available in a practice, the variability among the instruments may be considerable.[6] Thus, different readings from different instruments can reflect instrument variability rather than a change in the patient's status.

All of these possibilities must be taken into consideration, together with a general evaluation of the animal's condition, in judging how much credence to place on oximetry readings in a particular patient. The ideal situation is a well-perfused, tolerant (or unconscious) patient in which arterial blood gas samples can also be obtained periodically.

Although studies have not focused specifically on feline patients, two case series that included cats appeared to reflect more difficulty in obtaining reliable measures in cats than in dogs.[4,7] Nonetheless, because arterial blood samples are also much more difficult to obtain in cats, the pulse oximetry reading may provide the only possible source of objective information about oxygenation in feline patients. No commercial probe that is suitable for placing on a cat's lip is available, so that the less accurate probe locations (e.g., tail, digits, and skinfolds) are the only choices in conscious cats. The tongue is available only in unconscious patients but provides the most reliable values.

Cleaning the skin with alcohol swabs can improve readings, probably because this also increases circulation. However, once a good reading is obtained, it is usually not necessary to repeatedly prepare the surface before each application. After applying the probe, it is left in place while the instrument makes its determination of saturation and perfusion. After a few seconds, a reading of pulse rate, saturation, and perfusion level should appear on the screen. If the reading is unstable, if the pulse rate is different from the actual pulse rate, or if error signals appear, moving the probe to another location or increasing the perfusion of the tissue (e.g., by rubbing with an alcohol swab) may provide a better reading.

Interpretation of Results

Possible sources of error include sources of false pulsations (e.g., movement or respiratory movement artifact); abnormalities in the blood itself (e.g., severe anemia, icterus, and methemoglobinemia); and the possibility of light contamination from ambient lighting (e.g., fluorescent versus incandescent light sources). In fact, different models appear to suffer variably from these sources of error. In at least some studies, movement artifact rarely was a problem and neither icterus nor anemia produced false readings.[7] Room lighting has not been a problem in any studies. Very thick or darkly pigmented skin can be a problem, so that, for example, reading from the footpads of most dogs is not possible. However, studies have shown few problems in actual use.[4,7] Although perfusion abnormalities such as thromboembolism lead to grossly inaccurate readings, such conditions are generally rare or easily detected. In one study, a grossly inaccurate value was obtained from a dog undergoing CPR for cardiac arrest, as might be expected.[7]

The reference range for Spo_2 is 95% to 99% in animals breathing room air. Spo_2 results of 90% to 94% may represent moderate hypoxia, often corresponding with Pao_2 values of 60 to 80 mm Hg. Spo_2 values less than 90%, obtained with a strong pulse signal, are of significant concern; they may represent severe hypoxia and the need for aggressive measures to diagnose and treat the problem. Results of pulse oximetry must also be interpreted in relation to the Fio_2; an Spo_2 value of 92%, although adequate to support life, is of significant concern if it is obtained while an animal is anesthetized and breathing 100% oxygen. Animals with normal respiratory function receiving 100% oxygen should have Pao_2 values of up to 500 mm Hg. If errors related to probe pressure and tissue dessication are ruled out, a decrease in saturation to 92% potentially corresponds with a much lower Pao_2 value of 70 mm Hg, indicating profoundly abnormal respiratory function if the animal is breathing 100% oxygen.

Uses

There have been a number of attempts to use pulse oximetry to reflect tissue perfusion (e.g., of intestines during surgery to determine viability or of tissue perfusion during CPR); however, we review here only the applications for monitoring pulmonary function.

ANESTHESIA

Pulse oximetry was first described in anesthetized normal animals. Readings from the tongue of normal dogs, and then from the tail or penis, were found to be reliable and useful for monitoring trends when hypoxia was experimentally induced.[3] Lingual or rectal probes reflected Sp_{O_2} accurately over a mean blood pressure range from 40 to 100 mm Hg.[9] All placements and studies tend to underestimate Sa_{O_2} at values greater than 95%. A review of the recent literature shows numerous studies of additional species, including ferrets[10] and species of interest for zoo and wildlife medicine (e.g., an Asian elephant[11] and gazelles[12]). These studies have all concluded that pulse oximetry is safe, efficient, and reasonably accurate, and therefore improves the safety of anesthesia in these species. An evaluation of the utility of pulse oximetry in avian species, however, concluded that it is grossly inaccurate and will not be useful until a specific avian calibration curve is generated.[13]

DIAGNOSIS OF HYPOXIA

With all of the limits and caveats mentioned above, the detection of intermittent hypoxia in critically ill patients has been one of the most common applications of pulse oximetry. Of course, the sickest patients are often those in which perfusion is compromised, so that questioning the accuracy of Sp_{O_2} readings in sick patients is particularly important.[7]

MONITORING RESPIRATORY FUNCTION

The first report of pulse oximetry in unanesthetized dogs was its use for monitoring desaturation associated with sleep-disordered breathing in English bulldogs.[5] Continuous pulse oximetry to detect intermittent hypoxia in conscious ICU patients[4] and in ventilated patients[14] has also been reported, and these uses are routine in the author's ICU.

CONCLUSION

There is now no question that pulse oximetry has an important place in monitoring patients that are at risk for drops in oxygenation. Additional applications may also be discovered. For example, monitoring of neonatal cats and dogs has not been reported, but Sp_{O_2} values in newborn lambs correlated with vitality scores.[15] Forty-two lambs were tested after normal deliveries and 27 after dystocia.

In spite of the clear usefulness of pulse oximetry, we close with a cautionary note. Although veterinary medicine was relatively slow to develop a reliance on pulse oximetry, especially for unanesthetized patients, it now appears that pulse oximetry has a well-established role for monitoring anesthesia, ventilation, and oxygenation in veterinary patients. The flood of studies in nontraditional pet species (e.g., ferrets and avians) attests to a

recognition of the potential of a quick, noninvasive method for assessing respiratory function. However, pulse oximetry clearly has inherent limits. Recent pulse oximetry studies in humans conclude that clinicians should remain aware of the limits of the device and not be overly reliant exclusively on pulse oximetry and should use complementary methods of evaluating oxygen and pulmonary function and be wary of uncritically extending its use to novel applications. Veterinarians should maintain their traditional critical approach to this useful but relatively limited new technology.

REFERENCES

1. Grosenbaugh DA, Alben JO, Muir WW: Absorbance spectra of inter-species hemoglobins in the visible end-near infrared regions, J Vet Emerg Crit Care 7:36-42, 1997.
2. Rossing RG, Cain SM: A nomogram relating PO2, pH, temperature and hemoglobin saturation in the dog, J Appl Physiol 21:195-201, 1966.
3. Grosenbaugh DA, Muir WW: Accuracy of noninvasive oxyhemoglobin saturation, end-tidal carbon dioxide concentration, and blood pressure monitoring during experimentally induced hypoxemia, hypotension, or hypertension in anesthetized dogs, Am J Vet Res 59:205-212, 1998.
4. Fairman NB: Evaluation of pulse oximetry as a continuous monitoring technique in critically ill dogs in the small animal intensive care unit, Vet Emerg Crit Care 2:50-56, 1992.
5. Hendricks JC, Kline LR, Kovalski RJ et al: The English bulldog: A natural model of sleep-disordered breathing, J Appl Physiol 53: 1344-1350, 1987.
6. Matthews NS, Sanders EA, Hartsfield SM et al: A comparison of 2 pulse oximeters in dogs, J Vet Emerg Crit Care 5:115-120, 1995.
7. Hendricks JC, King LG: Practicality, usefulness, and limits of pulse oximetry in critical small animal patients, J Vet Emerg Crit Care 3: 5-12, 1993.
8. Fudge M, Anderson JG, Aldrich J et al: Oral lesions associated with orotracheally administered mechanical ventilation in critically ill dogs, J Vet Emerg Crit Care 7:79-87, 1997.
9. Barton LJ, Devey JJ, Gorski S et al: Evaluation of transmittance and reflectance pulse oximetry in a canine model of hypotension and desaturation, J Vet Emerg Crit Care 6:21-28, 1996.
10. Olin JM, Smith TJ, Talcott MR: Evaluation of noninvasive monitoring techniques in domestic ferrets (Mustela putorius furo), Am J Vet Res 58:1065-1069, 1997.
11. Mihm FG, Machada C, Snyder R: Pulse oximetry and end-tidal CO_2 monitoring of an adult Asian elephant, J Zoo An Med 19:106-109, 1988.
12. Schumacher J, Heard DJ, Young L et al: Cardiopulmonary effects of carfentanil in dama gazelles (Gazella dama), J Zoo & Wildlife Med 28:166-170, 1997.
13. Schmitt PM, Gobel T, Trautvetter E: Evaluation of pulse oximetry as a monitoring method in avian anesthesia, J Avian Med & Surg 12:91-99, 1998.
14. King LG, Hendricks JC: Positive pressure ventilation in dogs and cats: 41 cases (July 1990-January 1992), J Am Vet Med Assoc 204: 1045-1052, 1994.
15. Norton JR, Jackson PGG, Taylor PM: Measurement of arterial oxygen-haemoglobin saturation in newborn lambs by pulse oximetry, Vet Rec 142:107-109, 1998.

CHAPTER 27

End Tidal Capnography

Marc R. Raffe

Respiratory gas analysis has become a standard of care in human anesthesia and critical care medicine.[1] Information gained from respiratory gas measurement and blood gas analysis assists the clinician in determining global physiology and health of the pulmonary system.[2] Evaluating changes in carbon dioxide levels during inspiration and expiration can help the clinician assess dynamic pulmonary physiology. Graphically displaying this information provides additional information useful in determining appropriate support measures. The goal of this presentation is to review the current status of respiratory gas monitoring with a focus on carbon dioxide as a critical element in patient evaluation.

Background

Spectroscopy is an analytical technique that uses light absorption to quantify molecular concentration. In clinical medicine, spectroscopy is based on passage of a known light source through an optical measurement chamber. A photodetector located directly opposite the light source measures the amount of light that transverses the chamber.[3] Under baseline conditions, all emitted light transverses the detection chamber and is measured by the photodetector.[1,3] When molecules are introduced into the measurement chamber, they absorb part of the incident light, thereby reducing the quantity of light measured by the detector. The quantity of light absorbed is proportional to the concentration of molecules present in the measurement chamber.[3] Molecules best absorb light at certain wavelengths based on their structural characteristics. Absorptive wavelengths generally are in the infrared and ultraviolet regions of the light spectrum.

Capnometry is the spectroscopic technique for measuring carbon dioxide in respiratory gases.[1,3] Currently, two methods of measurement are commercially available: infrared spectrometry and Raman spectrometry.

Infrared Spectrometry

Infrared spectrometry is a quantitative method for measurement of carbon dioxide concentration in gas and liquid media.[1,3] A key factor in accurate measurement is to identify a light wavelength that provides quantitation without interference from other molecular species. A wavelength of 4.28 to 4.29 μm provides accurate carbon dioxide measurement without interference from other gases (e.g., nitrous oxide).[1,3]

The apparatus design includes a light-emitting diode that generates a steady 4.28- to 4.29-μm light beam that passes through an optical measuring chamber. A photo detector positioned on the opposite side of the chamber measures light intensity after transmission through the chamber. The presence of carbon dioxide molecules produces light absorption that is proportional to the carbon dioxide concentration. The quantity of light measured by the photodetector is, therefore, inversely proportional to the concentration of carbon dioxide in the analyzed gas sample.[1,3] The light detected is quantitated, signal processed, and displayed.[1,3]

Raman Spectrometry

Raman spectrometry works on a principle that is conceptually similar to infrared spectrometry. Raman spectrometry uses a helium-neon laser light source.[3] Light of a specific wavelength is emitted into a photodetection chamber. Molecules of interest (e.g., carbon dioxide) that interact with the light beam absorb photons. Due to the high energy imparted to the carbon dioxide molecule, a small fraction of absorbed light is reemitted at angles to the primary beam.[3] The reemitted photons have a lower energy than light emitted in the primary beam, thus creating a different light wavelength than the primary light beam.[3] The percent of reflected wavelength compared with the incident light source wavelength is proportional to the molecular concentration of gas in the photodetection chamber. In current designs, the photodetector is positioned at right angles to the axis of the light beam.[3]

Design Principles for Sample Collection

There are two different locations for carbon dioxide measurement relative to the patient. A mainstream analyzer uses an optical chamber that is interfaced to the patient's face or breathing circuit.[1,3] A light-emitting diode and photo detector unit surround the optical chamber to measure gas concentration. This design has the advantage of maintaining a closed breathing system to the patient without loss of gas volume. The main disadvantage is moisture condensation in the optical chamber, which can affect light absorption and produce inaccurate carbon dioxide measurement.

A side-stream analyzer incorporates a sampling port into the breathing circuit, nasal catheters, or face mask.[1,3,4] The sampling port is connected to a remotely located optical chamber via small bore tubing. Gas is continuously withdrawn for analysis from the sampling port into the optical chamber. A suction pump housed in the analyzer base unit provides the vacuum source used for gas withdrawal. Before introduction into the measurement chamber, gas passes through a moisture trap/desiccation chamber to remove condensation. Gas is then introduced into the measurement chamber, analyzed, and purged to the atmosphere. Measurements are displayed on the front panel of the analyzer. Although side-stream analyzers largely avoid the problem of moisture condensation in the measurement chamber, they have two potential disadvantages. The amount of gas drawn from the anesthetic circuit per minute may have a significant effect on minute ventilation in small patients unless efforts are made to compensate for the withdrawn gas volume. Secondly, the gas purged into the atmosphere will contain anesthetic gases if inhalants are in use, and care must be taken to vent the gases safely.

Two types of carbon dioxide monitors are available. Hand-held devices that display a digital value for carbon dioxide concentration are suitable for spot checks and general monitoring. Stationary patient monitors that display digital information and also have a waveform display are used in anesthesia and critical care settings. The ability to visualize and interpret the carbon dioxide waveform provides additional information to the clinician.

Colorometric Carbon Dioxide Detection

A device that colorometrically detects carbon dioxide is commercially available.[2] The device is composed of a plastic housing with molded fittings to interface with an endotracheal tube and breathing circuit. The center part of the plastic housing contains a filter paper disk that is impregnated with a color-sensitive pH indicator. A liquid film on the paper hydrates exhaled respiratory gas; the resulting pH is detected and displayed as a color in the disk section. The zone surrounding the disk contains a ring with different colored areas that represent carbon dioxide concentration. The color ranges from purple (0%) to yellow (>2%). The color shades are not accurate for predicting end tidal carbon dioxide levels; the major use for this device is to confirm airway placement of an endotracheal tube.

The system is easy and accurate except in low perfusion and respiratory states.[2] The detector is not accurate in patients with cardiopulmonary arrest because carbon dioxide levels are essentially zero until spontaneous circulation is reestablished. Patients with gastrointestinal gas associated with carbonated beverages may demonstrate a false positive. Despite these shortcomings, the device is easy to use and accurate under most conditions.

Capnogram

The carbon dioxide concentration measured by the photo detector can be graphically displayed on a monitor screen. A graphical plot of the changes in carbon dioxide concentrations over time is called a *capnogram* (Figure 27-1).[2,3,5-7] The shape of a normal capnogram has been well described. Under conditions of normal lung physiology, the graphical point on the plateau just before downward inflection represents the mixed alveolar carbon dioxide level.[5-7] This value is referred to as *end tidal carbon dioxide* ($ETCO_2$, $PETCO_2$). $ETCO_2$ values approximate blood CO_2 levels; however, the gradient between the two is species dependent.[5-7]

Analysis of Capnogram Waveforms

Capnogram waveforms can be useful in diagnosis and management of acute changes in respiratory function. An individual breath waveform is composed of component areas (see Figure 27-1). Several nomenclatures have been used to describe components of the waveform. Recently, an attempt to standardize the nomenclature has been reported.[5,6] The present description will use the traditional nomenclature followed by the proposed nomenclature in parentheses.[5,6] A zero baseline at the beginning of exhalation represents exhaled gas that has been in the anatomical dead space of the large conducting pathways, oropharynx, and nasopharynx. This part of the waveform tracing is the A-B (I) region. The rapid upstroke representing gas from the intermediate airways containing both fresh and exhaled gases is the B-C (II) region. The flat plateau area representing mixed alveolar gas is the C-D (III) region. The distinct end point of the plateau that represents true end tidal gas is the D point. The rapid downstroke of the curve associated with inspiration is the D-E (0) region. The D-E portion of the

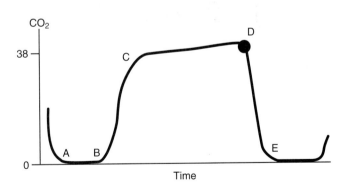

Figure 27-1. *Components of a normal capnograph waveform. Segment A-B represents the zero baseline. Segment B-C represents the rapid, sharp rise associated with gas from the intermediate airways. Segment C-D represents the flat alveolar plateau associated with alveolar gas detection. Point D is the end-tidal carbon dioxide concentration found in the alveolus. Segment D-E represents inspiration of fresh gas devoid of carbon dioxide.*

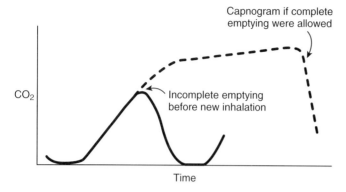

Figure 27-2. *Change in alveolar waveform indicating incomplete alveolar emptying. Incomplete emptying may be associated with asthma, upper airway obstruction, partial endotracheal tube obstruction, or chronic obstructive pulmonary disease. This is one example of a waveform change indicating a clinical problem.*

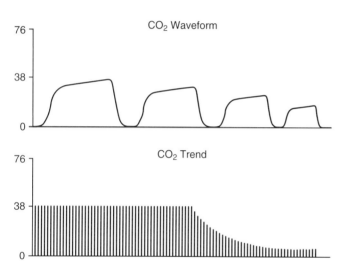

Figure 27-3. *Exponential fall in end tidal CO_2 indicating pulmonary embolism, severe pulmonary hypoperfusion, or cardiopulmonary arrest.*

waveform has a small carbon dioxide concentration due to the low carbon dioxide level in atmospheric gas.

Changes in capnogram waveform fall into one of two categories: (1) change in individual waveform characteristics and (2) change in waveform over time (trend monitoring). Changes may be noted in any phase of the capnogram waveform (Figure 27-2). In most cases, the point of change involves the plateau (C-D [III]), end tidal (D [IIIβ]), and expiratory (D-E [0]) phases.[5,6] Several characteristic patterns have been noted. Waveforms with a normal appearance but a higher scalar plateau represent elevated $ETco_2$, reflecting hypercapnia.[5,6] A gradual rise in $ETco_2$ may be noted with increased metabolism, hyperthermia, sepsis, hypoventilation, neuromuscular weakness, and reduced alveolar gas exchange. A stable, sustained rise in $ETco_2$ reflects sedative or anesthetic drugs, metabolic alkalosis, or hypoventilation. A gradual rise in both baseline and $ETco_2$ reflects rebreathing of carbon dioxide gas.

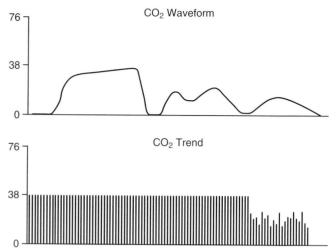

Figure 27-4. *Sudden fall in end tidal CO_2 indicating mechanical airway leak. Possible reasons include breathing circuit leak or disconnection, accidental extubation, partial airway obstruction, and ventilator leak.*

TABLE 27-1. **Conditions Producing an Increased $Paco_2$—$ETco_2$ Gradient**	
Increased Anatomical Dead Space	**Increased Physiological Dead Space**
Open ventilator circuit	Obstructive lung disease
Hypoventilation	Low cardiac output
Excessive endotracheal tube length	Pulmonary thromboembolism
	Excessive lung inflation

A decreased $ETco_2$ with a stable plateau phase reflects hyperventilation, hypothermia, and metabolic acidosis.[5-7] A sudden fall in $ETco_2$ to low values reflects airway leak, partial airway obstruction, and disconnection from a breathing circuit or mechanical ventilator malfunction.[5,6] A sudden fall in $ETco_2$ to zero may indicate a dislodged endotracheal tube, breathing circuit disconnection, mechanical ventilator malfunction, complete airway obstruction, pulmonary thromboembolism, severe pulmonary hypoperfusion, or cardiopulmonary arrest (Figure 27-3).[5-7] A low $ETco_2$ without alveolar plateau may reflect partial airway obstruction, bronchospasm, small airway mucous plugs, or incorrect ventilator settings (Figure 27-4).[5-7]

Comparison of $Paco_2$ and $ETco_2$ Values

In small animal species, a difference between arterial blood gas and $ETco_2$ values ($Paco_2$−$ETco_2$) of 5 torr or less is reported to be normal. $ETco_2$ values are lower than arterial values due to intrapulmonary dead space ventilation.[1,2,4,7]

When pulmonary gas exchange is impaired, less carbon dioxide is eliminated during each breath. In these cases, the $Paco_2$–$ETco_2$ gradient increases due to the decreased $ETco_2$. Many cardiac or respiratory disease states produce an increased $Paco_2$–$ETco_2$ gradient (Table 27-1). In these cases, arterial blood gas analysis remains the definitive method for evaluating carbon dioxide dynamics. Once the $Paco_2$–$ETco_2$ gradient is established, continued monitoring using $ETco_2$ might be practical.

Additional Information from ETco_2 Measurement

Trends in $ETco_2$ can be used to monitor cardiac output.[2,4] Studies have shown that $ETco_2$ measurement correlates well with cardiac output measurements during resuscitation from shock and cardiopulmonary arrest.[2,4] It is also useful in monitoring ventilator management by reporting ventilator related mishaps and monitoring controlled hyperventilation.[2,4] Finally, $ETco_2$ is helpful for monitoring patients during discontinuation of ventilatory support (weaning).[2,4]

REFERENCES

1. Lake CL, Hines RL, Blitt CD: Clinical monitoring: *Practical applications for anesthesia and critical care*, Philadelphia, 2001, WB Saunders.
2. Marino PL: *The ICU book*, ed 2, Baltimore, 1998, Williams & Wilkins.
3. Parbrook GD, Davis PD, Parbrook EO: *Basic physics and measurement in anaesthesia*, ed 3, Oxford, 1992, Butterworths, Heinneman.
4. Hendricks JC, King LG: Practicality, usefulness, and limits of end-tidal carbon dioxide monitoring in critical small animal patients, *J Vet Emerg Crit Care* 4:29-39, 1994.
5. Lynn-McHale DJ, Carlson KK: *AACN procedure manual for critical care*, ed 4, Philadelphia, 2001, WB Saunders.
6. Bhavani-Ahankar K, Kumar AY, Moseley HS et al: Terminology and the current limitations of time capnography: A brief review, *J Clin Monitor* 11:175-182, 1995.
7. Hightower CE, Kiorpes AL, Butler HC et al: End-tidal partial pressure of carbon dioxide as an estimate of arterial partial pressure of carbon dioxide during various ventilatory regimens in halothane-anesthetized dogs, *Am J Vet Res* 41:610-612, 1980.

CHAPTER 28

Transcutaneous Oxygen and Carbon Dioxide Monitoring

F. A. Mann

Physiology, Background, and Definition

Transcutaneous oxygen and carbon dioxide monitoring refers to measurement of partial pressures of oxygen ($Ptco_2$) and carbon dioxide ($Ptcco_2$) on the skin surface as a continuous estimation of arterial partial pressures of oxygen (Pao_2) and carbon dioxide ($Paco_2$) that would be obtainable by arterial sampling and blood gas analysis.

Transcutaneous movement of gases was recognized in the late 1700s.[1-3] In 1851, von Gerlach at the Royal Veterinary School in Berlin, Germany studied the transcutaneous movement of gases by gluing an air-filled horse bladder to the thoracic skin of horses, dogs, and humans, and by comparing the initial oxygen and carbon dioxide content of the bladder to the content 24 hours later.[1,2] One hundred years later, in 1951, Baumberger and Goodfriend demonstrated that the oxygen content in a phosphate-buffered solution surrounding a human finger would nearly equal the subject's Pao_2 within 15 minutes regardless of the starting oxygen content of the solution.[1-6] Development of the Clark polarographic electrode in 1956 made measurement of transcutaneous oxygen more practical, and in 1967 a correlation between $Ptco_2$ and Pao_2 was demonstrated.[1,4,5] Clinical devices for measuring $Ptco_2$ became available in the mid-1970s; clinical devices for measuring $Ptcco_2$ followed in the early 1980s.[7]

The basis for using $Ptco_2$ and $Ptcco_2$ to monitor Pao_2 and $Paco_2$ lies in the gas exchange between blood and skin that takes place at the level of the dermal capillaries. Oxygen diffuses out of the dermal capillaries in exchange for carbon dioxide that is generated during cellular metabolism. The dermis consumes little of the oxygen itself, but the dermal capillaries supply the epidermis, which consumes oxygen at a very high rate. The outer layer of the skin, the stratum corneum, functions as a diffusion membrane and provides a surface where the blood gases (oxygen and carbon dioxide) that diffuse upward from the dermis can be measured.[4,8] The accuracy of the measurement depends on sufficient skin permeability. Consistent permeability is achieved by heating the skin at the sampling site (usually to 43° to 45° C) to induce local vasodilation and thereby eliminate variations in vascular tone that would cause spurious P_{TCO_2} and P_{TCCO_2} readings.[1-3,5-7] Skin thickness also affects the accuracy of measurement, particularly with P_{TCO_2}. The partial pressure of oxygen falls as oxygen diffuses through the skin toward the stratum corneum; therefore P_{TCO_2} is lower in subjects with thicker skin. As a result, P_{TCO_2} more closely approximates Pa_{O_2} in human neonates than in adults.[1,3,4,9] Likewise, veterinary species with thin skin may have P_{TCO_2} readings that more closely approximate Pa_{O_2} than species with thicker skin; however, there is lack of data to substantiate this speculation.

Indications

Transcutaneous blood gas monitoring is well established in human critical care (especially neonatal critical care) as a method of continuously monitoring oxygenation and ventilation status.[2,3,6,7,11] Transcutaneous monitoring is less invasive than arterial blood draws (particularly in small neonates) and provides continuous assessment that cannot be achieved by intermittent arterial sampling for blood gas analysis.[2,12-14] Although pulse oximetry provides a means of continuous oxygenation assessment, it does not provide monitoring for hyperoxemia, which can only be monitored by measuring Pa_{O_2}. Hyperoxemia has serious consequences in neonates (e.g., retrolental fibroplasia and blindness) and potentially fatal consequences (i.e., oxygen toxicity) in all patients.[5,12,15] Monitoring P_{TCO_2} should be useful for recognizing dangerous elevations in Pa_{O_2} but has not consistently contributed to the prevention of these untoward effects.[16] Compared with pulse oximetry, P_{TCO_2} is more useful for monitoring oxygenation when the color of blood does not accurately represent hemoglobin saturation (e.g., in carbon monoxide poisoning), and it is more sensitive for detecting decreases in oxygen content and oxygen delivery due to hypovolemia, hypotension, and anemia when the pulse oximeter will not read and when hemoglobin saturation may be normal.[13] Transcutaneous blood gas monitoring has been shown to provide earlier detection of decreased respiratory function than pulse oximetry in human beings undergoing fiberoptic bronchoscopy.[17] Capnometry provides a noninvasive and continuous measurement of end-tidal carbon dioxide (ET_{CO_2}) to estimate Pa_{CO_2} but typically requires interfacing with a breathing circuit. Measurement of P_{TCCO_2} may be preferred over ET_{CO_2} and arterial blood gas sampling in nonintubated patients that require continuous Pa_{CO_2} assessment.[18] In human infants and neonates with respiratory failure, P_{TCCO_2} has been shown to provide a more accurate estimation of Pa_{CO_2} than ET_{CO_2}.[19]

Transcutaneous blood gas monitoring has had limited application in veterinary medicine. One P_{TCO_2}/P_{TCCO_2}

monitoring system (P_{TCO_2}/P_{TCCO_2} Monitor Model 840, Novametrix Medical Systems Inc., Wallingford, Conn.) was shown to be useful in assessing skin graft viability in experimental dogs and was accurate in evaluating oxygenation and ventilation status in two dogs being treated for respiratory abnormalities.[1,10,20] However, a different transcutaneous blood gas monitoring system (TINA™, Radiometer America Inc., Westlake, Ohio) yielded unobtainable or inaccurate results in one normal dog and 23 critically ill animals.[21] The former monitoring system was evaluated experimentally in anesthetized cats with some promising results.[22] In that study, P_{TCO_2} closely approximated Pa_{O_2} during normoxia and hypoxia but not during hyperoxia[22]; therefore the monitor has potential to be useful for detecting hypoxia, but it would not be a dependable means of monitoring for risk of oxygen toxicity. Although P_{TCCO_2} did not match Pa_{CO_2}, the correlations were good, suggesting that the unit might be valuable as a trend monitor for ventilatory status, particularly if individual animal or species-specific conversion equations could be derived to make P_{TCCO_2} more closely match Pa_{CO_2}.[22] Additional work will be necessary to adapt this useful human clinical tool to clinical veterinary medicine.

Contraindications

There are no specific contraindications for transcutaneous blood gas monitoring, but there are certain limitations of the technology that could result in patient morbidity if not addressed. Specific limitations that warrant emphasis are the necessity to heat the skin, drift in readings, the effect of patient movement, and other patient factors.

Heating the skin to 42° C or greater predisposes the skin to thermal burns, particularly with prolonged exposure. Usually a small hyperemic area of skin is the only evidence of thermal burn when the transcutaneous monitor's sensor is removed from the subject, and this hyperemia resolves without consequence. Serious burns are prevented by moving the sensor to a new skin site every 3 to 6 hours, especially in patients with thin or sensitive skin.*

Drift, a positive or negative change in baseline value, occurs over time and can result in significantly erroneous P_{TCO_2} results.[4,15] The only way to avoid erroneous readings due to drift is to periodically move the sensor and recalibrate the system. The interval of replacement for prevention of thermal burns should be sufficient for drift correction. Periodic arterial blood gas analysis should be performed to detect whether drift has occurred and to determine if appropriate correction has been achieved.[2,13]

Patient movement can interrupt readings and displace sensors from the skin. Caution should be exercised in interpreting readings in patients that are active; however, accurate readings have been acquired in mobile humans.[23-25] If the sensor becomes dislodged from the skin

*References 1, 2, 4, 7, 8, and 15.

it must be reattached and the unit must be recalibrated and equilibrated before readings can be once again obtained, a process that may take as long as 30 minutes.

Other patient factors include alterations to skin blood flow or permeability that may pose a barrier to oxygen and carbon dioxide diffusion (e.g., edema, inflammation, and external pressure).[1,3,7,13,15] To avoid inaccurate results, sensors should not be placed on edematous or inflamed skin or on skin that may be subject to external pressure (e.g., dependent or bandaged areas). Bandages over the sensor may create pressure at the sampling site and therefore should be avoided. Hyperventilation has been demonstrated to decrease skin blood flow resulting in erroneous P_{TCO_2} readings (decreased P_{TCO_2}/P_{aO_2} ratio); therefore caution should be exercised when interpreting P_{TCO_2} readings during hypocapnia.[26]

Instrumentation

Transcutaneous blood gas monitors are designed to measure P_{TCO_2} or P_{TCCO_2} individually or simultaneously. Three product lines of transcutaneous monitors* are readily available in the United States.[3] The monitors reported in veterinary medicine (i.e., the Novametrix and Radiometer monitors) measure both P_{TCO_2} and P_{TCCO_2} simultaneously. Combination P_{TCO_2}/P_{TCCO_2} monitors have a single sensor that contains a modified Clark polarographic electrode (for measuring oxygen), a Severinghaus pH electrode (for measuring carbon dioxide), an electrolyte solution, a semipermeable membrane, and a heating element. The sensor is attached to the subject with an adhesive ring and via a cable to the monitor (Figure 28-1)

Technique

The technique of application may vary somewhat among commercially available systems. Typically (e.g., in the Novametrix monitor) the sensor cable is connected to the monitor and, with the monitor turned off, a new membrane is applied to the sensor, if necessary, according to manufacturer specifications. A new membrane is required: (1) after extended periods of non-use; (2) if the membrane is damaged or loosened from the sensor; (3) if a significant amount of air (i.e., greater than 50% of the annulus) is noted under the membrane; or (4) after 7 days of continuous usage. After the membrane is applied the monitor is turned on and allowed to heat to, and stabilize at, the chosen operating temperature (usually 44° C). The process of applying a new membrane and stabilizing at operating temperature takes 25 to 30 minutes.[22] Once stabilized at operating temperature, and before attachment to the subject, a two-point calibration is performed using a calibration unit supplied by the manufacturer. Two gas canisters are attached to the calibration unit; one contains a low gas consisting of 95%

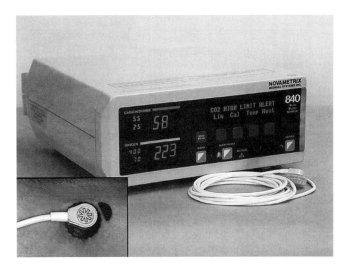

Figure 28-1. *Transcutaneous oxygen and carbon dioxide monitor with cable and sensor. The cable interfaces with the monitor on the rear of the monitor (not shown). The insert illustrates attachment of the sensor to feline skin using an adhesive ring.*

nitrogen, 5% carbon dioxide, and 0% oxygen; and the other contains a high gas consisting of 78% nitrogen, 10% carbon dioxide, and 12% oxygen. Calibration is performed each time the sensor is moved to a new site or reattached to the current site.[1,4,13,14]

The skin is prepared by clipping the area free of hair and cleansing/defatting the site with isopropyl alcohol, acetone, or ether. In addition, the skin may be stripped of some of the dead cells in the stratum corneum by repeated application and removal of transparent adhesive tape.[4,27] Application of tincture of benzoin to the skin can also be used to increase adhesiveness.[28] The sensor is attached to the skin with a two-sided O-ring adhesive patch. Some newer models of transcutaneous monitors (e.g., the Radiometer monitor) have a snap-on adhesive ring that allows multiple rings to be left in place for ease of rotating sensor sites; however, use of the snap-on sensor has not been reported in veterinary patients.

The site chosen should allow the sensor to lie flat against the skin surface without indenting or compressing the skin.[4] A well-perfused, centrally located site is preferred to the limbs; therefore trunkal skin, usually the chest or abdomen, is chosen.[13] In an experimental study in cats, there did not appear to be a significant difference in readings between dorsolateral thoracic and dorsal pelvic sites of sensor attachment.[22]

Once the sensor is attached to the skin an equilibration period is required to allow the readings to stabilize.[14] A period of at least 15 minutes is required for calibration, sensor attachment, and equilibration.[22] Therefore, at least 15 minutes of monitoring will be missed each time a sensor must be reapplied. The instrument with snap-on sensor adhesive rings mentioned above also has the advantage of snap-on membraning and high-speed, one-point calibration that minimizes set-up and calibration time.

During use the sensor must be protected from premature dislodgement. Bandaging should be avoided, but

---

*P_{TCO_2}/P_{TCCO_2} Monitor Model 840, Novametrix Medical Systems Inc., Wallingford, Conn.; TINA™, Radiometer America Inc., Westlake, Ohio; and HP 10181A, Hewlett Packard Company, Andover, Mass.

strategically placed butterfly tapes can serve to anchor the cable to the skin and distribute tension away from the sensor. Tilting of the sensor, which can lift the sensor from the skin, can be counteracted by placing appropriately sized gauze between the sensor cable and the skin near the sensor.

Sensors are relocated every 3 to 6 hours (usually, every 4 hours) to avoid thermal burn and to compensate for drift in readings. Periodic arterial blood gas analysis is necessary to thoroughly assess the patient's acid-base status and to evaluate how closely the P_{TCO_2} and P_{TCCO_2} correlate with the respective Pao_2 and $Paco_2$ in each individual patient.

REFERENCES

1. Rochat MC, Mann FA: Transcutaneous blood gas monitoring, *Compend Cont Ed Pract Vet* 16(9):1181-1186, 1994.
2. Rithalia SVS: Developments in transcutaneous blood gas monitoring: A review, *J Med Eng Technol* 15(4-5):143-153, 1991.
3. Robertson PW, Hart BB: Assessment of tissue oxygenation, *Respir Care Clin North Am* 5(2):221-263, 1999.
4. Malley WJ: Noninvasive blood gas monitoring. In Malley WJ, editor: *Clinical blood gases: Application and noninvasive alternatives,* Philadelphia, 1990, WB Saunders:
5. Huch A: Transcutaneous blood gas monitoring, *Acta Anaesthesiol Scand* 39(Suppl 107):87-90, 1995.
6. Sheffield PJ: Measuring tissue oxygen tension: A review, *Undersea Hyper Med* 25(3):179-188, 1998.
7. Hess D: Noninvasive respiratory monitoring during ventilatory support, *Crit Care Nurs Clin North Am* 3(4):565-574, 1991.
8. Severinghaus JW: Transcutaneous blood gas analysis, *Respir Care* 27(2):152-159, 1982.
9. Harrington GR, Hnatiuk OW: Noninvasive monitoring, *Am J Med* 95(2):221-228, 1993.
10. Rochat MC, Payne JT, Pope ER et al: Evaluation of skin viability in dogs using transcutaneous carbon dioxide and sensor current monitoring, *Am J Vet Res* 54(3):476-480, 1993.
11. Tobias JD, Wilson WR, Meyer DJ: Transcutaneous monitoring of carbon dioxide tension after cardiothoracic surgery in infants and children, *Anesth Analg* 88(3):531-534, 1999.
12. Brouillette RT, Waxman DH: Evaluation of the newborn's blood gas status, *Clin Chem* 43(1):215-221, 1997.
13. Benaron DA, Benitz WE, Ariagno RL et al: Noninvasive methods for estimating in vivo oxygenation, *Clin Pediatr* 31(5):258-273, 1992.
14. Rennie JM: Transcutaneous carbon dioxide monitoring, *Arch Dis Child* 65(4 Spec No):345-346, 1990.
15. Wahr JA, Tremper KK: Noninvasive oxygen monitoring techniques, *Crit Care Clin* 11(1):199-217, 1995.
16. Flynn JT, Bancalari E, Snyder ES et al: A cohort study of transcutaneous oxygen tension and the incidence and severity of retinopathy of prematurity, *N Engl J Med* 326(16):1050-1054, 1992.
17. Evans EN, Ganeshalingam K, Ebden P: Changes in oxygen saturation and transcutaneous carbon dioxide and oxygen levels in patients undergoing fibreoptic bronchoscopy, *Respir Med* 92(5):739-742, 1998.
18. Reid CW, Martineau RJ, Miller DR et al: A comparison of end-tidal and transcutaneous PCO_2 measurements during anaesthesia (abstract), *Can J Anaesth* 37(4 Pt 2):S89, 1990.
19. Tobias JD, Meyer DJ: Nonivasive monitoring of carbon dioxide during respiratory failure in toddlers and infants: End-tidal versus transcutaneous carbon dioxide, *Anesth Analg* 85(1):55-58, 1997.
20. Rochat MC, Pope ER, Payne JT et al: Transcutaneous oxygen monitoring for predicting skin viability in dogs, *Am J Vet Res* 54(3):468-475, 1993.
21. Hendricks JC, King LG, Moreau RE: Transcutaneous PO_2 and PCO_2 measurements in dogs. (abstract). In *Proceedings of the Third International Veterinary Emergency and Critical Care Symposium,* San Antonio, TX, 1992, Veterinary Emergency and Critical Care Society.
22. Mann FA, Wagner-Mann CC, Branson KR: Transcutaneous oxygen and carbon dioxide monitoring in normal cats, *J Vet Emerg Crit Care* 7(2):99-109, 1997.
23. Brudin L, Berg S, Ekberg P et al: Is transcutaneous PO_2 monitoring during exercise a reliable alternative to arterial PO_2 measurements? *Clin Physiol* 14(1):47-52, 1994.
24. Hoffmann U, Essfeld D, Stegemann J: Comparison of arterial, end-tidal and transcutaneous PCO_2 during moderate exercise and external CO_2 loading in humans, *Eur J Appl Physiol* 61(1-2):1-4, 1990.
25. Nayal W, Schwarzer U, Klotz T et al: Transcutaneous penile oxygen pressure during bicycling, *BJU International* 83(6):623-625, 1999.
26. Barker SJ, Hyatt J, Clarke C et al: Hyperventilation reduces transcutaneous oxygen tension and skin blood flow, *Anesth* 75(4):619-624, 1991.
27. Takiwaki H, Nakanishi H, Shono Y et al: The influence of cutaneous factors on the transcutaneous PO_2 and PCO_2 at various body sites, *Br J Dermatol* 125(3):243-247, 1991.
28. Warren RG, Webb AI, Kosch PC et al: Evaluation of transcutaneous oxygen monitoring in anaesthetized pony foals, *Equine Vet J* 16(4):358-361, 1984.

PART FOUR

Nonspecific Management of Respiratory Disease

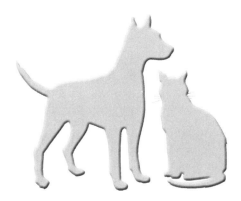

CHAPTER 29

Oxygen Supplementation and Humidification

Laura W. Tseng • Kenneth J. Drobatz

Oxygen (O_2) therapy plays a critical role in the treatment of hypoxemia and respiratory failure, but patient response to oxygen therapy varies significantly depending on the underlying cause of respiratory compromise. Furthermore, several potential complications can be associated with oxygen supplementation. A thorough understanding of the physiology and pathophysiology of oxygen supplementation is essential to ensure the optimal use of this drug.

Indications for Oxygen Therapy

Oxygen supplementation is a simple method of increasing the inspired oxygen concentration (FiO_2) in an attempt to increase the arterial partial pressure of oxygen (PaO_2) and hemoglobin saturation, thus increasing arterial oxygen content and, consequently, oxygen delivery to the tissues. Oxygen delivery to the tissues depends on hemoglobin concentration, oxygen saturation of hemoglobin, and cardiac output. The total oxygen content of the blood is equal to the hemoglobin content and the oxygen saturation of the hemoglobin, plus the amount of oxygen dissolved in the blood (PaO_2). As long as intrapulmonary shunting is not occurring, oxygen supplementation should increase both the dissolved oxygen and the oxygen saturation of the hemoglobin.[1]

CLINICAL SIGNS

Clinical signs of respiratory distress and hypoxemia may include anxiety, an extended head and neck, open mouth breathing, abducted elbows, increased respiratory effort or abdominal effort, and tachypnea. Clinical signs of hypoxia may also include tachycardia, psychomotor incoordination, gastrointestinal upset, and restlessness. Assessment of mucous membrane color should quickly detect cyanosis. Cyanosis is not a sensitive indicator of hypoxemia, however, because it is not evident until the Pao_2 is less than 50 mm Hg and because it cannot be detected in patients with severe anemia (i.e., packed cell volume less than 15%), carbon monoxide poisoning, or if the membranes are white due to hypoperfusion.[2,3] Arterial blood gas analysis, pulse oximetry, and calculation of alveolar-arterial oxygen tension (A–a) gradients can help document the severity of hypoxemia and the requirement for oxygen supplementation.

HYPOXEMIA

Hypoxia is defined as decreased levels of oxygen in air, blood, or tissue.[4] An inadequate supply of oxygen to the tissues can result from hypoxemia (subnormal oxygenation of arterial blood),[4] reduced oxygen carrying capacity of red cells, decreased tissue blood flow, increased tissue demand for oxygen, or impaired tissue extraction of oxygen. Hypoxemia can be caused by a low fraction of inspired oxygen (Fio_2); hypoventilation; or venous admixture due to diffusion impairment, intrapulmonary shunt, or ventilation-perfusion (V/Q) mismatch. The most common causes of impaired pulmonary gas exchange are ventilation-perfusion mismatch and physiological shunt secondary to alveolar collapse. Low Fio_2 values have been associated with oxygen delivery failure during anesthesia and the use of nitrous oxide. Low barometric pressure at high altitudes also results in decreased inspired oxygen.

The decision to supplement oxygen should be based on the complete clinical picture of the patient. In general, oxygen supplementation should be considered in patients with a Pao_2 of less than 70 mm Hg or an arterial hemoglobin saturation (Sao_2) of less than 93%. Although an animal in respiratory distress due to acute pulmonary disease with a Pao_2 of 60 mm Hg requires oxygen supplementation, another patient with a similar Pao_2 that has acclimatized to chronic lung disease and is breathing comfortably likely does not require additional oxygen.

DECREASED OXYGEN DELIVERY TO TISSUES

Oxygen delivery to the tissues is affected by anemia, hemoglobin abnormalities (e.g., carboxyhemoglobin or methemoglobin), and decreased tissue perfusion (e.g., as occurs in patients with shock). Increased tissue oxygen demand occurs in animals with increased body temperature or metabolic rate, which can be caused by fever, heat stroke, malignant hyperthermia, sepsis, and seizures. Oxygen therapy attempts to maximize hemoglobin saturation, thereby increasing oxygen delivery to the tissues in patients with poor blood flow or increased oxygen demand.

Oxygen therapy may be helpful in treating patients with head trauma because many suffer from cerebral ischemia secondary to increased intracranial pressure and reduction in cerebral perfusion. Oxygen supplementation is essential in these patients to maximize cerebral oxygen delivery. Patients with head trauma may not show the typical signs of respiratory distress due to altered mentation. Therefore, additional diagnostics may

be necessary to document the need for oxygen therapy in these patients.

Oxygen Administration Techniques

FACE MASK

The face mask is a short-term method of oxygen delivery that can be initiated quickly, requires minimal set up, and allows convenient access to patients (Figure 29-1). It is a useful and effective technique for short-term oxygen therapy while physical examination or diagnostics and therapeutics are performed. In anesthetized healthy dogs, this technique was a very efficient way of increasing inspired oxygen concentrations at a flow rate of 0.5 L/min.[5] The mean Fio_2 achieved with the mask held tightly to the face was 46.5%, with a range of 30% to 70.6% (Figure 29-2).[5] These studies were per-

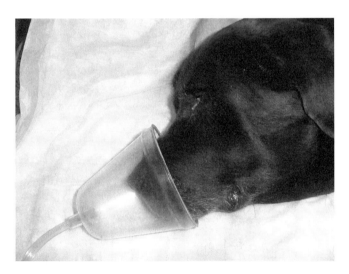

Figure 29-1. Face mask oxygen is a noninvasive method of oxygen delivery to a patient.

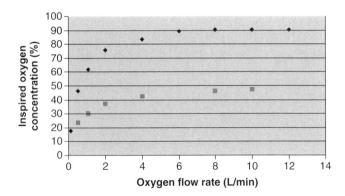

Figure 29-2. Oxygen concentration at the bifurcation of the trachea with face mask oxygen therapy at varying flow rates (diamonds) compared with flow-by oxygen 2 cm from the nose (squares). (Modified with permission from Loukopoulos P, Reynolds W: Comparative evaluation of oxygen therapy techniques in anaesthetized dogs: Face mask and flow by technique, Aust Vet Practit 27:34-39, 1997.)

formed in dogs weighing 15 to 29 kg and the results were reported as a mean $+/-$ standard deviation. Obviously, a flow rate of 1 L/min may be adequate for a small dog, whereas a giant breed dog with a much higher minute ventilation will require a much higher flow rate to obtain similar results. In large breed dogs, flow rates of 5 to 10 L/min should be used.

The stress of holding a face mask on a dyspneic, nonanesthetized animal may preclude optimal use of this technique, thus leading to a lower than expected Fio_2.

FLOW-BY OXYGEN

Flow-by oxygen is a simple, quick, and easy method of short-term oxygen supplementation in emergencies (Figure 29-3). It is less effective than mask oxygen but may be tolerated better by dyspneic animals. Flow-by oxygen supplementation is used at a flow rate of 2 to 5 L/min with the hose held 2 to 4 cm from the nose (or mouth in panting animals). In healthy, anesthetized dogs weighing 15 to 29 kg, flow-by oxygen was supplied 2 cm from the nose with a flow rate of 2 L/min.[5] A mean Fio_2 at the tracheal bifurcation of 37.2% (range 29.5% to 48%) was obtained with this method (see Figure 29-2).[5] No complications are seen with flow-by oxygen, but it is unlikely that dyspneic animals will tolerate and maintain oxygen flow 2 cm from the nose at all times. Disadvantages of this technique include the requirement for constant supervision, the inability to achieve high enough inspired oxygen concentrations in some cases,[5] and its wastefulness.

NASAL OXYGEN

Nasal O_2 administration is a practical and effective way of raising tracheal O_2 concentration and Pao_2. It is useful for tolerant patients that are anticipated to require several days of oxygen therapy. Passing a nasal catheter can be stressful for the patient, so severe respiratory distress may preclude its safe placement. Patients with upper

respiratory signs attributable to the nares, and brachycephalic breeds, should not be considered for nasal catheterization. There is an almost linear relationship between nasal oxygen flow rate and tracheal oxygen concentration, and therefore between nasal oxygen flow rate and Pao_2.[6] It is also clear that changes in tracheal oxygen concentration are greatest in smaller patients for each given flow rate (Figure 29-4). Low nasal flow rates of 50 to 100 ml/kg/min should be adequate to increase the mean tracheal O_2 concentration to 40% to 50%.[6] A nasal catheter flow rate of 0.75 L/min has been shown to produce a mean Fio_2 of 50% at the tracheal bifurcation in healthy anesthetized dogs.[6]

To place a nasal oxygen catheter, topical anesthetic (e.g., 2% lidocaine or proparacaine) should be instilled into one nostril at least 10 minutes prior to the placement of the catheter. A lubricated, soft rubber catheter (5 to 10 Fr, depending on the size of the patient), with multiple fenestrations at the distal end to prevent jet lesions in the mucosa, is introduced through the nares into the ventral nasal meatus. The catheter is gently but quickly advanced to the level of the carnassial tooth or of the medial canthus of the eye. It should then be sutured to the skin as close to the exit from the nares as possible. The remainder of the catheter is attached to the dorsolateral aspect of the nose and to the head with sutures or an adhesive agent (e.g., cyanoacrylate) and then attached to the oxygen source (Figure 29-5, A). The shortest, widest tubing possible for the animal should be utilized to maximize oxygen delivery. Poiseuille's law states that flow is directly proportional to the radius of the tube raised to the fourth power and inversely proportional to its length[8]; therefore the internal radius of the tube will have the greater effect on resistance to air flow.[9]

In very ill, sedated, or tolerant patients that are not moving around, nasal prongs designed for human beings can be used to supply oxygen directly into the nares, eliminating the stress of placing and securing an intranasal catheter. The prongs are only about 1 cm long and fit into each nare of the dog. They can be cut shorter

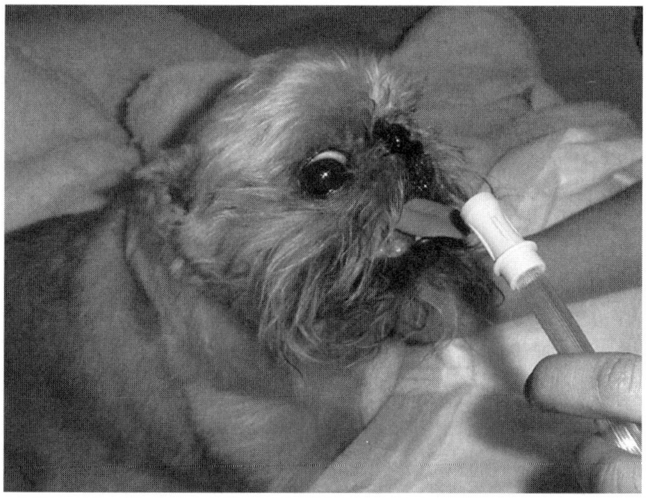

Figure 29-3. Oxygen delivered by the flow-by method.

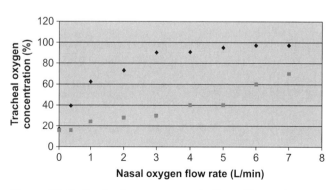

Figure 29-4. Tracheal oxygen concentration with nasal oxygen supplementation at varying flow rates in 10 kg (diamonds) and 40 kg (squares) dogs. (Modified with permission from Fitzpatrick RK, Crowe DT: Nasal oxygen administration in dogs and cats: Experimental and clinical investigations, JAAHA 22:296, 1986.)

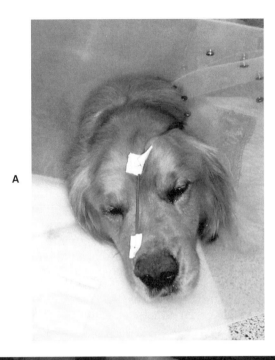

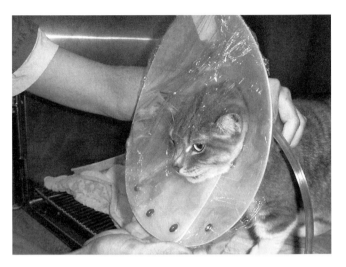

Figure 29-6. *Oxygen tubing is connected to a plastic-covered Elizabethan collar to increase the inspired oxygen concentration.*

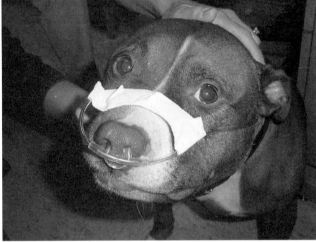

Figure 29-5. *Nasal oxygen can be provided **A**, through nasal catheters or **B**, prong cannulas.*

to fit the patient, and the tubing can be tightened behind the head to help secure the cannulas in the nares. A bridge of tape across the nose may help stabilize the cannula (Figure 29-5, *B*). Nasal prongs are easily dislodged if the patient moves and should not be used without close supervision. However, they provide an easy and noninvasive means to supply oxygen for short-term use (e.g., during anesthesia recovery).

Nasal oxygen therapy offers several advantages. The patient has freedom of movement and is accessible for monitoring without discontinuing oxygen supplementation. Nasal oxygen is also relatively inexpensive and not as wasteful as flow-by oxygen and oxygen cages.

Side effects include the possibility of nasal mucosal hemorrhage in coagulopathic animals, gastric distension at very high flow rates (greater than 5 L/min),[9] nasal dis-

charge, epistaxis,[6] and sneezing. If local irritation or inflammation occurs, the nasal catheter should be removed and replaced in the opposite nare to avoid pressure necrosis, lesions on the mucosa due to the jet of oxygen, and nasal or tube occlusion due to the accumulation of mucus.[9]

ELIZABETHAN COLLAR OR HOOD OXYGEN

An Elizabethan collar is applied snugly to the neck with the tip of an oxygen line placed inside the collar on the animal's neck. The front circle of the collar is then covered with a piece of clear plastic wrap and a small opening is made at the top of the canopy to allow the escape of CO_2 and humid and warm air (Figure 29-6). Alternatively, commercially available plastic hoods that snap in place around the patient's neck can be used.

The Fio_2 obtained inside the canopy depends on a variety of factors including the tightness of the collar, the size of the vent hole, the size of the patient, and the respiratory rate. Oxygen should be administered at a high flow rate for the first 1 to 2 minutes to fill the canopy quickly, then a maintenance rate of 0.75 to 1 L/minute can be used. An oxygen concentration of 40% was achieved at the bifurcation of the trachea with a flow rate of 1 L/minute in normal, healthy, anesthetized dogs.[10] In this study, a stable plane of anesthesia was attempted for all patients, but respiratory rate and other potential ventilatory variables were not measured. As minute ventilation may vary greatly between patients, especially when anesthetized, the Fio_2 values obtained in this study may not be accurate for an awake, dyspneic animal with a higher minute ventilation.

The oxygen concentration at the tracheal bifurcation has been compared using intranasal and Elizabethan collar methods of supplementation at similar oxygen flow rates. A flow rate of 0.75 L/min provided tracheal oxygen concentrations of 34.8% to 79.5% with the intranasal catheter and 30.5% to 48.6% with an Elizabethan collar.[10] Intranasal supplementation consistently provides a slightly higher Fio_2 than the Elizabethan collar method.

Another study of the Elizabethan collar method showed that an FiO_2 of 95% could be achieved with a 300 ml/kg/min flow rate.[11]

The advantages of canopy or hood oxygen include the accessibility of the patient, its effectiveness, the potential for long-term use, and lack of humidification requirements because the airways are not bypassed.[10] Although this method is economical and easy to set up, there are several disadvantages including oxygen leakage, hyperthermia, high humidity, potential CO_2 retention, and lack of patient cooperation. Another disadvantage is the potential variability in oxygen concentration within the hood, depending on the size of the vent hole, minute ventilation of the patient, and the exact placement of the oxygen hose within the hood.

INTRATRACHEAL OXYGEN

Intratracheal oxygen can be delivered through an endotracheal tube, tracheostomy tube, or transtracheal catheter. To place a transtracheal catheter, a large-gauge over-the-needle catheter is placed between two tracheal rings close to the larynx. The needle is removed, leaving the catheter in place.[12]

Intratracheal oxygen supplementation is highly effective in producing desired FiO_2 and PaO_2 levels. Higher FiO_2 and PaO_2 values are obtained when oxygen is delivered directly into the trachea than into intranasal catheters, even when lower flow rates are used. An intratracheal flow rate of 10 ml/kg/minute should ensure 97% hemoglobin saturation, compared with a required intranasal flow rate of 50 ml/kg/min.[12] The advantages of this method include higher oxygen concentration with a lower flow rate than intranasal routes. Disadvantages include the stress of placing the catheter; possible tracheal irritation leading to discomfort; kinking of the catheter at the skin entry point; and displacement of the catheter, resulting in the potential for subcutaneous insufflation of oxygen. Percutaneous placement of tracheal catheters should be avoided in patients with collapsing trachea or in those with coagulopathies.

OXYGEN CAGE

An oxygen cage provides a sealed compartment with mechanisms to regulate oxygen concentration, ambient temperature, humidity, and elimination of expired CO_2. This is a noninvasive, nonstressful method of supplementing oxygen that allows accurate monitoring and control of the environment. Disadvantages include the expense of purchasing the cage, oxygen waste, and isolation of the patient from the clinician. Examination of the patient with the door open results in disruption of the desired inspired oxygen concentration and may cause deterioration of the patient's condition. Ambient temperature should be maintained at approximately 22° C (70° F) with a relative humidity of 40% to 50%, but it can be altered to assist hypo- or hyperthermic patients reach and maintain normothermia.

In general, oxygen flow into the cage should be set to provide an FiO_2 of 40% to 60%. Severely dyspneic patients may require higher concentrations of oxygen to help attain stability.

MECHANICAL VENTILATION

Ventilatory support is usually required in patients with either ventilatory failure or failure of pulmonary oxygen exchange due to lung disease. Patients with high FiO_2 requirements for extended periods, respiratory fatigue or arrest, coma, increased intracranial pressure, or failure to respond to oxygen supplementation may require positive pressure ventilation.[7]

Humidification and Nebulization

Absolute humidity is defined as the weight of water vapor actually present per unit volume of gas or air.[4] The amount of water vapor carried in inspired gas is temperature dependent: warm air carries more water vapor than cold air. With many methods of oxygen supplementation, the upper airway of the animal, which is the natural area of humidification, is bypassed. Unhumidified oxygen causes drying of the mucous membranes and impairs mucociliary clearance.[6] Dry oxygen therapy also increases the viscosity of mucosal secretions, causes degeneration of respiratory epithelium, and increases the risk of infection.[6]

Humidification can be accomplished by bubbling oxygen through a polyethylene tube submerged in a bottle partially filled with sterile water. Sterile water should be used to prevent contamination of the respiratory tract with nosocomial organisms. The humidified oxygen from the space above the water is collected by a second polyethylene tube and delivered to the patient.[6] Commercially available humidifiers designed for insertion into the ventilator circuit warm, as well as humidify the inspired gas. In order to achieve a physiological level of humidification, the liquid and the inspired gas should be at a relatively high temperature (e.g., 30° C for 30 mg/L water vapor), which may lead to overheating of the patient.

Under experimental conditions, dry oxygen at a flow rate of 2 L/min into a mixing chamber reduced the measured relative humidity of the air-oxygen mixture from 40% to 37%.[13] Therefore humidification of supplemental oxygen administered via nasal cannula may not be necessary when the oxygen flow rate is 2 L/min or less.[13]

The airways can be hydrated either by increasing the humidity of the inspired air or by introducing particulate water droplets into the inhaled gas, termed nebulization. Airway nebulization therapy has minimal effect in a dehydrated animal. Therefore, maintenance of systemic hydration is essential for liquefaction of airway secretions. The water content of humidified air is limited by the saturated water vapor content of the air, which depends on temperature. The water content of nebulized air depends on the density of mist and size of water droplets produced by the nebulizer.[13]

Nebulization is most commonly carried out using an ultrasonic or gas-pressure-driven nebulizer that produces tiny droplets of water, allowing the water content of the gas to reach levels greater than could be achieved using evaporation. Commonly used nebulizers can generate water contents from 50 mg to 200 mg/L, with particle sizes in the 0.5- to 10-μm range. The larger particles are primarily deposited in the upper airways (i.e., trachea and bronchi), whereas the smaller particles are deposited in the terminal and respiratory bronchioles and alveoli.[14]

Monitoring the Response to Oxygen Therapy

Clinical signs are important tools for monitoring a patient's response to oxygen therapy. Serial assessments of respiratory rate, respiratory effort, auscultation, mucous membranes, capillary refill time, and pulses are vital. Several more objective tests can be performed to evaluate a patient's response to oxygen therapy, including arterial blood gas analysis, calculation of oxygen tension based indices, and pulse oximetry. As the patient's respiratory disease improves, trials without oxygen supplementation should be performed to confirm whether weaning should begin. At all times, the minimum possible Fio_2 that is consistent with adequate oxygenation and patient comfort should be used.

Arterial blood gas analysis is the most objective technique to monitor the oxygenation and ventilatory function of a patient. Ideally, arterial samples for blood gas analysis should be obtained while the patient is breathing room air. In oxygen-dependent patients, it is essential that the Fio_2 is maintained during arterial blood gas sampling because the Pao_2 will fall to reflect the new Fio_2 in 10 to 20 breaths. Disconnection from the oxygen source causes the tracheal oxygen concentration to fall to baseline in 10 seconds.[9]

In animals breathing room air, normal values for Pao_2 and $Paco_2$ are 85 to 100 mm Hg and 35 to 45 mm Hg, respectively. Animals with Pao_2 values less than 70 mm Hg may require oxygen supplementation, whereas those with a persistently elevated $Paco_2$ of 50 mm Hg or greater may require mechanical ventilation. The decision to supply oxygen or ventilate a patient should never be made based solely on numbers but must include full assessment of the clinical status of the patient. Results for Pao_2 and Sao_2 must be interpreted in light of the Fio_2 at the time of measurement. Based on the alveolar gas equation, if the arterial $Paco_2$ and respiratory exchange ratio remain constant, every mm Hg rise in inspired partial pressure of O_2 produces a corresponding rise in alveolar partial pressure of O_2. Therefore a patient with normal lungs breathing 100% oxygen should have a Pao_2 of approximately 600 mm Hg.[15]

Various oxygen tension–based indices can be used to further evaluate arterial blood gas results. The A–a gradient is calculated from arterial blood gas results and is a sensitive measure of the efficiency of pulmonary gas exchange. It estimates the adequacy of oxygen transfer from the alveolus to the pulmonary capillary blood and is derived using the alveolar gas equation:

$$PAo_2 = Fio_2 \ (P_b - PH_2O) - \frac{Paco_2}{RQ}$$

where PAo_2 is the alveolar Po_2; P_b is barometric pressure; PH_2O is water vapor pressure, and RQ is the respiratory quotient. For clinical use in animals at sea level, breathing room air, the alveolar gas equation can be abbreviated as follows:

$$PAo_2 = 150 - \frac{Paco_2}{RQ}$$

Respiratory quotient is estimated at 0.9 in dogs eating commercial diets, therefore:

$$PAo_2 = 150 - Paco_2$$

The alveolar gas equation is used to calculate the alveolar partial pressure of oxygen, and the Pao_2 is known from the blood gas analysis. The A–a gradient can then be calculated[8]:

$$P(A-a)o_2 = PAo_2 - Pao_2$$

The published reference range for the A–a gradient is less than 10 mm Hg,[3] but one recent study documented that the gradient could be as much as 20 mm Hg in normal dogs.[16] Gradient values greater than 30 mm Hg suggest clinically significant impairment of gas exchange.[3]

Gas exchange abnormalities can also be reflected by the Pao_2:Fio_2 ratio, which is a clinically relevant estimate of intrapulmonary shunt. This oxygen tension–based index is most useful in animals that are oxygen dependent, particularly patients being supported by positive pressure ventilation. In normal humans, the Pao_2:Fio_2 ratio should be greater than 300, and the published reference range in normal dogs is 432 to 564.[16] In animals, a ratio of less than 200 suggests serious lung disease and an animal that might be expected to have a positive response to oxygen supplementation. Values less than 100 indicate profound failure of gas exchange, a potentially poor response to oxygen therapy, and the probable need for positive pressure ventilation.

Pulse oximetry is a noninvasive method of monitoring the oxygen saturation of hemoglobin (Sao_2). Based on the oxyhemoglobin saturation curve, an Sao_2 of 90% is equivalent to a Pao_2 of approximately 60 mm Hg, indicating severe hypoxemia that warrants immediate oxygen supplementation.[2,3]

Arterial oxygen content (Cao_2) is a calculated value derived from Sao_2, hemoglobin concentration, and Pao_2. Because dissolved oxygen contributes less than 2% to the oxygen content of blood, Cao_2 is determined primarily by Sao_2 and hemoglobin concentration. Thus, maintenance of an acceptable Cao_2 requires not only adequate pulmonary function (Sao_2 greater than 90%) but also a satisfactory hemoglobin concentration.[3]

Complications of Oxygen Therapy

OXYGEN TOXICITY

Oxygen toxicity is thought to be caused by lipoperoxidation of essential intracellular sulfhydryl groups and polymorphonuclear cell infiltration.[17] Formation of oxygen radicals causes direct endothelial and epithelial cell damage, leading to increased endothelial permeability, cytotoxicity, and inflammatory activity.[18] Studies of oxygen toxicity in rats have confirmed that exposure to high concentrations of oxygen is damaging to the lungs. Changes are seen in the airway epithelium, the arterial vascular bed, the alveolar septa, and in the pleural space. Atelectasis, interstitial and alveolar edema, pleural effusion, and changes in cell function and structure occur.[19]

The sequence of morphological changes that occurs in the lungs in response to hyperoxia can be divided into several phases. The degree of oxygen exposure (i.e., lethal compared with sublethal doses) alters the end result. In cases of lethal exposure, initiation, inflammatory, and destructive phases result in the patient's death due to fulminant respiratory failure. In cases of sublethal exposure, the initiation, inflammatory, proliferative, and fibrotic phases result in varying degrees of permanent parenchymal change.[20]

Lethal Exposure

The initiation phase of lethal exposure occurs in the first 24 to 72 hours after exposure to 100% oxygen. Most animal species do not demonstrate significant morphological changes in the alveolar septa at this time. Augmentation of the production of partially reduced species of oxygen overwhelms the cell repair process and other metabolical functions, causing cell injury.[20]

The earliest morphological changes in the lung occur during the inflammatory phase. Subtle changes in endothelial cell structure result in pericapillary accumulation of fluid. Cell injury is amplified by release of inflammatory mediators and attraction of inflammatory cell elements into the lung microvasculature and interstitium.[21] After exposure to 100% oxygen for 48 hours, the volume of platelets retained in the pulmonary capillary bed almost doubles.[22] Following platelet accumulation, neutrophils are rapidly recruited to the lung, where they initiate the final stage of pulmonary oxygen toxicity by releasing further mediators of inflammation and by producing toxic oxygen species.[21,22] Morphological studies of pulmonary oxygen toxicity suggest that neutrophils accumulate in the pulmonary vasculature and in the lung interstitium as part of the inflammatory response but do not accumulate to a significant degree within the alveolar spaces.[23]

The destructive phase begins shortly after the inflammatory phase and involves the overt destruction of the pulmonary capillary endothelium. The capillary endothelial cells that remain at the time of the animal's death show cell membrane injury, margination and clumping of nuclear chromatin, dilation of perinuclear cisternae and cisternae of the endoplasmic reticulum, intracellular edema, swelling, and frank necrosis.[21]

Although similar morphological changes occur in all species, the severity of pulmonary pathology is variable. In rats at the time of death, there are no significant changes in the numbers of type I or type II epithelial cells. In primates after 4 days in 100% oxygen, the alveolar type I epithelium is almost completely destroyed. Hyperplasia of type II pneumocytes leads to almost total replacement of the alveolar lining with type II cells by the seventh day of exposure.[21]

In dogs, the primary injury is to the membranous pneumocytes, with endothelial cells being affected later.[24] Exposure of dogs to 100% oxygen produced alterations in lung function within the first 24 hours and death within an average of 50 to 60 hours.[25] Dogs exposed to 80% oxygen concentrations developed clinical signs of lung dysfunction but survived, whereas exposure to 50% O_2 concentration failed to produce any clinical signs or lung pathology.[26] Therefore, for long-term oxygen administration in dogs, the FiO_2 should be maintained less than 50% to prevent O_2 toxicity. An FiO_2 of 30% to 40% should be adequate for hemoglobin saturation in most cases.[27]

Sublethal Exposure

Exposure to sublethal doses of oxygen delays the onset of the inflammatory stage, compared with that induced by a lethal dose, and also blunts the magnitude and duration of the inflammatory response.[21,22] The length of the initiation phase varies inversely with the dose of oxygen, and the dose-response curve is steep. Exposure to 60% oxygen for up to 7 days results in almost no detectable morphological lung injury in normal animals. In contrast, rats exposed to 85% oxygen had prolongation of the initiation phase, so that at 72 hours only the early initiation changes were seen, with an increase in platelets in the lung vasculature.[20] The number of neutrophils found in the lung interstitium paralleled the changes in the lung microvasculature, with a transient increase in interstitial neutrophils on the fifth day of exposure to 85% oxygen. In the destructive phase, the rate of destruction of capillary endothelium following sublethal oxygen exposure is substantially slower than that resulting from exposure to 100% oxygen. In rats exposed to 85% oxygen, 40% to 50% of the endothelial cells were destroyed by the seventh day, but further net destruction did not occur.[21]

Following sublethal exposure, the cell proliferative response blunts the destructive phase and is responsible for the survival of the animal. Rats exposed to 85% oxygen showed an almost fourfold increase in the number of interstitial cells, predominantly a fibroblast and monocyte response.[21] The relative absence of polymorphonuclear leukocytes, and a high concentration of monocytes in the lung interstitium, are important characteristics in differentiating the morphological changes associated with sublethal and lethal pulmonary oxygen toxicity. Type II cells become larger in mean size and their ultrastructure is altered.[21] Finally, long-term exposure to hyperoxia or acute exposure, followed by a recovery period in air, is associated with a fibrotic reaction in the lung interstitium. Histopathological findings include increased deposition of collagen in the lung interstitium,[23] increased thickness of the alveolar interstitial space,[23] and an increased number of interstitial cells.[21] Enlargement of airspaces and destruction of large segments of the alveolar septal wall may also occur.[23]

In normal human subjects, substernal discomfort was reported after breathing 100% oxygen for 24 hours.

Patients that were mechanically ventilated with 100% oxygen for 36 hours showed a progressive fall in PaO_2 compared with a control group ventilated with air. Oxygen concentrations of 50% or higher for more than 2 days may produce toxic changes.[15]

Hyperoxia increases intracellular production of O_2 and H_2O_2, but tolerance can develop following repeated exposure. Adult rats exposed to 85% oxygen for 7 days are tolerant to a subsequent prolonged exposure to 100% oxygen, whereas normal adult rats uniformly die within 72 hours during exposure to 100% oxygen.[28] The development of oxygen tolerance correlates with an increase in lung superoxide dismutase activity. Up-regulation of superoxide dismutase varies between species and allows some animals to develop tolerance.[28]

There is a striking difference in the response of the neonate to hyperoxia, compared with that of the adult animal. Neonatal rats, mice, and rabbits are much more resistant to the oxygen-induced lung injury seen in adult animals. They can rapidly mount a protective lung biochemical response to high oxygen exposure (i.e., increased pulmonary antioxidant enzyme activities), an adaptive response that adult animals have lost the ability to manifest.[29] Rapid and significant increases in superoxide dismutase, catalase, and glutathione peroxidase are seen in response to hyperoxia.[30]

HYPERCARBIA

Injudicious use of oxygen therapy in human patients with chronic respiratory disease and chronic hypercapnia can lead to hypercarbia. In patients with chronic lung disease and a chronically high work of breathing, ventilatory drive results from hypoxic stimulation of peripheral chemoreceptors. If this patient is then treated with high concentrations of oxygen, a serious complication may develop. As the hypoxemia is relieved with oxygen supplementation, decreased ventilatory drive may result in a dramatic decrease in ventilation and severe hypercarbia may occur.[15] If the oxygen supplementation is then stopped, profound hypoxemia follows, and it may take many minutes to unload the large amount of CO_2 retained in the tissues. Mechanical ventilation may be necessary while diagnostic tests are performed to determine the underlying disease process. Although this phenomenon has been well documented in people with chronic lung disease, it has not been confirmed to occur often in small animals.

Another lesser cause of CO_2 retention in these patients may be the release of hypoxic vasoconstriction in poorly ventilated areas of lung due to the increased alveolar PO_2. The result is an increased blood flow to low V/Q areas and a worsening of the V/Q mismatch that exaggerates CO_2 retention.[15]

ABSORPTION ATELECTASIS

If an airway becomes totally obstructed, absorption atelectasis of the lung distal to the airway obstruction may occur. Since the sum of the partial pressures of gas in venous blood is less than atmospheric pressure, the trapped gas is gradually reabsorbed, resulting in collapse of alveoli and atelectasis. Nitrogen slows the absorption process because of its relatively low solubility compared with oxygen. Therefore in patients breathing high oxygen concentrations, the rate of absorption is accelerated. Atelectasis is most common in dependent regions of the lung because secretions tend to collect there due to gravity and the airways and alveoli are relatively poorly expanded for the same reason.[15]

OTHERS

Prolonged O_2 therapy has also been associated with suppression of erythropoiesis, pulmonary vasodilation, and systemic arteriolar vasoconstriction.[3]

Hyperbaric Oxygen

Hyperbaric oxygen therapy (HBOT) has limited uses and is rarely used in the treatment of primary respiratory disease. However, it has been used for treatment of severe carbon monoxide poisoning, in which most of the hemoglobin is unavailable to carry oxygen and the amount of dissolved oxygen is critically important. The high PaO_2 accelerates the dissociation of carbon monoxide from hemoglobin.[15]

In HBOT, 100% oxygen is pumped into a pressurized chamber at a pressure greater than 760 mm Hg, or 1 atmosphere (atm). Most treatments are administered at 2 atm.[31] This therapy promotes rapid healing of injured tissues, stimulates leukocyte and macrophage function, provides the oxygen necessary for cellular function, stimulates wound healing, and has direct antibacterial effects.[31,32]

MECHANISM OF ACTION

Hyperbaric oxygen therapy increases the amount of dissolved oxygen in plasma to 10 to 15 times normal concentrations.[31] HBOT increases oxygen tension in the capillaries surrounding ischemic tissue and promotes oxygen diffusion from the capillaries to the tissues, by two- to threefold. Therefore, in conditions of poor perfusion, HBOT may sustain cells until circulation is restored. Further, increased tissue oxygen levels facilitate the oxidative white blood cell–killing mechanism in ischemic areas of the body. Anaerobic bacteria are inhibited and toxin formation is reduced.[31] Treatment effects are therefore achieved by means of hyperoxygenation, antimicrobial effects, neovascularization, and vasoconstriction.

Common indications for use of HBOT include skin flaps and grafts, refractory osteomyelitis, clostridial infections, crush and drag injury, and decubital ulcers.

Complications can occur with HBOT. Because any gas under pressure expands, gas-containing cavities such as the lungs, sinuses, ears, and gastrointestinal tract must be evaluated before therapy begins. Other side effects include pneumothorax due to rupture of undiagnosed lung bullae, rupture of the tympanic membrane, and generalized discomfort from the increased pressure. Finally, formation of oxygen-derived free radicals, which have been implicated as mediators of microvascular damage, is a potential negative effect of hyperoxygenation.[31] However, HBOT enhances host enzyme activity to degrade free radicals.[31,32]

Conclusion

There are numerous indications for oxygen supplementation. Once the usefulness of oxygen supplementation is established, the appropriate method of oxygen delivery and humidification should be chosen on a patient–by-patient basis. Monitoring the response of the patient to oxygen therapy is accomplished through assessment of clinical signs, arterial blood gas analysis, pulse oximetry, and calculation of the A–a gradient and Pao_2-Fio_2 ratio. Major complications of oxygen therapy include oxygen toxicity and absorption atelectasis. Hyperbaric oxygen therapy in veterinary medicine is uncommonly used but theoretically is indicated in cases of carbon monoxide poisoning and to facilitate wound healing.

REFERENCES

1. Ganong WF: *Review of medical physiology,* Norwalk, Conn, 1995, Appleton & Lange.
2. Tseng LW, Waddell LS: Approach to the patient in respiratory distress, *Clin Tech Sm Anim Pract* 15(2):53-62, 2000.
3. Camps-Palau M, Marks S, Cornick J: Small animal oxygen therapy, *Compendium* 21(7):587-598, 1999.
4. Hensyl WR, editor: *Stedmans medical dictionary,* ed 1, Baltimore, 1987, Williams & Wilkins.
5. Loukopoulos P, Reynolds W: Comparative evaluation of oxygen therapy techniques in anaesthetized dogs: Face-mask and flow by technique, *Aust Vet Practit* 27:34-39, 1997.
6. Fitzpatrick Robert K, Crowe DT: Nasal oxygen administration in dogs and cats: Experimental and clinical investigations, *JAAHA* 22:293-300, 1986.
7. Mensack S, Murtaugh R: Oxygen toxicity, *Compendium* 21(4):341-351, 1999.
8. West JB: *Respiratory physiology: The essentials,* ed 6, Baltimore, 2000, Williams & Wilkins.
9. Pascoe PJ: Oxygen and ventilatory support for the critical patient, *Seminars in Vet Med and Surg (Small Animal),* 3(3):202-209, 1998.
10. Loukopoulos P, Reynolds W: Comparative evaluation of oxygen therapy techniques in anaesthetized dogs: Intranasal catheter and Elizabethan collar canopy, *Aust Vet Practit* 26:199-204, 1996.
11. Crowe DT: Use of an oxygen collar, *Vet Practice* 7(4):27-28, 1995.
12. Mann FA, Wagner-Mann C, Allert JA et al: Comparison of intranasal and intratracheal oxygen administration in healthy awake dogs, *Am J Vet Res* 53(5):856-860, 1992.
13. Cugell DW, Paleczney M: Nasal oxygen administration and humidification, *JAMA* 250(20):2859-2860, 1983.
14. Court MH, Dodman NH, Seeler DC: Oxygen administration, humidification and aerosol therapy, *Vet Clin North Am Small Anim Pract* 15:1041-1059, 1985.
15. West JB: *Pulmonary pathophysiology,* ed 5, Baltimore, 1998, Williams & Wilkins.
16. Beal MW, Paglia DT, Griffin GM et al: Ventilatory failure, ventilator management, and outcome in dogs with cervical spinal disorders: 14 cases (1991-1999), *JAVMA* 218:1598-1602, 2001.
17. Deneke SM, Fanburg BL: Normobaric oxygen toxicity of the lung, *N Engl J Med* 303:76-86, 1980.
18. Hitt ME: Oxygen derived free radicals: Pathophysiology and implications, *Compendium* 10(8):939-946, 1988.
19. Freeman BA, Crapo JD: Hyperoxia increases oxygen radical production in rat lungs and lung mitochondria, *J Biological Chemistry* 256(21):10986-10992, 1981.
20. Crapo JD: Morphologic changes in pulmonary oxygen toxicity, *Am Rev Physiol* 48:721-731, 1986.
21. Crapo JD, Barry BE, Foscue HA et al: Structural and biochemical changes in rat lungs occurring during exposures to lethal and adaptive doses of oxygen, *Am Rev Respir Dis* 122:123-143, 1980.
22. Barry BE, Crapo JD: Patterns of accumulation of platelets and neutrophils in rat lungs during exposure to 100% and 85% oxygen, *Am Rev Respir Dis* 132(3):548-555, 1985.
23. Bonikos DS, Bensch KG, Northway WH: Oxygen toxicity in the newborn, *Am J Pathol* 85:623-650, 1976.
24. Katzenstein AL, Bloor CM, Leibow AA: Diffuse alveolar damage: The role of oxygen, shock and related factors, *Am J Pathol* 85(1):210-228, 1976.
25. Paine JR, Lynn D, Keys A: Observations on effects of prolonged administration of high oxygen concentration to dogs, *J Thoracic Surg* 11:151-168, 1941.
26. Haskins SC: Physical therapeutics for respiratory disease, *Seminars in Vet Med and Surg (Small Animal)* 1(4):276-288, 1986.
27. Kirk RW, Bistner SI: Oxygen therapy. In Kirk RW, Bistner SI: *Handbook of veterinary procedures and emergency treatment,* ed 4, Philadelphia, 1985, WB Saunders.
28. Freeman BA, Crapo JD: Hyperoxia increases oxygen radical production in rat lungs and lung mitochondria, *J Biological Chemistry* 256(21):10986-10992, 1981.
29. Frank L, Bucher JR, Roberts RJ: Oxygen toxicity in neonatal and adult animals of various species, *J Applied Physiol* 45(5):699-704, 1978.
30. Frank L: Developmental aspects of experimental pulmonary oxygen toxicity, *Free Radical Biology and Medicine* 11:463-494, 1991.
31. Elkins AD: Hyperbaric oxygen therapy: Potential veterinary applications, *Compendium* 5:607-612, 1997.
32. Hosgood G, Elkins AD: Hyperbaric oxygen therapy: Mechanism and potential applications, *Compendium* 12(11):1589-1597, 1990.

CHAPTER 30

Airway Hygiene

Joan C. Hendricks

Patients with diseases of the respiratory system commonly suffer from airway irritation accompanied by reduced defenses, leading to the accumulation of secretions. In some patients this process is caused by the primary disease, as is the case when infectious or other inflammatory conditions lead to increased mucus production. In other animals, therapeutic interventions are the cause of airway irritation and increased secretions (e.g., when the upper airway is bypassed by tracheostomy or long-term intubation for ventilation). Furthermore, patients may not be able to defend their own airways against accumulated secretions when the normal upper airway defenses are bypassed; when the patient is too weak or compromised to cough or expel secretions; or when sedation or general anesthesia prevents normal coughing, sneezing, or grooming. The aims, general principles, and specific techniques of airway hygiene are discussed in this chapter.

Aims of Airway Hygiene

Good airway hygiene contributes to both the comfort and the health of the patient. For the patient that is too ill to groom, upper airway hygiene as part of nursing care can increase the sense of well-being and may improve appetite if the patient can smell the food. Throughout the respiratory system, removal of inflammatory secretions from mucosal surfaces where they can be irritating improves comfort. If possible, it is preferable to prevent accumulation and drying of secretions, after which removal can be irritating. Exudates from animals that have contagious diseases may carry infectious viral or bacterial particles, so that attentive removal and cleansing may help to contain the spread of disease from infected secretions that the patient would otherwise expel by coughing or sneezing.

The most urgent goal of airway hygiene is to prevent airway obstruction from accumulated secretions in airway passages from the nares to the bronchi. At the level of the pulmonary parenchyma, preventing or dislodging secretions can assist ventilation by removing alveolar material or by unblocking obstructed bronchi, thereby allowing re-expansion of areas of absorption atelectasis. Finally, in the case of infectious pneumonia, assisting the patient to expel purulent material with infectious particles and inflammatory mediators may reduce the load of toxic bacterial products and inflammatory medi-

ators. Even when the patient does not have a primary infectious cause for its lung disease, removing secretions and reducing irritation should reduce the risk of acquired infections that could result from pooling of secretions on irritated mucosal surfaces.

Principles of Airway Hygiene

The first general principle of airway hygiene is to *liquify secretions*, making it easier for the patient to expel the secretions by coughing or sneezing, or for the caretaker to remove the secretions. Toward this goal, the patient should be systemically well hydrated. Increasing external moisture at the nasal and oral passages through direct application of saline (e.g., on a saline-soaked gauze pad) and ensuring that the oral cavity is moist and clean can prevent irritation of these surfaces and also aid in the humidification of air passing through these passages.

Humidification is defined as saturation of the inhaled gas with water vapor.[1,2] In general, it is mandatory to humidify all air provided to the patient, whether through the normal upper airway or through an endotracheal tube or tracheostomy site. This is especially true when the ambient air is dry. Supplemental oxygen is usually humidified by bubbling it through a chamber filled with sterile water before its administration to the patient. Specially designed humidifiers that insert into the ventilator circuit are also available for use in animals that are being ventilated. Because the water vapor–carrying capacity of air increases with warming, these humidifiers both warm and moisten the inhaled gas to ensure that it contains the maximum possible amount of water vapor. All of these products add moisture to the inhaled gas by exposing it to a liquid interface. Alternatively, heat and moisture in exhaled air can be "recycled" using disposable heat and moisture exchangers (termed "artificial noses"*) that can be attached to the end of the endotracheal tube of animals that are being intubated for a short time, (e.g., a few hours).

Nebulization of sterile saline is a more sophisticated method of moistening the airways. Nebulizers generate tiny spherical droplets of water that are inhaled by the patient. The droplets then shower out at various levels

_____

*Humid-Vent 1, Glbeck Respiration, P.O. Box 711, 27 Upplands Vasby, Sweden.

of the respiratory tract, depending on their size. Droplets greater than 10 μm are unable to pass further than the upper airway and trachea. In the range of 1 to 10 μm, the smaller the droplet, the deeper it is able to penetrate into the respiratory tract. Droplets less than 0.5 μm reach the alveoli and are exhaled rather than showering out on the surface of the airways.[3] Most ultrasonic nebulizers create droplets in the 2- to 5-μm range, and there is always some variability in size of the droplets that are produced. The droplets impact the walls of the bronchi as a result of changes in direction of airflow, Brownian motion, and gravity.[3,4] Various bland solutions are commonly administered by nebulization, typically either consisting of sterile water or 0.9% saline.[5]

When viscous secretions are accumulating, the use of acetylcysteine has been advocated (e.g., instilled or aerosolized into a tracheostomy site). Acetylcysteine acts by breaking down disulfide bonds that are present in the mucoproteins of airway mucus, thereby making it less viscous. However, because this drug also increases the volume of secretions and may further irritate the mucosa resulting in bronchospasm, this approach should be undertaken with caution. The author does not use inhaled acetylcysteine as part of routine airway hygiene.

A second principle is that removal of secretions should produce *minimal irritation.* At the external nares, gentle physical removal with saline-soaked gauze pads may be effective. For the lower airways, suction may be the only effective means, but suction catheters and the barotrauma of applying negative pressure directly to the airways can produce considerable damage. Thus if at all possible, it is preferable to enable the animal to expel secretions on its own through the use of postural drainage and coupage. The "milking action" of coughing assists in movement of material into the pharynx, where it can be swallowed or expectorated. A variety of techniques are used to stimulate the cough reflex and improve mobilization of secretions. The simplest method is to stimulate an increased tidal volume during respiration; this is best achieved using mild exercise. Mild to moderate exercise often stimulates productive coughing, which should be encouraged by coupage. Coupage is the action of firmly striking the chest wall of the patient with a cupped hand, thereby stimulating the cough reflex.[6] Coupage should be performed several times daily, especially in patients that are unable to stand and move around. It is usually well tolerated, except in patients that have experienced thoracic trauma or thoracic surgery.

A third principle is the recognition that the accumulation or sudden movement of secretions can lead to profound changes in pulmonary function if the airways become obstructed. *Constant and attentive monitoring* for signs of upper airway obstruction is therefore mandatory. Animals that are anesthetized, sedated, or nearing respiratory failure may not exhibit overt signs of respiratory distress when the airways are progressively narrowed by secretions. Thus observation of respiratory patterns and respiratory muscle changes; auscultation for changes in airway turbulence that reflect narrowing airways; and, of course, monitoring for hypoxia or hypoventilation may alert the caretaker that airway hygiene may require attention. Routine but judicious inspection of artificial airways (e.g., endotracheal or tracheostomy tube) is necessary as part of good nursing care, even when no obvious changes in breathing pattern or pulmonary function are apparent, because the accumulation of secretions can be insidious.

As a final general principle, *patient excitement and respiratory compromise should be minimized.* Direct contact with irritated airways to remove secretions, brief obstruction of the airways to apply suction, the removal of ventilatory support to inspect or change endotracheal tubes, and even coupage, all risk exciting or compromising the patient. These manipulations may be life-saving, but the impact on the patient should not be underestimated. Preoxygenation, maintaining optimal sedation where appropriate, and simply keeping the procedures brief and calming the patient as much as possible are always considerations. Efficient, calm, and competent caretakers provide the best means of obtaining this ideal.

Techniques

NOSE AND NASAL PLANUM

Keeping the nose and nasal planum clear of secretions is generally simple and straightforward because these tissues are accessible. However, keeping the area moist and clean by gently using saline-moistened gauze pads and preventing accumulation and drying by applying petroleum jelly can be very helpful to maintain a patent airway. The impact on patient well-being, especially in cats, can be gratifying.

OROPHARYNX

The oropharyngeal passages are ordinarily clean and moist in conscious, well-hydrated patients, but in anesthetized or unconscious patients these tissues can become dry or secretions may pool. The author moistens the tongue of ventilated patients every 2 to 4 hours with glycerine and rinses the oral cavity and pharynx (after ensuring that the endotracheal tube cuff is fully inflated) using dilute chlorhexidine. The tongue and oropharyngeal surfaces are then gently swabbed with moistened gauze as needed.

TRACHEOSTOMY SITES

Tracheostomies present specific responsibilities and difficulties because the natural upper airway is bypassed. The nasal passages normally humidify and warm the inspired air and also remove particulate matter including bacteria and other infectious particles.

Temporary Tracheostomies

When a temporary stoma has been created, the tracheostomy tube should ideally have both an inner and an outer cannula. To aid in keeping the opening free of external obstructions, any excess skinfolds should be retracted at the time of surgery, and hair clipped away from the opening. Ideally, surgically placed stay sutures are left in place both to retract the skin and to pull the tracheal stoma open in the event that the tube needs to be removed and replaced.

Care must be taken that the tube does not become mechanically obstructed by patient movement. The intraluminal opening can be apposed to the tracheal wall and occluded when the patient moves, especially if it flexes its neck. Cats are especially inclined to ventroflex their heads in adopting the species-typical "sphinx" posture. Some patients will also obstruct the external opening by resting the neck on bedding or even putting paws over the stoma.

The patient must be watched conscientiously for signs of obstruction. Because the patient that requires a tracheostomy already suffers from some degree of respiratory compromise (and perhaps respiratory muscle fatigue resulting from its primary disorder), caretakers should be alert to insidious progression of an occlusion, sometimes without premonitory signs of respiratory distress. Even in the absence of signs of obstruction, the inner cannula should be routinely removed and cleaned of secretions with sterile saline. Ideally, a second sterile inner cannula should be kept on hand and placed inside the outer cannula to allow time for the first cannula to be cleaned. This process may be necessary as frequently as every 2 hours or as infrequently as every 6 hours, depending on how quickly secretions accumulate. At least four times daily, steps should be taken to humidify the inspired air, either by nebulization or by instilling sterile saline into the clean inner cannula if nebulization is not available.

Finally, in spite of the presence of an inner cannula, a coating of accumulated mucus may harden onto the intraluminal end of the outer cannula and can eventually plug the artificial airway. Thus there should not be a false sense of security just because an artificial airway is present. If the patient shows signs of respiratory distress or obstruction that are not relieved by cleaning the inner cannula, the possibility of removing and replacing the entire tracheostomy tube must be considered. This is always risky. In the conscious patient, the resulting excitement may be deleterious, and sedation, despite its inherent risks, may be required to calm the animal. Ensuring that a stoma can be maintained patent and a new tube placed correctly and efficiently requires planning and coordination. If stay sutures were not left in place around the tracheal rings, it is prudent to be prepared to induce general anesthesia and explore the neck to identify the opening and maintain an airway promptly. Peroral intubation may even be necessary to maintain an airway while the stoma is located and reopened.

Chronic/Permanent Tracheostomies

Somewhat paradoxically, even though a permanent tracheostomy is an unusual and somewhat heroic procedure usually undertaken for veterinary patients only when other measures have failed to maintain a patent airway, maintenance of a chronic tracheostomy is relatively straightforward compared with that of a temporary tracheostomy. The risk of airway obstruction is greatest early after surgery and is particularly great in smaller animals and those with large amounts of airway secretions. Reports of permanent tracheostomy in cats suggest a high incidence of sudden death because of obstruction by mucous plugs.[7,8]

As in all patients at risk, vigilance is necessary to note signs of respiratory obstruction. The external stoma should be kept free of secretions by cleaning with a saline-soaked gauze pad and applying petroleum jelly to the skin to prevent accumulation, if necessary. In the course of the operation, skinfolds and hair should have been removed as necessary to prevent occlusion of the opening. When the opening is new, the patient must be observed to determine whether it tends to occlude the site by behaviors such as folding the paws over the opening, flexing the neck excessively, or resting the neck on bedding. Initially, the air should be humidified by nebulization or instilling saline. With the passage of time, the tracheal mucosa will epithelialize so that irritation from dry air is no longer a problem, and there is reduced production of mucus by the tracheal mucosa. After healing is complete, the vigil for airway obstruction continues, with the risk of stenosis as the wound contracts.

LOWER AIRWAY HYGIENE

When the lower airways are at risk of accumulating secretions, the first line of defense is to aid the patient to mobilize and expel the secretions on its own. The patient should be well-hydrated and the inspired air well-humidified. If the patient is conscious and ambulatory, coughing can be stimulated and aided by coupage. To prevent pooling of secretions, the patient should be encouraged to stand and to move. Depending on the patient's overall condition, brief periods of exercise may be beneficial. In part by increasing tidal volume, and thereby stretching airways, exercise tends to induce coughing. In addition, exercise provides changes in posture that can aid in the mechanics of expelling secretions and may increase bloodflow and increase ventilation, normalizing ventilation:perfusion ratios and aiding in the mobilization of secretions. For many patients, the mental stimulation also seems to provide psychological benefit.

The patient that cannot cough or exercise is ordinarily turned every 2 to 6 hours as part of routine recumbent patient care. Turning is beneficial to prevent pooling of secretions in one location in the airways or parenchyma. In addition, turning helps to ameliorate compression atelectasis of the dependent lung lobe in large or overweight animals. Coupage and elevating the hindquarters after nebulization may free up secretions and allow them to flow into the larger airways where they can be accessible for suction. Suction through an endotracheal or tracheostomy tube can then be used to remove the secretions. Compared with natural cough, suction is inefficient and problematic. The necessarily narrow tubing is often quickly occluded by viscous secretions so that only a disappointingly small volume is actually removed. The necessity of partially obstructing the airway by the tubing interferes with spontaneous ventilation, if present. Suctioning a ventilated patient may necessitate interrupting positive pressure ventilation to apply suction. In most cases this is accomplished by breaking the ventilation tubing circuit, introducing the possibility of bacterial contamination. Even if tubing with a side port to allow suctioning without breaking the circuit is used,* the abrupt change from positive to negative pressure can lead to trauma because of the effect of shear forces on the mucosa and alveoli. Finally, the tip of the suction catheter may abut the mucosa and directly traumatize the mucosal surfaces of the airways, increasing inflammation and the risk of infection. If the catheter is introduced deeply into the lower airways, bronchospasm may be triggered. In spite of all of these caveats, suction may be the only means of removing secretions when the patient is not competent to do so. The negative impact can be minimized by following general principles, by ensuring that the patient is well-humidified and oxygenated before and after the suction, and by keeping the procedure brief and as infrequent as possible.

---

*Trach Care Pediatric Elbow Closed Tracheal Suction System,® Ballard Medical Products, Draper, Utah.

Conclusion

Whereas airway hygiene is conceptually simple, excellent hygiene is a gratifying and helpful component of managing respiratory conditions. Considerable finesse is often required to provide maximal benefit and minimal risk. Adapting the procedures carefully to the specific patient and to a specific patient's changing condition can allow high-tech and sophisticated procedures to be fully effective. Conversely, a lack of attention to these inexpensive, sensible measures may jeopardize the success of even the most intensive respiratory therapies.

REFERENCES

1. Branson RD: Humidification for patients with artificial airways, *Respiratory Care* 44(6):630-641, 1999.
2. Branson RD: The effects of inadequate humidity, *Resp Care Clin N Am* 4(2):199-214, 1998.
3. Court MH, Dodman NH, Seeler DC: Inhalation therapy: Oxygen administration, humidification, and aerosol therapy, *Vet Clin North Am Small Anim Pract* 15:1041-1058, 1985.
4. Rebuck AS, Braude AC: Assessment of drug disposition in the lung, *Drugs* 28:544-553, 1984.
5. Wanner A, Rao A: Clinical indications for and effect of bland, mucolytic and antimicrobial aerosols, *Am Rev Respir Dis* 122:79-87, 1980.
6. Selsby D, Jones JG: Some physiological and clinical aspects of chest physiotherapy, *Brit J Anaesth* 64:621-631, 1990.
7. Costello MF, Keith D, Hendrick M et al: Acute upper airway obstruction due to inflammatory laryngeal disease in 5 cats, *JVECC* 11(3):205-210, 2001.
8. Tasker S, Foster DJ, Corcoran BM et al: Obstructive inflammatory laryngeal disease in three cats, *J Fel Med and Surg* 1:53-59, 1999.

CHAPTER 31

Positive Pressure Ventilation

Steve C. Haskins • Lesley G. King

Ventilator Terminology

A few terms that will be used throughout this chapter have very specific meanings. *Ventilation* is the process involved in the movement of air in and out of the alveoli. Ventilation is important in the regulation of carbon dioxide, and arterial partial pressure of carbon dioxide ($Paco_2$) is commonly used as an index of alveolar minute ventilation. The term *oxygenation* refers to the process of oxygenation of blood as it flows through the lung and is defined by arterial partial pressure of oxygen (Pao_2). *Spontaneous ventilation* occurs when the animal is breathing entirely on its own, under its own power and totally in control of both breathing rate and the volume of each breath. *Assisted ventilation* is occurring when the patient determines the breathing rate, but an external device determines the tidal volume. During mechanical ventilation, assisted ventilation could be used for animals with normal neuronal responses but with diminished muscular ability to take an adequate breath.

Controlled ventilation is occurring when an external device controls both breathing rate and tidal volume. This is a common mode of mechanical ventilation when the patient has problems with both ventilation and oxygenation. External devices used to power a breath can be manual or mechanical. *Manual ventilation* occurs when a human squeezes a rebreathing bag or self-inflating manual resuscitator (AMBU® resuscitator) or otherwise causes gas to flow into the patient. Manual ventilation is commonly employed in emergency and short-term situations and when timing of the breath is crucial (e.g., cardiopulmonary resuscitation and tachypnea). *Mechanical ventilation* occurs when a machine takes the place of a human to power inspiration. Mechanical ventilation is commonly employed for prolonged positive pressure ventilation.

Inspiratory time is the length of time from the beginning of an inspiration to the end of that inspiration (the beginning of exhalation), including any inspiratory pause or plateau. Inspiratory flow time is the time during which gas is flowing into the lungs. Inspiratory pause time is the time during which gas is neither flowing into nor out of the lungs. *Expiratory time* is the length of time from the end of an inspiration to the beginning of the next inspiration. Expiratory flow time is the time during which gas is flowing out of the lungs. Expiratory pause time is the time during which gas is neither flowing into nor out of the lungs.

Peak airway pressure is the highest proximal airway pressure during an inspiration. Distal airway pressure is normally lower than proximal airway pressure because of resistance to airflow through the airways. If the airway is briefly occluded at peak inspiration, preventing any air movement into or out of the lungs, the proximal airway pressure decreases as gas equilibrates throughout the lung. This equilibrated upper airway pressure is termed the *pause pressure.* The difference between the peak and the pause pressure is directly proportional to airway resistance. In most ventilated dogs and cats, there is little difference between peak and pause pressure, suggesting that airway resistance is not usually increased. Pause pressure, rather than peak pressure, should be used in compliance calculations because it minimizes the airway resistance component of the measured upper airway pressure and better represents static compliance. *Positive end-expiratory pressure* (PEEP) is present when the airway pressure is purposely or inadvertently maintained at a level above atmospheric during the expiratory pause. PEEP is used to help keep small airways and alveoli open and functioning between breaths and to facilitate a more uniform distribution of the next tidal volume.

Functional residual capacity (FRC) is the amount of air remaining in the lung at the end of a passive exhalation (Figure 31-1). *Critical closing pressure or volume* is the transpulmonary pressure or lung volume below which spontaneous closure of the small airways occurs (usually during the expiratory pause). This normally occurs at the junction between expiratory reserve volume and residual volume. An increase in airway fluid in-

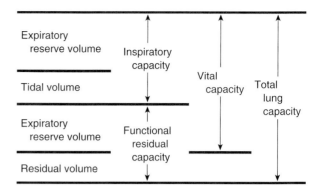

Figure 31-1. *Lung volumes and capacities.*

creases surface tension and the tendency for small airways and alveoli to collapse. The critical closing point moves upward, toward and into the normal tidal volume range; expiratory reserve volume is diminished and FRC is reduced. The open or closed status of small airways is the balance between the collapsing forces (mostly surface tension) and the expanding forces (mostly transpulmonary pressure). PEEP increases transpulmonary pressure and keeps FRC above critical closing pressure/volume. To the extent that small airways and alveoli collapse, they are not recruited in the next tidal volume, and the inspiratory reserve volume and total lung capacity are reduced.

Compliance is the change in expired tidal volume divided by the change in pressure (pause pressure minus end-expiratory pressure) that it took to create the tidal volume. Thoracic compliance is a measure of lung and chest wall stiffness or resistance to inflation. A decrease in compliance is implicit whenever a higher-than-normal pressure is required to ventilate a patient.

Mechanical ventilators come in many different configurations, broadly categorized by:
- Their power source
- The mechanism by which they push gas into the patient
- The mechanism by which they terminate an inspiration

Ventilators are powered either by a compressed gas source or by electricity. The tidal volume is driven either pneumatically via a compressed gas source or mechanically by an electrically operated compressor. Inspiration is terminated in one of three ways. *Pressure cycled ventilators* terminate inspiration when a preset peak pressure is reached. In this case tidal volume is determined by the peak pressure, inspiratory time, and the lung/chest wall compliance. *Volume cycled ventilators* terminate inspiration when a preset volume has been expelled from the ventilator; tidal volume is determined by the ventilator controls, and peak pressure is a dependent variable. *Time cycled ventilators* terminate inspiration after a preset time; tidal volume is determined by flow rate from the ventilator and time, and peak airway pressure is a dependent variable.

Indications for Positive Pressure Ventilation

Positive pressure ventilation (PPV) is indicated whenever an animal cannot ventilate adequately because of neuromuscular disease or pulmonary parenchymal disease. Hypoventilation may be associated with slow, shallow, or irregular breathing patterns in animals with neuromuscular disease, but it may also be associated with an exaggerated breathing effort in those with pulmonary parenchymal disease. An arterial Pco_2 in excess of 45 mm Hg in the dog defines hypoventilation, and a $Paco_2$ in excess of 60 mm Hg defines severe hypoventilation that warrants treatment. End-tidal CO_2 ($ETco_2$) estimates $Paco_2$; it is normally slightly lower than $Paco_2$ but can be variably lower in the presence of pulmonary disease and tachypnea and should be interpreted with caution. $ETco_2$ values greater than 50 mm Hg suggest hypoventilation.[1]

PPV is also indicated when hypoxemia does not respond to oxygen therapy. An arterial Po_2 below 80 mm Hg (at sea level) defines hypoxemia and a Pao_2 below 60 mm Hg defines hypoxemia that is serious enough to warrant treatment. Oxygen therapy is administered first in the treatment of hypoxemia. If the Pao_2 is not restored to at least 60 mm Hg, PPV should be considered. Inspired oxygen concentrations above 60% can be safely administered for short periods of time (i.e., less than 24 hours) but have deleterious pulmonary effects when administered for longer than 48 hours. PPV improves blood oxygenating efficiency of the lungs, which allows for reduction of the inspired oxygen concentration.

Blood oxygenation can also be assessed via pulse oximetry (Spo_2). An Spo_2 of 96% corresponds to a Pao_2 of 80 mm Hg, and 91% corresponds to 60 mm Hg. Pulse oximeters, like all indirect techniques, do not always accurately reflect hemoglobin saturation. When in error, they almost always indicate a value lower than the true value. It is recommended to check the reading at several different locations and take the highest measured value. A common cause of inaccuracy is poor peripheral pulse quality. The pulse oximeter measurement should not be believed if the indicated heart rate does not match that of the patient.

The most subjective indication for PPV is when the animal has to work excessively hard to breathe. Increased muscular activity is required to overcome the increased airway resistance and the decreased lung elasticity often associated with pulmonary disease. This increased work of breathing increases oxygen consumption to fuel the increased energy expenditure. In humans, the metabolic cost of breathing can increase from a normal of about 2% of total oxygen consumption to as high as 25% to 50%.[2] Much of any benefit, in terms of oxygen uptake, accrued by the increased breathing is negated by the increased oxygen consumption required to obtain it. The increased work of breathing also increases heat production and these animals often become hyperthermic, which further drives the breathing effort.

There is a limit to how much work muscles can sustain. This depends on a complex interaction between oxygen delivery, energy production (aerobic and anaerobic), and energy consumption. Muscle fatigue occurs when energy production cannot keep up with the energy consumption that is required to support the breathing effort. Exhaustion causes these patients to deteriorate rapidly with hypoventilation, hypoxemia, hypercapnia, and respiratory arrest. They are very difficult to resuscitate. Because ventilator therapy is a labor-intensive, cost-intensive endeavor, there is a common tendency to wait too long to apply it. If the animal's condition is serious enough to incite concern about the breathing effort, it is probably serious enough to warrant PPV.

Goals of Positive Pressure Ventilation

The goals of positive pressure ventilation are to stabilize ventilation ($Paco_2$ 35 to 60 mm Hg) and oxygenation (Pao_2 80 to 120 mm Hg) at modest inspired oxygen concentrations (e.g., less than 60%) while minimizing the deleterious effects of the procedure.

Getting the Animal on the Ventilator

Airway access is usually accomplished with an orotracheal tube. Unless the central nervous system is severely depressed, heavy sedation or light general anesthesia is usually required to introduce and maintain an endotracheal tube. In addition, few animals will tolerate PPV without disease or drug-induced CNS depression. Notwithstanding coexisting cardiovascular disease, any fast-acting anesthetic (e.g., ketamine/diazepam, propofol, etomidate, or thiopental) would suffice for the introduction of the tube. An opioid/diazepam combination can be used in animals with cardiovascular compromise, but it is a relatively slower induction process and care must be taken to avoid hypoxemia from the time of first drug administration to the time of intubation and ventilation. Mask induction with a gaseous anesthetic agent should be avoided.

A tracheostomy tube is used if the animal is quadriplegic or centrally depressed and there is reason to believe that the ventilation procedure can be accomplished without the use of drugs. Assessment of neurologic recovery and weaning from ventilator support is facilitated if the animal is not receiving sedative drugs. A commercial tracheostomy tube with an inner cannula is superior to a single lumen endotracheal tube because the inner cannula can be removed for easy cleaning.

General Guidelines for Ventilator Settings for Normal Lungs

The general guidelines for positive pressure ventilation of animals with relatively normal lungs, regardless of the method or brand of ventilator utilized, are:

- Peak proximal airway pressure of 10 to 20 cm H_2O
- Tidal volume of 8 to 12 ml/kg
- Inspiratory time of about 1 second (or just long enough to achieve a full tidal volume)
- Ventilatory rate of about 10 to 20 times per minute
- Minute ventilation of about 150 to 250 ml/kg/minute
- End-expiratory pressure of 0 to +2 cm H_2O
- Some ventilated patients may require a deep breath (sigh) at an airway pressure of 30 cm H_2O at regular intervals (30 minutes) to minimize small airway and alveolar collapse.

Guidelines for Ventilator Settings for Diseased Lungs

Diseased lungs are stiffer (less compliant) than normal lungs and are therefore much more difficult to ventilate. The above recommended guidelines are usually insufficient to adequately oxygenate or ventilate a patient with diffuse pulmonary parenchymal disease. Whenever ventilator settings do not seem to meet the needs of the patient or the aforementioned goals, it is first important to make sure that the ventilator settings, including the inspired oxygen, are indeed what you had planned. Next, evaluate patient synchrony and ensure that the patient is not "fighting the ventilator." Finally, it is important to ensure that other untoward problems are not present (e.g., hyperthermia or pneumothorax). After these conditions are met, the ventilator settings should be adjusted. To improve ventilation (in no particular order):

- The proximal airway pressure could be increased in a stepwise fashion up to 60 cm H_2O or to the limit of the ventilator, although current recommendations suggest that efforts should be made to maintain proximal airway pressures less than 35 cm H_2O.
- The tidal volume should probably not be increased in an animal with diffuse lung disease. Pulmonary disease is associated with a reduced vital capacity (see Figure 31-1) because of a reduced inspiratory and expiratory reserve volume. What would be a normal tidal volume for a normal lung could easily over-distend the reduced number of remaining lung units in a diseased lung, which would contribute to volutrauma. Protective lung strategies currently aim for smaller than normal tidal volumes, of 4-8 ml/kg.
- The ventilatory cycle rate could be increased in a stepwise fashion up to 60 breaths per minute.
- The inspiratory time or the inspiratory plateau could be increased. The inspiratory/expiratory (I/E) ratio must allow sufficient time for exhalation of all of the last breath, otherwise air trapping and auto-PEEP will occur.

- PEEP can be increased. Lung units are easier to ventilate when they are kept open after the last breath rather than having to start from a collapsed position. Current recommendations for lung protective ventilation strategies suggest that maintaining enough PEEP to hold open recruitable alveoli minimizes ventilator induced lung injury.

All of the above techniques to improve ventilation will also improve oxygenation. If oxygenation needs to be further improved, the inspired oxygen can be increased to 100% for short periods or to 60% for prolonged periods. Finally, the end-expiratory pressure can be increased to 20 cm H_2O or higher. PEEP increases transpulmonary pressure and functional residual capacity, keeps small airways and alveoli open during the expiratory phase, and thereby improves ventilation and oxygenation. PEEP also minimizes the repetitive collapse and reopening of small airways and alveoli, a process that contributes to ventilator-induced injury.

Positive end-expiratory pressure is available on most ventilators as an adjustable knob. PEEP can also be achieved by attaching a corrugated breathing tube to the exhalation port of the ventilator and placing the other end under water. The depth to which the end of the tube is submerged determines the airway pressure at the end of exhalation.

Choosing a Ventilator Mode

Ventilators come with many different capabilities and features, and there is much debate about which mode of ventilation is best. The objective, of course, is to match the ventilator settings to the needs of the patient. In this regard, there will always be more variation in patient needs than there ever will be in ventilator options. The best ventilator modes/settings should be those that are the least aggressive but that achieve the aforementioned goals of PPV. The various options can be broadly ordered with regard to the required work of breathing, but there is a great deal of overlap, depending on the actual ventilator settings used within each mode.

Controlled ventilation modes (pressure or volume) require no work from the patient. Assisted ventilation requires a little work because the patient has to initiate each breath, but the ventilator actually does all of the work of the breath. Pressure support, synchronized intermittent mandatory ventilation (SIMV), and continuous positive airway pressure (CPAP) ventilation will be discussed in more detail when it comes to weaning but, in general, represent a requirement for progressively increasing amounts of patient work. If a patient requires only a little help, it might be a good idea to start the ventilation procedure with one of these options.

There is no algorithm or magic in this decision. Many different combinations of ventilator modes and settings would suffice for most patients. To the limit of your ventilator, you are limited only by your imagination. If your first chosen ventilator settings do not suit the patient, change the mode/settings and keep changing them until you find one that works.

Open Lung Techniques/Lung Protective Ventilator Strategies

Positive pressure ventilation can induce lung injury ranging from alveolar septal rupture and pneumothorax to a diffuse respiratory distress syndrome that is indistinguishable from the disease for which PPV was implemented. This injury derives from various deleterious aspects of overinflation of individual lung units (volutrauma). *Open lung techniques* and *lung protective ventilation strategies* seek to recruit as many alveolar units as possible, to prevent their re-collapse, and to minimize alveolar overdistention.

These strategies involve high initial peak airway pressures (40 to 60 cm H_2O) for alveolar recruitment, applied for variable periods, one breath up to 1 minute. These recruitment maneuvers are usually accompanied by moderate to high PEEP (10 to 20 cm H_2O) to keep alveoli open. After the high pressure recruitment maneuver, peak pressures are reduced to a more moderate range (30 to 40 cm H_2O).[3-9]

The inevitable consequence of high PEEP pressures and moderate peak pressures is a small (compared with normal) tidal volume. A normal tidal volume in a lung with reduced vital capacity can cause volutrauma. The tidal volume needs to be appropriate for the patient, but unfortunately the magnitude of the disease-induced reduction in vital capacity cannot be predicted in advance. It needs to be assessed in each patient and then must be reassessed frequently because compliance and vital capacity can change over the course of a few hours. Protective lung strategies may also diminish the release of inflammatory mediators, which promote capillary endothelial and airway epithelial damage.[10]

Maintaining the Animal on the Ventilator

Managing a patient on a ventilator is very labor intensive, and knowledgeable personnel must be continuously present to deal with the various crises as they arise.

MANAGING THE VENTILATOR

The initial ventilator settings may not meet the ventilation and oxygenation needs of the patient and will need to be adjusted throughout the course of ventilation to keep pace with deteriorating or improving lung condition. Ongoing monitoring of the ventilator to make sure that it continues to operate properly is important. The gas source from which the ventilator operates should be checked at regular intervals and tanks changed as necessary. An alternative manual ventilation device should be available should the power source or the primary ventilator fail.

PATIENT-VENTILATOR SYNCHRONY

When a patient attempts to breathe out of phase with the ventilator, ventilation and oxygenation deteriorate rapidly. When patient-ventilator asynchrony occurs, check first for technical problems with the ventilator or the presence of worsening pulmonary or coexisting disease (e.g., pneumothorax, hypotension, or hyperthermia). Dyssynchrony may also result from too light a level of sedation because few animals will allow themselves to be ventilated unless they are significantly obtunded by disease or by drugs or unless they are tetraplegic. Try next to synchronize the ventilator to the patient by adjusting the commencement of inspiration to match that of the patient, by adjusting the inspiratory flow rate so that a full tidal volume can be achieved within the time preferred by the patient, or by trying different ventilator modes.

ANESTHESIA

Although any anesthetic can be used for short-term (e.g., 1- to 2-day) ventilation procedures, none of the available anesthetic agents are ideal for long-term (greater than 3-day) ventilation procedures (Table 31-1). The authors primarily use pentobarbital infusions (with and without diazepam) to maintain these patients. The initial infusion rate is 1 to 2 mg/kg/hr, and the drug is then titrated to maintain a light level of anesthesia. Alternative approaches, if pentobarbital induces hypotension, include

TABLE 31-1. Anesthetic Options for Ventilator Patients

Anesthesia/Immobilization Regime	Problem
Opioid/benzodiazepine	Tolerance, tachypnea, hyperthermia
Ketamine/benzodiazepine	Muscle hypertonus
Etomidate	Excessive propylene glycol administration, depression of endogenous cortisol
Propofol	Tolerance, lipemia
Pentobarbital	Recovery is prolonged and hyperreflexive after short-term use (2 days); associated with withdrawal dysphoria after medium-term use (3-7 days); and associated with seizures after prolonged use (longer than 1 week)
Inhalational agents	Environmental pollution
Sedative/neuromuscular blocking agents	No ability to self-breathe during disconnects or other complications; an occasional problem regaining neuromuscular function

the use of opioids such as continuous infusions of fentanyl (0.7 to 1 g/kg/min).

MANAGING THE VENTILATOR CIRCUITRY

The circuitry must be attached properly and securely (disconnects are a common problem). The ventilator circuitry must be supported so that it does not pull or torque the tracheal tube. The inspired air needs to be humidified, and excess water accumulating in the breathing circuit needs to be periodically drained. The authors recommend that ventilator tubing should be changed every 1 or 2 days.

MANAGING THE TRACHEAL TUBE AND CUFF

Accidental tube dislodgement is prevented by avoiding traction on the tube when the patient is moved or rotated (i.e., move the patient and the ventilator circuit in unison). Tubes should also be secured by tying around the maxilla, mandible, or the back of head (for orotracheal tubes) or around the neck (for tracheostomy tubes). The tie around the tube needs to be tight but not collapsing, and the tie around the face or neck needs to be snug but not tight. Ties around the face should be moved every 4 hours to minimize pressure points and lip necrosis. The tying material could be roll gauze, but this soaks up secretions and is not easily cleaned. The authors currently use a length of intravenous fluid extension tubing for this purpose. They recommend that the endotracheal tube should be replaced with a new sterile tube every 24 to 48 hours. A bacterial culture can be obtained from the removed endotracheal tube.

Endotracheal or tracheostomy tube cuffs are usually round, but the trachea is not. In order to seal some portions of the circumference, other portions are likely to be subjected to excessive cuff pressure. Asymmetric tube cuffs and overinflated cuffs magnify the problem. Since ventilation procedures can last for days, prevention of cuff pressure–induced tracheal damage is of paramount importance. Always inflate the cuff while simultaneously auscultating over the larynx for an air leak when pressure is applied to the airway. Inflate the cuff with just enough air to just barely stop the leak of air when positive pressure is applied to the airway (or to just barely *not* stop the leak—a small leak is acceptable as long as the lungs can be inflated). The pilot balloon is only used to indicate that there is air in the cuff; it bears no correlation whatsoever with the amount of pressure being applied to the tracheal wall and must not be used for this purpose. Use high-volume, low-pressure cuffs for long-term procedures whenever possible.

It may be advantageous to periodically change the cuff pressure point. This can be accomplished with endotracheal tubes by deflating the cuff every 4 hours and moving the tube slightly inward or outward. The cuff is then carefully reinflated. Prior to cuff deflation, flush the mouth, pharynx, and the lumen of the trachea rostral to the cuff with saline. All fluid should be removed by suctioning prior to deflating the endotracheal tube cuff. This procedure may predispose to nosocomial pneumonia, but the benefit of minimizing cuff-trachea pressure necrosis is deemed to outweigh the risk of potentiating nosocomial pneumonia.

MANAGING THE TRACHEAL TUBE LUMEN

Mucus and debris being elevated from the depths of the airways accumulate at the end of the endotracheal or tracheostomy tube. Intubated animals cannot cough effectively, and accumulated secretions can dry and obstruct the tracheal tube. The inner cannula of a tracheostomy tube can be easily removed and cleaned every 4 hours. Tracheal tubes without inner cannulas need to be suctioned and should be exchanged every 24 to 48 hours depending on the quantity and viscosity of secretions.

Tracheal suctioning should be done about every 4 hours irrespective of the tube type. It should be done more frequently if there are a lot of secretions and less frequently if there are scant secretions. Suction catheters should be soft and flexible and should have more than one hole in the tip to prevent sucking an epithelial plug into a single hole that would then be ripped away when the catheter is withdrawn. The suction catheter should have a proximal thumbhole so that suction can be applied in a controlled manner. The inside diameter of the catheter should be as large as possible to facilitate the removal of thick secretions. The outside diameter of the catheter should be no larger than 50% of the diameter of the endotracheal tube adapter. The air that is suctioned through the catheter must come from the room and must be able to flow freely down around the outside of the catheter in order to prevent excessive reduction in airway pressure and small airway and alveolar collapse.

The suctioning procedure must be atraumatic and aseptic. Closed tracheal suction systems* are available, thereby eliminating the need to disconnect the ventilator tubing. The airway should be well humidified before suctioning. The animal should breathe 100% oxygen for 5 minutes prior to suctioning to minimize the inevitable hypoxemia. Secretions can be mobilized into the central airways by chest coupage just before suctioning. Inject 0.2 ml/kg of saline into the tracheal tube and then manually hyperinflate the lungs several times. Gently insert the suction catheter into the trachea as far as it will advance. Suction is applied while the catheter is being withdrawn with a rotating and winding motion of the hand. Suction should not be applied to the airways for more than about 5 seconds so as to minimize small airway and alveolar collapse. The suctioning procedure should cease immediately if discomfort, restlessness, or changes in cardiac or respiratory rhythm occur. The animal should be manually hyperinflated with oxygen after suctioning to alleviate the small airway and alveolar collapse. The procedure should be repeated several times if it is productive.

Trach care pediatric Ballard Medical Products, Draper, Utah.

Tracheal suctioning should always net some airway secretions. If not, it is because they are too dry, and better humidification and secretion liquefaction are needed. The presence of blood in the aspirant indicates an excessively traumatic procedure. A more gentle aspiration technique with less pressure and lower flow rates and perhaps a smaller suction catheter should be tried.

AIRWAY HYDRATION

Air and oxygen supplied to and coming from the ventilator is anhydrous and must be humidified to minimize mucus production and epithelial desiccation. Humidification is the provision of water vapor to help prevent drying. Nebulization is the provision of particulate water droplets to therapeutically moisten already thick secretions. In-line humidifiers should be heated and sealed by a semipermeable membrane so that there is no water-air interface because warm water supports growth of infectious organisms, which are a source of nosocomial pneumonia. Unsealed humidifiers should be exchanged with sterile equipment every 24 hours. Cooling between the heated humidifier and the patient causes water to condense in the inspiratory tubing; it will need to be periodically drained. As an alternative to a commercial humidifier, sterile distilled water can be instilled into the inspiratory tubing and endotracheal tube about every 2 hours. Commercial condenser/humidifiers* are available that attach to the tracheal tube and function as an artificial nose. Systemic hydration is of paramount importance in ensuring adequate airway hydration; no airway humidification procedure will be very effective in a dehydrated patient.

REPOSITIONING

Immobility and positional stasis for prolonged periods predisposes to tissue necrosis and decubiti over bony protuberances, is associated with accumulated secretions and atelectasis in the lower regions of the lung, is associated with contracture and stiffening of muscles and ligaments, and may be associated with regional appendage edema because of poor lymphatic drainage. It is important to ensure that the body and all appendages are positioned comfortably and repositioned every 4 hours. The body and all appendages should be well padded, and legs should not be allowed to hang over the edge of the table. Passive range of motion exercises should be performed at 4-hour intervals.

The prone position seems to provide the most consistent and best lung function in ventilated animals. Lateral positions are easiest to maintain in animals and are usually associated with satisfactory lung function, but in some patients lateral positions may be associated with precipitous deterioration in lung function, especially when they are being turned from side to side.

*Humid-Vent 1,® Glbeck Respiration, P.O. Box 711, 5-194; 27 Upplands Vasby, Sweden.

MOUTH CARE

Comatose or anesthetized patients do not eat, drink, or swallow. The mouth and pharynx accumulate secretions, which soon become colonized with gram-negative organisms and predispose to nosocomial infection. The mouth and pharynx should be washed with sterile saline and suctioned every 4 hours. It is important to avoid torque or traction on the tracheal tube during this procedure. The pharynx and mouth should then be rinsed with a commercial chlorhexidine mouthwash solution.

The tongue will dry if it is allowed to flop out of the mouth, and it will develop pressure-induced ulcers if it is allowed to drape across teeth or if the pulse oximeter is left in one place for too long. The tongue should be cleaned along with the mouth. It should be left wholly within the mouth between cleanings. It can be wrapped in a saline and glycerin–soaked gauze sponge to keep it moist and to minimize sublingual edema.

EYE CARE

Corneal drying and ulceration is a common problem because of reduced lacrimal secretions and the absence of blinking. Artificial tears and bland ophthalmic ointments should be alternately placed into the conjunctival sac every 2 hours. The corneas should be fluorescein stained regularly to check for corneal ulcers, and if they develop, antibiotic ophthalmic ointment should be used.

OPTIMIZE FLUID THERAPY

The moistness and mobility of airway secretions depends a great deal on adequate systemic hydration. With exudative secretions (pneumonia), patients should be maintained on the high side of the range of normal hydration. Patients with transudative secretions (pulmonary edema) should be maintained on the low side of normal hydration to minimize fluid flux into the lungs. Animals on ventilators tend to retain sodium and water because of high aldosterone levels. Fluids in and out, body weight, and physical evidences of edema should be monitored closely.

BLADDER CARE

Recumbent, sedated patients often do not urinate normally, and when they do, it soils the skin. Human infant absorbent diapers, properly positioned, work very well for collecting the urine and preventing it from soaking the skin. The diapers can be weighed to quantitate the urine output. If the animal does not urinate, the bladder should be expressed; however, a urinary catheter is often placed to facilitate urine collection and sanitation and to quantitate urine output. Insertion must be accomplished in an aseptic fashion, and the urine collection system must be closed, aseptic, and below the horizontal level of the patient. Every 8 hours, flush the vestibule or prepuce with sterile saline and then a very dilute solution of betadine or 0.02% chlorhexidine solution.

COLON CARE

Recumbent, sedated patients often do not defecate normally. The colon should be palpated daily to assess its contents. An enema of warm saline may be indicated. Long hair around the anus should be clipped to facilitate the cleaning of feces.

MINIMIZING NOSOCOMIAL INFECTION

Ventilated patients are susceptible to the acquisition of a hospital-acquired infection, and every effort should be made to manage them aseptically. All patient circuits and nebulization equipment should be sterile when first connected and should be changed every 48 hours.

NUTRITION

Early nutrition is extremely important in supporting the animal's ability to fend off infection and to heal disordered tissues and organ dysfunctions. Ventilated animals can be fed via a nasogastric, esophagostomy, or gastrostomy tube if the stomach is motile or intravenously if it is not. Gastric stasis resulting in the accumulation of previous feedings is a common problem and with continued feeding will result in gastric distention and regurgitation. Gastric residuals must be checked prior to each feeding and should not be allowed to exceed about 10 ml/kg. Gastric motility may require augmentation by metoclopramide, erythromycin, or bethanechol.

BE PREPARED FOR EMERGENCIES

Emergency reintubation may be required if tubes become obstructed or accidentally dislodged. Options for alternate ventilation should be available: pneumatic in case the power goes out and manual in case the compressed gas supply becomes depleted. Suction equipment should also be readily available.

Problems and Precautions

THORACIC BLOODFLOW IMPAIRMENT

Positive pressure ventilation impairs intrathoracic bloodflow by increasing pleural pressure, which impedes venous return to both the right and the left side of the heart. To the extent that venous return is diminished, diastolic ventricular filling, stroke volume, cardiac output, and arterial blood pressure are also diminished. The degree of impairment of intrathoracic bloodflow is directly proportional to the magnitude of the increase in pleural pressure, the length of time that the pressure is applied per breath (the inspiratory time) and per minute (the cycle rate), and indirectly proportional to the baseline central venous pressure (the blood volume). The magnitude of circulatory impairment can be assessed by observing the effect of each inspiration on pulse quality or arterial blood pressure. If it is determined that excessive circulatory impairment is present,

the inspiratory pressure, the inspiratory time, or the breathing rate could be decreased or the blood volume could be increased. Diseased lungs are poorly compliant, and although it may require higher airway pressures to ventilate these lungs, less of the pressure is transmitted to the pleural space, and there is a decreased tendency to impair circulation.

ALVEOLAR SEPTAL RUPTURE

The use of high airway pressures and large tidal volumes in normal and abnormal lungs may be associated with alveolar septal rupture, pneumomediastinum, pneumothorax, pulmonary hemorrhage, air embolism, and lung inflammation. Alveolar septal rupture is reported to occur at a rate of between 3% and 40% of ventilated patients.[3,4,11-13] There is marked individual variation in susceptibility to this problem. Weg and colleagues reported that there was no airway pressure above which patients always developed alveolar septal rupture and no airway pressure below which it never occurred.[11] Preexisting parenchymal bullae or recent parenchymal rupture lower the threshold to ventilator-induced alveolar septal rupture. Airway pressure and tidal volume settings should only be as high as is minimally necessary to achieve acceptable ventilation and oxygenation. In diffuse pulmonary parenchymal disease, the total number of functional lung units is reduced. The introduction of normal tidal volumes causes overdistention of the remaining functional lung units. Lung protective strategies utilize smaller than normal tidal volumes to help prevent this volutrauma.

Monitoring for the development of a pneumothorax during positive pressure ventilation must be an ongoing endeavor. It should be one of the first rule-outs for patient-ventilator asynchrony or sudden hypoxemia. If a pneumothorax develops, a chest drain must be inserted and continuous chest drainage provided.

AUTO-PEEP

Whereas inhalation is an active process orchestrated by the ventilator, exhalation is a passive process that depends on lung and chest wall elastance. If exhalation is not complete prior to initiation of the next breath, the next tidal volume will be increased by the amount of air remaining in the lung from the preceding breath. This phenomenon, termed air trapping, breath stacking, or auto-PEEP, can result in overexpansion of lung units (volutrauma). Air trapping is more likely to occur if exhalation is delayed by narrowed lower airways because of chronic airway disease or bronchospasm, and with higher ventilator cycle rates. If the measured end-expiratory pressure exceeds that set on the ventilator, auto-PEEP is occurring.

Auto-PEEP is not necessarily bad unless it is excessive. PEEP, whether it comes intentionally from the ventilator or unintentionally from the patient-ventilator interaction, improves lung oxygenating efficiency. It is important to know when auto-PEEP is present, and then a decision can be made whether to keep it or treat it.

CAPILLARY ENDOTHELIAL DAMAGE

Airways and alveoli are tethered together by strands of collagenous and elastic fibers. When the airways are expanded, tangential and longitudinal traction is placed upon on the adjacent endothelium cell layers. This widens intercellular junctions, increases capillary permeability and the flux of fluids into the pulmonary interstitium. This phenomenon is exacerbated if there is concurrent generalized capillary endothelial injury as a consequence of release of inflammatory mediators.

AIRWAY AND ALVEOLAR EPITHELIAL DAMAGE

In animals with pulmonary disease, an increase in airway fluids increases surface tension and enhances the tendency for small airway and alveolar collapse. Reopening these units during the next breath requires breaking the surface tension seal between two adjacent epithelial cells. These tangential forces eventually damage the cell membranes. Adjacent lung units, for a variety of reasons, have different time constants and do not expand at the same time or rate. This causes a shear injury to the alveolar epithelium on each side of the thin septal membranes that form the common wall between two adjacent alveoli.

RELEASE OF INFLAMMATORY MEDIATORS

Positive pressure ventilation and, particularly, overdistention of lung units are thought to cause leuco-activation, resulting in the release of inflammatory mediators.[10] These at least enhance capillary permeability and can cause epithelial cell damage as well. Endothelial and epithelial damage worsens the magnitude of the diffuse parenchymal disease in a manner that is indistinguishable from the underlying disease process. PEEP, set above closing pressure, minimizes surface tension-induced airway/alveolar closure and asynchronous lung unit expansion.

PNEUMONIA

Pneumonia is a common consequence of long-term positive pressure ventilation. Positional stasis predisposes to atelectasis and decreased secretion clearance from the lower lung regions. The bacterial population proliferates in the mouth and pharynx, which become colonized by gram-negative organisms, and these microorganisms invariably migrate down the trachea past the inflated cuff and into the lower airways. Invasive procedures such as tracheal intubation and tracheal suctioning further predispose to the introduction of bacteria into the lower airways. If antibiotics are utilized, the patient is predisposed to colonization by resistant microorganisms. If histamine-2 blockers are utilized, the patient is predisposed to bacterial colonization in the stomach, and such fluids invariably find their way up the esophagus and into the airways.

The procedure of positive pressure ventilation, per se, is not considered to be an indication for prophylactic antibiotic therapy. In an unpublished experimental series (Haskins), all dogs needed to be placed on antibiotics by the end of 1 week. Regular repositioning, aseptic airway procedures, and regular mouth and pharynx care help minimize the development of pneumonia. Ventilated patients should be monitored for indications of infection and placed on appropriate antibiotics if and when the need arises.

Getting the Animal off the Ventilator

Weaning an animal off ventilatory support requires special attention because the patient may be slow to develop the ability to maintain its own ventilation and oxygenation requirements. Severe diffuse pulmonary parenchymal disease heals slowly; gradual withdrawal of support needs to mirror progressive improvement in oxygenating efficiency. The ventilatory muscles undergo disuse atrophy, and ventilatory support must be withdrawn slowly so that the animal has time to redevelop muscle strength. The objective of discontinuing ventilator support is to decrease the magnitude of ventilator support, requiring the patient to work harder to breathe, but at a rate that will not expose the patient to the recurrence of ventilation or oxygenation failure.

In a sense, the weaning process begins the moment an animal is set up and stable on the ventilator. That is to say, the animal is frequently being tested during the course of the ventilation procedure by trying slightly less aggressive ventilator settings and then assessing the animal's response. If there is no deterioration in lung performance, the ventilator settings are decreased a bit more, and so on. If there is an unacceptable deterioration in lung performance, the settings are returned to their previous level because it is apparent that the animal is not yet ready to be weaned. After a period in which one might expect measurable improvement (but not longer than 24 hours), the process is repeated.

The ability to safely discontinue ventilatory support is always a retrospective assessment. Prospective predictors of "weanability" are not very reliable and must address the reason for which the animal was initially placed on the ventilator (e.g., don't look at oxygenation parameters if the animal is being ventilated because of tetraplegia). Other considerations include:

- Respiratory center-mediated hypoventilation/apnea is usually associated with other signs of intracranial disease (e.g., coma). These animals do not require sedation to be maintained on the ventilator. When these patients regain sufficient consciousness that they no longer tolerate the ventilation procedure and endotracheal intubation, they probably will have regained sufficient function of their respiratory centers to maintain adequate ventilation. The ventilator settings are progressively decreased to see if the patient can maintain itself.

- Patients with spinal cord or peripheral neuromuscular disease–mediated hypoventilation should be ventilated via a tracheostomy tube so that they do not have to be sedated/anesthetized. Return of muscle function and strength can then be more easily assessed. Strength of the withdrawal reflex; resistance to appendage flexion; strength of the spontaneous breathing effort; ability to generate a subatmospheric pressure greater than 5 to 15 cm H_2O (cat to large dog, respectively) when inspiring against a closed airway; and ability to sit up or stand are all signs of possible weanability.

- Patients with pulmonary parenchymal disease may be ready to wean off mechanical ventilation when they require only minimal ventilator settings to generate acceptable arterial oxygenation. Oxygenation parameters do not need to be normal, just acceptable with inspired oxygen concentrations of 40% or less. The ability to maintain a Pao_2 of greater than 80 mm Hg with a PEEP less than 4 cm H_2O and an inspired oxygen of less than 40% is encouraging. The ability to maintain a $Paco_2$ of less than 45 mm Hg with a normal-range tidal/minute volume and peak airway pressures also suggests that the patient may be weanable.

A series of screening questions to assess potential weanability is suggested in Figure 31-2. A "no" answer to any question suggests that the patient may not be weanable at this time. If the answer to all questions is "yes," the ventilator settings should be decreased. An assessment of inspiratory muscle strength will help guide the direction of the process (Figure 31-3). If the patient has the muscle strength to decrease airway pressure more than 5 cm H_2O (for a cat), 10 cm H_2O (for a small dog), or 15 cm H_2O (for a large dog), it is assumed that the patient can tolerate a more aggressive weaning process. If not, a more gradual weaning process, which does not initially demand too much of the patient, should be implemented.

There are many different methods of weaning; all involve a gradual decrease in support and require a gradual increase in work by the patient. The method used is largely dependent on the capabilities of the ventilator and the patient. Weaning methods, in approximate order from least to most work required of the patient, include:

- Decreasing amounts of pressure support
- Intermittent mandatory ventilation, with decreasing mandatory breaths
- Spontaneous breathing with continuous positive airway pressure
- A gradual decrease in set ventilator cycle rate so that the animal has to trigger progressively more breaths on its own (assisted breathing with a gradual increase in the required trigger effort)
- Removing the patient from the ventilator for progressively longer spontaneous breathing trials

Combinations of these different weaning techniques are commonly used on individual patients. The endotracheal tube, the breathing circuit, and the ventilator generally increase the resistance to inspiratory flow. Several modes (e.g., SIMV and CPAP) require that the animal breathes through the ventilator. Without pressure support, this adds resistance to the inspiratory effort and increases the work of breathing for the patient.

PRESSURE SUPPORT

Pressure support is a spontaneous breathing mode offered on some ventilators. The patient determines when to start an inspiration, how fast to inspire, and when to terminate the inspiration. The ventilator applies a preselected amount of positive pressure to the airway throughout the inspiratory flow phase. Gas flow rate from the ventilator is initially very high in order to keep up with the patient's inspired gas flow rate while maintaining the preset proximal airway pressure. As the patient's lungs fill, the inspiratory flow rate decreases, and the fresh gas flow from the ventilator decreases proportionally. When the flow rate from the ventilator decreases to 20% of its peak, the ven-

Screen #1

NOTE: If the answer to any of the above questions is "no," do not try to wean.

- Is the Pao_2:Fio_2 above 300?

- Can oxygenation be maintained with an Fio_2 below 0.4 and a PEEP below 4 cm H_2O?

- Can ventilation and oxygenation be maintained with a peak airway pressure below 25 cm H_2O?

- Is there a light level of anesthesia and strong mandibular muscle tone?

- Does the animal cough during tracheal suctioning?

- Are there spontaneous breathing efforts?

Figure 31-2. *The initial determination of "weanability."*

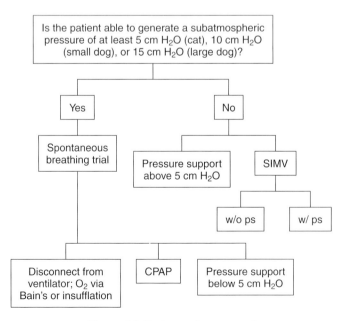

Figure 31-3. *A weaning protocol.*

tilator switches to the expiratory flow phase. This is a very patient-friendly mode of ventilation because the patient is in total control of each tidal volume, be it small or large or fast or slow. As the patient becomes stronger and capable of more of the work of breathing, the amount of pressure support can be decreased.

INTERMITTENT MANDATORY VENTILATION

Intermittent mandatory ventilation (IMV) modes provide a minimum number of controlled breaths from the ventilator but allow the animal to breathe spontaneously through the ventilator the rest of the time. Most IMV modes are synchronized to the patient's breathing efforts (SIMV) so that a mechanical ventilator breath coincides with the beginning of a spontaneous patient breath. As the intermittent controlled breaths are progressively decreased, the patient must breathe more on its own. The patient has to breathe through the resistance of the ventilator, breathing circuit, and tracheal tube unless pressure support is added.

CONTINUOUS POSITIVE AIRWAY PRESSURE

Continuous positive airway pressure (CPAP) is a spontaneous breathing mode at an elevated airway pressure. Both rate and tidal volume are controlled by the patient while the CPAP keeps small airways and alveoli open between breaths. This maximizes oxygenation and facilitates the distribution of the next breath to the lower airways.

DECREASING VENTILATOR RATE

In assist mode, a gradual decrease in the ventilator cycle rate requires the animal to trigger progressively more breaths of its own. Once triggered, however, the ventilator finishes the breath at the preset tidal volume, flow rate, and inspiratory time. The sensitivity control can be carefully adjusted to require progressively more effort from the patient to trigger a breath.

Screen #2

NOTE: A "yes" answer denotes failure to wean. Go back to the previous ventilator setting.

• Was it necessary to increase the FiO_2 above 0.4 to maintain oxygenation, or did the PaO_2:FiO_2 fall below 300?

• Was it necessary to increase the PEEP above 4 cm H_2O or peak pressure above 25 cm H_2O to maintain oxygenation?

• Did heart rate, blood pressure, or breathing rate increase more than 50%?

• Did the breathing effort increase or decrease appreciably?

Figure 31-4. How is the patient tolerating the discontinuance of ventilator support?

SPONTANEOUS BREATHING TRIALS

Ventilators without any type of weaning mode require that the patient be removed from the ventilator for short spontaneous breathing trials. The length of time off the ventilator is progressively increased as the patient's condition and strength allows.

A second series of questions (Figure 31-4) is aimed at determining how well the animal is tolerating the weaning process. A "no" answer to all questions suggests that the animal is tolerating the weaning process and that a trial of further reduction in the level of ventilator support is warranted. A "yes" answer to any question suggests weaning failure and that it is probably necessary to return to more supportive ventilator settings that require less work from the patient (Figures 31-5 and 31-6).

Getting the Animal off Sedative Drugs

Sedative drugs cause respiratory depression and muscle weakness. Sedated or anesthetized patients will not breathe as well as unsedated patients and therefore are more difficult to wean. Unfortunately, animals must

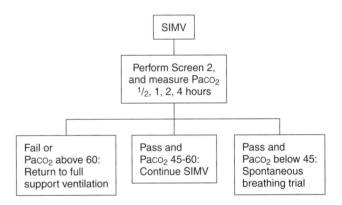

Figure 31-5. A course of action during the weaning process.

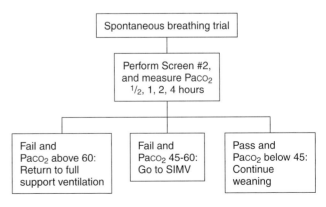

Figure 31-6. A course of action during the weaning process.

remain on sedative drugs throughout the weaning process, until such time that it is safe to disconnect them from the ventilator and extubate. It is especially important, therefore, during the weaning process, to be sure to utilize the least amount of sedation compatible with patient-ventilator synchrony and retention of the endotracheal tube. It is also desirable to use short-acting or reversible agents so that the sedative effects terminate as soon as possible following extubation.

Endogenous neurotransmitters accommodate to long-term sedation, and withdrawal of these drugs can be associated with excitation and, possibly, seizures. This is especially true for pentobarbital, which is a commonly used drug. Recovery from short-term pentobarbital anesthesia is often rough and hyperreflexive; adjunctive tranquilizers (e.g., diazepam or acepromazine) may be necessary to smooth out the recovery. Recovery from intermediate-length pentobarbital anesthesia (3 to 4 days) is associated with dysphoria and intolerance to handling; a diazepam infusion (0.2 to 0.5 mg/kg/hr) from the time the pentobarbital is turned off to 24 hours after weaning and extubation should minimize this effect. Recovery from prolonged anesthesia (longer than 1 week) may be associated with seizures. These patients should be started on phenobarbital (6 mg/kg q 12 hours) at least 4 days prior to stopping the pentobarbital infusion. Because it isn't known in advance when weaning will occur, it is better to start the phenobarbital early. It will help reduce the dose requirement of the other drugs during the procedure, and then will be there when the decision is made to start weaning the pentobarbital. Long-term pentobarbital infusions should not be stopped abruptly even with a phenobarbital background. Reduce the dose by half each day until the dose is below 1 mg/kg/hr, and then turn it off. An infusion of diazepam should be started if hyperexcitability or seizures occur. If more help is needed, keep the animal anesthetized with a propofol infusion (0.1 mg/kg/min) for 24 hours after the pentobarbital has been turned off (during which time a substantial proportion of the pentobarbital will have been metabolized and eliminated) and then let the animal recover from the propofol. Alternatively, continuous infusions of fentanyl can be used for sedation, and the effects of the narcotic can be reversed if necessary.

Neuromuscular blocking agents have been occasionally used in the management of ventilated animal patients, and they are commonly used in human intensive care units. Neuromuscular blocking agents remove all breathing capabilities, which might be protective should there be a ventilator malfunction or circuit disconnect. Withdrawal of the neuromuscular blocking agent is not always associated with reversal of the neuromuscular blockade. The reason for this is not known but may be associated with down-regulation of acetylcholine receptors at the neuromuscular junction. In general, neuromuscular blocking agents are not necessary for ventilating animals and, given their potential adverse effects, are not recommended for use by untrained individuals.

Conclusion

Positive pressure ventilation is labor-intensive and expensive. Successful endeavors require great attention to detail and virtually constant care. Patients require total care of all aspects of their well-being and there are many problematic roadblocks to success.

Long-term ventilation is, however, efficacious for some patients. A little over 50% of animals placed on the ventilator because of their inability to ventilate (neuromuscular disease) are successfully weaned from the ventilator, and a little less than 50% of these patients are discharged from the hospital. The success rate depends on the type of disease being treated. In one retrospective study of 14 dogs that required positive pressure ventilation to treat hypoventilation because of cervical spinal cord injury, 10 of the dogs were successfully weaned from the ventilator and recovered the ability to breathe, and 9 of the dogs recovered motor function and were eventually able to walk.[14] The average duration of PPV in that study was 4.5 days.[14]

About 25% of animals placed on the ventilator because of their inability to oxygenate (diffuse parenchymal disease) are successfully weaned from the ventilator, and about 15% are discharged from the hospital. Once again, outcomes depend on the type of lung disease; patients ventilated because of acute respiratory distress syndrome are likely to have a worse prognosis than those with other types of lung disease. In a retrospective study of 10 dogs that required PPV because of severe pulmonary contusions following trauma, 3 dogs recovered and were discharged from the hospital, 1 dog was euthanized at the owner's request despite significant improvement in lung function, 1 dog was weaned from the ventilator but died suddenly later during the hospitalization, and 5 dogs had progressively worsening lung dysfunction and died or were euthanized while on the ventilator.[15]

REFERENCES

1. Hendricks JC, King LG: Practicality, usefulness and limits of end-tidal carbon dioxide monitoring in critical small animal patients, *J Vet Emer Crit Care* 4(1):29-39, 1994.
2. Lumb AB: *Nunn's applied respiratory physiology*, ed 5, Butterworth-Heinemann, Boston, 2000.
3. Acute Respiratory Distress Syndrome Network: Ventilation with lower tidal volumes as compared with traditional tidal volumes for acute lung injury and the acute respiratory distress syndrome, *New Engl J Med* 342:1301-1308, 2000.
4. Amato MBP, Barbas CSV, Medeiros DM et al: Effect of a protective ventilation strategy on mortality in the acute respiratory distress syndrome, *N Engl J Med* 338:347-354, 1998.
5. Brochard L, Roudot-Thoraval F, Roupie E: Tidal volume reduction for prevention of ventilator-induced lung injury in acute respiratory distress syndrome: The multicenter trial group on tidal volume reduction in ARDS, *Am J Resp Crit Care Med* 158:1831-1838, 1998.
6. Brower RG, Shanholtz CB, Fessler HE et al: Prospective, randomized, controlled clinical trial comparing traditional versus reduced tidal volume ventilation in acute respiratory distress syndrome patients, *Crit Care Med* 27:1492-1498, 1999.
7. Kloot TE, Blanch L, Melynne-Youngblood A et al: Recruitment maneuvers in three experimental models of acute lung injury: Effect on lung volume and gas exchange, *Am J Respir Crit Care Med* 161:1485-1494, 2000.

8. Medoff BD, Harris RS, Kesselman H et al: Use of recruitment maneuvers and high-positive end-expiratory pressure in a patient with acute respiratory distress syndrome, *Crit Care Med* 28:1210-1216, 2000.
9. Stewart TE, Meade MO, Cook DJ et al: Evaluation of a ventilation strategy to prevent barotrauma in patients at high risk for acute respiratory distress syndrome, *N Engl J Med* 338:355-361, 1998.
10. Ranieri VM, Suter PM, Tortorella C et al: Effect of mechanical ventilation on inflammatory mediators in patients with acute respiratory distress syndrome: a randomized controlled trial, *JAMA* 282:54-61, 1999.
11. King LG, Hendricks JC: Use of positive-pressure ventilation in dogs and cats: 41 cases (1990-1992), *J Am Vet Med Assoc* 204:1045-1052, 1994.
12. Strieter RM, Lynch JP: Complications in the ventilated patient, *Clinics Chest Med* 9:127-139, 1988.
13. Weg JG, Anzueto A, Balk RA et al: The relation of pneumothorax and other air leaks to mortality in the acute respiratory distress syndrome, *New Engl J Med* 338:341-346, 1998.
14. Beal MW, Paglia DT, Griffin GM et al: Ventilatory failure, ventilator management, and outcome in dogs with cervical spinal disorders: 14 cases (1991-1999), *J Am Vet Med Assoc* 218(10):1598-1602, 2001.
15. Campbell VL, King LG: Pulmonary function, ventilator management and outcome of dogs with thoracic trauma and pulmonary contusions: 10 cases (1994-1998), *J Am Vet Med Assoc* 217(10):1505-1509, 2000.

CHAPTER 32

Drugs Affecting the Respiratory System*

Dawn Merton Boothe

Normal Respiratory Physiology

AIRWAY CALIBER CHANGES

Nervous innervation to the smooth muscle of the respiratory tract is complex. The parasympathetic system provides the primary efferent innervation, with acetylcholine as the primary neurotransmitter.[1,2] These fibers are responsible for the baseline tone of mild bronchoconstriction that characterizes the normal respiratory tract. The sympathetic system balances these effects by stimulating bronchodilation through beta-2-receptors.[3-5] In contrast, α-adrenergic stimulation can contribute to bronchoconstriction.[1,2,4] A third, poorly understood nervous system (referred to as the nonadrenergic, noncholinergic system, or the purinergic system), also innervates bronchial smooth muscle.[1,6] This system mediates bronchodilation via vagal stimulation. The afferent fibers of this system are probably irritant receptors, and although the neurotransmitter has not yet been conclusively identified, vasoactive intestinal peptide has been implicated in the cat.[7,8] Malfunction of this system has been associated with bronchial hyperreactivity, which often characterizes asthma.[6]

The intracellular mechanisms that transmit signals from the nervous system to smooth muscle depend, in part, on changes in the intracellular concentration of cyclic adenosine monophosphate (cAMP) and cyclic guanosine monophosphate (cGMP) (Figure 32-1). The effects of these two secondary messengers are reciprocal, such that the increased intracellular concentration of one is associated with a decreased concentration of the other. Cyclic AMP-induced bronchodilation is decreased by α-adrenergic stimulation and increased by beta-2-receptor stimulation.[3] In contrast, cGMP-induced bronchoconstriction is increased by stimulation of muscarinic (cholinergic) and, indirectly, histaminergic receptors (Figure 32-1). The relative sensitivity of bronchial smooth muscle to histamine-induced and acetylcholine-induced bronchoconstriction varies with the location and species.[5,9,10] For example, peripheral airways of dogs are more susceptible to acetylcholine than

*Portions of this chapter are found in Boothe DM: *Small animal clinical pharmacology and therapeutics*, Philadelphia, 2001, WB Saunders.

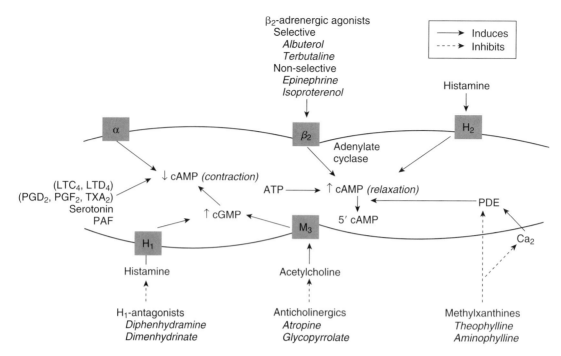

Figure 32-1. Factors determining bronchial smooth muscle tone. Reciprocal changes in cyclic adenosine monophosphate (cAMP) and cyclic guanosine monophosphate (cGMP) determine muscle tone. Contraction occurs when cAMP levels are decreased by events such as α-adrenergic stimulation, or when cGMP levels increase in response to muscarinic receptor (M3) stimulation by acetylcholine or H_1-receptor stimulation by histamine. Calcium (Ca^{2+}) and several other mediators can also induce bronchoconstriction. Increased cAMP levels induced by beta-2-adrenergic or histamine (H_2) receptor stimulation counteract muscle contraction. Inhibition of phosphodiesterase (PDE) also causes increased levels of cAMP. Although the effects of most inflammatory mediators are best counteracted by preventing their release, several drugs may be used to antagonize smooth muscle contraction regardless of the etiology. LTC, LTD = leukotrienes C and D; PAF = platelet-activating factor; PGD_2, PGF_2 = prostaglandins D_2 and F_2; TXA_2 = thromboxane. (Reprinted with permission from Boothe DM: *Small animal clinical pharmacology and therapeutics,* Philadelphia, 2001, WB Saunders.)

are those of cats. In general, cat airways are more sensitive to acetylcholine than histamine.[11] Smooth muscle receptors are also susceptible to stimulation by a variety of chemical mediators (Figure 32-1), which may also modulate cAMP and cGMP.[12-14]

Control of bronchial smooth muscle tone is very complex and depends on input from sensory receptors. At least five types of sensory receptors have been identified in cat lungs, which can be classified as irritant (or mechanoreceptor), stretch, or J-receptors.[6] All appear to be innervated by the parasympathetic system. Irritant receptors, located beneath the respiratory epithelium, occur in the upper airways[2] and, in cats, as far peripherally as the alveoli.[1] Physical, mechanical, or chemical stimulation of these receptors results in tachypnea, bronchoconstriction, and cough. Airflow velocity appears to be the most critical factor determining stimulation of irritant receptors in the upper airways.[1] Airway constriction that causes airflow velocity to exceed a specific threshold results in a vagally mediated cough reflex and bronchoconstriction. Airways can also be occluded by mucus and edema or by chemical mediators released during upper airway infections.[6]

RESPIRATORY DEFENSE MECHANISMS

The sneeze and cough reflexes are among the most important respiratory defense mechanisms in the respiratory tract. Two other systems provide major defense but also can contribute to the pathophysiology of disease: (1) the mucociliary apparatus and (2) the respiratory mononuclear phagocyte system.[2] The mucociliary apparatus (Figure 32-2) consists of the ciliary lining of the tracheobronchial tree and the fluid blanket surrounding the cilia. Two types of secretion form the fluid blanket of the respiratory tract. The cilia must be surrounded by a low-viscosity, watery medium to maintain their rhythmic beat. A more mucoid layer lies on top of the cilia and serves to trap foreign materials inspired with air. The synchronous motion of the cilia causes the cephalad movement of the mucous layer and any trapped materials. Nervous innervation to the cilia has not yet been identified. Although ciliary activity increases with beta-adrenergic stimulation, this may simply reflect the sequelae of beta-adrenergic stimulation and increased fluidity of respiratory secretions.[15] Changes in the viscoelastic properties of mucus such that it becomes ei-

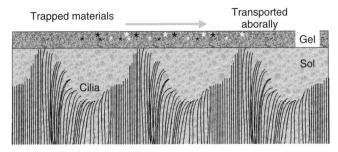

Figure 32-2. *The mucociliary apparatus represents the first line of defense for pathogens entering the respiratory tract. Cilia are bathed in a water or sol layer. When the cilia beat in synchrony, the movements send forward (orally) the mucoid or gel layer that lies on top of the cilia. Materials trapped in this layer also move forward to be swallowed or expectorated.* (Reprinted with permission from Boothe DM: *Small animal clinical pharmacology and therapeutics,* Philadelphia, 2001, WB Saunders.)

ther too watery or too rigid will result in mucous transport that is less than optimal.[2] Mucus released by goblet cells results from direct irritation[2] and is not amenable to pharmacological manipulation. Surface goblet cells, which are uniquely prominent in feline bronchioles,[16] increase in number with chronic disease.

Submucosal glands of the bronchi secrete both a serous and a mucoid fluid. The secretions tend to be more fluid than those of the goblet cells, but the degree varies with the stimulus. The normal consistency of the combined secretions of the tracheobronchial tree is 95% water, 2% glycoprotein, 1% carbohydrate, and less than 1% lipid.[2] Glycoproteins increase the viscosity of the secretions, providing protection and lubrication. Infection and chronic inflammatory diseases can have a profound effect on respiratory secretions. The glycoprotein component tends to be replaced by degradative products of inflammation such as DNA. Parasympathetic, cholinergic stimulation increases mucus secretion, whereas beta-adrenergic stimulation causes secretion of mucus, electrolytes, and water.[2,15]

The second major component of the pulmonary defense system is the respiratory mononuclear phagocyte system. In cats, calves, pigs, sheep, and goats, this includes both alveolar macrophages and the pulmonary intravascular macrophages (PIMs).[17] The PIMs are resident cells that are characterized by phagocytic properties and thus cause the release of inflammatory mediators. The clearance of blood-borne bacteria and particulate matter in these species is accomplished by PIMs rather than hepatic Kupffer cells and splenic macrophages, as in most other species.[17] The pharmacological significance of the mononuclear phagocyte system reflects its role in inflammation (Figure 32-3). A number of preformed (e.g., histamine and serotonin) and in situ (e.g., prostaglandins, leukotrienes, and platelet-activating factor) mediators are released by inflammatory cells.[12-14] Each is capable of inducing a variety of adverse effects that tend to decrease airway caliber (e.g., edema, chemotaxis, increased mucous production, and bronchoconstriction). The involvement of PIMs in both experimental and natural respira-

tory diseases of animals suggests that release of chemical mediators from these cells may be important in the pathogenesis of bronchial diseases.

SURFACTANT

Although its primary function is to decrease surface tension in alveoli, thus affecting both lung mechanics and gas exchange, pulmonary surfactant also contributes to pulmonary defense mechanisms.[18] Surfactant is synthesized and secreted by alveolar type II cells. Its complex mixture of lipids and proteins is fairly constant among mammalian species.[18] The primary components in human surfactant include phospholipids (80%), proteins (12%), and miscellaneous lipids (8%). The lipids, in turn, are composed principally of phosphatidylcholine (85%), with dipalmitoylated phosphatidylcholine (DPPC) contributing the most to the reduction in surface tension. Four surfactant-associated proteins (SP-A through SP-D) are active. Both SP-A and SP-D enhance phagocytosis of bacteria and viruses and regulate type II pneumocytes, whereas SP-B and SP-C reduce surface tension, particularly in terminal airways. A number of nonspecific host defense mechanisms have been attributed to surfactant.[18] Enhanced stability of the alveolar lining film appears to act as a nonspecific barrier to adhesion and subsequent pulmonary invasion by microorganisms. Mucociliary transport is improved by viscoelastic and rheological properties. Particle clearance is enhanced, in part because of an apparently stimulatory effect on chloride ion transport. Neutrophil superoxide production is reduced. In addition, surfactant may contain superoxide dismutase and catalase and thus may scavenge oxygen radicals.[18,19] Direct antibacterial and antiviral properties have also been attributed to surfactant. Both SP-A and SP-D appear to provide a first line of defense by acting as collectins that target carbohydrate structures on a variety of pathogens. Alveolar macrophage response is increased by SP-A and SP-D enhances macrophage release of oxygen radicals. Finally, cytokine (e.g., TNF-α, IL-1β, and IL-6) release is stimulated by SP-A.

Changes in surfactant have been associated with a number of respiratory diseases. In humans, acute respiratory distress syndrome (ARDS) is associated with changes in the biochemical and biophysical characteristics of surfactant. As a result, surface tension increases, and the phospholipid, fatty acid, and protein profiles change. Serum proteins and inflammatory mediators directly inhibit or degrade surfactant. Abnormalities in surfactant quantity and its content of phospholipids and proteins have been associated with infectious diseases of the lungs. The ability of surfactant to suppress immune-mediated lung injury has led to the suggestion that surfactant dysfunction may contribute to the pathophysiology of asthma. The surfactant system also has been postulated to contribute to the surface destruction that is associated with chronic obstructive pulmonary disease (COPD) and emphysema. Proposed factors include elastase-induced dysfunction of surfactant; reduction of type II cells responsible for surfactant synthesis and secretion; and impairment of SP-A and SP-D.[18]

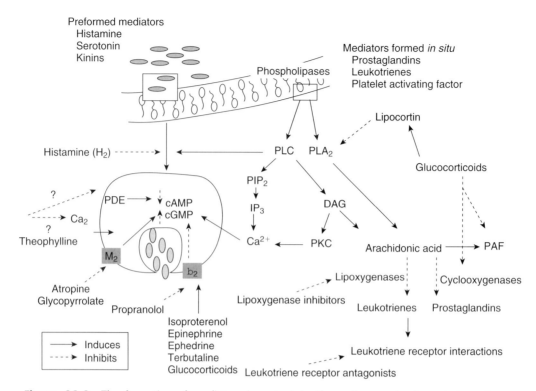

Figure 32-3. *The formation of mediators important in the pathogenesis of respiratory disease. Leukocytes and other cells release arachidonic acid metabolites and platelet-activating factor (PAF) after activation of phospholipases by a variety of stimuli. Mast cell degranulation induced by both immune and nonimmune stimuli is also accompanied by arachidonic acid metabolism as well as by the release of preformed mediators that are stored in the granules. Intracellular mechanisms that induce mast cell degranulation include increased calcium (Ca²⁺), increased cyclic guanosine nucleotide (cGMP) mediated by muscarinic (M3) receptors, and decreased cyclic adenosine nucleotide (cAMP) mediated by α-adrenergic receptor stimulation. Drugs used to prevent mediator release include glucocorticoids; this is one of the few classes of drugs that can prevent activation of phospholipases and therefore the release of arachidonic acid metabolites and PAF. Inhibition of prostaglandin synthesis by nonsteroidal antiinflammatory drugs may prove beneficial but also may lead to increased formation of leukotrienes by providing more arachidonic acid. Leukotriene actions can be blocked either by leukotriene receptor antagonists or by blockade of leukotriene receptors. Mast cell degranulation can be prevented by stimulation of beta-2-adrenergic receptors, inhibition of calcium influx or phosphodiesterase (PDE), or prevention of muscarinic (M3) receptor stimulation. Drugs that block beta-2-adrenergic receptors are contraindicated in most respiratory diseases. DAG = diacylglycerol; IP₃ = inositol triphosphate; PIP₂ = phosphatidylinositol; PKC, protein Kinase C; PLC, PLA₂ = phospholipases C and A₂.* (Reprinted with permission from Boothe DM: *Small animal clinical pharmacology and therapeutics,* Philadelphia, 2001, WB Saunders.)

Pathogenesis of Inflammatory Respiratory Diseases

Although not the only chronic disease of the respiratory tract, feline bronchial asthma provides a good model for discussing the pathophysiology of lung disease and the targets of drug therapy. The interaction of sensory receptors and mediators of bronchial tone is intricately balanced in the normal lung. In bronchial asthma, a series of pathologic disturbances severely disrupts the balance. Asthma is a pathologic state of the lungs characterized by marked bronchoconstriction and inflammation,[20-25] and inflammatory mediators are the major contributors to its pathogenesis.* Studies in several species have shown

that stimulation of mast cells, macrophages, and other cells lining the airways causes changes in mucosal epithelial permeability. Airways are often characterized by hypersensitivity to selected mediators (e.g., histamine and cholinergic stimulants).[5,9] As permeability increases, histamine and other inflammatory mediators are better able to reach and stimulate inflammatory cells located in the submucosa. Increased release of mediators is associated with stimulation of afferent nerve endings in the mucosa and reflex cholinergic bronchoconstriction. Mediators also increase microvascular permeability, induce chemotaxis, and stimulate mucus secretion. The release of cytotoxic proteins and toxic oxygen radicals further damages the respiratory epithelium, and the bronchial tree becomes hypersensitive. Mediators can also inhibit mucociliary function.[23] Bronchial smooth

_____

*References 20, 21, 23, 24, 26, and 27.

muscle often hypertrophies and undergoes spasms.[28] Airway obstruction in chronic disease reflects bronchoconstriction, bronchial wall edema, and accumulation of mucus and cells. As the disease progresses, airways eventually become plugged and ultimately collapse. Chronic inflammation leads to fibrosis, which contributes to the collapse, and air trapped within the alveoli can result in emphysema. Asthma is a disease of large and small (less than 2 mm) airways.[25] Previously considered "silent," studies in humans have revealed the importance of a therapeutic focus on airways beyond the 8th or 9th generation of the bronchial tree.

Recent advances in the treatment of human asthma are increasingly leading to its treatment as a systemic rather than simply a local allergic disease. In particular, the bone marrow response to allergens, and the subsequent release of eosinophils, is recognized to be an important systemic process in allergic inflammation.[25,29] Several cytokines, and interleukin-5 (IL-5) in particular, contribute to eosinophil movement from the bone marrow to local tissues. In humans, the number of eosinophil/basophil progenitors in the bone marrow declines with the peak allergy season, suggesting that the mature cells are circulating systemically. A central role of IL-5 has been supported through a number of studies documenting increased concentrations in asthmatics.[29] Eosinophilia, lung damage, and airway hyperresponsiveness are blunted in IL-5 deficient antigen-challenged mice.[29] Sources of IL-5 include TH_2 lymphocytes, mast cells, eosinophils, and bone marrow stroma. Among its actions are promotion of differentiation and maturation of progenitor cells, release of mature eosinophils, and promotion of survival and inhibition of apoptosis. T-cell recruitment to the lungs may play a key role in inflammation.[25] The role of leukotrienes (LTs) is not clear, although cysteinyl LTs are expressed on a number of bone marrow progenitor cells and appear to be involved (based on effects of antagonists) in eosinophil/basophil progenitor differentiation.

INFLAMMATORY MEDIATORS IN THE RESPIRATORY TRACT

Histamine

Histamine is a vasoactive amine stored in basophils and mast cells. Airway mast cells are located primarily beneath the epithelial basement membrane in dogs.[22] Histamine produces a variety of effects (e.g., chemotaxis, mucosal permeability, and edema) by interacting with specific receptors on target cells.[11,30] At least three histamine receptors have been identified,[20,31] two of which have been found in the trachea of the cat.[31,32] Interaction with the H_1 receptor causes an increase in intracellular calcium, and ultimately in cGMP (see Figure 32-3).[20] Histamine also stimulates cholinergic receptors in the airway.[20,22] Histamine causes constriction in both central and peripheral airways in dogs and cats.[11,22] The effects of histamine so closely mimic the pathophysiology of early asthma that, for many years, histamine was considered the major cause of the syndrome.[20] Lack of

clinical response to H_1-receptor antagonists, however, led to the realization that other factors are more important. In contrast to H_1 receptors, stimulation of H_2 receptors causes an increase in cAMP and bronchodilation.[20] Thus antihistamine drugs that block H_2 receptors may be contraindicated in asthma. Some studies have suggested that a defect in H_2 receptors may contribute to airway hyperreactivity.[20]

Histamine contributes to bronchial occlusion by mechanisms other than bronchoconstriction. Mucus secretion is mediated via H_2 receptors and by secretion of ions and water via H_1 receptors.[20] Microvascular leakage caused by contraction of endothelial cells also follows H_1-receptor stimulation.[20] Histamine is chemotactic to inflammatory cells, particularly eosinophils and neutrophils. Interestingly, histamine stimulates T-lymphocyte suppressor cells via H_2 receptors,[31] a function that also may be depressed in human patients with asthma.[20] Histamine also has a negative feedback effect on further histamine release mediated by IgE.[20] Both of these latter effects are mediated by H_2 receptors and would be inhibited by H_2-receptor antagonists.[31]

Serotonin

Serotonin (5-hydroxytryptamine [5-HT]) is released during mast cell degranulation.[20] Although serotonin does not appear to be an important mediator of either human or canine bronchial asthma, both the central and peripheral airways in cats are very sensitive to its bronchoconstrictive effects after aerosolization or intravenous administration.[11] Constriction may reflect interaction with serotonin receptors or enhanced release of acetylcholine. Serotonin may also cause profound vasoconstriction of the pulmonary vasculature and microvascular leakage.[20] Mast cells in feline airways have been documented to contain serotonin, and serotonin has been demonstrated to cause smooth muscle contraction in feline airways.[28]

Prostaglandins and Leukotrienes

Prostaglandins (PGs) and leukotrienes (LTs) are eicosanoids that are formed by phospholipases, activated in the cell membrane in response to a variety of stimuli (see Figure 32-3). Arachidonic acid (AA) is released from phospholipids and enters the cell, where it is converted by PGH synthase (commonly referred to as cyclooxygenase) to PGH_2, an inflammatory but unstable cyclic endoperoxide.[33] Various synthetases and isomerases produce the final PG products, including PGE_2, $PGF_{2\alpha}$, PGD_2, prostacyclin (or PGI_2), and thromboxane (TXA_2). Cyclooxygenase (COX) exists in two isoforms, which can be simplistically (but not totally accurately) described as constitutive (or basal) (COX-1) and inducible (COX-2). Inflammatory prostaglandins are generally recognized to be products of COX-2.[33] The amount of each PG produced in the lung varies with the cell type and species. The effects of the various PGs tend to balance one another. PGD_2, $PGF_{2\alpha}$, and TXA_2 cause bronchoconstriction, whereas PGE_1 and, to a lesser extent, PGI_1 cause bronchodilation.[1,20] Bronchoconstriction induced by PGD_2 is about 30 times as potent as that induced by histamine.

Imbalances between PGs may be important in the pathogenesis of bronchial disease. Both PGD_2 and TXA_2 have been implicated in immediate bronchial airway hyperreactivity.[20] Thromboxane A_2 appears to be the predominant AA metabolite produced by cat lungs, although other PG mediators are also important.[34] Prostaglandins are short lived, and actions occur close to the site of synthesis. Actions are mediated through one of at least nine receptors, each binding a specific PG. There are receptors for at least three subgroups: four relaxant receptors (bound by PGE_2, PGD and PGI_2), three contractile receptors (PGE, TXA_2, and $PGF_{2\alpha}$), and one chemotactant receptor (PGD_2).

Lipoxygenases in the lung catalyze the conversion of AA to hydroperoxyeicosatetraenoic acid (HPETEs), which are further metabolized to several hydroxy acids (HETEs) and LTs (see Figure 32-3). The predominant enzyme is 5-lipoxygenase,[33] which is selectively activated by antigenic challenge. The first product is LTA_4, the precursor to LTB_4 and LTC_4; in turn, LTC_4 is the precursor of LTD_4 and E_4. Eosinophils appear to preferentially activate 5-lipoxygenase.[20] All of these products, as well as the HETE intermediates, are biologically active in the respiratory tract,[20] and some are the most potent inflammogens known. LTs C, D_4, and E_4 make up the cysteinyl LTs, which are the components of slow reactive substance, an important mediator released in the lungs during anaphylaxis.[20,33] Bronchial smooth muscle contraction and microvascular permeability mediated by LTC_4 and LTD_4 is 100- to 1000-fold stronger than that induced by histamine. Both of these LTs are potent stimulators of mucus release in the dog but appear to be less potent in the cat.[20] LTD_4 is a potent chemotactant for eosinophils.[33] Leukotriene B_4, produced by macrophages, is the most potent chemotactant in the dog, causing neutrophil migration and increased airway responsiveness.[35] Leukotrienes act at distinct receptors, four of which thus far have been characterized.[33] Padrid has summarized the current status of LTs in cats with asthma.[28] Results are conflicting, but LTs (or their metabolic products) have been demonstrated in lavage fluid and urine of affected cats. Attributing a potentially significant role to LTs (including interaction with platelet activating factor) in the pathogenesis of feline asthma seems prudent, particularly with the recent emphasis in human medicine on the role of leukotrienes and other mediators at the level of the bone marrow.

Platelet-Activating Factor

Platelet-activating factor (PAF) is also formed after activation of phospholipase A_2 in all membranes. It is a potent, dose-independent constrictor of human airways, and it is the most potent agent thus far discovered in causing airway microvascular leakage.[20,21] PAF is also a potent chemotactant for platelets and eosinophils, both of which are a rich source of PAF. The effects of PAF may be mediated through LTs. PAF has been implicated as the cause of the sustained bronchial hyperresponsiveness that characterizes asthma.[21] The role of PAF in feline and canine respiratory diseases has not been addressed. Eosinophils are, however, a major cell type associated with feline bronchial disease and some canine diseases,[32] and it is likely that PAF is an important inflammatory mediator.

Reactive Oxygen Species

Reactive oxygen species (ROS) are constantly formed in the lung in order to contribute to pulmonary defense by assisting in the destruction of microorganisms and neoplastic cells, and stimulating the release of other inflammatory mediators.[19] Examples of ROS include free oxygen radicals, hydrogen peroxide, and hypochlorous acid. Inflammatory mediators such as TNF; interleukins 1, 6, and 8; and arachidonic acid derivatives (e.g., prostaglandins, leukotrienes, and platelet activating factor) contribute to the production of ROS. Hyperoxia also contributes to the generation of ROS.[19] The redox balance in the lungs is normally tightly controlled by endogenous antioxidants such that normal cells are protected. Endogenous antioxidant systems include enzymes (e.g., catalase, superoxide dismutase, and glutathione redox compounds [glutathione, glutathione peroxidase, and glutathione reductase]), fat-soluble compounds (vitamin E), water-soluble compounds (e.g., vitamin C, cysteine, reduced glutathione, and taurine) and high molecular weight antioxidants (e.g., mucus and albumin). The primary intracellular antioxidants are superoxide dismutase, catalase, and glutathione redox compounds.[19] Production of antioxidants in the lungs is enhanced by exposure to oxidants.[19]

Drugs Used to Modulate the Respiratory Tract

The syndrome of chronic bronchial disease is best treated by breaking the inflammatory cycle while immediately relieving bronchoconstriction. Thus antiinflammatory drugs and bronchodilators represent the cornerstone of therapy for many bronchial diseases. Other categories of drugs that are effective for the management of respiratory diseases, particularly in small animals, include antitussives, respiratory stimulants, and decongestants.

BRONCHODILATORS

Because of a shared mechanism of action, most drugs that induce bronchodilation also reduce inflammation. Bronchodilators reverse airway smooth muscle contraction by increasing cAMP, decreasing cGMP, or decreasing calcium ion concentration (see Figure 32-1). In addition, these drugs also decrease mucosal edema and are antiinflammatory because they tend to prevent mediator release from inflammatory cells (see Figure 32-3). Rapidly acting bronchodilators include beta-receptor agonists, methylxanthines, and cholinergic antagonists.

Beta-Receptor Agonists

Beta-receptor agonists are the most effective bronchodilators because they act as functional antagonists of airway constriction, regardless of the stimulus.[20,36-38] Large numbers of beta-2-receptors are located on several cell types in the lung, including smooth muscle and inflammatory cells.[3] The interaction between a beta-agonist and the receptor causes a conformational change in the receptor and subsequent activation of adenyl cyclase on the inner cell membrane (see Figure 32-1). Adenylate cyclase converts adenosine triphosphate to cAMP, which in turn serves as a second messenger for activation of specific protein kinases. The kinases activate the enzymes that cause relaxation of airway smooth muscle. Beta-receptor agonists are most effective in states of bronchoconstriction. In the inflammatory cell, increased cAMP inhibits mediator release (see Figure 32-3). Beta-receptors also stimulate secretion of airway mucus, resulting in a less viscous secretion and enhanced ciliary activity.[20,21,38] Drugs that block beta-2-receptors, such as propranolol, are contraindicated in animals with bronchial disease.

The nonselective beta-agonists (i.e., those capable of both beta-1 and beta-2 stimulation) such as epinephrine, ephedrine, and isoproterenol are used for acute and chronic therapy of respiratory diseases. Epinephrine and isoproterenol can be administered parenterally to achieve rapid effects. Drugs that can be given orally for chronic therapy include isoproterenol and ephedrine.[32] Both epinephrine and ephedrine have α-adrenergic activity, which may cause vasoconstriction and systemic hypertension and may contribute to airway constriction.[4] Nonselective beta-agonists may cause adverse cardiac effects because of beta-1-receptor stimulation. Aerosolization reduces the adverse effects of nonselective beta-adrenergic agonists by increasing beta-2 specificity, because only these beta-receptors appear to line the airways.

At appropriate doses, beta-2-selective agonists are not generally associated with the undesirable effects of beta-1-adrenergic stimulation. Few of these drugs have, however, been studied in dogs and cats. Metaproterenol, a derivative of isoproterenol; its analog, terbutaline;[32,37,39] and albuterol have all been used safely in small animals. Rapid first-pass metabolism of these drugs results in reduced systemic bioavailability after oral administration. Oral doses are thus higher than parenteral doses. All of these drugs, but particularly metaproterenol, can cause beta-1 side effects at high doses. Albuterol and isoetharine are examples of beta-2-selective agonists that have been administered by aerosolization to small animals.[37] Chronic use of beta-adrenergic agonists can result in refractoriness due to down-regulation (reduced numbers) of beta-receptors. This problem is largely avoided in humans by using proper doses.[38]

With the advent of metered dose inhalers in the 1960s, beta-adrenergics have become a common therapy for treatment of human asthma. Short-acting beta-2 agonists administered by aerosol include albuterol, pirbuterol, bitoleterol, and terbutaline, whereas longer-acting (in humans) products include salmeterol and formoterol.[25,39]

The drugs differ in their effects and uses. Short-acting products provide rapid symptomatic relief in human asthmatics when used at appropriate doses. The duration of onset of long-acting beta-adrenergics may be 1 hour or more. The use of short-acting beta-adrenergics at high doses has been associated with an increase in mortality in humans, leading to their recommended use on an "only as needed" basis.[25,39] On the other hand, improvement in pulmonary function in humans appears to be sustained with prolonged use of long-acting beta-adrenergics,[39] and their prolonged use does not appear to decrease symptomatic relief provided by short-acting drugs during bouts of exacerbation. Although minimally effective by themselves for control of inflammation, long-acting beta-adrenergics appear to enhance responsiveness to glucocorticoids. Rebound hyperresponsiveness does not appear to occur with rapid discontinuation of the long-acting drugs. Tolerance may occur to the effects of beta-adrenergics, probably caused by down regulation of receptors, particularly in the presence of triggering events (e.g., exercise in humans). Because beta-adrenergics do not provide as much antiinflammatory control, their efficacy may be reduced in the presence of inflammation, and combination therapy with an antiinflammatory drug such as an inhaled or systemic glucocorticoid, or use of theophylline, may be indicated.[25,39]

Methylxanthine Derivatives

Theophylline has been the cornerstone of long-term bronchodilatory therapy in animals. Its mode of action was originally attributed to inhibition of phosphodiesterase (PDE), and increased concentrations of cAMP (see Figure 32-1).[40] This mechanism is controversial, however, because theophylline does not inhibit PDE at therapeutic concentrations. Phosphodiesterase exists as various isoenzymes located at different sites within the cell, some of which are inaccessible to drugs.[20,21] Although theophylline may not affect total PDE, it may inhibit a specific isoenzyme, resulting in bronchodilation. Another possible mechanism is antagonism of the inhibitory neurotransmitter adenosine, which induces bronchoconstriction during hypoxia. Another mechanism (and perhaps the most plausible) by which theophylline induces bronchodilation is through interference with calcium mobilization.[20,21]

As with beta-agonists, theophylline is equally effective in large and small airways. Compared with beta-2 agonists, theophylline is considered a weaker relaxant of airway smooth muscle.[25] However, theophylline has other effects in the respiratory system that are important to its clinical efficacy.[20,21,40] In addition to its bronchodilatory effects, theophylline has significant antiinflammatory effects, including inhibition of mast cell degranulation and inflammatory mediator release (see Figure 32-3).[41] Theophylline increases mucociliary clearance and prevents microvascular leakage.[42] A major advantage of theophylline, compared with other bronchodilators, is increased strength of respiratory muscles and thus a decrease in the work associated with breathing.[40,43,44] This may be important to animals with chronic bronchopulmonary disease.

Theophylline is one of the few drugs active in the respiratory tract whose disposition has been effectively studied in dogs and, to a lesser degree, in cats. Because theophylline is not water soluble, it can only be given orally. Salt preparations of theophylline are available for either oral or parenteral administration. Dosing of the various salt preparations must be based on the amount of active theophylline (Table 32-1). Aminophylline, an ethylenediamine salt, is 80% theophylline, whereas oxtriphylline is 65% theophylline, and glycinate and salicylate salts are only 50% theophylline. Regular aminophylline is well absorbed (with a bioavailability of at least 90%) after oral administration in both dogs and cats.[45-47] In dogs, peak plasma drug concentrations for the theophylline base (approximately 8 µg/ml after a dose of 9.4 mg/kg) occur 1.5 hours after oral administration.[45] Interestingly, peak concentrations following intravenous (IV) or oral (sustained release) products are higher in cats when dosed in the evening compared with the morning.[48]

Slow-release preparations have been studied in dogs and cats.[48,49] The rate of oral absorption of slow-release products in dogs is apparently faster than in people. The extent of absorption varies with the preparation. The bioavailability of slow-release preparations varies from 30% (anhydrous theophylline 24-hour capsules*) to 76% (anhydrous theophylline tablets†).[49] The least variation among animals occurs for oxtriphylline enteric-coated capsules‡ and a 12-hour capsular anhydrous theophylline,§ which are approximately 60% bioavailable.

The minimum effective plasma concentration recommended for people (10 µg/ml) may not be reached by all slow-release products. Plasma drug concentrations during a 12-hour dosing interval vary, being almost 120% for the oxtriphylline product‡ but only 48% for the anhydrous tablet,† suggesting the latter may be the best product for use in dogs.[49] Thus, of the four preparations that have been studied in dogs, the anhydrous the-

---

*Theo-24 capsules, Searle Laboratories.
†Theo-Dor Tablets, Kay Pharmaceuticals.
‡Choledyl-SA Tablets, Parke-Davis.
§Slo-bid Gyrocaps, William H Rorer, Inc.

TABLE 32-1. Doses of Drugs Used to Treat Respiratory Diseases in Dogs and Cats

Drug	Route[a]	Dose[b]	Frequency
Beta-agonists[c]			
Epinephrine	IM,IV,SC	0.1mg (C) / or 20 µg/kg	
	SC	0.1 ml/kg of 0.001 solution	30 min[d]
Ephedrine	IM,PO	2-5 mg total (C)	
Isoproterenol	PO	0.44 mg/kg	q6-12h
	IM,SC,IV	0.1-0.2 mg total	q6h
	Aerosol	0.5 cc of 1:200 dilution	
Metaproterenol	PO	0.5 mg/kg	q6h
	Aerosol		
Albuterol	Aerosol	200 µg[e]	
	PO	50 µg/kg	q8h
Terbutaline	PO	0.625 to 1.25 mg total (C)	q12h
		1.25 to 5.0 mg (D)	q8-12h
Isoetharine	Aerosol	0.5-1.0 ml of 1:3 saline dilution	q8h
Anticholinergics			
Atropine	IV,IM,SC	0.02-0.04 mg/kg	PRN
Glycopyrrolate	IV,IM,SC	0.01-0.02 mg/kg	PRN
Methylxanthines			
Aminophylline	PO	10 mg/kg (D)	q6-8h (D)
		5-6 mg/kg (C)	q12h (C)
	IV infusion[i]	2-5 mg/kg	q8-12h over 30-60 min
Theophylline base	PO	4 mg/kg (C)[f]	q12h (C)
		5-10 mg/kg (D)	q6-8h (D)
Oxtriphylline	PO	10-15[g] mg/kg	q8-12h
Slow-release theophylline anhydrous	PO	20 [h] mg/kg	q12h (D) 24h (C)
Glucocorticoids and Other Antiinflammatories			
Prednisolone	PO	1-2 mg/kg	q6-12h[h]
Prednisolone sodium succinate	IV,IM[j]	2-4 mg/kg	q4-6h
Dexamethasone	IV,IM[j]	0.2-2.2 mg/kg	q24h
Triamcinolone	PO	0.25-0.5 mg total	q24h[h]
Beclomethasone dipropionate	Inhalant	200 µg total[e]	q6-8h

TABLE 32-1. **Doses of Drugs Used to Treat Respiratory Diseases in Dogs and Cats—cont'd**

Drug	Route[a]	Dose[b]	Frequency
Glucocorticoids and Other Antiinflammatories—cont'd			
Zafirlukast	PO	5-10 mg/cat	q12-24h
	PO	0.1-1 mg/kg (D)	q12-24h
Montelukast	PO	0.1 mg/kg	q24h
Cyproheptadine	PO	1.1 mg/kg (D)	q12h
	PO	2-4 mg (C)	q12h
Chlorpheniramine	PO	0.22 mg/kg (D)	q8h
	PO	2-4 mg total (C)	q24h
	PO	¼ to ½ slow release (C)	q24h
Diphenhydramine	PO	2-4 mg/kg (D)	q8h
Dimenhydrinate	PO	12.5 mg total (C)	q8h
	PO	8 mg/kg (D)	
Hydroxyzine	PO	2 mg/kg (D)	q6-8h
Antitussives			
Codeine	PO	1-2 mg/kg	q6-12h
Hydrocodone	PO	0.22 mg/kg	q6-12h
Butorphanol tartrate	SC,IM	0.055-0.11 mg/kg	PRN
	PO	0.5-1.0 mg/kg	q6-12h
	SC	0.55 mg/kg	
Dextromethorphan	PO	1-2 mg/kg	q6-8h
Morphine	IM,SC	0.1 mg/kg	q6-12h
Decongestants			
Pseudoephedrine	PO	15-60 mg (D)	q8h

[a] IV = Intravenous; IM = intramuscular; SC = subcutaneous; PO = orally; PRN = as needed.
[b] C = Cat, D = Dog.
[c] Use cautiously in cats with cardiac disease.
[d] Up to a total dose of 0.5 ml.
[e] Human dose.
[f] Based on 80% theophylline.
[g] Based on 65% theophylline.
[h] Note differences in bioavailability among slow release products may require monitoring to assure safe and effective dosing.
[i] Caution with IV infusion; reserve for emergency therapy.
[j] Taper doses to minimum effective dose.

ophylline tablet[†] is preferred. Although the mean residence time of the slow-release preparation was significantly longer (by 1 to 2 hours) than that of the regular preparation in dogs, the clinical significance of this difference is questionable.[49,50] The longer release time may, however, allow twice daily rather than three times daily dosing.

Two sustained-release theophylline products[†,§] have been evaluated in the cat.[48,51] Both products are reasonably (i.e., greater than 75%) bioavailable in the cat. Once daily administration has been recommended to achieve the human therapeutic range (see Table 32-1). Based on a chronopharmacokinetic study of these sustained-release products, dosing in the evening rather than in the morning appears to be associated with better bioavailability and less peak plasma theophylline concentration fluctuation.[48] A disadvantage of the use of the slow-release products for small animals is the limited dose sizes available. The product cannot

be divided for more accurate dosing without altering the kinetics of slow release.

Although it is not distributed to all body tissues, theophylline is characterized by a relatively large volume of distribution in dogs (0.7 to 0.8 L/kg) and a smaller volume in cats (0.41 L/kg).[45,49] Unlike in human beings, distribution of theophylline is not limited by binding to serum proteins in dogs; serum protein binding is less than 12%.[52,53] Elimination of theophylline is not dose dependent in dose ranges of 3 to 15 mg/kg.

Theophylline is metabolized by demethylation in the liver. Theobromine may be an active metabolite in some species. Different rates of metabolism result in variable clearance rates and drug elimination half-lives among animals, and doses consequently vary.[50,53] For example, the elimination rate constant of theophylline is less in cats (0.089/hour)[46] than in dogs (0.12/hour), resulting in a longer half-life in the cat (7.8 hours) compared with the dog (5.7 hours)[45,46] and thus necessitating a smaller dose in cats.[49] Theophylline concentrations can be affected—most commonly increased—by a number of drugs, including fluorinated quinolones,[54] erythromycin and its congeners,[55] and cimetidine.[56]

The side effects of theophylline limit its use in the management of human asthma.[25] Theophylline is associated with a wide range of adverse effects including central nervous system excitation (manifested as restlessness, tremors, and seizures);[53] gastrointestinal upset (nausea and vomiting); diuresis; and cardiac stimulation (tachycardia).[57] Therefore its intravenous use is limited to patients who have not responded to beta-agonist therapy. Compared with the salt preparations, theophylline is more irritating to the gastrointestinal tract than aminophylline.[37,40] Rapid infusions or infusions of undiluted aminophylline can cause cardiac arrhythmias, hypotension, nausea, tremors, and acute respiratory failure.[37] Treatment of toxicity is directed toward minimizing adverse effects and includes diazepam to control seizures, beta-blockers to control cardiac arrhythmias, and antiemetics (particularly metaclopramide) to treat nausea and vomiting.[57]

The application of therapeutic drug monitoring to guide therapy would assist in identifying the most appropriate dosing regimen. Although a therapeutic range has not been established for small animals, the range recommended for humans (i.e., 10 to 20 μg/ml) can be extrapolated until a more definitive range has been established. Dogs are apparently more tolerant of theophylline toxicity than are humans. In one study, toxicity (manifested as tachycardia, central nervous system stimulation [restlessness and excitement], and vomiting) did not occur until plasma theophylline concentrations reached 37 to 60 μg/ml. Doses of 80 to 160 mg/kg of a sustained-release preparation were required to induce toxicity.[58] In cats, concentrations as high as 40 μg/ml do not induce adverse reactions, although salivation and vomiting are common after administration of more than 50 mg/kg, and seizures may occur at doses greater than 60 mg/kg.[59]

The side effects of theophylline are dose dependent and might be avoided to a large degree by appropriate dosing. Therapeutic drug monitoring should facilitate the design of proper dosing regimens to avoid toxicity.

Anticholinergic Drugs

Anticholinergic drugs compete with acetylcholine at muscarinic receptor sites.[60] In the respiratory tract, they reduce the sensitivity of irritant receptors and antagonize vagally mediated bronchoconstriction. The site of action of these drugs in the respiratory tract is controversial. In some studies, bronchodilation is reported throughout the airways in asthmatic human patients and cats, whereas other investigators believe that the effects are confined to large airways.[60] Anticholinergic bronchodilators are less effective, compared with beta-2 adrenergic bronchodilators, in the treatment of human asthma. Additionally, they have a slower onset of action.[25] Thus despite their effect on bronchial airways, the anticholinergic drugs have not proved clinically effective in the treatment of bronchial diseases in animals, and their use is limited to treatment of bronchoconstriction associated with organophosphate toxicity or in animals in status asthmaticus unresponsive to bronchodilator therapy. The lack of clinical efficacy of anticholinergics may reflect nonselective drug-receptor interaction.[20,21] Thus far, three types of muscarinic receptors have been identified in airways. M3 receptors release acetylcholine, whereas M2 receptors block its release. Nonselective blockade of muscarinic receptors by atropine and ipratropium may actually potentiate acetylcholine release by antagonizing the effects of M2-receptor stimulation. Drugs specific for M3 receptors may ultimately lead to successful treatment of bronchial disease with anticholinergic drugs.[20,21]

Aerosolized atropine, a prototype anticholinergic drug, affects predominantly the central airways, whereas both central and peripheral airways are affected if the drug is administered intravenously.[20,21] Because atropine is highly specific for all muscarinic receptors, it causes a number of systemic side effects including tachycardia, mydriasis, and altered gastrointestinal and urinary tract function.[45] In the respiratory tract, atropine reduces ciliary beat frequency, mucus secretion, and electrolyte and water flux into the trachea. The net effect is decreased mucociliary clearance, which is undesirable in patients with chronic lung disease.[45] Aerosolization of atropine does not reduce the incidence of adverse reactions. Atropine is well absorbed (in humans) after oral administration. In humans, atropine has proved most useful for treatment of chronic bronchitis and emphysema, diseases that are characterized by increased intrinsic vagal tone.[60] A combination of atropine with either beta-adrenergic agonists or glucocorticoids will cause better bronchodilation than either drug alone.[60] Its adverse effects on respiratory secretions and ciliary activity, however, apparently negate its benefits to bronchial tone during long-term administration in animals. The primary indication for atropine in small animals is facilitation of bronchodilation in acutely dyspneic animals. It is the treatment of choice for life-threatening respiratory distress induced by anticholinesterases.[60]

Glycopyrrolate can also be used as a bronchodilator in small animals. Although its onset of action is slower than that of atropine,[37] its half-life is 4 to 6 hours compared with 1 to 2 hours for atropine. The potency after systemic therapy has apparently not been compared between the two drugs, although glycopyrrolate is twice as potent when aerosolized. The systemic side effects of glycopyrrolate are minimal.

Ipratropium bromide is a synthetic anticholinergic that is pharmacodynamically superior to atropine. Although the two drugs are equipotent, ipratropium does not cross the blood-brain barrier. It is not well absorbed after aerosolization, which limits the likelihood of adverse effects. Ipratropium has been studied in the dog but not in the cat.[60] Of the anticholinergic drugs studied in dogs, ipratropium appears to cause the greatest bronchodilation (twice as much as atropine) with the least change in salivation.[60] Unlike atropine, it does not alter mucociliary transport rates.

MAST CELL STABILIZERS

Drugs that stabilize mast cells are most effective in syndromes associated with marked mast cell activity. The stabilizing effects of beta-adrenergic agonists and methylxanthines on inflammatory cells have been discussed.

Cromolyn

Although the mechanism of action of cromolyn is not certain, it appears to inhibit calcium influx into mast cells, thus preventing mast cell degranulation and the release of histamine and other inflammatory mediators (see Figure 32-3).[20,21,61] At high concentrations, cromoglycate inhibits IgE-triggered mediator release from mast cells.[62] Some studies suggest that the activation of inflammatory cells other than mast cells (e.g., macrophages, neutrophils, and eosinophils) is also inhibited by cromoglycate.[63] Cromolyn is most useful as a preventative before activation of inflammatory cells. It is not significantly absorbed after oral administration and is characterized by a short half-life.[37] Thus effective therapy depends on frequent aerosolization, which limits its utility in the treatment of small animal diseases. Currently, cromolyn is among the safest of the drugs used to manage asthma in humans.[61] It is associated with only minor side effects, and its discovery has revolutionized the management of bronchial asthma in people. Inhaled cromones control the symptoms of asthma, including bronchospasms. However, because they are short acting and must be administered two to four times daily, their use is inconvenient.[25] Because of its wide therapeutic window and its apparent efficacy in the control of many inflammatory cells, its use in the control of small animal bronchial disease warrants further investigation.

Calcium Antagonists

The efficacy of calcium antagonists in the management of asthma has yet to be identified.[64] Their potential benefits include prevention of mediator release, smooth muscle contraction, vagus nerve conduction, and infiltration of inflammatory cells.[64,65] Most studies indicate that calcium antagonists have only a modest effect on airway smooth muscle contraction. Their effects as antiinflammatories may ultimately prove of greater benefit.

DRUGS THAT TARGET INFLAMMATORY MEDIATORS

Glucocorticoids

Glucocorticoids are most commonly used in clinical medicine for their antiinflammatory and immunosuppressive actions; however, glucocorticoids are reported to have "permissive" effects on beta-2-receptors, promoting bronchodilation.[21] The antiinflammatory and immunosuppressive effects of glucocorticoids reflect specific actions on white blood cells, and are inextricably linked. They generally occur only when the steroids are present in concentrations greater than those found in the normal physiologic state (pharmacological concentrations).

Glucocorticoids inhibit early and late phases of inflammation. Responses that are inhibited include edema formation, fibrin deposition, leukocyte migration, phagocytic activity, collagen deposition, and capillary and fibroblast proliferation. Many of these processes involve lymphokines and other soluble mediators of inflammation, and it is through these mediators that glucocorticoids exert their antiinflammatory actions. Specifically, glucocorticoids inhibit (via lipocortin) the enzyme phospholipase A_2, which converts arachidonic acid to prostaglandin and leukotriene metabolites. Glucocorticoids preferentially inhibit cyclooxygenase 2, the inducible form of cyclooxygenase.[66] Glucocorticoids also inhibit release of tumor necrosis factor and interleukin-2 (IL-2) from activated macrophages,[67] and the release of platelet-activating factor from leukocytes and mast cells. Platelet-activating factor induces vasodilation, platelet and leukocyte aggregation, smooth muscle contraction (especially in the bronchi), and increased vascular permeability.[68] The action of macrophage migration-inhibition factor (namely, to arrest the movement of macrophages at antigenic sites) is inhibited by glucocorticoids. Consequently, macrophages migrate away from the affected area. Glucocorticoids also alter synthesis of and biologic response to collagenase, lipase, and plasminogen activator. The antiinflammatory effects of glucocorticoids also may reflect inhibition of the inducible form of nitric oxide synthase (iNOS).[69] Synovial macrophage nitric oxide production and iNOS synthesis are inhibited by dexamethasone. The inhibitory effect appears to be mediated by lipocortin.

The immunosuppressive actions of glucocorticoids are more pronounced on the cellular arm than the humoral arm of the immune system. The immunosuppressive actions of glucocorticoids, like their antiinflammatory actions, involve disruption of intercellular communication of leukocytes via interference with lymphokine production, biologic action, or both. Glucocorticoids block the effects of the migration-inhibition factor-γ and interferon-γ (IFN-γ) on macrophages.[67] IFN-γ, which is released from activated T cells, plays an important role in facilitating antigen processing by macrophages. Glucocorticoids inhibit the synthesis and release of IL-1 by macrophages, thereby suppressing the activation of T cells. Glucocorticoids also inhibit IL-2 synthesis by activated T cells. Interleukin-2 plays a critical role in amplification of cell-mediated immunity. Additionally, glucocorticoids suppress the bactericidal and fungicidal actions of macrophages.

In 1997 the National Heart Lung Blood Institute Expert Panel Guidelines recommended control of mild persistent asthma in humans with a single, long-term control medication with antiinflammatory properties.[39] Glucocorticoid efficacy for treatment of respiratory inflammatory disease is dependent on achieving therapeutic concentrations in and below the epithelium of all diseased airways. However, whereas systemic therapy might provide the most consistent exposure to diseased airways, it also provides the greatest exposure to tissues other than the lungs, leading to adverse effects. Administration of glucocorticoids by aerosol has decreased many of the side effects associated with systemic glucocorticoid use in humans. Indeed, the current preferred treatment for humans with mild disease is low-dose inhaled glucocorticoids.[39] However, short courses (e.g., 5 to 7 days) of high doses of oral glucocorticoids are used to treat acute exacerbations of asthma.[25]

The addition of inhaled glucocorticoids has increased asthmatic control in humans. Beclomethasone was among the first aerosol glucocorticoid developed for inhalant therapy.[25] Systemic side effects associated with deposition of glucocorticoids on the pharynx and central airways, and local side effects in the upper airway (e.g., dysphonia in up to 50% of patients), led to the addition of "spacers" in inhalant devices that removed larger particles before they penetrated the pharynx.[25] Additionally, administration of glucocorticoids removed by first pass metabolism (e.g., budesonide or fluticasone) decreased the risk of systemic exposure to swallowed drug. However, poor compliance of inhaled glucocorticoids in human patients led to the development of combinations of steroids with long-acting beta-2 agonists (e.g., salmeterol/fluticasone or formoterol/budesonide). Although compliance has improved, concern has arisen that the beta-2 agonists will mask clinical signs that might otherwise indicate worsening of the disease.[25] In human asthmatics, deposition studies reveal that the majority of inhaled drug is deposited on central airways; yet, antiinflammatory therapy should target both large and small airways if inflammation is to be suppressed.[25,70] Thus systemic therapy should be considered either as sole therapy or in addition to systemic therapy in animals with moderate to severe disease. Note that the peak effect of inhaled glucocorticoids may not occur for 1 to 2 weeks after therapy has begun.

Drugs That Target Leukotrienes

Leukotrienes (LTs) are very potent causes of inflammation in the lungs, causing marked edema, inflammation, and bronchoconstriction.[33] The recent approval of drugs that specifically inhibit the formation of LTs or their actions has offered a new avenue for control of respiratory inflammatory disease (e.g., asthma) in human medicine.

Zafirlukast (Accolate®) is an LT receptor antagonist (LRA), whereas zileuton (Zyflo®) is a lipoxygenase inhibitor. Comparative studies in animals and humans suggest that, of the two, zafirlukast (0.15 to 0.2 mg/kg orally once daily) is more effective and less likely to increase hepatic enzymes (and thus is safer) among different species. It can be administered less frequently (every 8 to 12 hours compared with every 6 to 8 hours for zileuton). Zafirlukast is usually associated with very few side effects in human patients; however, recent reports delineate severe acute hepatopathy in 3 human patients receiving zafirlukast for at least 5 months.[71,72] Zafirlukast may inhibit some hepatic drug metabolizing enzymes.

In human clinical trials, LRA drugs inhibit early and late phase bronchoconstriction and increased bronchial hyperresponsiveness in response to allergens; accumulation of inflammatory cells and mediators in bronchial lavage fluid; and acute bronchospasm stimulated by exercise, cold air, and aspirin.[73] Their use has been associated with improvement of asthma either as sole therapy (in lieu of low dose inhaled glucocorticoids) in mild to moderate asthma, or as add-on therapy in patients that have not responded.[73] In humans, LRA drugs also appear to improve rhinitis, particularly in asthmatic patients.[74]

The role of LRA in the treatment of feline asthma has had some, albeit limited, attention. Because receptors for leukotrienes have not been found in the smooth muscle of airways in cats, the use of antagonists has been questioned. However, with the recent approach to asthma as a systemic response mediated at the level of the bone marrow, the use of LRA warrants further and strong consideration. The drug has shown some anecdotal efficacy in both dogs and cats. Although anecdotal reports of efficacy and safety exist for dogs and cats, no written report appears available.

Nonsteroidal Antiinflammatory Drugs

The role of nonsteroidal antiinflammatory drugs (NSAIDs) in the treatment of respiratory inflammatory diseases needs to be defined.[75,76] Both LTs and PGs are important in the pathophysiology of inflammatory diseases. Although NSAIDs effectively block PGs through inhibition of cyclooxygenase, they do not appear to have any effect on lipoxygenase and, therefore, production of LTs. They have no effect on other chemical mediators of inflammation. Additionally, NSAIDs nonselectively block all PGs, including those that provide some protection during periods of bronchoconstriction.[77] Some studies have shown that LT production increases in response to NSAID therapy, perhaps by providing more AA for lipoxygenase metabolism. Human asthmatic patients may suffer exacerbations of clinical signs when taking NSAIDs; treatment with LRA decreases clinical signs.[78]

Currently, the use of NSAIDs for the treatment of respiratory diseases in small animals is limited to aspirin therapy as treatment for thromboembolism associated with heartworm disease.[79,80] Aspirin is the preferred NSAID because at low doses it irreversibly inhibits TXA_2, an important contributor to pulmonary arterial vasoconstriction that accompanies thromboembolism. Current efforts in NSAID research are oriented toward identifying drugs that successfully inhibit both arms of the AA metabolic cascade or specific PG or LT inhibitors. The use of selective TXA_2 inhibitors for selected feline respiratory diseases is an example.[34]

Antihistamines

Antihistaminergic drugs have generally not proved clinically useful in the control of small animal or human respiratory diseases.[30,32,81] Several observations support their lack of efficacy. Although not proven, the number of histamine receptors located in the airways and the proportion of H_1 to H_2 receptors may not be sufficient to induce a response. Antihistaminergic drugs act to block target receptors from responding to histamine; however, until recently, the drugs have not prevented the release of histamine or other mediators from any inflammatory cell. Newer (H_1) antihistamines (e.g., loratadine, fexofenadine and cetirizine) are exceptions in that they also decrease histamine release from basophils.[82] Although well tolerated, these drugs apparently have not been studied for efficacy or safety in animals. The lack of efficacy of antihistamines also reflects the simultaneous release of other more potent mediators than histamine from degranulating mast cells or other inflammatory cells.[83] Finally, blockade of histamine receptors by antihistaminergic drugs is competitive and can be overwhelmed by high concentrations of histamine. The use of H_1 blockers may be detrimental in animals with chronic disease because of their effects on airway secretions.[20] The role of H_2 receptors in bronchodilation, mucus secretion, and inflammation suggests that H_2-receptor blockers should also be used with caution.[20,31] An exception to antihistamine use for treatment of respiratory inflammatory disease might be made for the use of cyproheptadine, an antiserotoninergic, antihistaminergic drug. Because feline airways are exquisitely sensitive to the constrictor effects of serotonin, this drug may prove particularly useful in cats either alone or as an adjunct to bronchodilators or glucocorticoids.[84]

ANTITUSSIVES

The goal of antitussive therapy is to decrease the frequency and severity of cough without impairing mucociliary defenses. Whenever possible, the underlying cause should be identified and treated. Cough suppressants should be used cautiously and are contraindicated if the cough is productive.[2] Irritant receptors, and perhaps chemoreceptors and stretch receptors, initiate the cough reflex.[2,46] Bronchoconstriction is another common and important cough stimulus.

Cough has been described as the most powerful (and in humans, most common) physiologic reflex. It acts to expel excess secretions and their trapped inhaled irritants from the airways.[85] The reflex is a multiphasic motor task involving motor drive to muscles (i.e., diaphragm, abdominal, and intercostal muscles) throughout the component phases of the cough cycle (i.e., inspiration, compression, expulsion).[85,86] Cough most commonly originates from the larynx and lower airways.[87] Cough is initiated by chemical or mechanical stimuli of epithelial sensory receptors. Three main groups of airway receptors stimulate cough: rapidly adapting or irritant receptors and bronchial C-fiber receptors located in the larynx and tracheobronchial tree, and slow adapting stretch receptors in the tracheobronchial tree.[85] Receptors are innervated by vagal and laryngeal nerves.[86] Cough can be suppressed either centrally or peripherally.

Centrally Acting Antitussives

Centrally acting drugs act at the cough center in the medulla (Figure 32-4).[2,88] Central drugs can inhibit cough frequency or motor (abdominal or diaphragmatic) activity,[86] and are classified as narcotic (opioid) and nonnarcotic drugs.[88,89] Most central antitussive drugs act to inhibit specific components of the cough motor pattern (in particular, the number of coughs) rather than causing general suppression.[86]

Opioid antitussives depress the sensitivity of the cough center to afferent stimuli. However, opioid receptors have been identified on the sensory arm of the vagus nerve, and thus they also appear to have a peripheral effect.[85] Opioids can be associated with strong sedative properties, and with constipation when administered chronically. Morphine, codeine, and hydrocodone are the narcotics most commonly used to control coughing. As Class II drugs, each is subject to the Controlled Substances Act of 1970. All can be used for cough suppression in both dogs and cats.

Codeine is the prototypical narcotic antitussive and is one of the most effective drugs available to suppress the cough reflex. Its antitussive effects are much greater than its analgesic effects. Codeine phosphate and codeine sulfate can be used either alone or in combination with peripheral cough suppressants or decongestants. Over-the-counter preparations are available for human use. Compared with morphine, codeine is equally effective as a cough suppressant but causes less central depression and less constipation. However, side effects of codeine include nausea and constipation.

Hydrocodone bitartrate is a hydrolysis product of dihydrothebaine. Hydrocodone is a more potent antitussive than codeine but causes less respiratory depression. It is probably the most commonly used antitussive in dogs.

The narcotic agonist/antagonist butorphanol tartrate is a potent antitussive when given orally or parenterally in dogs and cats.[90] Butorphanol is more commonly used as an analgesic, however. Reclassified as a Schedule IV drug, it is now subject to the Narcotics Act. It is approved for use as an antitussive for dogs. As an antitussive, it is 100 times more potent than codeine and 4 times more potent than morphine.[91] In dogs, after subcutaneous administration, butorphanol concentrations peak at 1 hour. Its mean half-life is 1.7 hours, with a duration of activity of 4 hours or more. Butorphanol is characterized by a wide safety margin. The LD_{50} in dogs after intramuscular administration is 20 mg/kg.[92] Therapeutic concentrations cause minimal cardiac or respiratory depression. Side effects include sedation, which can be significant and desirable; nausea; some diarrhea; and appetite suppression.

Dextromethorphan is a nonnarcotic opioid commonly found in over-the-counter cough preparations. It is a semisynthetic derivative of opium that lacks its narcotic properties, and sedation is unusual after its use. Only the L-isomer has antitussive activity, similar to that of codeine in potency. Its onset of action is rapid, being fully effective within 30 minutes after oral administration. It is used for small animals with minimal sedation, and its antitussive efficacy is equal to that of codeine. It can be used safely in cats. Studies in humans have shown that the combination of dextromethorphan with a bronchodilator is superior to dextromethorphan alone.[93]

Noscapine is a nonaddictive opium alkaloid (benzylisoquinolone) that has antitussive effects similar to codeine.[94] Its use for small animals appears to be limited.

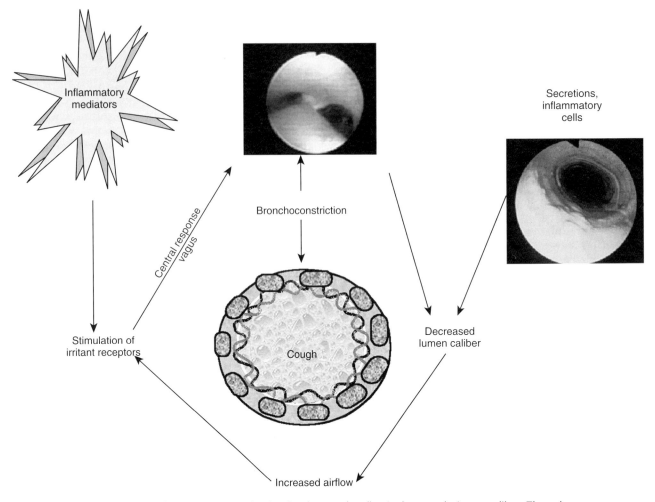

Figure 32-4. *The most potent stimulus for the cough reflex is decreased airway caliber. The subsequent increase in airflow velocity irritates stretch receptors. The vagus nerve serves as both the afferent and efferent limbs of the cough reflex, which is mediated centrally by the respiratory center in the medulla. Accumulation of debris and inflammatory mediators can either irritate receptors or decrease airway luminal caliber. Cough is accompanied by bronchoconstriction, which can further exacerbate coughing. (Reprinted with permission from Boothe DM:* Small animal clinical pharmacology and therapeutics, *Philadelphia, 2001, WB Saunders.)*

Peripherally Acting Antitussives

The cough reflex can be blocked peripherally via several mechanisms. Protussives facilitate removal of the irritant with mucolytics or expectorants. Bronchodilators act to increase airway caliber, although direct evidence that smooth muscle relaxation reduces cough does not exist.[87] Other peripherally-acting drugs act to block peripheral receptors or to decrease efferent nerves involved in the cough reflex.[85,87] Local anesthetics inhibit cough induced by a variety of stimuli when administered either topically or systemically, presumably because of a reduction of vagal nerve discharge.[87]

Bronchodilators relieve irritant receptor stimulation induced by mechanical deformation of the bronchial wall during bronchoconstriction. Ephedrine peripherally induces bronchodilation, and as both a bronchodilator and decongestant is a common constituent of over-the-counter cough preparations. Theophylline and isopro-terenol are also common ingredients found in some preparations. Other peripheral antitussives include mucokinetic agents and hydrating agents.[88]

PROTUSSIVES

Mucokinetics

Mucokinetic drugs facilitate the removal of secretions from the respiratory tree. They are indicated for conditions associated with viscous to inspissated pulmonary secretions. Mucokinesis can be induced by drugs that improve ciliary activity (e.g., beta-receptor agonists and methylxanthines) or by drugs that improve the mobility of bronchial secretions by changing their viscosity. The viscosity of bronchial secretions can be decreased by hydration (with sterile or bacteriostatic water or saline), increasing pH (with sodium bicarbonate), increasing

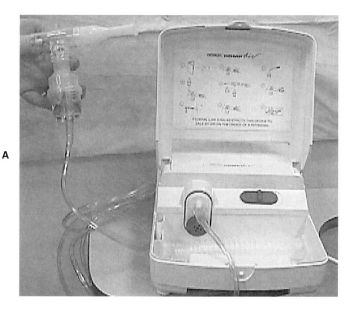

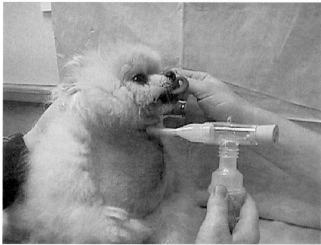

Figure 32-5. A, An example of a portable nebulizer compressor unit. Note that a rubber stopper has been placed in the nonpatient end of the aerosolization unit to increase the flow of the aerosol to the patient in the absence of inhalation. **B,** The aerosol is being delivered directly through the stoma of a tracheostomized patient. This unit cost $69.

ionic strength (with sodium bicarbonate and saline), or by rupture of sulfur (S-S) linkages in the mucus. Hydrating agents can be administered parenterally or by aerosolization. Home aerosolization can be easily achieved with a humidifier or steamed bathroom or with a commercially available aerosolizer (Figure 32-5). The efficacy of aerosolization in liquefying airway secretions is controversial,[24] with the greatest benefit occurring in the upper airways. The efficacy of ionic solutions or alkaline solutions on enhanced mucus mobility, compared with that of water, is controversial.[24]

Acetylcysteine (*N*-acetyl-L-cysteine) (NAC), the N-acetyl derivative of the naturally occurring amino acid L-cysteine, is the mucolytic drug most widely used by humans.[24,95] Although it appears to be efficacious after aerosolization, oral administration has become the preferred route.[95] In Europe, the drug is available in solid and powder dosing forms. Unfortunately, only the solution, which is unpalatable and malodorous, is approved for use in the United States. The powder is available as a chemical reagent from several chemical companies (search the Internet using the keywords "chemical companies" and "n-acetylcysteine"), and purchase for application to food or in a capsule might be considered.

Regardless of the route of administration, the mechanism of NAC reflects destruction of mucoprotein of the disulfide bonds by a free sulfhydryl group. Smaller molecules are less viscid and not able to efficiently bind to inflammatory debris. As a thiol compound, NAC is a radical scavenger because of its ability to directly interact with oxidants such as hydrogen peroxide, hydroxyl radicals, and hypochlorous acid.[19] In addition to its direct effects, as cysteine, NAC appears to promote cellular glutathione production.[96] A number of animal studies indicate efficacy of NAC in the prevention and therapy of lung injury associated with oxygen radicals.[96] Additionally, NAC also has antiinflammatory effects, yet has an apparent paradoxical effect on polymorphonuclear cells. Respiratory burst is suppressed but phagocytosis is increased in humans receiving 6 to 18 g of NAC by constant IV infusion.[96] The effects are dose dependent, with a low dose (300 mg three times daily in humans) being associated with an increase in respiratory burst. The impact of these effects can be beneficial in the presence of inflammatory disease or syndromes associated with ischemia/reperfusion or endothelial cell activation, but it can be detrimental in the presence of infectious diseases. Acetylcysteine appears to induce respiratory tract secretions, probably via a gastropulmonary reflex. At higher oral doses, NAC will also induce vomiting.[95,97] Acetylcysteine improved gas exchange in a study of dogs with experimentally induced methacholine bronchoconstriction.[98] The effects of NAC in human patients with COPD are not conclusive, with study results ranging from no effect to clinical effect.

In humans, NAC is rapidly absorbed from the gastrointestinal tract and extensively distributed to the liver, kidneys, and lungs, where it may accumulate. It is rapidly metabolized by the liver to the natural amino acids cysteine and cystine.[95,97] The indications for oral NAC therapy in humans include exposure to toxic inhalants (including tobacco smoke), bronchitis, chronic obstructive pulmonary disease, cystic fibrosis, asthma, tuberculosis, pneumonia and emphysema, and the acute respiratory distress syndrome. Installation of a 10% to 20% solution has also been used to clean and treat chronic sinusitis.[95] Acetylcysteine is often used in combination with aerosolized antimicrobials because it may improve antibacterial penetration of infected mucus.[95] Physiotherapy enhances the efficacy of NAC. The drug is usually dosed at 125 to 500 mg (about 5 to 10 mg/kg) in human patients. Higher doses (e.g., 144 mg/kg IV followed by 70 mg/kg 12 hours later) have been used safely by the author in life-threatening respiratory conditions. A twice or three times daily administration is recommended. Uses by the author have included pneumonia, chronic bronchial diseases, chronic sinusitis, electrical cord bites, chronic diaphragmatic hernia (before expansion of collapsed lung lobes), and other respiratory syndromes associated with inflammation.

Acetylcysteine therapy is associated with few adverse affects. Coughing may occur following aerosolization because NAC is acidic in solution[19] and it can cause reflex bronchoconstriction by irritant receptor stimulation. Its use should be preceded by administration of bronchodilators. In humans, doses as high as 500 mg/kg are well tolerated,[97] although vomiting and anorexia can occur. The median LD_{50} in dogs is 1 g/kg after oral use and 700 mg/kg after parenteral administration. Because it is metabolized to sulfur-containing products, it should be used cautiously in animals suffering from liver disease characterized by hepatic encephalopathy.

EXPECTORANTS

Expectorants such as potassium iodide are common ingredients in over-the-counter cough preparations. They increase the fluidity of respiratory secretions through several mechanisms, and are often used as adjuvants for the management of cough by facilitating removal of the inciting cause. Bronchial secretions are increased by vagal reflex after gastric mucosa irritation (iodide salts), directly through sympathetic stimulation, or by volatile oils that are partially eliminated via the respiratory tract. Although the combination of expectorants with antitussives in over-the-counter cough preparations may seem irrational, the antitussive drugs in these combination products do not appear to prevent stimulation of the cough reflex induced by liquified secretions. Their mechanism of action is unknown, and they may be ineffective at the doses used in cough preparations.[99] Demulcent expectorants (e.g., syrup) are often used as the vehicle for cough medicaments but have no apparent expectorant value. They may, however, be useful for treatment of cough caused by pharyngeal irritation.

Potassium iodide is a saline expectorant capable of increasing secretions by 150%. Ethylenediamine dihydroiodide, used as a nutritional source of iodine in cattle, may be useful for the treatment of mild respiratory diseases. Iodide preparations should not be used in pregnant or hyperthyroid animals or in milk-producing animals.

Stimulant expectorants are used for coughing associated with chronic bronchial diseases. Guaiacol and its glyceryl ether, guaifenesin (glyceryl guaiacolate), are wood tar derivatives. Neither the volume nor the viscosity of respiratory secretions appears to change after treatment with guaifenesin, although airway particle clearance increases in bronchitic human patients.

DECONGESTANTS

The indications for decongestants include sinusitis of allergic or viral etiology, and reverse sneezing or other complications of postnasal drip. Information regarding the use of decongestants in animals is largely based on extrapolation from human patients, for whom allergic rhinitis and the common cold are the most common indications. Often decongestants are administered as a single drug combined with expectorants.

The two major categories of drugs used as decongestants are the histamine (H_1) receptor antagonists (e.g., dimenhydrinate, diphenhydramine, chlorpheniramine, and hydroxyzine) and the sympathomimetic drugs (α-adrenergic agonists) such as ephedrine (EDE), pseudoephedrine (PSE), and phenylephrine (PNE).[100-102] These drugs can be given topically to avoid the systemic effects associated with oral therapy.

Stimulation of α-receptors concentrated on precapillary arterioles results in vascular smooth muscle vasoconstriction. Bloodflow to the nasal mucosal capillary bed is reduced; excess extracellular fluid and nasal discharge associated with congestion is thus decreased. α-Receptors are concentrated on the postcapillary venules; when stimulated, they reduce blood volume in the mucosa, reducing congestion. Sympathomimetic drugs mimic norepinephrine. Direct-acting agents stimulate one (PNE: α_1) or both types of α-receptors, depending on drug chemistry. Indirect-acting agents (PSE) displace norepinephrine from nerve terminals and sometimes block its reuptake, effectively increasing its action on postjunctional α-receptors. Some drugs (i.e., PSE and EDE) are both direct and indirect in their actions. Prolonged use of agents that act indirectly (e.g., EDE) may deplete storage granules, and the animal may become refractory to its effects. Alternatively, down-regulation of receptors (tachyphylaxis) may result in refractoriness.[101,102]

Topical agents containing sympathomimetic drugs (nasal sprays) act within minutes, with minimal side effects. Rebound hyperemia is common, particularly with extended use of the drugs. The mechanism of rebound hyperemia is not clear but may result from secondary beta-adrenergic effects because beta-receptors upregulate or desensitize α-receptors. Regardless of the cause, repeated contraction of the vasculature can result in ischemia and mucosal damage. Oral treatment with sympathomimetic drugs can be associated with a number of adverse reactions. Systemic vasoconstriction may cause hypertension; cardiac stimulation may result in tachycardia or reflex bradycardia. Stimulation of the central nervous system may also prove problematic, particularly with lipid-soluble agonists such as ephedrine. Stimulation of urinary sphincter α-receptors may result in urinary retention. Mydriasis may decrease aqueous humor exit and can prove detrimental in patients with glaucoma. These drugs should be avoided in patients with metabolic disorders such as thyroid disease and diabetes mellitus. There appears to be minimal relationship between plasma drug concentration and nasal decongestant efficacy, suggesting that topical therapy is as efficacious as other routes of administration. In addition, oral administration of some drugs (e.g., PNE) is limited by first-pass metabolism, which prevents therapeutic serum concentrations of the drug from being reached. Thus topical therapy may be the preferred route for sympathomimetic drugs. Note, however, that (in the United States) PSE is an "old drug," and as such is exempt from Food and Drug Administration (FDA) regulation.

Antihistamines are effective for the treatment of allergic rhinitis in human patients. In this scenario, they relieve and prevent itching and rhinorrhea but not nasal congestion. Thus antihistamines are commonly combined with sympathomimetic drugs. The efficacy of these drugs for the treatment of symptoms related to the common cold has not been proved, however. Sedation is the most common side effect of the first-generation antihistamines (diphenhydramine). Newer antihistamines (chlorpheniramine) are associated with minimal sedation. In contrast to other causes of rhinitis, topical decongestants may be more of a risk for patients with allergic rhinitis because of the risk of a drug reaction (rhinitis medicamentosa). Because the antihistamines are safer than the sympathomimetic drugs after oral use, this may be the preferred route of administration.[100]

Formulations of topical preparations can influence drug efficacy. Controlled-release polymers can decrease the rate of drug dissolution, and thus its ability to reach cellular targets. Although these differences may not be clinically relevant, bioequivalency of the topical decongestant products containing older drugs may vary. The major disadvantage of topical agents is their short duration of action.

Aerosolization as a Route of Drug Administration

Inhaled therapies were developed for humans in order to avoid side effects associated with systemically delivered drugs, particularly glucocorticoids. The goal of inhaled therapy was to provide long-term suppression of inflammation as well as to provide symptomatic relief.[25] Delivery of drugs to the respiratory tract via aerosolization (inhalation therapy) offers several advantages. Higher drug concentrations can be achieved in target tissues; lower doses can be administered to limit toxicity without compromising efficacy (e.g., anticholinergics, glucocorticoids, and beta-adrenergics). Response to aerosolized drug may be more rapid than systemic administration. Additionally, hepatic first-pass metabolism after oral administration is circumvented, prolonging the pharmacological effect of selected drugs such as beta-adrenergic agonists and beclomethasone.

In humans, aerosolization is a well-established route of administration for bronchodilators and antiinflammatories.[24,103] The development of effective inhalant devices in human medicine has led to the use of inhalant drug delivery as the primary route for treatment of asthma. In contrast, the primary indications for aerosolization in small animals have been direct delivery of drugs (antimicrobials) to the respiratory tract and facilitation of liquefaction and mobilization of respiratory secretions.[104] Indications in small animals include asthma, chronic bronchial disease, selected causes of tracheitis, and infections of both lower and upper airways.

Successful therapy with aerosolized drugs may depend more on adequate drug delivery than drug efficacy. The primary determinants of the amount of drug reach-

ing the airways are airway anatomy, ventilation rate and pattern, and aerosol characteristics.[70] The anatomy of the respiratory tract is designed to filter inhaled particles. Indeed, up to 90% of particles produced by pressurized meter dosed inhalers are removed before they reach the airways in humans.[70] The more tortuous the airways traversed by an aerosol, the smaller the percentage delivered. Variations in tidal volume; airflow rates; and respiratory rate, depth, and pattern will impact the amount of drug delivery. In humans, breath-holding is particularly important to ensure adequate drug delivery to the target sites.[70] With progression of chronic disease, or with moderate to severe acute disease, aerosol therapy may become less effective as the respiratory pattern of the animal becomes shallow and rapid. The depth of aerosol penetration decreases, and more drug is deposited in upper airways. The utility of aerosolization may be further limited because of stimulation of irritant receptors and reflex bronchoconstriction.[24,105] Resistance by the animal may further exacerbate respiratory distress and thus impact the site of particle deposition.

Among the characteristics of the aerosol that will influence airway deposition are the diameter, shape, electrical charge (for particles less than 1 μm in size), density, mass, hygroscopicity, and preparation type (e.g., solution versus suspension).[2,70,94,106] Larger particles generated by aerosol devices will impact on the pharynx and upper airways. The optimum particle size for particle (and drug) deposition in the trachea is 2 to 10 μm, and 0.5 to 5.0 μm in peripheral airways. Particle size produced differs among the different nebulizing devices. Jet and ultrasonic nebulizers tend to generate heterogenous particles that range from 1.2 to 6.9 and 3.7 to 10.5 μm in size, respectively. Spinning disk nebulizers produce particles ranging from 1.3 to 30 μm. The particle size generated by propellant-driven metered dose inhalers varies from 1 to 35 μm.[70] Penetration of small airways is best accomplished with particles that are 1.5 μm or less in size.[70] Aerosol deposition is also affected by the technique of delivery (e.g., mask versus endotracheal tube and nose versus mouth). Administration of an aerosol by mask may reduce drug delivery because particles will be deposited on the mask and face. Those deposited on the face may eventually be ingested during grooming.

NEBULIZERS

Aerosol delivery in animals is generally accomplished using nebulizers, although the use of metered dose inhalants is increasing, particularly in cats. A number of companies offer reasonably priced (i.e., $70 to more than $250) portable compressor-based nebulizing units (e.g., Omron Healthcare Inc.*). Compressors generate air at pressures (20 to 40 psi) and airflow rates (7 to 10 L/min) comparable to those produced by oxygen-based flow meters. Particle sizes generally range from 0.5 to 5 μm in diameter. The traditional nebulizer consists of a source of air or oxygen compressed to 10 to 15 psi, a well into which the drug is placed and through which the air flows

*Visit www.omronhealthcare.com.

at 7 to 10 psi, and a baffle upon which the drug impacts such that particles of aerosol are generated (Figure 32-6). Jet-enhanced nebulizers have the advantage of being "breath enhanced": an advanced valve system allows access by a second source of air to the drug well during inspiration. As a result, the number and size of particles is optimized for drug delivery, which is relatively rapid (7 to 10 minutes). The aerosol unit can be placed in an appropriately sized enclosed aquarium or, for large dogs, adapted to a mask. For tracheostomized patients, infant or adult tracheostomy masks are available; or, more simply, aerosol can be directed from the unit into the tracheostomy stoma. Aerosol units are generally reusable. However, great care must be taken to ensure that nebulizers remain free of microorganisms between uses. Adherence to cleansing procedures after each use of nebulizing equipment should be strict. Cold steriliza-

tion agents that are effective against *Pseudomonas* spp. should be selected. Note, however, that rinsing of the unit must be sufficient to avoid aerosolization of the disinfectant during therapy. Manufacturers' recommendations for cleansing of reusable equipment include washing in warm soapy water and rinsing well, followed by soaking for 30 minutes in a solution of 1 part vinegar and 3 parts water. Disposable equipment should be replaced frequently; replacement after use in patients with infection is particularly encouraged.

AEROSOL THERAPY IN ANIMALS

In order to optimize the site of particle deposition, animals to be aerosolized should be parenterally pretreated with a beta-adrenergic or methylxanthine bronchodilator 10 minutes before aerosolization. Alternatively, but po-

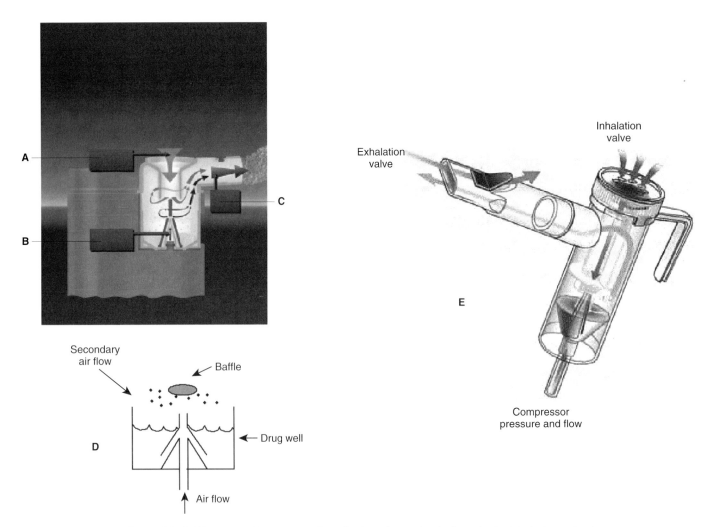

Figure 32-6. *Diagrammatic representation of a jet-enhanced nebulizer. **A,** An inhalation valve (open during patient inspiration) or open port increases airflow to the nebulizer. Air moves downward into the nebulizer cup or drug well, and mixes with air supplied by the compressor. **B,** Air supplied from the compressor moves upward under pressure and medication is nebulized at the top of cone. **C,** Nebulized aerosol is inspired by the patient. **D,** A breathing-enhanced jet nebulizer consists of airflow generated by the compressor or other source, the medicine cup or well and a baffle on which air plus drug impact to form the aerosol. The enhanced system allows additional air to reach the well during aerosolization. **E,** An example of a reusable aerosol unit. The valve system allows for additional air delivery during inspiration.*

tentially less ideal, a bronchodilator (e.g., 100 mg amino-phylline) should be included in the aerosolized solution. Care should be taken not to overhydrate and flood the respiratory tract. Treatments of approximately 30 to 45 minutes should be repeated every 4 to 12 hours.

The dose of drug to be nebulized is generally not scientifically derived. A general approach would be dilution of the calculated systemic dose in a sufficient volume of saline for a 30-minute aerosolization treatment. Drugs prepared by the manufacturer in irritating solutions (e.g., n-acetylcysteine) should always be diluted. The choice of antibiotic to be aerosolized should be based on efficacy against the targeted organism. The amount of drug that reaches the site can not easily be quantitated, and MIC based on aerosolized drugs have yet to be defined.[107] Although it is reasonable to anticipate that more drug can be delivered to the surface of the upper airways by aerosol than by systemic drug delivery, concurrent systemic therapy remains prudent, in the author's opinion, because of the questionable predictability of drug delivery by aerosol in animals. Systemic therapy is particularly indicated for treatment of small airway disease. Whether the aerosolized drug should be the same as that delivered systemically, or one that complements the action of the systemic drug, is difficult to answer without knowing how much drug will be delivered by aerosol. In general, if the systemic drug is water soluble (e.g., beta-lactams or aminoglycosides), the same drug should be aerosolized because systemic delivery to the site will be limited. If the systemic drug is lipid soluble, and particularly if it is one accumulated in white blood cells, drug delivery to the airways may reach effective concentrations and a complementary drug might be appealing.

INHALANT DEVICES

As inhalant devices have improved, inhalant therapy has become the predominant method of drug delivery to the lungs in humans. The most common device for aerosol drug delivery in humans is the metered dose inhaler.[108] These devices contain a suspension of drug in a propellant, the most common of which is a chlorofluorocarbon (CFC). Studies using radiolabeled aerosols in normal humans have documented that less than 20% (usually only 10%) of drug reaches the airways, even if the respiratory pattern is optimal.[25,108] The remaining drug is deposited orally and usually swallowed, leading (in humans) to undesired side effects.[108] The inclusion of spacers provides a "dead space" in which larger particles are deposited instead of in the oropharynx, thus decreasing systemic side effects of ingested drugs. Spacers also help minimize the difficulty in coordinating inhalation with the generation of the aerosol. The phasing out of CFC-based propellants (because of their effect on ozone) has led to alternative nonchlorine containing propellants such as hydrofluoroalkane (HFA). Particles of this propellant are referred to as extrafine, with an average of 1.1 μm in size compared to 3.5-4.0 μm in size for the CFC. The smaller size enhances deeper airway penetration.[25] The pattern of particle deposition with HFA propellants is reversed in humans compared with the CFC propel-

lants: the majority (up to 60%) of particles are deposited in the small airways rather than the oropharynx.[108] The HFA-based device appears to result in improved response in human asthmatics.

Even with extrafine particles and better small airway penetration, the smallest airways of the respiratory tract remain untreated with inhalant metered devices. Additionally, aerosol therapy is limited to the epithelial surface of the airways. Finally, compliance in humans with inhaled therapy is poor compared with systemic therapy.[25] Drug delivery in dogs and cats, using inhaled metered doses designed for humans, is further limited by species differences in airway anatomy as well as inability to control or direct intake in a manner that maximizes airway delivery. Adaptations of human inhalant devices to animal use include the use of masks modified with one-way valves that limit drug movement to inhalation,[28] or simple administration through an empty toilet paper roll. Cats breathe from the spacer 6 to 7 times after the medication is dispensed from the inhaler. The role of human inhalant metered devices for the long-term control of clinical signs related to asthma remains to be validated in animals. As such, systemic therapy might prudently be included in all but mildly affected patients. The use of inhalant devices might more wisely be used for exacerbations (e.g., short-acting beta-adrenergics or glucocorticoids), for animals for which systemic therapy is not sufficient (e.g., long-acting beta-adrenergics or glucocorticoids), or for those in which systemic therapy is contraindicated (e.g., animals with small airway disease accompanied by concurrent diabetes mellitus or heart disease).

Respiratory Tract Infections

PATHOPHYSIOLOGY

The bronchial-alveolar-blood barrier is a major barrier to passive drug movement from the blood to the site of infection in the respiratory tract.[109,110] Whereas drugs of a molecular weight up to 1000 Daltons can move easily through the open junctions of the capillaries, drugs must passively diffuse through the tight junctions between the alveolar epithelial cells.[109] Movement of drugs into bronchial secretions occurs primarily by passive diffusion, and is more likely to occur for drugs with favorable physicochemical characteristics such as high lipophilicity and low molecular weight (less than 450 Daltons). Few drugs achieve concentrations in respiratory tissues equal to concentrations in the plasma. Thus achieving only the MIC in the plasma against an organism infecting the respiratory tract is likely to result in therapeutic failure.[111,112] Rather, the targeted plasma drug concentration must be great enough to ensure that the MIC will be reached at the site of infection. The relationship between plasma and bronchial drug concentrations can be described by the partition ratio,[109,110] which is the area under the plasma drug concentration versus time curve in plasma divided by the same in bronchial secretions. Such a relationship would compare not only peak concentrations but also the time that drug stays in tissues, which generally is longer than in plasma. Collection of sequential bronchial secretion samples necessary for kinetic analysis is difficult, however, and such information currently is not available for many drugs. A more practical relationship is the ratio of bronchial drug concentrations to plasma drug concentrations. This ratio has been established for a number of antimicrobial drugs and is often available in package inserts or textbooks. The ratio can serve as a basis for antimicrobial selection and dose manipulation.[109,110]

Among the antimicrobial classes, the penicillin antibiotics are characterized by one of the poorest plasma-to-bronchial tissue drug concentrations (mean of 9%), although variation exists among the individual drugs. For example, amoxicillin reaches four to five times higher concentrations in bronchial secretions than ampicillin when given at the same dose, although this is probably because of higher plasma concentrations.[109,110] Only about 30% of either drug in plasma reaches bronchial secretions, however. The cephalosporins are distributed slightly better than the penicillins (mean of 15%), again with variation among the individual members. For example, cephalexin achieves only 15% of plasma concentrations, whereas cefoxitin and cefotaxime reach 25% of plasma concentrations. Selected third-generation cephalosporins may reach even higher concentrations. Imipenem also has one of the better distribution patterns of the beta-lactam antibiotics, reaching 20% of plasma concentrations in bronchial secretions.[109,110]

The aminoglycosides distribute into bronchial secretions somewhat better than the beta-lactams, generally reaching about 30% of plasma concentrations. Clindamycin achieves 61% of plasma concentrations. Tetracyclines, and particularly doxycycline (38%) and minocycline, can reach 30% to 60% of plasma concentrations after a single dose. Macrolides such as erythromycin generally distribute well into bronchial secretions (41% to 43%), although newer drugs such as azithromycin (which can accumulate up to 200-fold in pulmonary tissues) distribute much better than erthromycin.[109,110] The fluorinated quinolones reach 70% or more of plasma concentrations; they also accumulate over fiftyfold to 100-fold in alveolar macrophages. The potentiated sulfonamides have variable distribution. Whereas trimethoprim reaches 100% of serum concentrations in bronchial fluid, the sulfonamide component may achieve much lower concentrations. For example, sulfamethoxazole achieves only 18% of serum concentrations. Metronidazole, useful for anaerobic infections, achieves 100% of plasma concentrations in respiratory secretions.[109,110] For drugs with a long elimination half-life (e.g., doxycycline), the ratios of bronchial concentrations to plasma concentrations may increase with repetitive dosing as drugs accumulate.[109,110]

Inflammation generally increases concentrations of selected antibacterials (e.g., beta-lactams and aminoglycosides) in bronchial secretions because of local vasodilation and vascular permeability. Excessive inflammation can, however, preclude antibiotic distribution, particularly for drugs that do not accumulate in white blood cells.[109,110] Therefore, in the presence of inflammation, drugs that accumulate in phagocytic white blood cells should be considered. Aminoglycosides accumulate very slowly in cells, with several days elapsing before intracellular concentrations exceed extracellular levels. Although bioactivity against micoorganisms may be maintained, preferential distribution to lysosomes where the pH approximates 5.5 essentially precludes activity,[113,114] and aminoglycosides remain largely ineffective against intracellular organisms. Beta-lactams consistently fail to accumulate in phagocytic cells, with intracellular concentrations remaining below extracellular levels. Although the drug that does penetrate remains in the cytosol, it is ineffective against intracellular organisms unless extracellular concentrations are sufficiently high. Lincosamides accumulate into phagocytes very well, and are equally distributed between the cytosol and lysosomes.[113,114] Clindamycin remains only poorly active against intracellular organisms; however, macrolides also accumulate well into phagocytic cells, but uptake is markedly impaired in the presence of an acidic extracellular pH.[113] Efflux occurs rapidly (half-life 15 to 20 minutes) with the exception of azithromycin, which achieves and maintains very high intracellular concentrations with drug located in the cytosol.[113]

All of the fluorinated quinolones studied thus far accumulate fourfold to tenfold or more in phagocytic cells.[115-118] Although the majority of the studies have focused on fluorinated quinolones approved for human use, this effect has been confirmed for enrofloxacin and marbofloxacin. Originally reported[119] to concentrate up to eightfold in canine alveolar macrophages, in fact enrofloxacin (and its active metabolite, ciprofloxacin) was concentrated over 100-fold in these cells at 4 hours. Marbofloxacin accumulates approximately fiftyfold in canine alveolar macrophages.[120] Enrofloxacin and its active metabolite, ciprofloxacin, also accumulate to a ratio of eightyfold to 100-fold in peripheral white blood cells.[121] Subsequent studies have shown that enrofloxacin can be delivered to sites of inflammation following accumulation in circulating white blood cells.[122] Unlike the macrolides, uptake of fluorinated quinolones is not impaired by an acidic pH. Like the macrolides, efflux into a drug-free environment is rapid.[113,114] Uptake of the fluorinated quinolones does not appear to be associated with any detrimental changes in intracellular killing ability.[113,114,123-125] The fluorinated quinolones maintain intracellular antimicrobial efficacy against a number of organisms including *Chlamydia, Staphylococcus aureus, Legionella,* and *Salmonella.*

Mucus produced in response to a bacterial infection in the respiratory tract can also interfere with antimicrobial therapy.[109,110] Aminoglycoside efficacy may be decreased by chelation with magnesium and calcium in the mucus. Antibiotics may bind to glycoproteins, and mucus may present a barrier to passive diffusion. In addition, some antibiotics may alter the function of the mucociliary apparatus, either by increasing mucus viscosity or decreasing ciliary activity (e.g., tetracyclines). Because of these negative effects, drugs that decrease mucus viscosity or are mucolytic may facilitate antibiotic therapy.[109,110]

BACTERIAL TRACHEOBRONCHITIS

Bordetella bronchiseptica is the primary bacterial pathogen associated with infectious tracheobronchitis in dogs. This contagious disease, characterized by paroxysms of coughing, generally is mild and self-limiting but can become serious, particularly if multiple bacteria become involved. The respiratory tract has a very functional mucosal defense mechanism that generally is able to clear most organisms within 3 days of infection. *Bordetella*, however, persists for up to 14 weeks after infection.[126,127] Active attachment to cilia and ciliostasis induced by *Bordetella* appear to be important reasons for bacterial persistence. Whereas the disease generally is self-limiting to 7 to 10 days' duration, systemic signs of pneumonia indicate the need for antibiotic therapy.

Therapy should be based on culture and susceptibility data because organisms other than *Bordetella* commonly complicate infection. Antimicrobial therapy should, however, include a drug with known efficacy against *B. bronchiseptica*. It is likely that *Mycoplasma* spp. also play a role in infectious tracheobronchitis in dogs, and drug selection should include coverage for this organism. Systemic therapy should include a drug that penetrates bronchial secretions well. Because of the location of the organism and the difficulty of drug penetration into bronchial secretions, aerosolization of selected antimicrobials (e.g., aminoglycosides or polymyxin B) should be considered as an adjunct to systemic antibiotic therapy. Drugs with known *in vitro* efficacy against both *B. bronchiseptica* and *Mycoplasma* include the fluorinated quinolones, doxycycline or minocycline, chloramphenicol, and the macrolides. Among these, only the fluorinated quinolones typically are associated with bactericidal concentrations. Accumulation of the macrolides in lung tissue may, however, result in bactericidal concentrations of these otherwise bacteriostatic drugs.

BACTERIAL PNEUMONIA

Bacterial pneumonia is much more common in dogs than in cats. Although *B. bronchiseptica* and *Streptococcus zooepidemicus* are among the bacterial organisms commonly associated with pneumonia, many other organisms can cause infection, including *E. coli, Pasteurella, Klebsiella, Staphylococcus,* and *Pseudomonas.*[127] The potential for *Mycoplasma* spp. and anaerobic organisms (particularly in the presence of abscessation) as a cause of infection should not be ignored. Cytology and culture collected by tracheal wash, bronchoscopy, bronchial lavage, or lung aspiration should serve as the basis for treatment. Cultures of the pharyngeal area should not be the basis of antimicrobial selection for infections of the respiratory tract. Susceptibility data should be used to select the most appropriate antimicrobial. The more severe the infection, the more important lipid solubility becomes to drug selection. Doses should be sufficiently high to establish bactericidal concentrations of drug at the site of infection. Among the antimicrobials, fluorinated quinolones such as enrofloxacin should be considered because of their spectrum and lipid solubility. In addition, accumulation by

alveolar macrophages might enhance drug distribution at the site of inflammation.[119] Combination therapy should be considered, not only to broaden the spectrum of antimicrobials but also to enhance efficacy. Aerosolization should be considered in addition to (but never in lieu of) systemic antimicrobial therapy, particularly in severe cases. Aerosolization may be particularly important for infections associated with *B. bronchiseptica.*

Mobilization of respiratory secretions may be important to resolution of infection. In addition to physical techniques such as coupage, mucolytic and mucokinetic agents should be administered. Bronchodilators may also facilitate movement of respiratory secretions as well as facilitate airway movement. Their use is controversial, with some authors suggesting that their antiinflammatory effects may be detrimental. However, control of inflammation without the use of more direct immunosuppressants (e.g., glucocorticoids) may not be serious enough to outweigh the potential benefits of airway relaxation. Theophylline can cause ventilation perfusion mismatching, and oxygen therapy should be available to patients when this drug is administered in moderate to severe cases. Alternatively, beta-2-selective bronchodilators such as terbutaline should be considered. The author has used a combination of theophylline and terbutaline in severe cases of bronchopneumonia associated with hypoplastic trachea in a pediatric patient. Drug penetration through mucoid debris present at the site of infection will be decreased, and NAC (200 to 500 mg orally or IV twice daily) should be considered as adjuvant therapy in infections associated with marked inflammatory debris. Treatment should continue until resolution of radiographic signs of pneumonia, which may require up to 6 weeks.

PYOTHORAX

Pyothorax, otherwise known as *empyema,* refers to the accumulation of white blood cells in the pleural space.[27] Organisms reach the pleural space either by direct introduction (most commonly via a foreign body or penetrating wound) or by hematogenous or lymphatic spread. The physiologic forces that keep the pleural space essentially free of fluid are overcome by inflammation, resulting in an increase in regional bloodflow, capillary hypertension, increased capillary permeability, and increased oncotic draw (by inflammatory proteins) of fluid into the pleural space. Lymphatic drainage becomes progressively more important, but accumulation of inflammatory debris and fibrosis ultimately preclude lymphatic drainage of the pleural space. Gram stain of fluids collected via thoracocentesis can be the most rapid method of diagnosing the bacterial cause of infection. The incidence of anaerobic organisms either as sole agents (particularly in cats) or in combination with other bacteria is high. Thus samples submitted for culture should include both aerobic and appropriately collected anaerobic specimens. The presence of a foul smell (reflecting the production of organic matter by-products) is supportive of infection by anaerobic organisms. In order of incidence, causative species in the cat include *Bacteroides* (15%), *Actinomyces* (including *Nocardia*), *Peptostreptococcus, Pasteurella,*

Fusobacterium, and *Mycoplasma*. Causative organisms in the dog include *Fusobacterium*, *Actinomyces* (including *Nocardia*), *Corynebacterium*, *Streptococcus*, *Bacteroides*, *Pasteurella*, *E. coli*, *Klebsiella*, and *Peptostreptococcus*.[27] Fungal organisms also should be considered as a cause of pyothorax.

Removal of inflammatory debris is a critical component of effective antimicrobial therapy for the patient with pyothorax. Drainage by thoracocentesis alone is not likely to be effective; indeed, up to 80% mortality can be expected with this approach. Progression to a chronic stage can be expected in many patients in whom drainage has been inadequate, increasing both mortality and cost compared with the patient with adequate drainage. Thus therapy should include chest tube drainage (preferably by continuous water seal suction at 20 cm H_2O). Bilateral chest tube placement may be necessary in some patients. Effective removal of debris will not only remove inflammatory mediators but also will facilitate antimicrobial distribution. Response to antimicrobial therapy should be judged based on repeated cytology and Gram stains. Clinical signs and cytologic findings should improve once chest tube drainage is in place. Bacteria generally are nondetectable 2 to 3 days after therapy is begun; however, serial cultures should be used to confirm the absence of growth. Antimicrobial selection should be based on culture and susceptibility data. Unfortunately, growth often does not occur despite cytologic evidence of bacteria. An anaerobic environment should be assumed even if aerobes are cultured because many of these organisms are facultative anaerobes.

Antimicrobials that are not effective in an anaerobic environment (e.g., aminoglycosides) should not be used as sole agents in the treatment of pyothorax. Penicillins should be included in the initial therapy because their spectrum includes anaerobic organisms, and synergistic interactions occur with a number of other antimicrobials. An aminopenicillin (e.g., ampicillin or amoxicillin) is preferred to penicillin in order to extend the spectrum to include more gram-negative organisms. In severe cases, an extended beta-lactam (e.g., imipenem) should be considered. Because many of the organisms (including anaerobes) associated with pyothorax produce beta-lactamases, protected drugs or drugs inherently resistant to beta-lactamases should be selected. The use of cephalosporins for the treatment of pyothorax probably should be avoided because their efficacy against anaerobes is less than that of penicillins. The aminoglycosides (particularly amikacin) are among the drugs to which *Nocardia* and *Actinomyces* are very susceptible and should be considered in combination with a beta-lactam.

For initial therapy, particularly in serious cases, the author prefers a combination of amikacin (for *Nocardia*) and parenteral (IV) amoxicillin/ampicillin or ideally imipenem, if its cost is not prohibitive. Ampicillin should be given at a high dose at least every 6 hours and preferably every 4 hours. Amikacin should be given once daily. Therapy should be continued for 7 to 10 days. At that time, assuming improvement is evident, oral therapy can be implemented. In the absence of specific culture and sensitivity data, the author prefers high doses of amoxicillin/clavulanic acid (every 8 hours) and a sulfadiazine/trimethoprim combination (30 to 45 mg/kg twice daily). Synergistic actions against *Nocardia* have been documented (in vitro) with a number of antimicrobial combinations, including amikacin with imipenem and sulfadiazine/trimethoprim.[128] Other drugs that have shown efficacy against *Nocardia* or *Actinomyces* and are characterized by adequate distribution to the pleural space include clindamycin, minocycline, and doxycycline.[128] Caution is advised, however, when using these bacteriostatic drugs in combination with drugs dependent on rapid microbial growth for efficacy (e.g., beta-lactams).

REFERENCES

1. Moses BL, Spaulding GL: Chronic bronchial disease of the cat, *Vet Clin North Am Small Anim Pract* 15:929-949, 1985.
2. Slonim NF, Hamilton LH: Development and functional anatomy of the bronchopulmonary system. In Carson D, editor: Respiratory physiology, ed 5, St Louis, 1987, Mosby.
3. Scott JS, Berney CE, Derksen FJ et al: α-Adrenergic receptor activity in ponies with recurrent obstructive pulmonary disease, *Am J Vet Res* 52:1416-1422, 1991.
4. Gustin P, Dhem AR, Lekeux P et al: Regulation of bronchomotor tone in conscious calves, *J Vet Pharmacol Ther* 12:58-64, 1989.
5. Chand N, Deroth L: Responses to automatic and autacoid agents on horse lung strip, *J Vet Pharmacol Ther* 2:87-89, 1979.
6. Inque H, Masakazu I, Motohiko M et al: Sensory receptors and reflex pathways of nonadrenergic inhibitory nervous system in feline airways, *Am Rev Respir Dis* 139:1175-1178, 1989.
7. Altiere RJ, Diamond L: Comparison of vasoactive intestinal peptide and isoproterenol relaxant effects in isolated cat airways, *J Appl Physiol* 56:986-992, 1984.
8. Altiere RJ, Szarek JL, Diamond L: Neuronal control of relaxation in cat airway's smooth muscle, *J Appl Physiol* 57:1536-1544, 1984.
9. Derksen FJ, Robinson NE, Armstrong PJ et al: Airway reactivity in ponies with recurrent airway obstruction (heaves), *J Appl Physiol* 58:598-604, 1985.
10. Downes H, Austin DR, Parks CM et al: Comparison of drug responses in vivo and in vitro in airways of dogs with and without airway hyperresponsiveness, *J Pharmacol Exp Ther* 237:214-219, 1986.
11. Colebatch HJH, Olsen CR, Nadel JA: Effect of histamine, serotonin, and acetylcholine on the peripheral airways, *J Appl Physiol* 21:217-226, 1966.
12. Townley RG, Hopp RJ, Agrawal DK et al: Platelet-activating factor and airway reactivity, *J Allergy Clin Immun* 83:997-1011, 1989.
13. Soler M, Mansour E, Fernandez A et al: PAF-induced airway responses in sheep: Effects of a PAF antagonist and nedocromil sodium, *J Allergy Clin Immun* 67:661-668, 1990.
14. Gray PR, Derksen FJ, Robinson NE et al: The role of cyclooxygenase products in the acute airway obstruction and airway hyperreactivity of ponies with heaves, *Am Rev Respir Dis* 140:154-160, 1989.
15. Blair AM, Woods A: The effects of isoprenaline, atropine, and disodium cromoglycate on ciliary motility and mucus flow in vivo measured in cats, *Br J Pharmacol* 35:P379-P380, 1969.
16. Gallagher JT, Kent PW, Passatore M et al: The composition of tracheal mucus and the nervous control of its secretion in the cat, *Proc R Soc Lond* 192:49-76, 1975.
17. Winkler G: Pulmonary intravascular macrophages in domestic animal species: review of structural and functional properties, *Am J Anat* 181:217-234, 1988.
18. Frerking I, Gunther A, Seeger W et al: Pulmonary surfactant: Functions, abnormalities and therapeutic options, *Intensive Care Med* 27:1699-1717, 2001.
19. Gillisse A, Nowak D: Characterization of N-acetylcysteine and ambroxol in antioxidant therapy, *Respir Med* 92:609-623, 1998.
20. Barnes PJ, Chung KF, Page CP: Inflammatory mediators and asthma, *Pharmacol Rev* 40:49-84, 1988.
21. Barnes PJ: Our changing understanding of asthma, *Respir Med* 83(Suppl):17-23, 1989.

22. Gold WM, Meyers GL, Dain DS et al: Changes in airway mast cells and histamine caused by antigen aerosol in allergic dogs, *J Appl Physiol* 43:271-275, 1977.

23. Norn S, Clementson P: Bronchial asthma: Pathophysiological mechanisms and corticosteroids, *Allergy* 43:401-405, 1988.

24. Wanner A, Rao A: Clinical indications for and effects of bland, mucolytic, and antimicrobial aerosols, *Am Rev Respir Dis* 122:79-87, 1980.

25. Bjermer L: History and future perspectives of treating asthma as a systemic and small airways disease, *Respir Med* 95:703-719, 2001.

26. Barnes PJ: The drug therapy of asthma: Directions for the 21st century, *Agents Actions* 23(Suppl):293-313, 1988.

27. Bauer T, Woodfield JA: Mediastinal, pleural and extrapleural diseases. In Ettinger SJ, Feldman EC, editors: *Textbook of veterinary internal medicine*, ed 4, Philadelphia, 1995, WB Saunders.

28. Padrid PA: Feline asthma: Diagnosis and treatment, *Vet Clin North Amer Small Anim Prac* 30(6):1279-1293, 2000.

29. Cyr MM, Denburg JA: Systemic aspects of allergic disease: The role of the bone marrow, *Curr Opin Immunol* 13:727-732, 2001.

30. Eiser NM, Mills J, Snashall PD et al: The role of histamine receptors in asthma, *Clin Sci* 60:363-370, 1981.

31. Chand N: Reactivity of isolated trachea, bronchus, and lung strip of cats to carbachol, 5-hydroxytryptamine and histamine: Evidence for the existence of methylsergide-sensitive receptors, *Br J Pharmacol* 73:853-857, 1981.

32. Moise NS, Spaulding GL: Feline bronchial asthma: pathogenesis, pathophysiology, diagnostic, and therapeutic considerations, *Compend Contin Educ Pract Vet* 3:1091-1103, 1981.

33. Funk CD: Prostaglandins and leukotrienes: Advances in eicosanoid biology, *Science* 294:1871-1875, 2001.

34. McNamara DB, Harrington JK, Bellan JA et al: Inhibition of pulmonary thromboxane A_2 synthase activity and airway responses by CGS 13080, *Mol Cell Biochem* 85:29-41, 1989.

35. Ristimaki A, Narko K, Hla T: Down-regulation of cytokine-induced cyclo-oxygenase-2 transcript isoforms by dexamethasone: Evidence for post-transcriptional regulation, *Biochem J* 318 (Pt 1):325-331, 1996.

36. Daemen MJAP, Smits JFM, Thijssen HHW et al: Pharmacokinetic considerations in target-organ directed drug delivery, *TIPS* 9:138-141, 1988.

37. Papich MG: Bronchodilator therapy. In Kirk RW, editor: *Current veterinary therapy, vol 9: Small animal practice*, Philadelphia, 1986, WB Saunders.

38. Reed MT, Kelly HW: Sympathomimetics for acute severe asthma: Should only beta-2-selective agonists be used? *DICP Ann Pharmacother* 24:868-873, 1990.

39. Nelson HS. Combination therapy of bronchial asthma, *Allergy and Asthma Proc* 22(4):217-220, 2001.

40. Hendeles L, Weinberger M: Theophylline: a state of the art review, *Pharmacotherapy* 3:2-44, 1983.

41. Mizus I, Summer W, Farrkuhk I et al: Isoproterenol or aminophylline attenuate pulmonary edema after acid lung injury, *Am Rev Respir Dis* 131:256-259, 1985.

42. Short CE: Telazol: A new injectable anesthetic, *Cornell Fel Health Cent Info Bull* 2:1-3, 1987.

43. Murciano D, Aubier M, Lecocguic Y et al: Effects of theophylline on diaphragmatic strength and fatigue in patients with chronic obstructive pulmonary disease, *N Engl J Med* 311:349-353, 1984.

44. Viires N, Aubier M, Murciano D et al: Effects of aminophylline on diaphragmatic fatigue during acute respiratory failure, *Am Rev Respir Dis* 129:396-402, 1984.

45. McKiernan BC, Davis CAN, Koritz GD et al: Pharmacokinetics studies of theophylline in dogs, *J Vet Pharmacol Ther* 4:103-110, 1981.

46. McKiernan BC, Koritz GD, Davis LE et al: Pharmacokinetics studies of theophylline in cats, *J Vet Pharmacol Ther* 6:99-104, 1983.

47. McKiernan BC: Principles of respiratory therapy. In Kirk RW, editor: *Current veterinary therapy, vol 8: Small animal practice*, Philadelphia, 1983, WB Saunders.

48. Dye JA, McKiernan BC, Jones SD: Sustained-release theophylline pharmacokinetics in cats, *J Vet Pharmacol Ther* 13:278-286, 1990.

49. Koritz GD, McKiernan BC, Davis CAN et al: Bioavailability of four slow-release theophylline formulations in the beagle dog, *J Vet Pharmacol Ther* 9:293-302, 1986.

50. Errecalde JO, Baggot JD, Mulders MSG et al: Pharmacokinetics and bioavailability of theophylline in horses, *J Vet Pharmacol Ther* 7:255-263, 1984.

51. Dye JA, McKiernan BC, Neft Davis CA et al: Chronopharmacokinetics of theophylline in cats, *J Vet Pharmacol Ther* 12:133-140, 1989.

52. Munsiff IJ, Koritz GD, McKiernan BC et al: Plasma protein binding of theophylline in dogs, *J Vet Pharmacol Ther* 11:112-114, 1988.

53. Larsson CI, Kallings P, Persson S et al: Pharmacokinetics and cardio-respiratory effects of oral theophylline in exercised horses, *J Vet Pharmacol Ther* 12:189-199, 1989.

54. Rybak MJ, Bowles SK, Chandrasekar PH et al: Increased theophylline concentrations secondary to ciprofloxin, *Drug Intell Clin Pharmacol* 21:879-881, 1987.

55. Rodvold KA: Clinical pharmacokinetics of clarithromycin, *Clin Pharmacokinet* 37:385-398, 1999.

56. Cremer KF, Secor J, Speeg KV: The effect of route of administration on the cimetidine-theophylline drug interaction, *J Clin Pharmacol* 29:451-456, 1989.

57. Henderson A, Wright DM, Pond SM: Management of theophylline overdose patients in the intensive care unit, *Anaesth Intens Care* 20(1):56-62, 1992.

58. Munsiff IJ, McKiernan BC, Davis CAN et al: Determination of the acute oral toxicity of theophylline in conscious dogs, *J Vet Pharmacol Ther* 11:381-389, 1988.

59. Persson CGA, Ergefalt I: Seizure activity in animals given enprofylline and theophylline, two xanthines with partly different mechanisms of action, *Arch Int Pharmacodyn* 258:267-282, 1982.

60. Gross NJ, Skorodin MS: Anticholinergic, antimuscarinic bronchodilators, *Am Rev Respir Dis* 129:856-870, 1984.

61. Murphy S, Kelly HW: Cromolyn sodium: a review of mechanisms and clinical use in asthma. *DICP Ann Pharmacother* 21:22-35, 1987.

62. Holgate ST: Reflections on the mechanisms of action of sodium cromoglycate (Intal) and the role of mast cells in asthma, *Respir Med* 83(Suppl):25-31, 1989.

63. Kay AB, Walsh GM, Moqbel R et al: Disodium cromoglycate inhibits activation of human inflammatory cells in vitro, *J Allergy Clin Immunol* 80:1-8, 1987.

64. Massey KL, Hendeles L: Calcium antagonists in the management of asthma: Breakthrough or ballyhoo? *DICP Ann Pharmacother* 21:505-508, 1987.

65. Creese BR: Calcium ions, drug action and airways obstruction, *Pharmacol Ther* 20:357-375, 1983.

66. Crofford LJ, Wilder RL, Ristimaki AP et al: Cyclooxygenase-1 and -2 expression in rheumatoid synovial tissues. Effects of interleukin-1 beta, phorbol ester, and corticosteroids, *J Clin Invest* 93(3):1095-1101, 1994.

67. Haynes RC Jr.: Adrenocorticotropic hormone: Adrenocortical steroids and their synthetic analogs; inhibitors of the synthesis and actions of adrenocortical hormones. In Gilman AG, Rall TW, editors: *The pharmacological basis of therapeutics*, ed 8, New York, 1990, Pergamon Press.

68. Campbell WB: Lipid-derived autocoids: Eicosanoids and platelet activating factor. In Gilman AG, Rall TW, editors: *The pharmacological basis of therapeutics*, ed 8, New York, 1990, Pergamon Press.

69. Yang YH, Hutchinson P, Santos LL et al: Glucocorticoid inhibition of adjuvant arthritis synovial macrophage nitric oxide production: Role of lipocortin 1, *Clin Exp Immunol* 111:117-122, 1998.

70. Thompson PJ: Drug delivery to the small airways, *Am J Respir Crit Care Med* 157:S199-S202, 1998.

71. Reinus JF, Persky S, Burkiewicz JS et al: Severe liver injury after treatment with the leukotriene receptor antagonist zafirlukast, *Ann Intern Med* 133:964-968, 2000.

72. Danese S, De Vitis I, Gasbarrini A: Severe liver injury associated with zafirlukast, *Ann Intern Med* 135(10):930, 2001.

73. Tashkin DP: The importance of control in asthma management: Do leukotriene receptor antagonists meet patient and physician needs? *Allergy and Asthma Proc* 22(5):311-319, 2001.

74. Wilson AM, White PS, Gardiner Q et al: Effects of leukotriene receptor antagonist therapy in patients with chronic rhinosinusitis in a real life rhinology clinic setting, *Rhinology* 39(3):142-146, 2001.

75. Parratt JR, Sturgess RM: The effect of indomethacin on the cardiovascular and metabolic responses to *E. coli* endotoxin in the cat, *Br J Pharmacol* 50:177-183, 1974.

76. Wasserman MA: Modulation of arachidonic acid metabolites as potential therapy of asthma, *Agents Actions* 23(Suppl):95-111, 1988.

77. Walker BR, Voelkel NF, Reeves JT: Pulmonary pressor response after prostaglandin synthesis inhibition in conscious dogs, *J Appl Physiol* 52:705-709, 1982.

78. Dahlen SE, Malmstrom K, Nizankowska E: Improvement of aspirin-intolerant asthma by montelukast, a leukotriene antagonist: A randomized, double-blind, placebo-controlled trial, *Am J Respir Crit Care Med* 165(1):9-14, 2002.

79. Keith JC: Pulmonary thromboembolism during therapy of dirofilariasis with thiacetarsamide: Modification with aspirin or prednisolone, *Am J Vet Res* 44:1278-1283, 1983.

80. Rawlings CA, Keith JC, Lewis RE et al: Aspirin and prednisolone modification of radiographic changes caused by adulticide treatment in dogs with heartworm infection, *J Am Vet Med Assoc* 183:132, 1983.

81. Zenoble RD: Respiratory pharmacology and therapeutics, *Compend Contin Educ Pract Vet* 2:139-147, 1980.

82. Chyrek-Borowska S, Siergiejko Z, Michalska I: The effects of a new generation of H_1 antihistamines (cefirizine and loratadine) on histamine release and the bronchial response to histamine in atopic patients, *J Invest Allergol Clin Immunol* 5:103-107, 1995.

83. Krauer B, Krauer F: Drug kinetics in pregnancy, *Clin Pharmacokinet* 2:167-181, 1977.

84. Padrid PA, Mitchell RW, Ndukwu IM et al: Cyproheptidine-induced attenuation of type I immediate hypersensitivity reactions of airway smooth muscle from immune sensitized cats, *Am J Vet Res* 56:109-115, 1995.

85. Adcock JJ: Peripheral opioid receptors and the cough reflex, *Respir Med* 85(Suppl A):43-46, 1991.

86. Bolser DC, Hey JA, Chapman RW: Influence of central antitussive drugs on the cough motor pattern, *J Appl Physiol* 86(3):1017-1024, 1999.

87. Bolser DC: Mechanisms of action of central and peripheral antitussive drugs, *Pulmon Pharmacol* 9:357-364, 1996.

88. Roudebush P: Antitussive therapy in small companion animals, *J Am Vet Med Assoc* 180:1105-1107, 1982.

89. Irwin RS, Curlye FJ, Bennett FM: Appropriate use of antitussives and protussives: A practical review, *Drugs* 46:80-91, 1993.

90. Hosgood G: Pharmacologic features of butorphanol in dogs and cats, *J Am Vet Med Assoc* 196:135-136, 1989.

91. Gingerich DA, Rourke JE, Strom PW: Clinical efficacy of butorphanol injectable and tablets, *Vet Med Small Anim Clin* 78:179-182, 1983.

92. Christie GJ, Strom PW, Rourke JE: Butorphanol tartrate: A new antitussive agent for use in dogs, *Vet Med Small Anim Clin* 75:1559-1562, 1980.

93. Tukianinen H, Silvasti M, Flygare U et al: The treatment of acute transient cough: A placebo-controlled comparison of dextromethorphan and dextromethorphan-beta-2-sympathomimetic combination, *Eur J Respir Dis* 69:95-99, 1986.

94. Brain JD: Factors influencing deposition of inhaled particles, *Proc Third Ann Comp Respir Soc Symp* 3:232, 1983.

95. Ziment I: Acetylcysteine: A drug that is much more than a mucokinetic, *Biomed Pharmacother* 42:513-520, 1988.

96. Heller AR, Groth G, Heller SC et al: N-acetylcysteine reduces respiratory burst but augments neutrophil phagocytosis in intensive care unit patients, *Crit Care Med* 29(2):272-276, 2001.

97. Ziment I: Acetylcysteine: A drug with an interesting past and a fascinating future, *Respiration* 50(Suppl 1):26-30, 1986.

98. Ueno O, Lee L-N, Wagner PD: Effect of N-NAC on gas exchange after methacholine challenge and isoprenaline inhalation in the dog, *Eur Respir J* 2:238-246, 1989.

99. Papich MG: Current concepts in pulmonary pharmacology, *Semin Vet Med Surg* 1:289-301, 1986.

100. Hendeles L: Selecting a decongestant, *Pharmacotherapy* 13:129S-134S, 1993.

101. Johnson DA, Hricik JG: The pharmacology of alpha-adrenergic decongestants, *Pharmacotherapy* 13:110S-115S, 1993.

102. Kanfer I, Dowse R, Vuma V: Pharmacokinetics of oral decongestants, *Pharmacotherapy* 13:116S-128S, 1993.

103. Johnson CE: Aerosol corticosteroids for the treatment of asthma, *Drug Intell Clin Pharmacol* 21:784-790, 1987.

104. Bemis DA, Appel MJG: Aerosol, parenteral, and oral antibiotic treatment of *Bordetella bronchiseptica* infections in dogs, *J Am Vet Med Assoc* 170:1082-1086, 1977.

105. Malik SK, Jenkins DE: Alterations in airway dynamics following inhalation of ultrasonic mist, *Chest* 62:660-664, 1972.

106. Newhouse MT, Ruffin RE: Deposition and fate of aerosolized drugs, *Chest* 73(Suppl):936-943, 1978.

107. Todisco T, Eslami A, Baglioni S et al: Basis for nebulized antibiotics: Droplet characterization and in vitro antimicrobial activity versus *Staphylococcus aureus, Escherichia coli,* and *Pseudomonas aeruginosa, J Aerosol Med* 13:11-16, 2000.

108. Leach CL: Improved delivery of inhaled steroids to the large and small airways, *Respir Med* 92(Suppl A):3-8, 1998.

109. Bergogne-Bérézin E: Pharmacokinetics of antibiotics in respiratory secretions. In Pennington JE, editor: *Respiratory infections: Diagnosis and management,* ed 2, New York, 1988, Raven Press.

110. Braga PC: Antibiotic penetrability into bronchial mucus: Pharmacokinetic and clinical considerations, *Curr Ther Res* 49(2):300-327, 1989.

111. Levin S, Karakusis PH: Clinical significance of antibiotic blood levels. In Ristuccia AM, Cunha BA, editors: *Antimicrobial therapy,* New York, 1984, Raven Press.

112. Bergan T: Pharmacokinetics of tissue penetration of antibiotics, *Rev Infect Dis* 3:45-66, 1981.

113. Tulkens PM: Accumulation and subcellular distribution of antibiotics in macrophages in relation to activity against intracellular bacteria. In Fass RG, editor: *Ciprofloxacin in pulmonology,* San Francisco, 1990, W. Zuckschwerdt Vering Munchen.

114. Donowitz GR: Tissue-directed antibiotics and intracellular parasites: Complex interaction of phagocytes, pathogens and drugs, *Clin Infect Dis* 19(5):926-930, 1994.

115. Easmon CSF, Crane JP: Uptake of ciprofloxacin by human neutrophils, *J Antimicrobial Chemotherapy* 16:67-73, 1985.

116. Garraffo R, Jambou D, Chichmanian RM et al: In vitro and in vivo ciprofloxacin pharmacokinetics in human neutrophils, *Antimicrobial Agents and Chemotherapy* 35:2215-2218, 1991.

117. Memin E, Panteix G, Revol A: Is the uptake of pefloxacin in human blood monocytes a simple diffusion process? *J Antimicrob Chemotherapy* 38:787-798, 1996.

118. Schuler P, Zemper K, Borner K et al: Penetration of sparfloxacin and ciprofloxacin into alveolar macrophages, epithelial lining fluid and polymorphonuclear leucocytes, *Eur Respir J* 10:1130-1136, 1997.

119. Hawkins EC, Boothe DM, Guinn A et al: Concentration of enrofloxacin and its active metabolite in alveolar macrophages and pulmonary epithelial lining fluid of dogs, *J Vet Pharmacol & Therap* 21(1):18-23, 1998.

120. Jones SA, Boothe HW, Boothe DM et al: Concentration of marbofloxacin in canine alveolar macrophages, *Proc ACVIM* 18(110):732, 2000.

121. Boeckh A, Boothe DM, Wilkie S et al: Time course of enrofloxacin and its active metabolite in peripheral leukocytes of dogs, *Vet Therap* 2:334-344, 2001.

122. Boeckh A, Boothe DM, Boothe H: Effect of WBC accumulation of enrofloxacin on its concentration at the site of inflammation, *Proc ACVIM* 19, 2002.

123. Carlier M, Scorneaux B, Zeneberghe A et al: Cellular uptake, localization and activity of fluoroquinolones in uninfected and infected macrophages, *J Antimicrob Chemo* 26(Suppl B):27-39, 1990.

124. Bailly S, Fay M, Roche Y et al: Effects of quinolones on tumor necrosis factor production by human monocytes, *Int J Immunopharmac* 12:31-36, 1990.

125. Garcia I, Pascual A, Slavador J et al: Effect of paclitaxel alone or in combination on the intracellular penetration and activity of quinolones in human neutrophils, *Antimicrobial Chemotherapy* 38:859-863, 1996.

126. Thayer GW: Canine infectious tracheobronchitis. In Greene C, editor: Clinical microbiology and infectious diseases of the dog and cat, Philadelphia, 1984, WB Saunders.

127. Hawkins EC: Pulmonary parenchymal diseases. In Ettinger SJ, Feldman EC, editors: *Textbook of veterinary internal medicine,* ed 5, Philadelphia, 2000, WB Saunders.

128. Eliopoulos GM, Moellering RC: Antimicrobial combinations. In Lorian V, editor: *Antibiotics in laboratory medicine,* Baltimore, 1996, Williams & Wilkins.

CHAPTER 33

Anesthesia of the Patient with Respiratory Disease

Sandra Z. Perkowski

Effect of Anesthesia on Gas Exchange

Patients with respiratory disease include those with airway disease and inability to ventilate, and those with primary lung disease and inability to oxygenate. Some patients have difficulty both ventilating and oxygenating. During anesthesia, a number of clinically significant effects on both the respiratory and cardiovascular systems can exacerbate the impact of the underlying disease process on gas exchange. Decreases in ventilation, increases in ventilation/perfusion (V/Q) mismatching, and changes in shunt fraction may all contribute to the development of hypoxemia (arterial oxygen tension [Pao_2] less than 60 mm Hg), hypercarbia (arterial carbon dioxide tension [$Paco_2$] greater than 45 mm Hg), or both. In addition, mechanical failure of oxygen delivery may occur. The overall impact of anesthesia on the animal will depend on preexisting disease conditions and specific interactions with the anesthetic drugs being used. Adjustments in anesthetic technique must be made accordingly.

Hypoventilation commonly occurs in the anesthetized patient breathing spontaneously because of the ability of most anesthetic agents to depress central control mechanisms in a dose dependent manner. This can aggravate decreases in ventilation caused by conditions such as airway disease (e.g., laryngeal paralysis, neoplasia, and collapsing trachea); thoracic trauma; and diaphragmatic hernia. Increases in airway resistance caused by relaxation of pharyngeal muscles in the unintubated patient, progressive or acute obstruction of the endotracheal tube from airway secretions or kinking in the intubated patient, or drug-induced bronchospasm, may exacerbate the inability to ventilate.

Normal tidal volumes average 10 to 15 ml/kg in the awake small animal patient.[1] Respiratory minute ventilation, which depends upon both tidal volume and respiratory rate, averages 150 to 350 ml/kg/min. Gas exchange, however, depends on the volume of *fresh* gas reaching the alveoli each minute. Alveolar ventilation is always less than respiratory minute ventilation because part of each tidal volume fills the upper airway and tracheobronchial tree where gas exchange does not occur.

Normally, this *dead space* volume averages 25% to 40% of the tidal volume. With respiratory disease, however, this value may increase significantly because fresh gas reaches alveoli that receive no bloodflow. During anesthesia, decreases in cardiac output and pulmonary artery pressures, as well as positive pressure ventilation, can cause compression of pulmonary capillaries within portions of the lung and contribute to further increases in dead space ventilation. The use of excessively long endotracheal tubes or large face masks for anesthesia, or the use of bronchodilators for treatment of respiratory disease, can also add to dead space ventilation. The impact of changes in dead space volume on alveolar ventilation is exacerbated in the anesthetized patient breathing spontaneously, where tidal volumes are often lower than in the awake patient. In addition, inadequate mechanical ventilation can result in hypoventilation in any anesthetized patient.

Changes in ventilation under anesthesia can affect the amount of oxygen that reaches the alveoli, as described by the alveolar gas equation. Fortunately, administration of oxygen concentrations greater than 30% to 35% in the anesthetized patient generally prevents the development of hypoxemia caused solely by hypoventilation.[2] The increase in arterial CO_2 caused by hypoventilation can, however, have other effects. For example, a moderate increase in arterial CO_2 (permissive hypercapnia) stimulates the sympathetic nervous system and has been advocated by some to help support blood pressure during the anesthetic period.[3] However, this approach may also result in tachycardia, hypertension, and cardiac arrhythmias. In addition, the ensuing respiratory acidosis can lead to myocardial depression. Cerebral bloodflow increases in a linear fashion in response to the increase in CO_2. Although respiration is initially stimulated, central nervous system depression and respiratory depression may become evident as CO_2 continues to increase.

In addition to changes in ventilation, anesthesia also increases the dispersion between areas of ventilation and perfusion in the lung (i.e., increases V/Q mismatch). A greater percent of ventilation is distributed to the nondependent portions of the lung that receive less bloodflow (increased dead space), and a relatively greater percent of bloodflow is distributed to dependent areas that are poorly ventilated. Inhalant anesthetics can exacerbate this mismatch by attenuating hypoxic pulmonary vasoconstriction,[4] which normally decreases perfusion through poorly ventilated areas of the lung. Administration of inspired oxygen concentrations greater than 35% generally minimizes the hypoxemia caused by perfusion of alveoli with decreased V/Q ratios, although arterial oxygen tensions may remain lower than expected.[2]

The most common cause of hypoxemia in anesthetized patients receiving supplemental oxygen is the presence of a shunt (venous admixture), either anatomic in origin (rarely) or caused by bloodflow to areas of the lung receiving little to no ventilation (V/Q approaching zero). Shunts may occur in animals with congenital heart disease with right- to left-shunting (e.g., Tetralogy of Fallot). They may also occur in animals with pulmonary disease, including alveolar collapse secondary to pneumothorax, pyothorax, or lung lobe torsion; alveolar collapse from compression by neoplasms, diaphragmatic hernia, or abdominal distension; and alveolar filling caused by pneumonia, pulmonary edema, or pulmonary hemorrhage. The presence of a shunt results in the return of mixed venous blood directly to the arterial side of the circulation. Hypoxemia caused by a shunt is relatively unresponsive to the administration of 100% oxygen, because as blood from various parts of the lung meet and mix, oxygen contents (dependent primarily on hemoglobin saturation) rather than oxygen tensions are averaged. Supplemental oxygen has a minimal effect on the oxygen content of blood leaving nonshunted portions of the lung, because the hemoglobin is already more than 98% saturated with oxygen on room air. Blood leaving shunted portions of the lung continues to contribute mixed venous blood to the arterial circulation. Because of the sigmoid shape of the oxygen-hemoglobin dissociation curve, the addition of mixed venous blood (with an average saturation of approximately 75%) will have a significant impact in decreasing overall oxygen content.

Anesthesia causes an increase in the shunt fraction because of changes in functional residual capacity (FRC), the volume of gas remaining in the lung after a normal expiration. During anesthesia, FRC decreases because of recumbent positioning, thoracic and diaphragmatic muscle relaxation, and forward displacement of the diaphragm by abdominal contents. The decrease in FRC is often associated with a decrease in lung compliance and an increase in atelectasis and small airway closure, especially in the dependent lung areas (compression atelectasis). Continued perfusion of these areas contributes to an increase in shunt fraction from 1% to 10% of the cardiac output under anesthesia.[2] When ventilating the anesthetized patient, a larger breath or sigh should be occasionally administered to help decrease the degree of small airway closure.

Preoperative Evaluation

Although patients with a decreased ability to ventilate are handled somewhat differently from those with oxygenation problems, preoperative manipulation of both should incur a minimum of stress or excitement. Oxygen supplementation is often required while the patient is being assessed. Administration of at least 30% to 35% oxygen using a face mask, nasal cannula, or oxygen cage is recommended to prevent hypoxemia secondary to hypoventilation.

Recognition of hypoventilation is often difficult clinically but includes changes in respiratory rate and effort, hyperemia because of peripheral vasodilation, and signs associated with sympathetic stimulation. Patients commonly at risk include those with upper airway disease, as well as brachycephalic breeds undergoing anesthesia for any reason. Accurate assessment of ventilatory status requires measurement of arterial P_{CO_2}, normal values being 35 to 45 mm Hg in most species. A venous blood gas ($P_{V_{CO_2}}$ should be less than 45 to 50 mm Hg) can be helpful in ruling out a diagnosis of hypoventilation, although increases in $P_{V_{CO_2}}$ can be caused by decreased tissue perfusion as well as hypoventilation. Noninvasive estimates of ventilatory status can also be made by measuring end-tidal CO_2 using a capnograph. There is some variability in the correlation between end tidal and arterial CO_2, especially in patients that are hemodynamically unstable, but end-tidal CO_2 generally runs 5 to 10 cm H_2O lower than arterial CO_2.[5]

Recognition of hypoxemia also can be difficult clinically. An increase in respiratory rate and effort is often present in the awake animal because peripheral chemoreceptors in the carotid bodies stimulate respiration at Pa_{O_2} values less than 60 mm Hg. This response is markedly attenuated by low levels of inhalant anesthetics.[6] Heart rate initially increases in an attempt to increase cardiac output and oxygen delivery to the tissues, but as hypoxemia becomes more severe, myocardial depression and bradycardia follow. Cyanosis of the mucous membranes is not usually detected until arterial oxygen saturation falls to approximately 85%, equivalent to a Pa_{O_2} of approximately 50 mm Hg.[2] Although accurate assessment of PO_2 requires an arterial blood gas, changes in oxygen saturation can be measured with a pulse oximeter. Pulse oximetry is a noninvasive monitoring technique that measures oxygen saturation of hemoglobin in the arterial blood by detecting the differential transmission (or absorption) of light at two wavelengths, 660 nm (red) and 940 nm (infrared). Oxygen saturation should remain greater than 95% in patients with a Pa_{O_2} of 85 mm Hg or greater. An oxygen saturation of 90% is roughly equivalent to an arterial oxygen tension of 60 mm Hg.

Effects of Anesthetic Drugs on Gas Exchange

All anesthetic agents affect ventilation to some degree. Anticholinergic drugs (e.g., atropine and glycopyrrolate) cause dilation of the smooth muscle within the larger airways, decreasing airway resistance and increasing dead space volume. The viscosity of airway secretions also increases. Phenothiazine tranquilizers (e.g., acepromazine) and benzodiazepine tranquilizers (e.g., diazepam and midazolam) have minimal effects on ventilation at lower doses. Respiratory rate may decrease, but is usually compensated by an increase in tidal volume.[7,8] Respiratory depression may become more pronounced at higher doses or in combination with other drugs. Alpha 2 agonists (e.g., xylazine and medetomidine) do not generally depress ventilation at lower doses, although hypoxemia has been reported after their use.[9]

Although opioids directly depress central chemoreceptors in a dose dependent manner,[10] clinically significant respiratory depression does not occur as readily in small animals as it does in humans.[11,12] Care should still be taken with their use in patients at risk for hypoventilation. Panting is not considered effective ventilation because tidal volumes are quite low relative to dead space volumes. Mixed opioid agonist/antagonists (e.g., butorphanol) or partial agonists (e.g., buprenorphine) may cause less respiratory depression, with a ceiling effect at higher doses.[7,11]

Barbiturates (e.g., thiopental) and propofol can be potent respiratory depressants, acting in a dose- and rate-dependent manner to decrease the sensitivity of the central chemoreceptors to CO_2.[13,14] Apnea can occur after administration of an induction dose of either drug. Respiratory depression from barbiturates may persist into the postanesthetic period. Etomidate causes minimal respiratory depression at clinical doses.[15] Dissociative agents (e.g., ketamine and tiletamine-zolazepam) can cause transient decreases in respiratory rate, although tidal volumes usually remain normal.[8,16] Bronchodilation results both from direct effects and from catecholamine release and subsequent β-2 receptor mediated effects.[17] Laryngeal and pharyngeal function are well maintained after administration of ketamine, and animals may be more prone to laryngospasm.

The potent inhalants (e.g., halothane, isoflurane and sevoflurane) all decrease ventilation in a dose dependent manner. Ventilatory responses to both hypercarbia and hypoxemia are decreased;[6] therefore, all patients maintained on inhalant anesthesia, especially those with poor pulmonary reserve, should receive supplemental manual ventilation. Bronchodilation and inhibition of hypoxic pulmonary vasoconstriction can also contribute to changes in gas exchange. Nitrous oxide has minimal effects on ventilation, but can contribute to hypoxemia and should be avoided in animals with a closed gas space such as pneumothorax.

Ventilatory Support

Anesthesia of patients with respiratory disease should include intubation and delivery of supplemental oxygen. Mechanical ventilation, usually in the form of intermittent positive pressure ventilation, is often required. Usually, a rate of 8 to 15 breaths per minute is used, although higher rates may be required. Tidal volumes are generally set at 10 to 20 ml/kg, with maximum airway pressures usually limited to 15 to 20 cm H_2O. In patients with pulmonary disease, adjustment of tidal volume and

peak airway pressures may be necessary to prevent barotrauma. Higher pressures may be required in some conditions to provide adequate tidal volumes. Positive pressure delivered to the thoracic cavity can decrease venous return and cardiac output, especially if the patient is volume depleted. Therefore, the ratio of inspiratory time to expiratory time is generally limited to a ratio of 1:2 or 1:3. If the patient resists mechanical ventilation, an increase in anesthetic depth, or use of a neuromuscular blocker (e.g., atracurium) may be required.

Treatment of hypoxemia includes delivery of 100% oxygen and discontinuation of nitrous oxide if it is being used. Positive end-expiratory pressure (PEEP) may be necessary in patients that remain hypoxemic on 100% oxygen. Maintenance of airway pressure at end-expiration improves oxygenation by increasing alveolar volumes and recruiting collapsed alveoli, changing areas receiving no ventilation (shunt) to areas of low V/Q, which are then responsive to the delivery of supplemental oxygen. Positive end-expiratory airway pressures of 5 to 15 cm H_2O are usually used, although higher pressures may be required. Purpose-made PEEP valves are available or, alternatively, the scavenging hose from the pop-off valve may be restricted (e.g., by insertion of a syringe casing) to produce the desired pressure. Administration of PEEP may cause hypotension from decreased venous return and cardiac output. The decrease in blood pressure, in conjunction with the increase in alveolar pressure, can lead to increased dead space ventilation; therefore, the effects of PEEP on oxygenation can be optimized by concurrent administration of an inotrope such as dobutamine.[2]

Anesthesia for Patients with Airway Disease

UPPER AIRWAY OR TRACHEAL DISEASE

Patients with upper airway disease or tracheal obstruction caused by neoplasia, foreign material, or collapsing trachea are commonly anxious, with increased respiratory effort that often results in a vicious cycle of increased airway obstruction and patient distress. An exaggerated abdominal effort may be seen, with the chest demonstrating paradoxical inward movement on inspiration. Patients may become hyperthermic because of the increased work of breathing and poor thermoregulation. A complete preoperative examination is often difficult to perform without additional patient stress. Supplemental oxygen should be provided to prevent hypoxemia from hypoventilation. Postobstruction pulmonary edema may also contribute to hypoxemia.

Premedication with acepromazine can be useful to calm the patient without causing significant respiratory depression, although deep sedation should be avoided. Acepromazine can result in vasodilation and hypotension; therefore, care should be taken in patients that are cardiovascularly unstable. In brachycephalic breeds presenting with respiratory distress, premedication may result in relaxation of the pharyngeal musculature, causing severe upper airway obstruction. Ketamine may be useful in cats requiring premedication. Because keta-mine acts as a bronchodilator, it may be especially useful in cats with feline asthma. In patients with tracheal lacerations, butorphanol may be helpful as an adjunct to acepromazine, acting as an antitussive agent to decrease coughing that could introduce air into the mediastinum or thoracic cavity. Every animal presenting with upper airway obstruction should be closely monitored after administration of any anesthetic agent.

Induction of animals that are having difficulty venti-lating because of airway obstruction generally involves a rapid sequence intravenous technique and intubation. A mask induction can lead to unwanted excitement and additional respiratory distress. Preoxygenation is extremely important because it increases the time available until hypoxemia will occur, should difficulty be encountered during intubation. Never assume that intubation will be possible. An assortment of endotracheal tubes should be available, and achieving a secure airway may also require some ingenuity. Premeasurement of endotracheal tube length is important to ensure proper positioning of the tube beyond the lesion, if the site of the obstruction is

TABLE 33-1. Suggested Anesthetic Drug Doses for Sedation and Anesthesia of Patients with Respiratory Disease

Drug	Dose (mg/kg)	Comments
Premedication		
Acepromazine and/or	0.02-0.05 IM	Larger doses may cause hypotension
Oxymorphone*	0.05-0.2 IM	Good CV stability, respiratory depression
Hydromorphone*	0.05-0.2 IM	Good CV stability, respiratory depression
Butorphanol*	0.1-0.6 IM	Kappa agonist/Mu antagonist
Midazolam	0.1-0.5 IM	Good CV stability, may be used in place of acepromazine with any of the above opioids
Ketamine	4-8 IM	Do not use alone in dogs (seizures) Can be combined with midazolam +/− opioids in cats
Induction	All of the following doses titrated to effect	
Thiopental	2-8 IV	Rapid induction, respiratory depression
Propofol with/without	1-6 IV	Rapid induction and recovery, dose dependent respiratory and cardiovascular depression
Diazepam	0.2-0.5 IV	
Midazolam or	0.1-0.5 IV	
Oxymorphone	0.05-0.2 IV	Good cardiovascular stability, respiratory depression
Hydromorphone and	0.05-0.2 IV	Slow titrated induction
Diazepam	0.2-0.5 IV	
Midazolam with/without	0.1-0.5 IV	
Lidocaine with/without	1(cats)/2(dogs) IV	Lowers requirements for other drugs
Etomidate	1-2 IV	Excellent CV stability. Changes the above opioid/ benzodiazepine induction to a rapid sequence technique. May cause vomiting. Thiopental or propofol may be substituted for etomidate.
Ketamine and	1-8 IV	
Diazepam	0.2-0.5 IV	
Midazolam	0.1-0.5 IV	
Maintenance		
Propofol	1-6 IV (loading)	See comments above
	0.1-0.5 mg/kg/min constant rate infusion (CRI)	
Fentanyl	2-5 μg/kg IV (loading)	Good cardiovascular stability
	20-80 μg/kg/hr CRI	Respiratory depression

*May be reversed with naloxone 0.02 mg/kg IV, IM, SC.

known. Tubes may need to be of much smaller diameter than those usually required for the size of the animal. Orotracheal intubation using a tube with a high-volume, low-pressure cuff is preferred because it allows the airway to be sealed, protecting from aspiration and allowing administration of positive pressure ventilation. Ideally, a laryngoscope is used to visualize the airway and reduce trauma associated with intubation. A tracheostomy set should be readily available in case intubation is not possible. Commercially available cuffed tracheostomy tubes are preferred. Tracheostomy is only useful if the distal airway is patent. Most patients will spontaneously ventilate once the endotracheal or tracheostomy tube has been placed, bypassing the site of obstruction.

Opioids or other respiratory depressants should be used judiciously for induction in patients with airway obstruction, when intubation may be difficult or impossible. In these patients, induction with low doses of propofol and diazepam or ketamine and diazepam may be preferred (Table 33-1). Application of 2% lidocaine to the laryngeal area using an aerosolizer or syringe may help decrease laryngospasm and trauma on intubation. Inhalants are used for anesthetic maintenance, if providing a sealed airway is possible. If the site of obstruction or tracheal rupture cannot be bypassed, oxygen may be provided using a small diameter tube and high flows of oxygen (1 to 7 L/min). In dogs, intratracheal oxygen flow rates of 50, 100, 200, or 250 ml/kg/min produce inspired oxygen concentrations of 47%, 67%, 78%, and 86%, respectively.[18] Anesthetic maintenance in these cases is achieved with low doses of an intravenous anesthetic agent (e.g., propofol or ketamine and diazepam), titrated slowly to effect in an attempt to minimize respiratory depression.

BRONCHOSCOPY

General anesthesia is used for patients undergoing bronchoscopy to allow examination of the airway with minimal trauma to the patient and to the bronchoscope. Preoxygenation is recommended before induction. Recommended drugs for induction are the same as those discussed above for any patient with airway disease. In cats, topical laryngeal administration of 2% lidocaine, using an aerosolizer or syringe, may help prevent laryngospasm on introduction of the scope. If the patient can be intubated with a large enough endotracheal tube (e.g., a 7- or 8-mm tube), the bronchoscope can be introduced through a rubber valve in a special T-shaped endotracheal tube adapter, and inhalant anesthetics may be used. However, it is critical that enough space remains between the bronchoscope and the endotracheal tube to allow the escape of expiratory gases and prevent hypercarbia and overinflation of the lungs. The patient must be extubated to allow visualization of the upper airway. A mouth gag is usually inserted to protect the bronchoscope if the depth of anesthesia should suddenly decrease.

Alternatively, bronchoscopy may be performed in patients using total intravenous anesthesia. Short-acting or reversible drugs that cause minimal respiratory depression are recommended, to allow close control of the depth of anesthesia and to optimize ventilation (e.g.,

propofol or ketamine and diazepam [see Table 33-1]). Oxygen is usually supplied via the biopsy channel of the endoscope, although excessive flows must be avoided to prevent overinflation of the small airways and barotrauma. Placement of a catheter to the side of the bronchoscope, or use of jet ventilation for oxygen administration, have also been recommended.[19]

Rapid respiratory and/or cardiovascular decompensation can occur in these patients. Continuous cardiovascular monitoring using an EKG and Doppler ultrasonic flow probe is recommended. Pulse oximetry is routine, although if the probe is placed on the tongue, dislodgement commonly occurs during the procedure. Use of the Doppler device allows a continuous auditory signal during the procedure; changes in sound quality, in addition to changes in heart rate or rhythm, may signal sudden cardiovascular compromise from oxygen desaturation or pneumothorax. Communication between the anesthetist and the endoscopist must be clear, and the bronchoscope may need to be frequently removed in smaller patients to allow escape of trapped gas.

POSTOPERATIVE CARE AND MONITORING

Any patient at risk for upper airway obstruction must be closely monitored during recovery. Airway obstruction commonly occurs from postoperative laryngeal swelling, brachycephalic syndrome, or collapsing trachea. The airway must be supported until the patient demonstrates the ability to maintain an unobstructed airway. Recovery should be as quiet and stress free as possible. Acepromazine in the immediate postoperative period may be helpful for many of these patients to minimize excitement and possible obstruction.

Ventilation is generally depressed for some time in the postoperative period because of hypothermia and the persistence of anesthetic drugs, including inhalants and opioids. Oxygen should be administered until extubation, and often needs to be supplemented postextubation until the patient demonstrates the ability to maintain ventilation. Suctioning of blood and other material from the pharyngeal area before extubation may decrease the risk of aspiration. The risk may be further decreased by slow removal of the endotracheal tube with the cuff partially deflated and the head placed down, in order to remove any secretions that have accumulated in the trachea above the cuff. Relaxation of the pharyngeal area may hinder ventilation in some brachycephalic patients. Extension of the neck and exteriorization of the tongue may help to maintain a patent airway in some cases.

Anesthesia for Patients with Intrathoracic Disease

Patients presenting with primary lung disease are commonly hypoxemic and have poor pulmonary reserve. The choice of anesthetic agent depends on the patient's current physical status, underlying disease process, and ability to oxygenate and ventilate. Stress during patient handling should be avoided if possible. Administration of supplemental oxygen is recommended throughout the perioperative period.

Neoplasia can result in airway obstruction and increases in V/Q mismatching and shunt fraction. Similarly, pulmonary edema or pneumonia can lead to alveolar flooding and associated increases in V/Q mismatch and shunt fraction. Pulmonary embolism can result not only in increases in dead space ventilation, but also increases in V/Q mismatch and shunt fraction because of release of inflammatory mediators and bronchoconstriction. Torsion of a lung lobe causes venous and bronchial obstruction, resulting in decreased venous outflow and atelectasis, and may be associated with sanguineous or chylous pleural effusion. Atelectasis of the lung lobe may contribute to V/Q mismatching and increased shunt fraction, resulting in hypoxemia. Necrosis of the lung lobe may predispose to systemic inflammatory distress syndrome, with associated release of myocardial depressant factors and cardiovascular instability.

Patients with pleural space disease include those with pleural effusion (e.g., hemothorax, pyothorax, chylothorax); pneumothorax; or space-occupying masses in which the normal association between parietal and visceral pleurae is disrupted, resulting in decreased lung expansion and lung collapse. Clinical signs include increased respiratory rate and effort with rapid and shallow breathing, and occasionally coughing. Lung sounds will be decreased on thoracic auscultation of the affected areas. In patients with respiratory distress, aspiration of the pleural space (thoracocentesis) or placement of a thoracostomy tube will allow removal of some of the pleural fluid and help stabilize the respiratory system before induction. A rapid sequence induction using an intravenous technique to allow prompt intubation and control of the airway is preferred.

Preoxygenation of patients with poor pulmonary reserve should be routine, using a face mask to deliver high oxygen flows for 3 to 5 minutes before induction. Premedication is not required if an intravenous catheter can be placed with minimal stress to the patient. In patients with hypoxemia, but no airway obstruction, a slow titrated induction using a combination of an opioid agonist (e.g., oxymorphone, hydromorphone or fentanyl) and a benzodiazepine tranquilizer (e.g., diazepam or midazolam) is preferred. Additional opioids may be given until intubation is possible. This allows a closely controlled induction with minimal cardiovascular side effects. Lidocaine may be added to this combination, and helps to desensitize the airway and smooth the induction. If a rapid sequence induction is preferred, propofol, thiopental, ketamine, or etomidate may be used in place of, or in addition to, the opioid (see Table 33-1).

Anesthesia is generally maintained by intubation and administration of inhalational anesthesics in 100% oxygen. Airway pressures may require adjustment to prevent barotrauma in patients with pulmonary disease. Isoflurane, sevoflurane, or desflurane cause less myocardial depression than halothane. Hypotension may occur, however, because of vasodilation. Nitrous oxide should be avoided in patients that are hypoxemic.

Patients presenting with pneumothorax require special consideration if a chest tube is not in place because positive pressure ventilation may lead to an increase in air accumulation within the thoracic cavity and rapid deterioration of respiratory and cardiovascular parameters. Under these conditions, induction agents causing minimal respiratory depression should be selected so that spontaneous ventilation is maintained. Nitrous oxide is avoided to prevent accumulation of gas in the thorax over time.

Some patients may not tolerate inhalational anesthesia and become profoundly hypotensive. In these patients, a continuous infusion of fentanyl (starting at 0.7 µg/kg/min) may be used. Alternatively, small IV boluses of opioids such as hydromorphone or fentanyl and/or etomidate may be given. Neuromuscular blockade may be used as an adjunct to general anesthesia. Maintenance fluid rates for anesthetized patients are generally 6 to 12 ml/kg/hr, although more rapid rates may be given as necessary. Cardiovascular support using dobutamine, dopamine, or other sympathomimetic agents may be required.

SPECIAL CONSIDERATIONS FOR THORACIC SURGERY

Positive pressure ventilation (PPV) is required when the thorax is opened to prevent hypoxemia, hypoventilation, and respiratory acidosis. Many patients also require PPV before entering the thorax. Close monitoring of the cardiovascular system is important. Arterial blood pressure may fall with PPV because of the effect of changes in intrathoracic pressures on venous return and cardiac output. Heart rate, peripheral pulse quality, mucous membrane color, and capillary refill time should all be observed closely. An esophageal stethoscope may be useful for monitoring heart rhythm. Use of an electrocardiogram is helpful, especially in patients with cardiac arrhythmias. Blood pressure may be measured indirectly with a Doppler ultrasonic flow probe or an oscillometric measuring device. Direct measurements are made using an arterial catheter, usually placed in the dorsal metatarsal or femoral artery.

Close monitoring of the respiratory system is also important, not only while the chest is open, but also as the chest is being closed because pneumothorax is a potential complication. Respiratory rate and depth, and mucous membrane color, should be watched carefully. Pulse oximetry may be used, and oxygen saturation should remain greater than 95% in patients on 100% oxygen. Measurement of end-tidal CO_2 with a capnograph is also helpful to ensure adequate ventilation. Placement of a spirometer on the expiratory limb of the anesthetic circuit allows measurement of tidal volume and helps to assess the adequacy of ventilation. Blood gas analysis may be very helpful to evaluate respiratory status.

POSTOPERATIVE MONITORING AND ANALGESIA

Continued evaluation of respiratory function is critical in the postoperative period. Lungs are normally reinflated before thoracic closure unless compression has been present for several days. Aspiration of fluid and air from the pleural cavity is important as the thoracotomy site is closed. Normally, therefore, a chest tube is inserted before closure, which also allows repeated aspiration as needed in the postoperative period. Supplemental oxygen should be provided until the patient demonstrates the ability to maintain both ventilation and oxygenation.

Thoracotomy is considered a highly painful procedure, and effective postoperative analgesia is essential to encourage adequate ventilation. Patients with inadequate pain relief may breathe with smaller tidal volumes, predisposing to small airway closure, atelectasis and hypoxemia, as well as hypoventilation. A multimodal approach, including the use of analgesics from several classes, is recommended to optimize pain relief (Table 33-2). Preemptive analgesia (i.e., institution of the anesthetic protocol before surgery) is preferred. Protocols may include the administration of an opioid, local anesthetic, N-methyl-D-aspartate (NMDA) receptor antagonist such as ketamine; and/or nonsteroidal antiinflammatory agent (assuming that the patient is cardiovascularly stable).

Systemic opioids are usually given as part of the preoperative or intraoperative anesthetic protocol and may be continued in the postoperative period, but higher doses may contribute to hypoventilation. Opioid agonist-antagonists such as butorphanol may cause less respiratory depression than pure opioid agonists[11] but are unlikely to provide adequate analgesia. Buprenorphine, a partial mu agonist, may provide relatively effective analgesia postthoracotomy.[20] Administration of a partial agonist may partially reverse the effects, including the analgesic effects, of previously administered pure agonists. Alternatively, epidural administration of morphine (0.1 mg/kg of a preservative-free solution diluted to 0.3 ml/kg in sterile saline and administered at the lumbosacral junction) may be used. Pain relief is comparable to that with systemic opioids, with fewer systemic side effects.[21]

Intercostal nerve blocks using 2% lidocaine (total dose up to 4 mg/kg) or 0.5% bupivacaine (total dose of 1.5 mg/kg) may be used after lateral thoracotomy.[9] Bupivacaine is preferred because it provides a longer duration of analgesia (6 to 8 hours) than lidocaine (1 to 2 hours). Normally, two intercostal spaces on either side of the incision are blocked because of overlap of the nerve supply. The block is ideally performed on entry into the chest to assist with analgesia throughout the anesthetic period, al-

TABLE 33-2. **Suggested Analgesic Drug Doses for Postoperative Management of Patients with Respiratory Disease**

Drug	Dose (mg/kg)	Route	Duration (hr)	Comments
Opioids*				
Morphine	0.1-0.3	IV	2-4	Causes excitement IV; may cause hypotension IV (histamine release)
	0.2-1.0	IM,SQ	2-6	Vomiting may occur
Oxymorphone	0.02-0.2	IV	1-4	Good CV stability
	0.05-0.2	IM,SQ	2-6	
Hydromorphone	0.05-0.2	IM,IV	2-4	CV effects similar to oxymorphone
Meperidine	2.0-8.0 (dog)	IM	0.5-2	Do not give IV (histamine release)
Fentanyl	2-5 μg/kg (loading) CRI: 20-80 μg/kg/hr (intraop) CRI: 2-5 μg/kg/hr (postop)	IV		Constant rate infusion required
Butorphanol	0.1-0.6	IV,IM,SC	1-4	Kappa agonist, mu antagonist; more effective for mild/moderate pain/visceral pain
Buprenorphine	0.006-0.02	IV,IM,SC Sublingual	4-12	Mu partial agonist, may be difficult to reverse
Nonsteroidal Antiinflammatory Agents†				
Ketoprofen	2.0 (dog)	IV,IM,SC	Once (postop)	May cause clinically significant increases in bleeding if given preoperatively
Carprofen	4.0 (dog)	IV,IM,SC	At induction	May cause GI ulceration, idiopathic hepatotoxicity
Deracoxib	3.0-4.0 (dog)	PO	q 24 hr	Targeted COX-2 inhibitor; may cause GI irritation
Adjunct Therapy				
Ketamine	0.1-0.5 (loading)	IV		NMDA receptor antagonist
	2-10 μg/kg/min	CRI		
Lidocaine	2 mg/kg (loading)	IV		Use 1/4-1/2 the dose in cats
	25-100 μg/kg/min	CRI		CNS toxicity as higher doses

*NOTE: Cat doses are generally half that used in dogs for any of the opioids. Cats may be more prone to excitement after opioid administration.
†NOTE: Renal perfusion MUST be maintained when using any of the above NSAIDs in the perioperative period. Intravenous fluids and intraoperative blood pressure monitoring are recommended. Do not use in patients with renal disease.

though it may be done at the time of incision closure. Intercostal nerve blocks are difficult to repeat once the incision is closed and the patient is awake because of the risk of lacerating an intercostal vessel or causing pneumothorax. Alternatively, interpleural lidocaine (2% lidocaine, 2 to 4 mg/kg) or bupivacaine (0.5% bupivacaine, 1.5 mg/kg) may be infused via the chest tube.[20] The patient is positioned with the incision side down as the local anesthetic is infused and left in that position for up to 5 minutes, so that the anesthetic can diffuse across the parietal pleura and block the intercostal nerves. Ideally, the dorsal aspect of the intercostal nerves is blocked, to inhibit transmission from the more ventral aspects.

Low-dose ketamine infusion has recently been advocated as an adjunct to other analgesic techniques for postthoracotomy patients.[22] Ketamine, an NMDA receptor antagonist, given as a loading dose at the start of the procedure, and followed by a continuous infusion throughout the intraoperative and immediate postoperative period (see Table 33-2 for doses), may help reduce central sensitization of the pain response and decrease the amount of other analgesics required in the postoperative period.

New information and the availability of new COX-2 preferential drugs such as carprofen and deracoxib have increased the use of nonsteroidal antiinflammatory agents (NSAIDs) as part of the multimodal approach to pain relief in the perioperative period. NSAIDs, which inhibit the cyclooxygenase (COX) pathway of arachidonic acid metabolism, have antiinflammatory, antipyretic, and analgesic effects without causing sedation, excitement, respiratory depression, or hypotension when used at therapeutic doses. Although inhibition of the COX-1 isoform of the enzyme can result in gastric ulceration and prolonged bleeding times, preferential inhibition of the COX-2 isoform can provide effective antiinflammatory and analgesic effects while minimizing side effects.[23] Care must still be taken when using the newer COX-2 preferential drugs in the perioperative period, however, to ensure adequate renal perfusion, especially in patients in which hypotension and hypovolemia may be a concern. Administration of fluids and monitoring of blood pressure during the anesthetic period should be routine with their use.

Thoracoscopy

Thoracoscopy, or endoscopic surgery of the thorax, is currently being used as an alternative to thoracotomy for lung biopsy or lobectomy, pericardectomy, thoracic duct ligation, and general thoracic exploration. Advantages of this technique include minimal surgical invasiveness, decreased postoperative pain, and more rapid recovery. However, in addition to occasional difficulty with intrathoracic visualization, disadvantages include decreased gas exchange and a potential for cardiovascular compromise. These depend upon whether one-lung or two-lung ventilation is being used, and whether or not interpleural insufflation is required.

Patients are preoxygenated before induction. Induction techniques vary depending on the reason for thoracic exploration, but generally a rapid intravenous technique

causing minimal respiratory depression is selected, followed by intubation and ventilation with 100% oxygen. One-lung ventilation may be accomplished by selective bronchial intubation using a cuffed endotracheal tube placed under fiberoptic visualization into the unaffected lung, or by placement of a bronchial blocker in the affected lung.[24] Collapse of the surgical lung lobe can cause an increase in shunt fraction from continued perfusion of the nonventilated lung, which can result in significant hypoxemia. V/Q mismatch is exacerbated by the use of inhalant anesthetics to maintain anesthesia because of attenuation of hypoxic pulmonary vasoconstriction.

Bilateral hemithorax (two-lung) ventilation with intrathoracic insufflation of air or carbon dioxide to aid in collapse of the lungs on the surgical side has been recommended and may provide better support of pulmonary function.[25] Ventilation using smaller tidal volumes (i.e., 10 ml/kg or less) is usually necessary when using two-lung ventilation to allow adequate visualization of the thoracic cavity. Respiratory and cardiovascular parameters must be closely monitored no matter which technique is chosen because overinflation of the thoracic cavity can lead to signs associated with a tension pneumothorax.

Diaphragmatic Hernia

Patients requiring surgical repair of a diaphragmatic hernia often exhibit hypoxemia, hypercarbia, and respiratory acidosis caused by lung compression and collapse, decreases in FRC, and impaired diaphragmatic function. In the case of traumatic diaphragmatic hernia, pneumothorax and hemothorax can further contribute to respiratory compromise. Pulmonary contusions associated with the trauma may not be evident on radiographs until 6 hours after the event and may result in deterioration of oxygenation over that time. Animals are often painful, resulting in rapid, shallow respiration and further respiratory compromise. Cardiovascular instability is common because of compression of the heart and vena cava by the displaced viscera and release of inflammatory mediators from ischemic tissues. Ventricular arrhythmias associated with traumatic myocarditis may be present and may require antiarrhythmic therapy (e.g., 1 to 2 mg/kg lidocaine) before anesthesia, depending on their frequency and malignancy. Stress or poor positioning of the patient during induction can easily precipitate a crisis.

Cardiovascular stabilization with appropriate fluid resuscitation before anesthesia is extremely important. Aspiration of air and fluid before induction is indicated in animals with pleural effusion or pneumothorax and respiratory distress. Premedication is rarely required. If necessary, low doses of an opioid may be given, followed by close monitoring. Acepromazine is usually avoided. Preoxygenation is routine, if tolerated with a minimum of restraint. Respiratory function may become severely compromised as the patient moves into lateral recumbency, and care should be taken to keep the least affected side uppermost, or to maintain sternal recumbency, to optimize ventilation.

Induction is accomplished using a smooth, rapid intravenous technique and should include endotracheal intubation to ensure a secure airway and allow controlled, positive pressure ventilation. Thiopental, propofol, or ketamine and diazepam may be used in patients without cardiovascular compromise, although arrhythmogenic drugs such as thiopental and ketamine should be avoided in patients with traumatic myocarditis. A combination of opioid and benzodiazepine with or without etomidate, or a low dose of propofol to allow more rapid intubation, should be used in the unstable patient. Higher doses of propofol, depending on the total dose given and the rate of administration, may result in significant cardiovascular compromise. Lidocaine may be added to lower the required dose of other anesthetics and to treat ventricular arrhythmias. Because of lung compression by the viscera, tidal volumes may need to be decreased to avoid excessive airway pressures and barotrauma to damaged portions of the lung. Positioning the patient so that the body is tilted with the head higher may help pulmonary function.

Anesthesia is maintained with an inhalant (preferably isoflurane, sevoflurane, or desflurane) in 100% oxygen. Nitrous oxide should be avoided. In patients that do not tolerate inhalant anesthetics, repeated boluses or continuous infusion of an opioid (e.g., fentanyl at a rate starting at 0.7 μg/kg/min) may be preferred.

Positive pressure ventilation is required throughout surgery because disruption of the diaphragm results in communication between the interpleural and peritoneal spaces and lung collapse once the abdomen is open. Lung reinflation can result in ischemia/reperfusion injury and noncardiogenic pulmonary edema, especially in patients with chronic diaphragmatic hernia. Hyperinflation of the lung using excessive (i.e., greater than 30 cm H_2O) or prolonged airway pressures during lung reexpansion should be avoided because rapid reexpansion of the lungs may predispose to reexpansion pulmonary edema.[26] Lung lobes that do not reinflate at the time of surgery generally reinflate over a period of days once negative interpleural pressure is reestablished.

POSTOPERATIVE CARE AND MONITORING

Considerations are similar to those for postthoracotomy patients. Close monitoring and evaluation of both respiratory and cardiovascular parameters are required in the postoperative period. Many patients have both impaired ventilation and oxygenation postoperatively, and adequate analgesia is extremely important to optimize ventilation. Supplemental oxygen may be needed for some time, especially in patients with pulmonary contusions or edema. Arrhythmias usually do not require treatment in the recovery period unless they are increasing in frequency or affecting blood pressure. Most patients require continuous cardiovascular monitoring and intravenous fluid support in the postoperative period.

REFERENCES

1. McDonnell W: Respiratory System. In Thurmon JC, Tranquilli WJ, Benson GJ, editors: *Veterinary anesthesia*, ed 3, Baltimore, 1996, Williams & Wilkins.
2. Nunn JF: *Nunn's applied respiratory physiology*, ed 4, Jordan Hill, Oxford, 1993, Butterworth-Heinemann.
3. Fiehl E, Perret C: Permissive hypercapnia: How permissive should we be? *Am J Respir Crit Care Med* 150:1722-1737, 1994.
4. Marshall C, Lindgren L, Marshall BE: Effects of halothane, enflurane, and isoflurane on hypoxic pulmonary vasoconstriction, *Anesthesiology* 60:304, 1984.
5. Hendricks JC, King LG: Practicality, usefulness, and limits of end-tidal carbon dioxide monitoring in critical small animal patients, *JVECC* 4:29-39, 1994.
6. Steffey EP: Inhalation anesthetics. In Thurmon JC, Tranquilli WJ, Benson GJ, editors: *Veterinary anesthesia*, ed 3, Baltimore, 1996, Williams & Wilkins.
7. Stepien RL, Bonagura JD, Bednarski RM et al: Cardiorespiratory effects of acepromazine maleate and buprenorphine hydrochloride in clinically normal dogs, *Am J Vet Res* 56(1):78-84, 1995.
8. Haskins SC, Farver TB, Patz JD: Cardiovascular changes in dogs given diazepam and diazepam-ketamine, *Am J Vet Res* 47(4):795-798, 1986.
9. Venugopalan CS, Holmes EP, Fucci V et al: Cardiopulmonary effects of medetomidine in heartworm-infected and noninfected dogs, *Am J Vet Res* 55:1148-1152, 1994.
10. Weil JV, McCullough RE, Kline JS et al: Diminished ventilatory response to hypoxia and hypercapnea after morphine in normal man, *N Engl J Med* 292:1103-1107, 1976.
11. Berg RJ, Orton EC: Pulmonary function in dogs after intercostal thoracotomy: Comparison of morphine, oxymorphone, and selective intercostal nerve block, *Am J Vet Res* 47(2):471-474, 1986.
12. Campbell VL, Drobatz KJ, Perkowski SZ: Postoperative hypoxemia and hypercarbia in healthy dogs undergoing routine ovariohysterectomy or castration and receiving butorphanol or hydromorphone for analgesia, *JAVMA* 2003 (in press).
13. Turner DM, Ilkiw JE: Cardiovascular and respiratory effects of three rapidly acting barbiturates in dogs, *Am J Vet Res* 51:598-604, 1990.
14. Morgan DWT, Legge K: Clinical evaluation of propofol as an intravenous anaesthetic agent in cats and dogs, *Vet Rec* 124:31-33, 1989.
15. Nagel ML, Muir WW, Nguyen K: Comparison of the cardiopulmonary effects of etomidate and thiamylal in dogs, *Am J Vet Res* 40:193-196, 1979.
16. Hellyer P, Muir WW, Hubbell JAE et al: Cardiorespiratory effects of the intravenous administration of tiletamine-zolazepam to cats, *Vet Surg* 17:105-110, 1988.
17. Lin HC: Dissociative anesthetics. In Thurmon JC, Tranquilli WJ, Benson GJ, editors: *Veterinary anesthesia*, ed 3, Baltimore, 1996, Williams & Wilkins.
18. Mann FA, Wagner-Mann C, Allert JA et al: Comparison of intranasal and intratracheal oxygen administration in healthy awake dogs, *Am J Vet Res* 53:856-860, 1992.
19. Johnson L: Small animal bronchoscopy, *Vet Clin North Am Small Anim Pract* 31:691-705, 2001.
20. Conzemius MG, Brockman DJ, King LG et al: Analgesia in dogs after intercostal thoracotomy: A clinical trial comparing intravenous buprenorphine and interpleural bupivacaine, *Vet Surg* 23:291-298, 1994.
21. Pascoe PJ, Dyson DH: Analgesia after lateral thoracotomy in dogs: Epidural morphine vs. intercostal bupivacaine, *Vet Surg* 22:141-147, 1993.
22. Wagner AE, Walton JA, Hellyer PW et al: Use of low doses of ketamine administered by constant rate infusion as an adjunct for postoperative analgesia in dogs, *JAVMA* 70:3-12, 2002.
23. Budsberg S: Nonsteroidal antiinflammatory agents. In J Gaynor, Muir W, editors: *Veterinary pain management*, St Louis, 2002, Mosby.
24. Cantwell SL, Duke T, Walsh PJ et al: One-lung versus two-lung ventilation in the closed-chest anesthetized dog: A comparison of cardiopulmonary parameters, *Vet Surg* 4:365-373, 2000.
25. Faunt KK, Cohn LA, Jones BD et al: Cardiopulmonary effects of bilateral hemithorax ventilation and diagnostic thoracoscopy in dogs, *Am J Vet Res* 59(11):1494-1498, 1998.
26. Ray RJ, Alexander CM, Chen L et al: Influence of the method of reexpansion of atelectatic lung upon the development of pulmonary edema in dogs, *Crit Care Med* 12:364-366, 1984.

CHAPTER 34

Fluid Therapy in Animals with Lung Disease

Dez Hughes

Introduction

The choice of intravenous fluids, and the choice of rates and volumes administered, remain contentious issues despite decades of clinical experience and thousands of experimental studies. The deleterious effects of fluid overload are especially severe in animals with brain, lung, or heart disease; and in those with anuric renal failure. Some side effects (e.g., subcutaneous interstitial edema) are not immediately life threatening, although it has been suggested that fluid-induced edema may compromise tissue oxygenation,[1] and there is evidence that edema impedes wound healing.[2,3] In contrast, cerebral and pulmonary edema can be fatal. The effects of edema in other organs such as the heart[4] and gastrointestinal tract[5] remain to be fully elucidated; however, it seems likely that edema could result in decreased myocardial performance and gastrointestinal dysfunction.

It is well established in certain human patient populations that higher fluid resuscitation volumes and rates[6-9] and fluid retention[10,11] can be associated with increased morbidity and lower survival rates, and that negative fluid balance can be associated with improved survival.[12] It is still unclear whether the link between fluid retention and mortality is a cause and effect relationship. It is also not surprising that people who develop pulmonary edema during resuscitation from circulatory shock have a higher mortality.[13] On the other hand, there are also studies that document improved survival with more aggressive fluid rates.[14] These results may seem contradictory, but the simple explanation is that aggressive fluid therapy is beneficial in some patients but harmful in others. Inappropriate fluid restriction in some patients with hypoperfusion may increase the likelihood of organ failure or disseminated intravascular coagulation. Hence the potential benefits of intravenous fluid therapy must be weighed against its risks, depending upon the characteristics of each individual case. There is no single best intravenous fluid, rate, or volume.

A rational approach to fluid therapy necessitates an appreciation of the distribution of water, electrolytes, and proteins among different body compartments; the factors involved in maintenance of intracellular, extracellular, and intravascular fluid volume; the homeostasis

of body osmolality (i.e., water balance); and the regulation of arterial blood pressure and tissue perfusion. Appreciation of the potential effects of fluid therapy on the lung also requires knowledge of how fluid homeostasis in the lung differs from that of the rest of the body with respect to normal and abnormal water, solute, and protein fluxes in the lung; the processes involved in edema formation; the defenses that protect against pulmonary fluid accumulation; and the mechanisms responsible for clearance of water, solute, and protein from the pulmonary interstitium and alveoli. A review of lung fluid balance is presented in Chapter 66.

Fluid therapy is not administered as a primary treatment for lung disease. Rather, a patient with concurrent lung disease usually requires fluid therapy for treatment of hypoperfusion, dehydration, or acid base and electrolyte disturbances. The aim of fluid therapy in animals with lung disease is to treat these other abnormalities while minimizing potential respiratory complications.

Overview of Intravenous Fluid Therapy

Intravenous fluids should not be regarded as a single entity; rather they should be viewed as a range of pharmacological products, each with its own indications and contraindications, much like the choices of antibiotics for different bacterial infections. The most appropriate fluid varies with the existing disease processes and fluid deficits. The main groups of fluids are crystalloids; artificial colloids; and blood products, including the hemoglobin-based oxygen carriers (HBOCs). Crystalloids are electrolyte solutions that can pass freely out of the vascular space, whereas colloids contain macromolecules that are retained within the vascular space for a longer time.

CRYSTALLOIDS

Crystalloids can be hypotonic, isotonic, or hypertonic; the tonicity of the solution will determine its distribution following intravenous infusion. Because free water rapidly passes out of the intravascular space and distributes across the total body water, it is ineffective as an intravascular volume expander and should not be used for the treatment of hypoperfusion. Rapid infusion of hypotonic solutions can also cause severe dilution of serum electrolytes, cerebral edema, and death.

The isotonic solutions most commonly available are normal (0.9%) saline and balanced electrolyte replacement solutions (e.g., Ringer's solution, lactated Ringer's solution, Plasmalyte, Normosol R, and Hartmann's solution). Intravascular crystalloid rapidly extravasates into the interstitial space, and 1 hour following infusion only 10% to 25% of the infused volume remains within the intravascular space.[15,16]

This means that relatively large fluid volumes of crystalloids are required for the resuscitation of hypovolemic patients, compared with the volumes of colloids, blood products, or hypertonic saline needed. Animals in severe hypovolemic shock may require crystalloid doses up to or in excess of 60 to 90 ml/kg/hr (dogs) and 40 to 60 ml/kg/hr (cats). In patients with parenchymal lung disease these volumes may cause significant reduction in plasma colloid osmotic pressure and increases in hydrostatic pressure, resulting in dangerous accumulation of extravascular lung water and pulmonary edema. Consequently, infusion volumes should be reduced according to the severity of heart or lung disease present. It is impossible to give general guidelines as to the appropriate fluid rate reduction in patients with lung and/or heart disease. For example, a dog with mild mitral regurgitation and a normally functioning myocardium may be able to tolerate aggressive intravenous fluid rates, whereas even slow infusion rates may be fatal in a cat with hypertrophic cardiomyopathy or endomyocarditis.

Intravenous infusion of hypertonic crystalloid creates a large osmotic gradient; water is drawn from the interstitial and intracellular compartments, producing a rapid expansion of intravascular volume. Hypertonic saline is most commonly used to treat hypovolemia at a concentration of 7.5% (2400 mOsm/L). A dose of 4 to 7 ml/kg (dogs) or 2 to 4 ml/kg (cats) is given over 5 minutes, and produces a hemodynamic response similar to 60 to 90 ml/kg of crystalloid. Excessively rapid infusion of hypertonic saline can cause acute hypotension.[17] Because sodium rapidly diffuses out of the vasculature, the effects wane only 30 minutes after infusion. To prolong the duration of action, hypertonic saline may be administered with a colloid such as dextran 70, hydroxyethyl starch (HES), or pentastarch.

Hypertonic saline is useful when extremely rapid intravascular volume expansion is required, such as in patients with severe hypovolemia when death is imminent. It is also useful in very large dogs and in hypovolemic animals with inappropriately small intravenous catheters. Hypertonic saline appears to be the most appropriate fluid for intravascular volume expansion in the patient at risk for increased intracranial pressure.[18,19] A combination of colloid and hypertonic saline may also be used in these cases to raise arterial blood pressure and to minimize the increase in intracranial pressure, thereby optimizing cerebral perfusion pressure.

Hypertonic saline is contraindicated in animals with hyperosmolality or dehydration.[20] Hypertonic saline resuscitation raises arterial blood pressure rapidly and should therefore be avoided in patients in which aggressive volume expansion would be dangerous (e.g., patients with heart or lung disease). It can also cause ventricular arrhythmias,[21] especially when given rapidly, so an electrocardiogram should be monitored during infusion. Although hypertonic saline resuscitation has been suggested for patients with pulmonary contusions,[22] experimental studies have demonstrated no benefit,[23] and actually it is probably too aggressive a resuscitation protocol for these patients. In fact, this author would suggest that hypertonic saline be avoided in all patients with parenchymal lung disease.

COLLOIDS

Because of their large molecular size, colloids are retained within the intravascular space; as a consequence, intravascular volume expansion is greater and lasts longer using colloids compared with crystalloids.[15,24,25] Colloids also maintain intravascular colloid osmotic pressure (COP), thereby reducing fluid extravasation. Tissue perfusion may also be better following colloid infusion compared with crystalloids.[26] There are three common types of artificial colloid: (1) gelatins, (2) dextrans, and (3) hydroxyethyl starches. Gelatins are produced from mammalian collagen, dextrans are prepared from bacterial fermentation of sucrose, and hydroxyethyl starches are derived from plant starch. The molecules of different artificial colloids vary in size and weight. Hydroxyethyl starches are the largest, followed by dextrans, then gelatins. The range of molecular weights in a particular colloid preparation vary widely (e.g., hydroxyethyl starch, 2 to 5000 kD; dextran 70, 20 to 200 kD). Albumin molecules, by comparison, are all the same size (molecular weight, 69 kD). A hydroxyethyl starch with a molecular weight of 100 to 300 kD provides the best compromise between colloid osmotic volume expansion and duration of action. This molecular weight range also causes fewer effects on coagulation and is the best size to reduce the increases in permeability seen in vascular leak states.[27] This particular molecular weight distribution is best provided by pentastarch.

The main indication for colloids is hypoproteinemia, especially in disease states associated with increased microvascular permeability, provided that the increase in permeability is insufficient to allow significant extravasation of colloid. During vascular leak states, the dilemma is the determination of the magnitude of the increase in microvascular barrier permeability. In some vascular leak states, permeability increases may be very large, especially in the lungs. Unfortunately there are no clinically applicable methods to assess microvascular permeability. An insufficient response to a colloid bolus, or an inappropriately short duration of action, may be the only way to suspect increased colloid extravasation.

Clinical experience and experimental studies suggest that animals with severe hypoproteinemia may exhibit peripheral edema but rarely develop pulmonary edema.[28] This is not surprising because increased lung lymph flow is remarkably effective in protecting the lung against edema.[28] However, cardiogenic (high pressure) pulmonary edema occurs at lower hydrostatic pressures when hypoproteinemia is present.[29-31] In dogs with hypoalbuminemia, hydroxyethyl starch treatment results in clinical improvement of peripheral edema and ascites.[32] In hypoproteinemic patients, it is most important to diagnose and treat the underlying cause because if there are large, ongoing losses, colloid support at standard doses may be ineffective.

The manufacturers' recommended dose for hydroxyethyl starch and dextran 70 is 20 ml/kg/day; however, there is no single correct dose or administration rate for colloid, just as there is no single correct dose for packed red blood cells. The rate and dose depend upon the reason for colloid therapy and the risks for volume overload. An extremely rapid rate (e.g., 20 ml/kg/hr) may be appropriate when treating hypovolemia in a dog with septic peritonitis; however, a normovolemic dog with chronic, severe hypoalbuminemia could appropriately receive 10 to 20 ml/kg over 12 to 24 hours. The dose of 20 ml/kg is a theoretical maximum daily dose because at higher doses clinicopathologic abnormalities of coagulation reliably occur. However, larger doses can be given in many cases without apparent ill effects. Because 20 ml/kg represents one quarter of a dog's blood volume, the underlying cause (usually bleeding or sepsis) should be aggressively pursued if repeated doses of this magnitude are necessary to maintain arterial blood pressure. In patients with parenchymal lung disease, colloids should be administered with caution because of the risk of increasing intravascular hydrostatic pressure and fluid extravasation into the lung. In general, except in exceptional circumstances (e.g., life-threatening hypovolemia), colloid infusion rates should be no more than 5 ml/kg/hr. Even this rate could be dangerous in patients with severe parenchymal disease.

The volume and duration of intravascular expansion seen with colloids is influenced by many factors including the species of animal, the dose administered, the specific colloid formulation, the pre-infusion intravascular volume status, and the permeability of the microvasculature. Initial plasma volume expansion for hydroxyethyl starch and dextran 70 varies from about 70% to 170% of the infused volume, then falls exponentially to approximately 50% of the infused volume after 6 hours.[15,33-36] With hydroxyethyl starch, volume expansion then declines gradually from 60% to 40% of the infused volume over the next 12 to 18 hours, whereas with dextran 70, it falls to 20% of the infused volume.[37] Gelatins have a shorter duration of action than other colloids. In an experimental study in rats, 1 hour after a 60-minute infusion, intravascular expansion with polygeline was only 23% of the infused volume[38]; hence the benefits of gelatins as a colloidal volume expander are questionable. The duration of volume expansion with colloids can be much shorter than expected, especially with capillary leak syndromes.

Reported complications of colloid therapy include volume overload, coagulopathy, allergic reactions, renal dysfunction, and interference with clinical biochemistry.

Because colloids are retained within the vasculature to a greater extent than crystalloids, there is a greater likelihood of volume overload. Most clinicians are familiar with crystalloid infusion rates, so a helpful method to ensure a safe colloid infusion rate is to estimate the equivalent crystalloid rate. Because only 20% to 25% of crystalloid remains within the intravascular space 1 hour following infusion (compared with approximately 100% of infused colloid), multiplying the colloid infusion rate by 4 to 5 affords an appreciation of the volume-expanding effects of the colloid in terms of an equivalent crystalloid rate. This approach can be especially helpful in patients with cardiac disease, pulmonary parenchymal disease, or oliguria. If a cat would not be expected to tolerate 50 ml/hr of crystalloid, then it should not be given 10 ml/hr of colloid.

All commonly used artificial colloids can cause hypocoagulability; however, this is often not clinically significant unless the animal has ongoing bleeding (e.g., with pulmonary contusions) or has a preexisting coagulopathy or thrombocytopathia. Coagulation is more affected after larger doses or repeated administration. Following colloid administration there is a reduction in Factor VIII and von Willebrand factor (greater than that expected by dilution alone) and weakened clot formation.[39-43] In animals with a coagulopathy or thrombocytopathia it seems wise to avoid artificial colloids or to supplement clotting factors using fresh frozen plasma. Desmopressin, which increases factor VIII:C activity following hydroxyethyl starch infusion, can also be used as adjunct therapy.[44]

The low molecular weight dextrans, such as dextran 40, have been reported to cause renal failure.[45,46] Glomerular filtration of a high concentration of small dextran molecules is postulated to cause blockage of the renal tubules and/or osmotic nephrosis.[45,46] The major route of excretion for all artificial colloids is the kidney, so these should be used with caution in patients with renal failure. In contradistinction, in patients with capillary leak syndrome and oliguria caused by hypovolemia and hypotension, colloids may be the most effective means of increasing intravascular volume. A recent study has raised the possibility that the use of hydroxyethyl starch may be a risk factor for acute renal failure in people with sepsis or septic shock[47]; however, clinical experience in small animals suggests that this is very rare.

Dextrans, hydroxyethyl starches, and gelatins can all cause anaphylactic or anaphylactoid reactions;[48] however, the incidence of serious complications is extremely low.[49] Hydroxyethyl starch has also been associated with pruritus in as many as one third of people receiving long-term infusions. Deposits of hydroxyethyl starch in cutaneous nerves[50] and histiocytic skin infiltrates[51] have been identified. Colloid-induced immune dysfunction has also been postulated because large colloid molecules are taken up by the monocyte phagocytic system[52] and decreased plasma concentrations of fibronectin are seen following treatment with artificial gelatins[53] and hydroxyethyl starch.[54]

Measurement of refractometric total solids is no longer accurate after colloid therapy.[55] Hydroxyethyl starch and dextran 70 both yield refractometric total solids concentration (RTS) of 4.5 g/dL. During in vitro dilution studies, as plasma is replaced by artificial colloid, RTS should tend toward that of the colloid. If the initial plasma RTS is greater than 4.5 g/dL, colloid should cause a decline, whereas if the starting plasma RTS is less than 4.5 g/dL, colloid should cause an increase. Unfortunately, the situation in vivo is more complicated because of other influences (e.g., extravasation and excretion of colloid and fluid shifts into the vasculature following administration). Virtually all clinical patients with a pre-infusion RTS higher than 4.5 g/dL experience a fall in RTS following colloid administration. Increases in RTS following colloid seem very uncommon irrespective of the starting RTS reading. Failure to recognize the potential fall in RTS because of dilution by the colloid itself can mislead the clinician to misinterpret the fall in RTS as an indication for more colloid. Objective measures of hemodilution (e.g., plasma albumin concentration) almost invariably fall after colloid infusion. Serum amylase may be increased by 200% to 250% following hydroxyethyl starch administration because of complex formation and reduced excretion.[56,57] Hydroxyethyl starch can also cause potentially misleading results in blood typing and cross-matching because of increased rouleaux formation.[58]

Albumin has a molecular weight of approximately 69,000 Daltons and a molecular radius of 3.5 nm. In addition to its role in maintaining plasma COP, it also carries a wide range of substances such as bilirubin, fatty acids, metals and other ions, hormones, and drugs. Albumin is most commonly given to small animal patients as stored or fresh frozen plasma, stored whole blood, or fresh whole blood. Although intravascular albumin is the main determinant of COP, it equilibrates with the interstitial space more rapidly and to a greater extent than artificial colloids. This means that large volumes must be given to achieve a sustained rise in plasma COP. For example, two liters of plasma are required to raise the serum albumin from 1.5 g/dL to 2.5 g/dL in a 20-kg dog.

At least three meta-analyses have questioned the effectiveness of artificial and natural colloids for resuscitation of critically ill people.[59-61] Indeed, in certain patient populations there was a higher overall mortality with colloids compared with crystalloids. In one study involving trauma patients, a 12.3% difference in mortality rate in favor of crystalloid therapy was demonstrated.[59] Conversely, when data from studies of nontrauma patients were pooled, there was a 7.8% difference in mortality rate in favor of colloid treatment.[59] The authors concluded that colloid therapy was potentially deleterious in patients with sepsis, capillary leak syndrome, and adult respiratory distress syndrome following trauma.[59]

OXYGEN CARRYING SUPPORT

Maintaining adequate oxygen delivery to tissues is of paramount importance. Oxygen delivery is the product of the amount of bloodflow (proportional to cardiac output) and the total oxygen content of the blood. Oxygen is carried in two ways in the bloodstream: (1) bound to

hemoglobin and (2) dissolved in plasma. However, the vast majority of oxygen (approximately 98.5%) is carried by hemoglobin. Hemoglobin can therefore be viewed as the oxygen reservoir for the tissues. Hence it is vital in animals with lung disease, when PaO_2 may be lower than normal, that adequate hemoglobin levels are maintained. This can be achieved by transfusion of whole blood; packed red blood cells; or the hemoglobin-based, oxygen-carrying solution, Oxyglobin (Biopure, Cambridge, MA). Packed cell volume (PCV) should not be allowed to fall below 20% and ideally should be kept nearer 30%. If HBOCs are used, the PCV will be diluted and is no longer an accurate indicator of total blood hemoglobin levels. In this instance, if a hemoglobinometer is not available, then the clinician must rely on clinical signs and clinical judgment. Whereas Oxyglobin provides temporary oxygen-carrying support, it should be used with caution in patients with lung disease. It is a potent colloid and can be associated with volume overload.[62] It is also a nitric oxide scavenger[63] and can cause increases in pulmonary and systemic vascular resistance that could contribute to pulmonary edema and compromise cardiac function in animals with cardiac insufficiency.[64,65] The increases in systemic vascular resistance could potentially be beneficial in patients with systemic inflammatory response syndrome and inappropriate peripheral vasodilation.

Transfusion-related lung injury is a little-known complication of blood transfusion. In humans and in experimental studies in dogs, blood transfusion has been associated with increased permeability edema.[66,67] Transfusion-related acute lung injury in humans carries a mortality rate of 5% to 14%, making it the third leading cause of transfusion-related mortality. Although this phenomenon has not been reported to the author's knowledge in clinical veterinary medicine, it seems likely that it may occur.

Fluid Therapy in Animals with Lung Disease

All patients with lung disease are not at risk of developing pulmonary edema. Rather, pulmonary edema can worsen, or can develop in addition to another primary lung disease, if the patient's lungs are susceptible to elevations in pulmonary capillary hydrostatic pressure that may occur with higher rates of intravenous fluid administration. Susceptibility to increases in pulmonary hydrostatic pressure can be expected in animals with conditions that predispose to high pressure pulmonary edema (e.g., left-sided heart failure or insufficiency) or the various forms of increased permeability pulmonary edema (see Table 66-1).

The likelihood of fluid extravasation, and the subsequent development of pulmonary edema, therefore depends on the magnitude of the fluid therapy-induced increase in hydrostatic pressure and the permeability of the microvascular barrier. Marked increases in hydrostatic pressure (i.e., intravascular volume overload) will result in pulmonary edema even when microvascular permeability is normal, irrespective of the type of fluid used. When pulmonary microvascular permeability is increased, the fluid-retaining effect of the intravascular colloid osmotic pressure is reduced or lost, and relatively small rises in pulmonary capillary hydrostatic pressure can then result in extensive fluid loss into the lung.

The importance of the hydrostatic pressure gradient in both high-pressure and increased permeability edema cannot be overemphasized. Hydrostatic pressure is by far the major force acting to cause fluid extravasation into the lung parenchyma. Whereas the importance of minimizing hydrostatic pressure in high pressure edema is self evident, its role in increased permeability edema is less intuitive but even more important. With high-pressure edema, increases in lung weight do not occur until pulmonary capillary pressures reach approximately 25 mm Hg. In contrast, with increased permeability edema, lung weight increases at pulmonary capillary pressures of 12 mm Hg. In normal lungs the pulmonary endothelium is relatively permeable to protein compared to other tissues,[68] and albumin[69] and hetastarch[70] molecules equilibrate rapidly with the interstitial space. If the increase in permeability is small, then colloid molecules will remain within the intravascular space and reduce lung water or limit its increase.[71] If the increase in endothelial permeability is sufficient so that the majority of colloid molecules can pass through the pulmonary capillary endothelium, then colloid therapy may worsen pulmonary edema.[72] When administering colloid to a patient with the potential for increased pulmonary microvascular permeability it therefore makes sense to use hydroxyethyl starch, the colloid with the largest average molecular weight.

The effects of increases in hydrostatic pressure and microvascular permeability on the development of pulmonary edema after fluid therapy have been borne out in experimental and clinical studies. In dogs with experimental increased permeability pulmonary edema, aggressive infusions of saline and dextran 70 caused no increase in lung weight when left atrial pressure was kept constant.[73] In contrast, when left atrial pressure was allowed to increase, lung weight increased with both crystalloid and colloid infusion.[70] In an experimental study of smoke inhalation, dogs were given 50 ml/kg/hr of lactated Ringer's solution for 2 hours.[74] The control group without lung injury had no increase in extravascular lung water; the group with smoke inhalation that received fluids had a 50% increase in lung water compared with those exposed to smoke but not treated with fluids.[71] In a clinical study of blood products and colloids in human ARDS patients, those in the early stages of ARDS experienced improvement in cardiorespiratory function providing that wedge pressures of 18 mm Hg were not exceeded.[75] In patients in the later stages of ARDS, presumably with worsening pulmonary microvascular permeability, colloids worsened lung function.[72]

Nevertheless, patients with mild to moderate increases in pulmonary microvascular permeability may benefit from colloid infusion, especially if there is concurrent hypoproteinemia. It therefore seems prudent to evaluate the response of the animal to a cautious test infusion of colloid. If respiratory signs worsen after colloid infusion, then it is probably inadvisable to continue colloid therapy. Once pulmonary edema is established, the weight of evidence derived from experimental and clinical studies leans towards careful fluid restriction. This is especially important if positive pressure ventilation is not available, when serious deterioration of Pao_2 may be fatal. Restriction of fluid therapy in the patient with pulmonary edema must be weighed against the potential risks (e.g., compromised renal or cardiovascular function and multiple organ failure). Although aggressive fluid therapy can worsen lung function, under-resuscitation has been associated with an increased likelihood of people developing ARDS.[76] Therefore it appears that a very fine line exists between giving too much fluids and not enough.

Attention has been focused on the factors involved in the formation of pulmonary edema (i.e., increased hydrostatic pressure and increased permeability) whereas the concept that reduced drainage of fluid from the lung may contribute to pulmonary edema has largely been overlooked. Fluid is cleared from the pulmonary parenchyma via the bronchial circulation, pulmonary lymphatics, and by drainage into the pleural space and visceral pleural veins. Because the former two drain into the right side of the heart, increased cranial vena caval pressure may retard pulmonary fluid clearance. This potential effect seems to be more significant with increased permeability edema than with high-pressure edema. In dogs with experimental increased permeability pulmonary edema, increasing the cranial vena caval pressure while controlling right and left atrial pressure at baseline resulted in a large increase in extravascular lung water.[77] This is obviously relevant to fluid therapy because increases in central venous pressure are an expected result of receiving intravenous fluids.

Experimental evidence and clinical experience supports the view that aggressive volume expansion in patients with uncontrolled hemorrhage is associated with increased bleeding and a higher mortality rate.[78-85] This is likely because of increased volumes of hemorrhage and loss of red blood cells, platelets, and clotting factors. The most common situation in which uncontrolled hemorrhage is encountered is following vehicular trauma. Intraabdominal hemorrhage and pulmonary contusions are the most common sites of bleeding. Pulmonary hemorrhage appears to be exquisitely sensitive to volume expansion. Aggressive fluid resuscitation almost always worsens pulmonary bleeding, and this author considers aggressive volume expansion to be absolutely contraindicated in this patient population. The concept of hypotensive resuscitation, where gradual intravascular volume expansion is performed over a longer period, has been gaining support in recent years and may be particularly relevant in the management of animals with pulmonary contusions.

When most animals first present in left-sided heart failure, it is usually safest to treat with cage rest, oxygen supplementation, and diuresis, and not to administer any intravenous fluids for at least the first 12 to 24 hours. Subsequently, animals that will not voluntarily drink sufficient amounts and that become dehydrated may be placed on low intravenous fluid rates (e.g., half of normal maintenance fluid rates) using half strength (0.45%) saline. Sodium overload must be avoided in these patients because they are likely to avidly retain sodium as a result of reduced effective circulating blood volume and activation of the renin, angiotensin, aldosterone system. Although administration of fluids by the subcutaneous route has less immediate effects on the intravascular compartment, it can still be associated with volume overload in susceptible patients such as those with heart disease or oliguric renal failure. Some authors have suggested that hypotonic fluids such as half strength saline should not be given by the subcutaneous route. They postulate that there is the potential for electrolytes to diffuse into the subcutaneous fluid pocket, thereby worsening hypovolemia. Whether this is actually clinically significant remains unclear.

Patients with heart disease that results in diastolic dysfunction (e.g., those with hypertrophic cardiomyopathy) may be more preload dependent. In these cases, dehydration and reduced preload may precipitate life-threatening reductions in cardiac output; therefore avoidance of dehydration by use of judicious fluid therapy may be necessary. If possible, patients with heart disease that require intravenous fluid therapy should have a central venous catheter placed to allow monitoring of central venous pressure. This is especially useful in animals with concurrent heart disease and hypovolemia, when higher fluid rates might be necessary. Central venous pressure reflects right-sided rather than left-sided cardiac filling pressures. Therefore, in some cases, a pulmonary arterial catheter may be used to measure pulmonary capillary wedge pressure (pulmonary artery occlusion pressure), which is more representative of left-sided cardiac pressures.

Fluid therapy in animals with pulmonary edema secondary to left-sided heart failure is potentially dangerous because of the risk of increasing the already elevated pulmonary hydrostatic pressure, and worsening pulmonary edema. However, it is well established that a lower intravascular COP reduces the hydrostatic pressure at which high-pressure edema occurs.[29-31] In dogs with a plasma protein concentration reduced to 47% of normal, lung water begins to accumulate at left atrial pressures of only 11 mm Hg, compared with 24 mm Hg in dogs with a normal plasma protein concentration.[29] Hence hypoproteinemic animals in heart failure may benefit from carefully increasing the intravascular COP via colloid administration. This should be done with extreme caution to avoid increases in pulmonary capillary hydrostatic pressure. Because of the opposing effects of intravascular hydrostatic pressure and COP, the gradient between pulmonary artery occlusion pressure and COP has been used in the management of pulmonary edema.[13,86] Colloid support in the patient with left-sided heart failure should only be considered in animals with significant hypoproteinemia in a critical care environment with invasive monitoring capabilities.

REFERENCES

1. Heughan C, Ninikoski J, Hunt TK: Effect of excessive infusion of saline solution on tissue oxygen transport, *Surg Gynecol Obstet* 135(2):257, 1972.
2. Pai MP, Hunt TK: Effect of varying oxygen tensions on healing of open wounds, *Surg Gynecol Obstet* 135(5):756, 1972.
3. Armstrong DG, Nguyen HC: Improvement in healing with aggressive edema reduction after debridement of foot infection in persons with diabetes, *Arch Surg* 135(12):1405, 2000.
4. Dean DA, Amirhamzeh MM, Jia CX et al: Reversal of iatrogenic myocardial edema and related abnormalities of diastolic properties in the pig left ventricle, *J Thorac Cardiovasc Surg* 115(5):1209, 1998.
5. Prien T, Backhaus N, Pelster F et al: Effect of intraoperative fluid administration and colloid osmotic pressure on the formation of intestinal edema during gastrointestinal surgery, *J Clin Anesth* 2(5):317, 1990.
6. Kollmorgen DR, Murray KA, Sullivan JJ et al: Predictors of mortality in pulmonary contusion, *Am J Surg* 168(6):659, 1994.
7. Sakano T, Yamayoshi S, Higashi K et al: The effect of blood volume replacement on the mortality of head-injured patient, *Acta Neurochir Suppl (Wien)* 60:482, 1994.
8. Vassar MJ, Moore J, Perry CA et al: Early fluid requirements in trauma patients: A predictor of pulmonary failure and mortality, *Arch Surg* 123(9):1149, 1988.
9. Shah KJ, Chiu WC, Scalea TM et al: Detrimental effects of rapid fluid resuscitation on hepatocellular function and survival after hemorrhagic shock, *Shock* 18(3):242, 2002.
10. Lowell JA, Schifferdecker C, Driscoll DF et al: Postoperative fluid overload: Not a benign problem, *Crit Care Med* 18(7):728, 1990.
11. Sauven P, Playforth MJ, Evans M et al: Fluid sequestration: an early indicator of mortality in acute pancreatitis, *Br J Surg* 73(10):799, 1986.
12. Alsous F, Khamiees M, DeGirolamo A et al: Negative fluid balance predicts survival in patients with septic shock: A retrospective pilot study, *Chest* 117(6):1749, 2000.
13. Rackow EC, Fein IA, Siegel J: The relationship of the colloid osmotic-pulmonary artery wedge pressure gradient to pulmonary edema and mortality in critically ill patients, *Chest* 82(4):433, 1982.
14. Mock C, Visser L, Denno D et al: Aggressive fluid resuscitation and broad spectrum antibiotics decrease mortality from typhoid ileal perforation, *Trop Doct* 25(3):115, 1995.
15. Lamke LO, Liljedahl SO: Plasma volume changes after infusion of various plasma expanders, *Resuscitation* 5(2):93, 1976.
16. Shoemaker WC: Comparison of the relative effectiveness of whole blood transfusions and various types of fluid therapy in resuscitation, *Crit Care Med* 4:71-78, 1976.
17. Kien ND, Kramer GC, White DA: Acute hypotension caused by rapid hypertonic saline infusion in anesthetized dogs, *Anesth Analg* 73(5):597, 1991.
18. Prough DS, Johnson JC, Poole GVJ et al: Effects on intracranial pressure of resuscitation from hemorrhagic shock with hypertonic saline versus lactated Ringer's solution, *Crit Care Med* 13(5):407, 1985.
19. Schmoker JD, Zhuang J, Shackford SR: Hypertonic fluid resuscitation improves cerebral oxygen delivery and reduces intracranial pressure after hemorrhagic shock, *J Trauma* 31(12):1607, 1991.
20. Malcolm DS, Friedland M, Moore T et al: Hypertonic saline resuscitation detrimentally affects renal function and survival in dehydrated rats, *Circulatory Shock* 40(1):69, 1993.
21. Muir WW: Small volume resuscitation using hypertonic saline, *Cornell Vet* 80(1):7, 1990.
22. Duval D: Use of hypertonic saline solution in hypovolemic shock, *Compendium Contin Educ Pract Vet,* 17(10):1228-1231, 1995.
23. Cohn SM, Fisher BT, Rosenfield AT et al: Resuscitation of pulmonary contusion: Hypertonic saline is not beneficial, *Shock* 8(4): 292, 1997.
24. Dawidson IJ, Willms C, Sandor ZF et al: Lactated Ringer's solution versus 3% albumin for resuscitation of a lethal intestinal ischemic shock in rats, *Crit Care Med* 18:60-66, 1990.
25. Shoemaker WC, Schluchter M, Hopkins JA et al: Comparison of the relative effectiveness of colloids and crystalloids in emergency resuscitation, *Am J Surg* 142:73-84, 1981.

26. Funk W, Baldinger V: Microcirculatory perfusion during volume therapy: A comparative study using crystalloid or colloid in awake animals, *Anesthesiology* 82:975-982, 1995.

27. Zikria BA, King TC, Stanford J et al: A biophysical approach to capillary permeability, *Surgery* 105:625-631, 1989.

28. Zarins CK, Rice CL, Peters RM et al: Lymph and pulmonary response to isobaric reduction in plasma oncotic pressure in baboons, *Circ Res* 43:925-930, 1978.

29. Guyton AC, Lindsay NW: Effect of elevated left atrial pressure and decreased plasma protein concentration on the development of pulmonary edema, *Circ Res* 7:649-657, 1959.

30. Gaar KAJ, Taylor AE, Owens LJ et al: Effect of capillary pressure and plasma protein on development of pulmonary edema, *Am J Physiol* 213:79-82, 1967.

31. Kramer GC, Harms BA, Bodai BI et al: Effects of hypoproteinemia and increased vascular pressure on lung fluid balance in sheep, *J Applied Physiol: Respir, Environ & Exercise Physiol* 55:1514-1522, 1983.

32. Smiley LE, Garvey MS: The use of hetastarch as adjunct therapy in 26 dogs with hypoalbuminemia: a phase two clinical trial, *J Vet Intern Med* 8:195-202, 1994.

33. Rieger A: Blood volume and plasma protein. Changes in blood volume and plasma proteins after bleeding and immediate substitution with Macrodex, Rheomacrodex and Physiogel in the splenectomized dog, *Acta Chirurgica Scandinavica* (Suppl) 379:22-38, 1967.

34. Gollub S, Kangwalklai K, Schaefer C: Treatment of experimental hemorrhage with colloid-crystalloid mixtures, *J Surg Res* 9:311-317, 1969.

35. Hempel V, Metzger G, Unseld H et al: The influence of hydroxyethyl starch solutions on circulation and on kidney function in hypovolaemic patients, *Anaesthetist* 24:198-201, 1975.

36. Korttila K, Grohn P, Gordin A et al: Effect of hydroxyethyl starch and dextran on plasma volume and blood hemostasis and coagulation, *J Clin Pharmacol* 24:273-282, 1984.

37. Thompson WL, Fukushima T, Rutherford RB et al: Intravascular persistence, tissue storage, and excretion of hydroxyethyl starch, *Surg, Gynecol & Obstet* 131:965-972, 1970.

38. Ostgaard G, Onarheim H: Retention and distribution of polygeline (Haemaccel) in the rat, *Acta Anaesthesiol Scand* 40(1):96, 1996.

39. Gollub S, Schaefer C: Structural alteration in canine fibrin produced by colloid plasma expanders, *Surg, Gynecol & Obstet* 127:783-793, 1968.

40. Aberg M, Arfors KE, Bergentz SE: Effect of dextran on factor VIII and thrombus stability in humans: Significance of varying infusion rates, *Acta Chirurgica Scandinavica* 143:417-419, 1977.

41. Aberg M, Hedner U, Bergentz SE: Effect of dextran 70 on factor VIII and platelet function in von Willebrand's disease, *Thrombosis Research* 12:629-634, 1978.

42. Gollub S, Schaefer C, Squitieri A: The bleeding tendency associated with plasma expanders, *Surg, Gynecol & Obstet* 124:1203-1211, 1967.

43. Jones PA, Tomasic M, Gentry PA: Oncotic, hemodilutional, and hemostatic effects of isotonic saline and hydroxyethyl starch solutions in clinically normal ponies, *Am J Vet Res* 58:541-548, 1997.

44. Conroy JM, Fishman RL, Reeves ST et al: The effects of desmopressin and 6% hydroxyethyl starch on factor VIII:C, *Anesthesia & Analgesia* 83:804-807, 1996.

45. Mailloux L, Swartz CD, Capizzi R et al: Acute renal failure after administration of low-molecular weight dextran, *New Eng J Med* 277:1113-1118, 1967.

46. Ferraboli R, Malheiro PS, Abdulkader RC et al: Anuric acute renal failure caused by dextran 40 administration, *Renal Failure* 19:303-306, 1997.

47. Schortgen F, Lacherade JC, Bruneel F et al: Effects of hydroxyethyl starch and gelatin on renal function in severe sepsis: A multicentre randomised study, *Lancet* 357(9260):911, 2001.

48. Ring J: Anaphylactoid reactions to plasma substitutes, *Int Anesthesiol Clin* 23:67-95, 1985.

49. Ring J, Messmer K: Incidence and severity of anaphylactoid reactions to colloid volume substitutes, *Lancet* 1:466-469, 1977.

50. Metze D, Reimann S, Szepfalusi Z et al: Persistent pruritus after hydroxyethyl starch infusion therapy: A result of long-term storage in cutaneous nerves, *Brit J Dermatol* 136:553-559, 1997.

51. Cox NH, Popple AW: Persistent erythema and pruritus, with a confluent histiocytic skin infiltrate, following the use of a hydroxyethyl starch plasma expander, *Brit J Dermatol* 134:353-357, 1996.

52. Schildt B, Bouveng R, Sollenberg M: Plasma substitute induced impairment of the reticuloendothelial system function, *Acta Chirurgica Scandinavica* 141:7-13, 1975.

53. Brodin B, Hesselvik F, von SH: Decrease of plasma fibronectin concentration following infusion of a gelatin-based plasma substitute in man, *Scand J Clin Lab Invest* 44:529-533, 1984.

54. Treib J, Haass A, Pindur G et al: Decrease of fibronectin following repeated infusion of highly substituted hydroxyethyl starch, *Infusionstherapie und Transfusionsmedizin* 23:71-75, 1996.

55. Bumpus SE, Haskins SC, Kass PH: Effect of synthetic colloids on refractometric readings of total solids, *J Vet Emerg Crit Care* 8(1):21-26, 1998.

56. Boon JC, Jesch F, Ring J et al: Intravascular persistence of hydroxyethyl starch in man, *Eur Surg Res* 8:497-503, 1976.

57. Kohler H, Kirch W, Horstmann HJ: Hydroxyethyl starch-induced macroamylasemia, *Int J Clin Pharmacol Biopharm* 15:428-431, 1977.

58. Daniels MJ, Strauss RG, Smith-Floss AM: Effects of hydroxyethyl starch on erythrocyte typing and blood crossmatching, *Transfusion* 22:226-228, 1982.

59. Velanovich V: Crystalloid versus colloid fluid resuscitation: A meta-analysis of mortality, *Surgery* 105:65-71, 1989.

60. Schierhout G, Roberts I: Fluid resuscitation with colloid or crystalloid solutions in critically ill patients: A systematic review of randomised trials, *Brit Med J* 316:961-964, 1998.

61. Cochrane Injuries Group Albumin: Human albumin administration in critically ill patients: Systematic review of randomised controlled trials, *BMJ* 317(7153):235, 1998.

62. Gibson GR, Callan MB, Hoffman V et al: Use of a hemoglobin-based oxygen-carrying solution in cats: 72 cases (1998-2000), *JAVMA* 221(1):96, 2002.

63. Rooney MW, Hirsch LJ, Mathru M: Hemodilution with oxyhemoglobin: Mechanism of oxygen delivery and its superaugmentation with a nitric oxide donor (sodium nitroprusside), *Anesthesiology* 79(1):60, 1993.

64. Maxwell RA, Gibson JB, Fabian TC et al: Resuscitation of severe chest trauma with four different hemoglobin-based oxygen-carrying solutions, *J Trauma* 49(2):200, 2000.

65. Muir WWIII, de Morais HS, Constable PD: The effects of a hemoglobin-based oxygen carrier (HBOC-301) on left ventricular systolic function in anesthetized dogs, *Vet Surg* 29(5):449, 2000.

66. Bennett SH, Geelhoed GW, Aaron RK et al: Pulmonary injury resulting from perfusion with stored bank blood in the baboon and dog, *J Surg Res* 13(6):295, 1972.

67. Popovsky MA: Transfusion and lung injury, *Transfus Clin Biol* 8(3):272, 2001.

68. Parker JC, Perry MA, Taylor AE: Permeability of the microvascular barrier. In Staub NC, Taylor AE, editors: *Edema*, New York, 1984, Raven Press.

69. Vaughan TRJ, Erdmann AJ, Brigham KL et al: Equilibration of intravascular albumin with lung lymph in unanesthetized sheep, *Lymphology* 12:217, 1979.

70. Korent VA, Conhaim RL, McGrath AM et al: Molecular distribution of hetastarch in plasma and lung lymph of unanesthetized sheep, *Am J Respir Crit Care Med* 155:1302, 1997.

71. Tanaka H, Dahms TE, Bell E et al: Effect of hydroxyethyl starch on alveolar flooding in acute lung injury in dogs, *Am Rev Respir Dis* 148(4 Pt 1):852, 1993.

72. Holcroft JW, Trunkey DD, Carpenter MA: Extravasation of albumin in tissues of normal and septic baboons and sheep, *J Surg Res* 26:341, 1979.

73. Rutili G, Parker JC, Taylor AE: Fluid balance in ANTU-injured lungs during crystalloid and colloid infusions, *J Appl Physiol: Respir, Envir & Exercise Physiol* 56(4):993, 1984.

74. Clark WRJ, Nieman GF, Goyette D et al: Effects of crystalloid on lung fluid balance after smoke inhalation, *Ann Surg* 208(1):56, 1988.

75. Appel PL, Shoemaker WC: Evaluation of fluid therapy in adult respiratory failure, *Crit Care Med* 9(12):862, 1981.

76. Bishop MH, Jorgens J, Shoemaker WC et al: The relationship between ARDS, pulmonary infiltration, fluid balance, and hemodynamics in critically ill surgical patients, *Am Surg* 57(12):785, 1991.

77. Ando F, Arakawa M, Kambara K et al: Effect of superior vena caval hypertension on alloxan-induced lung injury in dogs, *J Appl Physiol* 68(2):478, 1990.
78. Sakles JC, Sena MJ, Knight DA et al: Effect of immediate fluid resuscitation on the rate, volume, and duration of pulmonary vascular hemorrhage in a sheep model of penetrating thoracic trauma, *Ann Emerg Med* 29(3):392, 1997.
79. Solomonov E, Hirsh M, Yahiya A et al: The effect of vigorous fluid resuscitation in uncontrolled hemorrhagic shock after massive splenic injury, *Crit Care Med* 28(3):749, 2000.
80. Abu-Hatoum O, Bashenko Y, Hirsh M et al: Continuous fluid resuscitation and splenectomy for treatment of uncontrolled hemorrhagic shock after massive splenic injury, *J Trauma* 52(2):253, 2002.
81. Abu-Hatum O, Bashenko Y, Hirsh M et al: Continuous fluid resuscitation for treatment of uncontrolled hemorrhagic shock following massive splenic injury in rats, *Shock* 18(6):574, 2002.
82. Krausz MM, Bashenko Y, Hirsh M: Crystalloid or colloid resuscitation of uncontrolled hemorrhagic shock after moderate splenic injury, *Shock* 13(3):230, 2000.
83. Krausz MM, Bashenko Y, Hirsh M: Crystalloid and colloid resuscitation of uncontrolled hemorrhagic shock following massive splenic injury, *Shock* 16(5):383, 2001.
84. Bickell WH, Wall MJ Jr., Pepe PE et al: Immediate versus delayed fluid resuscitation for hypotensive patients with penetrating torso injuries, *New Eng J Med* 331(17):1105, 1994.
85. Hambly PR Dutton RP. Excess mortality associated with the use of a rapid infusion system at a level 1 trauma center, *Resuscitation* 31(2):127, 1996.
86. Weil MH, Henning RJ, Morissette M et al: Relationship between colloid osmotic pressure and pulmonary artery wedge pressure in patients with acute cardiorespiratory failure, *Am J Med* 64(4):643, 1978.

PART FIVE

Disorders of the Respiratory Tract:

A. Nasal Cavity and Sinuses

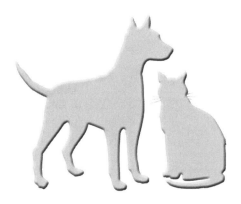

CHAPTER 35

Feline Viral Upper Respiratory Disease

Alan D. Radford • Rosalind M. Gaskell • Susan Dawson

Definition

Feline calicivirus (FCV) and feline herpesvirus (FeHV, also called feline rhinotracheitis virus) remain the two major causes of infectious upper respiratory tract disease in cats. Despite the widespread use of vaccines over some 30 years, respiratory disease caused by these two viruses remains a significant clinical problem. In general, the disease is most commonly seen where cats are grouped together (e.g., in boarding catteries or breeding establishments), particularly in young kittens as they lose their maternally-derived antibody.

When considering a case of apparently infectious respiratory disease in cats, it is important to remember that other pathogens may be involved, and it may be appropriate to include diagnostic testing for these as part of a diagnostic work-up. In addition to FCV and FeHV, there is in-

creasing evidence that *Bordetella bronchiseptica* is an important cause of respiratory disease in cats. *Chlamydophila felis* (previously *Chlamydia psittaci var felis*) may also cause respiratory disease, although it is predominantly associated with conjunctivitis. Other agents that have also been associated with feline respiratory disease include feline reovirus, cowpox virus, and various bacteria and mycoplasmas.

Etiology

FELINE CALICIVIRUS

Feline calicivirus is a small, nonenveloped, single-stranded RNA virus belonging to the *Caliciviridae*. This virus family contains a large number of important pathogens of man and animals including the Norwalk-like and Sapporo-like viruses (both important causes of diarrhea in man and other animals) and rabbit hemorrhagic disease virus (a generally fatal disease of rabbits). However, the viruses most closely related to FCV are vesicular exanthema of swine virus (no longer isolated), San Miguel sea lion virus, and canine calicivirus (CaCV). These have been grouped together in the vesivirus genus, reflecting a general ability of viruses in this genus to induce vesicles as a prominent part of their pathology.

FCV infects both domestic cats and other members of the Felidae.[1,2] Although CaCV is genetically distinct from FCV,[3] other caliciviruses have also been detected in dogs that antigenically cross-react and genetically cluster with FCV.[3-5] This raises the possibility that dogs may be infected by FCV-like viruses, and that if they are, these viruses may be transmitted between dogs and cats. However, the significance of these canine FCV-like viruses to either dogs or cats remains largely uncertain.

When the genetic sequences of different FCV isolates are compared with each other, they show a considerable amount of variability. This heterogeneity is often a feature of RNA viruses and is a reflection of the low accuracy or fidelity of the viral encoded polymerase. This leads to plasticity of the viral genome and the potential to generate variants at relatively rapid rates in comparison with organisms whose genetic material is based on DNA. Despite the observed variability of FCVs, comparative genetic analysis has failed to separate isolates of FCV into distinct clusters or genogroups. There appears to be no clear correlation between the sequence of a virus and either its year or location of isolation, or with the particular disease with which it is associated.[6-10] The genetic diversity of FCV has been used to develop typing methods based largely on sequence analysis to differentiate between isolates. These methods have been used to explore the epidemiology of FCV-related disease and the role of live vaccine virus in disease in recently vaccinated animals.[11-13]

This variability of the FCV genome has important implications to the antigenicity of this virus. The sequence variability has been shown to be particularly pronounced in key regions of the capsid protein that are responsible for the antigenic structure of the virus. It is therefore perhaps not surprising that most strains of FCV can be distinguished from one another on the basis of their antigenicity. However, there is sufficient cross-reactivity between FCV strains to allow them to be grouped together in a single serotype and to allow some degree of cross-protection between the majority of strains. This has important implications in relation to vaccine design.

FELINE HERPESVIRUS

Feline herpesvirus is a member of the herpesvirus family and has a double-stranded DNA genome with a glycoprotein-lipid envelope. It is classified in the alphaherpesvirus subfamily, which contains most of the herpesviruses of veterinary interest and is very closely related genetically and antigenically to canine herpesvirus-1 and phocine (seal) herpesvirus-1.[14-17] Although the domestic cat appears to be the main host for FeHV, isolates have also been obtained from nondomestic felids such as cheetahs.

When compared with the variability that is a feature of FCV, FeHV isolates are generally much more similar to one another. Slight differences between some biotypes do exist, however, with some attenuated strains used in vaccines and some apparently more virulent challenge strains. Antigenically, all isolates of FeHV are very similar and belong to one serotype. The virus also appears relatively homogenous at the genetic level although some differences between isolates have been found.[18-20] The overall homogeneity of feline herpesvirus means there is currently no easy method to study the role of individual isolates in the epidemiology of the disease.

Pathogenesis and Pathology

FELINE CALICIVIRUS INFECTION

Cats can be infected with FCV via the nasal, oral, or conjunctival routes. The virus replicates mainly in the oral and respiratory tissues, although some strains vary in their tissue tropism and pathogenicity. Thus some have a predilection for the lung and others have been found within macrophages in the synovial membrane of joints.[21,22] Virus has also been found in visceral tissues; feces; and, occasionally, in urine. The significance of this in transmission is unknown but is likely to be minimal.

Perhaps the most consistent pathological feature of FCV infection is oral ulceration. These ulcers begin as vesicles that subsequently rupture, with necrosis of the overlying epithelium and infiltration of neutrophils at the periphery and base. Healing generally takes place over a period of 2 to 3 weeks. Pulmonary lesions occur more rarely and appear to result from an initial focal alveolitis, leading to areas of acute exudative pneumonia and then to the development of a proliferative, interstitial pneumonia. Although primary interstitial pneumonia may occur with FCV, especially with the more virulent strains, it is possible that its importance in natural cases of disease has been overemphasized in the past. This is because many early experimental studies used aerosol challenge to infect cats, rather than the more natural oronasal route of infection. Lesions seen in FCV-infected joints consist of an acute synovitis with thickening of the synovial membrane and an increase in quantity of synovial fluid within the joint.[22]

FELINE HERPESVIRUS INFECTION

As with FCV, cats are infected with FeHV by nasal, oral, or conjunctival exposure. The virus primarily targets a number of tissues in the upper respiratory tract including the soft palate; tonsils; turbinates; conjunctivae; and, sometimes, the trachea. Virus shedding occurs as early as 24 hours after infection and generally persists for 1 to 3 weeks. Although it appears to be a rare sequel to infection, viremia has been reported, and generalized disease can be seen, particularly in young kittens or immunosuppressed individuals.

Infection with FeHV leads to areas of multifocal epithelial necrosis with neutrophilic infiltration and fibrin exudation. Intranuclear inclusion bodies are present in infected cells. Replication of the virus can also lead to osteolytic changes in the turbinate bones. Acute lesions normally take between 2 and 3 weeks to resolve, although turbinate destruction may be permanent and may predispose affected cats to chronic rhinitis. Primary lung involvement may occur but as with FCV infection, is rare. Although disease is not dependent on the presence of other organisms, secondary bacterial infection can enhance the pathology leading to bacterial pneumonia and sinusitis.

Clinical Signs

The clinical signs following infection with FCV or FeHV depend on a number of factors including those associated with the agent (e.g., strain and infecting dose), and those associated with the host (e.g., general health, age, and genetic make-up). Differences in microbial flora, in husbandry conditions, and the presence of any preexisting immunity may also affect the course of infection. Concurrent infections with immunosuppressive viruses such as feline ¬immunodeficiency virus and feline leukemia virus may lead to more severe disease.[23-25]

FELINE CALICIVIRUS

Following a short incubation period of 2 to 5 days, early signs of infection with most strains of FCV include depression and pyrexia. Affected cats generally appear brighter than those infected with FeHV. Perhaps the most characteristic clinical sign associated with FCV infection is ulceration of the tongue (Figure 35-1). Ulcers may also occasionally be seen on the lips or the nose. Cats with ulcerated mouths may show excessive salivation with wetness around the mouth. However, affected cats often show few other clinical signs, and it is likely that many cases in which oral ulceration is the main or only clinical sign go unrecognized. Sneezing, conjunctivitis, and ocular and nasal discharges typically occur but are usually less prominent than following FeHV infection. In most typical cases, clinical signs resolve over 7 to 10 days.

As well as this typically mild oral and respiratory disease, a wide range of other clinical presentations may also be observed following FCV infection. This pathogenic variability is again likely to be a reflection of the genetic variability of this virus. Therefore, although most strains induce fairly mild disease, some appear to be nonpathogenic, whereas others are capable of inducing more severe disease.

Skin ulceration on other parts of the body may be seen but occurs rarely and is generally mild. Some of the more virulent strains of FCV may cause pneumonia with associated dyspnea, particularly in younger animals when the disease becomes much more serious. FCV has also been reported in occasional cases of abortion.[26,27]

An acute lameness and pyrexia syndrome has also been described following FCV infection; it may or may

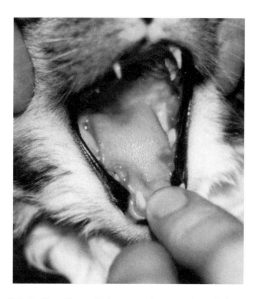

Figure 35-1. *Two lingual ulcers on the margins of the tongue of a cat acutely infected with FCV.*

not be associated with respiratory disease.[22,28,29] The lameness is usually described as shifting, affecting more than one leg, and is often accompanied by pyrexia. Affected cats are often dull and anorexic. Most cases recover within 1 to 2 days, and there are no known long-term effects on the joints. It is likely that such cases of lameness and the more typical cases associated with respiratory disease are not entirely distinct clinical entities. Instead, it has been suggested that most "limping" strains of FCV may cause some degree of respiratory disease, and vice versa.[29]

Lameness associated with FCV infection has also been seen after vaccination.[30-32] Sequence analysis of virus isolated from affected cats has shown that in most cases, the lameness appears to be caused by coincidental infection with field virus in young kittens as they lose their maternally-derived antibody. However, in some cases, virus originating from live vaccines appears to be involved.[11,12]

A potential worrying clinical development in the repertoire of FCV induced disease has recently been reported in the United States. In 1998, the first of several outbreaks of disease was described in which affected cats presented variably with facial and paw edema (50%), pyrexia (90%), upper respiratory tract infection (50%), icterus (20%), and hemorrhage from the nose and in the feces (30% to 40%).[9] Necrosis with ulceration was also seen in areas of earlier edema. The mortality rate associated with infection often reached 50%, with both kittens and adults succumbing to infection. Necropsy findings included pneumonia (80%), hepatomegaly (50%), pancreatitis (10%), and pericarditis (10%). The disease has been recreated experimentally by infection with FCV isolated from affected cats, further confirming the role of FCV in this serious disease. The variability of FCV means we should perhaps not be surprised by the occasional new and distinct manifestation of clinical disease. To date, most of these outbreaks have been relatively well controlled with strict quarantine and disinfection.

The chronic oral disease lymphoplasmacytic gingivitis stomatitis complex (LPGS) has also been associated with FCV infection. In some studies, approximately 80% of cats with LPGS have been shedding FCV, compared with 20% of controls.[33,34] However, these shedding rates may depend on the criteria used for the selection of clinical cases.[35] Chronic stomatitis developed following the accidental introduction of FCV into one cat colony, further suggesting a role for FCV in this disease.[36] However, chronic oral disease has not been reproduced experimentally in cats,[23,37-39] and attempts to identify consistent differences between FCV isolates from cats with LPGS and those from cats with other FCV-associated diseases have so far been unsuccessful.[6,7,39] It is therefore likely that factors not associated with FCV, including other pathogens and host factors, may also play a role in this complex and serious syndrome.

There has also been some debate about the role of FCV in feline urinary tract disease. Although virus can be visualized in and isolated from urine, there are currently no studies demonstrating a clear association between infection and disease.[8]

FELINE HERPESVIRUS

FeHV infection generally causes more consistent and severe upper respiratory and conjunctival disease than FCV, particularly in younger susceptible animals. The incubation period is usually 2 to 6 days but may vary depending on the challenge dose, with a higher dose inducing more rapid and severe clinical signs.

Initially, infected cats develop depression, marked sneezing, inappetence, pyrexia, and serous ocular and nasal discharges (Figure 35-2). In the earlier stages of infection, cats may also show excessive salivation and ptyalism (drooling of saliva). Conjunctivitis typically develops, and the ocular and nasal discharges change from serous to mucopurulent. In severe cases, dyspnea and coughing may also occur. Although oral ulceration can occur with FeHV infection, it is relatively rare compared with that following FCV infection. Occasionally, primary viral pneumonia or generalized disease may occur, particularly in young or debilitated animals. Other manifestations of infection include ocular disease such as ulcerative or interstitial keratitis and a possible association with uveitis.[40] Improved diagnosis (e.g., using the polymerase chain reaction) has led to greater recognition of such conditions.[41-43] Skin ulcers and dermatitis syndrome in domestic cats and cheetahs,[44-46] and neurological signs have also been reported, but these are likely to be rare sequels to FeHV infection.

Unlike many other alphaherpesviruses (e.g., canine herpesvirus-1), FeHV does not appear to have a significant role in reproductive tract disease. Experimental studies have suggested that abortion, when it occasionally occurs, is caused by the severe systemic nature of the illness rather than being a direct effect of the virus itself. Indeed, in an investigation of a natural outbreak of FeHV in specific pathogen-free cats, no

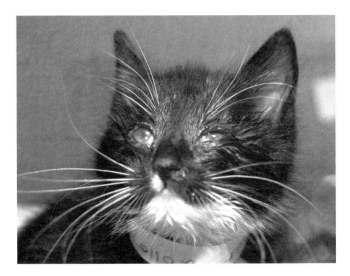

Figure 35-2. A kitten with early FeHV infection showing marked serous ocular and nasal discharges.

cases of abortion were seen, even in severely affected pregnant queens.[47]

As with classic FCV infection, the mortality rate with FeHV infection is generally low. In very young kittens or immunosuppressed cats, the mortality rate may be higher because of secondary bacterial infections and, more rarely, generalized viral infection. Clinical signs generally resolve over a period of 2 to 3 weeks. However, in some animals, permanent damage of the mucosa and turbinates may occur, leaving affected cats prone to chronic upper respiratory bacterial infections of the nose, paranasal sinuses, and conjunctiva.

Diagnosis

In many individual cases, it may not be necessary to determine the precise cause of infectious upper respiratory tract disease. However, there are some circumstances where a diagnosis is advisable. These include outbreaks of disease in colonies, where specific control measures may be required; and disease in vaccinated cats, where questions may arise concerning the safety and efficacy of a vaccine.

Whereas many of the clinical signs that occur in viral upper respiratory disease are common to both FCV and FeHV infection, a presumptive diagnosis in some cases may be possible based on clinical signs alone. FCV tends to cause a relatively mild disease in which oral ulceration is a relatively consistent feature. Lameness, if present, particularly in young kittens, is also suggestive of FCV infection. In contrast, FeHV tends to cause a more consistent and severe disease than FCV, associated with copious ocular and nasal discharges and sneezing.

Laboratory diagnosis is necessary where a definitive diagnosis is required. For both viruses, this has classically involved virus isolation in feline cell cultures. A plain oropharyngeal swab is taken from the cat and placed into suitable viral transport medium, then sent within 24 hours to an appropriate laboratory. For viral culture, results may take up to 2 weeks to confirm, particularly if the result is that no virus is isolated. Serology is generally not helpful for the diagnosis of acute FCV or FeHV infection because of widespread immunity from vaccination or earlier infection. The polymerase chain reaction (PCR) is also increasingly being used for the diagnosis of FeHV.[48-53] PCR and sequencing has also been used to distinguish between FCV isolates, where it has been particularly useful in the investigation of vaccine failures[11,12] and in dissecting the epidemiology of the disease.[54,55] The inherent variability of FCV strains has meant that the development of PCRs with high enough sensitivity to be used for the routine diagnosis of all FCV strains has been very problematic. Whereas some PCRs may show a high sensitivity with some strains, the sensitivity is likely to be lower with others, in some cases leading to false negative results. Recently, a real-time reverse-transcriptase PCR that targets relatively conserved regions of the virus genome has been described.[56] This method has been shown to be able to successfully amplify a broad range of FCV strains detecting 100% of 60 laboratory strains tested.

When diagnosing acute disease, results of virus isolation must be interpreted with care. False positives may occur because of the presence of clinically normal carriers in the population. False negatives may also occur particularly when only low levels of the infecting organism are shed, such as may occur in the later stages of acute disease. Other infections, particularly *Bordetella bronchiseptica* and *Chlamydophila felis*, may also be associated with upper respiratory tract disease in the cat, and therefore it may be appropriate to include testing for these as part of a diagnostic work-up.

Treatment

Currently no antiviral drugs are in widespread use for the treatment of FeHV or FCV. Drugs such as acyclovir, given in human herpesvirus infection, do not seem to have good activity against FeHV.[57,58] However, antiviral treatments are available for topical use in cases of ulcerative keratitis associated with FeHV infection.[43] Interferon has been suggested to be useful for treatment of acute viral infections. Some have advocated the use of human interferon orally, but the rationale for this is unclear because the majority of orally administered interferon may be expected to be degraded in the stomach. Recently, a commercial recombinant feline interferon has been licensed for parenteral administration in some countries, including the United Kingdom. However, there is currently little documented evidence for its success in the treatment of feline upper respiratory infections.

Broad-spectrum antibiotic treatment is generally recommended in cases of viral respiratory disease to minimize potential complications associated with secondary bacterial infection. Because swallowing may be painful, antibiotics can be given either as syrups (if available) or parenterally. In severe cases, bacterial culture and sensitivity testing may be required. Good nursing care, with regular cleansing of discharges, is essential. The cat should be encouraged to eat by offering strongly flavored, aromatic foods. If eating is painful, liquidized or specialized proprietary foods may be of some help. In some cases, the use of appetite stimulants such as diazepam or cyproheptadine may also be of some benefit. Some severely affected cases may require fluid therapy, and where anorexia is prolonged, a nasogastric esophagostomy or gastrostomy tube may be indicated.[59] In cases of chronic rhinitis, mucolytic drugs such as bromhexine hydrochloride may help clear mucus from airways. However, conventional steam inhalation (e.g., placing the cat in a steamy room) is probably of as much use.

Epidemiology

In the past, both FCV and FeHV were isolated from approximately equal numbers of cats with respiratory disease. Recently, however, FCV appears to be isolated more commonly.[60-62] This may be because of the antigenic diversity of FCV isolates compared with the single serotype of FeHV, which may affect the relative efficacy of the two vaccines. Both viruses remain fairly widespread in the general cat population, with an increased prevalence when cats are kept together. The viruses circulate and maintain themselves in the cat population in one of three ways. Firstly, there may be direct transmission of virus from acutely infected cats. Clearly, for the virus to persist in this way, there must be a sufficient number of susceptible animals within the population and opportunities for contact between them. Secondly, because FCV (and, to a lesser extent FeHV) can remain infectious for relatively short periods outside a host, viral contamination of the environment may lead to fomite transmission. This is particularly relevant within the close confines of a cattery or hospital, where secretions may contaminate cages, feeding and cleaning utensils, or personnel.[63] Finally, for both FCV and FeHV, animals that recover from acute disease may remain infected and develop persistent infections. Despite vaccination, such carriers are common in the population and are probably the main reason why these viruses remain so widespread.

There are no known reservoir or alternative hosts for FeHV, and in utero transmission does not generally seem to occur. The role of dogs in maintaining FCV in the population is not known, although as stated previously, FCV-like viruses have occasionally been recovered from dogs.

THE FCV CARRIER STATE

Following acute infection with FCV, clinical signs generally resolve in 7 to 10 days. However, most cats still shed FCV in oropharyngeal secretions for 30 days after infection, and such cats are defined as carriers (Figure 35-3). Subsequently, experimental studies have suggested that there is an exponential decline in the proportion of animals remaining infected, with approximately 50% of the cats still shedding virus 75 days later.[64] Although this most likely represents an over-simplification of the true dynamics of the FCV carrier state, it is a useful guide.

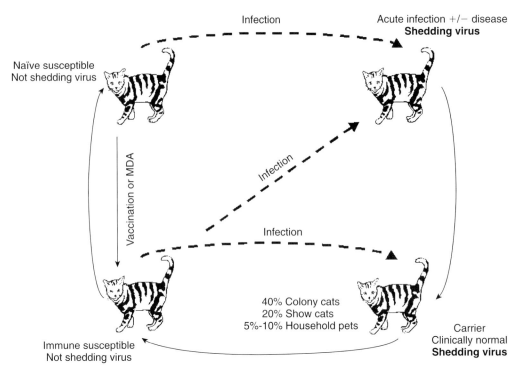

Figure 35-3. *FCV cycle of infection including the carrier state. Generally, clinically normal carriers develop following a period of acute clinical disease. However, carriers may develop in the absence of previous clinical disease under protection from maternally- or vaccine-derived immunity. (Modified from Gaskell RM, Radford AD, Dawson S: Feline infectious respiratory disease. In Chandler EA, Gaskell CJ, Gaskell RM, editors: Feline medicine and therapeutics, ed 3, Oxford, 2003, Blackwell Publishing.)*

Individual FCV carriers may shed virus for life, but most cats appear to spontaneously eliminate the virus. The mechanism by which some cats clear infection is not known. However, it is likely that in the field, reinfection is common. Concurrent infections with other pathogens may impact on the dynamics of the FCV carrier state. For example, there is some evidence that pre-existing FIV infection may potentiate FCV shedding either in terms of the duration of shedding,[23] or the titer of virus shed.[25]

FCV carriers shed virus more-or-less continuously. Individual cats seem to vary in the quantity of virus they shed,[65] and it is likely that those animals that shed the higher amounts of virus will transmit infection most readily. In contrast, low-level shedders are probably not as infectious and may also be more difficult to detect because the level of virus shed may intermittently fall below the sensitivity of virus diagnosis. Therefore when trying to detect FCV carriers, it is advisable to take a series of swabs over several weeks before an individual is believed to be FCV negative.

The mechanism of persistence for FCV is not fully elucidated. Viruses recovered from carrier cats have been shown to change antigenically over time.[66,67] This antigenic evolution correlates with sequence changes in key antigenic domains of the virus capsid, and has led to the suggestion that antigenic variants generated within carriers allow FCV to escape neutralization by the cat's im-

mune response.[67,68] Such a process is common among RNA viruses that cause persistent infections and is associated with the low accuracy of virally-encoded RNA polymerases.

Despite the use of vaccines for approximately 30 years, the prevalence of FCV infection in the general cat population remains high. Before vaccines were introduced in the 1970s, surveys showed that approximately 8% of household pets, 25% of cats attending cat shows, and 40% of colony cats were shedding the virus.[69] However, in recent years, approximately 20% to 25% of cats in a variety of husbandry situations still shed FCV.[60,61,70] In one rescue shelter, FCV prevalence was approximately 25% despite the regular use of vaccination to control clinical disease.[55] Molecular epidemiology studies showed that within this particular shelter, most isolates were distinct, unless the isolates were obtained from cats that were housed in the same pen. This suggests that the high prevalence within the rescue shelter was because of the high prevalence of FCV in cats arriving at the shelter rather than significant transmission within the shelter. In contrast, a single viral strain often seems to predominate in household colonies with a high prevalence of infection, although evolution of the individual colony isolates may occur over time.[71] Molecular studies should enable a clearer understanding of the epidemiology of FCV and the role of the carrier state in the continued high prevalence of this virus.

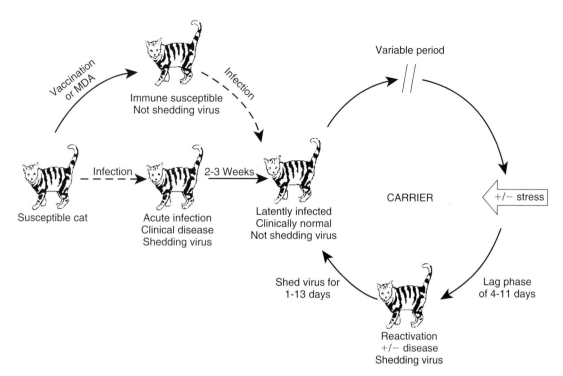

Figure 35-4. *FeHV cycle of infection including latency. Generally, latently infected carriers develop following a period of acute clinical disease. However, latency may also develop in the absence of previous clinical disease under protection from maternally or vaccine-derived immunity.* (Modified from Gaskell RM, Radford AD, Dawson S: Feline infectious respiratory disease. In Chandler EA, Gaskell CJ, Gaskell RM, editors: *Feline medicine and therapeutics,* ed 3, Oxford, 2003, Blackwell Publishing.)

Preexisting immunity, acquired either naturally as maternally derived antibody or artificially following parenteral vaccination, does not prevent infection with FCV. Animals may become carriers following subclinical infection with field virus, thereby maintaining infection in the population (see Figure 35-3). There is no evidence that vaccination will cure an existing carrier state.

THE FeHV CARRIER STATE

As with other alphaherpesviruses, cats become latently infected with FeHV following acute disease (Figure 35-4). During latency, no infectious virus is detectable; however, periodical episodes of virus reactivation occur, during which times infectious virus is present in oronasal and ocular secretions. In some cases, carriers show mild clinical signs while they are shedding (recrudescence) which may act as a useful indicator that such individuals are likely to be infectious to other cats.

Although latently infected carriers all have the potential to shed FeHV, some cats appear to do so more frequently, and as such are likely to be of greater epidemiological significance. Reactivation may occur spontaneously but is most likely to occur following a stress (e.g., after parturition) or a change of housing (e.g., going into a boarding cattery, to a cat show, or to stud).[72] Shedding does not occur immediately after stress: there is a lag period of approximately 1 week, followed by a shedding episode of up

to 2 weeks. Thus carrier cats are most likely to be infectious from 1 to 3 weeks following a stress (see Figure 35-4). Corticosteroid treatment can also induce shedding, and care should be taken when using these drugs in carriers because some of these cats may develop severe recrudescent disease.

As with some other herpesvirus infections, FeHV remains latent in carriers in trigeminal ganglia, although there is evidence to show that other tissues may also be involved.[51,73,74] Latency is almost certainly lifelong, but there is a refractory phase of several months after a period of shedding when animals are less likely to experience another episode.

The importance of latent FeHV carriers lies in their ability to transmit infection. Therefore any animal with a history of FeHV-associated respiratory disease, or with persistent or recurrent signs, should be considered potentially infectious. Similarly any queen who repeatedly produces litters that develop respiratory disease is probably a carrier and it may be advisable not to use such queens for breeding.

As with FCV, immunity to FeHV, whether vaccine-induced or maternally-derived, does not prevent infection, and cats may become carriers even though they have no history of clinical disease (see Figure 35-4). In latently infected queens, virus shedding that may be induced by the stress of parturition and lactation provides a source of infectious virus to kittens. Such a mechanism favors virus spread to the next generation without harming its host. In the case of vaccination, there is no evidence that vaccination will eliminate an existing latent infection, although it is theoretically possible that it may reduce episodes of virus shedding.

Transmission

FCV and FeHV are shed mainly in oral, nasal, and conjunctival secretions in both acutely infected and carrier cats. Transmission mostly occurs by direct contact between cats, but indirect transmission may occur. Thus cats may also be infected through contact with contaminated secretions on cages, feed bowls, cleaning utensils, and personnel.[63] However, because both viruses are relatively short-lived outside the cat, the environment is not usually a long-term source of infection.

Unlike many respiratory pathogens in other species, true aerosol transmission is not thought to be of major importance for the spread of feline respiratory viruses. This is thought to reflect the small tidal volume of the cat such that infectious aerosols are not generally produced during normal respiration. However, macrodroplets produced by sneezing may travel over a distance of 1 to 2 meters, allowing virus transmission to occur.

Transmission is most successful in overcrowded conditions where cats are more likely to have prolonged, close contact. Poor ventilation and hygiene may also lead to a build up of pathogens in the environment. Transmission is thought to be more easily achieved from acutely infected cats rather than carriers, as discharges are more copious and the amount of virus higher. However, carriers are undoubtedly important sources of virus, particularly in transmission between queens and kittens, and in the close contact seen between cats in multi-cat colonies.

Immunity

Most cats develop some degree of immunity to FCV following natural infection; however, it may not always be complete or of long duration. In addition, the many different strains of FCV show varying degrees of cross-protection. Immunity following the use of modified live or inactivated vaccines is similarly incomplete, though this may depend on the strains or challenge system used.[75-78]

After vaccination, protection against FCV disease has been reported to last for 10 to 12 months.[79] More recent work has suggested that partial protection may last considerably longer. Moderate levels of virus neutralizing antibody have been shown to persist in a group of vaccinated cats for at least 4 years, although after 7.5 years, titers had declined to low or nondetectable levels.[80,81] Protection against FCV challenge decreased from 85% at 3 weeks after vaccination to 63% after 7.5 years.

Virus-neutralizing antibody levels to FCV tend to be higher than with FeHV, and in general there is reasonable correlation with protection against disease.[82] However, protection has also been seen with lower levels of virus neutralizing antibody, suggesting cell-mediated and possible local immunity may also play a role.[38,76,83]

Following primary infection with FeHV, most cats are generally resistant to subsequent reinfection. However, protection is not necessarily complete in all animals and may only be of relatively short duration. By 6 months after infection, cats may only be partially protected from subsequent challenge, and carrier cats may also develop recrudescent disease. Low levels of virus neutralizing antibody develop following initial infection or vaccination, suggesting that, as for other alphaherpesviruses, cell-mediated and local immunity play a significant role in protection. However, after reactivation or field virus challenge, virus-neutralizing antibody titers generally rise to more moderate levels and thereafter remain reasonably stable, independent of virus shedding episodes.

Most cats are protected following the use of modified live or inactivated FeHV vaccines. Again, however, immunity is not necessarily complete in all animals, even if challenge takes place within 3 months of vaccination.[78,84,85] Similar levels of protection have been reported after a year.[86] More recent studies have shown that the relative efficacy of an inactivated vaccine decreased from 83% shortly after primary vaccination to 52% after 7.5 years.[81]

In kittens, maternally derived antibody (which is essentially colostral) may persist for 10 to 14 weeks and 2 to 10 weeks for FCV and FeHV, respectively.[87,88] However, for both viruses, low levels of maternally derived antibody do not necessarily protect against subclinical infection, and kittens infected at this time may become carriers without showing clinical disease (see Figures 35-3 and 35-4).

Prevention and Control

A number of vaccines against FCV and FeHV are available, and have been used relatively successfully for many years. Nevertheless, because of the epidemiology of the disease, respiratory disease may still occur, particularly where cats are housed together in breeding, boarding, or rescue catteries. Therefore, prevention and control is best achieved by a combination of vaccination and cattery management.

VACCINATION

The majority of vaccines marketed against FCV and FeHV are either live and attenuated or inactivated and adjuvanted, and are licensed for parenteral administration. Modified live intranasal vaccines are also marketed in some countries, including the United States.

Most vaccines induce reasonable protection against *disease.* However, it is worth restating that vaccination does not, in general, protect against *infection* and the development of the carrier state of either FCV or FeHV. Therefore, vaccinated animals may be subsequently infected with field viruses and develop persistent infections without clinical disease. Such vaccinated, field virus carriers are important sources of infection to other naïve cats and are likely to be partly responsible for the continued high prevalence of FCV and FeHV in the general cat population.

The differences in relative efficacy of FCV and FeHV vaccines are partly explained by the different level of strain variation shown by each of these viruses. For FeHV, there is only one serotype, and it is likely that vaccines protect equally against all field isolates. In contrast, the antigenic differences between FCV isolates mean that no single vaccine strain is likely to protect equally against all field viruses. The strains of FCV chosen for use in vaccines, such as F9 and more recently 255, have largely been selected on the basis of being broadly cross-reactive in virus neutralization tests in cell culture.[31,76,89] Recently, companies have sought market advantage through claims of broader cross-reactivity for their vaccine strains. Indeed, the ability of a company's vaccine to neutralize a high proportion of field isolates will probably play an increasingly important role in vaccine marketing. However, it is likely that strains of FCV will always exist that show limited neutralization by individual vaccines. It is also possible that the widespread use of vaccines may select for these "vaccine-resistant" strains.[76,89] In the authors' opinion it would be desirable, therefore, for the efficacy of commercially available vaccines to be regularly monitored against panels of contemporary field viruses. However, this is not currently routinely performed.

Despite designing vaccines to be broadly cross-reactive, the antigenic diversity of FCV means that in some groups of cats, FCV-related disease may still occur despite regular vaccination. In this situation, it may be appropriate to consider changing vaccines to one based on a different strain. However, vaccine changes should be approached with care because any new vaccine may show either increased or reduced protection against the predominant colony virus. Any decision to change vaccine may be informed by determining the neutralization profile of vaccine-induced antisera against the predominant colony virus. However, this test is only available at specialist laboratories, is expensive and time-consuming, and can be difficult to interpret. Rational choice of vaccines also requires information on the strains of FCV used in vaccines; however, this information is not often included in data sheet information for marketed vaccines.

Although live parenteral vaccines are generally considered to be safe, clinical signs have been reported following their use, particularly in young kittens after their first vaccination (Box 35-1).[30,32] Clinical signs may be induced if the vaccine reaches the oral or respiratory mucosa (e.g., if the cat or a littermate licks the injection site, or if an aerosol is made at the time of injection). In addition, in rare cases, vaccine virus may be able to generalize to the oropharynx even if it is correctly administered.[21,76]

For FCV, molecular typing has confirmed that the majority of vaccine reactions are associated with field virus infection.[11,12] However, in some cases, vaccine virus does seem to be involved. It is interesting to speculate what happens to such vaccine viruses once individual cats start shedding them. Vaccine safety studies required before live vaccines are marketed would suggest they are unlikely to spread and persist in the population and, until recently,

---

BOX 35-1
Major Reasons for Vaccine Failures

Vaccine Reactions (Clinical Signs Occurring Within 3 Weeks of Vaccination)

Operator Factors
- Vaccine virus gains access to the respiratory mucosa from modified live systemic vaccines through incorrect administration (e.g., aerosolization, licking the injection site).

Vaccine Factors
- Incomplete attenuation: spread of vaccine virus to the respiratory mucosa from modified live systemic vaccines through generalization of vaccine virus from the site of injection.
- Intranasal vaccines may cause mild clinical symptoms in some individuals.

Host and Viral Factors
- Infection with field virus prior to development of complete vaccine-induced protection. Most frequently seen after the first kitten vaccine.
- Respiratory disease due to pathogens not vaccinated against.
- Recrudescent disease in carrier cats associated with stress of vaccination (FeHV).

Vaccine Breakdowns (Clinical Signs Occurring 3 Weeks or More Following Vaccination)

Vaccine/Operator Factors
- Incorrect storage, handling or administration of vaccine.

Host Factors
- Failure to respond to vaccine due to immunosuppression (e.g., infection with feline leukemia or immunodeficiency viruses, corticosteroid treatment).
- Nonspecific factors that may either reduce the response to vaccine or increase an individual's disease susceptibility (e.g., age, genotype, general health and intercurrent disease).
- Failure to respond to vaccine due to maternally derived antibody.
- Respiratory disease due to pathogens not vaccinated against.
- Recrudescent disease in carrier cats (FeHV).

Viral Factors
- Infection with strains of virus not protected against by the vaccine (FCV).
- Overwhelming challenge dose due to overcrowding, poor hygiene.

Reprinted from Gaskell RM, Radford AD, Dawson S: Feline infectious respiratory disease. In Chandler EA, Gaskell CJ, Gaskell RM, editors: *Feline medicine and therapeutics,* ed 3, Oxford, 2003, Blackwell Publishing.

vaccine-type viruses have only been identified in recently vaccinated cats. More recently, however, FCV isolates closely related to those used in live vaccines have been found in the general cat population, raising the possibility that, in rare cases, vaccine virus may persist in individual cat populations, possibly causing disease.[9,10,54]

In contrast to live vaccines, inactivated vaccines have the advantage of not being able to spread or revert to virulence, and are therefore particularly useful in virus-free colonies. Some inactivated vaccines have also been used during pregnancy in queens as a useful control measure aimed at prolonging the persistence of maternally derived antibody in kittens[90]; however, individual data sheets should be checked for this indication. Although inactivated vaccines are classically considered less efficacious than live vaccines, modern adjuvants have led to improvements in immunogenicity. Indeed, a long duration of immunity and reasonable levels of protection in most cats has recently been shown for an adjuvanted, inactivated FCV and FeHV vaccine.[80,81]

Adjuvants may, however, cause clinical problems following vaccination in some individual cats. Both local injection site reactions and systemic reactions including pyrexia and lethargy have been observed. Most of these signs are transient, but local reactions may persist for several weeks. In recent years it has become apparent that in rare cases such reactions may progress to sarcomas.[91] Although adjuvants, particularly those based on aluminum, have been implicated in the etiology of vaccine-associated sarcomas, their precise role in the process remains unclear.

Live intranasal vaccines induce local mucosal immunity, and this is probably more effective than immunity induced by parenteral vaccines. However, because the virus replicates at the site of inoculation, clinical signs such as mild sneezing may be seen after several days in some individuals. Data sheets often state that oral lesions may also be observed following the use of intranasal vaccines, and that these tend to heal rapidly. Intranasal vaccines are particularly useful when a rapid onset of protection is required (e.g., for a cat going into a boarding cattery or in the face of an outbreak of disease). In contrast to parenteral vaccines, only a single dose of intranasal vaccine is generally required to induce immunity following primary vaccination. Complete protection has been shown 4 days after intranasal vaccination and partial protection after 2 days. These vaccines may also overcome maternally derived antibody better than parenteral vaccines, although in general their use is only licensed in kittens from 12 weeks of age. Live intranasal vaccines have shown an increase in popularity among some veterinarians, in part because of public concerns about the role of inactivated vaccines in vaccine-associated sarcomas. At the time of writing, no intranasal vaccines are marketed in the United Kingdom.

Boosters for FCV and FeHV vaccines are traditionally recommended every year. However, concerns about vaccine site reactions have led to the suggestion that, in some circumstances, vaccination frequency may be reduced based on an informed risk assessment of the likelihood of infection in each individual case.[92-94]

DISEASE CONTROL IN DIFFERENT SITUATIONS

The methods used to control disease caused by FCV and FeHV vary somewhat depending on the husbandry situation in which the cat is housed. In most cases, routine vaccination for FCV and FeHV is recommended unless there are strong indications that the risk of infection is negligible. Disinfection is also an important mainstay of control. Because of its lipid envelope, FeHV is highly susceptible to the effects of all common disinfectants. In contrast, FCV shows some degree of resistance to certain disinfectants. Both viruses, however, are inactivated by a number of proprietary products.

Household pets are most likely to be exposed to respiratory pathogens when entering a high-risk situation such as a boarding cattery or a veterinary hospital. Although transmission may also occur between cats within a neighborhood, the extent to which this occurs will depend on the level and opportunities for contact between them. Cats are mainly territorial animals and with neutered animals, once their territory is established, any contact with other cats is usually brief and does not encourage extensive transmission of pathogens. In addition, FCV and FeHV are relatively fragile outside their hosts, reducing the impact of indirect transmission. Therefore in order to reduce the risk of respiratory disease, individual cats should be routinely vaccinated and should avoid stress and social contact as far as possible.

Boarding catteries may be associated with high levels of virus challenge because of the large numbers of cats, the high prevalence of FCV and FeHV carriers, and reactivation of FeHV shedding induced by stress. Therefore all cats admitted to a boarding cattery should have an up-to-date vaccination record for both FCV and FeHV. This means that young kittens should have completed the full vaccination course, and adult cats should have had their annual booster, at least 7 days before admission. Where the booster vaccination interval has lapsed to 18 months, it might be advisable to revaccinate. In situations where rapid protection is required, intranasal vaccination may be used if available. However, clients should be aware that such vaccines themselves may induce mild clinical signs. Although vaccination is helpful in controlling disease, the owners of catteries should not rely on it solely for disease control. Indeed, even fully vaccinated animals may succumb to disease if the viral challenge is high enough. Precautions must be taken to minimize the risk of transmission within the cattery and to reduce the concentration of respiratory pathogens in the environment (Box 35-2).

Shelter facilities should apply the same measures as boarding catteries. However, it is often impossible to guarantee levels of vaccination before admission, and it may also be impossible to separate cats to the same extent. As far as possible, individual cats should be segregated or batched and quarantined, and those with clinical signs isolated. Unless animals can be quarantined on arrival for 3 to 4 weeks, systemic vaccines may not have time to become effective. In these circumstances it may be advisable to use intranasal vaccines if available.

BOX 35-2
Recommendations to Prevent Spread of Respiratory Viruses in a Boarding Cattery

- Make sure all incoming cats are fully vaccinated.
- Keep cats separate unless they are from the same household.
- Build catteries with solid partitions between pens. Ensure frontages are at least 1 meter apart and the surface of the pen is made of nonporous material that is easily washable.
- Arrange the pen so the food and water bowls and the litter tray are easily accessible without having to enter the pen.
- Either wash hands in disinfectant between visiting each pen, or have a set of disposable gloves on a peg by each pen. Dedicate gloves for use in that pen only; dispose of or thoroughly disinfect them before use with a new boarder.
- Wear rubber boots, and if it is necessary to enter the pen, step into a disinfectant bath before and after entering.
- Either use disposable food trays or have two sets of feed bowls used on alternate days. Soak the used set in a recommended disinfectant for several hours, thoroughly rinse, and leave to dry until next use.
- Prepare food in a central area.
- If necessary to replace a badly soiled litter tray, follow a similar system to the feed bowls.
- Between residents, thoroughly disinfect the pen; allow to dry; and, preferably, leave empty for 2 days before reusing.
- Put those cats that have signs of respiratory disease, or are known to have had respiratory disease, or are suspected from previous experience of being carriers, in a separate section or at one end of the cattery, and feed/clean last.
- Feed cats in the same order every day, and attend to each pen completely before moving to the next.
- Reduce concentration of infectious diseases in the environment by adequate ventilation, low relative humidity, and optimal environmental temperature.
- In mixed boarding catteries and kennels, be aware of possible transmission of *Bordetella bronchiseptica* between cats and dogs. Disinfect between areas, use separate staff if possible, and avoid visiting coughing dogs before cats (or coughing cats before dogs).

Reprinted from Gaskell RM, Radford AD, Dawson S: Feline infectious respiratory disease. In Chandler EA, Gaskell CJ, Gaskell RM, editors: *Feline medicine and therapeutics,* ed 3, Oxford, 2003, Blackwell Publishing.

In disease-free breeding catteries, cats should be vaccinated routinely if there is any contact at all with other cats, and in these situations, inactivated vaccines may be preferable. Great care should be taken to avoid bringing respiratory pathogens into the colony: any cat with a history of respiratory disease, or from a household with a history of respiratory disease, may be a carrier. It should be remembered that cats may become infected subclinically under cover of maternally derived antibody or vaccine-induced immunity. The greatest risk of infection to disease-free households is likely to be from stud cats and new breeding stock, where exposure is prolonged. Where possible, these cats should come from colonies free of respiratory disease. There is also a slight risk of infection from cat shows, where approximately 25% of cats are shedding FCV.[70] However, direct contact between cats at shows is limited and hygiene measures are usually good. Cats entering the colony should be quarantined for 3 weeks to identify animals incubating disease. During quarantine, oropharyngeal swabs should be taken for viral diagnosis at least twice a week in order to have the best chance of detecting carriers. Even so, there is still the risk of importing both latent FeHV carriers or low-level FCV carriers. The necessity to screen for other infectious causes of respiratory disease such as *B. bronchiseptica* and *C. felis* may also be considered.

In breeding colonies with endemic disease, attempts to control disease can be made by taking the following measures:
- Provide regular vaccination against FCV and FeHV.
- Give booster vaccinations to queens either before mating or during pregnancy to boost levels of ma-

ternally derived antibody in kittens. (If the latter, use an inactivated vaccine, and only if it has a data sheet supporting such use.)
- Avoid the use of particular queens with a history of respiratory disease in their kittens.
- Minimize stressful situations and employ good management practices.
- Move queens into isolation at least 3 weeks before term so that the kittens are not exposed to carriers in the colony, and so that any FeHV shedding episode from the queen induced by the move will be over before parturition.
- Wean kittens early into isolation as soon as it is feasible (ideally at 4 to 5 weeks) if it is likely the queen is a carrier.
- Vaccinate all kittens as soon as maternally derived antibody is at a noninterfering level (normally 9+ weeks) and keep them in strict isolation until a week after the second dose (normally at 12 weeks).
- Use earlier vaccination schedules: a recent field study has shown that kittens may respond to parenteral vaccination against FCV and FeHV given at 3-week intervals from 6 weeks of age.[95] Intranasal vaccines have also been advocated 7 to 10 days before disease normally occurs in a colony, and then again at 12 weeks of age. However, it should be kept in mind that such vaccines are not generally licensed for this use.
- In some circumstances it may be feasible to restock the colony with virus-free cats and to employ a barrier system to keep the viruses out. A commercial or institutional colony could achieve this using specific

pathogen-free animals. A pedigree cat breeding unit could hand-rear kittens of existing stock in isolation, bearing in mind that the viruses are very widespread and that it might be difficult to ensure that the colony remains virus free, even with vaccination.

REFERENCES

1. Kadoi K, Kiryu M, Iwabuchi M et al: A strain of calicivirus isolated from lions with vesicular lesions on tongue and snout, *New Microbiol* 20:141-148, 1997.
2. Hofmann-Lehmann R, Fehr D, Grob M et al: Prevalence of antibodies to feline parvovirus, calicivirus, herpesvirus, coronavirus, and immunodeficiency virus and of feline leukemia virus antigen and the interrelationship of these viral infections in free-ranging lions in east Africa, *Clin Diagn Lab Immunol* 3:554-562, 1996.
3. Roerink F, Hashimoto M, Tohya Y et al: Genetic analysis of a canine calicivirus: Evidence for a new clade of animal caliciviruses, *Vet Microbiol* 69:69-72, 1999.
4. Hashimoto M, Roerink F, Tohya Y et al: Genetic analysis of the RNA polymerase gene of caliciviruses from dogs and cats, *J Vet Med Sci* 61:603-608, 1999.
5. Martella V, Pratelli A, Gentile M et al: Analysis of the capsid protein gene of a feline-like calicivirus isolated from a dog, *Vet Microbiol* 85:315-322, 2002.
6. Geissler K, Schneider K, Platzer G et al: Genetic and antigenic heterogeneity among feline calicivirus isolates from distinct disease manifestations, *Virus Res* 48:193-206, 1997.
7. Glenn M, Radford AD, Turner DC et al: Nucleotide sequence of UK and Australian isolates of feline calicivirus (FCV) and phylogenetic analysis of FCVs, *Vet Microbiol* 67:175-193, 1999.
8. Rice CC, Kruger JM, Venta PJ et al: Genetic characterization of 2 novel feline caliciviruses isolated from cats with idiopathic lower urinary tract disease, *J Vet Intern Med* 16:293-302, 2002.
9. Pedersen NC, Elliott JB, Glasgow A et al: An isolated epizootic of hemorrhagic-like fever in cats caused by a novel and highly virulent strain of feline calicivirus, *Vet Microbiol* 73:281-300, 2000.
10. Horimoto T, Takeda Y, Iwatsuki-Horimoto K et al: Capsid protein gene variation among feline calicivirus isolates, *Virus Genes* 23:171-174, 2001.
11. Radford AD, Bennett M, McArdle F et al: The use of sequence analysis of a feline calicivirus (FCV) hypervariable region in the epidemiological investigation of FCV related disease and vaccine failures, *Vaccine* 15:1451-1458, 1997.
12. Radford AD, Dawson S, Wharmby C et al: Comparison of serological and sequence-based methods for typing feline calicivirus isolates from vaccine failures, *Vet Rec* 146:117-123, 2000.
13. Sykes JE, Studdert VP, Browning GF: Detection and strain differentiation of feline calicivirus in conjunctival swabs by RT-PCR of the hypervariable region of the capsid protein gene, *Arch Virol* 143:1321-1334, 1998.
14. Gaskell R, Willoughby K: Herpesviruses of carnivores, *Vet Microbiol* 69:73-88, 1999.
15. Harder TC, Harder M, Vos H et al: Characterization of phocid herpesvirus-1 and -2 as putative alpha- and gammaherpesviruses of North American and European pinnipeds, *J Gen Virol* 77:27-35, 1996.
16. Lebich M, Harder TC, Frey HR et al: Comparative immunological characterization of type-specific and conserved B-cell epitopes of pinniped, felid and canid herpesviruses, *Arch Virol* 136:335-347, 1994.
17. Willoughby K, Bennett M, McCracken CM et al: Molecular phylogenetic analysis of felid herpesvirus 1, *Vet Microbiol* 69:93-97, 1999.
18. Grail A, Harbour DA, Chia W: Restriction endonuclease mapping of the genome of feline herpesvirus type 1, *Arch Virol* 116:209-220, 1991.
19. Horimoto T, Limcumpao JA, Xuan X et al: Heterogeneity of feline herpesvirus type 1 strains, *Arch Virol* 126:283-292, 1992.
20. Maeda K, Kawaguchi Y, Ono M et al: Comparisons among feline herpesvirus type 1 isolates by immunoblot analysis, *J Vet Med Sci* 57:147-150, 1995.
21. Bennett D, Gaskell RM, Mills A et al: Detection of feline calicivirus antigens in the joints of infected cats, *Vet Rec* 124:329-332, 1989.
22. Dawson S, Bennett D, Carter SD et al: Acute arthritis of cats associated with feline calicivirus infection, *Res Vet Sci* 56:133-143, 1994.
23. Dawson S, Smyth NR, Bennett M et al: Effect of primary-stage feline immunodeficiency virus infection on subsequent feline calicivirus vaccination and challenge in cats, *AIDS* 5:747-750, 1991.
24. Reubel GH, George JW, Barlough JE et al: Interaction of acute feline herpesvirus-1 and chronic feline immunodeficiency virus infections in experimentally infected specific pathogen free cats, *Vet Immunol Immunopath* 35:95-119, 1992.
25. Reubel GH, George JW, Higgins J et al: Effect of chronic feline immunodeficiency virus infection on experimental feline calicivirus-induced disease, *Vet Microbiol* 39:335-351, 1994.
26. van Vuuren M, Geissler K, Gerber D et al: Characterisation of a potentially abortigenic strain of feline calicivirus isolated from a domestic cat, *Vet Rec* 144:636-638, 1999.
27. Ellis TM: Jaundice in a Siamese cat with in utero feline calicivirus infection, *Aus Vet J* 57:383-385, 1981.
28. Pedersen NC, Laliberte L, Ekman S: A transient febrile "limping" syndrome of kittens caused by two different strains of feline calicivirus, *Feline Practice* 13(1):26-35, 1983.
29. TerWee T, Lauritzen A, Sabara M et al: Comparison of the primary signs induced by experimental exposure to either a pneumotrophic or a "limping" strain of feline calicivirus, *Vet Microbiol* 56:33-45, 1997.
30. Church RE: Lameness in kittens after vaccination, *Vet Rec* 125:609, 1989.
31. Dawson S, McArdle F, Bennett M et al: Typing of feline calicivirus isolates from different clinical groups by virus neutralisation tests, *Vet Rec* 133:13-17, 1993.
32. Dawson S, McArdle F, Bennett D et al: Investigation of vaccine reactions and breakdowns after feline calicivirus vaccination, *Vet Rec* 132:346-350, 1993.
33. Knowles JO, Gaskell RM, Gaskell CJ et al: Prevalence of feline calicivirus, feline leukaemia virus and antibodies to FIV in cats with chronic stomatitis, *Vet Rec* 124:336-338, 1989.
34. Thompson RR, Wilcox GE, Clark WT et al: Association of calicivirus infection with chronic gingivitis and pharyngitis in cats, *JSAP* 25:207-210, 1984.
35. Tenorio AP, Franti CE, Madewell BR et al: Chronic oral infections of cats and their relationship to persistent oral carriage of feline calici-, immunodeficiency, or leukemia viruses, *Vet Immunol Immunopath* 29:1-14, 1991.
36. Waters L, Hopper CD, Gruffydd-Jones TJ et al: Chronic gingivitis in a colony of cats infected with feline immunodeficiency virus and feline calicivirus, *Vet Rec* 132:340-342, 1993.
37. Reubel GH, Hoffmann DE, Pedersen NC: Acute and chronic faucitis of domestic cats: A feline calicivirus induced disease, *Vet Clin North Am Small Anim Pract* 22:1347-1360, 1992.
38. Knowles JO, McArdle F, Dawson S et al: Studies on the role of feline calicivirus in chronic stomatitis in cats, *Vet Microbiol* 27:205-219, 1991.
39. Poulet H, Brunet S, Soulier M et al: Comparison between acute oral/respiratory and chronic stomatitis/gingivitis isolates of feline calicivirus: Pathogenicity, antigenic profile and cross-neutralisation studies, *Arch Virol* 145:243-261, 2000.
40. Maggs DJ, Lappin MR, Nasisse MP: Detection of feline herpesvirus-specific antibodies and DNA in aqueous humor from cats with or without uveitis, *Am J Vet Res* 60:932-936, 1999.
41. Nasisse MP, Glover TL, Moore CP et al: Detection of feline herpesvirus 1 DNA in corneas of cats with eosinophilic keratitis or corneal sequestration, *Am J Vet Res* 59:856-858, 1998.
42. Nasisse MP, Davis BJ, Guy JS et al: Isolation of feline herpesvirus 1 from the trigeminal ganglia of acutely and chronically infected cats, *J Vet Intern Med* 6:102-103, 1992.
43. Stiles J: Feline herpesvirus, *Vet Clin North Am Small Anim Pract* 30:1001-1014, 2000.
44. Flecknell PA, Orr CM, Wright AI et al: Skin ulceration associated with herpesvirus infection in cats, *Vet Rec* 104:313-315, 1979.
45. Junge RE, Miller RE, Boever WJ et al: Persistent cutaneous ulcers associated with feline herpesvirus type 1 infection in a cheetah, *J Am Vet Med Assoc* 198:1057-1058, 1991.

46. Hargis AM, Ginn PE: Feline herpesvirus 1-associated facial and nasal dermatitis and stomatitis in domestic cats, *Vet Clin North Am Small Anim Pract* 29:1281-1290, 1999.
47. Hickman MA, Reubel GH, Hoffman DE et al: An epizootic of feline herpesvirus, type 1 in a large specific pathogen-free cat colony and attempts to eradicate the infection by identification and culling of carriers, *Lab Anim* 28:320-329, 1994.
48. Stiles J, McDermott M, Bigsby D et al: Use of nested polymerase chain reaction to identify feline herpesvirus in ocular tissue from clinically normal cats and cats with corneal sequestra or conjunctivitis, *Am J Vet Res* 58:338-342, 1997.
49. Stiles J, McDermott M, Willis M et al: Comparison of nested polymerase chain reaction, virus isolation, and fluorescent antibody testing for identifying feline herpesvirus in cats with conjunctivitis, *Am J Vet Res* 58:804-807, 1997.
50. Sykes JE, Anderson GA, Studdert VP et al: Prevalence of feline Chlamydia psittaci and feline herpesvirus 1 in cats with upper respiratory tract disease, *J Vet Intern Med* 13:153-162, 1999.
51. Weigler BJ, Babineau CA, Sherry B et al: High sensitivity polymerase chain reaction assay for active and latent feline herpesvirus-1 infections in domestic cats, *Vet Rec* 140:335-338, 1997.
52. Vogtlin A, Fraefel C, Albini S et al: Quantification of feline herpesvirus 1 DNA in ocular fluid samples of clinically diseased cats by real-time TaqMan PCR, *J Clin Microbiol* 40:519-523, 2002.
53. Burgesser KM, Hotaling S, Schiebel A et al: Comparison of PCR, virus isolation, and indirect fluorescent antibody staining in the detection of naturally occurring feline herpesvirus infections, *J Vet Diagn Invest* 11:122-126, 1999.
54. Radford AD, Sommerville L, Ryvar R et al: Endemic infection of a cat colony with a feline calicivirus closely related to an isolate used in live attenuated vaccines, *Vaccine* 19:4358-4362, 2001.
55. Radford AD, Sommerville LM, Dawson S et al: Molecular analysis of isolates of feline calicivirus from a population of cats in a rescue shelter, *Vet Rec* 149:477-481, 2001.
56. Helps C, Lait P, Tasker S et al: Melting curve analysis of feline calicivirus isolates detected by real-time reverse transcription PCR, *J Virol Meth* 106:241-244, 2002.
57. Nasisse MP, Dorman DC, Jamison KC et al: Effects of valacyclovir in cats infected with feline herpesvirus 1, *Am J Vet Res* 58:1141-1144, 1997.
58. Nasisse MP, Guy JS, Davidson MG et al: In vitro susceptibility of feline herpesvirus-1 to vidarabine, idoxuridine, trifluridine, acyclovir, or bromovinyldeoxyuridine, *Am J Vet Res* 50:158-160, 1989.
59. Tennant B, Willoughby K: The use of enteral nutrition in small animal medicine, *Compendium of Continuing Education* 15:1054, 1993.
60. Binns SH, Dawson S, Speakman AJ et al: A study of feline upper respiratory tract disease with reference to prevalence and risk factors for infection with feline calicivirus and feline herpesvirus, *J Fel Med Surg* 2:123-133, 2000.
61. Harbour DA, Howard PE, Gaskell RM: Isolation of feline calicivirus and feline herpesvirus from domestic cats 1980 to 1989, *Vet Rec* 128:77-80, 1991.
62. Mochizuki M, Kawakami K, Hashimoto M et al: Recent epidemiological status of feline upper respiratory infections in Japan, *J Vet Med Sci* 62:801-803, 2000.
63. Wardley RC, Povey RC: Aerosol transmission of feline calicivirus: An assessment of its epidemiological importance, *Brit Vet J* 133:404-508, 1977.
64. Wardley RC, Povey RC. The clinical disease and patterns of excretion associated with three different strains of feline calicivirus, *Res Vet Sci* 23:7-14, 1977.
65. Wardley RC. Feline calicivirus carrier state: A study of the host/virus relationship, *Arch Virol* 52:243-249, 1976.
66. Johnson RP: Antigenic change in feline calicivirus during persistent infection, *Can J Vet Res* 56:326-330, 1992.
67. Radford AD, Turner PC, Bennett M et al: Quasispecies evolution of a hypervariable region of the feline calicivirus capsid gene in cell culture and in persistently infected cats, *J Gen Virol* 79:1-10, 1998.
68. Kreutz LC, Johnson RP, Seal BS: Phenotypic and genotypic variation of feline calicivirus during persistent infection of cats, *Vet Microbiol* 59:229-236, 1998.
69. Wardley RC, Gaskell RM, Povey RC: Feline respiratory viruses—their prevalence in clinically healthy cats, *J Sm Anim Pract* 15:579-586, 1974.
70. Coutts AJ, Dawson S, Willoughby K et al: Isolation of feline respiratory viruses from clinically healthy cats at UK cat shows, *Vet Rec* 135:555-556, 1994.
71. Radford AD: Unpublished observations, 2003.
72. Gaskell RM, Povey RC: Experimental induction of feline viral rhinotracheitis (FVR) virus re-excretion in FVR-recovered cats, *Vet Rec* 100:128-133, 1977.
73. Gaskell RM, Dennis PE, Goddard LE et al: Isolation of felid herpesvirus 1 from the trigeminal ganglia of latently infected cells, *J Gen Virol* 66:391-394, 1985.
74. Reubel GH, Ramos RA, Hickman MA et al: Detection of active and latent feline herpesvirus 1 infections using the polymerase chain reaction, *Arch Virol* 132:409-420, 1993.
75. Gaskell CJ, Gaskell RM, Dennis PE et al: Efficacy of an inactivated feline calicivirus (FCV) vaccine against challenge with United Kingdom field strains and its interaction with the FCV carrier state, *Res Vet Sci* 32:23-26, 1982.
76. Pedersen NC, Hawkins KF: Mechanisms of persistence of acute and chronic feline calicivirus infections in the face of vaccination, *Vet Microbiol* 47:141-156, 1995.
77. Povey RC, Koonse H, Hays MB: Immunogenicity and safety of an inactivated vaccine for the prevention of rhinotracheitis, caliciviral disease, and panleukopenia in cats, *J Am Vet Med Assoc* 177:347-350, 1980.
78. Scott FW: Evaluation of a feline viral rhinotracheitis-feline calicivirus disease vaccine, *Am J Vet Res* 38:229-34, 1997.
79. Bittle JL, Rubic WJ: A feline calicivirus vaccine combined with feline viral rhinotracheitis and feline panleukopenia vaccine, *Feline Pract* 5(6):13-15, 1975.
80. Scott FW, Geissinger CM: Duration of immunity in cats vaccinated with an inactivated feline panleukopenia, herpesvirus and calicivirus vaccine, *Feline Pract* 25(4):12-19, 1997.
81. Scott FW, Geissinger CM: Long-term immunity in cats vaccinated with an inactivated trivalent vaccine, *Am J Vet Res* 60:652-658, 1999.
82. Povey C, Ingersoll J: Cross-protection among feline caliciviruses, *Infect Immun* 11:877-885, 1975.
83. Tham KM, Studdert MJ: Antibody and cell-mediated immune responses to feline calicivirus following inactivated vaccine and challenge, *J Vet Med* 34:640-654, 1987.
84. Orr CM, Gaskell CJ, Gaskell RM: Interaction of a combined feline viral rhinotracheitis-feline calicivirus vaccine and the FVR carrier state, *Vet Rec* 103:200-202, 1978.
85. Povey RC, Wilson MR: A comparison of inactivated feline viral rhinotracheitis and feline caliciviral disease vaccines with live-modified viral vaccines, *Feline Pract* 8(3):35-42, 1978.
86. Bittle JL, Rubic WJ: Studies of feline viral rhinotracheitis vaccine, *Vet Med Small Anim Clin* 69:1503-1505, 1974.
87. Johnson RP, Povey RC: Transfer and decline of maternal antibody to feline calicivirus, *Can Vet J* 24:6-9, 1983.
88. Gaskell RM, Povey RC: Transmission of feline viral rhinotracheitis, *Vet Rec* 111:359-362, 1982.
89. Lauritzen A, Jarrett O, Sabara M: Serological analysis of feline calicivirus isolates from the United States and United Kingdom, *Vet Microbiol* 56:55-63, 1997.
90. Iglauer F, Gartner K, Morstedt R: Maternal protection against feline respiratory disease by means of booster vaccinations during pregnancy: A retrospective clinical study, *Kleintierpraxis* 34:235, 1989.
91. Morrison WB, Starr RM: Vaccine-associated feline sarcomas, *J Am Vet Med Assoc* 218:697-702, 2001.
92. Elston T, Rodan H, Flemming D et al: 1998 report of the American Association of Feline Practitioners and Academy of Feline Medicine Advisory Panel on Feline Vaccines, *J Am Vet Med Assoc* 212:227-241, 1998.
93. Gaskell RM, Gettinby G, Graham SJ et al: Veterinary Products Committee working group report on feline and canine vaccination, *Vet Rec* 150:126-134, 2002.
94. Gaskell RM, Gettinby G, Graham SJ et al: *Veterinary Products Committee (VPC) working group on feline and canine vaccination: Final report to the VPC* (PB 6432), London, 2002, Departmental for Environmental, Food and Rural Affairs.
95. Dawson S, Willoughby K, Gaskell RM et al: A field trial to assess the effect of vaccination against feline herpesvirus, feline calicivirus and feline panleucopenia virus in 6-week-old kittens, *J Feline Med Surg* 3:17-22, 2001.

CHAPTER 36

Fungal Rhinitis

Kyle G. Mathews

Aspergillosis

SIGNALMENT AND HISTORY

Canine fungal rhinitis is a common disease that primarily affects young to middle age dogs of mesaticephalic (e.g., Labrador retriever) and dolichocephalic (e.g., German shepherd) breeds. *Aspergillus fumigatus,* a ubiquitous soil saprophyte, is the most common pathogen, although *Penicillium* spp., and *Cryptococcus neoformans* have also been reported.[1-22] Nasal aspergillosis is rare in cats.[23] In one report of 60 dogs with nasal aspergillosis, the age of affected animals ranged from 3 months to 11 years (with a mean of 3.3 years).[9] In contrast, a major differential, nasal neoplasia, tends to occur in older animals.[24] A history of nasal trauma is uncommon, but has been reported in some dogs.[12] Nasal aspergillosis can occur concomitantly with, and probably secondary to, nasal tumors and nasal foreign bodies such as grass awns. Other differential diagnoses should include extension of dental disease; cleft palate; and lymphoplasmacytic, bacterial, and allergic rhinitis. It has been suggested that some dogs with nasal aspergillosis may have an underlying immunodeficiency that predisposes them to infection, and impaired lymphocyte blastogenesis responses have been reported.[4,15] However, it is unclear whether impaired lymphocyte function is a cause or a result of infection because *A. fumigatus* products have been shown to inhibit lymphocyte transformation *in vitro.*[25]

Clinical and historical signs consistent with nasal aspergillosis in dogs include mucopurulent nasal discharge, sneezing, signs of nasal pain (e.g., pawing at the face or pain on palpation), epistaxis, decreased appetite, lethargy, and nasal depigmentation or ulceration (Figure 36-1). Stertor, stridor, and/or open-mouth breathing may also be noted. Nasal discharge is initially unilateral in most cases, but often progresses to bilateral involvement. Facial deformity due to paranasal extension or inflammation can occur in advanced cases, and epiphora secondary to nasolacrimal duct obstruction occurs occasionally.

DIAGNOSIS

A thorough physical examination should include facial palpation for evidence of pain or asymmetry, evaluation of airflow through each nostril, and an oral examination.

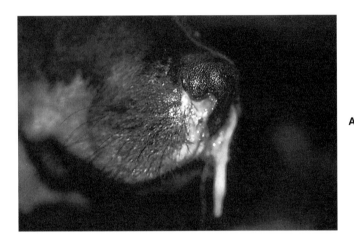

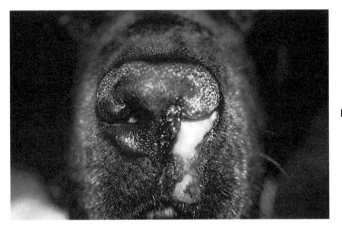

Figure 36-1. A, Typical mucopurulent nasal discharge; and *B,* nasal planum depigmentation/ulceration associated with nasal aspergillosis.

Established guidelines[1] used to make a definitive diagnosis include positive results on biopsy, a positive titer with positive culture results, or a positive titer with radiographic or computed tomography (CT) scan changes suggestive of fungal rhinitis (i.e., turbinate loss). Unfortunately, confirmation of the diagnosis often requires multiple tests because *Aspergillus fumigatus* may be found as endogenous flora in the nasal cavities of many animals.[13] Culture results may also be negatively impacted by secondary bacterial overgrowth.

Serology

Numerous techniques for determination of *Aspergillus* serum fungi-specific antibody titers have been evaluated, including agar gel double diffusion (AGDD), counterimmunoelectrophoresis (CIE), and enzyme-linked immunosorbent assay (ELISA) techniques. AGDD and CIE tests have been reported to be highly sensitive and specific, whereas ELISA appears to be less reliable.[18-20] However, negative AGDD results should be viewed with some skepticism if the clinical, radiographic, and rhinoscopic picture is consistent with fungal rhinitis. The author has obtained several false negative results using AGDD (Meridian Diagnostics, Inc., Fungal immunodiffusion system, Cincinnati, OH) early in the disease process from histologically confirmed cases of nasal aspergillosis. Many of these cases had positive titers when retested at a later date. Further, nasal *Penicillium* infection, which is clinically indistinguishable from aspergillosis, can result in a negative AGDD test if only *Aspergillus* antigens are used.[13] One should also remember that a positive result does not eliminate the possibility of a concurrent disease process such as neoplasia. Submission of an aspergillus titer followed by general anesthesia, a radiographic evaluation, and rhinoscopy with the intent to biopsy and culture is a logical diagnostic approach.

Imaging

Nasal and frontal sinus radiographs can be used as a screening tool to evaluate dogs with suspected fungal rhinitis. Rostral radiolucency due to turbinate lysis, and/or a mixed pattern of caudal lucency and opacity, are usually seen on dorsoventral views, whereas increased radioopacity and frontal bone thickening on rostrocaudal views is typical.[16] Studies have shown that CT is superior to nasal radiography for defining the extent of disease and for differentiating infectious from neoplastic rhinitis.[26,27] Fungal rhinitis is typified by loss of turbinates; however, significant accumulation of fluid can occur and obscure fungal granulomas, concomitant masses, and turbinate detail (Figure 36-2) with either imaging technique. Occlusion of the openings to the frontal sinuses by inflammatory tissue with secondary fluid accumulation in the sinuses may also occur. CT or magnetic resonance imaging (MRI) are required to evaluate the integrity of the cribriform plate.

Topical treatment may be performed without advanced imaging techniques if nasal radiographs and other diagnostic tests are suggestive of fungal infection. Referral for CT should be seriously considered, however, if there is evidence of caudal nasal involvement. Lysis of the cribriform plate may contraindicate the use of topical medications, although complications arising from leakage of antifungal medications into the central nervous system of dogs with fungal rhinitis have not been evaluated. Owners of affected dogs should be informed of this concern before topical administration of antifungal agents. If cribriform involvement is detected on CT, dogs may be treated with oral itraconazole.

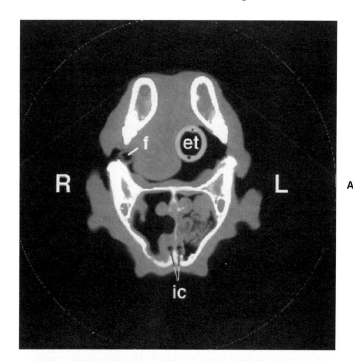
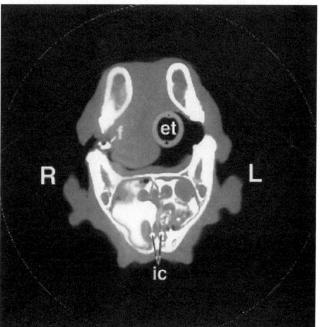

Figure 36-2. *Nonsurgical intranasal infusion in the dog.* ***A,*** *Preinfusion nasal CT scan (dorsal recumbency) showing position of infusion catheters (ic), Foley catheter (f), and endotracheal tube (et). Note the right-sided turbinate loss.* ***B,*** *Postinfusion CT scan showing widespread distribution of clotrimazole and contrast media.* (From Mathews KG, Koblik PD, Richardson EF et al: Computed tomographic assessment of noninvasive intranasal infusions in dogs with fungal rhinitis, *Vet Surg* 25:309-319, 1996.)

Rhinoscopy

Following radiographic or computed tomographic evaluation of the nasal cavity, rhinoscopy should be performed, preferably during the same anesthetic episode.[28] Nasal examination is never performed prior to radiography because hemorrhage induced by rhinoscopy will alter the results. General anesthesia is required, with a cuffed endotracheal tube in place to prevent aspiration of blood and lavage fluids. The external surface of the nasal cavity is examined for evidence of swelling, asymmetry, and ulceration. This includes a thorough oral examination and visualization of the nasopharynx with either a flexible fiberoptic scope or an angled dental mirror.[29] Precounted gauze sponges are then placed in the pharynx for further protection of the airways. Large laparotomy sponges with radioopaque markers should be used, if possible, because they are less easily swallowed by patients that respond to manipulation of the nasal tissues.

The distance from the nares to the area of interest on the nasal radiographs or other imaging studies is then measured to serve as a guide for sampling nasal biopsy specimens. In addition, prior to inserting any instrument in the nasal cavity, the distance from the nares to the medial canthus of the eye is noted and should not be exceeded at any time because penetration of the cribriform plate may result. Rhinoscopy can then be performed with the animal in sternal recumbency. Limited examination of the rostral nasal cavity may be performed with an otoscope, but this is generally inadequate for making a diagnosis of fungal rhinitis. A sterile rigid arthroscope with a 1.9- to 2.7-mm outside diameter and a 5- to 25-degree angle of view (Richard Wolf Medical Instruments Corp. Rosemont, IL) is commonly used for rhinoscopy. Evaluation of a lateral frontal sinus can also be performed with the rigid scope after creating a trephine hole in the dorsal wall of the sinus. A flexible bronchoscope with a 3.5- to 4.8-mm outside diameter (Olympus Corporation, Lake Success, NY) allows visualization of the nasopharynx by retroflexing the scope around the soft palate.

Light resistance is usually felt while inserting the scope through the nares. The scope can then be directed ventrally into the ventral nasal meatus toward the nasopharynx; or dorsally into the dorsal nasal meatus, toward the olfactory epithelium, the openings (ostia) of the frontal sinuses, and the cribriform plate. The advantages of direct visualization of the nasal cavity include a more thorough understanding of the nature of the disease process and the potential to place a biopsy instrument at the area of interest. Many scopes are equipped with biopsy ports or sleeves that simplify tissue sampling. In addition, a biopsy instrument such as uterine biopsy forceps may be inserted alongside the scope if room permits. Disadvantages of rhinoscopy include the need for expensive equipment, and poor visualization if excessive nasal discharge exists or if hemorrhage occurs.

Some degree of hemorrhage is inevitable. The nasal mucosa is richly endowed with blood vessels, which allow for efficient heat exchange. In addition, the neovascularization of mucosa that occurs with rhinitis results in a propensity for hemorrhage following biopsy or even light contact with the rhinoscope, in many cases. Coagulation profiles, cross matching, and blood transfusions should all be considered depending on the severity of the disease, history of epistaxis, and the invasiveness of the biopsy procedure about to be performed. Generally, hemorrhage from nasal biopsies obtained via the nares, although frustrating to the rhinoscopist, is self-limiting. Concurrent lavage of the nasal cavity with physiologic saline can improve visualization. To reduce hemorrhage, ice packs may be applied to the bridge of the nose and digital pressure may be placed on the rostral cartilaginous portion of the nasal cavity. Lavage of the nasal cavity with chilled saline, or instillation of epinephrine (1:100,000) may also be of benefit. Because of this propensity for hemorrhage, thorough examination of the entire nasal cavity should be performed prior to biopsy.

In some cases the nasopharynx is the primary area of interest based on the results of imaging studies, and nasopharyngeal examination should be performed with a flexible bronchoscope or dental mirror. Nasopharyngeal masses associated with cryptococcal infection have been reported in both cats and dogs. Tissue samples may be obtained from this area via a flexible scope; by surgical splitting of the soft or hard palate; or by retroflexion of a catheter dorsal to the soft palate, followed by lavage and suction.

Biopsy specimens are placed in formalin for histopathologic examination, in appropriate media for bacterial and fungal cultures, and rolled onto glass slides for immediate cytological examination. Following resolution of hemorrhage and prior to recovery from anesthesia, the pharyngeal gauze sponges are recounted and the pharynx is suctioned as needed.

Rhinoscopic evaluation of dogs with aspergillosis typically reveals areas of turbinate atrophy, mucopurulent discharge, and fungal plaques. Fungal plaques may be white, off-white, or have a greenish tint. The surface of a plaque may be fuzzy in appearance due to the presence of conidiophores (fruiting bodies). Collections of exudate, which are often easily dislodged by flushing, should not be mistaken for plaques. Cytologic evaluation of aspergillus plaques reveals septate hyphae with dichotomous branching at 45-degree angles. Conidia may also be present.[30]

If a diagnosis of nasal aspergillosis is rendered following nasal examination (based on consistent radiographic or CT findings, the presence of fungal plaques, and/or hyphae on cytological examination), topical treatment may be performed during the same anesthetic episode.

TREATMENT

Treatment of nasal aspergillosis with systemic antifungal medications (e.g., thiabendazole, ketoconazole and fluconazole) has been disappointing in that the reported response rate is only 43% to 60%.[1-5,12-14] Response to oral administration of itraconazole has been approximated at 60% to 70%,[30] but there are currently no large studies evaluating systemic treatment with itraconazole, and cost of the drug is often prohibitive. For example, treatment of a 30-kg dog for 2 months would cost over $1000 (Sporanox® 5 mg/kg BID PO). Hepatic toxicosis may mandate temporary or permanent discontinuation of itraconazole in 5% to 10% of dogs, and serial monitoring of serum ALT concentration is recommended.[30]

Topical administration of the imidazoles (e.g., enilconazole and clotrimazole) is more effective than orally administered antifungal medications.[4-7,9,10,14,31] Intranasal administration of enilconazole entails a surgical procedure to place indwelling catheters into the nasal cavity, the frontal sinuses, or both.[4-6] After catheter placement, small volumes (5 to 10 ml; 50 mg/ml = 10 mg/kg) of enilconazole are administered twice daily for 7 to 14 days. Larger volumes should be avoided because of risk of aspiration. In one study, nasal discharge resolved in 19 (80%) of 24 dogs treated solely with topical administration of enilconazole.[6] Common complications include premature removal of catheters, necessitating additional anesthetic episodes for catheter replacement; transient postoperative subcutaneous emphysema; inappetence; and ptyalism after administration of enilconazole.[4-6]

A 1-hour infusion of clotrimazole, administered to dogs that are under general anesthesia, also results in resolution of clinical signs in many dogs with nasal aspergillosis.[7,9,10] Clotrimazole at the high local concentrations achieved with topical administration causes direct damage to fungal membranes and inhibits fungal ergosterol synthesis.[32] Although a surgical procedure is initially used for catheter placement into the frontal sinuses, multiple treatments are not required, complications associated with indwelling catheters are eliminated, and hospitalization times are substantially reduced.[33]

In a study evaluating the distribution of dye injected into cadaver skulls of dogs without sinonasal disease, a noninvasive technique for intranasal infusion resulted in better distribution of infusate into the nasal cavity and frontal sinuses than techniques that used surgically placed catheters.[34] Larger volumes of infusate may be administered and leakage is minimal (thereby decreasing the risk of aspiration) if the nares and nasopharynx are occluded during intranasal infusion. With cadaver skulls placed in dorsal recumbency, bilateral administration of 50 ml (100 ml total) through the nares resulted in excellent distribution of infusate to the entire nasal cavity and frontal sinuses with minimal leakage into the pharynx.[34] This noninvasive intranasal technique resulted in good distribution of infusate to the nasal cavity and frontal sinuses, as determined by evaluation of pre- and postinfusion images on computed tomography (CT) in 12 dogs with confirmed fungal rhinitis (see Figure 36-2).[8] The percentage of the lateral sinus filled with infusate varied from 10% (enough to cover the roof of the lateral sinus) to 100% (mean 42%). The infusate mixed with exudate, if present, and outlined previously obscured fungal granulomas.[8]

One study evaluated 60 dogs with nasal aspergillosis treated with topical clotrimazole.[9] The goals of the study were to examine the clinical response to topical administration of clotrimazole in dogs with nasal aspergillosis, to compare the efficacy of surgical versus nonsurgical placement of catheters used for administration, and to examine whether subjective scoring of computed tomographic images can predict outcome. Topical 1% clotrimazole solution was infused during a 1-hour period via surgically placed frontal sinus and nasal catheters (27 dogs) and via nonsurgically placed intranasal catheters (18 dogs). An additional 15 dogs required and received 2 to 4 infusions by either route. Topical administration of clotrimazole resulted in resolution of clinical disease in 65% of dogs after one treatment and in 87% of dogs after one or more treatments. There was no difference in outcome between surgically and nonsurgically placed catheters. The CT images of the nasal cavity of each dog were divided into 8 anatomic regions and a radiographic score of 0 to 3 was assigned to each region depending on the severity of disease (0 = no detectable abnormalities; 1 = mild turbinate atrophy or fluid accumulation; 2 = moderate; 3 = severe). Anatomic regions included the right and left nasal turbinates (rostral to the maxillary recess), maxillary turbinates (at the level of the maxillary recess), ethmoid turbinates (caudal to the maxillary recess), and frontal sinuses. A total radiographic score was then calculated for each dog by summing the scores of the 8 regions (24 points = maximum score possible). Dogs with unfavorable responses were correctly predicted to do poorly 71% to 78% of the time (sensitivity) using a cutpoint of 8 or greater (total radiographic score). Dogs with favorable responses (i.e., elimination of clinical signs following one treatment) were correctly classified 79% to 93% of the time (specificity) using a total radiographic score of less than 8.

Topical administration of clotrimazole, using either technique, is therefore an effective treatment for nasal aspergillosis in dogs. The use of noninvasive intranasal infusion of clotrimazole eliminates the need for surgical trephination of the frontal sinuses in many dogs and is associated with fewer complications.[9,10] Preliminary information on the use of enilconazole administered in a similar fashion is not favorable. Of 4 dogs treated in this manner, 1 resolved after 2 treatments, 1 died from sepsis after the second treatment, and 2 developed profuse fungal growth in the face of therapy.[11]

Nasal discharge ceases in most dogs by 2 weeks after topical clotrimazole therapy.[9] A repeat treatment is recommended if nasal discharge continues without improvement 2 weeks after the initial treatment. Owners of affected dogs with high CT scores should also be advised that more than one treatment will probably be needed. Sequential evaluation of aspergillus titers does not aid in the decision to re-treat because titers may remain elevated for years despite resolution of disease.[4,17] Recurrent nasal discharge that resolved with empirical antibiotic therapy occurred in 7 of 60 dogs (within a mean of 4 months) following antifungal treatment.[9] Secondary bacterial rhinitis was suspected in these dogs, possibly because of destruction of the nasal anatomy by the fungal infection. Once nasal discharge ceases after clotrimazole treatment, it appears that a recurrence of rhinitis attributable to fungal infection is uncommon and was documented in only 1 of 60 dogs.[9]

The volume of the nasal cavity and frontal sinuses varies depending on the size of the dog, the extent of turbinate destruction, and the volume of accumulated exudate. Based on a study in cadavers, the average volume of the frontal sinuses in breeds predisposed to fungal rhinitis was 25 ml per side.[34] The nasal cavity and sinuses can be flooded with a larger volume of infusate (50 to 60 ml per side), resulting in distribution of the infusate to all areas of the nasal cavity and frontal sinuses (see Figure 36-2). A 1% formulation of clotrimazole in a polyethylene glycol base* is readily available in a 30-ml vial, which makes treatment with 2 vials per side convenient. Sixty ml per side is used in medium to large breed dogs regardless of head size. Thirty milliliters per side should be adequate for smaller breeds. Formulations that contain isopropyl alcohol and propylene glycol† should be used with caution because they may result in pharyngeal irritation and edema.[2]

Sinusotomy: Surgical Placement of Infusion Catheters

General anesthesia is induced and the dog is intubated with a cuffed endotracheal tube. Aseptic preparation and draping of the dorsal surface of the skull is performed with the dog in sternal recumbency. A hole is made in each frontal bone over the lateral frontal sinus using a Michelle's trephine or Steinman pin. Trephination is begun at a point halfway between the dorsal midline and the zygomatic process of the frontal bone. Penetration of the frontal bones caudal to these processes increases the risk of penetration through the floor of the frontal sinus or directly into the cranium. In the cat, the sinuses are much less extensive than in the dog, and there is less room for error when making this approach. In the dog, there are three separate frontal sinuses on each side of the midline—a large lateral frontal sinus, which is typically entered during sinusotomy; and the smaller rostral and medial frontal sinuses. In the cat, there is a single frontal sinus on each side of midline. Each sinus drains rostrally and ventrally into the nasal cavity via separate ostia. Exudate and necrotic material is removed by use of suction and curettage. Two 8 or 10 Fr polypropylene catheters are placed per side (4 catheters total) so that one catheter exits the sinus ostium with its tip in the caudal portion of the nasal cavity and the other catheter tip is within the lateral frontal sinus. The pharynx is packed with laparotomy sponges. A 12 Fr Foley catheter is placed through each nostril so that the inflated balloon slows leakage of medication. A single suture of 3-0 nylon placed across each nostril will prevent the balloon from migrating rostrally. One-percent clotrimazole solution is evenly divided between four 30-ml syringes and slowly infused through the surgically placed catheters during 1 hour. The dog is positioned so that its nose protrudes beyond the edge of the treatment table, thus allowing excess clotrimazole to drip into a disposable receptacle. After treatment, catheters and laparotomy sponges are removed and counted, excess medication is

allowed to drain rostrally, and the pharynx and proximal esophagus are suctioned to decrease the risk of aspiration. The skin is sutured to loosely appose the incisions. A single shortened catheter is often left protruding from each sinusotomy for 1 to 2 days, and held in place with a finger-trap suture pattern to decrease the risk of subcutaneous emphysema.

It has been shown that surgical damage to the ostia can result in granulation tissue and new bone formation that obstructs sinus drainage and results in fluid accumulation.[35] Fungal granulomas or associated inflammation can also result in ostia obstruction and subsequent fluid accumulation within the sinuses. Techniques that involve curettage of this area during biopsy, or placement of catheters through the sinus ostia for the treatment of fungal rhinitis (as above), could theoretically result in similar obstruction. In order to avoid this possibility, an alternative is to place a single infusion catheter in each lateral frontal sinus that does not penetrate the ostium.

Surgical placement of tubes is associated with more complications than nonsurgical intranasal catheter placement.[9] Two dogs have been reported to have serious complications with the surgical technique that eventually resulted in euthanasia. In neither case was a pretreatment CT scan performed. One dog developed neurologic signs consistent with a cortical encephalopathy and was euthanized 2 weeks after treatment. The second dog developed suppurative meningitis with seizure activity and was euthanized 6 weeks after clotrimazole therapy. The most common posttreatment complication in dogs treated by trephination of the frontal sinuses was subcutaneous emphysema. Subcutaneous and retrobulbar leakage, and nasolacrimal duct filling of clotrimazole have also occurred with no apparent adverse effects.

Nonsurgical Intranasal Placement of Infusion Catheters

General anesthesia is induced and the dog is intubated with a cuffed endotracheal tube. Catheters are placed with the dog in lateral recumbency. A 24 Fr Foley catheter is placed per os so that the tip of the catheter is dorsal to the soft palate. This process is aided initially by grasping the catheter tip with a pair of long-handled needle holders so that the catheter tip is directed rostrally. A mouth gag is placed and an assistant pulls the dog's tongue rostrally to improve exposure. The Foley catheter is advanced until its balloon is dorsal to the junction of the hard and soft palates. The balloon is inflated to occlude the nasopharynx, and is palpated through the soft palate to confirm its position. Precounted laparotomy sponges are placed in the pharynx so that the catheter cannot migrate caudally, and to absorb any infusate that might escape around the balloon. Smaller sponges are avoided because these are easily swallowed. The index finger of the operator's opposite hand is used to maintain balloon position during sponge placement. The mouth gag is removed. One 10 Fr polypropylene infusion catheter is advanced, beginning dorsomedially, through each nostril into the dorsal nasal meatus and to the level of the medial canthus of the ipsilateral palpebral fissure.

*Lotrimin® solution, Schering Corporation, Kenilworth, NJ.
†For example Canesten® solution, Miles Canada, Etobicoke, Ontario, Canada.

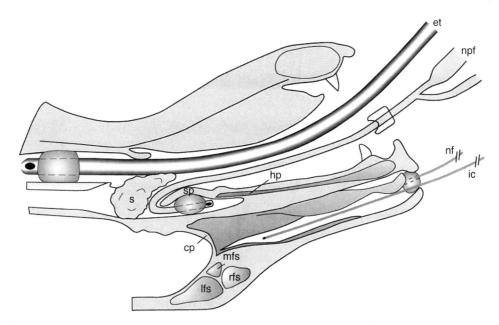

Figure 36-3. *Nonsurgical intranasal infusion in the dog. Sagittal section showing the position of the endotracheal tube* (et), *nasopharyngeal Foley catheter* (npf), *pharyngeal sponges* (s), *infusion catheter* (ic), *and rostral nasal Foley catheter* (nf) *in relation to the hard palate* (hp), *soft palate* (sp), *cribriform plate* (cp), *rostral frontal sinus* (rfs), *medial frontal sinus* (mfs), *and lateral frontal sinus* (lfs). (From Mathews KG, Koblik PD, Richardson EF et al: Computed tomographic assessment of noninvasive intranasal infusions in dogs with fungal rhinitis, *Vet Surg* 25:309-319, 1996.)

A 12 Fr Foley catheter is inserted into each nostril and the balloons are inflated so that they are positioned just caudal to and occluding the nostrils (Figure 36-3). A nylon suture is placed across each nostril to prevent rostral migration of the balloons. The balloons of the three Foley catheters (i.e., one nasopharyngeal, two nasal) serve to slow leakage of clotrimazole.

The dog is then placed in dorsal recumbency and an additional laparotomy sponge placed just caudal to the upper incisors, between the endotracheal tube and the incisive papilla, to control leakage of clotrimazole through the incisive ducts (Figure 36-4). One-percent clotrimazole solution is evenly divided between two 60-ml syringes and slowly infused during 1 hour. The polypropylene catheters are maintained parallel to the table throughout the infusion. The Foley catheters, in theory, allow air to escape the nasal chamber during the infusion. When fluid is noticed within the lumen of a Foley catheter, it is clamped. The dog is positioned so that its nose protrudes beyond the edge of the treatment table. The dog's head is rotated and maintained in the following positions to ensure drug contact with all nasal surfaces: dorsal recumbency (15 minutes), left lateral recumbency (15 minutes), right lateral recumbency (15 minutes), and dorsal recumbency (15 minutes). Posttreatment procedures are the same as for dogs treated via a sinusotomy.

Complications in dogs treated with intranasal infusion of clotrimazole are generally limited to leakage of clotrimazole through the incisive ducts during treatment, which is easily controlled with digital pressure; and transient increases in nasal drainage or sneezing immediately following recovery from anesthesia.

Given the good success rate with intranasal administration of clotrimazole, and the higher complication rate with sinusotomy, the intranasal route is generally used unless a fungal granuloma is detected within the frontal sinuses; this requires removal prior to therapy. If more extensive rhinotomy is required due to a large fungal mass, clotrimazole may be instilled directly into the nasal cavity prior to surgical closure.

Rhinotomy

Rhinotomy may be performed via either the dorsal or ventral approach, although a dorsal sinusotomy may be required to access granulomas within the frontal sinuses.[36] Rhinotomy should be limited to removal of fungal granulomas and grossly necrotic turbinates. Wholesale turbinectomy does not benefit the patient and may result in chronic serous nasal discharge.

Hemorrhage during rhinotomy may be diminished by temporary carotid artery ligation. This procedure requires a ventral midline surgical approach to the cervical region, with subsequent repositioning of the animal if dorsal rhinotomy is to be performed. Because of well-developed collateral circulation originating from the vertebral arteries in dogs, this procedure can be performed with no notable adverse effects. This is not true for the cat, where bilateral carotid ligation may result in death.[37-39] As previously stated, a minimalistic approach to rhinotomy as an adjunct to medical treatment of fungal rhinitis should be taken. Therefore the requirement for carotid artery ligation in affected animals is uncommon.

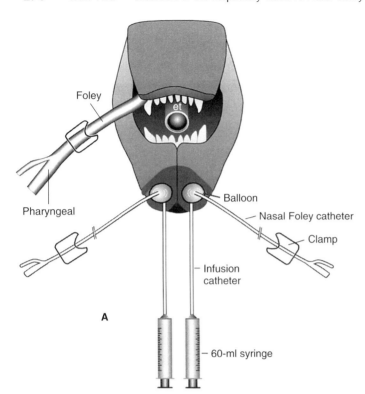
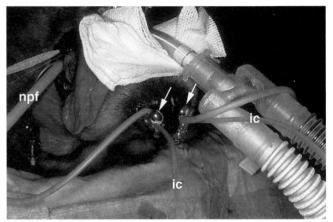

Figure 36-4. *Nonsurgical intranasal infusion in the dog.* **A,** *Catheter position with the dog in dorsal recumbency. A Foley catheter with the balloon inflated in the nasopharynx and pharyngeal gauze sponges (not shown) minimize leakage of infusate caudally. A cuffed endotracheal tube further diminishes the risk of aspiration. Two 60-ml syringes are used to inject infusate into the dorsal nasal meatus via polypropylene infusion catheters. Inflated Foley catheter balloons obstruct the nares to diminish leakage of infusate rostrally. Tubing clamps on Foley catheters are closed when fluid is observed within the catheter lumen.* **B,** *Photograph of clotrimazole intranasal infusion (dorsal recumbency). Nasopharyngeal Foley catheter (npf); polypropylene infusion catheters (ic); inflated Foley catheter balloons obstruct the nares to diminish leakage of infusate rostrally (arrows). Sponges placed between the endotracheal tube and rostral palate help diminish leakage of infusate through the vomeronasal organ.* (**A,** Modified from Mathews KG, Koblik PD, Richardson EF et al: Computed tomographic assessment of noninvasive intranasal infusions in dogs with fungal rhinitis, *Vet Surg* 25:309-319, 1996.)

Given the potential problems associated with dorsal rhinotomy (e.g., subcutaneous emphysema, the need to reposition the animal (twice) if carotid artery ligation is to be performed, and the relative dissatisfaction of owners with the appearance of their pets in the immediate postoperative period), ventral rhinotomy has also been investigated.[36,39] Dehiscence is rarely a problem following ventral rhinotomy, subcutaneous emphysema has not been reported, and cosmesis is improved in the immediate postoperative period. Access to caudal nasopharyngeal granulomas can be gained by incision of the soft palate alone. Access to the frontal sinuses is best achieved via the dorsal approach.

Cryptococcosis

Cryptococcus neoformans is the most commonly reported causative organism of feline fungal rhinitis.[40-52] Nasal cryptococcosis is not commonly reported in dogs.[22] Cryptococcus is a saprophytic budding yeast (5- to 15-µm diameter) with a polysaccharide capsule.[30] Avian ex-crement, and in particular that of the pigeon, is a common reservoir. Airborne Cryptococcus is presumably inhaled and deposited in the nasal cavity. In addition to causing nasal disease (e.g., granuloma formation, turbinate and bone lysis) it can result in lower respiratory tract disease. Extension to the central nervous system (meningoencephalitis) can occur either by direct invasion from the nasal cavity or by hematogenous spread. Cutaneous lesions and/or retinitis and anterior uveitis are also commonly reported.

As with dogs affected by nasal aspergillosis, an underlying immunodeficiency has been postulated.[43] Although the prevalence of FeLV or FIV infections has not been shown to be different between Cryptococcus-infected cats and the general population, FeLV or FIV seropositive status may affect the outcome of treatment.[40-42] In one study, FeLV or FIV-positive cats treated with itraconazole had a higher likelihood of treatment failure.[41] In another study, FIV positive cats tended to have more advanced disease and a slower response to therapy with fluconazole, although the outcome was still favorable.[40]

SIGNALMENT AND HISTORY

Cats with nasal cryptococcosis present with typical upper respiratory signs of sneezing and chronic nasal discharge (serous to mucopurulent) that is not responsive to antibacterial therapy. Chronic disease is often accompanied by anorexia and weight loss. Distortion of the nasal bridge and ulceration of the nasal planum are also commonly reported. Inspiratory stridor, snoring, dyspnea, and gagging may indicate nasopharyngeal involvement (nasopharyngeal granuloma).[44,46]

There is no age predilection in cats. Males and Siamese cats were overrepresented in one study,[40] as were young adult dogs, Great Danes, and Doberman pinschers in another study.[22] Differential diagnoses should include viral/bacterial rhinitis, neoplasia (e.g., lymphosarcoma, squamous cell carcinoma, and adenocarcinoma), lymphoplasmacytic rhinitis, dental disease, nasopharyngeal polyps, and foreign body.

DIAGNOSIS

Facial palpation and oral examination should be performed as for dogs with suspected aspergillosis. Ophthalmoscopic examination should be performed to determine if there is retinal or uveal involvement.

The diagnosis of nasal cryptococcosis is most readily made by cytologic evaluation of the nasal discharge. New methylene blue, Gram's, and India ink stains are typically used to highlight the organism and its refractile polysaccharide capsule (Figure 36-5). Identification of numerous budding yeasts on cytologic examination, or demonstration of the organism in nasal biopsy specimens, is considered diagnostic. Granulomatous masses should be submitted for histopathologic examination to rule out the possible differential diagnoses of neoplasia and nasopharyngeal polyps. A positive culture alone is not considered diagnostic because the organism has also been cultured in nasal flushes from clinically normal dogs and cats.[53]

Serologic testing with a latex agglutination test for capsular antigen* is also widely used and is highly sensitive and specific.[42,54] Serum latex cryptococcal antigen agglutination test (LCAT) titers correlate with disease severity, although high titers are not a predictor of poor response to therapy.[41,54] A titer of greater than or equal to 1:1 is considered positive.

Skull radiographs reveal increased radiodensity in the nasal cavity or sinuses consistent with a soft-tissue mass or fluid accumulation. Lysis of the turbinates and bone erosion may also occur. CT examination of the nasal cavity may be necessary to identify nasopharyngeal involvement and to evaluate cribriform plate integrity. As previously stated, CT has been shown to be superior to plain radiography in determining the extent of disease in dogs. Rhinoscopic examination of the nasal cavity and nasopharynx should also be considered to verify the extent of disease and for gathering tissue samples.

*Crypto LA, Wampole Laboratories, Cranbury, NJ.

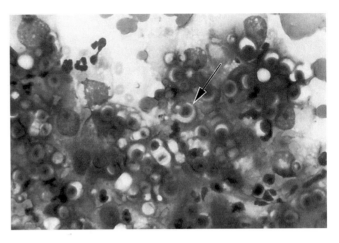

Figure 36-5. *Fine needle aspirate cytology from a nasal mass in a cat. Cryptococcal organisms are identified by their thick polysaccharide capsules* (arrow) *(Wright's Giemsa stain).*

TREATMENT

Treatment with a variety of enteral antifungal agents has been reported. The majority of cats respond favorably to fluconazole therapy administered at 50 mg/cat PO BID. Twenty-eight of 29 cats with nasal cryptococcosis had resolution of clinical signs.[40] The duration of treatment was 2 to 6.5 months. Side effects were limited to anorexia and minor increases in serum ALT concentration. Given these excellent results, fluconazole may be considered the drug of choice for treating feline nasal cryptococcosis.[32,40] Because fluconazole is primarily excreted through the kidneys, dosage adjustment or administration of itraconazole should be considered in cats with renal disease.

Diminution of LCAT antigen titer can be used to monitor response to therapy. Continuation of therapy has been recommended until the antigen titer falls to less than 1. This usually requires treatment for 1 to 2 months following resolution of clinical signs.[32,41,54]

Itraconazole has also been evaluated for the treatment of feline cryptococcosis.[41,52] Twenty-four of 28 cats with cryptococcosis (15 with nasal involvement) either improved (8 cats) or had resolution (16 cats) of their clinical signs.[52] The median itraconazole dose was 13.8 mg/kg/day for positive responders. Treatment was continued for a median of 8.5 months.[52] The authors recommended a dose of 50 mg/day in cats weighing less than 3.2 kg and 100 mg/day for cats weighing 3.2 kg or more.[52] Eight of the 28 cats had adverse reactions to itraconazole (e.g., anorexia, weight loss, and/or increased serum ALT concentration), and one cat died of itraconazole hepatotoxicity.[52]

Although the use of other antifungal drugs (e.g., ketoconazole, flucytosine, and amphotericin B) either alone or in combination has resulted in treatment success, they are in general associated with a higher rate of treatment failure and/or adverse side effects.[31,45,47-51]

In cats, trephination of the frontal sinuses has been performed[55] to allow instillation of medications for the treatment of bacterial rhinitis/sinusitis, but the use of topical medications for the treatment of feline nasal cryptococcosis has not been reported. If exploration of

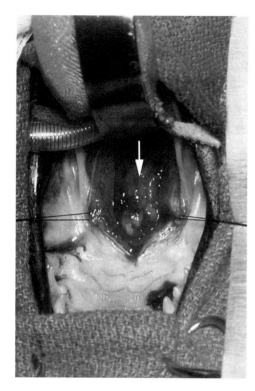

Figure 36-6. *Intraoperative ventral approach through the soft palate to remove a cryptococcal nasopharyngeal granuloma (arrow) in a cat.*

the sinuses is planned (e.g., for removal of a fungal granuloma), trephination and sinusotomy can be performed. In mature cats, a trephine hole is made just rostral to a line drawn between the zygomatic processes on either side of the midline. The trephine holes can then be connected with an osteotomy and a bone flap created for improved exposure. A ventral approach with surgical splitting of the soft and or hard palates may be required to remove nonpigmented nasopharyngeal granulomas that occur in some cases (Figure 36-6). Although the surgical removal of obstructive granulomas can lead to immediate clinical improvement, guidelines for surgery as an adjunct to medical management of nasal cryptococcosis have not been well established.[22,44]

REFERENCES

1. Harvey CE: Nasal aspergillosis and penicilliosis in dogs: Results of treatment with thiabendazole, *J Am Vet Med Assoc* 184:48, 1984.
2. Sharp NJH, Sullivan M: Use of ketoconazole in the treatment of canine nasal aspergillosis, *J Am Vet Med Assoc* 194:782, 1989.
3. Sharp NJH, Harvey CE, O'Brien JA: Treatment of canine nasal aspergillosis/penicilliosis with fluconazole, *J Small Anim Pract* 32:513, 1991.
4. Sharp NJH, Harvey CE, Sullivan M: Canine nasal aspergillosis and penicilliosis, *Compend Cont Ed* 13:41, 1991.
5. Sharp NJH, Sullivan M, Harvey CE: Treatment of canine nasal aspergillosis, *In Practice* 14:27-31, 1992.
6. Sharp NJH, Sullivan M, Harvey CE et al: Treatment of canine nasal aspergillosis with enilconazole, *J Vet Intern Med* 7:40, 1993.
7. Davidson AP, Pappagianis D: Treatment of nasal aspergillosis with topical clotrimazole. In Bonagura JD, editor: *Kirk's current veterinary therapy,* vol 12, Philadelphia, 1995, WB Saunders.
8. Mathews KG, Koblik PD, Richardson EF et al: Computed tomographic assessment of noninvasive intranasal infusions in dogs with fungal rhinitis, *Vet Surg* 25:309, 1996.
9. Mathews KG, Davidson AP, Koblik PD et al: Comparison of topical administration of clotrimazole through surgically versus nonsurgically placed catheters for treatment of nasal aspergillosis in dogs: 60 cases (1990-1996), *J Am Vet Med Assoc* 213:501, 1998.
10. Burbridge HM, Clark WT, Read R et al: Canine nasal aspergillosis: Results of treatment using clotrimazole as a topical agent, *Aust Vet Pract* 27:79, 1997.
11. Bray JP, White RAS, Lascelles BDX: Treatment of canine nasal aspergillosis with a new non-invasive technique: Failure with enilconazole, *J Small Anim Pract* 39:223, 1998.
12. Harvey CE, O'Brien JA: Nasal aspergillosis-penicilliosis. In Kirk RW, editor: *Current veterinary therapy,* vol 3, Philadelphia, 1983, WB Saunders.
13. Harvey CE, O'Brien JA, Felsburg PJ et al: Nasal penicilliosis in six dogs, *J Am Vet Med Assoc* 178:1084, 1981.
14. Sharp NJH: Aspergillosis and penicilliosis. In Greene CE, editor: *Infectious diseases of the dog and cat,* Philadelphia, 1998, WB Saunders.
15. Barrett RE, Hoffer RE, Schultz RD: Treatment and immunological evaluation of 3 cases of canine aspergillosis, *J Am Anim Hosp Assoc* 13:328, 1977.
16. Sullivan M, Lee R, Jakovljevic S et al: The radiological features of aspergillosis of the nasal cavity and frontal sinuses in the dog, *J Small Anim Pract* 27:167, 1986.
17. Sharp NJH, Harvey CE, Schwartzmann R et al: Sequential serology in canine nasal aspergillosis, *Proceedings of the 5th annual American College of Veterinary Internal Medicine forum,* 915, 1987.
18. Lane JG, Warnock DW: The diagnosis of *Aspergillus fumigatus* infection of the nasal chambers of the dog with particular reference to the value of the double diffusion test, *J Small Anim Pract* 18:169, 1977.
19. Richardson MD, Warnock DW, Bovey SE: Rapid serological diagnosis of Aspergillus fumigatus infection of the frontal sinuses and nasal chambers of the dog, *Res Vet Sci* 3:167, 1982.
20. Khan ZU, Richardson MD, Warnock DW et al: Evaluation of an enzyme linked immunosorbent assay (ELISA) for the diagnosis of *Aspergillus fumigatus* intranasal infection of the dog, *Sabaroudia* 22:251, 1984.
21. Caulkett N, Lew L, Fries C: Upper-airway obstruction and prolonged recovery from anesthesia following intranasal clotrimazole administration, *J Amer Anim Hosp Assoc* 33:264, 1997.
22. Malik R, Dill-Macky E, Martin P et al: Cryptococcosis in dogs: A retrospective study of 20 consecutive cases, *J Med Vet Mycol* 33:291, 1995.
23. Goodall SA, Lane JG, Warnock DW: The diagnosis and treatment of a case of nasal aspergillosis in a cat, *J Small Anim Pract* 25:627, 1984.
24. Henry CJ, Brewer WG Jr., Tyler JW et al: Survival in dogs with nasal adenocarcinoma; 64 cases (1981-1995), *J Vet Intern Med* 12:436, 1998.
25. Chaparas SD, Morgan PA, Holobaugh P et al: Inhibition of cellular immunity by-products of Aspergillus fumigatus, *J Med Vet Mycol* 24:67, 1986.
26. Codner EC, Lurus AG, Miller JB et al: Comparison of computed tomography with radiography as a noninvasive diagnostic technique for chronic nasal disease in dogs, *J Am Vet Med Assoc* 202:1106, 1993.
27. Park RD, Beck ER, LeCouter RA: Comparison of computed tomography and radiography or detecting changes induced by malignant neoplasia in dogs, *J Am Vet Med Assoc* 201:1720, 1992.
28. McCarthy TC, McDermaid SL: Rhinoscopy, *Vet Clin North Am Small Anim Pract* 20:1265, 1990.
29. Willard MD, Radlinsky MA: Endoscopic examination of the choanae in dogs and cats; 118 cases (1988-1998), *J Am Vet Med Assoc* 215:1301, 1999.
30. Larone DH:Yeast and Yeast-like organisms and thermallyl monomorphic molds. In Larone DH, editor: *Medically important fungi: A guide to identification,* ed 2, New York, 1987, Elsevier.
31. Legendre AM: Antimycotic drug therapy. In Bonagura JD, editor: *Kirk's current veterinary therapy,* vol 12, Philadelphia, 1995, WB Saunders.
32. Iwata K, Yamaguchi H, Hiratani T: Mode of action of clotrimazole, *Sabouraudia* 11:158, 1973.

33. Davidson A, Komtebedde J, Pappagianis D et al: Treatment of nasal aspergillosis with topical clotrimazole (abstract), *Proc 10th Am College Vet Intern Med Forum* 807, 1992.
34. Richardson EF, Mathews KG: Distribution of topical agents in the frontal sinuses and nasal cavity of dogs: Comparison between current protocols for treatment of nasal aspergillosis and a new non-invasive technique, *Vet Surg* 24:476, 1995.
35. Walsh TE: Experimental surgery of the ostium and nasofrontal duct in postoperative healing, *Laryngoscope* LIII(2):75, 1943.
36. Holmberg DL, Fries D, Cockshutt J et al: Ventral rhinotomy in the dog and cat, *Vet Surg* 18:446, 1989.
37. Clendenin MA, Conrad MC: Collateral vessel development after chronic bilateral common carotid artery occlusion in the dog, *Am J Vet Res* 40:1244, 1979.
38. King AS: Arterial supply to the central nervous system. In King AS: *Physiological and clinical anatomy of the domestic mammals,* vol 1, Oxford, 1987, Oxford University Press.
39. Holmberg DL: Sequelae of ventral rhinotomy in dogs and cats with inflammatory and neoplastic nasal pathology: A retrospective study, *Can Vet J* 37:483, 1996.
40. Malik R, Wigney DI, Muir DB et al: Cryptococcosis in cats: Clinical and mycological assessment of 29 cases and evaluation of treatment using orally administered fluconazole, *J Med Vet Mycol* 30:133, 1992.
41. Jacobs GJ, Medleau L, Calvert C et al: Cryptococcal infection in cats: Factors influencing treatment outcome, and results of sequential serum antigen titers in 35 cats, *J Vet Int Med* 11:1, 1997.
42. Flatland B, Greene RT, Lappin MR: Clinical and serologic evaluation of cats with cryptococcosis, *J Am Vet Med Assoc* 209:1110, 1997.
43. Jacobs GJ, Meleau L: Cryptococcosis. In Greene CE, editor: *Infectious diseases of the dog and cat,* Philadelphia, 1998, WB Saunders.
44. Malik R, Martin P, Wigney DI et al: Nasopharyngeal cryptococcosis, *Aust Vet J* 75:483, 1997.
45. Mikiciuk MG, Fales WE, Schmidt DA: Successful treatment of feline cryptococcosis with ketoconazole and flucytosine, *J Am Anim Hosp Assoc* 26:199, 1990.
46. Allen HS, Broussard J, Noone K: Nasopharyngeal diseases in cats: A retrospective study of 53 cases (1991-1998), *J Am Anim Hosp Assoc* 35:457, 1999.
47. Wilkinson GT, Bate MJ, Robins GM et al: Successful treatment of four cases of feline cryptococcosis, *J Small Anim Pract* 24:507, 1983.
48. Hansen BL: Successful treatment of severe feline cryptococcosis with long-term high doses of ketoconazole, *J Am Anim Hosp Assoc* 23:193, 1987.
49. Weir EC, Schwartz A, Buergelt CD: Short-term combination chemotherapy for treatment of feline cryptococcosis, *J Am Vet Med Assoc* 174:507, 1979.
50. Moore R: Treatment of feline nasal cryptococcosis with 5-flucytosine, *J Am Vet Med Assoc* 181:816, 1982.
51. Pentlarge VW, Martin RA: Treatment of cryptococcosis in three cats using ketoconazole, *J Am Vet Med Assoc* 188:536, 1986.
52. Medleau L, Jacobs GJ, Marks MA: Itraconazole for the treatment of cryptococcosis in cats, *J Vet Int Med* 9:39, 1995.
53. Malik R, Wigney DI, Muir DB et al: Asymptomatic carriage of *Cryptococcus neoformans* in the nasal cavity of dogs and cats, *J Med Vet Mycol* 35:27, 1997.
54. Malik R, McPetrie R, Wigney DI et al: A latex cryptococcal antigen agglutination test for diagnosis and monitoring of therapy for cryptococcosis, *Aust Vet J* 74:358, 1996.
55. Winstanley EW: Trephining frontal sinuses in the treatment of rhinitis and sinusitis in the cat, *Vet Rec* 95:289, 1974.

CHAPTER 37

Neoplasms of the Nasal Cavity

Margaret C. McEntee

Natural History and Incidence

Nasal and paranasal sinus tumors represent 59% to 82% of all canine respiratory tract tumors, but only 1% to 2% of all tumors in the canine, and are less commonly observed in the feline.[1-4] Nasal tumors occur most commonly in the nasal cavity, with secondary extension into the frontal and other paranasal sinuses; however, they occasionally arise initially in the paranasal sinuses. The majority of nasal tumors are malignant in both species.[1] They are primarily locally invasive and infrequently metastasize. The rate of metastasis at presentation in dogs has ranged from 0% to 12.5%.[5-7] Of 16 cats with nasal or paranasal sinus tumors, metastasis to the regional lymph nodes was documented in 2 cats (12.5%),

and one cat with nasal lymphoma had systemic involvement (i.e., kidney and lymph nodes).[8]

Some reports support a male predominance in the canine, with a male to female ratio of 1.3:1 to 3:1,[9-12] which may relate to behavior patterns as opposed to a hormonal influence.[10] Other studies do not support a sex predilection.[6,13] The male to female ratio in cats has ranged from 2:1 to 4:5.[1,14,15] Age at presentation in the dog ranges from 2 to 16 years,[7,13,16] with a median age of 10 years.[13] Dogs with nasal sarcomas may present at an earlier age than dogs with nasal carcinomas.[17] In one report of 35 dogs with nasal tumors the median age of dogs with carcinomas was 8.5 years, and for dogs with sarcomas was 5.8 years.[17] The mean age of cats with intranasal/paranasal sinus tumors is 8 to 10 years, with a range of 1 to 19 years.[8,14,15,18]

Epidemiology and Risk Factors, Including Environmental Influences

Certain canine breeds and skull conformations appear to be predisposed to the development of nasal cancer. Dolichocephalic and mesaticephalic dogs have a higher risk, whereas brachycephalic dogs have a lower risk of developing sinonasal cancer.[10] Brachycephalic breeds, with the associated malformations and nasal stenosis, are typically open mouth breathers with resultant decreased exposure of the nasal turbinates to potential environmental carcinogens. In one study, Boston terriers had a risk 2.3 times that of all brachycephalic breeds, although the reason for this is unknown.[10] Dogs have a very complex membranous turbinate structure with a large surface area compared with other species.[19] The nasal structures function as an efficient filter that may result in increased exposure to environmental airborne carcinogens. The risk of nasal cancer appears to correlate with the amount of surface area in the nasal passages and the efficiency of the filtering capability. Mixed-breed dogs have the same risk of developing nasal cancer as purebred dogs, suggesting an environmental influence. There is a marked significant effect of nasal length for both purebred and mixed breed dogs in the development of nasal cancer.[20]

Pet dogs have been investigated as sentinels for environmental cancer risks in people.[20] In one case control study, it was shown that environmental tobacco smoke was associated with no increased risk, whereas indoor kerosene or coal combustion was associated with an increased risk of neoplasia.[20] In contrast, data from another study supported an association between environmental tobacco and canine nasal cancer, although it did not hold up when an adjustment was made for use of flea control products.[21] The use of topical flea products, specifically flea spray, has been associated with increased sinonasal cancer risk.[20,21] It is not known what component of flea sprays (e.g., pyrethrins, organic solvents, or alcohol) may lead to the increased risk.

Breeds considered to be at increased risk of nasal neoplasms include Airedale terriers, basset hounds, old English sheepdogs, Scottish terriers, collies, Shetland sheepdogs, and German shorthaired pointers[10,22]; however, in a recent study, breed was not an independent predictor for risk of nasal cancer.[20]

Transmissible venereal tumor (TVT) is most commonly found on the external genitalia but has been reported to occur in the nasal cavity.[23-25] TVT is transmitted by contact with mucous membranes and occurs more readily if there are breaks in the integrity of a mucosal surface. TVT in the nasal cavity results from sniffing and licking.

In the feline there is some indication that chronic rhinitis/sinusitis may represent an initiating factor for the subsequent development of nasal neoplasia.[18] Feline leukemia virus (FeLV) may play a role in tumor development, but nasal lymphoma has been reported in FeLV-positive as well as FeLV-negative cats.[18,26,27] Although lymphoma is one of the most common nasal tumors in cats, other forms of lymphoma are more often observed.

In one report of 118 cats with lymphoma, only 5 (4%) had nasal lymphoma.[28]

Historical Findings, Clinical Signs, and Progression

Clinical signs in dogs with nasal tumors include respiratory, ocular, and nervous system–related signs. The duration of clinical signs prior to diagnosis ranges from 2 weeks to 2.5 years, with a mean duration of 2.5 to 4 months.[17,29,30] The most common clinical signs are decreased airflow through the affected nasal passage, epistaxis, and sneezing.[30] Other reported signs include reverse sneezing; stertorous breathing; serous, mucoid or mucopurulent nasal discharge; dyspnea; lethargy; weight loss; facial deformity or swelling; and pain.[17,30] In patients that have lysis of the hard palate there may be obvious deviation of the hard palate on oral examination, or a palpable palate defect. In a subset of dogs the tumor may be visible externally. Tumors on the nasal planum or in the nasal vestibule are typically localized to the rostral aspect of the nose. Ocular signs include discharge, exophthalmia, and blindness. On physical examination it may be possible to detect decreased retropulsion of the eye(s) if the tumor extends into the orbital region. Central nervous system signs include seizures, behavior changes, obtundation, and neurologic deficits.[31] Neurologic signs commonly occur only in the advanced disease state and following the development of nasal signs. A subset of dogs and cats present initially for neurologic signs and do not have nasal signs of disease.[31-34]

In cats there is variability in clinical signs depending whether a nasal or nasopharyngeal tumor is present.[35] Cats with nasal disease most commonly have a history of nasal discharge and sneezing. Cats with nasopharyngeal disease more often have stertorous respiration and change in phonation. In one report of nasopharyngeal disease in 23 cats in which soft palate digital palpation was performed, 19 cats (82%) had a palpable soft palate mass.[35] Other clinical signs include epiphora, epistaxis, and facial deformity.[14,15] The duration of clinical signs prior to presentation ranges from 1 week to 5 years.[8,18]

Differential Diagnosis

Approximately one third of all dogs with chronic nasal disease have nasal neoplasia.[36,37] Differential diagnosis for chronic nasal disease include aspergillosis, lymphoplasmacytic rhinitis, bacterial rhinitis (primary is rare; bacterial infection typically occurs secondary to another problem), foreign body (e.g., plant awn), oronasal fistulae, dental disease, inflammatory polyp, *Pneumonyssus caninum* (nasal mite), penicilliosis, rhinosporidiosis, and pythiosis.[38-40] There is one report of a dog with Cushing's disease that had a biopsy diagnosis of nasal chondrosarcoma and concurrently a definitive diagnosis of aspergillosis based on both culture and serology.[30] In patients with epistaxis, other differentials include primary coagulopathies, secondary coagulopathies (e.g., canine ehrlichiosis), and hyperviscosity syndrome (e.g., multiple myeloma). In cats, differential diagnoses include nasopharyngeal/inflammatory polyps, bacterial or viral rhinitis, lymphoplasmacytic rhinitis, and cryptococcosis.[35]

Diagnostic Tests

Initial evaluation includes a complete laboratory evaluation (e.g., hemogram, biochemical profile, and urinalysis), regional lymph node aspiration cytology, three view thoracic radiographs, nasal biopsy, and imaging of the nasal cavity (e.g., radiographs, computed tomography [CT], and/or magnetic resonance imaging [MRI]). In dogs with a history of epistaxis, a coagulation profile may be indicated to rule out an underlying coagulopathy. Blood work results are typically unremarkable, but there have been isolated reports of paraneoplastic syndromes associated with nasal tumors. One dog with a nasal fibrosarcoma had tumor-associated erythrocytosis with a hematocrit of 79%.[41] One dog had hypercalcemia (Ca^{++} = 19.4 mg/dl) associated with a nasal adenocarcinoma.[42] There is another report of a dog with an undifferentiated nasal carcinoma, hypercalcemia, and measurable serum levels of parathyroid hormone-related protein.[43] Immune-mediated thrombocytopenia was associated with recurrence of a nasal adenocarcinoma in another dog.[44]

Thoracic radiographs with three views are recommended to rule out pulmonary metastasis, but they are typically negative at the time of initial presentation. In studies reporting necropsy findings, 3% to 30% of dogs have had evidence of pulmonary metastasis.[1,10,12,45,46]

A number of different techniques have been described for obtaining cytology or tissue biopsy samples from the nasal cavity.[38,39,47-49] Techniques include nasal flush, traumatic core biopsy, blind pinch biopsy (Figure 37-1), and rhinoscopy-assisted biopsy. An alternative approach is endoscopic examination of the choanae using a flexible endoscope with the tip retroflexed caudal to the soft palate.[40] This approach is considered useful for caudally located tumors and is less traumatic and requires less time than rhinoscopy. Imprint and/or brush cytology can be diagnostic for canine nasal tumors, but biopsy and routine histopathology are recommended to obtain a definitive diagnosis prior to initiation of therapy.[30] The cytologic appearance of nasal tumors has been described.[38] The risk of significant hemorrhage after rhinoscopy-assisted biopsy is small with only 2 of 109 cases in one study experiencing protracted hemorrhage.[39] Biopsies obtained by blind procedures may result in nondiagnostic samples. The success rate is greater with endoscopic-guided biopsy procedures. CT-guided percutaneous biopsy has been reported in dogs with retrobulbar lesions, allowing a definitive diagnosis of nasal neoplasia.[50] On occasion it may be necessary to perform a dorsal or ventral rhinotomy to obtain sufficient material for histopathology and a definitive diagnosis of neoplasia.

There are a number of reports of the radiographic appearance of nasal disease in the dog.[51-54] Radiographic examination of the nasal cavity includes up to six different views. The two radiographic projections that are most useful are the dorsoventral (or ventrodorsal) intraoral

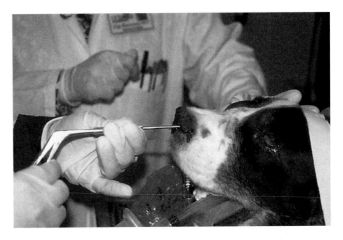

Figure 37-1. *A blind pinch biopsy is being performed on a dog with a history of epistaxis using cup biopsy forceps. The biopsy was diagnostic for nasal hemangiosarcoma.*

view of the nasal cavity (Figure 37-2) and the rostrocaudal view of the frontal sinuses. Of particular interest is the radiographic appearance of the cribriform plate and other boundaries of the nasal cavity[55-56] because evidence of involvement there warrants a poorer prognosis. Studies comparing the radiographic signs in dogs with rhinitis versus nasal tumors show that rhinitis is associated with a higher incidence of focal or multifocal lesions, localized soft tissue opacities, lucent foci, and a lack of frontal sinus involvement.[51,54] Nasal neoplasia is associated with soft tissue opacities and loss of turbinate detail affecting the entire ipsilateral nasal cavity, with signs of bony invasion, and with soft tissue/fluid opacities within the ipsilateral frontal sinus. The signs with the highest positive predictive value for rhinitis were absence of frontal sinus involvement and lucent foci in the nasal cavity, whereas invasion of bone was most predictive of neoplasia.[54] A presumptive diagnosis of carcinoma versus sarcoma cannot be made based on radiographic findings,[51] although there may be a greater tendency for carcinomas to cause bone lysis and facial swelling.[9,17] There is less information available about the radiographic differentiation of rhinitis from intranasal neoplasia in cats, and fewer descriptions of the radiographic appearance of feline nasal tumors.[8,15,18,57] Aggressive unilateral lesions are more suggestive of neoplasia than rhinitis in the cat.[57]

On both radiographic and CT examination of the nasal cavity a portion of the observed soft tissue opacification may be mucus, blood, or necrotic debris rather than tumor. Identification of a mass effect or associated turbinate or bone destruction lends support to soft tissue opacification being tumor. Frontal sinus involvement may be difficult to discern. Obstruction of the nasofrontal opening (the aperture between the frontal sinus and the nasal fossa) can result in mucus accumulation in the frontal sinus mimicking tumor involvement in the sinus. Without a biopsy from the frontal sinus region or evidence of a mass lesion or bone destruction, definitive evidence of frontal sinus involvement is often lacking.

Although routine radiography provides useful preliminary information, complete staging of nasal disease requires CT or MR imaging. There is substantial support for

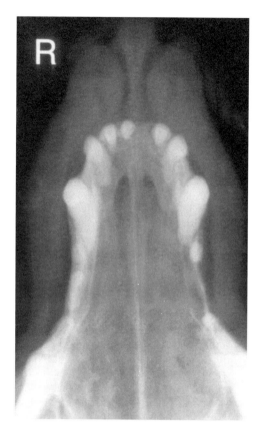

Figure 37-2. Intraoral radiographic view of a dog with an undifferentiated nasal carcinoma.

the utility of computed tomography in the evaluation of nasal tumors (Figure 37-3).[29,58-61] CT imaging is important both for staging (Table 37-1) and treatment planning (Figure 37-4). For radiation treatment planning CT, as opposed to radiography, has been shown to be critical for identification of the full extent of disease.[58] Furthermore, dorsal plane imaging may provide a more accurate assessment of the integrity of the cribriform plate in comparison with the standard transverse CT images.[59,63] Dorsal plane images can be obtained by reconstruction of the transverse slices, but direct acquisition provides better detail and is preferred. The normal CT anatomy of the canine[64,65] and feline[66] nasal passages has been reported.

TABLE 37-1. **Staging of Nasal Tumors**

Staging System	Stage	Description
WHO[62]	1	Ipsilateral tumor, no or minimal bone destruction
	2	Bilateral tumor, moderate bone destruction
	3	Extensive tumor with extranasal extension
MODIFIED[6]	1	Unilateral or bilateral neoplasm confined to the nasal passage(s) without extension into the frontal sinuses
	2	Bilateral neoplasm extending into the frontal sinuses with erosion of any bone of the nasal passages

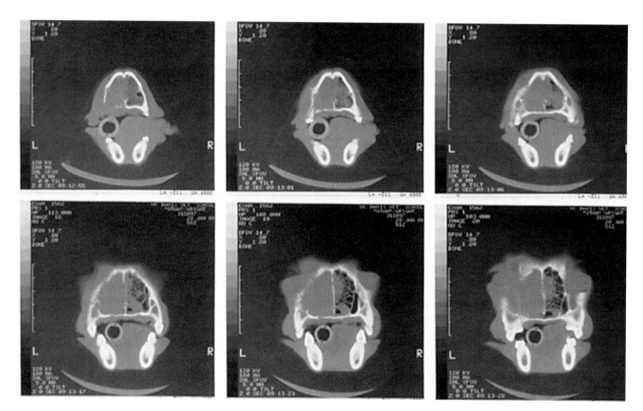

Figure 37-3. A series of CT images of the nasal cavity from the dog in Figure 37-2 showing the detail evident on CT as opposed to routine x-ray examination.

MR imaging has been used to a lesser extent than CT imaging but has been shown to be useful in imaging and identifying tumor extension into the brain.[34,67,68]

Pathological and Histopathological Findings

Tumors of epithelial origin are more commonly reported than mesenchymal tumors.[5,12,13] The most common epithelial tumors in dogs are adenocarcinomas, undifferentiated carcinomas, and squamous cell carcinoma.[12,13] Other epithelial tumors include transitional carcinoma, neuroendocrine tumors, and esthesioneuroblastoma.[6,12] Osteosarcoma and chondrosarcoma are the most common mesenchymal tumors.[69] In a retrospective study of 116 cases of canine axial skeletal osteosarcoma, 10 (8.6%) occurred in the nasal cavity and paranasal sinuses.[70] In another retrospective study of 97 dogs with chondrosarcoma, the most common site was the nasal cavity; 28.8% of the dogs had nasal involvement.[71] Other mesenchymal tumors that have been reported include fibrosarcoma, undifferentiated sarcoma, hemangiosarcoma, liposarcoma, leiomyosarcoma, myxosarcoma, rhabdomyosarcoma, malignant fibrous histiocytoma, and malignant nerve sheath tumor.[12,30,72-74] Round cell tumors reported to involve the nasal cavity include transmissible venereal tumor, lymphoma, and mast cell tumor.[17,25,73] Other nasal tumors include malignant melanoma and paranasal meningioma.[17,32] Benign nasal tumors are relatively uncommon. An oncocytoma was reported in one 15-month-old German shepherd,[30] a pleiomorphic adenoma in a 7-year-old boxer,[30] and an adenoma[40] and a leiomyoma[9] in two other reports. There is another report of a 1-year-old golden retriever with an angioleiomyoma of the nasopharynx that was treated successfully with surgery alone.[75] Other benign nasal tumors in the dog include papilloma, fibroma, and histiocytoma.[74]

The most common tumors in cats are lymphoma and carcinoma (e.g., adenocarcinoma and undifferentiated carcinoma). Other nasal and/or nasopharyngeal tumors that have been reported in cats include fibrosarcoma, anaplastic or undifferentiated sarcoma, squamous cell carcinoma, rhabdomyosarcoma, osteosarcoma, melanoma, esthesioneuroblastoma, chondrosarcoma, chondroma, adenoma, and hemangioma.* In one report the histopathologic diagnosis was altered substantially in 3 of 9 cats, with a diagnosis upon review of carcinoma instead of the original diagnosis of lymphoma in 2 cats, and a diagnosis of anaplastic carcinoma as opposed to fibrosarcoma in 1 cat.[18] Multiple osteochondromas of the turbinates and other bones were diagnosed in 2 young cats that were FeLV positive.[14]

Management and Monitoring

Surgery alone is ineffective, resulting in survival times comparable to that observed in untreated dogs. The mean survival time for 41 dogs undergoing surgery alone was 4 months, with a range of less than 1 month to 11.5 months.[2,45,79-83] Nevertheless, cytoreductive surgery is indicated before orthovoltage radiotherapy. Surgery may play a role in the treatment of nasal tumors after radiation therapy but this awaits additional investigation. Surgical approaches to the nasal cavity have been described.[84-88]

*References 8, 14, 15, 35, 57, 72, and 76-78.

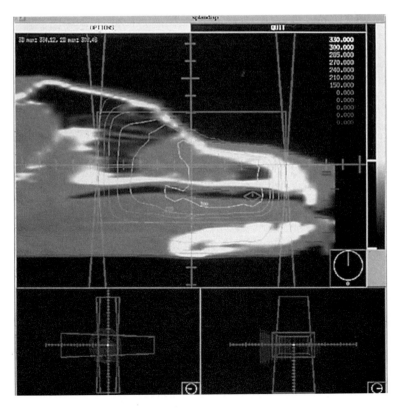

Figure 37-4. CT images, from a dog with a nasal carcinoma, used for 2½ D radiation treatment planning. The isodose curves showing the radiation dose distribution can be visualized in multiple planes (sagittal, coronal, and transverse) with 2½ D treatment planning as seen here in the sagittal view.

Surgery alone or in combination with radiation therapy is important in the management of squamous cell carcinoma of the rostral nasal cavity (i.e., the nasal planum, nasal vestibule) in the dog because radiation therapy alone is ineffective.[85,89,90]

Cryosurgery alone or in combination with radiation therapy has been reported but is not recommended. Survival time for 20 dogs treated with cryotherapy alone or in combination with radiation, surgery, or immunotherapy ranged from less than 1 month to 6 years with a median of 2.5 months.[45,80,91,92]

Iridium-192 brachytherapy has been used in the postoperative setting for the treatment of nasal tumors,[93-94] but teletherapy has been used to a far greater extent and is more widely available. Teletherapy sources used in the treatment of nasal tumors include orthovoltage,[5,46,95,96] and megavoltage using cobalt 60[6,7,46,97-99] or linear accelerator.[16,96] Radiation alone or after cytoreductive surgery has been the standard of care for treating nasal tumors. Cytoreductive surgery is recommended prior to orthovoltage radiation due to the difficulty in delivering dose at depth in dogs with nasal tumors. Information is available on the depth-dose characteristics and measurements for both orthovoltage and megavoltage irradiation of the nasal cavity.[100,101] Surgery has not been shown to result in improved survival in dogs treated with megavoltage radiation and in this setting is not recommended.[6,7,46,97]

The reported median survival times for dogs treated with orthovoltage radiation are 23 months[95] and 16.5 months.[5] The 1- and 2-year survival rates were 54% and 43%, respectively, in one report, which were equivalent to previously reported survival rates.[5,95] The mean and median survival with cobalt irradiation for 27 dogs was 20.7 and 12.8 months, respectively, with a 1-year survival rate of 59% and 2-year survival rate of 22%.[97] Comparable results were obtained in another study of 77 dogs treated with cobalt 60, with a mean survival of 21.7 months and median survival of 12.6 months, and a 1-year survival rate of 60.3% and 2-year survival rate of 25.1%.[6] A palliative radiation therapy protocol (e.g., 8 Gy per fraction once a week for 4 consecutive weeks) may be used in patients that are considered poor candidates for full course therapy due to extensive disease (e.g., intracranial extension) or in patients that cannot undergo multiple anesthesias or tolerate the local radiation side effects due to concurrent medical conditions. Information on response to palliative radiation protocols is currently lacking.

In early reports of irradiation of nasal tumors, a single dorsal port was used based on external landmarks (e.g., medial ocular canthi, caudal extent of the frontal sinuses, and nasal planum). With CT imaging it was determined that in 28 of 31 dogs, the external landmarks would have underestimated the tumor extent and resulted in a geographic miss.[58] Failure is usually due to local recurrence as opposed to metastasis. The mid- to caudal nasal cavity has been identified as the most common site of recurrence.[98] One study evaluated the efficacy of a boost technique to deliver additional dose to the expected site of recurrence.[99] The authors concluded that due to the extensive acute reactions and poorer survival (median survival of 177 days), the prescribed protocol could not be recommended.[99]

The median survival time for 13 dogs treated with a combination of external beam radiation therapy (6 MV linear accelerator; daily Monday through Friday; 3.3 Gy/fraction; median total dose of 49.5 Gy) and slow release cisplatin was 580 days.[16] Cisplatin in this setting is used as a radiation sensitizer, with a low level of cisplatin measurable in the serum for up to 3 weeks (i.e., throughout the course of radiation therapy). Drug delivery entails the use of an open-cell polylactic acid polymer impregnated with cisplatin and implanted intramuscularly at a distant site.[16] In contrast, the use of a combination of fluorouracil and cyclophosphamide or mitoxantrone alone in conjunction with cobalt 60 radiation therapy did not result in an improvement in survival over radiation alone.[7] Full dose carboplatin in conjunction with external beam radiation also did not improve survival.[13]

There is one report on the use of an altered fractionation scheme in conjunction with immunotherapy (liposome-encapsulated muramyltripeptide phosphatidylethanolamine) in 21 dogs, with a reported median survival of 428 days and a 1-year survival rate of 60%.[102]

Surgery alone in 4 cats with nasal adenocarcinoma or undifferentiated carcinoma resulted in a mean survival time of 2.5 weeks.[8] In another report the interval between surgery and euthanasia ranged from 2 to 8 months.[14] There are fewer reports of irradiation of feline nasal tumors.[8,15,18,27,76] One case report described a cat with a nasal osteosarcoma that was successfully treated with a combination of high dose per fraction (6 Gy weekly for 7 consecutive weeks) radiation therapy and the hypoxic cell sensitizer mctronidazole.[76] The cat was in remission for 2 years following treatment. Cytoreductive surgery prior to irradiation has been used prior to orthovoltage and cobalt 60 irradiation with minimal side effects.[8,18] However, due to the depth of the nasal cavity in the cat, radiation alone may be effective with orthovoltage as well as megavoltage radiation therapy.[15] The median and mean overall survival times (n = 16 cats; cobalt 60 radiotherapy in 13 cats; orthovoltage radiotherapy in 3 cats; surgery prior to irradiation in only 2 cats) in one study were 11.5 and 14.8 months respectively, with a 1- and 2-year overall survival rate of 44.3% and 16.7%.[15] Evans and colleagues reported a mean and median survival (n = 9 cats) of 27.9 and 20.8 months with 66.7% 1-year, 44% 2-year, and 33% 3-year survival rates.[18] Rhinotomy was performed in 6 of those 9 cats prior to orthovoltage irradiation.[18] Straw and colleagues reported a mean survival of 19 months and median survival of 13 months for 6 cats treated with megavoltage radiation alone.[27]

There is limited information on the response of nasal tumors to chemotherapy alone.[103-105] Documentation of response to single agent cisplatin[103] lends support to the application of chemotherapy in combination therapy protocols.[16] Cisplatin alone in a group of 11 dogs with nasal adenocarcinoma resulted in clinical improvement in all dogs, with two complete responses and one partial response for an overall response rate of 27%.[103] The median survival time, however, was 20 weeks, which is comparable to no treatment or surgery alone.[103] Doxorubicin has been used in 2 dogs with nasal adenocarcinoma with one partial response reported.[105] Chemotherapy alone may be effective in the management of select nasal tumors such as TVT.[22,106,107] Radiation therapy has also been shown to be efficacious in the treatment of transmissible venereal tumors.[20,108,109] In one study 7 of 8 dogs obtained a cure with a single 10 Gy dose.[108] Nasal lymphoma in cats has been treated with chemotherapy alone.[110] Two of three cats achieved a complete remission for 5 and 10 months with a combination of cyclophosphamide, vincristine, and prednisone.[110] Cats with nasal lymphoma can have long-term control with local irradiation alone, although a subset fail due to systemic disease. FeLV positive cats may have a greater likelihood of failure due to systemic involvement.[26] It is not currently possible to identify cats at risk for systemic failure, and the most aggressive treatment for feline nasal lymphoma would entail a combination of local radiation and systemic chemotherapy.[111] The optimal radiation protocol for feline nasal lymphoma is not known, but a number of different protocols are effective and a lower total dose of radiation may be equivalent to a fully fractionated full course of radiation in terms of response.[112]

Outcome and Prognosis

The majority of studies have shown that the extent of local disease based on the World Heath Organization staging system (Table 37-1) in dogs[5-7,46,97] and cats[15] does not have prognostic significance. A modified staging system (Table 37-1) has been shown to have prognostic significance for survival.[6] Dogs with stage 2 disease had a poorer prognosis than dogs with stage 1 disease, with a 2.3-fold higher relative risk of relapse.[6]

A scoring system was developed for radiological assessment of disease related to patient survival.[17] Six different parameters were scored to describe the extent of soft tissue opacification, bone involvement, and other parameters. This scoring system demonstrated significant increases in disease-free survival and survival for dogs with lower scores, with the caveat that proportionally more dogs with a lower score received treatment.[17]

Tumor histology has been shown to have prognostic significance in some studies, with sarcomas (primarily chondrosarcomas) having a better prognosis than carcinomas.[6] In contrast, a difference in survival between dogs with sarcomas versus carcinomas was not identified in another study.[97] Dogs with nasal squamous cell carcinoma and undifferentiated carcinomas have been shown to have significantly shorter survival times than dogs with adenocarcinoma or sarcoma.[46]

The acute side effects of radiation therapy typically are manifested during the latter part of therapy and continue for a number of weeks after the end of treatment. Acute effects include oral mucositis, halitosis, rhinitis, and moist desquamation of the skin. The use of oral antibiotics and antiinflammatory drugs (e.g., oral prednisone) can help to alleviate the acute side effects. Signs of nasal cavity disease often persist after a course of radiation therapy.[95] Damage to the nasal turbinates from the tumor, surgery or biopsy procedures, and radiation therapy result in persistent changes in the normal turbinates and resultant nasal discharge and/or rhinitis. Ophthalmic complications after radiation therapy can be significant in the dog.[113-115] In a histopathologic study of ocular damage from radiation, all dogs had evidence of chronic damage to the eye.[115] Ocular side effects include conjunctivitis, keratoconjunctivitis sicca, corneal damage, and cataracts. Close observation and monitoring can help to decrease the severity of the oc-ular side effects. When feasible, the ocular tissues are shielded from the primary radiation beam. There is less information available on ocular radiation side effects in cats. Three of 14 cats in one study had serious ocular complications from radiation with evidence of superficial corneal ulceration or keratitis.[15] One cat developed a cataract in an eye included in the radiation field at 48 months after radiation therapy.[18] In another report, 3 of 10 cats developed cataracts approximately 1 year after radiation therapy.[112] Other acute and chronic radiation side effects in cats irradiated for nasal tumors appear to be minimal.[15]

Compilation of data from 15 academic institutions indicated that the most common sites of metastasis in the dog are the lymph nodes, brain, and lung.[10] In one review of 285 canine sinonasal tumors (including 45 soft tissue tumors), only lymphomas and hemangiosarcomas had distant metastasis.[73] The highest rate of metastasis was reported in a study where 27 of 58 dogs irradiated for nasal tumors underwent necropsy examination and metastases were found in 41%, with the lung and regional lymph nodes the most common sites.[46] Although uncommon, metastasis to bone has been reported in dogs with nasal adenocarcinoma and carcinoma.[11,116] Other sites of metastasis include liver, adrenal glands, and testicle.[11]

Eight of 28 cats with nasal tumors were necropsied, and 3 had evidence of metastasis.[14] Two cats had metastasis to the retropharyngeal lymph nodes and lung. One young cat with a nasal fibrosarcoma had venous thrombi and metastasis to the lung, heart, and kidney.[14]

Overexpression of p53 tumor suppressor protein has been documented in canine nasal adenocarcinomas, but studies have not been done to correlate overexpression to prognosis.[117]

REFERENCES

1. Madewell BR, Priester WA, Gillette EL et al: Neoplasms of the nasal passages and paranasal sinuses in domestic animals as reported by 13 veterinary colleges, Am J Vet Res 37(7):851-856, 1976.
2. Bradley PA, Harvey CE: Intra-nasal tumors in the dog: An evaluation of prognosis, J Small Anim Pract 14(8):459-467, 1973.
3. Cotchin E: Neoplasms in small animals, Vet Rec 63:67-72, 1951.
4. Cotchin E: Some tumors of dogs and cats of comparative veterinary and human interest, Vet Rec 71:1040-1053, 1959.
5. Evans SM, Goldschmidt M, McKee LJ et al: Prognostic factors and survival after radiotherapy for intranasal neoplasms in dogs: 70 cases (1974-1985), J Am Vet Med Assoc 194(10):1460-1463, 1989.
6. Théon AP, Madewell BR, Harb MF et al: Megavoltage irradiation of neoplasms of the nasal and paranasal cavities in 77 dogs, J Am Vet Med Assoc 202(9):1469-1475, 1993.
7. Henry CJ, Brewer WG, Tyler JW et al: Survival in dogs with nasal adenocarcinoma: 64 cases (1981-1995), J Vet Intern Med 12(6):436-439, 1998.
8. Cox NR, Brawner WR, Powers RD et al: Tumors of the nose and paranasal sinuses in cats: 32 cases with comparison to a national database (1977 through 1987), J Am Anim Hosp Assoc 27(3):339-347, 1991.
9. Morgan JP, Suter PF, O'Brien TR et al: Tumours in the nasal cavity of the dog: A radiographic study, J Am Vet Radiol Soc 13(1):18-26, 1972.
10. Hayes HM, Wilson GP, Fraumeni JF: Carcinoma of the nasal cavity and paranasal sinuses in dogs: Descriptive epidemiology, Cornell Vet 72(2):168-179, 1982.
11. Moulton JE: Tumors of the respiratory system. In Mouton JE, editor: Tumors in domestic animals, ed 3, Berkeley, 1990, University of California Press.
12. Patnaik AK: Canine sinonasal neoplasms: Clinicopathological study of 285 cases, J Am Anim Hosp Assoc 25:103-114, 1989.

13. LaDue TA, Dodge R, Page RL et al: Factors influencing survival after radiotherapy of nasal tumors in 130 dogs, *Vet Radiol Ultrasound* 40(3):312-317, 1999.

14. Carpenter JL, Andrews LK, Holzworth J: Tumors and tumor-like lesions. In Holzworth J, editor: *Diseases of the cat: Medicine and surgery*, vol 1, Philadelphia, 1987, WB Saunders.

15. Théon AP, Peaston AE, Madewell BR et al: Irradiation of nonlymphoproliferative neoplasms of the nasal cavity and paranasal sinuses in 16 cats, *J Am Vet Med Assoc* 204(1):78-83, 1994.

16. Lana SE, Dernell WS, LaRue SM et al: Slow release cisplatin combined with radiation for the treatment of canine nasal tumors, *Vet Radiol Ultrasound* 38(6):474-478, 1997.

17. Morris JS, Dunn KJ, Dobson JM et al: Radiological assessment of severity of canine nasal tumours and relationship with survival, *J Small Anim Pract* 37(1):1-6, 1996.

18. Evans SM, Hendrick M: Radiotherapy of feline nasal tumors: A retrospective study of nine cases, *Vet Radiol* 30(3):128-132, 1989.

19. Schreider JP: Nasal airway anatomy and inhalation deposition in experimental animals and people. In Reznik G, Stinson SF, editors: *Nasal tumors in animals and man*, vol 3, Boca Raton, 1983, CRC Press.

20. Bukowski JA, Wartenberg D, Goldschmidt M: Environmental causes for sinonasal cancers in pet dogs, and their usefulness as sentinels of indoor cancer risk, *J Toxicol Environ Health* 54(7):579-591, 1998.

21. Reif JS, Bruns C, Lower KS: Cancer of the nasal cavity and paranasal sinuses and exposure to environmental tobacco smoke in pet dogs, *Am J Epidemiol* 147(5):488-492, 1998.

22. Madewell BR, Theilen GH: Tumors of the respiratory tract and thorax. In Theilen GH, Madewell BR, editors: *Veterinary cancer medicine*, ed 2, Philadelphia, 1987, Lea & Febiger.

23. Weir EC, Pond MJ, Duncan JR et al: Extragenital occurrence of transmissible venereal tumor in the dog: Literature review and case reports, *J Am Anim Hosp Assoc* 14:532-536, 1978.

24. Ginel PJ, Molleda JM, Novales M et al: Primary transmissible venereal tumour in the nasal cavity of a dog, *Vet Rec* 136(9):222-223, 1995.

25. Rogers KS: Transmissible venereal tumor, *Compend Cont Educ Pract Vet* 19(9):1036-1045, 1997.

26. Mooney SC, Hayes AA: Lymphoma in the cat: An approach to diagnosis and management, *Semin Vet Med Surg (Small Anim)* 1(1):51-57, 1986.

27. Straw RC, Withrow SJ, Gillette EL et al: Use of radiotherapy for the treatment of intranasal tumors in cats: Six cases (1980-1985), *J Am Vet Med Assoc* 189(8):927-929, 1986.

28. Gabor LJ, Malik R, Canfield PJ: Clinical and anatomical features of lymphosarcoma in 118 cats, *Aust Vet J* 76(11):725-732, 1998.

29. Park RD, Beck ER, LeCouteur RA: Comparison of computed tomography and radiography for detecting changes induced by malignant nasal neoplasia in dogs, *J Am Vet Med Assoc* 201(11):1720-1724, 1992.

30. Clercx C, Wallon J, Gilbert S et al: Imprint and brush cytology in the diagnosis of canine intranasal tumours, *J Small Anim Pract* 37(9):423-427, 1996.

31. Smith MO, Turrel JM, Bailey CS et al: Neurologic abnormalities as the predominant signs of neoplasia of the nasal cavity in dogs and cats: Seven cases (1973-1986), *J Am Vet Med Assoc* 195(2):242-245, 1989.

32. Patnaik AK, Lieberman PH, Erlandson RA et al: Paranasal meningioma in the dog: A clinicopathologic study of ten cases, *Vet Pathol* 23(4):362-368, 1986.

33. Foster ES, Carrillo JM, Patnaik AK: Clinical signs of tumors affecting the rostral cerebrum in 43 dogs, *J Vet Intern Med* 2(2):71-74, 1988.

34. Moore MP, Gavin PR, Kraft SL et al: MR, CT and clinical features from four dogs with nasal tumors involving the rostral cerebrum, *Vet Radiol* 32(1):19-25, 1991.

35. Allen HS, Broussard J, Noone K: Nasopharyngeal disease in cats: A retrospective study of 53 cases (1991-1998), *J Am Anim Hosp Assoc* 35(6):457-461, 1999.

36. Sullivan M: Rhinoscopy: A diagnostic aid? *J Small Anim Pract* 28(9):839-844, 1987.

37. Tasker S, Knottenbelt CM, Munro AC et al: Aetiology and diagnosis of persistent nasal disease in the dog: A retrospective study of 42 cases, *J Small Anim Pract* 40(10):473-478, 1999.

38. Rakich PM, Latimer KS: Cytology of the respiratory tract, *Vet Clin North Am Small Anim Pract* 19(5):823-850, 1989.

39. Lent SE, Hawkins EC: Evaluation of rhinoscopy and rhinoscopy-assisted mucosal biopsy in diagnosis of nasal disease in dogs: 119 cases (1985-1989), *J Am Vet Med Assoc* 201(9):1425-1429, 1992.

40. Willard MD, Radlinsky MA: Endoscopic examination of the choanae in dogs and cats: 118 cases (1988-1998), *J Am Vet Med Assoc* 215(9):1301-1305, 1999.

41. Couto CG, Boudrieau RJ, Zanjani ED: Tumor-associated erythrocytosis in a dog with nasal fibrosarcoma, *J Vet Intern Med* 3(3):183-185, 1989.

42. Wilson RB, Bronstad DC: Hypercalcemia associated with nasal adenocarcinoma in a dog, *J Am Vet Med Assoc* 182(11):1246-1247, 1983.

43. Anderson GM, Lane I, Fischer J et al: Hypercalcemia and parathyroid hormone-related protein in a dog with undifferentiated nasal carcinoma, *Can Vet J* 40(5):341-342, 1999.

44. Helfand SC, Couto CG, Madewell BR: Immune-mediated thrombocytopenia associated with solid tumors in dogs, *J Am Anim Hosp Assoc* 21:787-794, 1985.

45. Norris AM: Intranasal neoplasms in the dog, *J Am Anim Hosp Assoc* 15:231-236, 1979.

46. Adams WM, Withrow SJ, Walshaw R et al: Radiotherapy of malignant nasal tumors in 67 dogs, *J Am Vet Med Assoc* 191(3):311-315, 1987.

47. Withrow SJ: Diagnostic and therapeutic nasal flush in small animals, *J Am Anim Hosp Assoc* 13:704-707, 1977.

48. Withrow SJ, Susaneck SJ, Macy DW et al: Aspiration and punch biopsy techniques for nasal tumors, *J Am Anim Hosp Assoc* 21:551-554, 1985.

49. Smallwood LJ, Zenoble RD: Biopsy and cytological sampling of the respiratory tract, *Semin Vet Med Surg (Small Anim)* 8(4):250-257, 1993.

50. Tidwell AS, Johnson KL: Computed tomography-guided percutaneous biopsy in the dog and cat: Description of technique and preliminary evaluation in 14 patients, *Vet Radiol Ultrasound* 35(6):445-456, 1994.

51. Gibbs C, Lane JG, Denny HR: Radiological features of intra-nasal lesions in the dog: A review of 100 cases, *J Small Anim Pract* 20(9):515-535, 1979.

52. Harvey CE, Biery DN, Morello J et al: Chronic nasal disease in the dog: Its radiographic diagnosis, *Vet Radiol* 20:91-98, 1979.

53. Sullivan R, Lee R, Skae CA: The radiological features of sixty cases of intra-nasal neoplasia in the dog, *J Small Anim Pract* 28:575-586, 1987.

54. Russo M, Lamb CR, Jakovljevic S: Distinguishing rhinitis and nasal neoplasia by radiography, *Vet Radiol Ultrasound* 41(2):118-124, 2000.

55. Schwarz T, Sullivan M, Hartung K: Radiographic anatomy of the cribriform plate (lamina cribrosa), *Vet Radiol Ultrasound* 41(2):220-225, 2000.

56. Schwarz T, Sullivan M, Hartung K: Radiographic detection of defects of the nasal boundaries, *Vet Radiol Ultrasound* 41(2):226-230, 2000.

57. O'Brien RT, Evans SM, Wortman JA et al: Radiographic findings in cats with intranasal neoplasia or chronic rhinitis: 29 cases (1982-1988), *J Am Vet Med Assoc* 208(3):385-389, 1996.

58. Thrall DE, Robertson ID, McLeod DA et al: A comparison of radiographic and computed tomographic findings in 31 dogs with malignant nasal cavity tumors, *Vet Radiol* 30(2):59-66, 1989.

59. Koblik PD, Berry CR: Dorsal plane computed tomographic imaging of the ethmoid region to evaluate chronic nasal disease in the dog, *Vet Radiol* 31(2):92-97, 1990.

60. Burk RL: Computed tomographic imaging of nasal disease in 100 dogs, *Vet Radiol Ultrasound* 33(3):177-180, 1992.

61. Codner EC, Lurus AG, Miller JB et al: Comparison of computed tomography with radiography as a noninvasive diagnostic technique for chronic nasal disease in dogs, *J Am Vet Med Assoc* 202(7):1106-1110, 1993.

62. Owen LN: *TNM classification of tumours in domestic animals*, Geneva, 1980, World Health Organization.

63. Berry CR, Koblik PD: Evaluation of survey radiography, linear tomography, and computed tomography for detecting experimental lesions of the cribriform plate in dogs, *Vet Radiol* 31(3):146-154, 1990.

64. Burk RL: Computed tomographic anatomy of the canine nasal passages, *Vet Radiol Ultrasound* 33(3):170-176, 1992.

65. George TF, Smallwood JE: Anatomic atlas for computed tomography in the mesaticephalic dog: head and neck, *Vet Radiol Ultrasound* 33(4):217-240, 1992.

66. Losonsky JM, Abbott LC, Kuriashkin IV: Computed tomography of the normal feline nasal cavity and paranasal sinuses, *Vet Radiol Ultrasound* 38(4):251-258, 1997.

67. Voges AK, Ackerman N: MR evaluation of intra and extracranial extension of nasal adenocarcinoma in a dog and cat, *Vet Radiol Ultrasound* 36(3):196-200, 1995.

68. Kraft SL, Gavin PR, DeHaan C et al: Retrospective review of 50 canine intracranial tumors evaluated by magnetic resonance imaging, *J Vet Intern Med* 11(4):218-225, 1997.

69. Patnaik AK, Lieberman PH, Erlandson RA et al: Canine sinonasal skeletal neoplasms: Chondrosarcomas and osteosarcomas, *Vet Pathol* 21(5):475-482, 1984.

70. Heyman SJ, Diefenderfer DL, Goldschmidt MH et al: Canine axial skeletal osteosarcoma: A retrospective study of 116 cases (1986 to 1989), *Vet Surg* 21(4):304-310, 1992.

71. Popovitch CA, Weinstein MJ, Goldschmidt MH et al: Chondrosarcoma: A retrospective study of 97 dogs (1987-1990), *J Am Anim Hosp Assoc* 30(1):81-85, 1994.

72. Patnaik AK: Canine and feline nasal and paranasal neoplasm: Morphology and origin. In Reznik G, Stinson SF, editors: *Nasal tumors in animals and man*, vol 2, Boca Raton, 1983, CRC Press.

73. Patnaik AK: Canine sinonasal neoplasms: Soft tissue tumors, *J Am Anim Hosp Assoc* 25:491-497, 1989.

74. Berzon JL: Undifferentiated carcinoma in the nasal cavity of an Old English sheepdog, *Vet Med Small Anim Clin* 74(7):947-951, 1979.

75. Carpenter JL, Hamilton TA: Angioleiomyoma of the nasopharynx in a dog, *Vet Pathol* 32(6):721-723, 1995.

76. Lord PF, Kapp DS, Schwartz A et al: Osteogenic sarcoma of the nasal cavity in a cat: Postoperative control with high dose-per-fraction radiation therapy and metronidazole, *Vet Radiol* 23(1):23-26, 1982.

77. Anderson WI, Parchman MB, Cline JM et al: Nasal cavernous haemangioma in an American short haired cat, *Vet Rec* 124(2):41, 1989.

78. Legendre AM, Carrig CB, Howard DR et al: Nasal tumor in a cat, *J Am Vet Med Assoc* 167(6):481-483, 1975.

79. Delmage DA: Some conditions of the nasal chambers of the dog and cat, *Vet Rec* 92(17):437-442, 1973.

80. MacEwen EG, Withrow SJ, Patnaik AK: Nasal tumors in the dog: Retrospective evaluation of diagnosis, prognosis, and treatment, *J Am Vet Med Assoc* 170(1):45-48, 1977.

81. Cook WR: Observations on the upper respiratory tract of the dog and cat, *J Small Anim Pract* 5:309-329, 1964.

82. Hoerlein BF, Evans LE: Clinical diagnosis and surgical removal of nasal tumors in the dog, *Vet Med and Small Anim Clin* 2:65-73, 1962.

83. Spruell JSA: Surgery of the nasal cavity of the dog. In Kirk RW, editor: *Current veterinary therapy*, vol 4, Philadelphia, 1971, WB Saunders.

84. Holmberg DL, Fries C, Cockshutt J et al: Ventral rhinotomy in the dog and cat, *Vet Surg* 18(6):446-449, 1989.

85. Holt D, Prymak C, Evans S: Excision of tumors in the nasal vestibule of two dogs, *Vet Surg* 19(6):418-423, 1990.

86. Holmberg DL: Sequelae of ventral rhinotomy in dogs and cats with inflammatory and neoplastic nasal pathology: A retrospective study, *Can Vet J* 37(8):483-485, 1996.

87. Birchard SJ: Surgical diseases of the nasal cavity and paranasal sinuses, *Semin Vet Med Surg (Small Anim)* 10(2):77-86, 1995.

88. Hedlund CS: Nasal cavity: Rhinotomy techniques. In Bojrab MJ, editor: *Current techniques in small animal surgery*, ed 3, Philadelphia, 1990, Lea & Febiger.

89. Thrall DE, Adams WM: Radiotherapy of squamous cell carcinomas of the canine nasal plane, *Vet Radiol* 23(5):193-195, 1982.

90. Rogers KS, Helman RG, Walker MA: Squamous cell carcinoma of the canine nasal planum: Eight cases (1988-1994), *J Am Anim Hosp Assoc* 31(5):373-378, 1995.

91. Withrow SJ: Cryosurgical therapy for nasal tumors in the dog, *J Am Anim Hosp Assoc* 18:585-589, 1982.

92. Krahwinkel DJ, Merkeley DF, Howard DR: Cryosurgical treatment of cancerous and noncancerous diseases of dogs, horses, and cats, *J Am Vet Med Assoc* 169(2):201-207, 1976.

93. White R, Walker M, Legendre AM et al: Development of brachytherapy technique for nasal tumors in dogs, *Am J Vet Res* 51(8):1250-1256, 1990.

94. Thompson JP, Ackerman N, Bellah JR et al: 192Iridium brachytherapy, using an intracavitary afterload device, for treatment of intranasal neoplasms in dogs, *Am J Vet Res* 53(4):617-622, 1992.

95. Thrall DE, Harvey CE: Radiotherapy of malignant nasal tumors in 21 dogs, *J Am Vet Med Assoc* 183(6):663-666, 1983.

96. Morris JS, Dunn KJ, Dobson JM et al: Effects of radiotherapy alone and surgery and radiotherapy on survival of dogs with nasal tumours, *J Small Anim Pract* 35(11):567-573, 1994.

97. McEntee MC, Page RL, Heidner GL et al: A retrospective study of 27 dogs with intranasal neoplasms treated with cobalt radiation, *Vet Radiol* 32(3):135-139, 1991.

98. Thrall DE, Heidner GL, Novotney CA et al: Failure patterns following cobalt irradiation in dogs with nasal carcinoma, *Vet Radiol Ultrasound* 34(2):126-133, 1993.

99. Thrall DE, McEntee MC, Novotney C et al: A boost technique for irradiation of malignant canine nasal tumors, *Vet Radiol Ultrasound* 34(4):295-300, 1993.

100. Feeney DA, Johnston GR, Williamson JF et al: Orthovoltage radiation of normal canine nasal passages: Assessment of depth dose, *Am J Vet Res* 44(8):1593-1596, 1983.

101. Walker M, Durrer R, Weir V et al: A study to evaluate single port, central axis dosimetry and verification techniques for veterinary radiotherapy, using the canine nasal cavity as a model target, *Vet Radiol Ultrasound* 35(3):210-216, 1994.

102. Adams WM, Miller PE, Vail DM et al: An accelerated technique for irradiation of malignant canine nasal and paranasal sinus tumors, *Vet Radiol Ultrasound* 39(5):475-481, 1998.

103. Hahn KA, Knapp DW, Richardson RC et al: Clinical response of nasal adenocarcinoma to cisplatin chemotherapy in 11 dogs, *J Am Vet Med Assoc* 200(3):355-357, 1992.

104. Knapp DW, Richardson RC, Bonney PL et al: Cisplatin therapy in 41 dogs with malignant tumors, *J Vet Intern Med* 2(1):41-46, 1988.

105. Ogilvie GK, Reynolds HA, Richardson RC et al: Phase II evaluation of doxorubicin for treatment of various canine neoplasms, *J Am Vet Med Assoc* 195(11):1580-1583, 1989.

106. Brown NO, Calvert C, MacEwen EG: Chemotherapeutic management of transmissible venereal tumors in 30 dogs, *J Am Vet Med Assoc* 176(10):983-986, 1980.

107. Amber EI, Henderson RA, Adeyanju JB et al: Single-drug chemotherapy of canine transmissible venereal tumor with cyclophosphamide, methotrexate, or vincristine, *J Vet Intern Med* 4(3):144-147, 1990.

108. Thrall DE: Orthovoltage radiotherapy of canine transmissible venereal tumors, *Vet Radiol* 23(5):217-219, 1982.

109. Rogers KS, Walker MA, Dillon HB: Transmissible venereal tumor: A retrospective study of 29 cases, *J Am Anim Hosp Assoc* 34(6):463-470, 1998.

110. Cotter SM: Treatment of lymphoma and leukemia with cyclophosphamide, vincristine, and prednisone II: Treatment of cats, *J Am Anim Hosp Assoc* 19:166-172, 1983.

111. Elmslie RE, Ogilvie GK, Gillette EL et al: Radiotherapy with and without chemotherapy for localized lymphoma in 10 cats, *Vet Radiol* 32(6):277-280, 1991.

112. Meleo KA: The role of radiotherapy in the treatment of lymphoma and thymoma, *Vet Clin North Am Small Anim Pract* 27(1):115-129, 1997.

113. Roberts SM, Lavach JD, Severin GA et al: Ophthalmic complications following megavoltage irradiation of the nasal and paranasal cavities in dogs, *J Am Vet Med Assoc* 190(1):43-47, 1987.

114. Jamieson VE, Davidson MG, Nasisse MP et al: Ocular complications following cobalt 60 radiotherapy of neoplasms in the canine head region, *J Am Anim Hosp Assoc* 27(1):51-55, 1991.

115. Ching SV, Gillette SM, Powers BE et al: Radiation-induced ocular injury in the dog: A histological study, *Int J Radiat Oncol Biol Phys* 19(2):321-328, 1990.

116. Hahn KA, Matlock CL: Nasal adenocarcinoma metastatic to bone in two dogs, *J Am Vet Med Assoc* 197(4):491-494, 1990.

117. Gamblin RM, Sagartz JE, Couto CG: Overexpression of p53 tumor suppressor protein in spontaneously arising neoplasms of dogs, *Am J Vet Res* 58(8):857-863, 1997.

CHAPTER 38

Nasal Foreign Bodies

Lillian R. Aronson

Incidence

The nasal cavities of the dog and cat are responsible for warming and humidifying the air that passes through them and also for the removal of inhaled particulate matter. The sneeze reflex is a very important and usually very effective way of expelling foreign material from the nose; occasionally, however, foreign material can become lodged in either the external nares or in the nasal turbinates and cause chronic inflammation.

Nasal foreign bodies appear to be an uncommon occurrence in both the dog and the cat. One study of 119 dogs documented nasal foreign bodies in only 2 cases, an incidence of only 1.7% in dogs that required rhinoscopy because of nasal disease.[1] It is likely that the incidence of this problem in cats is even lower. Some of the more common foreign bodies that have been identified include grass awns (Figure 38-1); twigs; thorns; and porcupine quills (Figure 38-2), particularly in working and field type dogs. Other nasal foreign bodies that have been recognized include bullets, rocks, fishhooks, arrowheads, and needles (Figure 38-3).[2]

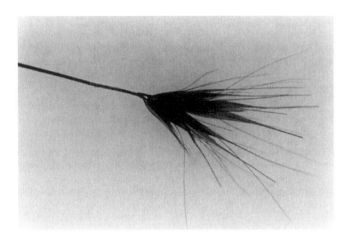

Figure 38-1. *Typical appearance of a grass awn.*

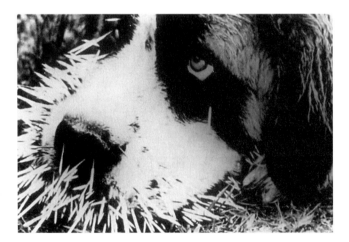

Figure 38-2. *A 1-year-old female Saint Bernard puppy following an encounter with a porcupine.*

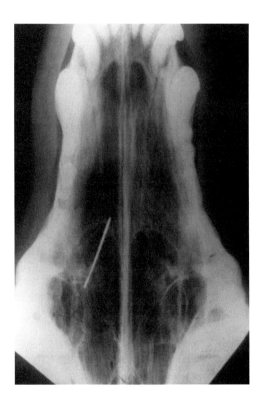

Figure 38-3. *Open mouth, dorsal ventral radiograph of a 3-year-old, female, spayed Labrador retriever identifying a needle foreign body in the right nasal cavity.*

Clinical Signs

Common clinical signs in patients with nasal foreign bodies include excessive sneezing, unilateral or bilateral epistaxis, and unilateral or bilateral mucopurulent nasal discharge. Because of the very vascular nature of the maxilloturbinates and of the mucous membranes in the rostral nasal cavity, the epistaxis is often caused by mechanical damage to this vasculature by the foreign object.[3] Additionally, excessive sneezing can often result in epistaxis secondary to vascular rupture. With time, inflammation and infection associated with the foreign body can result in chronic rhinitis and a unilateral or bilateral mucopurulent nasal dicharge.[3] Other clinical signs and physical examination findings that have been reported include head shaking, pawing the nose, snorting, enlarged mandibular lymph nodes, and a possible entrance wound.[2]

Because of the nonspecific clinical signs in many patients with nasal foreign bodies, and the infrequent occurrence of this problem, other differential diagnoses need to be considered in each case. Other causes of these clinical signs may include nasal neoplasia; acute and chronic rhinitis (e.g., viral, bacterial, and fungal); and other causes of epistaxis including an underlying coagulopathy, a diseased tooth, nasal polyps, trauma, polycythemia vera and other hyperviscosity syndromes, and drug toxicity (e.g., thrombocytopathia due to aspirin administration).

Diagnosis

In acute cases, clinical signs along with information offered by the owner may alert the veterinarian to the possibility of a foreign body. In chronic cases, the diagnosis of a nasal foreign body may be more difficult. Diagnostic tests that can be performed on a patient suspected of having a nasal foreign body include radiography; positive contrast rhinography; rhinoscopy; computed tomography (Figure 38-4); and if necessary, exploratory rhinotomy.

Radiopaque foreign bodies can readily be identified with plain radiography (Figure 38-5, A and B). For radiolucent foreign bodies, positive contrast rhinography is a simple, noninvasive procedure that can be performed to help outline nasal foreign bodies that cannot otherwise be identified using survey radiographs.[4] Barium sulfate can be administered at a dose of 1 ml/5 kg body weight through a catheter placed in the nasal passage.[5] With chronicity, an area of lysis caused by movement or infection often may be identified within the turbinates surrounding the radiopaque or radiolucent object.[3] Rhinoscopy can be performed using a small flexible bronchoscope or a rigid arthroscope. In patients with foreign bodies lodged in the rostral nasal cavity, an otoscope may be all that is necessary for visualization.[6] Typically, patients are anesthetized for the rhinoscopy procedure and for radiographic studies. If a foreign body cannot be identified using rhinoscopy, biopsies should be taken for histopathology, bacteriologic determination, and fungal cultures to rule out any underlying neoplasia or other causes of rhinitis.

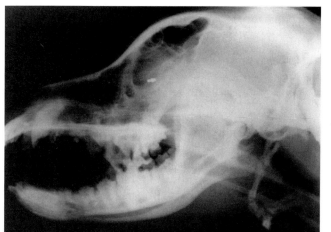

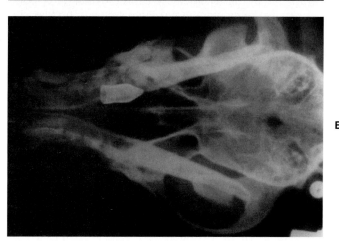

A

B

*Figure 38-5. **A,** Lateral skull radiograph of a 4-year-old, female, spayed Dalmatian with a 1-month history of sneezing and unilateral epistaxis. A Bic pen was removed from her left nasal cavity using a pair of forceps through the external nares. **B,** Dorsal ventral skull radiograph of an arrow foreign body in the left nasal cavity of a dog.*

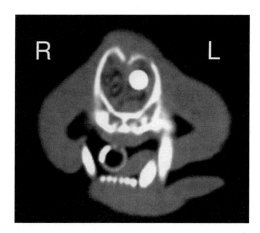

Figure 38-4. *Computed tomography scan of a 5-year-old mixed-breed dog that was shot with a BB gun. An intranasal BB is present in the left nasal cavity.*

Treatment

Treatment of nasal foreign bodies depends on the accessibility and location of the foreign body within the nasal cavity. Foreign bodies located in the rostral nasal passage (fish hooks and porcupine quills are common in this location) can often be removed using small alligator forceps. Occasionally, with foreign bodies located in the caudal nasal passage, the graspers of the bronchoscope or arthroscope can be used to facilitate removal. If the foreign body is located in the nasopharynx, this area can be visualized either through the nasal cavity or with a flexible bronchoscope through the oral cavity. Occasionally, the foreign body can be dislodged into the oropharynx where it can then be retrieved.[4] The flushing systems with these scopes can be beneficial in aiding visualization by removing excessive mucopurulent exudates.

Unfortunately, in some patients, the foreign body may be inaccessible using minimally invasive techniques, and a dorsal or ventral rhinotomy may be required. The approach chosen often depends on location of the foreign body and on the surgeon's preference. The rostral nasal passages can be exposed from either the dorsal or ventral approach; however the area caudal to the ethmoid turbinates is approached ventrally.[3] The dorsal approach is chosen when the frontal sinuses are involved.

DORSAL RHINOTOMY

To perform a dorsal rhinotomy, a dorsal midline incision is made through the skin and subcutaneous tissue from the medial canthi to the planum nasale. An incision is then made in the periosteum, and the periosteum is elevated and reflected laterally. If the frontal sinuses are going to be explored, the initial incision can be extended just caudal to a line connecting the dorsal orbital rims. Depending on the location of the foreign body, one or both sides of the nasal cavity can be explored. A bone saw is used to create either a large single bone flap, exposing both sides of the nasal cavity; or a smaller bone flap to expose one side of the nasal cavity. The surgeon should be careful to identify the nasolacrimal ducts and the infraorbital canal so that these structures can be avoided. The foreign body and any damaged tissue is removed and the cavity copiously lavaged. If appropriate, biopsy samples can be taken for histopathology and bacteriologic culture and sensitivity testing, or for fungal culture. Some surgeons reattach the bone flap and others choose to discard it. To reduce the incidence of subcutaneous emphysema, a tube can be placed through the rhinostomy for 2 to 3 days postoperatively to act as a vent. Prior to extubation, the oro- and nasopharynx are cleared of all fluid to prevent obstruction or aspiration of material into the airways.

VENTRAL RHINOTOMY

Depending on the location of the foreign body, an approach can be made to either the rostral or caudal nasal passage using a ventral rhinotomy. In the rostral approach, an incision is made in the mucoperiosteum and a periosteal elevator used to elevate the mucoperiosteum and retract it laterally. A section of the palatine bone is discarded, exposing the ventral aspect of the rostral nasal passage. The foreign body and any necrotic tissue can then be removed. The mucoperiosteum is closed in two layers using absorbable suture material.

To expose the caudal nasal passage, the midline incision is extended through the soft palate as well as the hard palate. The mucoperiosteum of the hard palate is elevated laterally as previously described, and the soft palate is incised full thickness. The incision through the hard and soft palate is held open with stay sutures and, if necessary, a section of palatine bone is removed. The foreign body and any necrotic tissue can then be removed. The nasal mucosa of the soft palate is closed with absorbable suture material. The periosteum of the hard palate is closed with absorbable sutures and then the oral mucosa of the hard and soft palate are closed with absorbable suture material. Similar to the dorsal approach, prior to extubation, the oro- and nasopharynx are cleared of all fluid to prevent any obstruction or aspiration.

Prognosis

In general, the prognosis for nasal foreign bodies in both dogs and cats is excellent. Typically, the foreign body is easily diagnosed and treated. In patients that present with a chronic history, the diagnosis and treatment can be more challenging. Patients that require a rhinotomy for foreign body removal tend to have a longer recovery period and need to be monitored for complications such as subcutaneous emphysema, wound dehiscence, and discomfort.

Although nasal foreign bodies are generally not life threatening, it is very important that the clinician differentiate nasal foreign bodies from more common and more serious conditions (e.g., neoplasia, rhinitis, or serious causes of epistaxis) because the prognosis for these conditions can be more guarded.

REFERENCES

1. Forbes Lent SE, Hawkins EC: Evaluation of rhinoscopy and rhinoscopy-assisted mucosal biopsy in diagnosis of nasal disease in dogs: 119 cases (1985-1989), *J Am Vet Med Assoc* 201(9):1425-1429, 1992.
2. Fallon RK, McCaw D, Lattimer J: Unusual nasal foreign body in a dog, *J Am Vet Med Assoc* 186(7):710, 1985.
3. Bright RM: Nasal foreign bodies, tumors, and rhinitis/sinusitis. In Bojrab MJ, editor: *Pathophysiology in small animal surgery*, Philadelphia, 1981, Lea & Febiger.
4. Nelson AW: Upper respiratory system. In Slatter D, editor: *Textbook of small animal surgery*, ed 2, vol 1, Philadelphia, 1993, WB Saunders.
5. Goring RL, Ticer JW: *Contrast rhinography: A radiographic technique for evaluating diseases of the nasal cavity and paranasal sinuses in the dog.* Presented at the annual meeting of the American College of Veterinary Surgery, San Diego, CA, 1982.
6. Goring RL, Ticer JW, Ackerman N et al: Contrast rhinography in the radiographic evaluation of diseases affecting the nasal cavity, nasopharynx, and paranasal sinuses in the dog, *Vet Radiol* 25(3):106, 1984.

CHAPTER 39

Lymphoplasmacytic Rhinitis

Andrew J. Mackin

Lymphoplasmacytic rhinitis is a relatively common cause of inflammatory nasal disease in the dog.[1] Lymphoplasmacytic rhinitis has also been reported, albeit less commonly, in cats.[2] The definitive etiology of lymphoplasmacytic rhinitis in small animals is as yet undetermined, although it is probable that the condition is a common response to multiple different precipitating factors. Lymphoplasmacytic rhinitis typically presents as a chronic and gradually progressive nasal disease associated with mild to moderate clinical signs such as sneezing, snorting, and a mucoid or mucopurulent nasal discharge. Although the clinical signs associated with lymphoplasmacytic rhinitis can often be distressing to both pet and owner, the condition is rarely life threatening. Lymphoplasmacytic rhinitis usually responds well to medical treatment, although ongoing maintenance therapy is often necessary to prevent recurrence of clinical signs.

Definition and Etiology

Lymphoplasmacytic rhinitis is one of the most common forms of chronic noninfectious rhinitis in the dog and cat.[1] Other chronic noninfectious nasal inflammatory diseases seen in small animals include eosinophilic rhinitis and hyperplastic rhinitis. In the veterinary literature, these conditions have often been grouped together and described as chronic rhinitis or, if there is a significant proliferative component, as chronic hyperplastic rhinitis.[3,4] Classification of chronic nasal inflammatory diseases into distinct categories based on the predominant inflammatory cell and the presence or absence of hyperplasia is somewhat arbitrary: histopathologically, many chronic rhinitides are composed of a mix of different inflammatory cell types associated with varying degrees of proliferative response.

The definitive causes of lymphoplasmacytic rhinitis and other chronic inflammatory nasal diseases in dogs and cats have not been established, although some clinicians believe that the condition is a chronic inflammatory response to an inhaled irritant or allergen. In people, there is a well-established link between chronic rhinitis and diseases known to be caused by airborne or inhaled allergens such as allergic conjunctivitis, hay fever, recurrent seasonal rhinitis, and asthma. Affected patients often have positive intradermal skin tests to a range of well-known inhalant allergens including seasonal pollens, molds and fungi, animal dander and feathers, and house dust mite. Chronic rhinitis in people is associated with a number of different inflammatory cell types (particularly eosinophils, lymphocytes, and plasma cells), and may eventually lead to marked hyperplastic and proliferative changes in the nasal mucosa. Nasal polyps are a relatively common end result of chronic rhinitis in humans.

Lymphoplasmacytic rhinitis in dogs and cats, in contrast to chronic rhinitis in people, typically occurs without concurrent conjunctivitis or allergic lower airway disease. However, despite the common lack of involvement of the eyes or lower airways, there is evidence that at least some cases of lymphoplasmacytic rhinitis in animals are caused by inhaled irritants or allergens. Experimentally, for example, long-term exposure to cigarette smoke has been shown to cause chronic rhinitis in dogs,[5] a finding supported by the anecdotal clinical observation that elimination of exposure to secondhand smoke is associated with a significant reduction of signs in some patients with lymphoplasmacytic or eosinophilic rhinitis. Chronic rhinitis has also, in individual canine patients, been associated with positive intradermal skin tests against a number of inhaled allergens,[6] although no large studies have been performed to determine whether this is a common finding in animals with chronic nasal inflammatory diseases. Dogs with chronic rhinitis have been shown to have higher concentrations of immunoglobulin (both IgM and IgG) within nasal secretions; although the pathophysiological significance of this finding has not been established, it has been suggested that the increased levels of IgG are consistent with an allergic etiopathogenesis.[7] Certainly, in people, there is a well-recognized spectrum of allergic nasal diseases ranging from acute allergic rhinitis (signs are often seasonal) to more chronic and hyperplastic rhinitis, and it is similarly feasible that dogs and cats with allergic nasal disease could have a comparable spectrum of clinical syndromes.

Some authors believe that lymphoplasmacytic rhinitis in dogs may have an immune-mediated (rather than allergic or irritant) pathogenesis.[8] Moreover, even though the condition is usually considered to be noninfectious, in some animals lymphoplasmacytic rhinitis may potentially have an infectious trigger. For example, some cats with chronic rhinitis associated with feline viral rhinotracheitis can have a significant lymphocytic and plasmacytic tissue response rather than the more typical neutrophilic inflammatory response.

Pathophysiology and Pathogenesis

Lymphoplasmacytic rhinitis is characterized by infiltration of the nasal mucosa with inflammatory cells of lymphoid origin (e.g., lymphocytes and plasma cells), although variable numbers of other inflammatory cells (e.g., neutrophils and eosinophils) are also often present. Inflammation of the nasal mucosa leads to vasodilation and increased vascular permeability with associated congestion and edema of the nasal tissues. Exudation of fluid from leaky vessel walls leads to both mucosal edema and accumulation of serous fluid in the nasal lumen. With chronic lymphoplasmacytic rhinitis, nasal secretions become progressively more mucoid as mucus-secreting glands within the nasal mucosa proliferate and become hypersecretory in response to chronic inflammation.

In the healthy animal, the mucus blanket that coats the nasal mucosa is pushed caudally via the coordinated beating of cilia on the luminal surface of nasal respiratory epithelial cells. This normal mucociliary clearance mechanism pushes nasal secretions (with associated inhaled particles and microbial organisms) back into the oropharynx, where typically the mucus and debris is swallowed. Chronic nasal inflammation, however, leads to destruction of cilia and squamous metaplasia of the respiratory epithelium,[8] causing disruption of mucociliary clearance and accumulation of nasal secretions. Stasis of the normal flow of secretions is compounded by narrowing and obstruction of the lumen of the nasal passages associated with mucosal congestion, edema, and hyperplasia.

Reduced mucociliary clearance of nasal secretions creates an ideal microenvironment for proliferation of bacteria, with a resultant increased susceptibility to secondary infection. Secondary nasal infection in patients with lymphoplasmacytic rhinitis leads to recruitment of neutrophils and the development of a purulent exudate. Secondary infections in patients with chronic rhinitis are typically caused by bacteria that are normally resident on the skin and within the oral and nasal cavities (e.g., *Staphylococcus intermedius*).

Unlike more aggressive nasal diseases such as fungal rhinitis and neoplasia, lymphoplasmacytic rhinitis rarely causes severe tissue destruction or lysis of bony nasal structures. Lymphoplasmacytic rhinitis is therefore uncommonly associated with major epistaxis, although nasal secretions can occasionally be slightly hemorrhagic.

Historical Findings, Clinical Signs, and Progression

Although lymphoplasmacytic rhinitis can be seen in animals of any age, the condition is most commonly seen in young adult and middle-aged small animals, and is more common in dogs than in cats.[1,4,8] Whippets and dachshunds may be more susceptible to the condition.[4] Initial clinical signs are often subtle and intermittent and may consist solely of occasional sneezing, reverse sneezing or snorting, and a mild serous nasal discharge.[1] Questioning of owners often reveals a long history of subtle signs of nasal disease.

The nasal discharge associated with lymphoplasmacytic rhinitis is often (but not invariably) bilateral.[1] With chronic disease, the nasal discharge tends to become more persistent and mucoid. Secondary nasal infections may cause the discharge to become mucopurulent or sanguineous. In some animals, excessive nasal secretions may not be obvious to owners, either because the secretions are passing caudally into the oropharynx or because the discharge is fastidiously licked up by the patient as soon as it appears at the anterior nares. Explosive sneezing in badly affected patients often expels long strings of mucoid or mucopurulent discharge. Excessive "postnasal drip" may also occasionally cause a mild cough as nasal secretions leak into the caudal pharyngeal region.

Although lymphoplasmacytic rhinitis is typically not a destructive disease, excessive nasal secretions and luminal narrowing because of mucosal edema, congestion, and proliferation sometimes leads to partial or complete obstruction of the nasal passages. Affected patients may therefore exhibit excessive nasal noise when breathing (particularly during inspiration) or, in extreme cases, be forced to breathe with an open mouth.

Physical examination typically reveals no significant abnormalities because the condition almost invariably does not affect the systemic health of the patient. Because lymphoplasmacytic rhinitis typically does not cause pain, tissue destruction, or bony proliferation, routine nasal examination often reveals only subtle abnormalities such as a serous, mucoid, or mucopurulent discharge; or increased inspiratory nasal noise. Thorough visual examination and palpation for asymmetry; deformity; or pain involving the nasal bones, frontal sinuses, hard palate, and teeth is essential in order to exclude destructive and proliferative nasal diseases (e.g., fungal rhinitis, neoplasia, or tooth root abscessation) but typically reveals no abnormalities in animals with lymphoplasmacytic rhinitis. Careful evaluation of nasal airflow may sometimes reveal partial or complete unilateral or bilateral obstruction of the passage of air in patients with severe lymphoplasmacytic rhinitis. Percussion of the nasal cavity and frontal sinuses may reveal hyporesonance in luminal spaces containing excessive secretions rather than air.[9] Submandibular lymph nodes may be mildly enlarged, particularly in patients with secondary bacterial nasal infections.

Differential Diagnosis

Many different chronic nasal diseases in the dog and cat can present with clinical signs that are very similar to those of lymphoplasmacytic rhinitis. In the dog, major differential diagnoses include fungal rhinitis, nasal neoplasia, dental disease, foreign bodies, nasal parasites (mites or nematodes), and ciliary dyskinesia. In the cat, major differential diagnoses include chronic viral upper respiratory tract infection, fungal rhinitis, nasal neoplasia, dental disease, foreign bodies, nasopharyngeal polyps, and nasopharyngeal stenosis.

Diagnostic Tests

A thorough diagnostic evaluation of nasal disease in the dog and cat is typically expensive and moderately invasive. Because lymphoplasmacytic rhinitis is not life threatening, and often causes only mild to moderate clinical signs, clinicians can be tempted to empirically treat patients with low-grade chronic nasal disease for lymphoplasmacytic rhinitis rather than commence extensive diagnostic evaluations. Unfortunately, however, small animals with many other common nasal diseases (e.g., fungal rhinitis, nasal neoplasia, foreign bodies, and tooth root abscessation) can present with identical clinical signs. Empirical therapy for lymphoplasmacytic rhinitis can therefore detrimentally delay the diagnosis and specific treatment of a number of other important nasal diseases. For this reason, a thorough diagnostic evaluation is preferable to empirical therapy.

Because secondary infection is common in patients with lymphoplasmacytic rhinitis, clinical signs often partially or completely resolve with antibiotic therapy, only to recur when antibiotics are discontinued. Antibiotic therapy immediately before commencing a diagnostic investigation in patients with suspected lymphoplasmacytic rhinitis can, however, sometimes be helpful in reducing an overlying suppurative inflammatory response that may complicate findings on endoscopy and biopsy.

The only diagnostic test that can provide a definitive diagnosis of lymphoplasmacytic rhinitis is histopathologic examination of nasal mucosal biopsies. Collection of nasal mucosal biopsies is typically one of the last steps in the standard diagnostic approach to nasal disease, primarily because the hemorrhage associated with biopsy collection can significantly obscure the diagnostic information that might be provided by nasal radiography and rhinoscopy. Because radiography and rhinoscopy can be vital tools for detecting neoplasia, fungal rhinitis, foreign bodies, and dental disease, imaging and endoscopy should always be performed before collecting biopsies. Patients with lymphoplasmacytic rhinitis therefore must undergo a standard step-wise diagnostic evaluation before a final diagnosis is obtained.

PRELIMINARY TESTING

Most of the major nasal diagnostic tests are performed under general anesthesia. Routine preanesthetic testing consisting of hematology, serum biochemistry, and urinalysis is therefore recommended early in the diagnostic investigation of lymphoplasmacytic rhinitis. Because collection of nasal biopsies can cause significant bleeding, prior evaluation of hemostasis (platelet count and either an activated clotting time or prothrombin and par-

tial thromboplastin times) is also recommended. In some canine patients, fecal flotation for the eggs of the nasal nematodes (*Eucoleus* and *Capillaria* spp.) may be indicated.

DIAGNOSTIC IMAGING

Nasal radiography under general anesthesia is indicated in most patients with chronic nasal disease. In patients with lymphoplasmacytic rhinitis, however, radiographic changes tend to be subtle, diffuse, and nonspecific. Most have normal nasal radiographs or a mild to moderate increase in fluid/tissue radiodensity associated with excessive intraluminal nasal discharge. Nasal discharge can cause a loss of air contrast in the nasal cavity and frontal sinuses, leading to obscuring of trabecular bony details; it is important not to overinterpret this loss of detail as evidence of tissue destruction and bone lysis. Some degree of symmetrical or asymmetrical trabecular destruction is relatively common in animals with lymphoplasmacytic rhinitis,[1,8,10] particularly in the rostral portions of the nasal cavity.[11] Radiographic changes are, however, typically mild compared with the bony destruction often seen with conditions such as neoplasia or fungal infection.[3,11]

Thoracic radiography may be indicated as part of the work-up of patients with nasal disease because some nasal conditions may, uncommonly, also affect the chest (e.g., metastatic nasal neoplasia). Thoracic radiographs are typically normal in patients with lymphoplasmacytic rhinitis. Affected animals may occasionally have increased bronchointerstitial pulmonary markings, which may indicate an inhaled irritant or allergic etiology concurrently affecting the lower airways.

Computed tomography is often superior to standard radiography for evaluating nasal disease in the dog and cat.[2,12,13] As computed tomography becomes more available, this modality may supercede standard radiography as the modality of choice for investigating lymphoplasmacytic rhinitis.

RHINOSCOPY

Endoscopic examination of the nasal passages of animals with lymphoplasmacytic rhinitis typically reveals relatively subtle and nonspecific abnormalities. In most animals, thorough examination of the nasal passages is possible with an appropriately-sized rigid or flexible endoscope. Because affected animals often have copious mucopurulent discharge filling most of the nasal cavity and hampering endoscopic visualization, generous flushing with saline before and during rhinoscopy is often necessary in order to perform an adequate examination. Rhinoscopy typically reveals diffuse mild mucosal hyperemia,[14] although hyperemia may be more marked in patients with secondary bacterial infections. Affected patients sometimes have proliferation or thickening of the nasal mucosa, and the mucosal surface in more severe cases may be excessively friable and have a granular or cobble-stoned appearance.[14] Uncommonly, severe proliferative or polypoid changes may obstruct passage of the endoscope.

Pathological and Histopathological Findings

Collection of nasal mucosal biopsies for histopathological analysis is necessary to establish a definitive diagnosis of lymphoplasmacytic rhinitis. Biopsies may be collected either with pinch biopsy forceps passed through an endoscope; or blindly using laparoscopic biopsy instruments, mare uterine biopsy instruments, alligator forceps, or other biopsy techniques. Because the histopathological changes associated with lymphoplasmacytic rhinitis are typically diffuse and distributed throughout the nasal cavity, blind biopsy specimens usually provide a definitive diagnosis. Collection of blind biopsies through the anterior nares may therefore be worth considering if an appropriate endoscope is not available. Collection of biopsies without prior rhinoscopy, however, although acceptable for diagnosing lymphoplasmacytic rhinitis, may lead to misdiagnosis of patients with focal diseases such as neoplasia or a nasal foreign body.

Biopsy specimens should be submitted for routine histopathological examination. Histopathological findings consistent with a diagnosis of lymphoplasmacytic rhinitis are a mixed inflammatory cell infiltration of mature lymphocytes and plasma cells within the nasal mucosa and submucosa.[8] Other inflammatory cells that may be present include eosinophils and, especially with secondary infection, neutrophils. The respiratory epithelium may exhibit hyperplasia, squamous metaplasia, or ulceration, and beneath the epithelial cells there may be submucosal fibrosis or glandular hyperplasia. Biopsy specimens should be collected from both sides of the nasal cavity; because lymphoplasmacytic rhinitis is usually (although not invariably) bilaterally symmetrical, a marked difference in histological appearance between specimens from the left and right sides suggests the possibility of a diagnosis other than typical lymphoplasmacytic rhinitis.

Nasal flush cytology is typically nondiagnostic in patients with lymphoplasmacytic rhinitis. Secondary bacterial infections often cause an overlying suppurative inflammation, and neutrophils may therefore be the predominant cell type in a nasal flush rather than the expected lymphocytes and plasma cells. Uncommonly, microscopic examination of nasal flushes may reveal nematode eggs or nasal mites. Bacterial cultures of nasal swabs, flushes, or biopsies are rarely of diagnostic value, and merely detect bacteria that are either normally present in nasal secretions or present in larger numbers because of secondary infection.

The final diagnosis of lymphoplasmacytic rhinitis is established when a thorough nasal diagnostic evaluation excludes other causes of nasal disease, and when nasal biopsy histopathology reveals a predominantly lymphoplasmacytic inflammatory process.[8,15]

Management and Monitoring

Because at least some cases of lymphoplasmacytic rhinitis are probably caused by a local reaction to inhaled substances, it is always worth trying to reduce exposure to potential irritants or allergens as part of the treatment of chronic rhinitis in dogs and cats. In the majority of cases, however, no underlying irritant or allergen can be identified, and drug therapy is needed to control clinical signs. Medical therapy can be either systemic or local, and may include glucocorticoids, immunosuppressive agents, antibiotics, and other symptomatic therapy. Lymphoplasmacytic rhinitis is more inconvenient and distressing than it is life threatening, and it is therefore important not to treat so aggressively that the animal is placed at significant risk of drug side effects. In many instances, partial alleviation of clinical signs with conservative therapy is more desirable than attempted complete resolution of signs with more aggressive and risky treatments.

GLUCOCORTICOIDS

The traditional primary treatment of choice for lymphoplasmacytic rhinitis is systemic glucocorticoids, started at immunosuppressive doses and tapered over time to antiinflammatory doses.[8,10] Oral prednisone or prednisolone is commenced at a starting dose of approximately 2 mg/kg daily for at least 1 to 2 weeks, and then gradually tapered to effect.[8] Although an aggressive induction course of glucocorticoid seems to promptly improve clinical signs, complete resolution of signs can take weeks to months. Excessive mucus production, in particular, may take a long time to resolve even if the underlying inflammatory disease is controlled. Eventually, long-term maintenance antiinflammatory doses of prednisone or prednisolone (0.5 to 1 mg/kg every other day) may be successful at controlling most clinical signs. The persistence of mild, tolerable signs of rhinitis (e.g., intermittent sneezing or a slight serous or mucoid nasal discharge) may be preferable to over-treatment with glucocorticoids and the resultant side effects.

Systemic glucocorticoids are rarely indicated in people with chronic noninfectious rhinitis, and have been superceded by nasal sprays containing topical glucocorticoids that have strong local effects and very little systemic absorption. Nasal medications are passed caudally by mucociliary clearance to the nasopharynx, and then swallowed. In order to avoid systemic side effects, nasal medications must therefore have very poor oral bioavailability. Fluticasone propionate, for example, is a powerful glucocorticoid that, once it enters the gastrointestinal tract and then the enterohepatic circulation, is almost completely eliminated via first pass metabolism. Nasal sprays containing fluticasone propionate have revolutionized the treatment of people with chronic rhinitis because aggressive local antiinflammatory glucocorticoid doses can be utilized with very little risk of systemic steroid side effects. The use of similar nasal sprays may not be as practical in veterinary medicine because dogs and cats cannot be trained to actively inhale at the precise time that a spray of medication is initiated.

Although nasal sprays are not feasible in dogs and cats, several other means of administering topical glucocorticoid therapy may have more promise. Attempted treatment with topical steroid eye drops (containing glucocorticoids such as prednisolone) administered through the anterior nares with the tip of the nose directed vertically upwards, is sometimes met with patient resistance and vigorous sneezing. Furthermore, following mucociliary clearance and passage of medication into the gastrointestinal system, steroids such as prednisolone can have significant systemic effects. Potentially, nasal drop instillation of a steroid with almost entirely local effects (e.g., fluticasone propionate) may be more efficacious.

Another method of administering steroids with predominantly local effects, the metered dose inhaler attached to a pediatric spacing device and face mask, may hold more promise. Over the past few years, the combination of an inhaler, a pediatric spacer, and a face mask to administer metered doses of fluticasone propionate has been used to manage feline asthma and canine chronic bronchitis.[16] Most cats and dogs appear to tolerate the administration of inhaled steroids via a face mask, and systemic side effects are few. Because with this method of administration, the inhaled fluticasone propionate typically passes through the nasal cavity when the patient's mouth is closed, the technique may have potential for treating nasal disease as well as lower airway disorders. A recommended starting dose of inhaled fluticasone propionate for both dogs and cats is 220 µg twice daily, with doses then titrated up or down to effect. To date, although anecdotal successes have been suggested regarding treatment of lymphoplasmacytic rhinitis with inhaled fluticasone propionate, there have been no published studies evaluating this method of administration.

It is unlikely that any topical therapy will adequately reach affected areas of the nasal cavity in patients with significant airway obstruction secondary to accumulation of discharge, congestion, and proliferation. In these patients, systemic glucocorticoid therapy (and antibiotics, if needed) should be used to get the condition under initial control, after which the patient may be able to be weaned onto topical steroid administration.

IMMUNOSUPPRESSIVE THERAPY

Uncommonly, immunosuppressive agents may be indicated in patients with severe lymphoplasmacytic rhinitis that fail to respond to systemic or topical glucocorticoids, or that exhibit unacceptable steroid side effects. In these animals, the concurrent use of glucocorticoids and oral immunosuppressive agents such as azathioprine or cyclosporine may be effective when steroids alone are ineffective.[10] The efficacy of immunosuppressive agents has not been evaluated in dogs and cats with lymphoplasmacytic rhinitis, and the benefits of aggressively treating a non–life-threatening local disease must be carefully weighed against the expense and side effects associated with the use of such agents.

ANTIBIOTIC THERAPY

Antibiotics are not a mainstay of the treatment of lymphoplasmacytic rhinitis. Secondary infections of the nasal passages, however, may benefit from selectively timed courses of antibiotics. A 1- to 2-week course of a broad spectrum oral antibiotic may be beneficial both during the initial treatment of lymphoplasmacytic rhini-

tis patients with excessive nasal discharge; and during any subsequent relapses that feature a mucopurulent, purulent, or sanguineous discharge. Although specific antibiotics such as clindamycin or azithromycin have been recommended for treatment of chronic rhinitis, there is little objective evidence that one antibiotic is preferable to another. Oral tetracycline or doxycycline have been anecdotally reported to be effective in some patients with lymphoplasmacytic rhinitis, either because of their antimicrobial effects or because of their immunomodulating properties.[10]

OTHER MEDICAL THERAPIES

Although topical and systemic decongestants and antihistamines are commonly used to treat chronic rhinitis in people, such medications have rarely proven to be efficacious in the treatment of lymphoplasmacytic rhinitis in dogs and cats. Symptomatic therapies designed to soften mucus and facilitate clearance of excessive nasal discharge (e.g., nasal saline drops, humidification, and nebulization) may be helpful in individual cases. Oral interferon-α has also been recommended by one author as an ongoing oral medication in animals with lymphoplasmacytic rhinitis.[10]

Outcome and Prognosis

Lymphoplasmacytic rhinitis usually responds well to appropriate and aggressive medical therapy. Clinical signs, however, can take many weeks or months to completely resolve.[8] Unless a triggering allergen or irritant can be identified and eliminated, the underlying processes leading to nasal disease may persist for many years, or even for the life span of the animal. Relapses are therefore common if treatment is tapered or discontinued. Affected animals may therefore require ongoing medical therapy, with drug doses titrated to maintain a fine balance between excessive signs of nasal disease and excessive drug side effects. In order to minimize drug side effects during long-term maintenance therapy, topical or local treatments (when feasible) are probably preferable to systemic medications.

REFERENCES

1. Tasker S, Knottenbelt CM, Munro EAC et al: Aetiology and diagnosis of persistent nasal disease in the dog: A retrospective study of 42 cases, *J Small Anim Pract* 40(10):473-478, 1999.
2. Allen HS, Broussard J, Noone K: Nasopharyngeal diseases in cats: A retrospective study of 53 cases (1991-1998), *J Am Anim Hosp Assoc* 35(6):457-461, 1999.
3. Gibbs C, Lane JG, Denny HR: Radiological features of intra-nasal lesions in the dog: A review of 100 cases, *J Small Anim Pract* 20(9): 515-535, 1979.
4. Sullivan M: Differential diagnosis of chronic nasal disease in the dog, *In Practice* 9(6):217-222, 1987.
5. Zwicker GM, Filipy RE, Park JF et al: Clinical and pathological effects of cigarette smoke exposure in beagle dogs, *Archives of Pathology and Laboratory Medicine* 102(12):623-628, 1978.
6. McDougal BJ: Allergic rhinitis: A cause of recurrent epistaxis, *JAVMA* 171(6):545-546, 1977.
7. Wolschrijn CF, Macri RM, Bernadina WE, et al: Immunoglobulin concentrations in nasal lavage fluids in dogs with non-specific rhinitis, *Vet Quarterly* 18:13-17, 1996.

8. Burgener DC, Slocombe RF, Zerbe CA: Lymphoplasmacytic rhinitis in five dogs, *J Am Anim Hosp Assoc* 23(5):565-568, 1987.
9. Forrester SD, Noftsinger MH: Initial approach in dogs with nasal discharge, *Vet Med* 97(7):521-528, 2002.
10. Gartrell CL, O'Handley PA, Perry RL: Canine nasal disease: Part II. *Compendium on Continuing Education for the Practicing Veterinarian* 17(4):539-547, 1995.
11. Codner EC, Lurus AG, Miller JB, et al: Comparison of computed tomography with radiography as a noninvasive diagnostic technique for chronic nasal disease in dogs, *JAVMA* 202(7):1106-1110, 1993.
12. Burk RL: Computed tomographic imaging of nasal disease in 100 dogs, *Vet Radiol Ultrasound* 33(3):177-180, 1992.
13. McCarthy TC, McDermaid SL: Rhinoscopy, *Vet Clin North Am Small Anim Pract* 20(5):1265-1290, 1990.
14. Forrester SD, Jones JC, Noftsinger MH: Identifying the cause of nasal disease in dogs, *Vet Med* 97(7):530-541, 2002.
15. Forrester SD, Jones JC, Noftsinger MH: Diagnostically evaluating cats with nasal discharge, *Vet Med* 97(7):543-550, 2002.
16. Padrid P: Feline asthma: Diagnosis and treatment, *Vet Clin North Am Small Anim Pract* 30(6):1279-1293, 2000.

B. Pharynx and Larynx
CHAPTER 40

Brachycephalic Airway Syndrome

Joan C. Hendricks

Definition

Brachycephalic airway obstructive syndrome is a consequence of the pharyngeal and nasal anatomy in brachycephalic, or "short-headed," dog breeds. The precise conformation that constitutes brachycephaly has not been rigorously defined. Breeds usually considered to be brachycephalic include bulldogs (e.g., English, French, and Boston bull terrier), Pekingese, pugs, and boxers, although beagles and Chinese shar-peis might be included. For the purposes of this chapter, brachycephalic breeds are those that have been described to have upper airway obstruction as a result of their anatomy. In the first case series reported,[1] bulldogs, pugs, boxers, and Pekingese dogs were disproportionately represented in the population receiving soft palate resections. In a recent review, breeds that developed brachycephalic airway syndrome requiring surgery were the English bulldog, pug, Boston bull terrier, and Cavalier King Charles spaniel.[2]

In the medical record database from 1986 to 2000 at the Veterinary Hospital of the University of Pennsylvania (VHUP), 72 dogs from 32 pure breeds were coded with a soft palate diagnosis and received surgery. During that time, only a single mixed-breed dog received surgery for a soft palate diagnosis. Dogs from five breeds (i.e., English bulldogs, pugs, Boston bull terriers, shar-peis and cocker spaniels) accounted for almost 50% (35/72) of the cases. Eight other dog breeds were represented more than once (i.e., boxers, Pekingese, Shih Tzus, Lhasa apsos, French bulldogs, King Charles spaniels, Maltese, and golden retrievers). Miniature dog breeds accounted for 19 of the 72 animals (25%), whereas large and giant breed dogs were in the minority. Only 4 giant-breed dogs (5%) were in the VHUP database; these were all dogs with distinctly short heads (i.e., a Saint Bernard, a Newfoundland, a rottweiler, and a mastiff). Although "short-headed" cat breeds are common and, at least subjectively, the distortion of their conformation is as extreme as that of many dog breeds, soft palate surgery to relieve upper airway obstruction in cats is extremely rare. Only a single Persian cat was found in the database with a soft palate diagnosis, although cats make up 25% of the caseload at VHUP.

Brachycephalic airway syndrome appears to arise from the increased airway resistance that results from airway narrowing at the nares, nasal turbinates, and nasopharynx at the caudal edge of the soft palate and hyoid apparatus. This narrowing requires that greater inspiratory effort is exerted by the diaphragm, intercostal, and extrinsic chest wall muscles. Therefore the decrease in airway pressure during inspiration is greater than in normal dogs with wider airways. Although the airway narrowing is present at multiple points, the impact of this negative pressure is greatest on the soft tissues of the pharynx, where the region of the caudal soft palate and hyoid is relatively unsupported by cartilaginous and bony structures.

The author has found, using imaging studies described in more detail below, that the midhyoid region is the narrowest point of the upper airway, even in normal dogs.[3] In brachycephalic dogs, there is commonly a large volume of soft tissue in this region, consisting of both the soft palate and the pharyngeal mucosa. This may be in part congenital (as certainly appears to be the case in shar-peis) or may be acquired as a result of soft tissue edema and inflammation caused by chronic barotrauma during respiration.

The single most common component of the brachycephalic airway syndrome is soft palate elongation, occurring in 101/118 patients in a recent review.[2] In the same study, 56/118 dogs also had stenotic nares conformation that required resection to increase the airway cross-sectional area. Another 54 dogs required resection of everted laryngeal saccules. Eversion of the mucosal lining of the laryngeal saccules is believed to be another acquired abnormality resulting from prolonged airway obstruction.[1]

Early descriptions of brachycephalic airway syndrome report that many of these breeds also have a narrow tracheal diameter and describe a method of quantifying the relative size of the tracheal lumen using thoracic radiographs.[4] Because the whole length of the trachea is affected, there is no treatment for this tracheal hypoplasia. Although it complicates upper airway surgery by making tracheostomy placement very difficult, it is not clear that tracheal hypoplasia correlates with signs of respiratory distress or with a poor surgical outcome.[4] In addition, the author has noted that an obviously narrowed trachea in a pup may increase in size proportionally more than the animal's thoracic size as the animal grows, so that the calculated ratio between the tracheal lumen and the thoracic inlet greatly increases over time. In other words, at least in growing animals, the degree of tracheal hypoplasia is not a static parameter.

Quantifying Brachycephaly

In clinical practice, the diagnosis of brachycephaly generally occurs during the preoperative visual inspection of the nares, pharynx, and larynx. The component of brachycephalic airway syndrome that is routinely identified on radiographs is the length of the soft palate and its overlap with the tip of the epiglottis. Objective means to define the degree of brachycephaly have also been applied to radiographs. A report of craniometry (the quantitative measure of angles of the bony structures of the head) in 50 dogs found that two brachycephalic breeds (i.e., the Pekingese and boxer) could be distinguished reliably from more normal or dolichocephalic breeds (e.g., greyhounds, pointers, and German shepherds).[5] Such measures are not routine but could be applied in future case series studies because they require no additional testing if good lateral radiographs of the head are available. It would be helpful to discover whether these objective measures correlate with clinical signs of respiratory obstruction or with long-term outcome.

Diagnosis

It would be ideal to have objective means to quantify the degree of brachycephaly and to correlate such quantitative measures with the need for surgery and with its outcome. However, the diagnosis is a clinical one that relies on a history of upper airway obstruction including snoring, syncope, and cyanosis with exercise; and occurring in a breed recognized to have a predisposition to the syndrome. Additionally, many brachycephalic dogs are prone to collapse during eating, perhaps because of transient airway obstruction while they swallow. Physical signs of airway narrowing include stenotic nares, recognizable on routine physical examination; and pharyngeal stertor that is easily auscultated, often without the aid of a stethoscope. Nonspecific signs of increased upper airway resistance include open mouth breathing, a behavioral adjustment to increase the size of the oropharyngeal lumen to compensate for the narrowed airways. Many brachycephalic dogs open their mouths to breathe throughout most of their waking time, which the owners may not find abnormal, but the clinician may observe or discover while eliciting the history. A marked sinus arrhythmia is another nonspecific sign that reflects increased thoracic pressure swings resulting from the narrowed upper airways.

Lateral radiographs of the head and neck can assist in predicting the extent of soft palate elongation and also allow measurement of the size of the trachea. The latter is important in planning for tracheal intubation and in determining the advisability of performing a tracheostomy. Pharyngoscopy and laryngoscopy under anesthesia provide the definitive diagnosis and are ordinarily part of a single anesthesia that includes surgery to relieve the obstruction.[1]

Simply stated, if the owner has observed signs of upper airway obstruction that seem to warrant surgery and if soft tissue that is present in the airway can be resected to provide a greater luminal cross-sectional area, then surgery to resect the tissue will be recommended. Such an animal then meets our definition of brachycephalic airway syndrome. The diagnosis is thus clearly influenced by the owner and clinician, as well as by the patient.

Auxiliary tests are advisable when considering anesthesia and surgery. Additional conditions that may be present as a direct result of the respiratory difficulty include esophageal and gastric dilation with air caused by aerophagia, hiatal hernias, and aspiration pneumonia. These can lead to retching, gagging, coughing, regurgitation, and sometimes even to abnormal gastrointestinal tract motility. Affected brachycephalic breeds are also commonly afflicted by unrelated conditions that should be assessed as part of a complete evaluation (e.g., skin disease; and ophthalmologic, dental, and musculoskeletal abnormalities).

Treatment

The mainstay of treatment is surgery. The first description of a surgical approach to relieve upper airway obstruction resulting from brachycephalic conformation was in 1929.[1] A series of articles describing the diagnosis, surgical approach, and follow-up of each component was published in 1982.[4] No new approaches have been described in the veterinary literature, and the specific surgical techniques are not described here. A general approach to upper airway obstruction, including tracheostomy, is described in Chapter 5.

Prognosis and Outcome of Standard Therapy

The outcome of surgery was reported to be excellent in 1982.[1] The age at surgery was related to the outcome, with dogs receiving surgery before 1 year of age having a more satisfactory outcome, based on owner assessment, than those receiving surgery at older ages. Outcome was also related to the type of surgery performed: 96% of dogs that required surgery for stenotic nares and overlong soft palate (often dogs younger than 1 year) were improved, whereas only 69% of those that required laryngeal saccule resection and palate surgery (often older dogs) were improved. A more recent report on 118 dogs identified specific complications and related outcome to breed, type of surgery, and the presence of complicating factors before surgery.[2] Aspiration pneumonia was identified in 15/118 dogs, occurring postoperatively in the majority of these dogs. Among the 56 dogs that had surgery, the outcome was excellent in 17, good in 16, and poor in 23.[1] Poor outcomes occurred disproportionately more often in English bulldogs, with 55% having a poor outcome compared with 33% of all other breeds. Overall, 8 of 56 dogs (14%) died, 6 due to aspiration pneumonia. Five of the 6 dogs that died of aspiration pneumonia were English bulldogs.[2]

Experimental Studies to Characterize Breathing in Brachycephalic Dogs

Some laboratory studies have pursued more extensive characterization of the impact of chronically narrowed upper airways on the organism. Amis and Kurpershock[6] used tidal breathing flow-volume loops to identify increased airway resistance in 16 English bulldogs and 3 Boston terriers. Although these measures were different from the loops in normal dogs, 11 brachycephalic dogs without clinical signs of obstruction had loop indices similar to those of 8 brachycephalic dogs with clinical signs of obstruction.

The English bulldog has been extensively studied because these dogs experience intermittent hypoxia during sleep, providing a natural animal model of sleep apnea, a serious and prevalent human disorder. These studies may provide the best hope for developing new therapeutic approaches to aid veterinary patients with chronic airway obstruction. Furthermore, insights into the pathophysiology and natural history of chronic airway obstruction are likely to be relevant to airway obstruction from any cause.

Sleep apnea affects at least 5% of the human population worldwide. This condition, which is easily diagnosed in a diagnostic sleep laboratory, was first recognized in the 1960s. The long delay in documenting a disorder that has almost certainly existed throughout human history is, in part, because sufferers are unaware of the events (i.e., pauses in breathing that can lead to profound hypoxia as frequently as 100 times per hour) that occur during sleep. During waking, respiratory function is generally completely normal, so that all pulmonary testing is nondiagnostic. The easily recognized historical signs of loud snoring and extreme sleepiness during the day may not be volunteered by patients. Following the discovery that sleep apnea is relatively common in humans, Adrian Morrison, a veterinarian and basic sleep researcher, proposed that brachycephalic dogs—animals with naturally occurring upper airway obstruction—might also suffer from the same disorder. This suggestion directly inspired the studies of the English bulldog as a model of sleep apnea.

Canine Sleep Apnea

In 1984 the first English bulldog was "volunteered" for study in the VHUP sleep lab. Wrapped with elastic belts to record chest wall motion, with an pulse oximeter taped to her ear and a video camera recording her every move, she dropped to sleep readily and immediately showed signs of sleep apnea. Subsequently, all bulldogs studied (to date, more than 30 dogs, some as young as 2 weeks of age) exhibit the hallmark signs that are found in human patients with sleep apnea. These include:

- *Hypersomnolence:* When tested in an unfamiliar laboratory situation, these dogs fall asleep in less than 15 minutes, whereas normal dogs have to be habituated for days before they will sleep.
- *Snoring:* When they are sleeping, these dogs snore, a manifestation of a narrowed upper airway that increases airway resistance.
- *Obstructive apneas* (detected by opposing, or paradoxical movements of the abdomen and ribcage) and *central apneas* (cessation of respiratory movements).
- Apneas result in *decreases of oxygenation* (as measured by pulse oximetry) and in microarousals documented by a waking pattern on the EEG.

We found these abnormalities as often as 100 times per hour during the rapid eye movement (REM) phase of sleep in some dogs, and as rarely as five times per hour of sleep in some bulldogs.

The severity of the disorder during the initial phase of sleep (slow wave sleep, [SWS]) is dramatically less in dogs than in people. One explanation for this marked difference may lie in the different physiology of SWS between the two species. Human SWS has four substages, with most apneas occurring during the lighter three stages, and virtually none during deep SWS. Dogs have only two substages of SWS, and the lighter stage is relatively brief.[7] Whatever the reason for this difference, dogs and humans are similar in that waking abnormalities in respiration are undetectable or minor compared to the sleep abnormalities, and that REM sleep is the time of most frequent and severe apnea. Unlike humans, where men show an increased risk, no gender difference in predisposition has been apparent in bulldogs. Although research efforts have focused on this breed because it is universally affected, the author has also seen clinical cases of shar-peis, Boston bull terriers, and obese dogs of several small breeds with typical histories indicating sleep apnea. Obesity is a major risk factor in human patients, for reasons that are still not well understood.

Since 1984 the author has studied the underlying abnormalities that lead to frequent pauses in breathing during sleep in English bulldogs. The first focus was on the neural control of respiratory muscles during sleep. Because the sleep-disordered breathing (SDB) events are often more prolonged and saturation measured by pulse oximetry (SpO_2) nadirs lower during REM, we began by investigating basic mechanisms of SDB during REM. It was predicted that the mechanisms of SDB in REM would be related to the normal phasic changes in respiratory control during REM. This is in contrast to the underlying mechanisms for SWS SDB, when homeostatic mechanisms are intact, and cyclic arousals are thought to be a response to hypoxia.

The pattern of respiratory muscle activity is related to, and controlled by, arterial blood gases during waking and SWS. SDB during SWS is thought to be the result of recurrent respiratory reflex and arousal responses that lead to cyclical relief of the obstruction, and then a recurrence. In contrast, the worst apneas during REM sleep occur relatively randomly. REM sleep is normally characterized by periods of quiet, when breathing is regular, punctuated by phasic periods that include apparently random fluctuations of muscle tone. Throughout REM, large postural muscles are actively suppressed to prevent excessive movements of the body during dreaming. We postulated that SDB during REM might be caused by excessive suppression of the respiratory muscles, especially during the phasic periods. Homeostatic mechanisms that keep blood gases within a normal range have been thought to be suspended during phasic REM, and respiratory muscle firing is aberrant. Recordings of the electrical activity (EMG) of the diaphragm (DIA) and the sternohyoid (SH), an upper airway dilating muscle, were made in 5 English bulldogs during sleep. The author found that, as predicted, SDB events were associated with phasic influences (i.e., SDB events occurred during periods of rapid eye movements) rather than with arousals or responses to hypoxia. The onset of SDB was significantly related to suppression of neural drive to both the DIA (p less than 0.01) and the SH (p less than 0.01). The mean drive of the DIA was suppressed to 42% of normal and of the SH to 17% of normal; the suppression of the SH was significantly greater than that of the DIA (p less than 0.05). SDB events were associated with changes in respiratory muscle EMG patterns typical of REM (p less than 0.01) for each muscle. Typical examples are displayed in Figures 40-1 and 40-2. When such aberrant respiratory muscle activity occurred in bulldogs, hypoxia resulted.[8] The

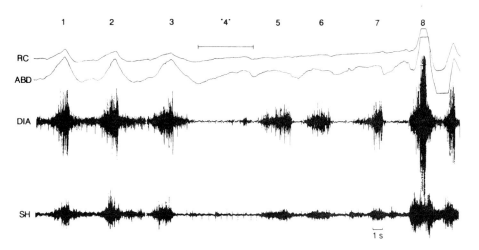

Figure 40-1. *A typical SDB event in an English bulldog with decreased muscle activity at the onset. In the three normal breaths (1 to 3), the ribcage (RC) and abdominal (ABD) movements are in phase. In breaths 4 to 7, the respiratory movements are decreased to less than 50% of normal, with RC movement virtually absent. Oxyhemoglobin saturation fell from 97% to 89%. The resolving breath 8 is characterized by an increase with synchronous excursions of both chest and abdomen. During the event (breaths 4 to 7), the DIA and SH activity are unmeasurable throughout the first breath (4) and reduced during breaths 5 to 7, with the SH suppression being relatively greater than the DIA suppression. (From Hendricks JC, Kovalski RJ, Kline LR: Phasic respiratory muscle patterns and sleep-disordered breathing during rapid eye movement sleep in the English bulldog,* Am Rev Respir Dis *144(5):1112-1120, 1991.)*

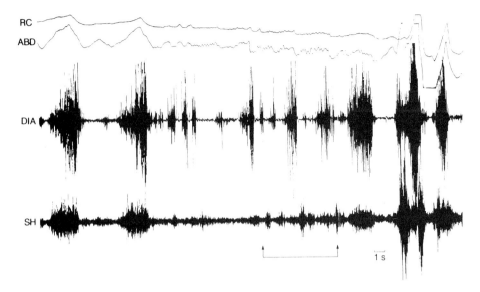

Figure 40-2. *An SDB event in an English bulldog characterized by disrupted respiratory muscle activity. After two normal breaths, as indicated by RC and ABD excursions, a period of reduced, irregular movements lasts 25 seconds before a large breath; the synchronous excursions of both body cavities signals the resolution of the event. Saturation fell from 93% to 85%. Overall, muscle activity decreased throughout the event, with the SH being more suppressed.* (From Hendricks JC, Kovalski RJ, Kline LR: Phasic respiratory muscle patterns and sleep-disordered breathing during rapid eye movement sleep in the English bulldog, *Am Rev Respir Dis* 144(5):1112-1120, 1991.)

events were not terminated by arousals in response to low SpO_2, as would be expected during waking or SWS. Rather, as would be expected of phenomena associated with REM, the onset and termination of events were unpredictable. The association of SDB in REM with randomly timed phasic REM influences, rather than a cyclical pattern of arousal in response to hypoxia, suggests new directions for therapeutic approaches, discussed further below.

The author next asked whether upper airway dilating muscle activity was related to abnormal mechanics of the airways in English bulldogs. The answer was found in a combination of imaging techniques and in careful analysis of EMG patterns throughout the animals' waking and sleep, in comparison with the same measures in normal dogs. We carefully quantified the size and movements of the bulldog's pharyngeal airway as he breathes, using rapid computer-assisted tomography (cine-CT).[3] By analyzing images collected several times per second and relating them to the respiratory cycle, we found that bulldogs have a nearly closed pharynx at the end of each breath (end-expiration). When the bulldog begins to inhale, the airway dilates to a larger cross-sectional area. This was in marked contrast to the pattern of normal dogs (and humans), whose airways are slightly smaller during inspiration (presumably because of the slightly negative forces during inspiration that tend to collapse the pharyngeal walls inward into the lumen) but wide open at end-inspiration and throughout expiration.

The author also compared the EMG activity of the DIA and the SH in 6 English bulldogs and in 5 control dogs.[9] The activity of the DIA was similar in the two groups of dogs throughout sleep, with the normal increased vari-

ability and altered recruitment patterns during REM sleep in all dogs. That is, whereas SDB events reliably followed decreases in respiratory muscle effort in bulldogs, the same decreases were observed in normal dogs but did not lead to SDB events. However, in the presence of the narrowed upper airway of bulldogs, the pattern of the upper airway dilator was dramatically different. In bulldogs, SH activity virtually always (96% to 100% of breaths) occurred during inspiration in both waking and SWS. In contrast, inspiratory increases in SH activity occurred in only a minority of breaths (32%) during SWS in control dogs (p less than 0.05). During REM sleep, SH drive fell in bulldogs, whereas it increased in control dogs (p less than 0.05). In control dogs without SDB, we found that central respiratory drive to the SH was highest but variable during waking and minimal during SWS and that it fluctuated with phasic events during REM sleep. In bulldogs, however, high levels of SH activity occurred during waking and throughout SWS, apparently preventing SDB in these states. These data support the proposition that compensatory pharyngeal dilator hyperactivity is necessary to maintain airway patency and normal breathing in bulldogs.

In summary, direct recordings of upper airway dilating muscles during waking and SWS confirmed that bulldogs use their upper airway muscles actively to maintain a patent pharyngeal airway, pulling the airway open during inspiration to counteract the collapsing forces. During REM sleep, when respiratory muscle activity is decreased, the mechanical forces prevail and airway collapse occurs. Subsequently, the same pattern of upper airway muscle hyperactivity has also been found in waking humans with sleep apnea. In contrast, normal dogs allow their muscles to be silent or to show only behavior-related activity (e.g., swallowing, head movements, or barking) for the vast majority of the time during waking or sleep; no airway muscle activity is necessary to maintain a patent airway. Thus, it appears that the primary abnormality in both species is anatomical airway narrowing. In order to maintain normal blood gas values, both canine and human sleep apneics increase their upper airway muscle activity to compensate for their narrow upper airways. This compensation is interrupted or overwhelmed by the normal changes in muscle control that occur during sleep, and apnea results. In order to breathe, the sleep apnea sufferer must awaken briefly, leading to severely fragmented sleep.

Pathophysiology of Progression of Sleep Apnea and Upper Airway Obstruction

The author speculated that the burden of using additional muscle effort throughout life might lead to muscle damage over time.[10,11] Full-thickness biopsies were obtained from two pharyngeal dilator muscles, the SH and the geniohyoid (GH), as well as a limb muscle, the anterior tibialis, in bulldogs (n = 5) and control dogs (n = 7). Immunohistochemical analysis of myosin heavy chain expression revealed an increased proportion of fast type II myosin heavy-chain fibers in the SH in bulldogs. The bulldog SH also demonstrated increased connective tissue content compared with control dogs, consistent with the presence of fibrosis. Both pharyngeal dilators in the bulldog exhibited an elevated proportion of morphologically abnormal fibers indicative of ongoing or prior injury. No differences in any of the above parameters were seen between bulldogs and control dogs in the anterior tibialis limb muscle.[10] The author hypothesizes that the chronic load and altered pattern of usage imposed on the upper airway dilators in SDB lead to myopathic changes that may ultimately impair the ability of these muscles to maintain pharyngeal patency.[11] This may account for the deterioration that is often noted clinically in adult bulldogs.

Anecdotal information and the author's own experience with both bulldogs housed in a colony and with clinical VHUP patients indicates that bulldogs tend to die relatively young (between 4 and 8 years of age) with signs of intractable upper respiratory obstruction, cardiovascular collapse, or sudden death. The author speculated that the strain of pulling the airway open repeatedly might result in accumulated muscle damage, with eventual decompensation in some individuals. Quantitative magnetic resonance imaging (MRI) was used to characterize the relaxation times of airway muscles (i.e., geniohyoid, sternohyoid, sternothyroid, thyropharyngeus, and hyopharyngeus) and nonairway muscles.[12] Quantitative differences between the medians and distributions of relaxation times of airway versus nonairway muscles were demonstrated. These differences were related to the de-

gree of sleep-disordered breathing. The changes observed are compatible with the hypothesis that there is increased edema and fibrosis in upper airway muscles of dogs with sleep apnea.

In summary, we found through biopsies and MRI of the upper airway dilating muscles, that English bulldogs have edema and fibrosis of the upper airway muscles. The extent of muscle damage correlates with the severity of sleep apnea. These findings have also been recognized in humans.[11,13]

Natural History of Sleep-Disordered Breathing in English Bulldogs

SDB appears to be acquired in bulldog puppies within the first few weeks of life. Specifically, we have found that neonatal (aged less than 2 weeks) pups show no SDB events (n = 3); slightly older pups (aged 6 to 12 weeks) exhibit disordered breathing events in waking and in both non-REM and REM sleep. By 16 weeks of age, the adult pattern of SDB is established with no waking events, with rare non-REM sleep events, and with a predominance of REM SDB events. Typically, up to 4 years of age the SDB indices are relatively stable; beyond 4 years, it appears that many but not all bulldogs begin to decompensate. Dogs demonstrated exercise intolerance or syncope when stressed. By age 6 to 7 years, oxyhemoglobin saturations in non-REM sleep are reduced from a range of 92% to 95% to a range of 87% to 90%. The author was able to measure arterial blood gases in four older bulldogs in the colony, all of which developed hypercapnia (resting $Paco_2$ 50 to 60 mm Hg). These older dogs with hypoventilation occasionally demonstrated snoring, paradoxical respiration, and stridor in waking. Five dogs in our colony less than 4 years of age (range, 4.5 to 6.5 years) have died or been euthanized due to severe signs of respiratory or cardiac failure. We also found, in a review of the ages of English bulldogs compared to mixed-breed dogs that were presented to VHUP by their owners, that the age of English bulldogs was significantly lower than that of mixed-breed dogs, with only 1 bulldog older than 8 years. This is an abnormally brief lifespan. Dogs are not generally considered geriatric until they are more than 10 years of age.[14]

IMAGING STUDIES OF AGING DOGS

The author hypothesizes that these overt signs of respiratory and cardiac disease in aging bulldogs are directly related to upper airway obstruction, and that the decompensation over time might be related, in part, to upper airway muscle damage from increased use. Preliminary analysis of the pharyngeal airway has been completed in 5 unanesthetized bulldogs and in 2 beagles using cine-CT. The author found that the lateral movement of the hyoid apparatus at the level of maximal collapse of the pharynx, and its relation to dilation of the airway lumen, was different in the bulldogs. In normal beagles, as in normal humans,[3] the airway size is adequate even during expiration, and there are minimal changes in airway lumen size throughout respiration (mean change in airway cross-sectional area [CSA] = 5.5 mm²). In contrast, in some bulldogs the end-expiratory airway was virtually obliterated by soft tissue, and the lateral bones of the hyoid apparatus were grossly abducted during inspiration such that the mean change in airway CSA within the hyoid bones was increased by more than 100 mm² in the five bulldogs. At the same time, the soft tissue contained within the hyoid bones expanded into the lumen by an average of 75 mm,² so that the net inspiratory dilation of the airway was only 25 mm.² The five bulldogs were affected with degrees of SDB ranging from mild (SDBI [number of hypoxic events per hour of sleep] = 4 to 17), to more severe (SDBI = 25 to 39). Interestingly, in the two minimally affected dogs, the large change in the hyoid apparatus (mean change = 83 mm²) greatly dilated the pharyngeal airway (mean change = 54 mm²). By contrast, even larger changes in hyoid CSA (mean change = 127 mm²) only produced

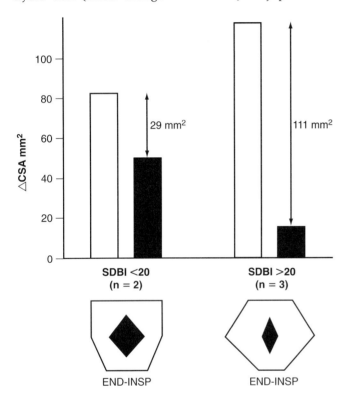

Figure 40-3. *Rapid cine-CT images of the mid-hyoid level of the pharynx were obtained in 5 bulldogs. The minimum (end-expiratory) and maximum (end-inspiratory) cross-sectional area contained within the hyoid apparatus* (white) *and the CSA of the airway lumen* (black) *were calculated on the digital images. The average differences between the minimum and maximum points are displayed for 2 dogs with mild SDB (less than 20 events/hour,* left), *and for 3 dogs with more severe SDB (greater than 20 SDB events/hour,* right). *As depicted in the schematic drawings below the graph, the maximal abduction of the hyoid bones accompanied effective airway dilation in the minimally affected dogs, whereas an even greater maximal abduction in more severely affected dogs did not produce effective dilation of the airway. The airway lumen is depicted schematically in black; the white area represents the soft tissue within the hyoid apparatus.*

minimal airway dilation (mean change = 16 mm²) in the 3 severely affected dogs (Figure 40-3). The author interprets these data to indicate that muscle hyperactivity during the compensated phase dilates the airway effectively; however, with progression of the disease, even greater contraction of the muscles is less effective in dilating the airway, setting the stage for muscle failure.

CARDIOVASCULAR CONSEQUENCES

Cardiovascular consequences of SDB have only begun to be explored in the bulldog. In the initial report, systemic arterial blood pressures measured in waking bulldogs were only slightly higher than control dogs;[8] however, acute direct blood pressures in untrained dogs are highly variable. The most appropriate method to monitor blood pressure is through chronically implanted catheters. When a chronically implanted femoral arterial catheter was used in one bulldog, the author found that arterial blood pressure actually increased during sleep onset, and furthermore that the pressures were higher during snoring than when the dog was not snoring. Interestingly, the pressure increased during each snoring inspiratory effort compared with the expiratory blood pressure, suggesting a neural rather than a mechanical cause.

The author has also sought evidence for cardiac effects of SDB. In most bulldogs, transthoracic echocardiograms do not reveal obvious differences in either ventricular sizes or wall thickness. Nonetheless, in 2 of the older dogs in our colony, dilated chambers and decreased wall motion were found; and 1 of these dogs developed clinical signs of cardiomyopathy (diagnosed by electrocardiography, radiography, and echocardiography) that was confirmed on postmortem. Regional variations in structure and thus contractility of the ventricles are thought to precede global alterations in cardiac function, but conventional imaging studies of the heart have several limitations for the study of regional heart wall motion. In studies of human patients with heart disease, the magnetic tagging method Spatial Modulation of Magnetization (SPAMM) allows the quantitative assessment of regional changes. SPAMM has demonstrated some consistent changes in regional heart wall motion in human patients, even when echocardiography was normal.[15] The author used the SPAMM technique to image the left ventricle, and analyzed these images to study function (motion and strain) of the cardiac wall in 1 bulldog, aged 4.5 years, who was showing no clinical signs of decompensation and whose echocardiogram was normal. Global measures were generally within a 95% confidence interval when compared with normal dogs using the same technique; however, the ejection fraction was low, at 32%. The regional contractility from end-diastole to end-systole was quite different from that of normal dogs. In several regions, longitudinal displacement was depressed, and maximal contraction varied regionally in the bulldog, with the midventricular and basal levels most affected. Vascular pathology, sympathetic nerve activity, and angiotensin-renin changes have not been explored in the bulldog. It seems likely that, if comprehensively investigated with suitable techniques, cardiovascular sequelae of SDB would be documented in bulldogs.

PROGRESSION OF HYPOXIA IN WAKING AND SLEEP

As in humans with SDB, the disease in dogs is a chronic process, and one that may progress over years. Figure 40-4, *A* shows the range of SDB values in dogs less than 4 years of age, compared with those greater than 4.5 years of age. The differences in both range and in the number of animals with increased values are obvious.

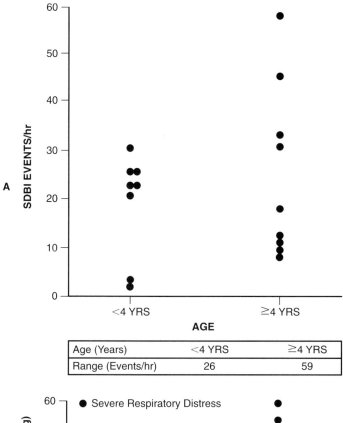

Age (Years)	<4 YRS	≥4 YRS
Range (Events/hr)	26	59

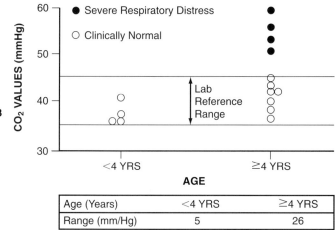

Age (Years)	<4 YRS	≥4 YRS
Range (mm/Hg)	5	26

***Figure* 40-4.** *Data from bulldogs of different ages.* **A,** *Sleep-disordered breathing indices (SDBI = number of hypoxic events/hour of sleep).* **B,** *Paco$_2$ levels from arterial blood gas samples.*

Furthermore, the SDB indices have increased with time in all but one individual bulldog observed in the colony over several years. Similarly, in Figure 40-4, *B,* carbon dioxide measurements of arterial blood gas samples tend to be higher in older dogs, and 4 of the older bulldogs demonstrated a progression to chronic hypoventilation.

THE SEARCH FOR AN IDEAL THERAPY

The author was interested in searching for a therapy for sleep apnea for several reasons. First, the present therapies are unsatisfactory. The surgical methods that are used for both humans and dogs are only partially effective. The author followed the SDB measures of 2 bulldogs that received soft palate, nares, and laryngeal surgery; 1 dog was greatly improved, whereas the second was not changed.[9] As described above, surgical treatments are also imperfect with regard to resolving clinical signs of respiratory distress noted by owners. The mechanical method that is widely used in humans (i.e., applying a nighttime constant positive airway pressure mask [CPAP]) is obviously not applicable to dogs, and actually is appropriately used by only about 50% of human patients.

Secondly, it is clear that the fundamental understanding of neurochemicals that control airway muscles and their changes during sleep should provide the basis for a drug therapy. The author has found that serotonin is the neurochemical that maintains the compensatory upper airway hyperactivity in English bulldogs.[3] Because basic research has shown that brainstem serotonin neuron activity is reduced during sleep, and especially during REM sleep, and results in the usual decrements in upper airway activity during REM, attention is now focused on identifying a safe and effective method to increase serotonin during sleep. The author has found that such a strategy can be effective, at least in the short-term.[16,17]

As work continues with more selective drugs, the author hopes to identify an approach that could be useful in dogs with upper airway obstruction from any cause. Such a drug would be especially helpful, for example, for brachycephalic dogs requiring sedation and anesthesia, which can be life-threatening because of the risk of airway obstruction during induction and recovery. The author currently expects that a new therapy will be investigated in human clinical trials within the next few years. For human sleep apnea, as for definitive treatment for the brachycephalic syndrome, long-term safety and efficacy will be imperative if a drug is to serve as an adjunct to CPAP or surgery or as an alternative for long-term therapy.

Unanswered Questions

Many similarities between dogs with sleep apnea and human patients have been noticed, as well as some important differences, as noted above. The long-term consequences of sleep apnea are largely still unexplored. In man, the consequence of pathological sleepiness is a higher risk of mortality because there is an increased risk of motor vehicle and industrial accidents. In dogs, this is not true. However, evidence is building that sleep apnea in humans also has medical sequelae, because it appears to put individuals at increased risk for death due to heart attack and stroke. Theoretically, repeated intermittent hypoxia could also alter neurological function and systemic immune responses. The author has not pursued these areas with rigorous studies in dogs, although there is considerable suggestive anecdotal information. If resources and effort were focused on studying these consequences in animals, we might identify additional pathology beyond the upper airway abnormalities that have been documented to date. We do not know the mechanisms that would lead from a primary disorder of upper airway narrowing to cardiovascular and immune disorders, nor whether such consequences might be species-variable.

The answers to these questions are likely to benefit humans by providing predictive and preventative measures. For dogs, this information would assist us in guiding owners in their expectations and in providing advice about whether their pet's condition warrants surgery or—if and when it becomes available—other less invasive therapies.

ACKNOWLEDGMENTS: These studies have been supported by a series of grants from the National Heart, Lung, and Blood Institute. We are also grateful to the Commonwealth of Pennsylvania for their generous support of the School of Veterinary Medicine. I thank Drs. Adrian Morrison, Richard O. Davies, and Allan I. Pack for their generous and important assistance throughout the years. The dogs studied benefited from the loving care of full-time research technicians Karen, Polina, and Jen. Finally, I am permanently indebted to English bulldogs, whose conformational flaws belie the nobility and purity of their spirits.

REFERENCES

1. Harvey CE: Upper airway obstruction surgery, *JAAHA* 18:535-567, 1982.
2. Lorison D, Bright RM, White RAS: Brachycephalic airway obstruction syndrome: A review of 118 cases, *Canine Practice* 22:18-21, 1997.
3. Veasey S, Panckeri K, Hoffman E et al: The effects of serotonin antagonists on upper airway muscle activity and breathing during wakefulness in an animal model of sleep-disordered breathing, *Am J Respir Crit Care Med* 153:776-786, 1996.
4. Harvey CE, Fink EA: Tracheal diameter: Analysis of radiographic measurements in brachycephalic and nonbrachycephalic dogs, *JAAHA* 18:571-576, 1982.
5. Regodon S, Vivo JM, Franco A et al: Craniofacial angle in dolicho-, meso-, and brachycephalic dogs: Radiological determination and applications, *Ann Anat* 175:361-363, 1993.
6. Amis TC, Kurpershock C: Pattern of breathing in brachycephalic dogs, *Am J Vet Res* 47:2200-2204, 1986.
7. Lucas EA, Powell EW, Murphree OD: Baseline sleep-wake patterns in the pointer dog, *Physiology & Behavior* 19:285-291, 1977.
8. Hendricks JC, Kline LR, Kovalski JA et al: The English bulldog: A natural model of sleep-disordered breathing, *J App Physiol* 53:1344-1350, 1987.
9. Hendricks JC, Petrof BJ, Panckeri K et al: Upper airway muscle hyperactivity during non-rapid eye movement sleep, *Am Rev Respir Dis* 148:185-194, 1993.
10. Petrof BJ, Pack AI, Kelly AM et al: Pharyngeal myopathy of loaded upper airway in dogs with sleep apnea, *J App Physiol* 76:1746-1752, 1994.
11. Petrof BJ, Hendricks JC, Pack AI: Does upper airway muscle injury trigger a vicious cycle in obstructive sleep apnea? A hypothesis, *Sleep* 19:465-471, 1996.
12. Schotland HM, Insko EK, Panckeri KA et al: Quantitative magnetic resonance imaging of upper airway musculature in an animal model of sleep apnea, *J App Physiol* 81:1339-1346, 1996.
13. Schotland HM, Insko EK, Schwab RJ: Quantitative magnetic resonance imaging demonstrates alterations of the lingual musculature in obstructive sleep apnea, *Sleep* 22:605-613, 1999.
14. Goldston RT: Preface, geriatrics and gerontology, *Vet Clin N Am* 19:ix, 1989.
15. Palmon LC, Relchek N, Yeon SB: Intramural myocardial shortening in hypertensive left ventricular hypertrophy with normal pump function, *Circulation* 89:122-131, 1994.
16. Veasey S, Panckeri K, Pack AI et al: The effects of trazodone with L-tryptophan on sleep-disordered breathing in the English bulldog, *Am J Resp Crit Care Med* 160:1659-1667, 1999.
17. Veasey SC, Chachkes J, Fenik P et al: The effects of ondansetron on sleep-disordered breathing in the English bulldog, *Sleep* 24(2):155-160, 2001.

CHAPTER 41

Laryngeal Paralysis

David E. Holt • Daniel Brockman

Definition and Etiology

Laryngeal paralysis is caused by a disruption of the innervation of the intrinsic laryngeal muscles that prevents normal abduction and adduction of the arytenoid cartilages and vocal folds. The most common form of laryngeal paralysis is the acquired idiopathic form seen in older dogs. Laryngeal paralysis can also be congenital; it can affect one or both sides of the larynx, to varying degrees; and it can progress at varying rates.

Congenital laryngeal paralysis has been reported in Bouvier des Flandres,[1,2] Siberian huskies,[3] dalmatians,[4] rottweilers,[5] English bull terriers, Labrador retrievers, and English setters.[6] In Bouviers, the disease has an autosomal dominant mode of inheritance.[2] Histologically, this form of the disease is associated with degeneration of the nucleus ambiguus and the recurrent laryngeal nerves, and with neurogenic atrophy of the dorsal cricoarytenoid muscles.[7] In dalmatians, the disease is associated with diffuse axonal degeneration in the recurrent laryngeal and appendicular peripheral nerves, with more severe changes in the distal parts of the nerves.[4] A similar polyneuropathy was found in rottweilers.[5]

Acquired canine laryngeal paralysis has been described secondary to foreign body penetration of the esophagus[8] and endotracheal intubation.[9] Masses in the neck or cranial mediastinum can disrupt recurrent laryngeal nerve function, as can surgical trauma[10,11] or excessive use of monopolar electrocautery in the neck. All of these conditions damage the recurrent laryngeal nerves either uni- or bilaterally, and result in denervation atrophy of the intrinsic laryngeal musculature. In the majority of dogs with acquired laryngeal paralysis, there is no identifiable cause of recurrent laryngeal nerve dysfunction. In some dogs, laryngeal paralysis has been seen in conjunction with central[12] and peripheral neuropathies,[13,14] but in most, recurrent laryngeal nerve dysfunction is the only neurologic abnormality that is clinically apparent. A variable percentage of dogs with laryngeal paralysis have had concurrent hypothyroidism in some reports,[13-16] although the nature of the association between these two diseases is not clear.

In cats, laryngeal paralysis has been reported secondary to vagus nerve neoplasia[17] and lead poisoning[18] and is associated with progressive neuromuscular disease.[19] In cats without evidence of concurrent disease, laryngeal electromyography was consistent with denervation of the dorsal cricoarytenoideus muscles.[20] One of the authors has also seen one cat develop bilateral laryngeal paralysis after bilateral thyroidectomy, presumably due to surgical or electrical (electrocautery) damage to the recurrent laryngeal nerves.

Pathophysiology and Pathogenesis

The larynx normally contributes only 6% of the total inspiratory resistance during nasal respiration in the dog. In normal animals, contraction of the paired dorsal cricoarytenoideus muscles during forceful respiration abducts the arytenoid cartilages and vocal folds, widening the glottis and minimizing resistance to airflow (Figure 41-1).[21-23] The dorsal cricoarytenoid muscles are normally innervated by the paired caudal laryngeal nerves, the terminal parts of the recurrent laryngeal nerves.[24] The recurrent laryngeal nerves also supply motor fibers to the remaining intrinsic muscles of the larynx, except the paired cricothyroideus muscles.[25] Denervation of the dorsal cricoarytenoideus muscles results in failure of abduction of the arytenoid cartilages and vocal folds, which subsequently take up a paramedian position during resting respiration.[26] Denervation atrophy is probably progressive in many dogs, and clinical signs may not be apparent until respiratory work increases.

With hot weather or exercise, a greater force of respiration is required. In animals with laryngeal paralysis, the narrowed rima glottidis increases the airflow velocity and turbulence, causing laryngeal edema and further resistance to airflow. Increased flow velocity through the narrowed area decreases lateral pressure on the larynx because of the Bernoulli effect.[27] Diaphragmatic and intercostal muscle efforts are increased to generate a lower intrapleural pressure and maintain airflow. In severe cases, this pressure gradient draws the arytenoid cartilages and vocal folds medially on inspiration, creating a dynamic collapse that obstructs the glottis. The increased muscular work of breathing generates heat that cannot be adequately dissipated because the airway obstruction prevents air movement over the surface of the tongue. Consequently, many animals with laryngeal paralysis present with both severe respiratory obstruction and moderate to severe hyperthermia.

Upper airway obstruction in canine laryngeal paralysis has been quantified using tidal breathing flow-volume loops,[27] and the severity of respiratory dysfunction has

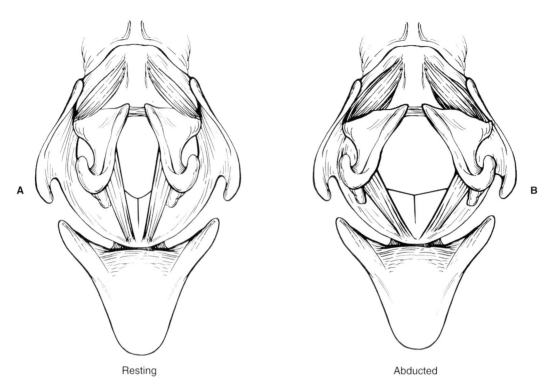

Figure 41-1. *Diagrammatic representation of laryngeal function.* **A,** *Normal resting larynx.* **B,** *The paired dorsal cricoarytenoideus muscles contract during inspiration, abducting the arytenoid cartilages and tensing the vocal folds. This minimizes airway resistance in the larynx.*

Resting   Abducted

been quantified by arterial blood gas analysis.[28] Tidal breathing flow loop analysis demonstrates that the airway obstruction can vary from minimal to dynamic inspiratory obstruction to a fixed obstruction affecting both inspiration and expiration. Presumably the latter pattern represents severe laryngeal inflammation and edema.[27] Sedated dogs with mild, moderate, and severe clinical signs of laryngeal paralysis had Pao_2 values of 85 ($\pm$7), 80 ($\pm$3), and 51 ($\pm$7) mm Hg respectively, compared to a control population mean value of 91 mm Hg.[28] These results show that severely affected animals can have substantial hypoxemia, even at rest.

During swallowing, the larynx is pulled cranially on the hyoid apparatus by the geniohyoideus and myelohyoideus muscles,[25] folding the epiglottis over the glottis.[29] The laryngeal adductor muscles also contract, closing the glottis and providing a second line of defense against aspiration of pharyngeal contents into the airway. The relative importance of each of these two parts of the swallowing reflex is uncertain; however, a variable percentage of dogs with laryngeal paralysis present with concurrent aspiration pneumonia, presumably due to failure of arytenoid adduction during swallowing.

Normal laryngeal function is also important for barking in dogs. Phonation is achieved by movement of air over the vocal and vestibular folds. The nature of the bark is influenced by the length and thickness of the folds and by changes in subglottic pressure.[30] Vocal fold length and thickness are dependent on contraction of the

paired vocalis and cricothyroideus muscles. Dogs with laryngeal paralysis often have a change in their bark.

Animals with severe laryngeal paralysis can develop pulmonary edema. The mechanisms of edema formation are incompletely understood. Proposed mechanisms include a gradient across the alveolar-capillary membrane favoring flux of fluid from the pulmonary capillaries to the alveoli and interstitium, created by the markedly low intrapleural pressure; mechanical disruption of the capillary walls caused by increased wall stress, which is proportional to the transmural capillary pressure; and increased capillary permeability secondary to severe hypoxia.[31-35]

The extremely low intrapleural pressure can also draw part of the stomach through the esophageal hiatus into the thoracic cavity, resulting in signs of regurgitation and nausea.[36]

Incidence

The incidence of congenital laryngeal paralysis seems low in the United States, with few cases cited other than those reported in the dalmatian[4] and rottweiler.[5] In one review, 21% of the cases of laryngeal paralysis presenting to a large veterinary teaching hospital were congenital.[37] The incidence of acquired laryngeal paralysis has not been defined in large studies; however, many referral surgeons consider this a condition they see relatively often in older dogs.[38]

Epidemiology and Risk Factors

The epidemiology of congenital laryngeal paralysis has been discussed earlier in this chapter. This diagnosis should be suspected in any puppy with significant dyspnea associated with an upper airway stridor, especially if it is one of the breeds predisposed to congenital laryngeal paralysis.

Acquired, idiopathic laryngeal paralysis generally occurs in older large or giant breed dogs,[39] although medium, small, and toy breeds also develop this condition.[13] Saint Bernards, Labrador and other retrievers, Afghan hounds, and setters seem to be more commonly affected.[11,37] Some studies state that males are more often affected than females,[11,13,37,40] although this finding is not consistent across all reports. The average age of affected dogs in several large studies varied from 7 to 12 years.[11,15,37,40-42] Perhaps more importantly, there is a wide age range for the onset of the acquired disease, varying from 2[15] to 16 years.[41]

Historical Findings, Clinical Signs, and Progression

Historical findings include decreased exercise tolerance, noisy respiration, and sometimes a change in bark. Some animals have a history of gagging, coughing, and perhaps vomiting or regurgitation. Physical examination findings vary depending on the severity of the respiratory compromise. Many dogs with laryngeal paralysis have mild clinical signs with slightly raspy, stridorous respiration when presented. Gentle external compression of the larynx will often worsen the stridorous respiration. More noticeably affected animals have moderate to marked inspiratory dyspnea. Severely affected animals present with marked respiratory distress, cyanosis, and collapse. Many dogs appear to have slowly progressive disease and compensate well, without showing marked clinical signs until stressed by exercise or hot weather. The sudden apparent worsening of respiratory distress then precipitates veterinary examination. In some instances, increased respiratory distress is caused by one or more episodes of aspiration, resulting in pneumonia.

Differential Diagnosis

In young animals, marked inspiratory dyspnea can be associated with brachycephalic airway syndrome in appropriate dog breeds. Congenital subglottic stenosis has also been reported.[43] Foreign body or insect inhalation, trauma, and abscess should all be considered. Laryngeal obstruction as an unusual manifestation of anticoagulant intoxication has also been described.[44]

In older dogs, neoplasms or abscesses that might affect recurrent laryngeal nerve function should be ruled out. Neoplasia of the pharynx, tonsil,[45] larynx,[46] and especially thyroid[47] can cause clinical signs compatible with laryngeal paralysis. Thyroid carcinomas can invade the cervical musculature, esophagus, trachea, and larynx, causing inspiratory stridor.[47] In cats, inflammatory or granulomatous laryngeal disease, pharyngeal polyps, and laryngeal or tracheal lymphosarcoma should be considered as possible causes of the clinical signs. Other tracheal neoplasms, foreign bodies, mediastinal neoplasia, and tracheal avulsions can cause signs similar to laryngeal paralysis.

In animals with a history of regurgitation, esophageal dysfunction should be considered. Megaesophagus[13] and gastroesophageal reflux associated with hiatal hernia[36] have been associated with laryngeal paralysis.

Pathological and Histopathological Findings

Gross pathological findings in dogs with laryngeal paralysis are often minimal and are confined to the larynx, where atrophy of the intrinsic musculature may be apparent. Pulmonary abnormalities such as aspiration pneumonia may also be visible. The histopathological findings associated with congenital laryngeal paralysis have been discussed earlier in this chapter. In acquired idiopathic laryngeal paralysis, histological changes include degenerative changes in the vagus and laryngeal nerves including loss of axons, beading of myelin, and perineural fibrosis.[12] Groups of small, eosinophilic myofibers with pyknotic nuclei and necrotic myofibers are found in the intrinsic laryngeal musculature, indicative of denervation atrophy.[12] In adult dogs with evidence of polyneuropathy, the main findings in nerve fiber studies were demyelination and remyelination.[14] Muscle changes included scattered angular atrophic fibers, small fiber atrophy, fiber hypertrophy, and necrosis.[14]

Preoperative Management

Management of an animal with suspected laryngeal paralysis is determined by the severity of respiratory distress at presentation. The majority of dogs present with mild to moderate respiratory stridor but do not have severe respiratory compromise at rest. These animals should have a careful physical examination that emphasizes oral examination, thorough cervical palpation to rule out neoplasia or other masses, and complete thoracic auscultation. The pattern of respiration should be observed, and the upper airway carefully ausculted to localize the site of airway obstruction. The animal's temperature should be monitored because even mildly affected animals may be hyperthermic. A complete neurologic examination is performed in stable animals to exclude the possibility of associated polyneuropathy or myopathy.

Ideally, radiographs of the thorax are made to rule out aspiration pneumonia, noncardiogenic pulmonary edema, and intrathoracic masses that may interfere with the recurrent laryngeal nerves. Three views of the thorax, including opposite laterals, are required to diagnose or rule out metastatic disease if neoplasia is suspected.[48] Dyspneic animals are often aerophagic, and the esophagus and stomach may appear to be full of air. This can be a confusing finding because some animals with diffuse neuropathies or myopathies may have concurrent megaesophagus. In addition, evidence of a hiatal hernia may be present on plain or contrast thoracic radiographs. Although hiatal hernia has been described in association with laryngeal paralysis,[36] in many cases the hiatus itself is anatomically normal. Presumably the lower intrapleural pressure generated as the animal tries to inspire against a dynamic upper airway obstruction pulls the cardia and part of the fundus of the stomach into the thorax. Because it is usually not possible to differentiate between aerophagia and true megaesophagus, or between primary versus secondary hiatal hernia, the upper airway obstruction should be definitively treated first. The possible megaesophagus or hiatal hernia is then reevaluated when the animal is no longer dyspneic.

If possible, the neck should be radiographed. Nonpalpable tracheal, laryngeal, pharyngeal, or retropharyngeal masses may be detected radiographically.[49,50] A lateral radiograph of the larynx may show soft tissue masses if they are surrounded by air; however, superimposition of the laryngeal cartilages may make radiographic diagnosis of primary laryngeal neoplasms difficult.[51]

Animals presenting with respiratory distress are true emergencies. These animals have severe hypoxemia (mean Pao_2 = 50 mm Hg in one study).[28] This Pao_2 corresponds to an 80% hemoglobin oxygen saturation. Any further respiratory compromise will rapidly result in desaturation of hemoglobin because of the steep slope of the oxygen/hemoglobin dissociation curve.[52] Clinically, many animals present on this threshold of disaster, and they have used up all of their compensatory mechanisms. Any further decrease in ventilation or increase in oxygen demand will cause complete decompensation. These animals must be handled with minimal restraint to prevent struggling that increases oxygen consumption. Procedures such as jugular venipuncture should be avoided because associated struggling and breath holding may further compromise oxygenation. However, vascular access is mandatory and a short peripheral intravenous catheter is placed using minimal restraint. Blood is collected from the catheter hub for an emergency database (i.e., packed cell volume, total solids, and dextrometer).

Immediate oxygen supplementation should be provided using a mask, cage, flow-by oxygen, or tent. Intravenous corticosteroids at antiinflammatory doses can decrease laryngeal swelling and edema. Sedation with acepromazine (0.025 to 0.05 mg/kg IV) may calm the animal and decrease its oxygen requirements. Sedation may also result in decreased respiratory drive, and therefore minimize the increased intrapleural pressure that results in further laryngeal collapse and edema. As previously discussed, many animals with severe respiratory distress are markedly hyperthermic. To cool the animal's core temperature, cold intravenous fluids are administered. If the rectal temperature is greater than 105° F, the animal may need to be soaked and/or packed with ice, and a fan may be used to blow air on the patient for further cooling. Efforts to decrease the animal's body temperature are a priority because hyperthermia contributes significantly to respiratory drive in dogs and therefore exacerbates respiratory distress when airway obstruction is present. Severe hyperthermia (greater than 106° F) may result in life-threatening disseminated intravascular coagulation and organ failure. The animal's temperature should be carefully monitored every 15 to 30 minutes, and cooling efforts should be terminated when the temperature has dropped to 103° F to prevent subsequent hypothermia.

Medical treatment should be given an extremely limited time to have an effect. If medical treatment (e.g., oxygen supplementation, sedation, antiinflammatory corticosteroids and cooling) does not alleviate severe respiratory distress within minutes, the animal should be anesthetized, the larynx rapidly examined, and the animal intubated. Once intubated, a more complete physical examination is performed. The lungs are carefully ausculted and thoracic radiographs made to rule out pneumonia or pulmonary edema secondary to upper airway obstruction. A tracheostomy is performed allowing the laryngeal swelling to decrease and the animal to stabilize before definitive surgery.

Laryngoscopy

The current gold standard for the diagnosis of laryngeal paralysis is laryngoscopy performed under light anesthesia. The amount of anesthetic agent must be carefully titrated to effect because moderate to deep planes of anesthesia result in cessation of all laryngeal movement.[53] Small amounts of ultra–short-acting barbiturate are normally administered, although more recently acepromazine, narcotics, and propofol have all been used. The relative effects of these agents on laryngeal function has not been clearly evaluated in dogs and cats. Ideally the animal should be light enough that it is intermittently gagging during the examination. In normal animals, abduction of the arytenoid cartilages should occur during inspiration. In animals with laryngeal paralysis, normal abduction does not occur. In some animals, the negative intrapleural pressure generated during inspiration can pull the vocal folds and arytenoid cartilages medially; at expiration they are pushed out to a paramedian position by the expired air. This paradoxical movement gives a false impression of normal function and emphasizes the importance of correlating laryngeal movement with the phase of respiration.[53] Once the larynx has been evaluated, the animal is intubated. In animals with suspected aspiration pneumonia, an endotracheal lavage performed through a sterile endotracheal tube provides samples for culture and sensitivity testing.

When the diagnosis is in doubt, electromyographic studies on the intrinsic laryngeal musculature may be useful.[54] The exact time required for electromyographic changes to become apparent in idiopathic laryngeal paralysis is unknown.[37] Electrodes may be inserted percutaneously or per os.[1] Recently, ultrasonographic examination of the pharynx and larynx of normal dogs has been described.[55] The laryngoscopic diagnosis of laryngeal paralysis is sometimes clouded by different anesthetic agents used for sedation and the depth of anesthesia. Ultrasound is a technique that allows evaluation of laryngeal function in the awake animal.

Surgical Treatment

Surgery is the treatment of choice for animals with confirmed laryngeal paralysis. The issue of timing of surgery is not always clear. Some animals have one episode of dyspnea associated with mild laryngeal paralysis that responds well to medical treatment. The disease may then progress slowly with minimal clinical signs over months or even years. Other dogs may primarily present with illness caused by aspiration pneumonia but with minimal evidence of upper airway obstruction despite the presence of laryngeal paralysis. In these cases, surgery to open the larynx may only exacerbate the tendency to aspirate.

However, the majority of laryngeal paralysis patients with moderate to marked clinical signs are repeatedly subject to the same initiating stresses (e.g., exercise, heat) that precipitated the initial episode of respiratory distress and will have repeated episodes of dyspnea. Hence surgery is recommended as soon as the animal is clinically stable. In severely affected animals, stabilization using tracheostomy is recommended to allow laryngeal edema and swelling to decrease before definitive surgery. The aims of surgery are to widen the glottis so that the animal can adequately ventilate when performing nonathletic functions, simultaneously maintaining the relatively normal laryngeal anatomy during swallowing to allow the epiglottis to completely cover the glottis and prevent the aspiration of food and water. Many surgical techniques have been described to treat laryngeal paralysis in dogs and cats. These tend to fall into one of three groups:

1. Surgical procedures that widen mainly the dorsal glottis: These procedures include unilateral[11,42,56] and bilateral arytenoid lateralization[40,57] and an experimental cricoarytenoid re-innervation procedure.[58]
2. Surgical procedures that widen mainly the ventral glottis: These procedures include vocal fold resection,[15,59] partial laryngectomy,[13,41,60,61] and castellated laryngofissure including vocal fold resection[62] and a modified arytenoid lateralization.[63]
3. Surgical procedures that widen both the dorsal and ventral glottis: One experimental study described a procedure that is a combination of castellated laryngofissure and bilateral arytenoid cartilage lateralizations.[64]

Laryngeal paralysis is a less common clinical entity in cats, and so large studies on surgical techniques to treat this disease in cats are not available. Both partial laryngectomy[19,20] and arytenoid lateralization[19] have been performed successfully in cats.

ARYTENOID LATERALIZATION

Arytenoid lateralization procedures have become the accepted treatment for laryngeal paralysis in dogs. Using one or two sutures, these procedures abduct one or both arytenoid cartilages to a position similar to that of the arytenoid during normal inspiration.

After clipping, the animal is placed in right lateral recumbency with the neck extended over a sandbag or rolled towel and the area prepared for aseptic surgery (Figure 41-2). The skin incision is made over the larynx ventral to the junction of the maxillary and jugular veins. The platysma muscle is incised and adipose tissue overlying the larynx dissected. In obese dogs, the cricoid cartilage can be used as a landmark to guide the surgeon to the thyroid cartilage, which is palpated under the thyropharyngeus muscle. The maxillary and jugular veins are retracted dorsally and the dorsal aspect of the thyroid cartilage rotated laterally using a Senn retractor. The thyropharyngeus muscle is transected along the dorsal wing of the thyroid cartilage to expose the fascial membrane of the larynx, which is also incised (Figure 41-3). The cricothyroid articulation is palpated medial to the caudal

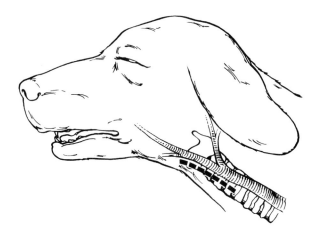

Figure 41-2. Surgical approach for left arytenoid lateralization. The animal is placed in left lateral recumbency and an incision is made over the lateral aspect of the larynx ventral to the maxillary and jugular veins.

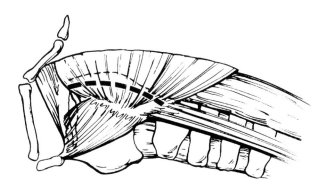

Figure 41-3. The thyropharyngeus muscle is transected along the dorsal wing of the thyroid cartilage to expose the fascial membrane of the larynx, which is also incised.

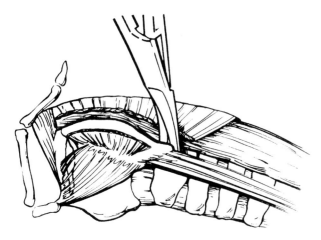

Figure 41-4. *The cricothyroid articulation is palpated medial to the caudal aspect of the thyroid cartilage and is transected with a scissor.*

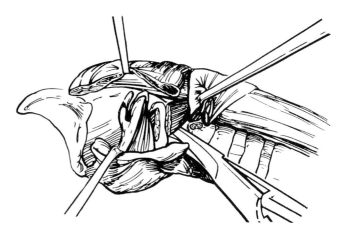

Figure 41-6. *The cricoarytenoid articulation is carefully incised with scissors or a scalpel to expose the articular surfaces of this joint.*

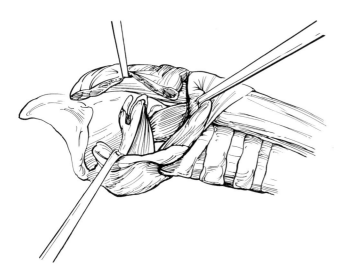

Figure 41-5. *The dorsal cricoarytenoid muscle is transected just caudal to its insertion on the muscular process.*

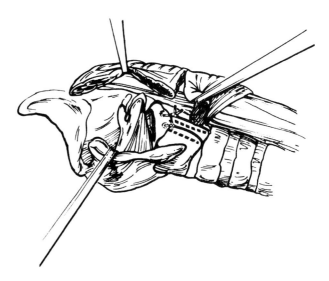

Figure 41-7. *Two sutures of 2/0 or 0 polypropylene or monofilament nylon are then placed from the caudodorsal edge of the cricoid cartilage through the articular face of the muscular process of the arytenoid cartilage.*

aspect of the thyroid cartilage and is transected with a scissor, allowing greater retraction of the thyroid cartilage and visualization of the muscular process of the arytenoid cartilage (Figure 41-4). The muscular process of the arytenoid cartilage is initially identified by palpation, and the dorsal cricoarytenoid muscle is transected just caudal to its insertion on the muscular process (Figure 41-5). The residual insertion of the dorsal cricoarytenoid muscle can be used to retract the muscular process laterally, and the cricoarytenoid articulation is carefully incised with scissors or a scalpel to expose the articular surfaces of this joint (Figure 41-6).

The dorsal interarytenoid sesamoid band is then severed by passing a scissor dorsally and slightly rostrally, medial to the muscular process of the arytenoid carti-

lage. Care must be taken not to enter the laryngeal lumen during this part of the dissection. Two sutures of 2/0 or 0 polypropylene or monofilament nylon are then placed from the caudodorsal edge of the cricoid cartilage through the articular face of the muscular process of the arytenoid cartilage (Figure 41-7). Gentle traction on the sutures should result in free caudodorsal movement of the arytenoid. The larynx is already partially abducted by the endotracheal tube, so the sutures should only be gently tightened. The surgeon should not expect the muscular process to approximate to the cricoid cartilage; over-tightening the sutures in this manner will cause excessive abduction. Arytenoid abduction may be checked by extubating the animal and examining the larynx with a laryngoscope. The thyropharyngeus muscle, subcutaneous tissue, and skin are closed in a routine manner.

Several variations of this procedure have been described and deserve discussion.

Dissection of the Cricothyroid Articulation

This has been recommended to increase exposure of the muscular process of the arytenoid cartilage.[56] The cricothyroid articulation provides lateral support to the cricoid cartilage, however, and experimentally, bilateral disarticulation of the cricothyroid articulation resulted in significant collapse of the dorsoventral height of the rima glottidis.[65] The concern raised by the anatomy of the larynx and the experimental study is that cutting the articulation may result in medial collapse of the cricoid or dorsoventral collapse of the rima glottidis. Because dissection of the cricothyroid articulation has been used successfully in a large number of clinical cases,[11,57] this concern may be unwarranted when unilateral dissection is performed. It may be possible, however, to induce unilateral cricoid cartilage medial collapse if the cricoarytenoid sutures are placed laterally rather than dorsally on the cricoid cartilage and overtightened.

Dissection of the Cricoarytenoid Cartilage

One report describes placement of a suture from the cricoid cartilage through the muscular process of the arytenoid without dissecting the process from the cricoid cartilage.[42] Although this procedure was successful, the majority of reports describe cricoarytenoid disarticulation.[11,40,56,57] Dissecting the articulation frees the arytenoid from the cricoid cartilage, allowing it to be pulled caudodorsally with less tension on the muscular process and the sutures.

Cutting the Interarytenoid Sesamoid Band

Cutting the sesamoid band results in a significant increase in mobility of the arytenoid cartilage.[56] At the same time, this dissection is difficult because it is performed blindly, and the lumen of the larynx can be inadvertently penetrated. Although there are no experimental studies on suture tension with the various dissection procedures, empirically, cutting the sesamoid band seems to minimize tension on the laryngoplasty sutures. Experimentally, cricoarytenoid disarticulation and cutting the sesamoid band resulted in significant dorsolateral displacement of the corniculate process of the arytenoid cartilage.[66] Although the authors of this study speculated that this glottic malalignment may result in aspiration pneumonia, clinical studies in which this technique was performed had the lowest rates of postoperative pneumonia reported.[11,56]

Placement of Suture in the Arytenoid Cartilage

The laryngoplasty suture may be placed either through the muscular process or through the articular facet of the arytenoid cartilage. Either a simple suture or a mattress suture can be used. Published[66] and anecdotal clinical experience tends to indicate a greater rate of cartilage fracture or splitting when the suture is placed through the muscular process. The majority of surgeons now place the suture through the articular facet of the arytenoid cartilage from medial to lateral.

Thyroarytenoid Sutures Versus Cricoarytenoid Sutures

Suturing the arytenoid cartilage to either the thyroid cartilage,[40] the cricoid cartilage,[11,56] or both,[11] has been described. Experimentally, cricoarytenoid lateralization provided a greater increase in the size of the glottic lumen than thyroarytenoid lateralization.[66]

Unilateral Versus Bilateral Laryngoplasty

Both unilateral[11,42,56] and bilateral lateralization[40,57] have been reported. There are no controlled trials comparing the procedures for efficacy in working dogs. However, bilateral lateralization has been recommended in working dogs to prevent collapse of the unstable side during heavy exercise.[40] Bilateral lateralization may result in excessive distortion of the dorsal glottis, predisposing to aspiration.

Dorsal cricoarytenoid lateralization has become the procedure of choice for treating canine laryngeal paralysis for several reasons. The procedure is very effective in most animals and has a low rate of complications attributable directly to the surgery. There is a low incidence of postoperative aspiration pneumonia; and because the procedure is performed outside the laryngeal lumen, the possibility for postoperative glottic scarring is eliminated. In general, a tracheostomy tube and the extensive postoperative nursing care associated with tube maintenance are not required. The procedure widens the dorsal glottis, preventing dynamic collapse in most dogs. However, the procedure is not as technically easy as vocal fold resection. It is *not* recommended to a surgeon unfamiliar with the technique because the learning curve is steep. The results of the initial 40 lateralization procedures performed at a veterinary teaching hospital showed that the incidence of nonfatal perioperative complications was 30%,[67] far higher than when the procedure was performed by an experienced surgeon (10%).[11] This clearly demonstrates that familiarity with the technique is vital for successful results.

Complications with the technique include seroma formation, fragmentation of the arytenoid cartilage, avulsion of the suture, inadequate lateralization, intralaryngeal hematoma formation, and aspiration pneumonia.[11,40,42] Animals with complications affecting the glottic opening (e.g., suture avulsion or hematoma formation) generally develop acute dyspnea within hours to days after surgery. These animals should be lightly anesthetized and the larynx examined. Intralaryngeal hematomas generally resolve with time; the larynx should be bypassed for several days using a tracheostomy tube. When lateralization fails because of cartilage fragmentation or suture pullout, either the original surgery site can be reexplored and salvage attempted or the lateralization can be performed on the opposite side.

NEUROMUSCULAR PEDICLE GRAFTING/REINNERVATION

Both neuromuscular pedicle grafting[58] and reinnervation[68] have been investigated to treat laryngeal paralysis in dogs. Although successful experimentally, both techniques have two major limitations in many clinical cases. First, many animals have significant respiratory distress when presented for surgery. Neuromuscular pedicle grafting or reinnervation would not be expected to improve laryngeal function for 4 to 6 months. Secondly, in many animals the dorsal cricoarytenoid muscles have undergone substantial denervation atrophy, and thus may not respond to either neuromuscular pedicle grafting or reinnervation.

VOCAL FOLD RESECTION

Vocal fold resection is generally performed through the mouth with the animal in sternal recumbency using either cup forceps[59] or scissors.[15] Some authors recommend placing the endotracheal tube into the trachea via a tracheostomy prior to vocal fold resection to minimize aspiration of blood[15]; others perform the procedure with the animal extubated.[59] The vocal folds are removed from the vocal process ventrally, leaving 3 to 5 mm of each vocal fold above the ventral floor of the larynx to prevent scar formation. The animal is then recovered either with[15] or without[59] a tracheostomy tube in place. Per oral vocal fold resection alone is an appealing procedure because it is simple to learn and does not distort the glottis; however, if a tracheostomy tube is used in the postoperative period, a substantial round-the-clock nursing commitment is required. When vocal fold resection is performed per os, the incised laryngeal mucosa heals by granulation and a ventral web of scar develops in some animals, necessitating a second surgery. In spite of the fact that the glottis is not distorted, aspiration occurs with some frequency in animals after vocal fold resection.[15,59]

PARTIAL LARYNGECTOMY

Partial laryngectomy is performed per os, generally with a tracheostomy tube in place. A uni-[41] or bilateral vocal fold resection[13,60,61] is performed, and part of the corniculate process of the arytenoid cartilage is unilaterally removed using laryngeal cup forceps. This procedure also generally requires a tracheostomy tube and the associated nursing care postoperatively. Ventral scarring of the larynx can occur. Removing part of the corniculate process potentially increases postoperative laryngeal irritation and causes loss of the epiglottic seal in this area during swallowing. Results with a unilateral vocal fold resection and partial arytenoidectomy were favorable in one report,[41] but the majority of reports on partial laryngectomy cite an unacceptable mortality rate in the postoperative period and high rates of aspiration pneumonia in the follow-up period.[13,60,61]

CASTELLATED LARYNGOFISSURE

Castellated laryngofissure is performed with the animal in dorsal recumbency with a tracheostomy tube in place. A stepped (castellated) incision is made in the ventral aspect of the thyroid cartilage, creating a central flap of cartilage.[62] The vocal folds are removed, and in one revision of the procedure, a modified arytenoid lateralization is performed.[63] When closing the thyroid cartilage incision, the created step is moved rostrally and sutured to the opposite edge of the thyroid cartilage incision, thus widening the ventral glottis. Whereas a ventral approach allows the suturing of the laryngeal mucosa after vocal fold resection, this procedure involves extensive laryngeal dissection. A tracheostomy tube is recommended after the surgery. Aspiration pneumonia has been reported after this procedure. In spite of the modified arytenoid lateralization, one of the authors has seen 3 dogs with recurrence of dyspnea following castellated laryngofissure. Dynamic collapse of the dorsal larynx in hot weather or after exercise was the presumed cause of this complication.

Postoperative Management

Animals should recover from surgery under close observation. Prior to extubation, the cuff on the endotracheal tube is deflated and then reinflated with a small volume of air (1 to 4 cc, depending on the size of the tube and cuff). As the tube is removed, the partially inflated cuff will prevent any blood that may have entered the larynx or trachea migrating further down the airway. The larynx is examined with a laryngoscope to ensure adequate arytenoid lateralization. The animal's respiration rate and effort are checked frequently. The animal's temperature is checked periodically. Balanced electrolyte solution should be administered intravenously at maintenance rates until the animal can drink comfortably. Water and food are withheld for a minimum of 12 hours after surgery. The animal is initially offered a small amount of water under close supervision. The clinician should watch for any difficulty swallowing or any coughing after drinking. If water is accepted uneventfully, the animal may then be offered a small amount of canned food.

The animal can be discharged once it is eating and drinking without difficulty. The owners should be instructed to restrict the animal's activity for 2 to 4 weeks. Walks are kept short and a harness rather than a collar is recommended. Skin sutures are removed in 7 to 10 days.

Aspiration pneumonia is a potentially devastating complication in animals with laryngeal paralysis. Regardless of the surgical technique used, dysfunction of the recurrent laryngeal nerves means that the inherent adductive mechanism of the larynx is lost, predisposing these animals to aspiration of pharyngeal contents into the airway. Aspiration can occur prior to presentation.

While the focus in severely dyspneic animals is often on the upper airway obstruction, failure to diagnose and treat preexisting pneumonia can be life threatening because cold, dry inhalant gases used during anesthesia can worsen the condition. Any crackles, wheezes, or dull areas found on thoracic auscultation should prompt thoracic radiographs. If an animal is so dyspneic that it requires intubation, radiographs are made under general anesthesia. An endotracheal lavage is performed on animals with suspected pneumonia, and the fluid obtained is submitted for Gram stain and culture and sensitivity testing. Animals are given broad-spectrum bactericidal antibiotics intravenously pending culture and sensitivity results. Nebulization and coupage are performed every 4 to 6 hours to assist airway clearance.

Outcome and Prognosis

The prognosis for dogs with idiopathic laryngeal paralysis is good. In the absence of aspiration pneumonia, over 90% of dogs treated with unilateral arytenoid lateralization have a good long-term clinical course.[11,56] Animals presenting with aspiration pneumonia have a more guarded prognosis. Many dogs presenting with laryngeal paralysis are older, and many reports describe concurrent diseases in a percentage of cases. Such animals and those with laryngeal paralysis associated with a more generalized polyneuropathy, myopathy, or true megaesophagus should also have a more guarded prognosis.

In one report of 3 cats, all did well following partial laryngectomy.[20] In a second report, 2 out of 4 cats were euthanized postoperatively because of progressive neuromuscular weakness, and one was euthanized because of continuing pneumonia.[20]

REFERENCES

1. Venker-van Haagen AJ, Hartman W, Goedegebuure SA: Spontaneous laryngeal paralysis in young Bouviers, J Am Anim Hosp Assoc 14:714, 1978.
2. Venker-van Haagen AJ, Bouw J, Hartman W: Hereditary transmission of laryngeal paralysis in Bouviers, J Am Anim Hosp Assoc 17:75, 1981.
3. O'Brien JA, Hendricks JC: Inherited laryngeal paralysis: Analysis in the husky cross, Vet Q 8:310, 1986.
4. Braund KG, Shores A, Cochrane S et al: Laryngeal paralysis-polyneuropathy complex in young dalmatians, Am J Vet Res 55:534, 1994.
5. Mahony OM, Knowles KE, Braund KG et al: Laryngeal paralysis-polyneuropathy complex in young rottweilers, J Vet Intern Med 12:330, 1998.
6. Lane JG: Canine laryngeal surgery, Vet Annual 183:239, 1978.
7. Venker-van Haagen AJ: Investigations of the pathogenesis of hereditary laryngeal paralysis in the Bouvier. PhD Thesis, Proefschrift University, Utrecht, Netherlands, 1980.
8. Salisbury SK, Forbes S, Blevins WE: Peritracheal abscess associated with tracheal collapse and bilateral laryngeal paralysis in a dog, J Am Vet Med Assoc 196:1273, 1990.
9. Dass LL, Sahay PN, Khan AA: Vocal cord paralysis following endotracheal intubation in a bitch, Vet Record 116:218, 1985.
10. Obradovich JE, Withrow SJ, Powers BE et al: Carotid body tumors in the dog: Eleven cases (1978-1988), J Vet Intern Med 6:96, 1992.
11. White RAS: Arytenoid lateralization: An assessment of technique, complications and long term results in 62 dogs with laryngeal paralysis, J Small Anim Pract 30:543, 1989.
12. O'Brien JA, Harvey CE, Kelly AM et al: Neurogenic atrophy of the laryngeal muscles of the dog, J Small Anim Pract 15:521, 1973.
13. Gaber CE, Amis TX, LeCouteur RA: Laryngeal paralysis in dogs: A review of 23 cases, J Am Vet Med Assoc 186:377, 1985.
14. Braund KG, Steinberg S, Shores A et al: Laryngeal paralysis in immature and mature dogs as one more sign of a more diffuse polyneuropathy, J Am Vet Med Assoc 194:1735, 1989.
15. Holt DE, Harvey CE: Idiopathic laryngeal paralysis: Results of treatment by bilateral vocal fold resection in 40 dogs, J Am Anim Hosp Assoc 30:389, 1994.
16. Harvey HJ, Irby NL, Watraus BJ: Laryngeal paralysis in hypothyroid dogs. In Kirk RW, editor: Current veterinary therapy, vol 8, Philadelphia, 1983, WB Saunders.
17. Schaer M, Zaki FA, Harvey HJ et al: Laryngeal hemiplegia due to neoplasia of the vagus nerve in a cat, J Am Vet Med Assoc 174:513, 1979.
18. Maddison JE, Allan GS: Megaesophagus attributable to lead toxicosis in a cat, J Am Vet Med Assoc 197:1357, 1990.
19. White RAS, Littlewood JD, Herrtage ME et al: Outcome of surgery for laryngeal paralysis in four cats, Vet Record 118:103, 1986.
20. Hardie EM, Kolata RJ, Stone EA et al: Laryngeal paralysis in three cats, J Am Vet Med Assoc 179:879, 1981.
21. Grandage J, Richardson K: Functional anatomy. In Slatter DH, editor: Textbook of small animal surgery, ed 2, Philadelphia, 1992, WB Saunders.
22. Harvey CE: Laryngeal surgery in the dog. FRCVS thesis, 1986.
23. Wykes PM: Canine laryngeal diseases part I: Anatomy and disease syndromes, Comp Cont Ed 5:8, 1983.
24. Ohnishi T, Ogura J: Partitioning of pulmonary resistance in the dog, Laryngoscope 79:1847, 1969.
25. Evans HE, Christensen GC: Muscles of the head. In Evans HE, editor: Miller's anatomy of the dog, ed 2, Philadelphia, 1979, WB Saunders.
26. Dedo HH: The paralyzed larynx: An electromyographic study in dogs and humans, Laryngoscope 80:1455, 1970.
27. Amis TC, Smith MM, Gaber CE et al: Upper airway obstruction in canine laryngeal paralysis, Am J Vet Res 47:1007, 1986.
28. Love S, Waterman AE, Lane JG: The assessment of corrective surgery for canine laryngeal paralysis by blood gas analysis: A review of 35 cases, J Small Anim Pract 28:597, 1987.
29. Harvey CE: The larynx. In Bojrab MJ, editor: Pathophysiology in small animal surgery, Philadelphia, 1981, Lea & Febiger.
30. O'Brien JA, Harvey CE: Diseases of the upper airway. In Ettinger SJ, editor: Textbook of veterinary internal medicine, Philadelphia, 1983, WB Saunders.
31. Lee KWT, Downes JJ: Pulmonary edema secondary to laryngospasm in children, Anesthesiology 59:349, 1983.
32. Kamal RS, Agha S: Acute pulmonary oedema: A complication of upper airway obstruction, Anesthesia 39:464, 1984.
33. Weissman C, Damask MC, Yang J: Noncardiogenic pulmonary edema following laryngeal obstruction, Anesthesiology 60:163, 1984.
34. Schwartz DR, Maroo A, Malhotra A et al: Negative pressure pulmonary hemorrhage, Chest 115:1194, 1999.
35. Mathieu-Costello O, Willford DC, Fu Z et al: Pulmonary capillaries are more resistant to stress failure in dogs than in rabbits, J Appl Physiol 79:908, 1995.
36. Burnie AG, Simpson JW, Corcoran BM: Gastro-esophageal reflux and hiatus hernia associated with laryngeal paralysis in a dog, J Small Anim Pract 30:414, 1989.
37. Greenfield CL: Canine laryngeal paralysis, Comp Contin Ed Pract Vet 9:1011, 1987.
38. Pardo AD: Laryngeal paralysis: Standards of diagnosis and treatment. In Proceedings of the 9th annual American College of Veterinary Surgeons' Symposium, San Francisco, 1999, p 197.
39. LaHue TR: Laryngeal paralysis, Sem Vet Med Surg Small Anim 10:94, 1995.
40. Burbidge HM, Goulden BE, Jones BR: Laryngeal paralysis in dogs: An evaluation of the bilateral arytenoid lateralization procedure, J Small Anim Pract 34:515, 1993.
41. Trout NJ, Harpster NK, Berg J et al: Long-term results of unilateral ventriculocordectomy and partial arytenoidectomy for the treatment of laryngeal paralysis in 60 dogs, J Am Anim Hosp Assoc 30:401, 1994.

42. Payne JT, Martin RA, Rigg DL: Abductor muscle prosthesis for correction of laryngeal paralysis in 10 dogs and one cat, *J Am Anim Hosp Assoc* 26:599, 1990.
43. Venker-van Haagen AJ, Engelse EJJ, van den Ingh ThSGAM: Congenital subglottic stenosis in a dog, *J Am Anim Hosp Assoc* 17:223, 1981.
44. Peterson J, Streeter V: Laryngeal obstruction secondary to brodifacoum toxicosis in a dog, *J Am Vet Med Assoc* 208:352, 1996.
45. MacMillan R, Withrow SJ, Gillette EL: Surgery and regional irradiation for treatment of canine tonsillar squamous cell carcinoma: Retrospective review of eight cases, *J Am Anim Hosp Assoc* 18:311, 1982.
46. Saik JE, Toll SL, Diters RW et al: Canine and feline laryngeal neoplasia: A 10-year survey, *J Am Anim Hosp Assoc* 22:359, 1986.
47. Ogilvie GK: Tumors of the endocrine system. In Withrow SJ, MacEwan EG, editors: *Small animal clinical oncology*, ed 2, Philadelphia, 1996, WB Saunders.
48. Lang J, Wortman JA, Glickman LT et al: Sensitivity of radiographic detection of lung metastasis in the dog, *Vet Radiol* 27:74, 1986.
49. Kealy KJ: *Diagnostic radiology of the dog and cat*, Philadelphia, 1987, WB Saunders.
50. Lee R: Radiographic examination of localized and diffuse tissue swellings in the mandibular and pharyngeal area, *Vet Clin N Am* 4:723, 1974.
51. Gaskell CJ: The radiographic anatomy of the pharynx and larynx of the dog, *J Small Anim Pract* 14:89, 1974.
52. West JB: *Pulmonary pathophysiology: The essentials*, ed 4, Baltimore, 1992, Williams & Wilkins.
53. Burbidge HM: A review of laryngeal paralysis in dogs, *Br Vet J* 151:71,1995.
54. Harvey CE, O'Brien JA: Treatment of laryngeal paralysis in dogs by partial laryngectomy, *J Am Anim Hosp Assoc* 18:551, 1982.
55. Bray JP, Lipscombe VJ, White RAS et al: Ultrasonographic examination of the pharynx and larynx of the normal dog, *Vet Radiol Ultrasound* 39:566, 1998.
56. LaHue TR: Treatment of laryngeal paralysis in dogs by unilateral cricoarytenoid laryngoplasty, *J Am Anim Hosp Assoc* 25:317, 1989.
57. Rosin E, Greenwood K: Bilateral arytenoid cartilage lateralization for laryngeal paralysis in the dog, *J Am Vet Med Assoc* 180:515, 1982.
58. Greenfield CL, Walshaw R, Kumar K et al: Neuromuscular pedicle graft for restoration of arytenoid abductor function in dogs with experimentally induced laryngeal hemiplegia, *Am J Vet Res* 49:1360, 1988.
59. Petersen SW, Rosin E, Bjorling DE: Surgical options for laryngeal paralysis in dogs: A consideration of partial laryngectomy, *Comp Contin Ed Pract Vet* 13:1531, 1991.
60. Harvey CE, O'Brien JA: Treatment of laryngeal paralysis in dogs by partial laryngectomy, *J Anim Hosp Assoc* 18:551, 1982.
61. Ross JT, Matthiesen DT, Noone K et al: Complications and long-term results after partial laryngectomy for the treatment of idiopathic laryngeal paralysis in 45 dogs, *Vet Surg* 20:169, 1991.
62. Gourley IM, Paul H, Gregory C: Castellated laryngofissure and vocal fold resection for treatment of laryngeal paralysis in the dog, *J Am Vet Med Assoc* 182:1084, 1983.
63. Smith MM, Gourley IM, Kurpershoek MS et al: Evaluation of a modified castellated laryngofissure for alleviation of upper airway obstruction in dogs with laryngeal paralysis, *J Am Vet Med Assoc* 188:1279, 1986.
64. Burbidge HM, Goulden BE, Jones BR: An experimental evaluation of castellated laryngofissure and bilateral arytenoid lateralization for the relief of laryngeal paralysis in dogs, *Aust Vet J* 68:268, 1991.
65. Lozier S, Pope E: Effects of arytenoid abduction and modified castellated laryngofissure on the rima glottidis in canine cadavers, *Vet Surg* 21:195, 1992.
66. Lussier B, Flanders JA, Erb HN: The effect of unilateral arytenoid lateralization on rima glottidis area in canine cadaver larynges, *Vet Surg* 25:121, 1996.
67. Holt DE, Brockman DJ: Diagnosis and management of laryngeal disease in the dog and cat, *Vet Clin N Am Small Anim* 24:855, 1994.
68. Brondbo K, Hall C, Teig E et al: Functional results after experimental reinnervation of the posterior cricoarytenoid muscle in dogs, *J Otolaryngol* 15:259, 1986.

CHAPTER 42

Nasopharyngeal Polyps

David E. Holt

Definition and Etiology

Nasopharyngeal polyps are non-neoplastic masses that arise in either the auditory tube or middle ear of cats, and grow into either the nasopharynx[1-11] or external ear canal (aural polyps)[12,13] or both.[3,13] Nasopharyngeal polyps may be unilateral or bilateral.[1,13] The majority of cases occur in young cats, indicating a possible congenital etiology. One report suggests that these polyps may arise from branchial arch remnants.[3] Viral infection was suggested as another possible etiology because feline calicivirus was isolated from 1 polyp in one report[8];

however, virus isolation was performed in 3 of 31 cats in another study and no growth was found.[1]

The role of otitis media in cats with nasopharyngeal polyps is not clear. The inflammation associated with otitis media in young cats might play a role in the genesis of the polyp. Conversely, there is convincing circumstantial evidence that the presence of a nasopharyngeal polyp leads to otitis media. The auditory tube normally acts as a drainage conduit for the middle ear.[14] Obstruction of the auditory tube and its nasopharyngeal opening causes negative pressure within the middle ear and a serous otitis media.[1]

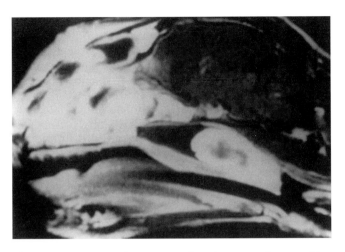

Figure 42-1. *Magnetic resonance imaging scan of a cat with a large nasopharyngeal polyp that obstructed the nasopharynx and caused nasal discharge and stertor.*

Pathophysiology and Pathogenesis

Nasopharyngeal polyps are an uncommon[1] but important differential diagnosis for young cats presenting with clinical signs of upper respiratory disease. Growth of the polyp into the nasopharynx obstructs the normal flow of air from the nose to the larynx. The physiologic drainage of respiratory secretions from the nasal passages to the nasopharynx is also disrupted if the mass becomes big enough (Figure 42-1). A serous rhinitis develops, which may be complicated by secondary bacterial infection resulting in the development of a mucopurulent rhinitis. The large mass in the nasopharynx makes swallowing uncomfortable for affected animals.

Concurrent otitis media can be sterile or associated with bacterial infection. In the largest reported study of feline nasopharyngeal polyps, cultures taken during bulla osteotomy in 23 cats were positive for bacteria in only 3 cats.[1] However, the otitis media is often severe and chronic enough to cause radiographically visible changes in the petrous temporal bone.* Extension of the polyp through the tympanic membrane into the external ear canal is associated with a ceruminous, purulent, and/or bloody otic discharge.[10,12]

Epidemiology and Risk Factors

The majority of cats with nasopharyngeal polyps are young. In the largest report (n = 31 cats), the mean age of affected cats was 13.6 months, with a range of 3 months to 8 years.[1] In another review, information on 73 cats with aural and/or nasopharyngeal polyps was summarized. Affected cats had a mean age of 3.8 years (median age 2.5 years) and an age range of 3 months to 15 years.[16] We should bear in mind that the diagnosis of this condition depends on both veterinary examination and

*References 1, 5, 6, 8, 10, and 15.

an awareness of the disease. Evaluation of nasopharyngeal polyp reports indicates that many of the affected animals had clinical signs for months to years before presentation,[1] potentially skewing the reported age of the affected cats away from very young animals.

There are no studies comparing the population of cats affected with nasopharyngeal polyps to the control population. Affected cat breeds include the domestic shorthair, Abyssinian, Persian, Himalayan, Siamese, Maine coon, and rex.[16] There is no apparent sex predilection.

To date, only one case of a nasopharyngeal polyp has been reported in a dog. The mass was removed from the nasopharynx of a 7-month-old female Chinese shar-pei via an incision in the soft palate.[17]

Historical Findings, Clinical Signs, and Progression

Historical findings are dependent on the direction of growth of the polyp. Cats with nasopharyngeal polyps may have a history that includes difficult, noisy respiration; nasal discharge; dysphagia; and poor weight gain or weight loss. Occasionally, severely affected animals are syncopal. Animals previously examined and treated for upper respiratory tract infections have often exhibited a poor long-term response to medication. Cats with polyps extending into the external ear canal have histories that include head shaking, ear scratching, head tilt, and, occasionally, dysequilibrium.

Clinical signs are often present for months before veterinary attention is sought.[1] Cats with nasopharyngeal polyps often have stertorous respiration and serous to purulent nasal discharge on physical examination.[1] Sneezing is uncommon.[2] Severely affected animals may have episodic dyspnea[7] and cyanosis.[6] Young kittens with poor appetites may be listless and have poor hair coats.[6] The clinical signs are often progressive as the polyp enlarges and causes greater interference with breathing and swallowing.

Differential Diagnosis

A nasopharyngeal polyp should be suspected in any cat that presents with upper respiratory signs. In young cats, these signs are also compatible with calicivirus and feline herpesvirus-1 infections.[18] In kittens and younger cats, congenital anomalies (e.g., choanal atresia or nasopharyngeal stenosis) are other possible diagnoses.[19,20] In cats with an acute onset of coughing and gagging, a nasopharyngeal grass foreign body should be considered.[21]

In older cats, neoplastic disease of the nasopharynx is a more likely diagnosis. In a retrospective study of nasopharyngeal disease in 53 cats, 26 (49%) had lymphosarcoma; 15 (28%) had nasopharyngeal polyps; and the remaining cats had other diseases including squamous cell carcinoma, adenocarcinoma, lymphoplasmacytic rhinitis/pharyngitis, rhabdomyosarcoma, spindle cell carcinoma, and melanoma.[11] The mean age of the cats with lymphosarcoma was 10.7 years (range 5 to 19 years) and the mean age of the cats with polyps was 3 years (range 4 months to 7 years). In cats with signs of aural disease, other causes of chronic otitis externa (including aural neoplasia[22]) should be considered.

Pathological and Histopathological Findings

Grossly, nasopharyngeal polyps are smooth, grey-pink masses visible dorsal to the soft palate. Their large size (up to 2.5 cm diameter, even in kittens) is often surprising in small cats. In the majority of cats, both compartments of the bony middle ear contain polyp, which is associated with a variable degree of thickening of the petrous temporal bone. In the external ear canal, polyps appear as smooth, red-to-pink masses in the horizontal canal.

Histologically, polyps are composed of well-vascularized, loose fibrous connective tissue.[4,12] They are covered by a thin layer of either ciliated columnar or stratified squamous epithelium with variable numbers of mucous glands and goblet cells.[1,4,12] In some areas, submucosal infiltration with lymphocytes and plasma cells is visible.

Management

DEFINITIVE DIAGNOSIS

Any young cat with signs of upper airway disease should be examined for a nasopharyngeal polyp. Rapid palpation of the hard and soft palate can be performed in most cats during a routine physical examination. As the index finger slides caudally along the hard palate, in normal cats the finger should be able to move dorsally at the junction of the hard and soft palate. A nasopharyngeal polyp displaces the soft palate, and hence the veterinarian's finger, ventrally.

In fractious animals, general anesthesia is recommended for oropharyngeal examination. Prior to anesthesia, a complete blood count and feline leukemia virus and feline immunodeficiency virus serology are obtained. A laryngoscope must be available to aid in visualizing the larynx because the polyp may significantly distort the normal pharyngeal anatomy. Premedication with atropine or glycopyrrolate is recommended because laryngeal and pharyngeal manipulation can result in vagal stimulation. Preoxygenation for 5 to 10 minutes is recommended before anesthetic induction. Anesthesia is rapidly induced, and a cuffed endotracheal tube is placed in the trachea and secured in place by tying it to the mandible. At least moderate anesthetic depth is required because oropharyngeal examination stimulates gagging in animals under light planes of anesthesia.

The hard and soft palates are palpated as previously described. Under general anesthesia, the paired, ventrally projecting hamular processes of the pterygoid bones should be easily palpable. They delineate the lateral borders of the cranial nasopharynx. Nasopharyngeal polyps are often palpated as a swelling displacing the soft palate ventrally in this area. The soft palate is retracted cranially with a small spay hook or stay suture placed through the caudal edge of the soft palate. The polyp(s) is visible as a smooth, grey-pink mass dorsal to the soft palate. Otoscopy is performed in all cats because polyps can extend into one or both horizontal ear canals.

Radiographs of the skull, with lateral, ventrodorsal, and open mouth views, are necessary for adequate evaluation of the bullae. Computerized tomography has also been described in cats with polyps.[15] The polyp is often visible as a mass in the pharynx. The affected bulla is thickened, with an increased fluid or soft tissue density in the lumen. Changes may be present bilaterally on radiographs. The more severely affected side is usually the site of the polyp's origin, but this is not always the case.[1] As previously mentioned, both middle ears can contain polyps. It is also important to remember that radiographic changes are not always present in animals with middle ear disease.[4,5,8,23,24]

POLYP REMOVAL AND BULLA OSTEOTOMY

The polyp(s) are removed from the pharynx by grasping either the stalk or the body of the polyp and applying gentle, increasing traction. The polyp should come away as a single large mass with a trailing stalk (Figure 42-2). Occasionally, small polyps cannot be adequately exposed without splitting the soft palate. The author prefers to partially incise the soft palate, leaving the caudal 5 mm of the palate intact. The incised edges are retracted laterally with stay sutures to facilitate exposure. After polyp removal, the palate is sutured with a single layer of single interrupted 5/0 PDS sutures. Polyps in the ear canal(s) are removed by grasping them with forceps and applying traction. Some surgeons prefer to do this after ventral bulla osteotomy when the polyp's attachment in the middle ear has been disrupted. In some cats a lateral wall resection may be necessary for adequate exposure to remove an aural polyp.[12]

Ventral bulla osteotomy[25,26] should be performed on the side from which the polyp originates, even if there

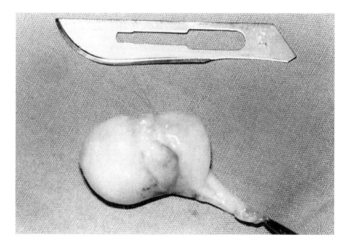

Figure 42-2. *Nasopharyngeal polyp and stalk. A No. 20 scalpel blade provides size comparison.*

are no radiographic changes indicating otitis media.[1] The surgery is performed with the cat in dorsal recumbency. Hair is shaved from the rostral mandible to the midcervical region. The bulla can often be palpated medial to the junction of the body and the vertical ramus of the mandible. A skin incision is made cranial to caudal between the midline and the mandible, centered at the junction of the body and the vertical ramus of the mandible. The platysma muscle is incised and the mandibular salivary gland identified. Dissection is continued medial to the salivary gland between the digastricus muscle laterally and the styloglossus and hyoglossus muscles medially. The hypoglossal nerve should be visible on the lateral boarder of the hyoglossus muscle. The lingual artery and the external carotid artery are visualized medial and lateral to the bulla, respectively. The vital structures are gently retracted with Senn retractors. The hyoid apparatus attaches to the skull caudally and lateral to the bulla; the stylohyoid bone can be gently palpated and used as a landmark for the bulla.

The bulla is penetrated with a Steinman pin held in a hand chuck. The opening is then enlarged with rongeurs. Samples for culture and sensitivity are taken immediately. The tympanic bulla of the cat is divided into larger ventromedial and smaller dorsolateral compartments by a transverse bony septum. The larger ventromedial compartment is invariably entered first. All polyp tissue is removed, avoiding the cochlear (round) window and the promontory on the dorsomedial aspect of the bulla where the sympathetic fibers run. The transverse septum is then removed, and the polyp is removed from the dorsolateral compartment. The middle ear is thoroughly flushed and a Penrose drain is placed in the middle ear cavity. The incision is closed using fine absorbable material in the muscles and subcutaneous tissue. The Penrose drain exits through a separate, small incision.

POSTOPERATIVE MANAGEMENT

The nasopharynx is thoroughly cleaned before anesthetic recovery to remove blood or mucus that may accumulate after polyp removal. Cats should be watched constantly after extubation because pharyngeal swelling and discharge from the auditory tube can compromise normal nasal breathing. During the anesthetic recovery, the mouth is opened and the tongue is gently pulled out of the mouth to encourage mouth breathing if upper airway obstruction is noted. Horner's syndrome (i.e., miosis, ptosis, and third eyelid prolapse) is very common postoperatively even if traction avulsion of the polyp is performed without bulla osteotomy,[16] but this will resolve in the vast majority of cases within 4 weeks.[1] Facial nerve paralysis is rare and is reported to resolve.[1] Otitis interna is another occasional complication, with signs of head tilt, nystagmus, and circling or rolling developing postoperatively. Otitis interna can largely be prevented by avoiding overzealous curettage in the dorsal bulla.[16]

Cats with purulent otitis media found at surgery are placed on antibiotics pending culture and sensitivity results. The Penrose drain should remain in place for 2 to 3 days; cats may require an Elizabethan collar to prevent scratching at the drain or suture line. Skin sutures are removed in 7 days.

Outcome and Prognosis

The prognosis for cats with nasopharyngeal polyps is good. Cats in which polyp removal by traction was combined with a ventral bulla ostotomy had very low rates of polyp recurrence.[1] Veterinarians should expect a 25% to 50% polyp recurrence rate if bulla osteotomy is not performed in conjunction with polyp removal. Regrowth can occur months to years after the initial removal.[12]

REFERENCES

1. Kapatkin AS, Matthiesen DT, Noone KE et al: Results of surgery and long-term follow-up in 31 cats with nasopharyngeal polyps, *J Am Anim Hosp Assoc* 26:387, 1990.
2. Bedford PGC, Coulson A, Sharp NJH et al: Nasopharyngeal polyps in the cat, *Vet Record* 109:551,1981.
3. Baker G: Nasopharyngeal polyps in cats (letter), *Vet Record* 111:43, 1982.
4. Lane JG, Orr CM, Lucke VM et al: Nasopharyngeal polyps arising in the middle ear of the cat, *J Small Anim Pract* 22:511, 1981.
5. Bradley RL, Noone KE, Saunders GK et al: Nasopharyngeal and middle ear polypoid masses in five cats, *Vet Surg* 14:141, 1985.
6. Stanton ME, Wheaton LG, Render JA et al: Pharyngeal polyps in two feline siblings, *J Am Vet Med Assoc* 186:1311, 1985.
7. Brownlie SE, Bedford PGC: Nasopharyngeal polyp in a kitten, *Vet Record* 117:25, 1985.
8. Parker NR, Binnington AG: Nasopharyngeal polyps in cats: Three case reports and a review of the literature, *J Am Anim Hosp Assoc* 21:473, 1985.
9. Whittaker CJG, Dill-Macky E, Hodgson DR: Nasopharyngeal polyp in a cat, *Aust Vet Practit* 24:8, 1994.
10. Trevor PB, Martin RA: Tympanic bulla osteotomy for treatment of middle-ear disease in cats: 19 cases (1984-1991), *J Am Vet Med Assoc* 202:123, 1993.
11. Allen HS, Broussard J, Noone K: Nasopharyngeal disease in cats: A retrospective study of 53 cases (1991-1998), *J Am Anim Hosp Assoc* 35:457, 1999.
12. Harvey CE, Goldschmidt MH: Inflammatory polypoid growths in the ear canal of cats, *J Small Anim Pract* 19:669, 1978.
13. Faulkner JE, Budsberg SC: Results of ventral bulla osteotomy for treatment of middle ear polyps in cats, *J Am Anim Hosp Assoc* 26:496, 1990.
14. Sade J, Meyer FA, King M et al: Clearance of middle ear effusions by the mucociliary system, *Acta Oto-Laryngologica* 79:277-282, 1975.
15. Seitz SE, Losonsky JM, Marretta SM: Computed tomographic appearance of inflammatory polyps in three cats, *Vet Radiol Ultrasound* 37:99, 1996.
16. Pope ER: Feline inflammatory polyps, *Sem Vet Med Surg Small Anim* 10:87, 1995.
17. Fingland RB, Gratzek A, Vorhies MW et al: Nasopharyngeal polyp in a dog, *J Am Anim Hosp Assoc* 29:311, 1993.
18. August JR: Feline viral diseases. In Ettinger SJ, editor: *Textbook of veterinary internal medicine*, ed 3, Philadelphia, 1989, WB Saunders.
19. Mitten RW: Nasopharyngeal stenosis in four cats, *J Small Anim Pract* 29:341, 1988.
20. Novo RE, Kramek B: Surgical repair of nasopharyngeal stenosis in a cat using a stent, *J Am Anim Hosp Assoc* 35:251, 1999.
21. Riley P: Nasopharyngeal grass foreign body in eight cats, *J Am Vet Med Assoc* 202:299, 1993.
22. Kirpensteijn J: Aural neoplasms, *Sem Vet Med Surg Small Anim* 8:17, 1993.

23. Remedios AM, Fowler JD, Pharr JW: A comparison of radiographic versus surgical diagnosis of otitis media, *J Am Anim Hosp Assoc* 27:183, 1991.
24. Love NE, Kramer RW, Spodnick GJ et al: Radiographic and computed tomographic evaluation of otitis media in the dog, *Vet Radiol Ultrasound* 36:375, 1995.
25. Ader PL, Boothe HW: Ventral bulla osteotomy in the cat, *J Am Anim Hosp Assoc* 15:757, 1979.
26. Boothe HW: Surgery of the tympanic bulla (otitis media and nasopharyngeal polyps), *Problems Vet Med* 3:254, 1991.

CHAPTER 43

Laryngeal Trauma

David E. Holt

Definition and Etiology

There are few original references in the veterinary literature dealing with laryngeal trauma,[1] and the majority of information available about its treatment is derived from humans.[2] This paucity of specific veterinary information emphasizes the rarity of laryngeal trauma in veterinary patients. Laryngeal trauma can be caused by choke chain injuries,[1] by bite wounds, and by penetrating missiles (e.g., arrows and bullets). Occasionally, pharyngeal penetration by stick foreign bodies can cause severe perilaryngeal inflammation.[3]

Pathophysiology and Pathogenesis

The larynx is a cartilaginous box suspended by the hyoid apparatus. Cranially, the thyroid cartilage forms the ventral and lateral sides of the box; more caudally, the cricoid cartilage completely encircles the laryngeal lumen and articulates with both the thyroid cartilage and the trachea. The cranial and dorsal part of the larynx is delineated by the paired arytenoid cartilages[4,5] (Figure 43-1). Trauma to the larynx is uncommon because of its anatomically protected location. Choke chain injuries variably crush and fracture the thyroid cartilage, the cricoid cartilages, or both. Bite wounds can produce similar crushing injuries and can also penetrate the ventrally located cricothyroid membrane. Stick foreign bodies tend to damage the cranially located arytenoid cartilages. Penetrating missiles cause varying degrees of laryngeal trauma depending on the missile size and velocity and its path through the neck.

Narrowing of the laryngeal lumen caused by crushing, cartilage fractures, hemorrhage, and swelling due to inflammation or edema results in increased resistance to airflow. Animals have respiratory obstruction and airway compromise of varying severity. Graded degrees of hypoxemia result from laryngeal paralysis of increasing severity in dogs;[6] presumably these results can be extrapolated to animals with laryngeal trauma. Dogs with severe laryngeal paralysis had arterial partial pressures of oxygen (Pao$_2$) of 51 ± 7 mm Hg while maintaining normal Paco$_2$ levels.[6] Blood in the laryngeal lumen secondary to trauma can be aspirated into the lungs, increasing the risk for subsequent pneumonia. Airway obstruction can also result in the development of noncardiogenic pulmonary edema, further exacerbating abnormal gas exchange.[7,8]

Historical Findings, Clinical Signs, and Progression

Affected animals present with a history of acute-onset dyspnea associated with upper airway stridor. The history may be specific for airway trauma if the owner witnessed the traumatic event.

Clinical signs include either predominantly inspiratory or inspiratory and expiratory dyspnea; increased respiratory effort; and, possibly, paradoxical respiration, depending on the severity of the obstruction. Auscultation may be difficult because of loud referred sounds from the upper airway. Rectal temperature may be elevated, either because of hyperthermia due to inability to adequately thermoregulate as a result of the airway obstruction, or because of fever due to infection or tissue necrosis following penetrating trauma. Animals can also present with a change in bark quality and with difficulty swallowing. Subcutaneous emphysema and crepitus can be present if bite wounds or a projectile penetrated the larynx. Signs may worsen as hematomas enlarge and as the laryngeal mucosa and perilaryngeal tissues swell. The larynx may collapse if trauma has disrupted the cartilaginous framework of the larynx enough that it cannot resist the negative luminal pressures generated by increased respiratory effort.

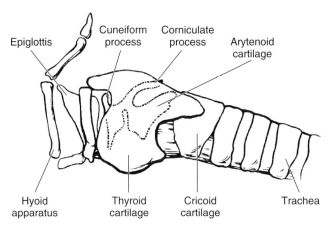

Figure 43-1. *Cartilages of the normal larynx.*

Labels: Epiglottis, Cuneiform process, Corniculate process, Arytenoid cartilage, Hyoid apparatus, Thyroid cartilage, Cricoid cartilage, Trachea

Severe upper airway obstruction can result in noncardiogenic pulmonary edema[7,8] or be associated with aspiration pneumonia; crackles in dorsal or ventral lung fields, respectively, in addition to the increased upper airway sounds expected as a result of the upper airway obstruction, may therefore be revealed by careful auscultation of the lungs.

Differential Diagnosis

Injury to the caudal pharynx, insect inhalation, allergic reaction, tracheal trauma, or foreign body obstruction of the airways are the other most likely differential diagnoses for acute-onset dyspnea associated with respiratory stridor. Animals with mild laryngeal paralysis can become acutely dyspneic in hot weather or when exercised. Acute laryngeal obstruction secondary to anticoagulant ingestion has also been described.[9] Subcutaneous emphysema that is most severe in the cervical area is usually caused by perforation of the larynx, esophagus or trachea, or severe cervical bite wounds. In the absence of subcutaneous emphysema, severe acute aspiration pneumonia, asthma, pneumothorax, diaphragmatic hernia, congestive heart failure, and other lower airway or lung parenchymal disorders should also be considered as differential diagnoses because not all animals with laryngeal trauma have obvious stridor.

A broad range of serious injuries can accompany missile perforation or bite wound injuries to the larynx. Fractures of the skull, intracranial injury, cervical fractures and spinal trauma, major vessel laceration, hypovolemic or septic shock, and bite wound injuries to other body areas should all be considered in these patients. In animals with severe multiple trauma, laryngeal crush injury is occasionally initially overlooked.

Management

STABILIZATION

Initial management depends on the degree of respiratory compromise and on the severity of concurrent injuries. A tracheostomy set and a variety of endotracheal tubes, including small diameter, noncuffed tubes, must be easily accessible. In animals in severe respiratory distress, an intravenous catheter is placed with minimal restraint. The animal is lightly anesthetized and the larynx rapidly inspected using a laryngoscope. Intubation is attempted with a small diameter, cuffed endotracheal tube. In animals with severe laryngeal deformity or fractures secondary to crushing injury, intubation is often possible with a small diameter, noncuffed tube or even a red rubber urinary catheter. A tracheostomy can then be performed with the airway secured. Rarely, an endotracheal tube cannot be passed and an emergency tracheostomy must be performed.

In less severely affected animals, oxygen supplementation provided by mask, oxygen cage, or tent may be beneficial prior to definitive management. Pulse oximetry or arterial blood gas analysis, if available and tolerated, can provide both a useful, objective measurement of hemoglobin saturation and an indication of the success of treatment. Stabilization should also include measurement of rectal temperature and aggressive efforts to cool the animal if the temperature is greater than 106° F. Because of the risk of disseminated intravascular coagulation, tests of coagulation may be appropriate in animals that have suffered severe hyperthermia. After appropriate samples have been obtained for bacterial culture and sensitivity testing, antibiotic therapy may be appropriate in animals with bacterial infection following penetrating trauma.

Concurrent injuries associated with the laryngeal trauma must be rapidly assessed and prioritized. Skull fractures and intracranial injury, cervical spinal injury, bite wounds penetrating the thorax, and major cervical vessel laceration and hemorrhage all constitute life-threatening problems. Initial emergency management should restore effective circulation, minimize intracranial pressure, and maintain effective ventilation and gas exchange. In animals with bite wounds to the neck and thorax this may involve intubation, assisted ventilation, thoracocentesis, and limited volume intravenous fluid resuscitation (i.e., incremental doses of 10 ml/kg of balanced electrolyte replacement solution) to minimize pulmonary capillary leakage and alveolar edema.

LARYNGOSCOPY

Once the animal is stabilized, the larynx, pharynx, and trachea can be further evaluated. Laryngeal evaluation in veterinary medicine has traditionally been performed with laryngoscopy and plain radiography. In cases with severe upper airway obstruction, laryngoscopy can be performed after a tracheostomy tube has been placed. The symmetry and function of the arytenoid cartilages are evaluated with the animal under light anesthesia. Evaluation of function is particularly important in animals with cervical bite wounds that might have damaged the recurrent laryngeal nerves. The clinician should also look for the presence of flaps of laryngeal mucosa that might indicate laryngeal disruption. The caudal pharynx is carefully examined for any evidence of foreign body penetration or hematomas that might indicate hyoid apparatus disruption. Esophagoscopy or a barium swallow (if tolerated) may be necessary to rule out pharyngeal or esophageal perforation.

RADIOGRAPHIC IMAGING

Plain radiographs of the larynx help evaluate the integrity of the hyoid apparatus. Computed tomographic evaluation of the larynx is routinely performed in human medicine when laryngeal or tracheal injury is suspected.[10] Computed tomographic scans are also used in humans to evaluate concurrent cervical spinal and vascular injuries.[11] Thoracic radiographs are made to evaluate animals for pulmonary edema secondary to upper airway obstruction[7,8] or for rib fractures, pulmonary contusions, and possible pneumothorax in animals with multiple bite wounds. However, lack of pneumothorax on thoracic radiographs does not rule out thoracic wall penetration by bite wounds. The author has seen several cases in which bites penetrated the thoracic wall but pneumothorax was not evident on radiographs.

SURGICAL MANAGEMENT

The indications for exploration of laryngeal injuries in veterinary patients have not been clearly established. Guidelines for exploration of laryngeal injury in humans include severe airway obstruction, subcutaneous emphysema, exposed cartilage in the laryngeal lumen, and laryngeal cartilage fractures.[12] The larynx is explored via a ventral midline cervical incision. In cases of laryngeal trauma secondary to bite wounds, the surrounding skin and subcutaneous fat and muscles are debrided back to healthy, bleeding tissue.[13] The laryngeal lumen is visualized via a midline ventral thyrotomy or through thyroid cartilage fractures.[2] Mucosal flaps are trimmed and mucosal edges are apposed with single interrupted sutures of 5/0 or 6/0 absorbable material. Mucosal apposition is vital to minimize the likelihood of granulation tissue formation, scar, and subsequent glottic stenosis. Laryngeal cartilage fractures must be reduced and immobilized to prevent stenosis. Recommendations for immobilization of cartilage fractures vary. Some references advocate predrilling cartilage fragments and using monofilament sutures for apposition.[2,12] A more recent study using a rabbit model advocates the use of miniplate fixation for thyroid cartilage fractures.[14] Intraluminal solid stents of silicone or rolled silastic sheet are used to hold the laryngeal mucosa apposed to the underlying cartilage.[2] The stent is held in place with sutures penetrating the lateral laryngeal walls and the stent. A tracheostomy tube must be maintained until the stent is removed. In animals with traumatic laryngeal paralysis but no mucosal damage or fracture of the laryngeal cartilages, unilateral cricoarytenoid lateralization is performed.

PERMANENT TRACHEOSTOMY

When bite wounds have irreparably crushed the larynx, a permanent tracheostomy can be made to salvage the airway. The midline incision over the larynx is continued

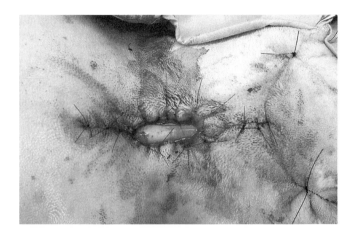

Figure 43-2. Postoperative permanent tracheostomy performed on a 6-year-old female spayed pug for laryngeal collapse. The cranial aspect is to the right of the picture, and the endotracheal tube is still visible in the trachea. The sutures lateral and cranial to the tracheostomy incision were placed to prevent excessive skin of the dog's jowls and neck from obstructing the tracheostomy.

caudally to expose the trachea to the level of the sixth or seventh tracheal ring. The midline sternohyoid muscles are separated, and approximately 3 cm of the trachea is dissected from its lateral attachments. The medial edges of the sternohyoid muscles are sutured together dorsal to this length of the trachea, elevating it toward the skin. The cartilage from the ventral third of three or four rings is removed, leaving the mucosa intact.[15] A piece of skin the size of the desired stoma is excised from the ventral cervical region. The skin and subcutaneous fat are trimmed and the skin is sutured to the peritracheal fascia lateral to the stoma, and to the annular ligaments proximal and distal to the stoma. The tracheal mucosa is then incised and sutured to the skin edges with simple interrupted sutures using 4/0 absorbable monofilament material. Precise apposition of the skin to the mucosa is important to minimize granulation tissue formation and stoma stenosis[15] (Figure 43-2).

Postoperatively, animals (especially cats) with permanent tracheostomies should be carefully monitored for respiratory distress or for sudden death due to acute airway obstruction with mucus. Tracheal mucus will be deposited at the stoma by the mucociliary apparatus and must be carefully removed to prevent stoma obstruction. Adequate hydration and nebulization at the stoma site prevents the mucus from becoming thick and tenacious. Applying ointments to the stoma site aids in removing accumulated mucus.

Outcome and Prognosis

No objective data exist on the outcome of laryngeal trauma in a large number of animals. Presumably the prognosis is dependent on the severity of the injury, appropriate emergency management, timing and skill of surgical intervention, and adept postoperative management.

REFERENCES

1. Manus AG: Canine epihyoid fractures, *J Am Vet Med Assoc* 147: 129, 1965.
2. Nelson AW: Upper respiratory system. In Slatter DH, editor: *Textbook of small animal surgery*, ed 2, Philadelphia, 1992, WB Saunders.
3. Lane JG: Canine laryngeal surgery, *Vet Ann* 183:239, 1978.
4. Evans HE, Christensen GC: The respiratory apparatus. In Evans HE, editor: *Miller's anatomy of the dog*, ed 2. Philadelphia, 1979, WB Saunders.
5. Grandage J, Richardson K: Functional anatomy. In Slatter DH, editor: *Textbook of small animal surgery*, ed 2, Philadelphia, 1992, WB Saunders.
6. Love S, Waterman AE, Lane JG: The assessment of corrective surgery for canine laryngeal paralysis by blood gas analysis: A review of 35 cases, *J Small Anim Pract* 28:597, 1987.
7. Kerr L: Pulmonary edema secondary to upper airway obstruction in dogs: A review of nine cases, *J Am Anim Hosp Assoc* 25:207, 1989.
8. Lang SA, Duncan PG, Shephard DAE et al: Pulmonary edema associated with upper airway obstruction, *Can J Anesth* 37:210, 1990.
9. Peterson J, Streeter V: Laryngeal obstruction secondary to brodifacoum toxicosis in a dog, *J Am Vet Med Assoc* 208:352, 1996.
10. Lupetin AR: Computed tomographic evaluation of laryngotracheal trauma, *Curr Prob Diag Radiol* 26:185, 1997.
11. LeBlang SD, Nunez DB Jr.: Helical CT of cervical spine and soft tissue injuries of the neck, *Radiology Clinics N Am* 37:515, 1999.
12. Brandenburg JH: Management of acute blunt laryngeal injuries, *Otolaryngol Clin North Am* 12:741, 1979.
13. Holt DE, Griffin G: Bite wounds in dogs and cats, *Vet Clin North Am Small Anim Pract* 30:669, 2000.
14. Dray TG, Coltrera MD, Pinczower EF: Thyroid cartilage fracture repair in rabbits: Comparing healing with wire and miniplate fixation, *Laryngoscope* 109:118, 1999.
15. Hedlund CS, Tangner CH, Montgomery DL et al: A procedure for permanent tracheostomy and its effects on the tracheal mucosa, *Vet Surg* 11:13, 1982.

CHAPTER 44

Laryngitis

Merilee Costello

Laryngitis in dogs and cats is a common clinical syndrome that often has an excellent prognosis. Laryngitis is characterized by inflammation; irritation; and, possibly, swelling and edema of the laryngeal tissue, which may be associated with generalized inflammation of the upper respiratory tract mucosa.[1] It may be acute or chronic, and the etiology is often multifactorial and varies between species. The clinical signs also vary between species and depend on the etiology, chronicity, and severity of the inflammation. In dogs, the most common cause is infectious tracheobronchitis, whereas viral diseases (e.g., rhinotracheitis or calicivirus) are causes of feline laryngitis.[1-3] The treatment for laryngitis varies depending on the etiology, duration of clinical signs, and severity of illness. The response to treatment is generally good, but rare, life-threatening complications can occur. In these cases, surgical intervention may be necessary.

Clinical Signs

The clinical presentation of laryngitis varies markedly between species. The clinical signs also vary with the duration of illness and the severity of laryngeal inflammation. In dogs, laryngitis is often mild and self-limiting, and the most common presenting complaint is a dry, hacking cough. The owners may also notice a change in voice,

gagging, stridor, or nasal discharge. Fever and dyspnea are rare in dogs, and there are rarely other signs of systemic illness. In contrast, feline laryngitis is often accompanied by fever, anorexia, dehydration, ptyalism, and lethargy. It is not uncommon for cats to present with dyspnea, and stridor or a change in voice may occur. Other clinical signs may include gingivitis, lingual ulceration, gagging, or retching.[2] Cats may occasionally have a history of coughing, although this is much less common than in dogs. As the disease progresses, secondary swelling, edema, and continued inflammation may lead to upper airway obstruction and increased dyspnea and respiratory distress. Pulmonary complications (e.g., pneumonia or noncardiogenic pulmonary edema secondary to upper airway obstruction) may also result in a more severe clinical presentation and a more critical patient.

Physical Examination

In dogs, physical examination often reveals an easily induced, dry, hacking cough, which may be more pronounced during periods of excitement. Dogs can also have episodes of paroxysmal coughing, which may lead to gagging or retching. Stridor is often noted and there may be a nasal discharge. These patients are generally in good health and rarely have evidence of other systemic disease. Fever is rare and, if present, may indicate secondary pneumonia, especially if accompanied by harsh lung sounds or crackles. Occasionally, dogs may present as cyanotic or severely dyspneic if there is concurrent pulmonary pathology or upper airway obstruction due to chronic inflammation or edema.

In contrast, cats often present with clinical signs of systemic illness. Physical examination findings may include stridor, fever, ptyalism, and dehydration. Dyspnea and open-mouthed breathing are not uncommon clinical findings in these cats, and gingivitis or oral ulceration may be seen if the laryngitis is associated with viral disease. As in dogs, crackles or increased bronchovesicular sounds may be heard if there is associated pulmonary pathology, and acute upper airway obstruction can occur secondary to edema or severe inflammation.

Etiology

The diversity of clinical findings associated with laryngitis suggests that multiple etiologies exist. In dogs, the most common clinical syndrome associated with laryngitis is infectious tracheobronchitis, or kennel cough, caused by a collection of viruses, bacteria, and *Mycoplasma* spp. *Bordetella bronchiseptica* is thought to be one of the primary pathogens. *Bordetella* is often associated with respiratory disease, and its predilection for ciliated airway epithelium results in a common association with laryngitis, tracheitis, and pneumonia. The bacterium is spread by aerosolization and direct contact, and does not usually survive for long periods outside of the animal. In areas of heavy contamination the bacteria may survive for extended periods on inert substances. Infectious tracheobronchitis has been diagnosed in animals of all ages, but young or debilitated animals are more susceptible and may have more severe manifestations such as pneumonia.[4]

Voice abuse is another common cause of laryngitis in dogs. Chronic irritation of the laryngeal tissue due to barking (e.g., during boarding) can lead to inflammation and loss of voice. Laryngitis also occurs secondary to intubation, inhalation of caustic gases, laryngeal abscess, trauma, foreign bodies, or insect bites in both dogs and cats. Although much less common than other causes of laryngitis, these etiologies can often be diagnosed based on history and physical examination. Finally, mild laryngitis can develop in both dogs and cats secondary to a primary respiratory disease process that results in coughing. Prolonged periods of coughing or gagging can result in mild laryngitis due to chronic physical irritation.

In cats, laryngitis is most often associated with generalized inflammation of the upper respiratory tract. The most common etiologic agents are viral, and include feline herpesvirus-I (rhinotracheitis) and calicivirus. Laryngitis in these cats is often associated with other clinical signs such as fever, nasal or ocular discharge, coughing or sneezing, anorexia, ptyalism, dehydration, and weight loss. Physical examination in these cats may also reveal oral or lingual ulceration.

Granulomatous or inflammatory laryngitis leading to upper airway obstruction has been reported in both dogs and cats.[5-8] The etiology of the inflammation and subsequent upper airway obstruction is unknown, although granulomas can develop in dogs secondary to laryngeal surgery such as vocal fold resection. It is important to note that the diagnosis of granulomatous or inflammatory laryngitis must be made on histopathology, because gross examination does not allow distinction between inflammation and neoplasia. In one report of inflammatory laryngeal disease in cats, eosinophilic granuloma complex was thought to be a possible underlying etiology leading to the formation of a laryngeal inflammatory mass.[8] In humans, the most common causes of laryngeal granulomas include intubation, chronic vocal fold abuse, and gastroesophageal reflux.[9]

Diagnostics

The diagnosis of laryngitis is often made based on history and a thorough physical examination. In cases where there is evidence of upper airway obstruction, sedation for a laryngeal examination is indicated (Figure 44-1). Whenever a patient with a potential upper airway obstruction is sedated or anesthetized, preparations should be made for a temporary tracheostomy, if needed. The laryngeal examination should include an evaluation of laryngeal function as well as observation of the gross characteristics of the vocal folds and laryngeal mucosa. If abnormal areas of the larynx or a mass lesion are identified, biopsy and histopathology should be performed for a definitive diagnosis. Chest radiographs may be performed to evaluate for any evidence of pneumonia or noncardiogenic pulmonary edema. If there is a suspicion of pneumonia, a transtracheal or endotracheal wash should be performed. Fluid from an endotracheal or transtracheal wash should be cytologically evaluated and submitted for microbiologic culture and sensitivity.

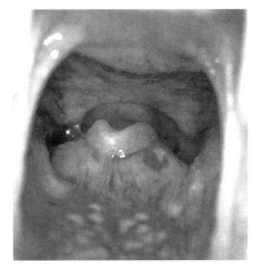

Figure 44-1. *Direct visualization of the laryngeal area in a cat with inflammatory laryngeal disease.*

Differential Diagnosis

There are many important differential diagnoses for patients who present with the generalized signs that often accompany laryngitis. In dogs, a cough may be due to primary airway, pulmonary, or cardiac disease. Pneumonia or chronic bronchitis can lead to laryngitis from chronic coughing and associated inflammation. Primary cardiac disease often leads to coughing, either by direct compression on the mainstem bronchus, or due to pulmonary edema. Thoracic radiographs are important to evaluate the pulmonary parenchyma, cardiac silhouette, and pulmonary vessels. Functional laryngeal or pharyngeal disease (e.g., laryngeal paralysis, elongated soft palate, or everted laryngeal saccules) can be evaluated under light anesthesia and laryngoscopy. Surgery is the treatment of choice in these cases. In cats, primary airway or pulmonary diseases such as asthma or pneumonia can also lead to coughing and associated laryngeal inflammation.

In patients with upper airway obstruction due to a mass lesion, the most common differential diagnosis is neoplasia. Inhaled foreign bodies leading to a granuloma or abscess should also be considered. The diagnosis of neoplasia must be made based on histopathology because neoplasia, inflammatory lesions, and granulomas are indistinguishable on gross examination.

Histopathology

There are multiple reports in the veterinary literature of severe inflammation of the larynx leading to a laryngeal mass effect. Biopsy and histopathology are imperative in these cases because the gross appearance of the lesions is indistinguishable from neoplasia. The histopathology of these lesions is variable and may show marked infiltration of the laryngeal tissue with inflammatory cells, including neutrophils, lymphocytes, plasma cells, macrophages, and mast cells (Figures 44-2 and 44-3). Histopathology may also reveal granulomatous laryngitis or a laryngeal granuloma.

Treatment and Prevention

The treatment of laryngitis varies based on the underlying etiology, as well as with the severity of the inflammation and the subsequent patient compromise. In dogs with *Bordetella* or laryngitis secondary to voice abuse or intubation, the disease is often self-limiting and resolves with time. Medical management in these cases may consist of voice rest or antitussives to reduce the amount of continued inflammation secondary to coughing. In cases of voice abuse, corticosteroids at an antiinflammatory dose may be helpful, but should be avoided if there is any indication of an infectious process. It is important to note that antitussives and corticosteroids are contraindicated in any animal with pneumonia. Antibiotics may be indicated if there is an associated fever, persistent cough (longer than 14 days), or radiographic evidence of pneumonia. The choice of antibiotic should ideally be based on microbiologic culture and sensitivity.

If laryngitis occurs secondary to an insect bite, antiinflammatory doses of corticosteroids during the acute phase are the treatment of choice in controlling the subsequent inflammation and edema, which if left untreated can lead to upper airway obstruction and death. Treatment of laryngitis due to inhalation of caustic gases is often aimed primarily at supportive care, maintenance of a patent airway, and management of injury to the tracheobronchial tree and lungs.

In cats, treatment of laryngitis is primarily supportive and includes intravenous fluids, nutritional support, and

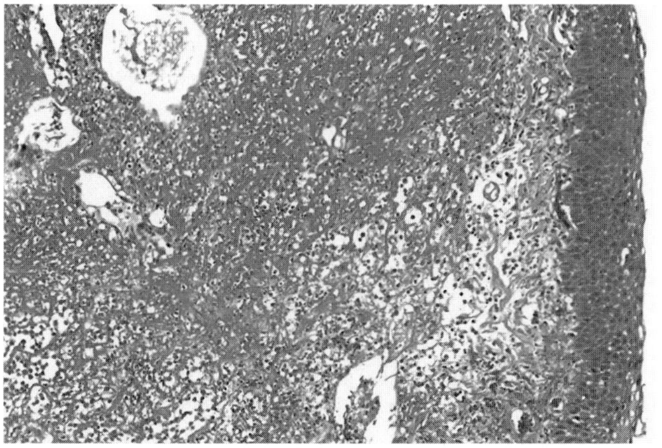

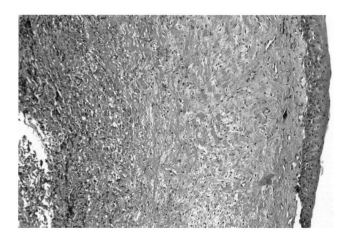

Figure 44-2. High magnification of the histopathology of a cat with acute inflammatory laryngitis. The stratified squamous epithelium is to the far right of the picture, followed by a layer of fibrin, and beneath that is the layer of inflammatory cells, consisting primarily of neutrophils and lymphocytes. (Courtesy of Dr. Mattie Hendrick, Department of Pathobiology, School of Veterinary Medicine, University of Pennsylvania.)

Figure 44-3. High magnification of the histopathology of a cat with chronic inflammatory laryngitis. The stratified squamous epithelium is to the far right of the picture, followed by a layer of fibrous connective tissue. Beneath that is the layer of inflammatory cells, consisting of a mixed population of cells. (Courtesy of Dr. Mattie Hendrick, Department of Pathobiology, School of Veterinary Medicine, University of Pennsylvania.)

symptomatic care. Antiviral drugs and immunostimulants may be considered in severely affected cats. Intravenous broad-spectrum antibiotics are indicated to help control secondary bacterial infections. Nutritional support should be instituted in cats that are anorexic or those in which oral lesions or laryngitis make it painful to eat. Nutritional support can be provided using a nasoesophageal or nasogastric tube, esophagostomy tube, or a gastrotomy tube.

In patients with upper airway obstruction due to severe inflammation, edema, or a laryngeal mass, a temporary tracheostomy may be required. A temporary tracheostomy should be performed early if indicated because prolonged breathing against an upper airway obstruction can lead to respiratory muscle fatigue and secondary noncardiogenic pulmonary edema.

In cases of severe inflammatory or granulomatous laryngitis, a temporary tracheostomy is often needed to provide a patent airway during diagnostics and initial treatment. The response of this condition to treatment is variable. A good long-term prognosis has been given for combined medical and surgical treatment in previous reports.[5,6,8] In two reports of this condition in cats, the response to corticosteroids and antibiotics was variable, but an excellent response was reported in some of the cases.[6,8]

If a temporary or permanent tracheostomy is required, it is imperative that the animal be monitored closely in the hospital. One study of inflammatory laryngitis in cats reported that post-mortem examination of a cat that had undergone a permanent tracheostomy revealed occlusion of the tracheostomy site by exudates.[8] In another report, a cat died acutely 15 weeks after a permanent tracheostomy, presumably due to acute upper airway obstruction, but a post-mortem examination was not permitted.[6] In a retrospective study of 34 cases of dogs and cats with permanent tracheostomy, few complications were reported; however, some authors suggest that because cats are more prone to develop thick airway secretions, they may be at increased risk for occlusion of the tracheostomy site by exudates.[10] While permanent tracheostomy may be necessary in some cases, owners should be advised of the associated risks; and care should be taken to monitor the stoma site carefully during the postoperative period.

Management of laryngitis should also be aimed at prevention and early treatment of the underlying etiology. Vaccinations are available for feline rhinotracheitis and calicivirus, as well as canine *Bordetella*. When intubating animals, care should be taken to minimize the laryngeal irritation associated with this procedure. Early identification and treatment of laryngitis can help prevent progression of the disease and also decrease the severity of the clinical presentation.

Complications

Complications associated with laryngitis are rare, but can be life threatening. Severe inflammation and edema can lead to upper airway obstruction and noncardiogenic pulmonary edema. Pneumonia can develop due to *Bordetella*, other viral organisms (e.g., calicivirus or rhinotracheitis), aspiration of gastrointestinal tract contents, or secondary bacterial pneumonia due to impaired respiratory defenses. Although rare, these complications can require aggressive medical or surgical intervention.

REFERENCES

1. Holt D, Brockman D: Diagnosis and management of laryngeal disease in the dog and cat, *Vet Clin North Am Small Anim Pract* 24:855-871, 1994.
2. Venker-Van Haagen A: Diseases of the larynx, *Vet Clin North Am Small Anim Pract* 22:1155-1172, 1992.
3. Willoughby K, Coutis A: Differential diagnosis of throat and ear disease in cats, *In Practice* 17:206-214, 1995.
4. Bemis D: *Bordetella* and *Mycoplasma* respiratory infections in dogs and cats, *Vet Clin North Am Small Anim Pract* 22:1173-1186, 1992.
5. Oakes M, McCarthy R: What is your diagnosis? (Granulomatous laryngitis), *J Am Vet Med Assoc* 204:1891-1892, 1994.
6. Tasker S, Foster D, Corcoran B et al: Obstructive inflammatory laryngeal disease in three cats, *J Feline Med Surg* 1:53-59, 1999.
7. Harvey C, O'Brien J: Upper airway obstruction surgery, *J Am Anim Hosp Assoc* 18:535-569, 1982.
8. Costello MF, Keith D, Hendrick M et al: Acute upper airway obstruction due to inflammatory laryngeal disease in 5 cats, *J Vet Emerg Crit Care* 11:205-210, 2001.
9. Emami AJ, Morrison M, Rammage L et al: Treatment of laryngeal contact ulcers and granulomas: A 12-year retrospective analysis, *J Voice* 13(4):612-617, 1999.
10. Hedlund C, Tangner C, Waldron D et al: Permanent tracheostomy: Perioperative and long-term data from 34 cases, *J Am Anim Hosp Assoc* 24:585-591, 1988.

CHAPTER 45

Tumors of the Larynx and Trachea

Craig A. Clifford • Karin U. Sorenmo

Primary tumors of the larynx and trachea in dogs and cats are rare; there is a paucity of information in the literature regarding incidence, tumor type, clinical signs, diagnosis, treatment, and survival. In an effort to provide further insight into these malignancies, the authors have reviewed cases with tumors of the larynx and trachea treated at the Veterinary Hospital of the University of Pennsylvania (VHUP) from 1990-2000. Diagnosis was made on the basis of cytology alone (n = 2), histopathology alone (n = 23), or both (n = 5). This retrospective study identified 30 cases of either laryngeal (n = 20) or tracheal (n = 10) tumors in dogs and cats. Data from this study will be used in addition to existing information from the literature in the following review.

The limited occurrence of tumors in the larynx and trachea of dogs and cats is in contrast to human oncology, where they represent over 3% of all tumors.[1-3] In humans, epidemiologic data suggest that the etiology and pathogenesis of laryngeal and tracheal carcinomas are influenced by environmental and lifestyle related factors (e.g., tobacco use, alcohol consumption, and exposure to toxic substances).[1-3] In addition, dietary factors, irradiation, papilloma virus infection, and laryngopharyngeal reflux seem to be significant carcinogenic cofactors.[1-3] In veterinary medicine, no such factors have been identified, with the exception of feline lymphosarcoma, which has been associated with feline leukemia virus infection.[4]

Tumor Types

A variety of both benign and malignant laryngeal tumors have been reported in dogs, with the majority of tumors being malignant.[5,6] Benign osteocartilagenous tumors occur in young animals with active osteochondral ossification centers.[7,8] Other benign canine laryngeal tumors include rhabdomyoma, chondroma, myxochondroma, fibropapilloma, leiomyoma, lipoma, and oncocytoma.[5,6,8-20] Reported malignant tumors include lymphosarcoma, plasma cell tumor, mast cell tumor, malignant melanoma, rhabdomyosarcoma, chondrosarcoma, granular cell myoblastoma, adenocarcinoma, un-

differentiated carcinoma, and squamous cell carcinoma (SCC).* In cats, lymphosarcoma (LSA) predominates, followed by SCC, adenocarcinoma, and undifferentiated carcinoma.[5,12,32,33]

Benign tracheal tumors in both dogs and cats include osteochondroma, oncocytoma, leiomyoma, ecchondroma, and chondroma.† The most common malignant tracheal tumors in both dogs and cats are LSA and SCC, followed by osteosarcoma, chondrosarcoma, mast cell tumor, and adenocarcinoma.[4,5,41-50] Tumor types identified in the retrospective survey of laryngeal and tracheal tumors at VHUP were similar to those noted in the literature, with the exception of a seromucinous gland tumor in the trachea of a cat, which has not been previously reported (Tables 45-1 and 45-2).

Signalment, History, and Clinical Signs

Tracheal and laryngeal tumors have been reported in various pure breeds as well as mixed breeds, and there does not appear to be any specific breed predilection.[5,6,8,12] Most animals with laryngeal and tracheal tumors are middle age to older.[5,6,12] In our evaluation of 20 laryngeal tumors (see Tables 45-1 and 45-2) the median age in dogs was 7 years (range 4 to 12 years) and the median age in cats was 11 years (range 3 to 16 years). The median age for both dogs and cats with tracheal tumors was 10 years (with ranges of 5 to 14 years and 7 to 15 years, respectively). This age distribution is similar to that seen in the literature, with the exception of benign laryngeal rhabdomyomas, which occur more often in younger dogs.[5,6]

Clinical signs associated with laryngeal and tracheal tumors are insidious in nature and include progressive exercise intolerance, dysphonia, stridor, stertor, dysphagia, coughing, halitosis, hemoptysis, oral hemorrhage, and pytalism.[5,6,8,17,31] A history of progressive worsening of clinical signs over days to months is commonly

---

*References 5, 6, 8, 10, 17, and 21-31.
†References 4, 5, 12, 20, and 34-40.

TABLE 45-1. Tumor Type, Signalment, Clinical Signs, Treatment, and Outcome in 20 Dogs and Cats with Laryngeal Tumors at VHUP

Species	Breed	Age (Years)	Sex	Tumor Type	Clinical Signs	Treatment	Outcome
Canine	Border terrier	6	FS	Rhabdomyoma	Dyspnea	None	Euthanized, not treated
Canine	Mix breed	12	MC	Rhabdomyoma	Coughing, gagging, choking, dyspnea	Excised	Still alive
Canine	Labrador retriever	4	MC	Rhabdomyoma	Stridor, dyspnea	Excised	Still alive
Canine	Bulldog	5	M	Round cell tumor	Wheezing, dyspnea	None	Euthanized, not treated
Canine	Golden retriever	10	FS	Thyroid carcinoma	Dyspnea	None	Euthanized, not treated
Canine	American pit bull terrier	10	FS	LSA	Gagging, coughing, dyspnea	None	Euthanized, not treated
Canine	Cocker spaniel	7	FS	SCC	Voice change, coughing, stridor	Piroxicam	Lost to follow-up
Canine	Springer spaniel	7	FS	SCC	Voice change, vomiting	Excised	Lost to follow-up
Feline	Domestic shorthair	16	MC	SCC	Stridor, increased RR/RE	Excised	Lost to follow-up
Feline	Domestic shorthair	16	FS	SCC	Dyspnea	None	Euthanized, not treated
Feline	Domestic shorthair	10	FS	SCC	Stridor, wheezing	None	Euthanized, not treated
Feline	Domestic shorthair	8	MC	LSA	Progressive dyspnea	Partial excision	Euthanized at surgery
Feline	Domestic shorthair	8	FS	LSA	Stridor, dyspnea	Partial excision, chemotherapy	Euthanized at 4 months
Feline	Domestic longhair	11	FS	LSA	Stridor, dyspnea	Chemotherapy, radiation	Lost to follow-up (last recheck at 6 months)
Feline	Domestic shorthair	14	FS	LSA	Stridor, increased RR/RE	None	Euthanized at 3 months
Feline	Siamese	15	FS	Adenocarcinoma	Voice loss, stridor	Partial excision, Prednisolone	Euthanized at 2 months
Feline	Domestic shorthair	14	FS	Adenocarcinoma	Increased RR/RE	None	Euthanized, not treated
Feline	Domestic shorthair	3	FS	Carcinoma	Dyspnea	None	Euthanized, not treated
Feline	Abyssinian	8	FS	Carcinoma	Snorting, dyspnea	None	Lost to follow-up
Feline	Domestic shorthair	8	MC	Undifferentiated sarcoma	Dyspnea	None	Euthanized, not treated

FS = Female spayed; MC = male castrated; M = male intact; LSA = lymphosarcoma; SCC = squamous cell carcinoma; RR/RE = respiratory rate/respiratory effort.

TABLE 45-2. Tumor Type, Signalment, Clinical Signs, Treatment and Outcome in 10 Dogs and Cats with Tracheal Tumors at VHUP

Species	Breed	Age (Years)	Sex	Tumor Type	Clinical Signs	Treatment	Response to Therapy
Canine	Labrador retriever	11	MC	Chondrosarcoma	Upper respiratory sounds	Excision	Still alive
Canine	Shih Tzu	14	FS	SCC	Coughing, dyspnea	Partial excision	Lost to follow-up
Canine	Beagle	10	M	Carcinoma	Increased RR/RE	Excision	Lost to follow-up
Canine	Rottweiler	5 months	F	Rhadomyosarcoma	Stridor	Excision	Still alive
Feline	Domestic shorthair	10	MC	LSA	Dyspnea	Excision, chemotherapy	Still alive
Feline	Domestic shorthair	7	MC	SCC	Wheezes	None	Euthanized, not treated
Feline	Domestic shorthair	9	FS	SCC	Coughing, dyspnea	None	Lost to follow-up
Feline	Domestic shorthair	15	MC	Carcinoma	Stridor	None	Euthanized, not treated
Feline	Domestic shorthair	15	FS	Seromucinous gland tumor	Wheezing	None	Euthanized, not treated
Feline	Domestic shorthair	9	MC	LSA	Stridor, wheezing, dyspnea	Excision, chemotherapy, radiation	Lost to follow-up

FS = Female spayed; MC = male castrated; M = male intact; F = female intact; LSA = lymphosarcoma; SCC = squamous cell carcinoma; RR/RE = respiratory rate/respiratory effort.

reported.* Some animals may present with signs of acute upper airway obstruction (e.g., severe dyspnea, tachycardia, and cyanosis).† Tumors of the larynx and trachea may also be noted as an incidental finding in stable patients during physical examination or intubation for routine general anesthesia.[5,6,8,10,12] Presenting clinical signs for dogs and cats with laryngeal and tracheal tumors at VHUP (see Tables 45-1 and 45-2) included dyspnea (n = 17), stridor (n = 9), coughing/gagging (n = 5), wheezing (n = 5), and voice change (n = 3).

Diagnosis

In patients with laryngeal and tracheal tumors, physical examination findings vary depending on the size and location of the primary tumor.‡ Auscultation of the cervical region may reveal stridor associated with a partial airway obstruction. Tachypnea, dyspnea, and crackles (presumably due to noncardiogenic pulmonary edema or aspiration pneumonia) may be present in animals with acute upper respiratory obstruction related to a tracheal or laryngeal tumor.§ Palpation of the larynx and proximal trachea may reveal a discrete palpable mass, asymmetry, or diffuse swelling due to inflammation.[19]

Plain survey radiographs may aid initial evaluation and diagnosis by providing information regarding the size and extent of both tracheal and laryngeal tumors.[5,6,12] Small tumors may appear as simple minor variations in the shape of normal structures, whereas larger tumors may compress associated structures.[5] Laryngeal tumors generally appear as a distinct, lobulated, soft tissue density (Figure 45-1). In cats with laryngeal LSA, a diffuse thickening of the larynx rather than a distinct mass may be found on

radiographs, whereas adenocarcinoma of the larynx may appear as an annular narrowing of the larynx.[5,12] If indicated, orally administered barium may provide additional information by delineating the esophagus.

Tracheal tumors are best visualized on a lateral cervical radiograph, and often appear as a distinct mass originating from the tracheal wall, extending into the lumen (Figure 45-2, A).[5,12] Other radiographic findings include mineralization of tumors of osteocartilagenous origin and annular narrowing of the trachea in tumors of epithelial origin.[5,12,46] Thoracic radiographs are also necessary for staging purposes in cases with malignant tumors, as well as to identify possible lung diseases (e.g., aspiration pneumonia and noncardiogenic pulmonary edema) that may be sequelae of partial airway obstruction.[12]

In our retrospective study, cervical radiographs were obtained in 20/30 cases (7 tracheal, 13 laryngeal). Of these, radiographs revealed a mass in nine cases (4 tracheal, 5 laryngeal). Two of the nine animals had mineralized laryngeal masses, both of which were diagnosed with carcinoma. None of the patients with thoracic radiographs (n = 20) had pulmonary metastatic disease at the time of diagnosis.

Ultrasonography has been used in human and veterinary medicine to investigate laryngeal function, and pro-

---

*References 5, 6, 8, 10, 12, and 17.
†References 5, 6, 8, 10, 12, 17, and 51.
‡References 5, 6, 8, 10, 12, and 17.
§References 5, 6, 8, 10, 12, 17, and 51.

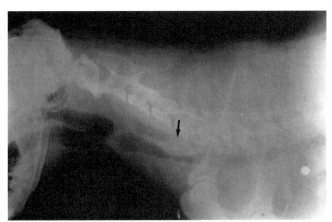

A

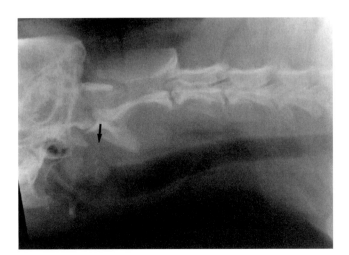

Figure 45-1. *Lateral cervical radiograph delineating a laryngeal rhabdomyosarcoma* (arrow) *in a mixed-breed dog.*

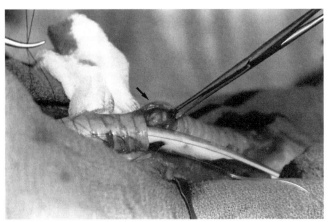

B

Figure 45-2. A, *Lateral radiograph of a tracheal chondrosarcoma* (arrow) *in a Labrador retriever.* **B,** *Surgical exploration revealing the tracheal chondrosarcoma* (arrow) *in the Labrador retriever.*

vides another noninvasive technique for identifying and diagnosing laryngeal tumors.[52,53] One study evaluated the usefulness of ultrasonography for diagnosis of laryngeal masses in 6 cats and 1 dog.[53] All seven animals had a narrowed laryngeal lumen, with either unilateral displacement of the laryngeal gas shadow or complete distortion of the normal laryngeal anatomy. Lymphosarcoma appeared as a well circumscribed, homogeneously hypoechoic mass in 3 of 4 cats. One dog and one cat had laryngeal squamous cell carcinoma, and in both cases the tumor appeared as a mixed echogenic mass. No normal structures were detected in the cat with SCC. Percutaneous biopsies were obtained via ultrasound guidance, with no reported complications noted.[53]

Computed tomography (CT) and magnetic resonance imaging (MRI) offer other sensitive diagnostic modalities that allow a more accurate determination of tumor margins, which may be beneficial for treatment planning if surgical resection is to follow. Both CT and MRI are commonly used in human medicine and are recently becoming more readily available in veterinary medicine.

Direct visual examination of the pharynx and larynx using a lighted laryngoscope provides crucial information in patients suspected to have laryngeal or pharyngeal tumors.[5,6,12,51] Laryngoscopy is performed under sedation or light general anesthesia, allowing proper examination of all associated anatomical structures; arytenoid movement; and determination of the size, location, and intraluminal extension of the mass.[5,6,12,17] When a biopsy of the mass is performed, the cuff of the endotracheal tube should be inflated to protect the airway and to assist in removal of secretions upon extubation of the animal.[12] Bronchoscopy provides another useful diagnostic tool for both laryngeal and tracheal tumors not visible via direct laryngeal examination.[8] With either approach, several biopsy samples should be obtained to ensure that specimens are diagnostic. Transtracheal or endotracheal lavage may provide cells for cytological evaluation in tumors that exfoliate easily. In selected patients, laryngeal and tracheal tumors may only be identified during surgical exploration (Figure 45-2, B).

Treatment

For both laryngeal and tracheal tumors, treatment options include surgical excision, chemotherapy, radiation therapy, or a combination thereof.* The type, location, and stage of the tumor influences which of these treatment modalities would be the most appropriate in an individual case.† There is limited information about the response to treatment in veterinary patients with laryngeal and tracheal tumors. Carcinoma is the most common laryngeal tumor in humans and the therapeutic choice is influenced mainly by the histologic differentiation, size, and location of the tumor.[1-3] Small tumors may be treated effectively with radiotherapy alone.

Small lesions can also be cured by functional endoscopic resection techniques (laser) or surgery.[61-65] Larger, more locally advanced tumors may require neoadjuvant chemotherapy followed by radiation therapy.[1,61-65] Patients with tumors infiltrating the laryngeal framework may need a total laryngectomy and radiotherapy.[61-65] Tracheal tumors, usually carcinomas, are often treated by surgical resection and anastomosis followed by radiotherapy.[66,67] Chemotherapy is used in patients with or at risk for distant metastasis or in conjunction with radiation therapy for the primary tumor.[1] The most common agents used in human oncology for the treatment of laryngeal or tracheal carcinomas are cisplatin, bleomycin, and fluorouracil (5-FU).[1] In humans, radiation therapy in conjunction with surgery generally yields a good prognosis for local cure and control in patients with early stage tumors.[1,66-69]

In veterinary medicine, surgery alone for malignant laryngeal tumors is often only palliative and does not usually provide a cure.[6,21] Complete surgical resection of laryngeal tumors may be attempted via partial laryngectomy, especially in cases where the tumor is confined to the glottic region.[9,12,15,19,43] A total laryngectomy and a permanent tracheostomy may be performed in patients with larger invasive tumors.[12,43,54-57] Small, pedunculated tumors may be excised either perorally using a laryngoscope or via a ventral neck incision.[6,12,43] Tracheal tumors are most often excised via tracheal ring resection and anastomosis.[12,43,51,58-60]

In our retrospective study, surgery was performed on seven patients (3 dogs, 4 cats) with laryngeal tumors (see Tables 45-1 and 45-2). A partial laryngectomy was performed on six patients (3 dogs, 3 cats), and surgical debulking was performed on one patient (see Table 45-1). Six patients with tracheal tumors underwent surgical resection, and a complete resection was obtained in five patients (see Table 45-2).

Chemotherapy, either alone or in conjunction with radiation therapy, may be a rational approach in cases with laryngeal or tracheal LSA.* Lymphomas are highly sensitive to chemotherapy, and there are several established protocols for treating canine and feline lymphomas.[4] The common chemotherapeutic agents used in lymphoma protocols include L-asparaginase, vincristine, cyclophosphamide, adriamycin, and prednisone.[4] Chemotherapy may also be indicated as an adjunct to surgery and radiation therapy in other tumors (e.g., plasmacytomas, mast cell tumors, or other high grade tumors) that are not treated effectively with local modalities.[6,12,48]

Radiation therapy provides a reasonable alternative to radical resection, or an adjunct to surgery.[12,70,71] In veterinary medicine, the efficacy of radiation therapy is unknown, and only a few case reports exist in the literature.[12,70,71] However, anecdotal evidence suggests that radiation therapy may provide good long-term control for selected laryngeal neoplasms. Radiation therapy has been associated with prolonged remission and even cure in some cats with Stage I LSA of the trachea.[12,71]

*References 5, 6, 12, 51, and 54-67.
†References 5, 6, 8, 12, 51, and 54-67.

*References 6, 8, 12, 35, 46, and 48.

Prognosis

The overall prognosis for laryngeal tumors is unknown and depends on tumor type, size, and local invasiveness.[5,6,8,12] Surgical excision of benign tumors can be curative, but for malignant tumors it is often only palliative and may be associated with a high postoperative morbidity.* Chemotherapy is generally limited to cases with lymphoreticular tumors, but may provide good long-term control.[6,12,48] Radiation therapy may provide good local tumor control and may also be curative in some cases.[12,70,71] Multimodal therapy combining surgical excision, chemotherapy, and/or radiation therapy may be necessary to provide optimal tumor control in most patients with nonlymphoreticular laryngeal or tracheal tumors.

In our study, overall prognosis was poor; and specific survival times associated with each treatment modality and tumor type were not determined because a high number of cases were lost to follow-up (see Tables 45-1 and 45-2). Ten patients with laryngeal tumors (4 dogs, 6 cats) were euthanized either at presentation (n = 9) or at surgery (n = 1) due to clinical judgment of a poor prognosis. Three cats with tracheal tumors were likewise euthanized at presentation due to poor prognosis. Two dogs with laryngeal tumors (rhabdomyoma) treated by surgical excision are still alive at 80 and 100 days postdiagnosis. One cat treated with surgery, chemotherapy, and radiation therapy for a laryngeal LSA was lost to follow-up at 6 months posttreatment. Two dogs with tracheal tumors (rhabdomyosarcoma, chondrosarcoma) treated by surgical resection and anastomosis are still alive at 40 and 700 days, respectively. One cat with tracheal LSA treated by surgical resection and anastomosis and chemotherapy is still alive over 1 year postdiagnosis.

Conclusion

Tumors of the larynx and trachea are rare and usually malignant. Clinical signs vary and are often insidious in nature; however, some animals may present as emergencies as a result of upper airway obstruction. Diagnostic modalities include palpation, pharyngeal/laryngeal examination, radiographs, bronchoscopy, ultrasonography, CT, and MRI. Prognosis depends on tumor type and completeness of surgical resection. For benign tumors, surgery may be curative, but for malignant tumors surgery is often only palliative. Chemotherapy and radiation therapy may provide good long-term control in cases of lymphoreticular tumors. Although the overall prognosis for both laryngeal and tracheal tumors is poor, a multimodal approach may be required to significantly improve survival in most cases.

*References 5, 6, 8, 12, 43, 51, and 56.

REFERENCES

1. Sessons RB, Harrison LB, Forastierre AA: Tumors of the larynx and hypolarynx. In DeVita VT, Hellman S, Rosenberg SA, editors: Cancer: Principles and practice of oncology, Philadelphia, 1997, Lippincott-Raven.
2. Ferlito A, Rinaldo A, Devaney KO: Malignant laryngeal tumors: Phenotypic evaluation and clinical implications, Ann Otol Rhinol Laryngol 104:587-589, 1995.
3. Cattaruzza MS, Maisonneuve P, Boyle P: Epidemiology of laryngeal cancer, Eur J Cancer B Oral Oncol 32:293-305, 1996.
4. Vonderhaar MA, Morrison WB: Lymphosarcoma. In Morrison WB, editor: Cancer in dogs and cats: Medical and surgical management, Baltimore, MD, 1998, Williams & Wilkins.
5. Carlisle CH, Biery DN, Thrall DE: Tracheal and laryngeal tumors in the dog and cat: Literature review and additional 13 patients, Veterinary Radiol 32:229-235, 1991.
6. Saik JE, Toll SL, Diters RW et al: Canine and feline laryngeal neoplasia: A 10-year survey, JAAHA 22:359-365, 1986.
7. Pass DA, Huxtable CR, Cooper BJ et al: Canine laryngeal oncocytomas, Vet Pathol 17:672-677, 1980.
8. Withrow SJ: Cancer of the larynx and trachea. In Withrow SJ, MacEwen EJ, editor: Small animal clinical oncology, Philadelphia, 2001, WB Saunders.
9. Calderwood-Mays MB: Laryngeal oncocytomas in two dogs, J Am Vet Med Assoc 185:677-679, 1984.
10. Gonzales JL, Rollan E: Garcia P et al: Laryngeal adenocarcinoma in a dog, J Small Anim Pract 34:146-148, 1993.
11. Clercx C, Desmecht D, Michiels L et al: Laryngeal rhabdomyoma in a golden retriever, Vet Rec 143:189-198, 1998.
12. Fox LE, King RR: Cancers of the respiratory system. In Morrison WB, editor: Cancer in dogs and cats: Medical and surgical management, Baltimore, MD, 1998, Williams & Wilkins.
13. Ligget AD, Weiss R, Thomas KL: Canine laryngopharyngeal rhabdomyoma resembling an oncocytoma: Light microscope, ultrastructural and comparative studies, Vet Pathol 22:526-532, 1985.
14. Lightfoot RM, Bedford PGC, Hayword AHS: Laryngeal leiomyoma in a dog, J Small Anim Pract 24:753-758, 1983.
15. Meuten DJ, Calderwood-Mays MB, Dillman RC et al: Canine laryngeal rhabdomyoma, Vet Pathol 22:533-539, 1985.
16. Rivera RYR, Carlton WW: Lingual rhabdomyoma in a dog, J Comp Pathol 106:83-87, 1992.
17. Stan SE, Bauer TG: Respiratory tract tumors, Vet Clin North Am 15:535-557, 1985.
18. Tang KN, Mansell JL, Herron AJ et al: The histologic, ultrastructural, and immunohistochemical characteristics of a thyroid oncocytoma in a dog, Vet Pathol 31:269-271, 1994.
19. Venker-van Haagen: Diseases of the larynx, Vet Clin North Am Small Anim Pract 22:1155-1171, 1992.
20. Berry KK, Wilson RW, Holscher MA et al: Oncocytoma in a cat, Compend Compan Animal Pract 2:16-18, 1988.
21. Clark GN, Berg J, Engler SJ et al: Extramedullary plasmacytomas in dogs: Results of surgical excision in 131 cases, J Am Anim Hosp Assoc 28:105-111, 1992.
22. Beaumont PR, O'Brien JB, Allen HJ et al: Mast cell sarcoma of the larynx of a dog: A case report, J Small Animal Pract 20:19-25, 1979.
23. Bright RM, Gorman NT, Calderwood-Mays MB: Laryngeal neoplasia in two dogs, J Am Vet Med Assoc 184:738-740, 1984.
24. Brodey RS, O'Brien J, Berg P et al: Osteosarcoma of the upper airway in the dog, J Am Vet Med Assoc 155:1460-1464, 1969.
25. Flanders JA, Castleman W, Carberry CA et al: Laryngeal chondrosarcoma in a dog, J Am Vet Med Assoc 190:68-70, 1987.
26. Hulland TJ: Tumors of the muscle. In Moulton JE, editor: Tumors in domestic animals, ed 3, Berkeley, CA, 1990, University of California Press.
27. Ladds PW, Webster DR: Pharyngeal rhabdomyosarcoma in a dog, Vet Pathol 8:256-259, 1971.
28. Madewell B, Lund J, Munn R et al: Canine laryngeal rhabdomyosarcoma: An immunohistochemical and electron microscopic study, Nippon Juigaku Zasshi 50(5):1077-1084, 1988.
29. McConnell EE, Smit JD, Venter HJ: Melanoma in the larynx of a dog, J South Afr Vet Med Assoc 42:189-191, 1971.
30. Ndikuwera J, Smith D, Obwolo MJ: Malignant melanoma of the larynx in a dog, J Small Anim Pract 30:107-109, 1989.

31. Wheeldon EB, Suter PF, Jenkeins T: Neoplasia of the larynx in the dog, *JAVMA* 180:642-647, 1982.
32. Vasseur PB, Patnaik AK: Laryngeal adenocarcinoma in a cat, *J Am Anim Hosp Assoc* 17:639-641, 1981.
33. Wheldon EB, Amis TC: Laryngeal carcinoma in a cat, *J Am Med Assoc* 186:80-81, 1985.
34. Bryan RD, Frame RW, Kier AB: Tracheal leiomyoma in a dog, *J Am Vet Med Assoc* 178:1069-1070, 1981.
35. Ogilvie GK, Moore AS: Tumors of the respiratory system. In Ogilvie GK, Moore AS, editors: *Managing the veterinary cancer patient: A practice manual,* Trenton, NJ, 1995, Veterinary Learning Systems.
36. Aron DN, Devires R, Short CE et al: Primary tracheal chondrosarcoma in a dog: A case report with description of surgical and anesthetic techniques, *J Am Anim Hosp Assoc* 16:31-37, 1980.
37. Black AP, Liu S, Randolph JF: Primary tracheal leiomyoma in the dog, *J Am Vet Med Assoc* 179:905-907, 1981.
38. Carb A, Halliwell WH: Osteochondral dysplasia of the canine trachea, *J Am Anim Hosp Assoc* 17:193-199, 1981.
39. Gourley IMG, Morgan JP, Gould DH: Tracheal osteochondroma in a dog, *J Small Anim Pract* 11:327-335, 1970.
40. Hough JD, Krahwinkle DJ, Evans AT et al: Tracheal osteochondroma in a dog, *J Am Vet Med Assoc* 170:1416-1418, 1977.
41. Cain GR, Manley P: Tracheal adenocarcinoma in a cat, *J Am Vet Med Assoc* 182:614-616, 1983.
42. Engle GC, Brodey RS: A retrospective study of 395 feline neoplasms, *J Am Anim Hosp Assoc* 5:21-31, 1965.
43. Fossum TW: Laryngeal and tracheal tumors. In Fossum TW, editor: *Small animal surgery,* St Louis, MO, 1997, Mosby Year Book.
44. Beaumont PR: Intratracheal neoplasia in two cats, *J Small Anim Pract* 23:29-35, 1982.
45. Hill JE, Mahaffey EA, Farrell RL: Tracheal carcinoma in a dog, *J Comp Pathol* 97:765-770, 1987.
46. Neer TM, Zeman D: Tracheal adenocarcinoma in a cat and review of the literature, *J Am Anim Hosp Assoc* 23:377-380, 1987.
47. Lieberman LL: Feline adenocarcinoma of the larynx with metastasis to the adrenal gland, *J Am Vet Med Assoc* 125:153-154, 1954.
48. Schneider PR, Smith CW, Feller DL: Histiocytic lymphosarcoma of the trachea in a cat, *J Am Anim Hosp Assoc* 15:485-487, 1979.
49. Veith LA: Squamous cell carcinoma of the trachea of a cat, *Feline Pract* 4:30-32, 1974.
50. Harvey HJ, Sykes G: Tracheal mast cell tumor in a dog, *J Am Vet Med Assoc* 180:1097-1100, 1982.
51. Holt D, Brockman D: Diagnosis and management of laryngeal disease in the dog and cat, *Vet Clin North Am* 24:855-871, 1994.
52. Rudorf H: Ultrasound imaging of the mouth and larynx in normal dogs, *J Small Anim Pract* 38:439-444, 1997.
53. Rudorf H, Brown P: Ultrasonography of laryngeal masses in six cats and one dog, *Vet Radiol Ultr* 39:430-434, 1998.
54. Block G, Clarke K, Salisbury SK et al: Total laryngectomy and permanent tracheostomy for the treatment of laryngeal rhabdomyosarcoma in a dog, *J Am Anim Hosp Assoc* 31:510-513, 1995.
55. Crowe DTJ, Goodwin MA, Greene CE: Total laryngectomy for laryngeal mast cell tumor in a dog, *J Am Anim Hosp Assoc* 22:809-816, 1986.
56. Henderson RA, Powers RD, Perry L: Development of hypoparathyroidism after excision of laryngeal rhabdomyosarcoma in a dog, *J Am Vet Med Assoc* 198:639-643, 1991.
57. Hedlund CS, Tanger CH, Montgomery DL et al: A procedure for permanent tracheostomy and its effects on tracheal mucosa, *Vet Surg* 11:13-17, 1982.
58. Hedlund CS: Tracheal resection and reconstruction, *Probl Vet Med* 3:210-228, 1991.
59. Withrow SJ, Holmberg DL, Doige CE et al: Treatment of tracheal osteochondroma with an overlapping end to end anastomosis, *J Am Anim Hosp Assoc* 14:469-473, 1978.
60. Yanoff SR, Fuetealba C, Boothe HW et al: Tracheal defect and embryonal rhabdomyosarcoma in a young dog, *Can Vet J* 37:172-173, 1996.
61. Davis RK: Endoscopic surgical management of glottic laryngeal cancer, *Otolaryngol Clin North Am* 30:79-86, 1997.
62. Moreau PR: Treatment of laryngeal carcinomas by laser endoscopic microsurgery, *Laryngoscope* 110:1000-1006, 2000.
63. Semczuk B, Szmeja Z, Janczewski G et al: Efficiency of surgical treatment in patients with laryngeal cancer in four clinical centers, *Otolaryngol Pol* 49:195-200, 1995.
64. Carew JF, Shah JP: Advances in multimodality therapy for laryngeal cancer, *Cancer J Clin* 48:211-228, 1998.
65. Keum KC, Kim GE, Suh CO et al: Role of definitive radiation therapy for larynx preservation in patients with advanced laryngeal cancer, *J Otolaryngol* 28:245-251, 1999.
66. Makarewicz R, Mross M: Radiation therapy alone in the treatment of tumours of the trachea, *Lung Cancer* 20:169-174, 1998.
67. Mathisen DJ: Tracheal tumors, *Chest Surg Clin N Am* 6:875-898, 1996.
68. O'Brien PC: Tumour recurrence or treatment sequelae following radiotherapy for larynx cancer, *J Surg Oncol* 63:130-135, 1996.
69. Cortesina G, De Stefani A, Cavalot A et al: Current role of radiotherapy in the treatment of locally advanced laryngeal carcinomas, *J Surg Oncol* 74:79-82, 2000.
70. Thrall DE, Dewhirst MW: Use of radiation and/or hyperthermia for treatment of mast cell tumors and lymphosarcoma in dogs, *Vet Clin North Am* 15:835-843, 1985.
71. Meleo KA: The role of radiotherapy in the treatment of lymphoma and thymoma, *Vet Clin North Am Small Anim Pract* 27:115-129, 1997.

C. Trachea and Bronchi
CHAPTER 46

Tracheal Collapse

Robert A. Mason • Lynelle R. Johnson

Definition and Etiology

The trachea is the flexible conduit connecting the upper airway (nasal, oral, pharyngeal and laryngeal portions) with the lower (bronchial and bronchiolar) airways. In the dog, the trachea is supported by a series of C-shaped cartilaginous rings connected by annular ligaments.[1,2] Dorsally, the open area of these rings is completed by the *dorsal trachealis* muscle, also referred to as the dorsal tracheal membrane.[1] The anatomy of the trachea allows it flexibility for wide excursions of the neck as well as rigidity to withstand external compressive forces without collapsing,[2] somewhat analogous to the structure and function of a vacuum cleaner hose. The trachea is unique among airways in that it spans both the extra- and intrathoracic portions of the respiratory tract, and as such, is exposed to both atmospheric and pleural pressure changes.[2] This concept becomes important when discussing the dynamic components of tracheal collapse.

Tracheal collapse has been associated with tracheal trauma, intraluminal masses, compressive extraluminal masses, tracheal hypoplasia, and tracheomalacia. In the dog, the term "tracheal collapse" generally refers to a condition of excessive collapsibility of the trachea,[2] usually resulting in dorsoventral flattening of the tracheal lumen.[2-7] The collapsed trachea has a wide, hypotonic, dorsal tracheal membrane[3,5-8] that may become flaccid, redundant, and sag into the lumen.[3,6] Weakened cartilage rings may form a shallow arc impinging on the tracheal lumen.[2,3,5,7-10]

Baumann originally described the condition of tracheal collapse (TC) in the dog in 1941.[11] The first definitive review was published by Dr. Joan O'Brien and colleagues in 1966,[6] in which 29 further cases from the University of Pennsylvania were reported. This group reported the first bronchoscopic examinations and descriptions of abnormal airway architecture in TC patients.[6] Done[12] in 1970 noted that only 2 cases had been reported in Great Britain at that point, whereas in 1994, White's study at Cambridge comprised 100 cases seen at that institution in just 4 years.[13]

Pathophysiology

Although tubular, the trachea is a dynamic structure, changing both size and shape in response to transmural pressure changes and to the effects of gas flow.[1] During expiration in the healthy lung at quiet tidal breathing, gas flows out of the lungs following a "downhill" pressure gradient caused by elastic recoil of the lung. During passive expiration, intraluminal airway pressure exceeds intrapleural pressure (Ppl), and dynamic collapse does not occur in the intrathoracic trachea. During forced expiration (e.g., during coughing, sneezing, a Valsalva maneuver, or conditions of increased small airway resistance), Ppl increases well above airway pressure. At some point along the airway, the airway pressure is equal to the Ppl. This is known as the equal pressure point (EPP). Any remaining intrathoracic trachea orad to the EPP tends to be compressed during expiration.[2] Any obstruction to airflow (e.g., bronchoconstriction or mucus accumulation) causes the EPP to move closer to the alveoli, creating a longer segment of intrathoracic airway collapse.[5] To simplify this, if the collapsing tracheal segment is intrathoracic, it tends to collapse during expiration, especially during increased Ppl[1,3] (e.g., with cough or forced expiration) and also when there is flow limitation in the small airways (e.g., with bronchoconstriction).

Conversely, during inspiration, Ppl is negative as the chest wall expands to create a negative alveolar pressure that draws air into the lungs.[1,2] Whereas this tends to hold the intrathoracic airways open during inspiration, the negative intraluminal pressures in the extrathoracic airways increase their tendency toward collapse during inspiration if they are weakened,[2,5] as in cases of TC of the cervical trachea.

Microscopic and ultrastructural changes in the organic matrix of the cartilage of affected rings is a striking feature of TC.[4,8,10,14] The affected cartilage is hypocellular with respect to chondrocytes, and there is loss of normal hyaline cartilage and replacement with fibrocartilage or fibrous tissue, compared with the tracheal cartilage from unaffected toy breed dogs.[8] There are decreased amounts of chondroitin sulfate and calcium in the cartilage matrix,[8] as well as decreased glycoproteins and glycosaminoglycans.[14] Ultrastructural examination with scanning electron microscopy revealed abnormal structure of the amorphous matrix of TC cartilage compared with that of normal dogs.[14] The lack of glycosaminoglycans (GAG) is of particular interest because they normally bind water electrostatically to confer structural rigidity to the cartilage.[2,14] This absence of GAG in TC cartilage may play a significant role in the weakness noted in these rings.

The etiology of tracheal collapse in the dog remains unclear.* Numerous theories on causation have been advanced, including genetic,[1,6,8] nutritional,[12] neurological,[16] and inflammatory causes.[11] In 1941, an inflammatory etiology of TC was first proposed, suggesting that deep-seated tracheitis led to weakening of tracheal support.[11] All 10 cases reported in 1976 had evidence of inflammation.[4] An association between chronic bronchitis and tracheal collapse has been suggested.[2,4,9] Full thickness tracheal wall inflammation has been reported in several cases of TC that had similar changes in the peripheral lung tissues.[4] Whether the inflammation that is seen in TC is cause, effect, or unassociated with the cartilaginous changes remains unclear.

The theory that there may be a genetic cause is supported by the prevalence of this disease among toy breeds. Affected breeds tend to favor chondrodystrophic body characteristics, and the ultrastructural changes in TC cartilage are reportedly consistent with chondrodystrophy.[17] Breeds commonly affected have relatively large or dome-shaped heads and are mildly brachycephalic,[6,8] as well as having narrow pointed muzzles, well-muscled necks, and narrow thoracic inlets.[6] However, tracheal collapse has also been reported in large-breed dogs.[18]

A neurologic deficiency of the trachealis muscle has been proposed[16]; however, histology of the dorsal trachealis muscle in TC failed to show any alteration in innervation compared with normal dogs.[8] Yamamoto reported that the microanatomy of the tracheal plexus of nerves is much more complex in the dog than in other species, and that this peritracheal nerve plexus is expected to play an important role in the pathogenesis of tracheal collapse.[19]

The nutritional basis of tracheal collapse is tenuous. It is interesting, however, to speculate on the potential benefits that some of the nutriceuticals being used in connective tissue disorders of the musculoskeletal system (e.g., methyl sulphonyl methane, glucosamine hydrochloride, chondroitin sulfate, and cetyl myristoleate) might have in a connective tissue disease such as chondromalacia and tracheal collapse.

Tracheomalacia is a syndrome similar to TC that has been described in humans. This is a structural abnormality of tracheal cartilage that allows collapse of its walls, leading to airway obstruction.[20] This abnormality includes hypoplasia, dysplasia, and absence of the normal cartilaginous framework.[21] The syndrome occurs in a primary or congenital form as well as a secondary or acquired form.[21,22] The primary form usually occurs as an isolated segmental tracheal defect[22] but may include proximal, distal or diffuse tracheal involvement.[20] Congenital tracheomalacia results from idiopathic disease or is associated with congenital tracheoesophageal fistula.[20] The acquired form may occur as a result of a variety of degenerative conditions.[20] Similarities to canine tracheal collapse exist, including reduced cartilage

throughout the trachea. Another feature of tracheomalacia is an excessively wide *pars membranacea* portion of the trachea, analogous to the pendulous dorsal tracheal membrane in dogs.[21,22] A severe form of inflammatory disease in man, called *relapsing polychondritis,* can result in acquired tracheomalacia.[23] The characteristic histologic findings in this condition include loss of chondrocytes; decreased basophilic staining; and a dense inflammatory infiltrate,[23] consisting mainly of polymorphonuclear cells or lymphocytes,[24] very similar to the histologic findings in canine TC cartilages.[4,5,6,8,14]

Epidemiology

In dogs, the condition most commonly affects middle age toy and miniature breeds.* There is a typical phenotype among breeds prone to TC: apple- or dome-shaped head; small, pointed, narrow muzzle; well-muscled neck; and a narrow thoracic inlet.[6] These characteristics of affected dogs are similar to chondrodystrophic dogs.[8] The most commonly affected breeds include Toy Poodles, Yorkshire Terriers, Pomeranians, Maltese, Pugs, and Chihuahuas.* The prevalence of TC among 2780 canine patients seen at the University of Queensland during a 2-year period was 0.5%.[5] Of the 521 toy breeds presented to this clinic, 14 (2.7%) had tracheal collapse; 2.9% of miniature or toy poodles and 9.3% of Pomeranians were affected.[5] In another study of 29 cases of tracheal collapse, 10% were Pomeranians and 41% were Chihuahuas.[6] Of all cases of TC in the literature between 1967 and 1979, 30 of 133 cases (22.5%) were Pomeranians,[7] although the Yorkshire terrier represented 65% of 100 cases recently reported from Britain.[13] The breed most often afflicted with TC seems dependent on the geographic location and the population density of those predisposed breeds in different countries. Tracheal collapse has also been occasionally reported in large-breed dogs.[18]

There appears to be a biphasic age distribution for TC, with most presenting in middle age and a subpopulation of affected dogs showing clinical signs during puppyhood.[3,4,12,13] Various studies report average ages of onset of 6.6 years (range 0.25 to 15),[13] 7.5 years,[2,3] 8 years (range 2 to 10.5),[6] and 3 to 8 years of age.[1,4,12] Most dogs have clinical signs for an extended period before presentation or diagnosis of TC, ranging from months to years, with an average of 2 years.[4,5,6,9,13]

Historical Findings and Clinical Signs

Cough is the classical presenting complaint in dogs with tracheal collapse, with or without exercise intolerance. The character of the cough is often described as dry, hacking, or "goose-honking"; however, moist and productive cough or the complete absence of a cough should not necessarily preclude a diagnosis of collapsed trachea. The cough may be mild initially, but often becomes severe, paroxysmal, or incessant as the disease advances. Coughing is usually

*References 1, 3, 5, 6, 13, and 15.

*References 1-3, 5, 6, 8, 9, 14, and 25.

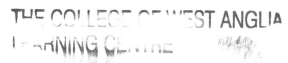

worse with excitement, exercise, tracheal compression by a neck collar, or eating and drinking. The degree of exercise intolerance is proportional to the severity of the collapse and activity of the dog. Individual dogs with a sedentary lifestyle may have no obvious exercise intolerance; or, conversely, their lack of activity may be caused by their tracheal collapse. Severe disease may cause dyspnea at rest, cyanosis, and collapse. Obesity is a commonly reported finding in tracheal collapse patients, with an incidence reported from 9% to 67%.[5,13]

Gagging may be reported, especially after eating or drinking. This may be related to laryngeal paresis or paralysis, a concurrent condition found in up to 30% of dogs with tracheal collapse.[3,9] Gagging after coughing may be caused by tracheal mucus that is expelled into the nasopharynx during the cough.[3] Inspiratory dyspnea or stridor is another commonly reported finding, especially during eating, drinking, excitement, or pulling on a neck leash. The stridor often leads to a bout of paroxysmal coughing, or vice versa. Stridor is consistent with a diagnosis of cervical tracheal collapse,[1-3,9] which has been reported to be the more common form.[1,3,9] The authors have observed, however, that both segments of the trachea are affected in the majority of cases undergoing endoscopic examination. Stridor may also be a manifestation of laryngeal paralysis/paresis noted in up to 30% of cases of TC.[9] Occasionally, expiratory dyspnea may be clinically apparent in animals with pure intrathoracic tracheal or tracheobronchial collapse.[1,3,7]

Physical Examination

Affected dogs may be completely normal on physical examination.[3] More often, the typical harsh cough occurs spontaneously or is easily induced by gentle tracheal palpation.[1-3,7,13] Flattened cartilaginous tracheal rings, with prominent dorsolateral angles, may occasionally be palpated in cases of cervical collapse, especially at the thoracic inlet.[1-3,5,6,7,12] Hyperextension of the occipitoatlantal joint may increase the level of dyspnea by worsening the dorsoventral tracheal flattening.[4,7] Tracheal and thoracic auscultation may reveal harsh wheezing sounds in dogs with concurrent bronchitis.[3] A characteristic "snap" that may be auscultated at the end of expiration is thought to result from the abrupt separation of opposing mucosal walls in the collapsed segment.[1-3] Lung sounds are usually normal, except in cases with concomitant lower airway disease such as chronic bronchitis, in which case adventitial sounds such as wheezes and crackles may be heard.[2,5]

Heart sounds vary from normal to systolic murmurs that may or may not be associated with significant heart disease.[3,9] Tangner's review of 20 surgical cases only included 1 dog with a pre-operative audible murmur.[9] *Cor pulmonale*, or right-sided heart failure secondary to pulmonary hypertension, may arise from the chronic dyspnea associated with chronic collapse of the major airways.[3,26] In cases of pulmonary hypertension secondary to chronic tracheal collapse, there may be delayed closure of the pulmonic valve, leading to a split second heart sound.

Hepatomegaly has also been reported in association with this syndrome, either as a result of chronic congestion from right heart failure, from fatty hepatic infiltrates in obese dogs, or caused by the steroid hepatopathy of hyperadrenocorticism, which has been reported in a percentage of tracheal collapse cases.[13] In the authors' experience, the trilogy of tracheal collapse, chronic small airway disease, and hyperadrenocorticism occurs much more commonly than is currently reported in the literature.

Differential Diagnosis

The list of differential diagnoses in the small breed dog with cough or dyspnea should include tracheal collapse; brachycephalic syndrome (including tracheal hypoplasia); laryngeal disease (e.g., collapse, paresis, or paralysis); chronic bronchitis; infectious tracheobronchitis; heartworm disease; primary pulmonary disease; primary cardiovascular disease; and intrinsic or extrinsic tracheal obstruction.[3] Besides the history and clinical examination, the most useful diagnostic tests include radiography (both inspiratory and expiratory), electrocardiography, tracheobronchoscopy, cytology and bacteriology of airway secretions, and pulmonary function testing.[1-3,5,6,9,25]

Diagnostic Tests

RADIOGRAPHY

Lateral radiographs of the neck and chest are commonly employed in the diagnosis and staging of TC.[1-3,5,6,9,25] Dorsoventral flattening of the tracheal lumen may be observed at the affected site.[1-7,9,12,13,25] In one group, normal thoracic radiographs were observed in 7 of 17 dogs with TC,[9] representing only a 60% sensitivity of standard radiographs in diagnosing TC. Another recent report found 84% sensitivity in 100 dogs radiographed with TC.[13] The clinical utility of standard radiography in diagnosing TC, especially in dogs with dynamic collapse, is only fair, at best.

Superimposition of overlying structures such as the esophagus, fat, or the *longus colli* muscles can lead to a false positive interpretation of TC.[1,2,6] Positioning of the head and neck during radiography is very important in this condition. Some authors advocate extreme dorsoflexion of the neck to augment the degree of collapse during radiography[5,6]; others feel this practice may lead to false positive interpretations.[2]

More objective criteria for assessing normal tracheal diameter on plain radiographs have been advocated.[27,28] On lateral survey radiographs of the neck and thorax, the normal trachea should be equal to the diameter of the laryngeal lumen at the level of the cricoid cartilage.[27] Alternatively, the trachea should be three times the diameter of the proximal one third of the third rib.[27] Harvey and Fink[28] proposed a modification of these measurements to correlate tracheal dimensions with body size, particularly thoracic inlet diameter. A ratio of the internal tracheal diameter to the distance between the ventral edge of the first thoracic vertebra and the dorsal edge of the manubrium can be calculated: 0.16 or greater is considered normal.[28] These criteria are more often, and more appropriately, used in the diagnosis of tracheal hypoplasia, where the trachea is narrow for its entire length.[7,27,28] In TC, the collapsed segment is often quite obviously narrower than the proximal or distal segments. One criticism of these measurements is that they do not take into account various other parameters that affect resistance to airflow. For example, dynamic collapse of the dorsal tracheal membrane might not be visible on radiographs but would have a dramatic influence on airway resistance. Factors such as intraluminal mucus or small airway disease can change the pulmonary mechanics in such a way that small changes in tracheal diameter become very significant.[5]

Because of the dynamic nature of the disease, both inspiratory and expiratory phases of respiration may be assessed radiographically.[2,3,7,13,29] In animals with cervical tracheal collapse, the cervical trachea should appear collapsed and the intrathoracic trachea should be normal to dilated on inspiration.[3,16,30] Accordingly, in cases of intrathoracic TC, cervical dilation and intrathoracic narrowing should occur on expiration. Evidence of collapse during both phases of respiration may be seen in more advanced cases.[3] Fluoroscopy has the obvious advantage of continuous documentation through all phases of the respiratory cycle, and is considered by many to be the diagnostic method of choice.[2,3,6,29] Another advantage of fluoroscopy is that dynamic tracheal collapse, which is only evident during dramatic elevations of intrapleural pressure (e.g., during coughing), may also be documented.[3] Fluoroscopic examination may have a higher specificity for diagnosis of TC than standard radiography alone, but these two modalities should not be relied upon for definitive diagnosis of tracheal collapse.[3,31] Radiographs of the chest are also useful in the diagnosis of concurrent problems such as cardiovascular, pulmonary, or small airway disease.[1,3,5,9,13] In one group of 20 dogs with TC, only 1 dog had a detectable heart murmur, yet 11 dogs had radiographic evidence of cardiomegaly.[9]

Early reports on the diagnosis of tracheal collapse included contrast radiography. One study in dogs cites the use of positive contrast barium esophagrams to delineate the weakened area of the trachea into which the barium-filled esophagus collapses.[6] Similar techniques are utilized in the diagnosis of tracheomalacia in human patients.[21] Positive contrast tracheobronchography has been employed,[7] but has been widely replaced by tracheobronchoscopy. Rudorf reported on the clinical utility of ultrasonography in the diagnosis of tracheal collapse in the awake dog, but this technique has yet to gain widespread acceptance.[32]

TRACHEOBRONCHOSCOPY

The advent of tracheobronchoscopy has had a major impact on the diagnosis, staging, and understanding of the pathophysiology of collapsing trachea in the dog. The healthy trachea is structurally rigid, and the size changes minimally during tidal breathing.[2] In dogs with tracheal

collapse, the dorsal tracheal membrane is often seen as pendulous, sagging, or redundant in the affected segment,[2,3,5-7,13] and the tracheal cartilages may be flattened, losing the normal C-shaped character.[3,5-7,13]

Tracheobronchoscopy was first used to diagnose tracheal collapse in 1966.[6] A rigid 3.5 mm × 30 cm bronchoscope was used. At the collapsing segment, the dorsal tracheal membrane was sagging into the lumen and had to be elevated by the bevel of the bronchoscope to permit its further passage.[6] The membrane was easily and freely movable. The tracheal lumen, at this point, was a flattened ellipse.[6] Numerous similar descriptions have followed since this pioneering work.[2,3,9,15] Advances in flexible fiberoptic and videobronchoscopy have made the availability and utility of this technique more widespread in veterinary medicine in recent years.

A grading system of TC has been proposed by Tangner and Hobson[9] based on the endoscopic appearance of the airway (Figure 46-1). **Grade I** collapse represents normal tracheal cartilage anatomy with slightly pendulous trachealis muscle impinging into the tracheal lumen with up to 25% loss of luminal diameter. In **grade II** collapse, the trachealis becomes wide and more pendulous, there

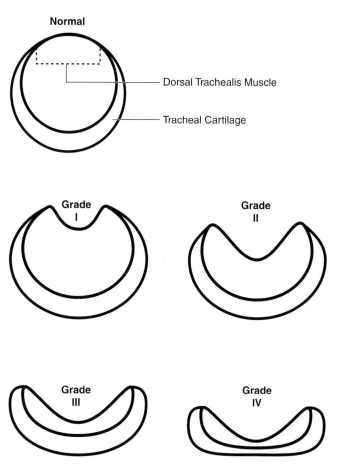

Figure 46-1. *A classification system for tracheal collapse using tracheobronchoscopy findings. (Reproduced with permission from Tangner CH, Hobson HP. A retrospective study of 20 surgically managed cases of collapsed trachea, Vet Surg 11:146-149, 1982.)*

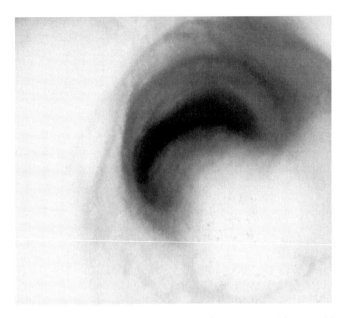

Figure 46-2. Grade II tracheal collapse in a 13-year-old Yorkshire terrier with dyspnea caused by concurrent severe pulmonary thromboembolism. (Photograph courtesy of Dr. Lesley King, University of Pennsylvania, Philadelphia, PA).

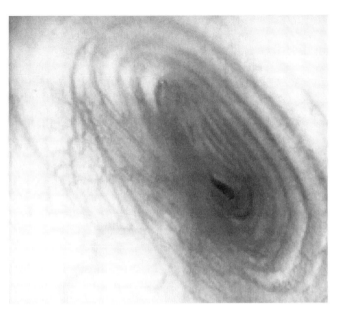

Figure 46-3. Grade IV tracheal collapse in a 5-year-old Pomeranian with no other apparent respiratory tract disease, and severe clinical signs of respiratory distress attributable to the airway obstruction. (Photograph courtesy of Dr. Lesley King, University of Pennsylvania, Philadelphia, PA).

is mild flattening of the tracheal cartilages, and the lumen is reduced by 50%. **Grade III** (Figure 46-2) manifests severe flattening of the cartilage rings such that the edges are clinically palpable. The dorsal tracheal membrane is almost in contact with the opposite tracheal wall, and the lumen diameter is 75% reduced. Finally, **grade IV** (Figure 46-3) represents total tracheal collapse: the trachealis muscle lies on the tracheal floor, the cartilage rings are completely flattened or occasionally inverted, and the lumen is completely obliterated.[9]

As with all clinical grading systems, this grading system may be useful to stage the severity of the disease and facilitate management decisions, allow case stratification for evaluation of treatment protocols, and it may have prognostic value. It has been suggested that animals with grade I disease can be successfully managed medically, whereas those with grades II to IV are surgical candidates.[9] In the authors' experience, grades I through III tend to respond well to medical management, with surgery reserved for those cases with severe grade IV collapse. Serial tracheoscopic re-evaluation and staging may aid the assessment of therapy and prognosis.

Endoscopic examination is performed under general anesthesia.[2,3,5,6,9] Because other forms of airway obstruction may be found concurrent with TC, pharyngoscopy, laryngoscopy, and bronchoscopy are often included as part of the complete airway examination.[2,3,7,13] Laryngeal function should be assessed for potential laryngeal paresis during anesthestic induction.[2,3,9,15] In one study, endoscopic examination was considered to provide the most significant diagnostic information.[13]

Anesthetic considerations include awareness of the increased vagal tone in these patients, the possibility of cor

pulmonale or secondary right heart disease, and possible concurrent small airway disease such as COPD and bronchoconstriction. Pre-oxygenation via face mask, if not too stressful to the patient, is recommended.[33] Narcotic antitussives, bronchodilators, and anticholinergics should be considered as part of the drug protocol. Extubation of these patients upon recovery can be a critical step, and prolonged intubation and oxygen supplementation postprocedure with the aid of narcotic sedation (e.g., butorphanol or meperidine), as well as strict and close patient monitoring during this period, is advised.[33] Short-acting glucocorticoids may be used to decrease airway swelling at the end of the procedure. If unfamiliar with these cases, consult a veterinary anesthesiologist regarding a safe induction, maintenance, and recovery protocol.

CYTOLOGY AND BACTERIOLOGY

Obtaining an airway wash for cytological and bacteriological examination is often advocated.[2,3,7,9,34] One study demonstrated that 36% of clinically healthy dogs had positive aerobic bacterial cultures from lower tracheal swabs.[34] In this study, samples were obtained under general anesthesia using guarded culture swabs passed through endotracheal tubes. Twenty-five of the swabs were premoistened with sterile saline, and 10 were dry. The moist swabs had a 48% growth rate, whereas the dry swabs had 0%, reducing the mean growth rate to 36%. Had all moistened swabs been used, it is conceivable that the overall bacterial recovery rate from these healthy dogs may have been closer to 48%. The common bacteria isolated included alpha-hemolytic *Streptococci* spp., *Pasteurella multocida*, *Klebsiella pneumoniae*, and coagulase-positive *Staphylococci* spp.[34] In light of this work, interpretation of the significance of positive bacterial cultures from individuals with tracheal collapse is difficult.[2]

Cytologic evaluation of tracheal secretions often yields nonspecific inflammatory changes; these findings rarely change the diagnosis, prognosis, or choice of therapy in tracheal collapse.[2] Bronchial fluid analysis may be helpful to assess small airway disease (chronic bronchitis). Small airway disease could produce dramatic changes in tracheal pressures and luminal diameter that would exacerbate tracheal collapse, especially during coughing[2] or forced expiration.[17] An association between chronic bronchitis and tracheal collapse has been suggested.[2,4,9] Pathologic examination of tracheal tissues from several cases of TC revealed full thickness tracheal wall inflammation that was similar to changes seen in the peripheral lung.[4] It has been suggested that part of the diagnostic evaluation of patients with TC should include an assessment of the lower airways.[3]

PULMONARY FUNCTION TESTING

Pulmonary function testing (PFT) has recently been employed to evaluate tracheobronchial obstruction in dogs.[2,17,31,35-41] Tidal breathing flow-volume loop (TBFVL) analysis has been adapted for this purpose.[35] In short, tracheal collapse represents a nonfixed, dynamic obstruction, and may result in flattening of either inspiratory or expiratory phases of the TBFVL loop depending on the location of the collapse site.[2] Because this is a noninvasive procedure that can be performed on the awake, untrained patient, it offers promise as an objective clinical measurement of the severity of dysfunction associated with tracheal collapse, as well as providing an objective measure of improvement or progression of the disease with therapy.

In summary, many tests are used in the diagnosis of collapsing trachea. Radiography has limited yield in dynamic collapse; fluoroscopy has a higher sensitivity than radiography but limited availability, especially in private practice; and tracheoscopy requires specialized equipment and training, as well as general anesthesia. Some investigators suggest: ". . . the recognition of both a persistent cough with response to tracheal palpation and endoscopic confirmation of the anatomic tendency to collapse, with inflammation and thickening of the dorsal tracheal membrane, as being essential criteria for the confirmation of a diagnosis of tracheal collapse."[13] Tracheobronchoscopy is ideal because it allows both diagnosis and grading of the severity of tracheal collapse, along with visual assessment of potential complications (e.g., laryngeal paresis or bronchial collapse), as well as assessing potential small airway disease through bronchoalveolar lavage for cytologic and microbiologic assessment of the lower airway.

Management and Monitoring

The controversy that embroils the etiology and diagnosis of tracheal collapse is trivial compared with that associated with the treatment of TC. The two major modes of

therapy are conservative medical management and surgical treatment. Some of the contention concerning therapeutic options has been clarified by Tangner and Hobson's endoscopic classification scheme,[9] although the majority of diagnosticians appear to use more empirical criteria.* There is a definite bias amongst surgeons to operate on all but the mildest cases early in the course of the disease,† whereas some medicine clinicians go as far as to question the need for surgery at all.[13]

MEDICAL MANAGEMENT

Medical therapy for TC is symptomatic[1] and palliative, not curative.[2] Classically, dogs are treated with a combination of antitussives, bronchodilators, corticosteroid antiinflammatories, antibiotics, and sedatives,[1-7,9] although no controlled clinical trials of any form of therapy have been reported. Very few animals require all of the above therapies, and treatment is tailored to the individual.

Although **antitussive** therapy is often advocated,[1-3,5,9,12] the choice of drug, dosage, and frequency of administration is variable. Narcotics are often prescribed, having both potent central antitussive and mild sedative effects that may help reduce dyspneic attacks induced by excitement.[1,2] Antitussives are indicated to break the cycle of cough-induced airway irritation. In addition, these agents help decrease the tussive increase in Ppl that further exacerbates intrathoracic collapse.[17] Butorphanol tartrate (Torbutrol) is a very effective antitussive with minimal sedative effects at antitussive dosages. The dosage range is very wide, with 0.55 mg/kg PO every 6 to 12 hours as a suggested starting point. The dosage can be adjusted upward for effect, or downward if the patient is too sedated. Hydrocodone (Hycodan) is another narcotic antitussive used at 0.22 mg/kg PO every 6 to 12 hours. Antitussives must be used judiciously in cases with concurrent small airway disease because there is a concern of decreasing small airway clearance of mucus and debris if the cough is productive. Antitussives are used to control excessive coughing—the definition of excessive is jointly made by the veterinarian and pet owner.[2]

Bronchodilators are often cited as a mainstay of medical therapy for TC,[1-3,5] although some authors cite that bronchoconstriction is rarely documented.[1,2] If bronchodilators affect the dorsal trachealis muscle, this already flaccid structure may further relax and impinge upon the airway.[1] Others believe that dilation of the smaller airways would decrease expiratory effort, leading to diminished intrathoracic pressure (i.e., Ppl) during expiration, thus decreasing subsequent tracheal narrowing[3] in dogs with intrathoracic tracheal collapse. In cases with concomitant small airway disease, where bronchoconstriction is suspected or possibly documented via pulmonary function testing, bronchodilation may be helpful.

Methylxanthines such as theophylline are often prescribed,[1,3] as well as β_2-agonists such as terbutaline and albuterol.[2] TheoDur®, a sustained release form of theophylline, has been extensively studied in the dog, and

_____

*References 1-3, 5, 7, 13, 30, and 42-44.
†References 3, 7, 9, 16, 29, 30, 42, and 44-46.

a dose of 20 mg/kg PO every 12 hours has been established.[47] TheoDur® is no longer available; however, other sustained release theophylline products can be used at a dose of 10 mg/kg PO BID. Other potential advantages of methylxanthines include enhanced mucociliary clearance, positive inotropism for respiratory muscles including the diaphragm, and purported antiinflammatory effects.[1] Oral forms may soon be unavailable as the pharmaceutical industry phases oral bronchodilators out in favor of inhalant aerosol forms. Alternatively, beta-2 agonists such as terbutaline (Bricanyl, 1.25 to 2.5 mg/dog PO every 12 hours) have been recommended. Inhalant bronchodilators, with the use of spacing chambers such as those used in asthmatic infants (Aero-Chamber), have been used in dogs and cats with bronchoconstrictive disease, but the dosages and recommended formulation are empirical. The authors have successfully used salbutamol inhalers in the treatment of chronic small airway disease, but not as yet in collapsing trachea.

Treatment with **glucocorticoids** is controversial.[1,2] Their use is often associated with abatement of clinical signs,[1,2,13] although continued usage may predispose the animal to bacterial tracheobronchitis, bronchopneumonia, and other side effects of corticosteroid therapy.[1,13] Drugs such as prednisone or dexamethasone are often advocated in severe acute clinical exacerbations when tracheal inflammation and edema have occurred because of mechanical trauma from the collapsing tracheal wall during coughing.[1-3,13,16] Generally, antiinflammatory dosages are used (prednisone 0.25 to 1 mg/kg PO every 12 to 24 hours). An association with allergic disease has been suggested in some cases of TC.[13] Glucocorticoids may also be advantageous in patients with concurrent small airway disease.

Antibiotics have been advocated based on the results of transtracheal wash cultures[1,2,29] and throat swabs,[9,16] or have been used empirically in many cases.[1,5,9,48] McKiernan's work in normal dogs clearly demonstrated that the results of pharyngeal swabs are not an accurate reflection of the flora from the lower trachea.[34] Furthermore, the results of that study cast doubt on the significance of culture results from the large airways or carina.[34] Routine use of antibiotic therapy in treatment of TC is not encouraged.[2]

Sedation is required in hyperactive animals that tend to have acute exacerbations of TC during times of excitement.[1-3,6] Sedation is often a beneficial side effect of narcotic antitussives.[2] Alternatively, mild sedatives such as diazepam or low dose oral acepromazine (0.5 to 2.0 mg/kg PO every 6 to 24 hours) have been used.

In a recent report of 100 cases of TC, a 71% success rate of medical management was reported, with success defined as owner satisfaction with the resolution of the severe coughing and return to adequate function.[13] All of the dogs were treated with Lomotil (diphenoxylate hydrochloride and atropine sulfate), prednisone, and treatment for concurrent disorders affecting the respiratory system.[13] Although not clearly explained in the report, presumably diphenoxylate, being a narcotic, has some degree of antitussive effect. The accumulation of mucus in the lower airway as a result of failure of the mucocil-

iary escalator has been proposed as a major mechanism of cough in dogs with TC.[6] The antisecretory effects of atropine may be advocated to reduce the volume of mucus secreted into the lower airway, and hence lessen the cough.[13] Others argue that anticholinergic therapy might dry out lower airway secretions, compounding the inspissation of mucus plugging the smaller airways.[11] The amount of atropine found in Lomotil is reported to have no clinical effect at these dosages.[49] In the above study, of the 71 dogs that responded well to this regimen, 51 were asymptomatic when medication was completely withdrawn, whereas another 20 dogs required ongoing medication to maintain remission.[13] This represents a substantial improvement in medical management of TC compared with previous reports.* The mechanism of action of this therapy is not completely understood, but it is an interesting alternative.

Controlling obesity,[1,3,6,13] improving the ventilation and air quality in the environment of affected individuals,[1,13] and using a chest harness instead of neck leashes[1] have all been reported as adjunct medical therapies, and may, in fact, play the biggest role in the success or failure of long-term management. Control of any associated endocrine disorders such as hypothyroidism or hyperadrenocorticism (that may predispose to obesity) or other complicating factors (e.g., chronic bronchitis and tracheomalacia with hyperadrenocorticism) may also play an important role in control.

SURGICAL MANAGEMENT

Equal numbers of surgical and medical therapies for tracheal collapse have been reported.† The first report of surgical management of TC in dogs appeared in 1964.[51] A rigid plastic tube that had been modified into a trough was sutured to the outer portion of the trachea at the collapse site, but no follow-up was provided.[51] The obvious disadvantage to this external splint was the inability of the rigid prosthesis to bend with the neck.[16,42]

In 1967, Knowles and Snyder presented the technique of corrective chondrotomy for TC.[30] In this procedure, transverse incisions through the ventral aspect of the tracheal cartilages are made in the area of the collapse. These cartilage rings were digitally compressed laterally, breaking the cartilage at the incision, changing the elliptical lumen to a pyramidal shape, and therefore significantly enlarging its collapsed calibre.[30,42] A modification to this technique was reported in 1971, in which alternate rings were incised.[26] Although 7 dogs were treated by this technique, there was no postoperative follow-up.[26] A further modification included multiple incisions made in the same ring to confer a more oval shape to the tracheal lumen.[15] The major limitation to these techniques was that they did not alleviate the stenosis caused by the redundant dorsal tracheal membrane.[15] There was an increased incidence of lateral TC postoperatively.[42] Chondrotomy, in general, is only effective if

---

*References 3, 5, 6, 9, 16, and 42.
†References 3, 5, 7, 9, 26, 42, 43, and 50.

the tracheal cartilages are rigid enough to support the new pyramidal lumen, and most dogs with TC are reported to have flaccid tracheal cartilage.[4,26,42]

A tracheoplasty with eversion of the pendulous dorsal trachealis muscle was mentioned in a report in 1966, but was not expanded upon.[6] Plication of the dorsal tracheal membrane was reported in detail in 1973.[48] This technique involves shortening the gap between the free ends of the tracheal rings by placing a horizontal mattress suture through the dorsal tracheal membrane, thus effectively improving the luminal diameter.[15,48] In the 9 dogs included in this report, 7 showed marked improvement and 2 showed no improvement with surgery.[48] In very small animals, it was felt that the plication technique would leave too narrow a tracheal lumen.[15,16,42]

In 1976, the first description appeared of a practical external prosthesis for the treatment of TC.[16] The total ring prosthesis (TRP) is prepared from 3-ml polypropylene syringe cases. Widths of 5 to 8 mm are cut transverse to the long axis of the syringe case, 4 to 6 holes are drilled in the loops of plastic, and each loop is cut open between 2 holes to form rings that can be threaded around the exposed trachea.[16] The trachea is approached at its collapsed segment, an area wide enough to accept the ring is isolated, and the ring is applied. It is sutured in place to the collapsed tracheal ring, drawing the cartilage and trachealis muscle out to the plastic ring in all directions.[16] The rings are placed every 10 to 15 mm until the entire collapsed segment has been supported. The major advantage over previous prostheses is that the TRP is segmental and thus flexible with movements of the neck.[16] The blood and nerve supplies to the trachea are not disrupted throughout its entire length, only at the area of the individual plastic rings.[16] Along with restoring the C-shape to the collapsed cartilaginous ring, the TRP also elevates the trachealis membrane from the lumen.[15] Although originally described for cervical and upper intrathoracic tracheal collapse via a ventral cervical approach,[16] the TRP has been used in conjunction with thoracotomy for intrathoracic TC.[7,9]

A retrospective study conducted on 20 dogs with TC repaired by the TRP revealed improvement in coughing (84%), dyspnea (80%), level of activity (55%) and a decrease in tracheal infections (60%), as documented by telephone follow-up from 4 months to 4 years postoperatively (average 1.5 years).[9] Others have reviewed this technique less favourably, noting that only 20% of these dogs were asymptomatic at 1 year after surgery.[13]

A modification of the TRP, the polypropylene spiral ring prosthesis (PSP), was introduced by Fingland and colleagues in 1986.[29,42] This prosthesis is also manufactured from 3-ml syringe cases, which in this case are cut in 15-degree spiral lengths to produce three 5.5-cm long, spring-like PSPs, each with 3-mm wide turns separated by 6-mm wide spaces.[42] This prosthesis is applied in much the same way as the TRP, with the exception that the trachea must be exposed and stripped of all fascial attachments for the entire length of the collapse to apply the PSP. The major advantages of the PSP over the TRP were reported to include: uniform support of the entire collapsed trachea including the sections between rings;

more inherent flexibility because the TRP may span 2 or 3 tracheal rings, resulting in minor inflexibility compared to the spring-like PSP which does not encircle the trachea at any one point; resistance to kinking between rings as may occur with the TRP, resulting in focal tracheal necrosis; speed and ease of application because the sutures are passed around spirals of the PSP, not through pre-drilled holes as in the TRP; and that the entire prosthesis is threaded or "screwed on," rather than individually applied one ring at a time.[42] Seven clinical cases repaired by this technique were evaluated postoperatively by a clinical scoring system based on coughing, dyspnea, and tracheal lumen diameter.[29] The combined score was rated as "excellent" for four of five cases and "good" for one of five cases that were followed 2 to 14 months after surgery; 2 dogs died, 1 and 8 months postoperatively.[29]

A prospective trial was conducted on 11 normal dogs to compare the TRP and PSP procedures.[45] By the parameters used in this study (i.e., clinical evaluation, radiography, tracheoscopy, necropsy, and histology), there were no detectable differences between the two techniques.[45] The major criticism of the PSP technique was the disruption of the tracheal vascular and nervous supply.[16,46] As Dr. Hobson had forewarned in 1976:

"Both vascular supply and innervation are extremely critical in the normal function of the tracheal mucosa and while you may 'get away' with complete isolation of long segments of the trachea during surgery, I can assure you, especially where the tracheal lumen is very small, early recovery following surgery will be difficult."[16]

This phenomenon was documented in a study on tracheal bloodflow conducted on normal dogs in 1991.[46] The trachea of 20 normal adult dogs was surgically exposed for PSP application; some had the prosthesis placed, others did not. Radio-labelled microspheres carrying 4 different marker isotopes were injected preoperatively, and then 3 and 7 days postoperatively, to assess tracheal bloodflow at these times.[46] Acutely, all dogs had significantly reduced bloodflow to all tracheal segments irrespective of PSP placement.[46] At day 3, bloodflow was dramatically reduced to the central portion of the trachea, and bloodflow was increased in the same area on day 7,[46] confirming suspicions that the central trachea has poor inherent collateral blood supply.[16] Further to these observations, 4 of 20 dogs died before day 3, all with transmural necrotizing tracheitis and vascular thrombosis.[46] The conclusions from this study were that the surgical approach for the application of the PSP, which involves complete isolation of the trachea and stripping of the lateral pedicles that contain tracheal vessels and nerves, results in significant diminution of blood supply during the immediate postoperative period, regardless whether the prosthesis is applied or not.[46] A second complication of surgery, disruption of the recurrent laryngeal nerve, may result in iatrogenic laryngeal paralysis in the postoperative period.

This study prompted the original authors of the PSP technique to develop a modified application procedure in 1993.[43] Although the same prosthesis is used, the approach to the trachea is similar to Hobson's TRP approach. Only the segments of the tracheal pedicle through which the prosthesis is to be threaded are stripped on one side, allowing for preservation of vascular supply to the trachea between turns of the spirals.[43]

Ayers reported a modified technique in 1999[50] involving a pliable, extraluminal, total ring prosthesis. In this technique, the prosthesis was styled from a polyvinyl chloride drip chamber from an intravenous fluid administration set. This technique provided stability to the weakened trachea, along with improved ease of creation and placement of the prosthesis. White reported decreased likelihood of catastrophic postoperative complications associated with iatrogenic laryngeal paralysis, a potential complication of extraluminal prosthesis placement, by performing prophylactic unilateral left laryngeal tie-back surgery at the same time.[52]

Other experimental techniques include endoscopic laser-assisted reshaping of collapsed tracheal cartilage.[53] An attempt to combine an autograft of the patient's own tissue over a synthetic prosthesis to reconstruct the trachea has been reported.[54] In this study, staged tracheal replacement was performed using polyethylene terephthalate (PET) tubular prostheses that had been previously cultured in the major omentum of the subject. In all cases, the anastomosis site failed.[54] Nonstented platysma myocutaneous door flaps have been used experimentally to reconstruct tracheal defects in dogs, but lack of structural integrity of the flaps resulted in 100% fatal luminal occlusion.[55]

The multiplicity of available surgical techniques is cited as evidence that there is an obvious lack of outright success of any one procedure.[13]

NONSURGICAL MANAGEMENT

Nonsurgical interventional techniques for severe TC have been investigated using several types of intraluminal prosthesis, or stents. Kirby's elegant study demonstrating the liability associated with surgical exposure of the trachea,[46] the early success of Dr. Dumon's silastic endoprosthesis in human patients with tracheal stenoses,[56-59] and its nonsurgical endoscopic placement, all make the Dumon stent an attractive alternative therapeutic modality for severe TC.

Mason conducted studies placing the Dumon silastic stent into the normal canine airway.[60] Normal dogs tolerated the stents fairly well for periods of up to 6 months. Coughing and bacterial colonization of the stents occurred in all cases, but these mild complications could all be controlled pharmacologically.[60] No long-term studies using the Dumon stent in clinical cases have yet been reported in dogs.

Radlinsky reported on the use of the Palmaz balloon expandable stent,[61] which is a metal mesh expandable stent. In normal dogs, this stent was associated with unacceptable migration, stent collapse, and deleterious changes to the epithelium. For these reasons, it was deemed inappropriate for placement in the cervical trachea of dogs, but may have better application in intrathoracic and mainstem bronchial collapse,[61] areas that are difficult to approach for surgical extraluminal prostheses.

At this time, until a more acceptable endoluminal prosthesis is developed, this procedure seems most useful as a short-term measure in acutely decompensating cases of severe, stage IV collapse. The other area of application may involve placement of stents in areas that are otherwise very difficult to access surgically, such as collapse of the intrathoracic trachea or the mainstem bronchi.

Prognosis

The prognosis for dogs with tracheal collapse is directly correlated to its clinical severity, as well as the presence of other risk factors such as the degree of obesity and concurrent disease status. Generally, grades I through III are amenable to medical management. The prognosis for more severe cases that require surgical management appears to be influenced by the skill of the operator.

REFERENCES

1. Spaulding GL: Medical management considerations for upper airway disease, *Respir Med* 4(2):419-428, 1992.
2. Padrid P, Amis TC: Chronic tracheobronchial disease in the dog, *VCNA* 22(5):1203-1229, 1992.
3. Hedlund CS: Tracheal collapse, *Prob Vet Med* 3(2):229-238, 1991.
4. Done SH, Drew RA: Observations on the pathology of tracheal collapse in dogs, *J Small Anim Pract* 17:783-791, 1976.
5. Amis TC: Tracheal collapse in the dog, *Austral Vet J* 50:285-289, 1974.
6. O'Brien JA, Buchanan KW, Kelly DF: Tracheal collapse in the dog, *J Am Vet Radiol Soc* 7:12-19, 1966.
7. Nelson AW: Lower respiratory system. In Slatter DH, editor: *Textbook of veterinary surgery*, Philadelphia, 1985, WB Saunders.
8. Dallman MJ, McClure RC, Brown EM: Histochemical study of normal and collapsed tracheas in dogs, *Am J Vet Res* 49(12):2117-2125, 1988.
9. Tangner CH, Hobson HP: A retrospective study of 20 surgically managed cases of collapsed trachea, *Vet Surg* 11:146-149, 1982.
10. Dallman MJ, Brown EM: Structural consideration in tracheal disease, *Am J Vet Res* 40(4):555-558, 1979.
11. Baumann R: Ueber die Dorso-Ventrale Abplastund der Luftrohre, *Berl Munch Lierarztl* 37:445-447, 1941.
12. Done SH, Clayton-Jones DG, Price EK: Tracheal collapse in the dog: A review of the literature and report of two new cases, *J Small Anim Pract* 11:743-750, 1970.
13. White RAS, Williams JM: Tracheal collapse in the dog—Is there really a role for surgery? A survey of 100 cases, *J Small Anim Pract* 35:191-196, 1994.
14. Dallman MJ, McClure RC, Brown EM: Normal and collapsed trachea in the dog. Scanning electronmicroscopy study, *Am J Vet Res* 46(10):2110-2115, 1985.
15. Walker TL: Upper respiratory obstruction, *Proc AAHA* 397-401, 1981.
16. Hobson HP: Total ring prosthesis for the surgical correction of collapsed trachea, *JAAHA* 12:822-828, 1976.
17. Robinson NE: Airway physiology, *VCNA* 22(5):1043-1064, 1992.
18. Spodnick GJ, Nwadike BS: Surgical management of extrathoracic tracheal collapse in two large-breed dogs, *J Am Vet Med Res* 211(12):1545-1548, 1997.
19. Yamamoto Y, Ootsuka T, Atoji Y et al: Tyrosine hydroxylase and neuropeptides immunoreactive nerves in canine trachea, *Am J Vet Res* 61(11):1380-1383, 2000.
20. Greenholz SK, Karrer FM, Lilly JR: Contemporary surgery of tracheomalacia, *J Pediat Surg* 21(6):511-514, 1986.
21. Vinograd I, Filler RM, Bahoric A: Long-term functional results of prosthetic airway splinting in tracheomalacia and bronchomalacia, *J Pediat Surg* 22(1):38-41, 1987.

22. Vinograd I, Filler RM, England SJ et al: Tracheomalacia: An experimental animal model for a new surgical approach, *J Surg Res* 42:597-604, 1987.

23. Sane DC, Vidaillet HJ, Burton CS: Saddle nose, red ears, and fatal airway collapse, *Chest* 91(2):268-270, 1987.

24. Schummacher HR: Relapsing polychrondritis. In Wyngaarden JB Smith LH, editors: *Cecil's textbook of medicine*, Philadelphia, 1988, WB Saunders.

25. Leonard HC: Collapse of the larynx and adjacent structures in the dog, *JAVMA* 137(6):360-363, 1960.

26. Leonard HC: Surgical correction of collapsed trachea in dogs, *JAVMA* 158(5):598-600, 1971.

27. Suter PF, Colgrove DJ, Ewing GO: Congenital hypoplasia of the canine trachea, *JAAHA* 8:120-127, 1972.

28. Harvey CE, Fink EA: Tracheal diameter: Analysis of radiographic measurements in brachycephalic and non-brachycephalic dogs, *JAAHA* 18:570-576, 1982.

29. Fingland RB, DeHoff WD, Birchard SJ: Surgical management of cervical and thoracic tracheal collapse in dogs using extraluminal spiral prostheses: Results in seven cases, *JAAHA* 23:173-181, 1987.

30. Knowles RP, Snyder CC: Chondrotomy for congenital tracheal stenosis, *Proc AAHA* 246-248, 1967.

31. McKiernan BC, Jones SD: Computerized tidal breathing flow-volume loop acquisition in the dog, *Proc of Sixth Vet Respir Symp*, 1987.

32. Rudorf H, Herrtage ME, White RA: Use of ultrasonography in the diagnosis of tracheal collapse, *J Small Anim Pract* 38(11):513-518, 1997.

33. Brock N: *Veterinary anesthesia update—Guidelines and protocols for safe small animal anesthesia*, Self-published 1994.

34. McKiernan BC, Smith AR, Kissil M: Bacterial isolates from the lower trachea of clinically healthy dogs, *JAAHA* 20:139-142, 1984.

35. McKiernan BC, Johnson LR: Clinical pulmonary function testing in dogs and cats, *VCNA* 22(5):1087-1099, 1992.

36. Amis TC, Kurpershock C: Tidal breathing flow-volume loop analysis for clinical assessment of airway obstruction in conscious dogs, *Am J Vet Res* 47(5):1002-1006, 1986.

37. Amis TC, Kurpershock C: Pattern of breathing in brachycephalic dogs, *Am J Vet Res* 47(10):2200-2204, 1986.

38. Amis TC, Smith MM, Gaber CE et al: Upper airway obstruction in canine laryngeal paralysis, *Am J Vet Res* 47(5):1007-1010, 1986.

39. Smith MM, Gourley IM, Amis TC et al: Management of tracheal stenosis in a dog, *JAVMA* 196(6):931-934, 1990.

40. Padrid PA, Hornof WJ, Kurpershock CJ et al: Canine chronic bronchitis—a pathophysiologic evaluation of 18 cases, *J Vet Int Med* 4:172-180, 1990.

41. McKiernan BC: Pulmonary function testing in dogs and cats: Techniques for clinical use, *Proc Tenth Vet Respir Symp*, 1991.

42. Fingland RB, DeHoff WD, Birchard SJ: Surgical management of cervical and thoracic tracheal collapse in dogs using extraluminal spiral prostheses, *JAHHA* 23:163-172, 1987.

43. Coyne BE, Fingland RB, Kennedy GA et al: Clinical and pathologic effects of a modified technique for application of spiral prostheses to the cervical trachea of dogs, *Vet Surg* 22(4):269-275, 1993.

44. Buback JL, Boothe HW, Hobson HP: Surgical treatment of tracheal collapse in dogs; 90 cases (1983-1993), *JAVMA* 208(3):380-384, 1996.

45. Fingland RB, Weisbrode SE, DeHoff WD: Clinical and pathologic effects of spiral and total ring prostheses applied to the cervical and thoracic portions of the trachea of dogs, *Am J Vet Res* 50(12):2168-2175, 1989.

46. Kirby BM, Bjorling DE, Rankin JH et al: The effects of surgical isolation and application of polypropylene spiral prostheses on tracheal bloodflow, *Vet Surg* 20(1):49-54, 1991.

47. Boothe DM, McKiernan BC: Respiratory therapeutics, *VCNA* 22(5):1231-1258, 1992.

48. Rubin GJ, Neal TM, Bojrab MJ: Surgical reconstruction for collapsed tracheal rings, *J Sm Anim Pract* 14:607-617, 1973.

49. Plumb DC: *Veterinary drug handbook*, ed 2, Ames, Iowa, 1995, Iowa State Press.

50. Ayers SA, Holmberg DL: Surgical treatment of tracheal collapse using pliable total ring prostheses: results in one experimental and 4 clinical cases, *Can Vet J* 40(11):787-791, 1999.

51. Schiller AG, Helper LC, Small E: Treatment of tracheal collapse in the dog, *JAVMA* 145(7):669-671, 1964.

52. White RN: Unilateral arytenoid lateralisation and extraluminal polypropylene ring prostheses for correction of tracheal collapse in the dog, *J Small Anim Pract* 36(4):151-158, 1995.

53. Wang Z, Perrault DF, Pankratov MM et al: Endoscopic laser-assisted reshaping of collapsed tracheal cartilage: A laboratory study, *Ann Otol Rhinol Laryngol* 105(3):176-181, 1996.

54. Villegas-Cabello O, Vazquez-Juarez JL, Gutierrez-Perez FM et al: Staged replacement of the canine trachea with ringed polyethylene terephthalate grafts, *Thorac Cardiovasc Surg* 42(5):302-305, 1994.

55. De Mello-Filho FV, Mamede RC, Sader AA et al: Use of the platysma myocutaneous flap for cervical trachea reconstruction: an experimental study in dogs, *Laryngoscope* 103(10):1161-1167, 1993.

56. Dumon JF: A dedicated tracheobronchial stent, *Chest* 97(2):328-332, 1990.

57. Colt HG, Dumon JF: A way to offer patients relief from persistent dyspnea? Airway obstruction in cancer; the pros and cons of stents, *J Respir Dis* 12(8):741-749, 1991.

58. Tsang V, Williams AM, Goldstraw P: Sequential silastic and expandable metal stenting for tracheobronchial strictures, *Ann Thorac Surg* 53(5):856-860, 1992.

59. Bollinger CT, Probst R, Tschopp K et al: Silicone endoprosthesis in the treatment of tracheobronchial stenosis. Report of the first 12 patients treated with this method, *Schweiz Med Wochenschr* 121(36):1283-1288, 1991.

60. Mason RA: *The installation of the Dumon silastic endotracheal stent in the normal canine airway and evaluation via pulmonary function testing*, DVSc Thesis, University of Guelph, 1994, Ontario Canada.

61. Radlinski MG, Fossum TW, Walker MA et al: Evaluation of the Palmaz stent in the trachea and mainstem bronchi of normal dogs, *Vet Surg* 26(2):99-107, 1997.

CHAPTER 47

Tracheal Hypoplasia

Robert A. Mason

Definition and Etiology

Tracheal hypoplasia is a condition of brachycephalic dogs in which the caliber of the tracheal lumen is congenitally undersized. This condition may occur as a separate problem or it may accompany other respiratory and cardiac congenital abnormalities. When it is present along with other anomalies, the combination may create a significant challenge to normal breathing.

Pathophysiology

Unlike segmental conditions such as collapsing trachea or tracheal stenosis, the trachea of dogs with tracheal hypoplasia (TH) is abnormally narrow for its entire length.[1] In the normal trachea, the cartilage rings are C-shaped. In contrast, tracheal cartilages in cases of hypoplasia form closed rings with virtually no dorsal tracheal muscle.[1]

In flow dynamics, the resistance to flow through a tube changes exponentially with the diameter of the tube, proportional to the radius to the fourth power. In other words, small decreases in the radius of a tube create massive increases in resistance to flow through that tube. For example, the difference between a 20-mm diameter trachea and an 18-mm diameter trachea represents a decrease of only 10% in diameter, but that small change results in a 56% increase in resistance to airflow.

When the tracheal diameter is decreased, the increased resistance to airflow requires the animal to increase both positive and negative intrapleural pressure (Ppl) during breathing to overcome that resistance. This can result in the classical breathing pattern of a *fixed upper airway obstruction*, with increased effort during both inspiratory and expiratory phases of respiration. Over time, these dramatic swings in Ppl can result in respiratory muscle fatigue, and eventually result in damage and scarring of the pleura and lung. End-stage changes (e.g., pulmonary fibrosis and emphysema) may result.[1] Patients with TH that develop clinical signs of respiratory disease typically tend to have other concurrent diseases, either other airway malformations or congenital cardiovascular anomalies.

Epidemiology

Affected breeds tend to favor chondrodystrophic body characteristics with brachycephalic conformation. One multi-institutional retrospective study of 103 dogs diagnosed with tracheal hypoplasia reported that 70% of cases occurred in two breeds; bulldogs accounted for 55% of cases, and Boston terriers for another 15%.[2] Suter reports that TH occurs with increased frequency in English bulldogs and bull mastiffs as an inherited familial abnormality.[1] The author has seen several affected miniature shar-peis. In the multi-institutional study, males were more often affected (66%) than females. The age range was 2 days to 12 years, with the median being 5 months.[2] Concurrent congenital brachycephalic airway anomalies included elongated soft palate (n=44) and stenotic nares (n=23). Nonrespiratory anomalies included cardiac defects in 12 cases, and megaesophagus in 10 cases.[2] Other affected breeds reported include Labrador retrievers, German shepherds, weimaraners, and bassett hounds.[1]

In humans, tracheal hypoplasia is rarely reported as a clinical entity. Tracheal agenesis/atresia is a rare congenital defect in human infants, characterized by respiratory distress, absence of crying, and impossible intubation in the newborn.[3] This syndrome has been reported only 87 times since its initial report in 1900,[3] and typically has fatal consequences.[4]

Historical Findings and Clinical Signs

Common presenting complaints include exertional expiratory and inspiratory dyspnea, decreased exercise tolerance, and recurrent respiratory tract infection.[1] Chronic bronchopneumonia may result in stunted body growth.[1] The individual dog with a sedentary lifestyle may have no obvious exercise intolerance, or conversely, the dog's lack of activity may be caused by its diminished tracheal caliber. In Coyne's report of 103 affected dogs, of the 42 reexamined more than 6 months after diagnosis, 25 dogs (60%) were clinically normal. Of the remaining 17 dyspneic cases, 15 of them (88%) had concurrent respiratory or cardiovascular disease that could account for all of their clinical signs.[2] The authors concluded that tracheal hypoplasia appears to be well tolerated in the absence of concurrent respiratory or cardiovascular disease.[2]

Physical Examination

Affected dogs may be completely normal on physical examination. *Cor pulmonale,* or right-sided heart failure secondary to pulmonary hypertension, may arise from chronic dyspnea associated with major airway narrowing.[5] In such cases, delayed closure of the pulmonic valve may lead to a split second heart sound on auscultation. Abnormal lung sounds may be present, caused by bronchopneumonia or chronic lung disease; and murmurs or dysrhythmias may accompany concurrent heart disease. Palpation of the trachea may reveal a decreased diameter and increased firmness.

Differential Diagnosis

The list of differential diagnoses in the brachycephalic dog with fixed upper airway obstruction should also include brachycephalic airway obstructive syndrome; laryngeal disease (e.g., collapse, paresis, or paralysis); tracheal collapse; chronic bronchitis; infectious tracheobronchitis; heartworm disease; primary pulmonary disease; primary cardiovascular disease; and intrinsic or extrinsic tracheal obstruction.[5] Besides the history and clinical examination, the most useful diagnostic tests include radiography (both inspiratory and expiratory) and pulmonary function testing.[5-9]

Diagnostic Tests

RADIOGRAPHY

Lateral radiographs of the neck and chest are commonly employed in the diagnosis and staging of TH. Objective criteria for assessing normal tracheal diameter on plain radiographs have been advocated.[1,10] On lateral survey radiographs of the neck and thorax, the normal trachea should be equal to the diameter of the laryngeal lumen at the level of the cricoid cartilage.[1] Because tracheal size varies with breed, an arbitrary guideline was proposed that a reduction of the tracheal diameter to one-half or less of the laryngeal airway should be considered abnormal.[1] Alternatively, the trachea should be three times the diameter of the proximal one-third of the third rib.[1]

Harvey and Fink proposed a modification of these measurements to correlate tracheal dimensions with body size.[10] A ratio of the internal tracheal diameter to the distance between the ventral edge of the first thoracic vertebra and the dorsal edge of the manubrium can be calculated: 0.16 or greater is considered normal (Figure 47-1).[10] Bulldogs have significantly smaller ratios than other breeds.[10]

Superimposition of overlying structures such as the esophagus, fat, or the *longus colli* muscles can lead to a false positive interpretation of the tracheal diameter.[6,7,11] Suter reports that the reduced tracheal lumen can be seen in both lateral and ventrodorsal projections extending from the cricoid cartilage through to the tracheal bifurcation.[1] In most affected dogs, the mainstem bronchi are larger than the trachea.[1]

These criteria are used in the diagnosis of tracheal hypoplasia, where the trachea is narrow for its entire length,[1,10,12] as opposed to focal tracheal narrowing (e.g.,

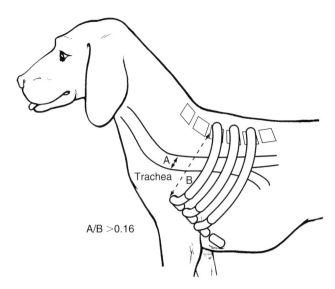

Figure 47-1. *Ratio of the internal tracheal diameter to the thoracic inlet proposed by Harvey and Fink,[10] based on the lateral thoracic radiograph. A = Tracheal diameter, B = distance from ventral edge of T1 to the dorsal edge of the manubrium. A/B greater than 0.16 is considered normal.*

because of tracheal collapse or stenosis). One criticism of these measurements is that they do not take into account various other parameters that affect resistance to airflow, such as concurrent airway disease. Dynamic narrowing of the trachea may occur in animals that are making efforts to inhale against a fixed upper airway obstruction (e.g., brachycephalic airway syndrome). This may cause some radiographic narrowing of the trachea that could result in overestimation of the severity of tracheal hypoplasia.

Interestingly, in Coyne's large retrospective study, neither ratio of tracheal luminal diameter (i.e., to the depth of the thoracic inlet or to the width of the third rib) correlated with the degree of dyspnea.[2]

Radiographs of the chest are also useful in the diagnosis of concurrent problems (e.g., cardiovascular, pulmonary, or small airway disease).[5,6,8,9,13] Associated lesions include aortic stenosis, mitral valve insufficiency, heart failure, pulmonic stenosis, and myocarditis.[1]

TRACHEOBRONCHOSCOPY

The advent of tracheobronchoscopy has had a major impact on the diagnosis, staging, and understanding of the pathophysiology of tracheal disease in the dog. Endoscopic examination is performed under general anesthesia.[5,7-9,11] Because other forms of upper airway obstruction may be found concurrent with TH, pharyngoscopy, laryngoscopy, and bronchoscopy are commonly included as part of the complete airway examination.[5,7,12,13] Laryngeal function should be assessed for potential laryngeal paresis during anesthetic induction.[5,7,9,14]

Anesthetic considerations include awareness of the increased vagal tone in these patients, the presence of possible *cor pulmonale* or secondary right heart disease, and concurrent small airway disease such as chronic bronchitis and bronchoconstriction. Preoxygenation via face mask, if not too stressful to the patient, is recommended.[15] Narcotic antitussives, bronchodilators, and anticholinergics should be considered as part of the drug protocol. Endotracheal intubation can be challenging because the tube size needed is generally much smaller than one would typically select for a patient of that size. Careful visual examination of the laryngeal structures with a laryngoscope is vital, and care must be taken not to traumatize the larynx in an attempt to intubate the airway. The step of intubation for routine procedures such as neuter surgery may, in fact, be the very first indication of decreased tracheal size in TH patients.

Extubation of these patients upon recovery can be a critical step. Prolonged intubation postprocedure with the aid of narcotic sedation (e.g., butorphanol or meperidine), and strict and close patient monitoring during this period is advised.[15] Short-acting glucocorticoids may be used to decrease airway swelling at the end of the procedure. If unfamiliar with these cases, consult a veterinary anesthesiologist regarding a safe induction, maintenance, and recovery protocol.[15]

PULMONARY FUNCTION TESTING

Pulmonary function testing has recently been employed to evaluate tracheobronchial obstruction in dogs.[7,16-24] In particular, tidal breathing flow-volume loop (TBFVL) analysis has been adapted for this purpose.[17] In short, tracheal hypoplasia represents a fixed, nondynamic obstruction and may result in blunting or flattening of both the inspiratory and expiratory portions of the flow loop (Figure 47-2).[17]

Because TBFVL analysis is a noninvasive procedure that can be performed on the awake, untrained individual, it offers promise as an objective clinical measurement of the severity of dysfunction associated with tracheal hypoplasia, as well as providing an objective measure of improvement or progression of the disease with therapy.

Management and Monitoring

MEDICAL MANAGEMENT

Medical therapy for tracheal hypoplasia is symptomatic and palliative, not curative. Because the hypoplastic trachea is a *physical* obstruction, medications are generally ineffective at addressing the root cause. Most clinically dyspneic patients have concurrent cardiorespiratory disease, and treatment strategies are often aimed at these issues rather than the TH. Diagnosis and management of concurrent heart disease may be a vital part of successful treatment in these patients. Classically, dogs with clinical signs may be treated with a combination of antitussives, bronchodilators, corticosteroid antiinflammatories, antibiotics, and sedatives,[5-9,11,13] although no controlled clinical trials of any form of therapy have been reported. Very few animals require all of the above therapies, and treatment is tailored to the individual.

Weight control may play a vital role in obese patients. Controlling obesity,[5,6,11,13] improving the ventilation and air quality in the environment of affected individuals,[6,13] and using a chest harness instead of neck leashes[6] have all been reported as adjunct medical therapies. Control of any associated endocrine disorders such as hypothyroidism or hyperadrenocorticism (that may predispose to obesity) or other complicating factors (e.g., chronic bronchitis and tracheomalacia with hyperadrenocorticism) may also play an important role in control of clinical signs.

SURGICAL MANAGEMENT

There are no surgical options for specific treatment of TH. Associated brachycephalic airway syndrome should be addressed surgically. Stenotic nares, elongated soft palate, and laryngeal eversion may all have excellent response to surgery. Laryngeal collapse, however, carries a grave prognosis even with surgery.[25]

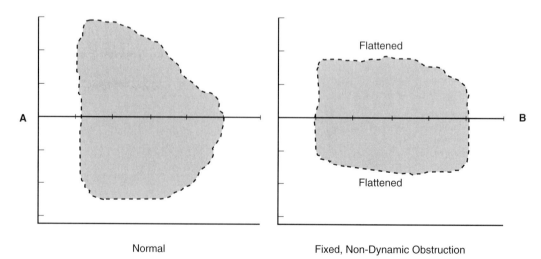

Normal — Fixed, Non-Dynamic Obstruction

Figure 47-2. Tidal breathing flow-volume loops (TBFVL) as a noninvasive pulmonary function test. *A,* Normal TBFVL in a dog. *B,* Fixed, nondynamic obstruction that results in "flattening" of both the inspiratory and expiratory portions of the TBFVL. Tracheal hypoplasia creates this latter pattern.

Prognosis

The prognosis for dogs with tracheal hypoplasia is directly correlated to its clinical severity, as well as to the presence of other risk factors such as the degree of obesity and concurrent cardiac or respiratory disease. Coyne reported that, of 42 of 103 affected dogs reexamined 6 months after diagnosis, 60% were clinically normal.[2] It is not clear whether the remaining 61 cases were lost to follow-up or did not survive. That study demonstrated, however, that there was no clear correlation between the measured radiographic ratios and the clinical severity of the disorder.[2]

REFERENCES

1. Suter PF: Diseases of the nasal cavity, larynx, and trachea. In Suter PF, editor: *Thoracic radiography, a text atlas of thoracic disease of the dog and cat,* Weltswil, Switzerland, 1984, Peter F. Suter.
2. Coyne BE, Finland RB: Hypoplasia of the trachea in dogs: 103 cases (1974-1990), *JAVMA,* 201(5):768-772, 1992.
3. Siala SG, Masmoudi A, Ben Hassine L et al: Tracheal atresia: A case report, *Tunis Med* 79(6-7):393-397, 2001.
4. Hill SA, Milam M, Manaligod JM: Tracheal agenesis: diagnosis and management, *Int J Pediatr Otorhinolaryngol* 31:59(1):63-68, 2001.
5. Hedlund CS: Tracheal collapse, *Prob Vet Med* 3(2):229-238, 1991.
6. Spaulding GL: Medical management considerations for upper airway disease, *Respir Med* 4(2):419-428, 1992.
7. Padrid P, Amis TC: Chronic tracheobronchial disease in the dog, *Vet Clin North Am Small Anim Pract* 22(5):1203-1229, 1992.
8. Amis TC: Tracheal collapse in the dog, *Austral Vet J* 50:285-289, 1974.
9. Tangner CH, Hobson HP: A retrospective study of 20 surgically managed cases of collapsed trachea, *Vet Surg* 11:146-149, 1982.
10. Harvey CE, Fink EA: Tracheal diameter: analysis of radiographic measurements in brachycephalic and non-brachycephalic dogs, *JAAHA* 18:570-576, 1982.
11. O'Brien JA, Buchanan KW, Kelly DF: Tracheal collapse in the dog, *J Am Vet Radiol Soc* 7:12-19, 1966.
12. Nelson AW: Lower respiratory system. In Slatter DH, editor: *Textbook of veterinary surgery,* Philadelphia, 1985, WB Saunders.
13. White RAS, Williams JM: Tracheal collapse in the dog—Is there really a role for surgery? A survey of 100 cases, *J Small Anim Pract* 35:191-196, 1994.
14. Hobson HP: Total ring prosthesis for the surgical correction of collapsed trachea, *JAAHA* 12:822-828, 1976.
15. Brock N: *Veterinary anesthesia update,* self-published, Dr. Nancy Brock, 1-800-338-9986, 10100 Westminster Highway, Richmond, BC, Canada, V6X 1B2.
16. Robinson NE. Airway physiology: *Vet Clin North Am Small Anim Pract* 22(5):1043-1064, 1992.
17. McKiernan BC, Johnson LR: Clinical pulmonary function testing in dogs and cats, *Vet Clin North Am Small Anim Pract* 22(5):1087-1099, 1992.
18. Amis TC, Kurpershock C: Tidal breathing flow-volume loop analysis for clinical assessment of airway obstruction in conscious dogs, *Am J Vet Res* 47(5):1002-1006, 1986.
19. McKiernan BC, Jones SD: Computerized tidal breathing flow-volume loop acquisition in the dog, *Proc of 6th Vet Respir Symp,* 1987.
20. Amis TC, Kurpershock C: Pattern of breathing in brachycephalic dogs, *Am J Vet Res* 47(10):2200-2204, 1986.
21. Amis TC, Smith MM, Gaber CE et al: Upper airway obstruction in canine laryngeal paralysis, *Am J Vet Res* 47(5):1007-1010, 1986.
22. Smith MM, Gourley IM, Amis TC et al: Management of tracheal stenosis in a dog, *JAVMA* 196(6):931-934, 1990.
23. Padrid PA, Hornof WJ, Kurpershock CJ et al: Canine chronic bronchitis—a pathophysiologic evaluation of 18 cases, *J Vet Int Med* 4:172-180, 1990.
24. McKiernan BC: Pulmonary function testing in dogs and cats: Techniques for clinical use, *Proc 10th Vet Respir Symp,* 1991.
25. Fossum T: Laryngeal collapse. In Fossum T, editor: *Small animal surgery,* St Louis, 1997, CV Mosby.

CHAPTER 48

Tracheal Trauma

David E. Holt

Definition and Etiology

Tracheal trauma occurs when compressive, tensile, or shearing forces either cause tracheal perforation or compromise the trachea's structural integrity. In both dogs and cats, tracheal trauma can result from crushing injuries or penetrating missiles.[1-4] In cats specifically, intrathoracic tracheal disruption has been associated with blunt trauma.[5-12] Bite wounds and missiles can generate both compressive and shearing forces on the trachea. Tensile forces are generated during avulsion injuries or by endotracheal tube cuff overinflation. Cervical and intrathoracic tracheal tears[13-15] and strictures[16] have been associated with intubation.

Pathophysiology and Incidence

The trachea is composed of many incomplete C-shaped hyaline cartilage rings connected dorsally by the tracheal muscle. The cartilages are lined with ciliated epithelium; mucosa; and a submucosa made up of elastic fibers, fat cells, and tubular seromucinous glands. Cartilages are connected to each other by fibroelastic annular ligaments.[17] The teeth of an attacking animal can penetrate the interannular ligaments or the cartilage. Bite wounds can also crush or fracture tracheal cartilage. Blunt trauma can result in segmental tracheal collapse.[3]

Intrathoracic tracheal rupture has been associated with blunt trauma episodes such as automobile accidents. It is theorized that hyperextension of the neck occurs during the traumatic episode and because the carina is fixed, the trachea ruptures just cranial to this point as it is violently stretched.[5,18] Some of these injuries (and other concurrent injuries) are probably fatal; however, in some cats, the peritracheal adventitia or mediastinum maintains the continuity of the intrathoracic airway, allowing the animal to breathe. Initially, many cats do not have marked dyspnea.[5] It is speculated that dyspnea develops several days after the trauma because of stenosis or displacement of the proximal and distal tracheal segments.[18]

Tracheal tears occur secondary to intubation because of overinflation of the endotracheal tube cuff.[13] Although other mechanisms of injury (e.g., improper tube placement, injury from the use of a stylet, and failure to deflate the cuff before repositioning or removing the tube) have been suggested as causes for iatrogenic tracheal rupture, only cuff overinflation produced tracheal rupture in cadavers similar to that seen in clinical cases.[13] Low-volume, high-pressure cuffs may be more prone to cause rupture than high-volume, low-pressure cuffs. In the majority of clinical cases reported, the tracheal ruptures occurred in animals after dental procedures.[13-15] Presumably ruptures occurred in these cases when cuffs were inflated excessively because of concern for fluid leakage around the endotracheal tube.

Historical Findings, Clinical Signs, and Progression

Cats with intrathoracic tracheal rupture can present with a known history of trauma (e.g., fall, motor vehicle accident) or return home after a variable period of absence. In animals with an uncertain history, a finding of avulsed or abraded nails indicates possible trauma. The clinical signs of tracheal trauma can be mild and masked by the signs of other injuries.[5] Clinical signs of shock or of neurologic and musculoskeletal injury are often present concurrently. Respiratory signs (e.g., increased respiratory effort, dyspnea, exercise intolerance, open-mouthed breathing with exertion, and cyanosis) can be present immediately[6] or develop days to weeks after the trauma.[5] Finding subcutaneous emphysema on examination is a strong indicator of tracheal trauma (Figure 48-1). Other respiratory injuries, including pneumothorax and pulmonary contusions, can also be present.[5]

Animals with tracheal collapse or stenosis secondary to trauma can present with dyspnea developing over

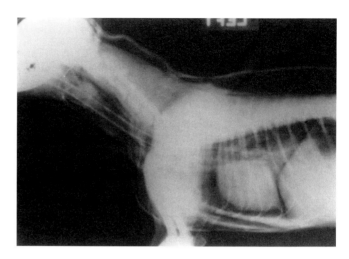

Figure 48-1. *Severe subcutaneous emphysema in a dog with a trachea that was lacerated by a bite.*

days to weeks.[2,3,11] The owner may or may not be able to relate a history of trauma. Stridor on inspiration, indicative of upper airway obstruction, is often audible. Affected animals may not tolerate exertion and may become cyanotic when stressed.[11]

Cats with tracheal rupture secondary to intubation invariably have moderate to marked subcutaneous emphysema,[13,14] which is usually apparent either during or immediately after the anesthetic episode. Other intermittent clinical signs include dyspnea, anorexia, coughing, and respiratory stridor.[13,14]

Differential Diagnosis

Subcutaneous emphysema after an anesthetic procedure can also be caused by barotrauma.[18] This can occur in anesthetized animals on high flows of oxygen when the anesthetic machine pop-off valve is closed. Overinflation of the lungs causes marginal alveoli to rupture; air escapes through the base of marginal alveoli into perivascular or peribronchial connective tissue sheaths and migrates into the mediastinum and cervical tissue planes.[19] Other causes of subcutaneous emphysema include perforation of the larynx or esophagus, and severe cervical bite wounds. Cervical subcutaneous emphysema and dyspnea have also been reported in association with tracheoesophageal fistulas.[20]

The inspiratory stridor seen in some animals with tracheal stenosis secondary to trauma could also be associated with laryngeal diseases (e.g., paralysis, trauma, and neoplasia), pharyngeal diseases (e.g., injury, foreign body, and neoplasia), insect inhalation or perhaps other allergic reactions, and foreign body obstruction of the trachea or bronchi.

Animals with intrathoracic tracheal rupture usually present dyspneic with little stridor and no subcutaneous emphysema. Similar clinical signs might be seen in animals with airway foreign bodies;[21] laryngeal, tracheal, or bronchial tumors;[22] eosinophilic tracheal granuloma;[23]

parasitic infestation of the trachea;[24,25] anticoagulant rodenticide intoxication;[26] tracheal polyps;[27] or tracheal cuterebriasis.[28] Intrathoracic tracheal compression by esophageal foreign bodies or mediastinal tumors, abscesses, or hematomas; pneumothorax; pleural effusion; and diaphragmatic herniation might also cause similar clinical signs.

Diagnostic Tests

In many cases, the diagnosis can be suspected from the history and physical examination findings. The tests used to confirm the diagnosis of tracheal trauma are often determined by the severity of the animal's respiratory distress. Plain lateral radiographs of the thorax and neck will often provide a clear indication of tracheal disruption, particularly in cats with intrathoracic tracheal avulsion (Figure 48-2). In these animals, either the interruption of the trachea or the bulging peritracheal or mediastinal tissues surrounding the rupture are clearly visible. However, in other cases, the subcutaneous emphysema and pneumomediastinum associated with the tracheal damage make identifying the specific area of tracheal rupture extremely difficult.

Animals that are extremely dyspneic require anesthesia and intubation. Although this is often a necessity, intubation must be performed with extreme care if tracheal disruption is suspected. A tube substantially smaller than the tracheal lumen should be used. In animals with cervical or cranial thoracic tracheal disruption, passage of a large endotracheal tube could cause complete disruption and separation of the tracheal ends, leaving the animal with no means of ventilating. The larynx and pharynx should be quickly inspected at intubation for evidence of trauma, perforation, neoplasia, or laryngeal paralysis and the tube passed only into the larynx and proximal trachea. Ideally, the plane of anesthesia should be light enough for the animal to maintain spontaneous respiration. Positive pressure ventilation should be avoided if possible, but if the animal is not spontaneously breathing, assisted breaths should be given with minimal pressure. In cats with complete intrathoracic tracheal disruption, positive pressure ventilation can "blow out" the tenuous membrane of mediastinum that has been maintaining airway continuity; thus effective ventilation of the lungs ceases and a rapidly worsening pneumothorax develops. Respiratory failure and death ensue.

Pharyngoscopy, laryngoscopy, esophagoscopy, and tracheobronchoscopy may be necessary to confirm a diagnosis of tracheal rupture and rule out other possible causes of the clinical signs. The larynx and laryngeal function can only be briefly inspected before intubation of dyspneic animals. Once the animal is intubated and breathing spontaneously a gentle, thorough examination of the pharynx is performed, initially using a laryngoscope blade with a bright light source. The area dorsal to the soft palate can be inspected using either a small spay hook to retract the palate rostrally, or a flexible fiberoptic endoscope. Esophagoscopy is performed if a perforation of the esophagus is the suspected source of pneu-

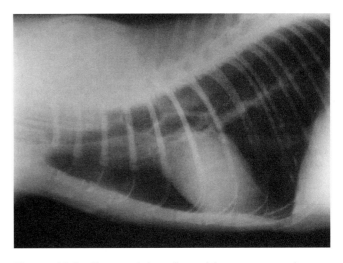

Figure 48-2. *Characteristic radiographic appearance of a ruptured intrathoracic trachea in a cat. Note the discontinuity of the trachea and the interposed "bubble" of mediastinal tissue.* (Courtesy of Dr. Daniel Brockman, Royal Veterinary College, London, England.)

momediastinum, or if an esophageal foreign body is suspected as a cause of tracheal compression.

In medium and large breed dogs, the trachea can be examined by passing an endoscope through the endotracheal tube. In small breed dogs and cats, the animal must be briefly extubated to allow passage of a small bronchoscope or cystoscope. Anesthesia must therefore be maintained with injectable agents in these animals. The endoscope must be passed down the trachea carefully to avoid worsening a tracheal tear or creating a pneumothorax. Positive contrast tracheography has been performed during tracheoscopy to radiographically delineate a tracheal stricture.[11,29]

Management and Monitoring

Anesthesia and intubation concerns in animals with tracheal tears are mentioned above. High frequency jet ventilation has been used to manage two cases of segmental tracheal stenosis,[10] but this technology is not widely available. In animals in which tracheal disruption is confirmed prior to anesthesia, the ventral cervical area and right thoracic wall should be clipped prior to induction of anesthesia, if this can be accomplished without further stressing a dyspneic animal. As soon as the animal is intubated, the anesthetist and surgeon should watch carefully for thoracic wall movement and spontaneous respiration. If the animal breathes spontaneously and pulse oximetry or arterial blood gas analysis indicates effective blood oxygenation, the tracheal tear can be approached as a more elective procedure.

If, however, the animal is not spontaneously ventilating and the thoracic wall does not move with gentle positive pressure ventilation, the correct position of the endotracheal tube in the larynx should be quickly checked. If the endotracheal tube is correctly placed in the larynx, but the animal is unable to ventilate effectively, an endotracheal tube must be immediately surgically placed distal to the tracheal tear.

In animals with confirmed cervical tears, the trachea is approached by a midline ventral cervical incision. In animals with intrathoracic tracheal avulsion, the trachea is approached via a right lateral third or fourth intercostal space thoracotomy. The distal end of the trachea is located; this is often difficult in intrathoracic tears because the mediastinum obscures the trachea. A sterile endotracheal tube is placed in the distal trachea, connected to the anesthetic machine, and ventilation is reestablished.

Cervical tracheal tears are most often associated with bite wounds, penetrating missile injuries, or endotracheal tube cuff overinflation. In animals with bite wounds and penetrating missile injury, tracheal repair is combined with culture, debridement, lavage, and repair of the associated soft tissue injuries. During surgical exploration, vital cervical structures (e.g., the recurrent laryngeal nerves, carotid arteries, and vagosympathetic trunks) must be identified and preserved. The trachea is carefully examined along its length. In animals with small tracheal lacerations, the endotracheal tube is passed beyond the damaged segment under direct surgical visualization and guidance. Small lacerations are debrided back to healthy, bleeding tissue and closed using 5/0 to 3/0 monofilament absorbable suture, depending on the animal's size.

In animals with extensive tracheal injury, a sterile endotracheal tube is placed into the trachea via a tracheostomy made at the expected distal site of tracheal resection. The tube is connected to the anesthetic machine using sterile tubing. The orally placed endotracheal tube is left in place and is used during closure. The devitalized segment of trachea is resected, leaving proximal and distal ends to be anastomosed. In medium and large breed dogs, a split cartilage technique should be used for anastomosis. The tracheal cartilage at the proximal and distal ends of the anastomosis is split circumferentially using a number 11 scalpel blade. The two remaining tracheal cartilage halves are apposed by preplacing 8 to 12 sutures of 4/0 to 3/0 monofilament absorbable material around the opposite cartilage halves and through the dorsal tracheal membrane on either side of the anastomosis. A split cartilage anastomosis technique is preferred because it results in better alignment and apposition of the tracheal ends, and in less long-term luminal stenosis than the annular ligament and cartilage technique.[30] In smaller dogs and cats, the tracheal cartilages may not be wide enough to be split without fragmentation. In these animals, the trachea is resected by incising the annular ligament between the cartilage rings. Sutures are pre-placed around the proximal and distal cartilage rings. The orally placed endotracheal tube is advanced across the anastomosis site if it is long enough, and the tracheostomy tube removed. If the orally placed tube is not long enough, the tracheostomy tube remains in place while the dorsal anastomosis sutures are tied. It is then removed and the ventral sutures are rapidly tied, re-establishing airway continuity and al-

lowing effective ventilation through the orally placed endotracheal tube.

In cats with tracheal tears secondary to intubation, both surgical and conservative management have been reported.[13-15] In one report, all cats (n = 7) that were treated conservatively with cage rest survived; clinical signs took 2 days to 5 weeks to resolve.[13] The majority of cats treated surgically (6/9) in the same report also survived.[13] Attempted surgical repairs of tears extending to the carina were unsuccessful. In a second report, 15 cats with moderate dyspnea were successfully treated with medical management.[14] This included cage rest in all cats, and supplemental oxygen (n = 3), sedatives (n = 2), and respiratory monitoring (n = 6) in some cats. Cats with severe respiratory distress, cyanosis unresponsive to oxygen supplementation, and worsening subcutaneous emphysema were treated surgically.[14] Surgical treatment was successful in 3 of 4 cats. All ruptures treated surgically in the second report were identified at the thoracic inlet on the dorsolateral aspect of the trachea at the junction of the tracheal rings and the trachealis muscle.[14] Definitive indications for surgical management of tracheal tears secondary to intubation have not been developed. From these reports, however, potential indications for surgery would include severe dyspnea and dyspnea worsening with conservative management. The possibility of clinically significant tracheal stricture formation with conservative management is not known, but seems minimal from the information available.[13,14]

Surgical repair of cervical tracheal tears is performed via a ventral midline cervical incision. Splitting the first several sternebrae may also be required for access.[13,14] Tears associated with intubation invariably involve the trachealis muscle. The trachea should be exposed and rotated so that the dorsal tracheal membrane is visible. The tissues are sutured using 5/0 or 4/0 monofilament absorbable suture.

Intrathoracic tracheal disruptions are approached via a right lateral thoracotomy. The third or fourth intercostal space is normally used; for more exposure, the third or fourth rib can be resected. Ideally, the animal should breathe spontaneously until the pleural space is opened, then breaths should be given with the minimum amount of positive pressure needed to maintain effective ventilation. The trachea lies dorsal to the cranial vena cava in the mediastinum. It may not be visible because of scarring and hemorrhage in the mediastinum. Sterile endotracheal tubes of several appropriate sizes should be available on the surgery table before dissecting the mediastinum.

As soon the mediastinum is opened, the distal trachea must be located and intubated as quickly as possible. The thoracic endotracheal tube is connected to the anesthetic machine with sterile hoses. The ends of the trachea are debrided and apposed using single interrupted 5/0 to 3/0 monofilament absorbable sutures, depending on the size of the animal. The sutures should be pre-placed, and the medial sutures tied first. The thoracic endotracheal tube is removed and the lateral sutures rapidly tied. The orally placed endotracheal tube is used to assist ventilation. A chest tube is placed and the thoracotomy closed in a routine manner.

Tracheal strictures have been reported in the cervical,[2] thoracic inlet,[12] and intrathoracic[10,11,16,29] sections of the trachea. Stricture resection has been described; the approaches and anastomosis techniques are similar to those described previously for tracheal tears and avulsions. Tracheal resection and anastomosis is also described to treat traumatic tracheal collapse.[3] The length of the stenotic area should be carefully considered when planning a resection. Puppies and adult dogs can tolerate resection of 20% to 25%, and 25% to 50% of the trachea, respectively.[31,32]

Successful balloon dilation of a tracheal stricture involving the carina of a cat has been described.[11] The balloon dilation catheter was passed through the lumen of the endotracheal tube and dilation was accomplished under direct visualization via a thoracotomy. Balloon dilation may also be performed using fluoroscopic or endoscopic guidance.

Outcome and Prognosis

The success of treating tracheal trauma depends largely on appropriate emergency and anesthetic case management. The majority of cases in which the trachea is repaired will recover well and breathe normally. Stenosis after resection and anastomosis is an uncommon complication.[2] The results of conservative versus surgical management of tracheal tears caused by overinflation of the endotracheal tube cuff have been discussed earlier. Such injuries are far better prevented than treated. The use of an appropriately sized endotracheal tube; high-volume, low-pressure cuffs; and the minimum volume of air in the cuff necessary to create an airtight seal (0 to 3 ml in cats)[13] should prevent this iatrogenic injury.

REFERENCES

1. Kellagher REB, White RAS: Tracheal rupture in a dog, *J Small Anim Pract* 28:29, 1987.
2. Smith MM, Gourley IM, Amis TC et al: Management of tracheal stenosis in a dog, *J Am Vet Med Assoc* 196:931, 1990.
3. Bradley RL, Schaaf JP: Tracheal resection and anastomosis for traumatic tracheal collapse in a dog, *Comp Contin Educ Pract Vet* 9:234, 1987.
4. Caylor KB, Moore RW: What is your diagnosis? (Severed trachea in cat attacked by dogs), *J Am Vet Med Assoc* 205:561, 1994.
5. Lawrence DT, Lang J, Culvenor J et al: Intrathoracic tracheal rupture, *J Feline Med Surg* 1:43, 1999.
6. White RN, Milner HR: Intrathoracic tracheal avulsion in three cats, *J Small Anim Pract* 36:343, 1995.
7. Jorger VK, Fluckiger M, Geret U: Ruptur der trachea bei drei katzen, *Berl Munch Tierarztl Wschr* 101:128, 1988.
8. Brouwer GJ, Burbidge HM, Jones DE: Tracheal rupture in a cat, *J Small Anim Pract* 25:71, 1984.
9. Kennedy RK: Traumatic tracheal separation with diverticuli in a cat, *Vet Med Sm Anim Clin* 71:1384, 1976.
10. Whitfield JB, Graves GM, Lappin MR et al: Anesthetic and surgical management of intrathroracic segmental tracheal stenosis utilizing high-frequency jet ventilation, *J Am Anim Hosp Assoc* 25:443, 1989.
11. Berg J, Leveille CR, O'Callaghan MW: Treatment of posttraumatic carinal stenosis by balloon dilation during thoracotomy in a cat, *J Am Vet Med Assoc* 198:1025, 1991.
12. Corcoran BM: Posttraumatic tracheal stenosis in a cat, *Vet Rec* 124:342, 1989.
13. Hardie EM, Spodnick GJ, Gilson SD et al: Tracheal rupture in cats: 16 cases, *J Am Vet Med Assoc* 214:508, 1999.
14. Mitchell SL, McCarthy R, Rudloff E et al: Tracheal rupture associated with intubation in cats: 20 cases (1996-1998), *J Am Vet Med Assoc* 216:1592, 2000.
15. Wong WT, Brock KA: Tracheal laceration from endotracheal intubation in a cat, *Vet Rec* 134:622, 1994.
16. McMillan FD: Iatrogenic tracheal stenosis in a cat, *J Am Anim Hosp Assoc* 21:747, 1985.
17. Hare WCD: Carnivore respiratory system. In Getty R, editor: *The anatomy of the domestic animals*, Philadelphia, 1975, WB Saunders.
18. Nelson AW: Lower respiratory system. In Slatter DH, editor: *Textbook of small animal surgery*, ed 2, Philadelphia, 1993, WB Saunders.
19. Brown D, Holt DE: Subcutaneous emphysema, pneumothorax, pneumomediastinum and pneumopericardium in a cat: A case of barotrauma, *J Am Vet Med Assoc* 206:997, 1995.
20. Freeman LM, Rush JE, Schelling SH et al: Tracheoesophageal fistula in two cats, *J Am Anim Hosp Assoc* 29:531, 1993.
21. Lotti U, Niebauer GW: Tracheobronchial foreign bodies of plant origin in 153 hunting dogs, *Comp Cont Ed Pract Vet* 14:7, 1992.
22. Carlisle CH, Biery DN, Thrall DE: Tracheal and laryngeal tumors of the dog and cat: Literature review and 13 additional patients, *Vet Radiol* 32:229, 1991.
23. Brovida C, Castagnaro M: Tracheal obstruction due to an eosinophilic granuloma in a dog: Surgical treatment and clinicopathological observations, *J Am Anim Hosp Assoc* 28:8, 1992.
24. Metcalfe SS: Filaroides osleri in a dog, *Aust Vet Pract* 27:65, 1997.
25. Cobb MA, Fischer MA: Crenosoma vulpis infection in a dog, *Vet Rec* 130:452, 1992.
26. Blocker TL, Roberts BK: Acute tracheal obstruction associated with anticoagulant rodenticide intoxication in a dog, *J Small Anim Pract* 40:577, 1999.
27. Sheaffer KA, Dillon AR: Obstructive tracheal mass due to an inflammatory polyp in a cat, *J Am Anim Hosp Assoc* 32:431, 1996.
28. Fitzgerald SD, Johnson CA, Peck EJ: A fatal case of intrathoracic cuterebriasis in a cat, *J Am Anim Hosp Assoc* 32:353, 1996.
29. Hauptman J, White JV, Slocombe RF: Intrathoracic tracheal stricture management in a dog, *J Am Anim Hosp Assoc* 21:505, 1985.
30. Hedlund CS: Tracheal anastomosis in the dog: Comparison of two end-to-end techniques, *Vet Surg* 13:135, 1984.
31. Maeda M, Grillo HC: Effect of tension on tracheal growth after resection and anastomosis in puppies, *J Thoracic Cardiovasc Surg* 65:658, 1973.
32. Cantrall JR, Folse JR: The repair of circumferential defects of the trachea by direct anastomosis: Experimental evaluation, *J Thoracic Cardiovasc Surg* 42:589, 1961.

CHAPTER 49

Infectious Tracheobronchitis

Richard B. Ford

Introduction

Infectious tracheobronchitis (ITB), also called kennel cough, canine cough, or canine croup, is an acute, highly contagious respiratory infection of dogs characterized by paroxysmal cough, typically without signs of pneumonia. Fever, anorexia, and lethargy are commonly observed among infected dogs during outbreaks. Knowledge of recent contact with dogs, especially coughing dogs, becomes an important historical feature in establishing a clinical diagnosis. Dogs with complicated infections may develop a purulent to mucopurulent nasal and ocular discharge; pneumonia; respiratory distress; and, occasionally, death.

First associated with canine distemper infection in the early 1900s, it is only since the 1970s that new information on the pathogenesis of this complex respiratory infection has been described and that significant improvements in treatment and vaccination have been made. Despite these advancements, infectious tracheobronchitis continues to pose a threat to susceptible dogs, particularly those residing in shelters, boarding kennels, and veterinary hospitals. Although sporadic in nature, outbreaks of ITB are still most likely to occur among dogs housed in groups or clusters. Clinical infections are attributed to one or a combination of bacterial and/or viral agents capable of colonizing the epithelium of the upper respiratory tract, trachea, bronchi, bronchioles, and even the pulmonary interstitium. *Bordetella bronchiseptica,* parainfluenza virus, and canine adenovirus-2 are the pathogens that pose the greatest risk of causing clinical signs in susceptible dogs. To a limited extent, *B. bronchiseptica* also has a role in the pathogenesis of infectious respiratory disease in cats, especially kittens. The prognosis for recovery is excellent in dogs with uncomplicated infections. Isolation combined with administration of antitussive medication and a broad-spectrum antibiotic is the cornerstone of therapy among dogs with clinical signs. Hospitalization is not usually indicated unless there is evidence of respiratory distress and pneumonia.

Today, approximately 11 vaccines are licensed for protection of dogs against the principal viral and bacterial agents associated with infectious tracheobronchitis. One vaccine is licensed for protection of cats against *B. bronchiseptica.* Not surprisingly, vaccination protocols for both dogs and cats are inconsistently applied in clinical practice. This is due, in part, to the wide choice of parenteral and topical products available; and also to the lack of information about the duration of immunity derived from the constituent antigens, both viral and bacterial, in available multivalent products. Although vaccination of dogs against ITB is regarded to be widespread, the experience of veterinarians and dog owners suggests that current vaccines do not provide complete protection against this respiratory syndrome.

Recent introduction of an avirulent live vaccine for feline *B. bronchiseptica** infection has raised questions among practitioners about the occurrence of this clinical disease in cats as well as about the appropriate vaccination guidelines. Paradoxically, it was the introduction of the vaccine, rather than the occurrence of infection, that drew attention to the role of *B. bronchiseptica* infection in feline respiratory disease. Although *B. bronchiseptica* resides in the respiratory tract of cats and has been isolated from kittens (and occasionally adult cats) with clinical signs of lower respiratory disease, the role of *B. bronchiseptica* as a primary agent of respiratory disease in cats has not been clearly elucidated. In the absence of reports describing risk factors and disease prevalence, feline vaccination recommendations for *B. bronchiseptica* are generally limited to multiple cat households in which the bacterium is believed to be associated with clinical signs of respiratory disease (especially cough).

Etiology

It is important to emphasize that *Bordetella bronchiseptica* is not the sole etiological agent of ITB. In fact, various bacteria and viruses, acting either alone or in combination, contribute to the various signs associated with canine ITB. Single-agent infections, particularly viral, are generally mild and often self-limiting; however, in the clinical setting, concurrent bacterial and viral infections may actually predominate. Canine parainfluenza virus (CPiV) and *B. bronchiseptica* are the two most common organisms isolated from dogs with signs of ITB.[1-5] Although canine adenovirus-2 (CAV-2), canine distemper virus (CDV), reovirus, and canine herpesvirus are all capable of infecting the upper respiratory tract of dogs and causing acute-onset cough, their roles in the etiopathogenesis of ITB are less important than those of *B. bronchiseptica* and CPiV.[1,4]

---

*PROTEX®-Bb, Intervet, Inc. Millsboro, Del.

VIRUSES

Canine parainfluenza virus (CPiV) is the most common and perhaps the most significant virus associated with acute onset of ITB. CPiV is a single-stranded RNA virus known to have worldwide distribution. Canine infections with CPiV are typically restricted to the nasal cavity and trachea because the virus does not replicate in macrophages. CPiV is often considered to be an inciting viral agent in ITB that damages the tracheal epithelium, thereby predisposing the patient to secondary bacterial infection, especially with resident *B. bronchiseptica*. Transmission of CPiV between dogs occurs predominantly following direct contact with aerosolized microdroplets, subsequent to sneezing or coughing episodes in an infected dog. Clinical signs are characterized by an acute onset, high-pitched, honking cough associated with swollen vocal cords and restriction of airflow through the glottis during coughing. Dogs infected with CPiV alone are typically healthy, remain afebrile, and are expected to maintain a normal appetite. Generally, infections are short-lived. After a 3- to 10-day incubation period, cough and viral shedding typically occurs for 6 to 8 days postinfection.[6] Recovery is regarded to be complete because a carrier state does not appear to develop.

Canine adenovirus-2 (CAV-2) has infrequently been reported as a cause of respiratory infection in dogs and, in the clinical setting, is not regarded to be a predominant factor in the etiopathogenesis of canine ITB. The role of CAV-2 in canine respiratory disease becomes more important in dogs co-infected with *B. bronchiseptica* or other respiratory viruses such as CPiV. Infection with CAV-2 occurs following oronasal contact with infected dogs. The virus replicates in the epithelium of the nasal mucosa, pharynx, tonsillar crypts, trachea, and bronchi, as well as in nonciliated bronchiolar epithelium. Infections are typically short-lived. The virus is usually not isolated beyond day 9 of the infection.[7] Infection of type 2 alveolar cells has been associated with interstitial pneumonia in some dogs.[7] Clinical signs of CAV-2 infection include cough. Unless the patient is co-infected with other organisms associated with ITB, infections are generally mild. Subclinical infections have been reported. There are no known reports of CAV-2 infections in the cat.

Other viruses (e.g., canine distemper virus [CDV], canine adenovirus-1 [CAV-1], and reoviruses-1, -2, and -3) are occasionally isolated from coughing dogs. Although CDV acts synergistically with CPiV and *B. bronchiseptica,* it is generally not regarded as a primary pathogen in the etiology of ITB. CAV-2, canine herpesvirus, and the various reoviruses are considered to be minor agents in the etiopathogenesis of ITB.

BORDETELLA BRONCHISEPTICA

B. bronchiseptica is a gram negative, aerobic coccobacillus regarded as one of the principal causative agents of canine ITB. Although either CPiV or CAV-2 may cause mild clinical infections, clinical disease is expected to be more severe in dogs co-infected with *B. bronchiseptica*

than in dogs infected with any of these agents alone. *B. bronchiseptica* is transmitted through aerosolization of respiratory secretions. Bacteria can also be transmitted by contaminated dishware, human hands, and other fomites. Because *B. bronchiseptica* possesses several intrinsic mechanisms for evading host defenses[3,4] it is recognized for its role as a significant complicating factor in dogs with multiple-agent respiratory infections. For example, fimbriae, which are hairlike appendages extending from the cell membrane of *B. bronchiseptica,* recognize specific receptors within the respiratory tract. This allows *B. bronchiseptica* to colonize the surface of ciliated epithelial cells, where it then releases various exotoxins and endotoxins that impair the function of the respiratory epithelium and therefore compromises the ability of the infected host to eliminate the infection.[3,5] Additionally, *B. bronchiseptica* is regarded as an extracellular pathogen that has the unique ability to invade host cells. Once contained within the intracellular environment, bacteria are able to avoid immunologic defense mechanisms and establish a persistent infection or carrier state. The pathogenesis of *B. bronchiseptica* has recently been reviewed.[3,4]

MYCOPLASMA

Mycoplasmas are prokaryotic microbes distinguished from bacteria by the fact that they are enclosed in a cytoplasmic membrane but lack a distinct cell wall. Although various groups of mycoplasmas, acholeplasmas, and ureaplasmas have been recovered from the nasopharyngeal mucosa of healthy dogs and cats, their roles in the pathogenesis of ITB remain unclear. Mycoplasmas isolated from the lower respiratory tract of dogs *(M. cynos)* and cats *(M. felis)* are usually associated with pneumonia. Mycoplasmas are known to colonize both ciliated and nonciliated epithelia. Infections are characterized by purulent bronchitis and bronchiolitis. Systemic infection is rare; however, once the lower respiratory epithelium is colonized, chronic shedding of several months' duration is possible.[5]

Clinical Signs

Characteristically, the clinical signs of canine infectious tracheobronchitis (ITB) include paroxysmal coughing episodes, often associated with retching and expectoration, in an otherwise healthy, active dog. Swelling of the vocal folds, associated with laryngitis, can result in a loud, high-pitched cough often described as a goose honk or seal honk. Expectoration of mucus following an episode of retching or hacking behavior may be misinterpreted by the owner as vomiting. Anorexia, fever, and lethargy may be observed among infected dogs during an outbreak. The onset of clinical signs typically ranges from 3 to 10 days following exposure. In most clinical cases, the onset of signs can be associated with recent exposure to other dogs or to general anesthesia and endotracheal intubation. The ability to elicit a cough on manipulation of the trachea is an inconsistent and nonspecific clinical finding that should not be used exclusively to rule canine ITB in or out.

A second, more severe respiratory syndrome has been observed in dogs residing within kennel environments during an outbreak of ITB. Although cough may be present, the predominant clinical sign is associated with mucoid to mucopurulent nasal and ocular discharge. Pneumonia is likely to be a complicating factor that in some cases may become life threatening, particularly in puppies. In these cases, *B. bronchiseptica* has been isolated from the pharynx and trachea as a pure culture. Affected dogs are characteristically febrile, lethargic, anorexic, and may show some degree of respiratory distress or even dyspnea. The author has observed outbreaks at any time of the year, which may affect more than 50% of dogs in a densely populated environment. Puppies are more severely affected and are at significant risk of dying if not treated.

Diagnosis

A clinical diagnosis of infectious tracheobronchitis is based on historical or physical examination findings that meet the clinical criteria described above. In addition, a history of exposure to other dogs (whether or not they have signs of coughing) is helpful in establishing the diagnosis. A favorable and rapid response to empiric antibacterial and antitussive treatment supports the diagnosis of uncomplicated ITB. Routine thoracic radiography, hematology, and biochemistry profiles are neither diagnostic nor prognostic in uncomplicated cases. An inflammatory leukogram with a significant leukocytosis or left shift may develop in dogs with a complicated infection associated with pneumonia.

Although fluid collected during transtracheal wash/aspiration may reveal a neutrophilic exudate and bacteria, this procedure is rarely indicated in establishing a diagnosis of uncomplicated ITB. Bacterial culture of aspirated fluid specimens may be helpful in identifying specific types of bacteria in patients with infections complicated by bacterial pneumonia, and antibiotic sensitivity testing may help direct treatment in these patients. It should be noted that because of the large number of indigenous microflora in the canine respiratory tract, bacterial isolates from the nasal and oral cavities do not provide information about bacteria in the trachea and bronchi, and will not distinguish a primary infection from a secondary or opportunistic infection.

In dogs with uncomplicated ITB, thoracic radiographs are typically unremarkable. Dogs with respiratory complications associated with ITB may have radiographic signs of pulmonary hyperinflation, interstitial pneumonia, and segmental atelectasis.[1,3,4] To rule out pneumonia, thoracic radiography should be considered in any dog with ITB that is showing signs of systemic illness, fever, or anorexia.

Acute and convalescent serum neutralizing or hemagglutinin inhibition (HI) antibody titers can be used to establish exposure to various viral agents involved in canine ITB. However, the ability to demonstrate a rising titer has little clinical application because of the relatively short duration of viral infection.

Treatment

In the absence of confirmation of infection with any of the agent(s) associated with canine ITB, it is appropriate to administer empiric supportive therapy to dogs with clinical signs. The cornerstone of treatment is the oral administration of an antimicrobial. However, it may be in the patient's best interest to administer cough suppressants in the form of antiinflammatory and/or antitussive drugs. In cases with demonstrable evidence of pneumonia, the addition of short-term aerosol therapy may be helpful.

ANTIMICROBIALS

Most cases of uncomplicated ITB can be regarded as self-limiting and do not necessarily require antimicrobial therapy; however, conventional practice standards include empiric, short-term administration of an antimicrobial to prevent opportunistic infections. Whether or not dogs with clinical signs of ITB are at significant risk of developing bacterial pneumonia has not been definitively established. On the other hand, evidence of a mucoid to mucopurulent nasal and/or ocular discharge justifies administration of an antimicrobial. Doxycycline, administered orally at 5.0 to 10.0 mg/kg, once daily for a minimum of 2 weeks, is the first choice of antibiotic due to its efficacy against *B. bronchiseptica.* However, the ability of *B. bronchiseptica* to persist in the respiratory tract of infected dogs for as long as 3 months justifies a treatment duration of up to 30 days, particularly when attempting to manage simultaneous infections in multiple dogs living in the same environment. Depending on the severity of the outbreak, administration of an antimicrobial to all dogs in the environment, whether or not they are manifesting clinical signs, is justified when practical. Alternative antibiotic regimens for the treatment of both dogs and cats with *B. bronchiseptica* infection are listed in Table 49-1.[8,9]

GLUCOCORTICOIDS

Short-term administration of glucocorticosteroids, administered concurrently with an antimicrobial, is safe and effective in attenuating severe cough in dogs with uncomplicated infections but should be avoided in animals that might have pneumonia. Prednisolone can be administered at antiinflammatory doses (0.25 to 0.5 mg/kg) orally once or twice daily for up to 5 days as needed to control cough. Because some of the antimicrobials recommended in the treatment of canine ITB are bacteriostatic, concurrent use of glucocorticoids should not be extended beyond 5 days. It is recommended that antimicrobial therapy be continued for at least 5 to 7 days beyond the day that the corticosteroid is discontinued. Glucocorticoids are effective in reducing cough associated with inflammation of the respiratory mucosa

TABLE 49-1. **Antibiotic Recommendations for the Treatment of *B. bronchiseptica* Infection in Dogs and Cats**

Drug	Dosage	Treatment Duration	Comments
Doxycycline	5-10 mg/kg, orally, twice daily	2-4 weeks	**Caution:** Orally administered capsules have been associated with focal esophagitis and esophageal stricture in cats. Liquid preparations are available and are recommended.
Azithromycin	5 mg/kg, orally, once every 3 to 5 days	Repeat once or twice as needed	Capsule and liquid preparations are available.
Amoxicillin-clavulanate	15 to 20 mg/kg, orally, 2 or 3 times daily	2-4 weeks	
Enrofloxacin	5 mg/kg, orally, once daily (**dog only**)	3-4 weeks	**Caution:** Enrofloxacin has been associated with retinopathy and irreversible blindness in cats and is therefore not recommended at any dose in this species.
Trimethoprim-sulfonamide	30 mg/kg, orally, once or twice daily	3-4 weeks	

All doses are based on oral administration.

but they do not shorten the clinical course of the infection.[1] There are no controlled studies that substantiate the value of intratracheal administration of glucocorticoids in controlling cough.

ANTITUSSIVES

Antitussives, alone and in combination with bronchodilators, have been recommended in the treatment of canine ITB. Treatment with either hydrocodone or butorphanol is recommended. In the clinical setting, over-the-counter cough suppressant drugs (e.g., dextromethorphan) are not recommended because they appear to provide little or no relief from cough associated with ITB. Administration of narcotic cough suppressants (e.g., hydrocodone) will suppress cough and induce sedation; however, prolonged use of narcotic antitussives at high doses can lead to retention of respiratory secretions and diminished clearance of bacteria. In cases of ITB that are complicated by bacterial pneumonia, administration of narcotic antitussives is therefore not recommended.

BRONCHODILATORS

The benefits of bronchodilator therapy in dogs and cats with bronchitis remain unclear. At issue is whether or not the airway response to bacteria and viruses increases airway hyperactivity and baseline resistance to airflow. Two categories of bronchodilators are used: methylxanthine derivatives and beta$_2$-agonists. The methylxanthine bronchodilators theophylline and aminophylline (theophylline-ethylenediamine) prevent bronchial constriction and therefore may be used as supportive treatment in dogs with complicated infections associated with respiratory difficulty. However, methylxanthine bronchodilator therapy alone does not significantly suppress the cough associated with canine ITB. The use of methylxanthine bronchodilators is generally limited to patients with respiratory distress believed to be attributable to bronchoconstriction. Dogs receiving bronchodilators may experience increased gastrointestinal motility (diarrhea), tachycardia, and hyperexcitability.

The beta$_2$-agonists terbutaline and albuterol have been shown to be of benefit when administered to dogs with chronic bronchitis.[10] These drugs have the advantage of reducing cough as well as reducing pulmonary infiltrates associated with uncomplicated bronchitis. Excitability or tremors may be encountered during the first few days of treatment. The role of bronchodilators in treating cats with *B. bronchiseptica* infection has not been described, and their use is not recommended.

AEROSOL THERAPY

In contrast to humidification therapy, aerosol therapy, also called nebulization, refers to the production of a liquid particulate suspension within a carrier gas, usually oxygen. Dogs and cats with ITB that derive the most benefit from aerosol therapy are those with excessive accumulations of bronchial and tracheal secretions and those with bacterial bronchial or pulmonary infections. Small, disposable, hand-held jet nebulizers (Figure 49-1) are inexpensive and readily available through hospital supply retailers. Experience has shown that patients benefit from aerosol therapy when 6 to 10 ml of sterile saline is nebulized over 15 to 20 minutes one to four times daily. Oxygen must be delivered at flow rates of 3 to 5 liters per minute to effectively nebulize saline. Aerosol therapy must be administered in the hospital and is generally administered over 1 to 4 days as needed to control respiratory signs. Most dogs tolerate aerosol therapy administered through a facemask attached over the nose, and generally acclimatize quickly to the mask. Administration of aerosol therapy to cats generally requires confining the cat within a specially designed chamber modified with necessary ports through which aerosolized liquid can be delivered (Figure 49-2). There

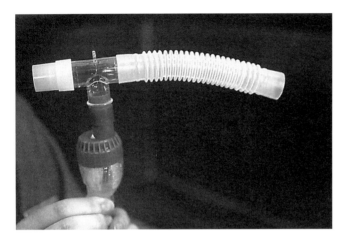

Figure 49-1. Hand-held jet nebulizer adaptable for use in managing respiratory infections in dogs and cats.

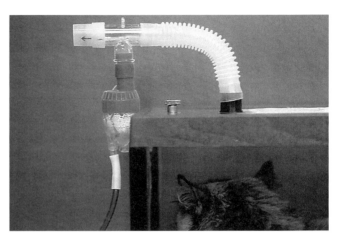

Figure 49-2. Plexiglass nebulizing chamber used to treat cats with complicated respiratory infections associated with respiratory distress.

is no value in nebulizing mucolytic agents (e.g., acetylcysteine), which can be irritating and induce bronchospasm. Nebulization of glucocorticoid solutions (e.g., methylprednisolone sodium succinate) has not been critically studied in veterinary medicine; however, patients with acute paroxysms of cough that lead to or predispose to airway obstruction may derive short-term benefits from nebulized steroid solutions.

Dogs unresponsive to oral or parenteral administration of antibiotics may respond to nebulized antibiotics. Aerosolized kanamycin, gentamicin, and polymyxin B have each been shown to be effective in reducing the population of *B. bronchiseptica* in the trachea and bronchi of infected dogs for up to 3 days after discontinuation of treatment.[5] Although clinical signs are not eliminated, the severity of signs may be significantly reduced. Administration of antibiotic solutions by aerosolization does not result in the development of significant blood levels; therefore administering aminoglycoside antibiotics in nebulized saline does not pose a risk of nephrotoxicity.

SUPPORTIVE CARE

Additional supportive treatment is not necessary in dogs with uncomplicated ITB. Most patients may be effectively treated on an outpatient basis depending on the risk posed to other pets in the household. However, dogs and cats with lower respiratory tract infections benefit from supportive treatment directed at maintaining adequate caloric and fluid intake during the acute infection. Dehydrated patients should receive the benefit of intravenous fluid therapy as the preferred means for maintaining hydration within the respiratory tract and preventing the formation of excessively thick respiratory secretions. When feasible, fluid therapy may be administered on an outpatient basis to avoid hospitalization of dogs with highly contagious infections. Administration of fluids by the subcutaneous route is only indicated when intravenous fluid administration is not feasible or possible.

TREATMENTS NOT RECOMMENDED

Considering the fact that canine ITB represents a significant percentage of the total cases of infectious upper respiratory disease in dogs, creative therapeutic modalities have been administered in an attempt to shorten the course of disease and minimize the clinical signs. The treatments listed below are largely anecdotal, have not been subjected to scientific scrutiny, and at this time are not recommended in the treatment of canine ITB:

Antiviral therapy: Because at least three agents associated with canine ITB are viruses (i.e., canine parainfluenza virus, canine adenovirus-2, and canine distemper virus), administration of various antiviral drugs approved for use in humans has been suggested for dogs with ITB. However, antiviral therapy is highly specific and is generally targeted at specific viruses. In veterinary medicine, antiviral therapies directed against the viruses associated with canine ITB are not available. At this time, no human antiviral therapy is recommended for use in either the dog or the cat with ITB.

Intranasal vaccination: Unpublished and anecdotal reports have suggested that some dogs with ITB may derive therapeutic benefit from administration of a single dose of an intranasal *B. bronchiseptica* vaccine. Experience with this treatment modality in outbreaks of canine ITB within a shelter environment has not shown a diminished intensity of clinical signs or a shortened course of the disease. It has also been suggested that dogs experiencing chronic or persistent cough beyond the expected recovery time for acute ITB may benefit from therapeutic vaccination. To date, there are no controlled studies to support this recommendation.

Expectorants: A variety of over-the-counter expectorants have been used in canine ITB to facilitate the clearance of mucous secretions within the trachea and bronchi. Saline expectorants, guaifenesin, and volatile oils that can be inhaled as a vapor are intended to stimulate secretion of less viscous bronchial mucus and, thereby, enhance clearance of respiratory secretions. However, the value of expectorant therapy in dogs with

ITB has not been established and it is currently not recommended. Numerous over-the-counter cough suppressant medications are available and are occasionally administered to coughing dogs. The author's experience with these products suggests that they offer little to no physical benefit in ameliorating the clinical signs associated with ITB.

Prevention

MATERNAL IMMUNITY

Maternal (colostral) immunity to the viruses associated with canine ITB provides variable levels of protection. Maternally derived CPiV antibody does not appear to interfere with parenteral vaccine administered to puppies that are aged 6 weeks and older. Maternal antibody to CAV-2 does not protect against infection, but may interfere with parenteral CAV-2 vaccination for as long as 12 to 16 weeks.[7] Antibody derived in utero will likely protect colostrum-deprived puppies from 1 to 4 weeks of age. Colostral antibody represents approximately 97% of the initial titer in nursing newborn puppies, an amount that is equal to approximately 77% of that in the bitch. Maternal (colostral) antibodies are usually absent by 12 to 14 weeks of age. Neither the quality nor duration of maternally derived immunity to B. bronchiseptica is known.

NATURAL IMMUNITY

The duration of immunity following recovery from CPiV and CAV-2 infection has not been thoroughly studied; however, one report documented the presence of CPiV neutralizing antibody 2 years after infection in dogs not reexposed to virus.[11] The greater question, perhaps, is the duration of immunity derived following recovery from B. bronchiseptica infection. Studies have shown that dogs are resistant to infection for at least 6 months following recovery from the acute infection.[6] However, the level of protection derived by dogs following active infection varies depending on the individual animal, number and type of viruses and bacteria involved in the infection, and the opportunity for reexposure.

VACCINATION

Several commercially licensed canine vaccines are available for protection against B. bronchiseptica, CAV-2, and CPiV. At this time, only one vaccine is licensed for protection against feline B. bronchiseptica infection. Canine vaccines are available for topical (intranasal) as well as parenteral administration, whereas the feline B. bronchiseptica vaccine is approved for topical (intranasal) administration only. The various vaccine types used in dogs and cats are summarized in Table 49-2.

Although intranasal vaccines are generally considered less convenient to administer, the ability of the vaccine to evoke local immunity in the presence of maternal antibody may be an advantage in protecting young dogs (aged 8 weeks or less) living in high-risk environments.

Avirulent live B. bronchiseptica cultures are believed to stimulate local secretory antibodies; however, there is little information about the specificity of the immune response stimulated by those products. It appears that avirulent live B. bronchiseptica vaccine strains are genetically distinct from field isolates and, therefore, may express altered levels, or immunologically distinct variants, of critical antigens.[3]

The efficacy of vaccination administered by either the topical or the intranasal route is well documented. Regardless of the route of administration, vaccinated dogs experience substantially less coughing than control dogs following challenge with a virulent strain of B. bronchiseptica. Vaccination is not expected to completely eliminate the risk of infection or the development of subclinical to mild infection following exposure. Fever, anorexia, and lethargy have been shown to be minimal among vaccinates following experimental challenge. At issue, however, is whether or not sequential vaccination (i.e., administering both a topical B. bronchiseptica vaccine and a parenteral vaccine during the same appointment) provides superior protection compared to either vaccine given alone. This issue was addressed in a recent study in which puppies were vaccinated either by the parenteral (intramuscular) or the topical (intranasal) routes alone, or by both routes sequentially.[12] Serological and clinical responses to challenge with virulent B. bronchiseptica were evaluated following challenge.[12] The authors concluded that sequential administration of both types of vaccine afforded greater protection than that derived from vaccination by either route alone. Their conclusion was based on the fact that dogs receiving both vaccines had less or no growth of B. bronchiseptica in postmortem specimens collected from both the upper and lower respiratory tract. Interpreting the results of this study to mean that all dogs should routinely receive sequential B. bronchiseptica vaccination is inappropriate. It is most important to acknowledge that vaccination by either route is effective and indicated for administration to dogs at risk.

With regard to the onset of immunity, it is recommended that dogs be vaccinated at least 5 days prior to a known (or potential) exposure to ITB (e.g., being housed in a boarding kennel). Despite the assumption that topically administered vaccine provides the most rapid onset of immunity, it is not known whether intranasally administered vaccine will immunize a susceptible dog in less than 5 days. Vaccination recommendations pertaining to route and earliest age vary considerably depending on the particular vaccine manufacturer. Generally, puppies inoculated by the intranasal route can be immunized from as early as 2 to 3 weeks of age. Parenteral B. bronchiseptica vaccines should not be given to dogs under 6 weeks of age due to the potential for interference by circulating maternal antibodies. Most manufacturers recommend initial parenteral vaccination at 6 to 8 weeks of age or older. All dogs should receive two initial doses 3 to 4 weeks apart. Among dogs over 16 weeks of age, booster vaccination with B. bronchiseptica is still recommended on an annual basis for dogs at risk of exposure.

TABLE 49-2. Vaccine Types Licensed for Protection Against *B. bronchiseptica*, Canine Parainfluenza virus, and Canine Adenovirus-2

Canine Vaccines

Vaccine	Volume/Route	Minimum Age at First Dose	Initial Series
Bordetella bronchiseptica (killed-extracted cellular antigens)	1 ml **Parenteral** (SC only)	8 weeks	2 doses, 2-4 weeks apart
Bordetella bronchiseptica (avirulent live culture) PLUS Canine Parainfluenza virus (modified-live virus) PLUS Canine Adenovirus-2 (modified-live virus) (combined with Canine Distemper Virus)	1 ml **Parenteral** (SC or IM)	Not stipulated (8 weeks recommended)	2 doses, 2-4 weeks apart. Dogs vaccinated prior to the age of 4 months should receive a single dose on reaching 4 months of age.
Bordetella bronchiseptica (avirulent live culture) PLUS Canine Parainfluenza virus (modified-live virus)	0.4 or 1.0 ml, depending on manufacturer **Topical** (intranasal only)	**2 or 3** weeks, depending on manufacturer	1 dose (NOTE: Some manufacturers stipulate a 2nd dose at 6 weeks of age in puppies that receive the first dose between 3 and 6 weeks of age.)
Bordetella bronchiseptica (avirulent live culture) PLUS Canine Parainfluenza virus (modified-live virus) PLUS Canine Adenovirus-2 (modified-live virus)	0.4 or 1.0 ml, depending on manufacturer **Topical** (intranasal only)	**3 or 8** weeks, depending on manufacturer	1 dose

Feline Vaccine

Vaccine	Volume/Route	Minimum Age at First Dose	Initial Series
Bordetella bronchiseptica (avirulent live culture)	0.2 ml **Topical** (intranasal only)	8 weeks	1 dose

IM = Intramuscular; *SC* = subcutaneous.
Routes of administration as stipulated by the manufacturer are **not** optional.

DURATION OF IMMUNITY FOLLOWING VACCINATION

The minimum duration of immunity following vaccination with a modified-live viral vaccine is expected to be quite different from that of a *B. bronchiseptica* bacterin. Yet, CAV-2 and CPiV vaccines are available in combination with *B. bronchiseptica,* in products that are recommended for annual revaccination (booster). In fact, individual antigens (bacterial and viral) may respond quite differently depending on the route of administration. No studies are available that define the maximum duration of immunity following vaccination with either the parenteral or topical *B. bronchiseptica* vaccine. Likewise, the maximum duration of immunity following administration of topical CPiV or CAV-2 is not known. The conventional recommendation for annual boosters of multivalent vaccines seems quite inappropriate considering the fact that most ITB vaccines combine a bacterial vaccine with a parenterally administered modified-live virus vaccine.

Generally speaking, the minimum duration of immunity derived from modified-live virus vaccines CPiV and CAV-2 is expected to be 3 years following vaccination in adult dogs. On the other hand, the duration of immunity against *B. bronchiseptica* following vaccination by either parenteral or intranasal routes is likely to be considerably shorter. Estimates range from 3 months to 10 months depending on the field strain used in the vaccine and the route of administration. Because the duration of immunity against *B. bronchiseptica* following intranasal vaccination is generally considered to be less than 12 months, a single booster vaccination is recommended at least 5 days before possible exposure (e.g., boarding, shipping, showing) in dogs that have not been vaccinated within the preceding 6 months.

VACCINE ADVERSE EVENTS

The occurrence of vaccine reactions and outbreaks of pertussis among infants vaccinated against *Bordetella pertussis* has led researchers to question the safety and efficacy of standard wholesale whooping cough vaccines. As a result, a new group of acellular whooping cough vaccines, based on highly purified antigens, has been pursued. Studies of these newer vaccines have shown greater efficacy and safety than standard whole cell pertussis bacterin. The relationship between *B. pertussis* and *B. bronchiseptica* suggests that similar improvements in the canine vaccine should be considered.

Adverse events reported to occur following administration of parenteral vaccine for canine ITB are generally limited to local irritation at the injection site with occasional granuloma formation. There are no known reports that postvaccinal granuloma formation has resulted in development of neoplasia in dogs. All vaccines approved for topical (intranasal) administration to dogs and cats contain live, avirulent *B. bronchiseptica,* which is occasionally associated with postvaccination sneezing, nasal discharge, and/or cough. Postvaccinal signs generally develop 2 to 5 days postinoculation. Rarely, postvaccinal signs are sufficiently severe or persistent that administration of an antimicrobial is indicated. In the event that clinical signs become severe, antimicrobial therapy should be administered orally for a period of 7 days. It is generally not recommended that intranasal vaccine be administered to dogs receiving antimicrobials at the time of vaccination. The immunizing dose of *B. bronchiseptica* could be significantly attenuated if the vaccine is given during a time in which the patient is receiving antibiotics.

Management of Outbreaks

Dogs housed in high-density populations (e.g., commercial kennels, shelters, dog shows), particularly those in which new animals are frequently introduced into the environment, are at considerable risk of exposure to one or more of the agents known to cause canine ITB. Although important in minimizing the severity of signs associated with infection in the individual dog, vaccination does not guarantee protection against development of clinical signs or the spread of infection to susceptible dogs. Dogs living in kennel/shelter environments should be isolated if clinical signs consistent with ITB develop. Thorough, routine cleaning of housing facilities (preferably using fresh sodium hypochlorite, chlorhexidine, or benzalkonium solution) is helpful in containing the spread of ITB. Kennels and shelter facilities should ensure adequate ventilation that includes 12 to 20 air exchanges per hour.

There is no evidence to support simultaneous administration of intranasal vaccine to all dogs within a kennel environment at the first sign of infection, in an attempt to alter the course of an impending outbreak. A reduction in the incidence of ITB has been observed in dogs whose vaccinations for all infections were current; however, attempts to prevent outbreaks through routine, widespread intranasal vaccination may be ineffective if vaccination and exposure are likely to occur within the same day. Furthermore, postvaccinal coughing or nasal discharge may preclude adoption of otherwise healthy dogs from impoundment facilities. In addition to vaccination, adequate housing, proper cleaning, and adequate ventilation are critical factors in preventing outbreaks of ITB whenever dogs are housed within crowded environments. General vaccination recommendations for kennel/shelter environments, however, do include vaccinating by way of the intranasal route using a product that contains vaccines for at least *B. bronchiseptica* and CPiV.

Once an outbreak has developed, restricting the movement of all dogs into and out of the facility for up to 4 weeks may be the most cost-effective measure to control the spread of organisms among susceptible dogs. In addition to extensive cleaning, treating all of the dogs in the facility with antibiotics, whether or not they manifest clinical signs of ITB, may be important in managing clinical signs associated with *B. bronchiseptica.*

Public Health Considerations

The potential for canine *B. bronchiseptica* infections to infect humans has been reviewed.[1,13] Human infection with *B. bronchiseptica* is most likely to occur in children and immunocompromised adults.[14] Although infections are uncommon, at greatest risk are individuals whose immunosuppression is related to alcoholic malnutrition, hematologic malignancy, long-term glucocorticoid therapy, concurrent HIV infection, splenectomy, and pregnancy.[13] As expected, individuals subjected to tracheostomy or endotracheal tube intubation are also at risk for infection. Humans infected with preexisting respiratory disease (e.g., chronic bronchitis and pneumonia) may also be at greater risk. Although human infection with *B. bronchiseptica* has been associated with contact with a variety of domestic and wildlife animal species, presumptive evidence of transmission of disease from dogs to humans is generally based on a history of exposure to dogs; dog-to-human transmission has seldom been confirmed.

It has been estimated that up to 40% of immunocompromised adults living in the United States today have pets. While it may seem logical to assume that the incidence of respiratory infection associated with *B. bronchiseptica* among populations of immune compromised people would be significantly higher compared to the general population, there are no reports to suggest that this is true. The risk of a child or immunocompromised adult becoming infected with pet-associated *B. bronchiseptica* infection must be considered small, particularly when exposure to high concentrations of dogs (e.g., kennels and animal shelters) can be avoided.

Feline Bordetella Bronchiseptica Infection

The introduction of a topical (intranasal) vaccine against feline *B. bronchiseptica* has prompted concerns about the actual prevalence of feline respiratory infections caused by or associated with *B. bronchiseptica* and the indications for vaccinating. Unfortunately, there are few published reports that describe the clinical features and pathogenesis of *B. bronchiseptica* infection in cats.[15-21] Among cats with confirmed infections, cough is the predominant presenting complaint. Unlike the dog, the character of the cough is neither unique-sounding nor inordinately loud. Age and housing may be important risk factors for infection. Most reports of severe respiratory infections associated with *B. bronchiseptica* involve multiple kittens (less than 6 months of age) housed together. However, there is a paucity of literature describing the risk factors for infection and the incidence in the general population of cats.

Whereas the occurrence of *B. bronchiseptica* infection is likely to be greater among cats maintained in multiple cat households with a history of respiratory disease, the overall prevalence of infection within the cat population is not known. Serological surveys have shown rates of seropositivity that range from 30% to as high as 85% in multiple cat households.[15] Over 130 isolates of *B. bronchiseptica* examined by pulse field gel electrophoresis have been recovered from cats.[22] Cats housed together were found to carry similar or identical strains and subtypes. The fact that there were no reported differences in the electrophoresis patterns in isolates from carrier cats and those with clinical infections implies that active infections are likely to be opportunistic. Furthermore, the likelihood that a particular isolate will produce disease is probably related to host or environmental factors such as crowding and stress.[22]

It's important to note, however, that the presence of *B. bronchiseptica* antibody in an individual cat is not indicative of active infection. Furthermore, *B. bronchiseptica* may be one of many resident bacteria in the oral cavity of healthy cats. Until additional information can be made available, specific recommendations for vaccination of cats against *B. bronchiseptica* will be difficult to make. Recommendations by the American Association of Feline Practitioners indicate that *B. bronchiseptica* vaccination is not required in all cats.[23] Use of the vaccine is generally limited to cluster households and shelters where *B. bronchiseptica* is known to be associated with lower respiratory infection in cats. As occurs in dogs, transient postvaccinal sneezing or cough is expected in some cats within 24 hours postvaccination.

REFERENCES

1. Ford RB, Vaden SL: Canine infectious tracheobronchitis. In CE Greene, editor: *Infectious diseases of the dog and cat*, ed 2, Philadelphia, 1998, WB Saunders.
2. Ellis JA, Haines DM, West KH et al: Effect of vaccination on experimental infection with *Bordetella bronchiseptica* in dogs, *JAVMA* 218:367-375, 2001.
3. Keil DJ, Fenwick B: Role of *Bordetella bronchiseptica* in infectious tracheobronchitis in dogs, *JAVMA* 212(2):200-207, 1998.
4. Keil DJ, Fenwick B: Canine respiratory bordetellosis: Keeping up with an evolving pathogen. In Charmichael LE, editor: *Recent advances in canine infectious diseases*, International Veterinary Information Service (www.ivis.org Document No. A0104.0100), accessed 13 January 2000.
5. Bemis DA: *Bordetella* and *Mycoplasma* respiratory infection in dogs and cats, *Vet Clin North Am Small Anim Pract* 22:1173-1186, 1992.
6. Appel M, Binn LN: Canine parainfluenza virus. In Appel M, editor: *Virus infections of carnivores,* Amsterdam, 1987, Elsevier.
7. Appel M: Canine adenovirus type 2 (infectious laryngotracheitis virus). In Appel M, editor: *Virus infections of carnivores,* Amsterdam, 1987, Elsevier.
8. Greene CE: Respiratory infections. In Greene CE, editor: *Infectious diseases of the dog and cat,* Philadelphia, 1998, WB Saunders.
9. Booth DM: Principles of drug selection for respiratory infections in cats, *Suppl Comp Cont Educ Pract Vet* 19:5-15, 1997.
10. Johnson L: CVT update: Canine chronic bronchitis. In Bonagura JD, editor: *Kirk's current veterinary therapy XIII: Small animal practice,* Philadelphia, 2000, WB Saunders.
11. Appel M, Binn LN: Canine infectious tracheobronchitis: Kennel cough. In Appel M, editor: *Virus infections of carnivores,* Amsterdam, 1987, Elsevier.
12. Ellis JA, Krakowka GS, Dayton AD et al: Comparative efficacy of an injectable vaccine and an intranasal vaccine in stimulating *Bordetella bronchiseptica*-reactive antibody responses in seropositive dogs, *JAVMA* 220:43-48, 2002.
13. Ford RB: *Bordetella bronchiseptica* has zoonotic potential, *Topics in Vet Med* 6:18-22, 1995.
14. Dworkin MS, Sullivan PS, Harrington RD et al: *Bordetella bronchiseptica* infection in human immunodeficiency virus-infected patients, *Clin Infect Dis* 28:1095-1099, 1999.
15. Hoskins JD, Williams J, Roy AF et al: Isolation and characterization of *Bordetella bronchiseptica* from cats in southern Louisiana, *Vet Immunol Immunopathol* 65:173-176, 1998.
16. Welsh RD: *Bordetella bronchiseptica* infections in cats, *JAAHA* 32:153-158, 1998.
17. Speakman AJ, Dawson S, Binns SH et al: *Bordetella bronchiseptica* infection in the cat, *J Small Anim Pract* 40:252-256, 1999.
18. Jacobs AAC, Chalmers WSK, Pasman J et al: Feline bordetellosis: Challenge and vaccine studies, *Vet Rec* 133:260-263, 1993.
19. Willoughby K, Dawson S, Jones RC et al: Isolation of *Bordetella bronchiseptica* from kittens with pneumonia in a breeding cattery, *Vet Rec* 129:407-408, 1991.
20. Elliot H: *Bordetella bronchiseptica* in a closed cat colony, *Vet Rec* 132:474-475, 1991.
21. Coutts AJ, Dawson S, Binns SH et al: Studies on the natural transmission of *Bordetella bronchiseptica* in cats, *Vet Microbiol* 48:19-27, 1996.
22. Binns SH, Speakman AJ, Dawson S: The use of pulsed-field gel electrophoresis to examine the epidemiology of *Bordetella bronchiseptic* isolated from cats and other species, *Epidemiology and Infection* 120:201-208, 1998.
23. *2000 Report of the American Association of Feline Practitioners and Academy of Feline Medicine Advisory Panel of Feline Vaccines,* Nashville, 2000, AAFP/AFM.

CHAPTER 50

Primary Ciliary Dyskinesia

Carol R. Norris

The respiratory tract is protected from insult by a variety of defense mechanisms including mechanical filtration; cough and sneeze reflexes; the mucociliary apparatus; humoral and cell-mediated immunity; phagocytic cells; and antimicrobial substances such as alpha-1-antitrypsin, lysozyme, and lactoferrin.[1] Primary ciliary dyskinesia (PCD), a congenital disorder associated with defective ciliary motility with or without ultrastructural abnormalities, results in impairment of the mucociliary apparatus.[2-4] The mucociliary apparatus protects the respiratory tract from the effects of inhaled inorganic and organic particulate and gaseous materials that impinge on the conducting airways.[5] It is composed of a ciliated epithelial lining surface, a periciliary fluid layer (sol), and mucus-secreting glands and cells that produce the superficial mucus layer (gel). The ciliated epithelium is found in the nasal cavity and the tracheobronchial tree to the level of the terminal bronchioles.[6] The mucociliary apparatus mechanically traps inhaled debris and clears it from the lung by ciliary action, moving mucus and foreign material cranially to the pharynx for expectoration. Deficient clearing of mucus from the airways results in chronic mucous plugging; inflammation and infection; and, ultimately, in clinical manifestations of rhinosinusitis, bronchitis, bronchiectasis, and bronchopneumonia.

Primary ciliary dyskinesia has also been termed immotile cilia syndrome[6-8] and congenital ciliary dysfunction.[9,10] Kartagener's syndrome, a triad of situs inversus (lateral transposition of visceral organs), rhinosinusitis, and bronchiectasis, is considered a subgroup of PCD.[8] Kartagener's syndrome has been described in approximately 50% of humans with primary ciliary dyskinesia. This syndrome is believed to be due to either a defect in the ultrastructure of the cilia or a functional abnormality that cannot be detected by ultrastructural examination, either of which causes ciliary dysmotility or immotility.[11] Situs inversus is speculated to result from ciliary dysfunction affecting embryonic rotation, allowing for random determination of visceral organs. Rhinosinusitis and bronchiectasis are sequelae of impaired mucociliary clearance in the nasal passages, sinuses, and tracheobronchial tree.[7]

Ciliary Ultrastructure

The complex ultrastructure of cilia enables a coordinated ciliary beat in normal individuals. Each cilium is a fin-gerlike projection that extends from the surface of the respiratory epithelial cell, is anchored by a basal body, and is covered by the cell membrane. Approximately 200 cilia cover the surface of each columnar epithelial cell of the respiratory tract.[12] The axoneme (core) of the cilium is composed of two central single microtubules surrounded by nine peripheral doublets (Figure 50-1). The doublets are interconnected by inner and outer dynein arms that, when ATP is hydrolyzed for energy, allow for a sliding motion during ciliary movement.[12] Other interconnections important in normal ciliary function include nexin links and radial spokes.[8]

In PCD in the dog, a variety of ultrastructural defects of the cilia have been described. These defects include a lack of inner dynein arms, abnormal radial spokes and nexin links, microtubule doublet displacement, subnumerary or supernumerary microtubule doublets or central microtubules, shortened outer dynein arms, disoriented cilia, and fibrous rings between the circle of doublets and the cell membrane.[3,6-8] Some people and dogs appear to lack ultrastructural defects.[4,11] The mode of inheritance of PCD in dogs is speculated to be autosomal recessive.[13]

Patients with ultrastructural or functional defects may have associated clinical abnormalities in other organs with ciliated epithelial cells. In dogs, these defects have included hydrocephalus;[1,4,6,10] renal fibrosis and dilated distal renal tubules;[7] male infertility due to abnormal spermatozoa;[7,14] and abnormal sternebrae, vertebrae, and ribs.[7,14] Although microtubules are also important components of the neutrophil cytoskeleton and allow for phagocytosis and killing of organisms,[2] studies in dogs with PCD have not established significant impairment of neutrophil function.[2,9] Ultrastructural examination from the airways of healthy dogs shows a prevalence of ciliary abnormalities ranging from 0.4% to 6.8%.[7] In dogs with ciliary dyskinesia, the prevalence of abnormalities may be as high as 100%.[15]

Clinical Presentation

The many different breeds of dogs that have been diagnosed with PCD include the English pointer, English springer spaniel, English setter, Border collie, Old English sheepdog, Doberman pinscher, Chihuahua, golden retriever, rottweiler, chow chow, Chinese Shar-Pei, Newfoundland, dalmatian, bullmastiff and bichon

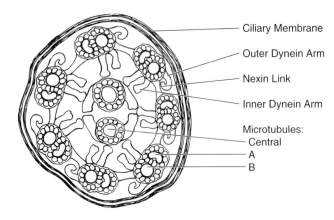

Figure 50-1. *Diagram of a normal cilium in cross-section.* (From Morrison W, Wilsman N, Fox L et al: Primary ciliary dyskinesia in the dog, *J Vet Intern Med* 1:67-74, 1987.)

frise.[1,3,4,6-9,13-18] A presumptive diagnosis of PCD was made in one cat based on ultrastructural ciliary defects in oviductal cilia (the respiratory epithelial cilia were not examined) and widened bronchi on computed tomography, although this cat was asymptomatic for respiratory disease.[19,20] Most affected dogs are young,[12] although PCD was presumptively diagnosed in one 11-year-old dog.[21] Because it lacked respiratory symptoms for the first 10 years of its life, it is possible that this dog had secondary ciliary dyskinesia.[3]

Young dogs with PCD present with signs of chronic recurrent upper and lower respiratory tract infections including mucopurulent nasal discharge and cough.[1,6,7,13,16] Dyspnea has occasionally been reported.[13,17] Respiratory symptoms are generally antibiotic responsive but tend to recur after discontinuation of therapy. Clinical signs relating to dyskinetic cilia in other organs may also be apparent; these include mental depression and seizures due to hydrocephalus caused by dysfunctional ependymal cells in the ventricles, and hearing loss and otitis media due to abnormalities of the ciliated eustachian tube.[12,14] Male dogs may be infertile.

Differential Diagnosis

Primary ciliary dyskinesia must be differentiated from secondary ciliary dyskinesia (SCD); and from congenital immunodeficiency syndromes such as selective IgA deficiency, complement deficiency, and congenital abnormalities of cell-mediated immunity or neutrophil function, all of which may present with recurrent upper and lower respiratory tract infections.[3,12] Reversible ultrastructural lesions of the respiratory cilia as a result of a variety of acquired diseases (e.g., chronic bronchitis; chronic respiratory tract infections; and toxic injuries, including secondhand cigarette smoke) are the hallmark of SCD.[3,12,22] Serial mucociliary clearance studies may document resolution of SCD if the underlying disorder is appropriately treated, but mucociliary clearance studies remain abnormal in dogs with PCD.[12] Many of the

congenital immunodeficiency syndromes predispose to more generalized infections and are not localized solely to the respiratory tract. Evaluation of some of these syndromes can be performed by the use of immunoglobulin quantitation; total hemolytic complement assay; lymphocyte mitogenesis; and neutrophil chemotaxis, adhesion, ingestion, and nitroblue tetrazolium reduction assays.[1,9]

Diagnostics

Hematological findings are nonspecific and may reflect secondary infection: leukocytosis, due to a mature neutrophilia, is therefore common.[6,13,14] Thoracic radiography is useful in identifying abnormalities of the tracheobronchial tree and pulmonary parenchyma. Radiographic findings may include situs inversus, a peribronchial pattern, interstitial or alveolar infiltrates, and bronchiectasis.[1,6-8,12,13,15] The peribronchial pattern reflects bronchitis, and chronic bronchial inflammation and infection can lead to bronchiectasis, defined as abnormal irreversibly dilated airways caused by chronic inflammatory damage to the airway walls.[23] Interstitial and alveolar infiltrates can occur with secondary bacterial pneumonia due to poor mucociliary clearance.

Tracheobronchial lavage (i.e., endotracheal, transtracheal, or bronchoalveolar lavage) may be used to obtain specimens for cytologic examination and culture. Cytologic findings often include purulent inflammation with or without intra- or extracellular bacteria.[6,8,17] Microorganisms isolated from nasal swabs or tracheobronchial lavages include *Streptococcus* spp., *Mycoplasma* spp., *Pasteurella* spp., *Acinetobacter* spp., *Staphyloccus* spp., *Actinomyces* spp., *Corynebacterium* spp., *Flavobacterium* spp., *Pseudomonas* spp., and *Escherichia coli.** Growth of fungal organisms has not been reported to date. One report noted simultaneous nasal and tracheal cultures yielded growth of the same microorganisms from both sites.[14] The authors of that study suggested that respiratory flora might be monitored by culturing nasal exudate; however, few animals were studied, quantitative data was not shown, and tracheal rather than bronchial lavages were performed. Therefore, further studies must be performed before this can be routinely recommended.

In male dogs, collection of spermatozoa has been performed to evaluate for microtubular anomalies because the spermatozoal flagellum[4] is a modified cilium. The arrangement of microtubules in sperm tails is the same as for the cilia of respiratory epithelial cells.[14] In dogs with PCD, sperm have been reported to be immotile[15] or to have decreased progressive motility[4,13] resulting in sterility. Normal motile spermatozoa have been described in humans with dyskinetic respiratory cilia.[14]

Mucociliary scintigraphy using 99-technetium-macroaggregated albumin (99Tc-MAA) can be used to evaluate the in-vivo functional status of the mucociliary apparatus. The mucociliary transport droplet test is performed by anesthetizing and intubating the patient, instilling a radioactive droplet through a sleeved polystyrene

---

*References 4, 6, 8, 10, 12, and 17.

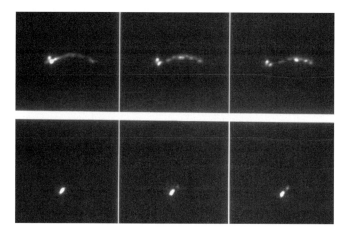

Figure 50-2. *Mucociliary scintigraphy in a normal dog (top) and in a dog with PCD (bottom). The dog in the top row demonstrates effective mucociliary clearance of the radioactive droplet from the carina towards the pharynx. The dog in the bottom row shows no movement of the radioactive droplet. Serial images are obtained 5 minutes apart.* (Photo courtesy of Ned K. Waters, University of California, Davis.)

catheter, withdrawing both the catheter and the endotracheal tube as a unit, and monitoring the velocity of the particle using a gamma camera.[22] Static images can be obtained every 5 minutes for a total of 30 minutes. With PCD, there is no movement of the droplet from the carina cranially during the 30-minute period (Figure 50-2). This test has been successfully employed to support a diagnosis of PCD in clinically affected dogs.[1,3,4,13] False positives can occur with secondary ciliary dyskinesia or with deposition of the radiopharmaceutical in the secondary bronchi.[22] In animals with normal mucociliary clearance rates, PCD can be eliminated from the differential list.

Documentation of ultrastructural abnormalities in PCD relies on electron microscopic examination of tissue. Biopsies of nasal and tracheal mucosa are often the easiest tissues to obtain, and should be immediately fixed in glutaraldehyde. Quantitation and description of ciliary defects can then be performed.

Ciliary beat frequency and synchrony have been evaluated on biopsy specimens using computerized microscope photometry.[3,13] This technique has demonstrated that the majority of cilia in dogs with PCD and in normal dogs are actually motile; thus the term "immotile cilia syndrome" is probably a misnomer.[4,13-15] An uncoordinated (dyskinetic) ciliary beat has been correlated with ultrastructural lesions[3] and can result in severe mucociliary dysfunction.

Ciliogenesis is an *in vitro* culture technique using epithelial cells from nasal, tracheal, or bronchial mucosal biopsies.[3] Cells are allowed to grow on a monolayer until they become confluent, squamous, and lose their cilia. The deciliated cells are then brought about in suspension, where they may regenerate their cilia. These cells are evaluated for ultrastructural changes using electron microscopy. Patients with PCD retain their ultrastructural abnormalities after ciliogenesis. In contrast, the acquired lesions of SCD are lost after ciliogenesis.

Treatment

Recurrent secondary bacterial infections of the nasal passages, paranasal sinuses, and tracheobronchial tree require treatment with antibiotics; the choice of antibiotic should be based on culture and sensitivity testing. With an impaired mucociliary apparatus, coughing becomes one of the most important protective mechanisms to clear particulate debris and microbes from the lung, and cough suppressants should therefore be avoided.[12] Minimizing environmental exposure to irritants such as cigarette smoke, dust, or aerosols can also minimize the load on the dysfunctional mucociliary apparatus.

Prognosis

The severity of ciliary dysfunction is variable from mild to severe, and mildly affected dogs may require minimal treatment. In more severely affected animals, management of secondary bacterial pneumonia is the key to successful management of PCD. Many dogs develop bronchiectasis from repeated infections and chronic inflammation; this further predisposes them to the development of pneumonia. Although some animals die or are euthanized because of severe bacterial bronchopneumonia at an early age, with appropriate treatment of secondary bacterial infections, dogs may live several years with this disease.

REFERENCES

1. Dhein C, Prieur D, Riggs M et al: Suspected ciliary dysfunction in Chinese shar-pei pups with pneumonia, *Am J Vet Res* 51:439-446, 1990.
2. Morrison W, Frank D, Roth J et al: Assessment of neutrophil function in dogs with primary ciliary dyskinesia, *J Am Vet Med Assoc* 191:425-430, 1987.
3. Clercx C, Peeters D, Beths T et al: Use of ciliogenesis in the diagnosis of primary ciliary dsykinesia in a dog, *J Am Vet Med Assoc* 217:1681-1685, 2000.
4. Edwards D, Kennedy J, Toal R et al: Kartagener's syndrome in a chow chow dog with normal ciliary ultrastructure, *Vet Pathol* 26:338-340, 1989.
5. Wanner A, Salathe M, O'Riordan T: Mucociliary clearance in the airways, *Am J Respir Crit Care Med* 154:1868-1902, 1996.
6. Edwards D, Patton C, Bemis D et al: Immotile cilia syndrome in three dogs from a litter, *J Am Vet Med Assoc* 183:667-672, 1983.
7. Afezelius B, Carlsten J, Karlsson S: Clinical, pathologic, and ultrastructural features of situs inversus and immotile-cilia syndrome in a dog, *J Am Vet Med Assoc* 184:560-563, 1984.
8. Randolph J, Castleman W: Immotile cilia syndrome in two Old English sheepdog litter-mates, *J Small Anim Pract* 25:679-686, 1984.
9. Maddux J, Edwards D, Barnhill M et al: Neutrophil function in dogs with congenital ciliary dyskinesia, *Vet Pathol* 28:347-353, 1991.
10. Daniel G, Edwards D, Harvey R et al: Communicating hydrocephalus in dogs with congenital ciliary dysfunction, *Dev Neurosci* 17:230-235, 1995.
11. Herzon F, Murphy S: Normal ciliary ultrastructure in children with Kartagener's syndrome, *Ann Otol* 89:81-83, 1980.
12. Crager C: Canine primary ciliary dyskinesia, *Comp Contin Ed* 14:1440-1444, 1992.
13. Edwards D, Kennedy J, Patton C et al: Familial immotile-cilia syndrome in English springer spaniel dogs, *Am J Med Genet* 33:290-298, 1989.
14. Morrison W, Wilsman N, Fox L et al: Primary ciliary dyskinesia in the dog, *J Vet Intern Med* 1:67-74, 1987.

15. Wilsman N, Morrison W, Farnum C et al: Microtubular protofilaments and subunits of the outer dynein arm in cilia from dogs with primary ciliary dyskinesia, *Am Rev Respir Dis* 135:137-143, 1987.
16. Carrig C, Suter P, Ewing G et al: Primary dextrocardia with situs inversus, associated with sinusitis and bronchitis in a dog, *J Am Vet Med Assoc* 164:1127-1134, 1974.
17. Hoover J, Howard-Martin M, Bahr R: Chronic bronchitis, bronchiectasis, bronchiolitis, bronchiolitis obliterans, and bronchopneumonia in a rottweiler with primary ciliary dyskinesia, *J Amer Anim Hosp Assoc* 25:297-304, 1989.
18. Watson P, Herretage M, Sargas D: Primary ciliary dyskinesia in Newfoundland dogs, *Vet Rec* 143:484, 1998.
19. Roperto F, Saviano R, Guarino G: Atypical basal bodies in a cat with immotile-cilia syndrome, *J Submicrosc Cytol Pathol* 26:565-567, 1994.
20. Roperto F, Brunetti A, Saviano L et al: Morphologic alterations in the cilia of a cat, *Vet Pathol* 33:460-462, 1996.
21. Killingsworth C, Slocombe R, Wilsman N: Immotile cilia syndrome in an aged dog, *J Am Vet Med Assoc* 12:1567-1571, 1987.
22. Toal R, Edwards D: Mucociliary scintigraphy. In Berry C, Daniel G, editors: *Handbook of veterinary nuclear medicine*, Raleigh, NC, 1996, North Carolina State University.
23. Norris C, Samii V: Clinical, radiographic, and pathologic features of bronchiectasis in cats: 12 cases (1987-1999), *J Am Vet Med Assoc* 216:530-534, 2000.

CHAPTER 51

Bronchiectasis

Carol R. Norris

Bronchiectasis is defined as a pathological destruction of the elastic and muscular components of the bronchial wall leading to chronic abnormal dilation and distortion of the bronchi.[1] A variety of congenital and acquired conditions have been described in humans, dogs, and cats that lead to a cycle of chronic airway infection and inflammation and resulting bronchiectatic changes.[2-6] Damage to the epithelial cells lining the airways induces squamous metaplasia and ciliary loss, which leads to impairment of the mucociliary apparatus.[2] Clearance of both normal and abnormal pulmonary secretions is dependent on transport of mucus and associated particulate materials by the ciliated epithelial cells of the mucociliary apparatus. Dysfunction of the mucociliary apparatus allows pooling of mucus, exudate, and microbes in the distal airways. Obstruction of the airways can occur due to accumulation of mucus, hemorrhage, inflammatory cells, and necrotic tissue; or due to a mass effect from neoplasia or enlarged lymph nodes.[2] Secondary infection stimulates a host inflammatory response, creating a vicious cycle of further damage to the airway walls.[7-9] Neutrophil lysosomal enzymes (e.g., elastase, collagenase, and cathepsin G) and oxygen radicals play a role in this damage,[1,4] as does the recruitment and activity of other inflammatory cells such as macrophages, T cells, and eosinophils.[10]

Reversible dilation of the bronchi has been described in acute pulmonary diseases in humans (e.g., pneumonia, tracheobronchitis, and atelectasis) and must be differentiated from true bronchiectasis.[1] True bronchiectasis is permanent; this fact has important implications in the management of the condition. Reversible or pseudo-bronchiectasis has also been described in the dog.[11]

Etiology

Bronchiectasis may be congenital or may develop secondary to acquired disease, with the latter etiology being much more common. In humans, congenital causes of bronchiectasis include congenital anatomical defects (e.g., developmental arrest of the tracheobronchial tree or cartilage deficiency), immunodeficiency states (e.g., panhypogammaglobulinemia; antibody subclass deficiency; and defects of neutrophil adhesion, respiratory burst and chemotaxis), cystic fibrosis, α_1-antitrypsin deficiency, and primary ciliary dyskinesia.[1,6,12-14] In dogs, bronchiectasis is a common sequela of primary ciliary dyskinesia,[15] and markedly dilated bronchi have been seen in dogs with bronchial cartilage aplasia[16] and bronchial hypoplasia.[17] Bronchiectasis was detected by thoracic radiography in a 10-month-old miniature dachshund with *Pneumocystis carinii* pneumonia,[18] an infection affecting dogs of this breed less than 1 year of age. Recently, these dogs were found to have a primary immunodeficiency called common variable immunodeficiency (CVID).[19] Despite the young age of the dogs affected, CVID is considered an acquired or adult onset deficiency of B and T cells.[19] Congenital bronchiectasis was reported in a cat with bronchial dysgenesis,[20] and computed tomographic evidence of bronchiectasis was found in a cat with presumptive primary ciliary dyskinesia.[21]

Acquired causes of bronchiectasis in humans include diseases that cause bronchial obstruction (e.g., asthma, chronic bronchitis, panbronchiolitis, neoplasia, foreign body, hilar lymphadenopathy, recurrent aspiration pneumonia, and broncholiths) and necrotizing or suppurative pneumonia.* In dogs, acquired bronchiectasis usually develops as a result of eosinophilic bronchitis, chronic bronchitis, bronchiolitis, or bronchopneumonia.[2,3,24-30] Interestingly, although allergic bronchitis (feline asthma) and chronic bronchitis are common clinical disorders in the cat, bronchiectasis is rarely found in association with these diseases. In studies evaluating cats with bronchial disease, thoracic radiographic evidence of bronchiectasis was not reported in any cat.[31,32] Histologic evidence of bronchiectasis was not detected in an experimental model of feline asthma.[33] In a recent retrospective study evaluating cats with a histological diagnosis of bronchiectasis, only 12 cases were found over a 12-year period.[5] Although bronchiectasis in the cat is a rare sequela to bronchopulmonary disease, the most commonly identified underlying diseases included chronic bronchitis and bronchiolitis, neoplasia, and bronchopneumonia.[5] Bronchiectasis was also reported in a cat with miliary broncholithiasis.[34]

Clinical Presentation

Most dogs and cats with bronchiectasis are middle age or older, consistent with the higher incidence of acquired versus congenital bronchiectasis. In one study, 92% of dogs were age 7 years or older,[3] and in another, the mean age was 7 years (range 2 to 17 years).[25] A study of cats with bronchiectasis reported a mean age of 12 years (range 7 to 16 years).[5] There appear to be breed predispositions for American cocker spaniel dogs and Siamese cats.[3,5,25] No sex predisposition has been reported in dogs, but a trend for male overrepresentation was noted in cats.[5]

Clinical signs associated with bronchiectasis likely reflect the underlying disease process. In humans these signs include chronic cough; purulent or mucopurulent sputum production; wheezing; dyspnea; recurrent fever; hemoptysis; and, in advanced stages, anorexia and weight loss.[1,14,23] Clinical signs in dogs include cough; gag; tachypnea; dyspnea; and, occasionally, fever.[2,35,36] In the retrospective study of bronchiectasis in cats, only 5 of 12 cats had clinical signs referable to the respiratory system (i.e., cough, tachypnea, and dyspnea).[5] Four of the cats had chronic respiratory symptoms (range 1 to 8 years duration).

Diagnostic Tests

There are two key components in the diagnostic evaluation of patients with bronchiectasis. First, the dilated airways must be recognized and localized because this pathologic process by itself is responsible for ongoing bronchopulmonary inflammation. Second, the underlying disease process that led to the development of bronchiectasis must be identified. Bronchiectasis can be detected by survey thoracic radiography, bronchography, high resolution computed tomography (HRCT), bronchoscopy, and

histology. In humans, HRCT is considered the gold standard because it is highly sensitive and noninvasive.[1,6] The utility of HRCT to specifically demonstrate bronchiectatic airway changes in dogs and cats has not been evaluated to date, aside from a single case report in a cat with presumptive primary ciliary dyskinesia.[21]

Different radiographic patterns can be seen in patients with bronchiectasis. The major forms include cylindrical, saccular, cystic, and varicose bronchiectasis.[2,11] Cylindrical bronchiectasis appears as dilated bronchi with nontapering ends of approximately the same diameter that terminate in consolidated or atelectatic lung tissue.[2,11] This form tends to affect the larger, thick-walled bronchi. Saccular bronchiectasis has the appearance of a cluster of grapes and results from circumscribed sacculations of bronchial walls at their terminal end, separated by inflamed or indurated lung tissue.[2,25] In contrast to saccular bronchiectasis, which affects the intermediated-sized bronchi, cystic bronchiectasis is believed to be a severe form of saccular bronchiectasis that involves terminal bronchi.[2] The varicose form of bronchiectasis consists of beaded, widened bronchi with irregular contours.[11] Most cases of bronchiectasis in dogs and cats are of the cylindrical form, with saccular bronchiectasis being the next most common form.[5,25] Cystic bronchiectasis has been described in the dog but not in the cat.[2,5] Varicose bronchiectasis has not been reported in either dogs or cats.

Thoracic radiography is also useful in determining whether bronchiectasis is focal or diffuse. In the retrospective study of cats with bronchiectasis,[5] thoracic radiography demonstrated a nearly equal distribution of focal and diffuse lesions; this was similar to one report in dogs[3] but contradictory to another study that found the diffuse form of bronchiectasis to be more common.[25] Focal lesions tend to correspond to the presence of solitary masses (e.g., neoplasms) or regional infection (e.g., aspiration pneumonia) causing localized obstruction. Diffuse lesions are usually seen with generalized inflammatory processes such as chronic bronchitis, bronchiolitis or bronchopneumonia. Thoracic radiographs should be thoroughly examined for the presence of other underlying disease processes.

Survey thoracic radiography may not be a sensitive test for bronchiectatic changes because imaging of the bronchial walls is dependent on inflammation and fibrosis of the airways, conditions typical of advanced disease.[25] In humans, thoracic radiography has been shown at times to be unremarkable in the early stages of disease. In both dogs and cats, bronchiectasis has been documented by other diagnostic modalities (e.g., histology) in patients with normal thoracic radiography.[24,37]

The technique for bronchography has been previously described in small animals,[36,38] and this tool has been used successfully to document and localize bronchiectasis in the dog.[36] Visual examination of the airways using bronchoscopy can also help in the recognition of bronchiectatic lesions. Bronchoscopy has the advantages of being able to grossly visualize the airways for evidence of an obstructive lesion and enabling collection of samples for cytological examination and culture.

---

*References 1, 6, 9, 12, 14, 22, and 23.

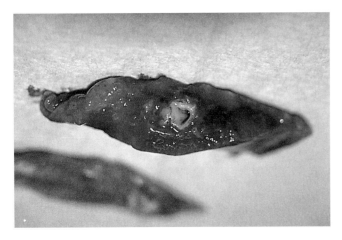

Figure 51-1. *A lung biopsy from a dog demonstrating a grossly dilated airway (bronchiectasis) with intraluminal mucopurulent exudate. This dog had severe diffuse bronchiectasis secondary to chronic eosinophilic bronchitis.*

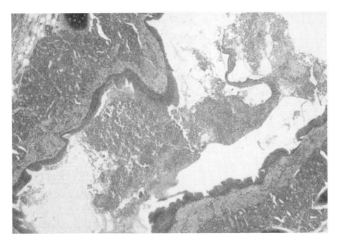

Figure 51-2. *A histologic specimen of the lung from a cat with bronchiectasis secondary to bronchopulmonary dysplasia. Note the widely dilated airway with accumulation of intraluminal cells (neutrophils). Hematoxylin and eosin stain; 40×.* (Courtesy of Stephen M. Griffey, University of California, Davis).

Gross examination of bronchiectatic airways reveals prominent dilation and luminal filling with purulent secretions (Figure 51-1). Histological examination of the lungs reveals dilation of the affected airways and various degrees of airway wall remodeling with granulation tissue and fibrosis. Microscopically, the lumen of the airways is usually filled with mucus, proteinaceous material, and inflammatory cells (Figure 51-2).[1,2,4] The types and quantity of cellular infiltrates in the lung parenchyma are dependent on the underlying cause of disease. Inflammation in the peribronchial tissues is common.[1,2,4]

Ancillary tests used in the diagnosis of bronchiectasis in humans include sputum examination and pulmonary function testing.[7,8,13] These tests are not routinely employed in the diagnosis of bronchiectasis in dogs or cats.

Treatment

Because bronchiectasis is irreversible, the goal of therapy is to control clinical signs and slow the progression of disease.[1] Patients with focal bronchiectasis are the exception; in these animals' surgical removal of the affected lung lobe may be curative.[1,2,39] Most cases of bronchiectasis in dogs and cats are acquired secondary to an underlying disease. Addressing the primary pathological process is vital to attempt to halt the progression of destruction of the bronchial walls. Treatment of recurrent bacterial infections (ideally based on culture and sensitivity) is critical in breaking the cycle of the host inflammatory response to microorganisms and further damage to the bronchial walls. Airway humidification may help loosen secretions and avoid inspissation and subsequent airway obstruction.[1,2] If the underlying disease is inflammatory (e.g., chronic bronchitis, canine idiopathic eosinophilic bronchitis, or feline asthma), antiinflammatory drugs such as corticosteroids are indicated. However, systemic corticosteroids must be administered with caution because of the risk of further infection. A beneficial role of inhaled steroids has been shown in humans with bronchiectasis[10]; similar studies using metered dose inhaled steroids delivered through a valved holding chamber* are warranted in dogs and cats with inflammatory airway disease.

Prognosis

In humans, bronchiectasis can lead to bronchopneumonia, pulmonary hemorrhage, bronchiolitis obliterans and emphysema, chronic respiratory insufficiency, and cor pulmonale.[1] Focal bronchiectasis treated with surgical lobectomy is associated with a good prognosis.[2] The prognosis for patients with diffuse bronchiectasis depends on the underlying disease process, the severity of pulmonary lesions and their resultant clinical manifestations, and the response to antimicrobial and/or antiinflammatory therapy.

REFERENCES

1. Swartz M: Bronchiectasis. In Fishman A, editor: *Fishman's pulmonary diseases and disorders,* ed 3, New York, 1998, McGraw-Hill.
2. Hamerslag K, Evans S, Dubielzig R: Acquired cystic bronchiectasis in the dog: A case history report, *Vet Radiol* 23:64-68, 1982.
3. Hawkins E, Ferris K, Berry C: Risk factors and objective radiographic criteria associated with bronchiectasis in dogs, *Proceedings 15th ACVIM Forum* 688, 1997.
4. Dungworth D: The respiratory system. In Jubb K, Kennedy P, Palmer N, editors: *Pathology of domestic animals,* ed 4, Orlando, FL, 1993, Academic Press.
5. Norris C, Samii V: Clinical, radiographic, and pathologic features of bronchiectasis in cats: 12 cases (1987-1999), *J Am Vet Med Assoc* 216:530-534, 2000.
6. Pasteur M, Helliwell S, Houghton S et al: An investigation into causative factors in patients with bronchiectasis, *Am J Respir Crit Care Med* 162:1277-1284, 2000.

*OptiChamber,® Respironics, Cedar Grove, NJ.

7. Wilson C, Jones P, O'Leary C et al: Systemic markers of inflammation in stable bronchiectasis, *Eur Respir J* 12:820-824, 1998.
8. Tsang K, Ho P, Lam W et al: Inhaled fluticasone reduces sputum inflammatory indices in severe bronchiectasis, *Am J Respir Crit Care Med* 158:723-727, 1998.
9. Keistinen T, Saynajakangas O, Tuuponen T et al: Bronchiectasis: An orphan disease with a poorly-understood prognosis, *Eur Respir J* 10:2784-2787, 1997.
10. Gaga M, Bentley A, Humbert M et al: Increases in CD4+ lymphocytes, macrophages, neutrophils and interleukin 8 positive cells in the airways of patients with bronchiectasis, *Thorax* 53:685-691, 1998.
11. Suter P: Lower airway and pulmonary parenchymal diseases, *Thoracic diseases of the dog and cat,* Wettswil, Switzerland, 1984, PF Suter.
12. Robbins S: *Robbins' pathologic basis of disease,* ed 4, Philadelphia, 1989, WB Saunders.
13. De Gracia J, Rodrigo M, Morell F et al: IgG subclass deficiencies associated with bronchiectasis, *Am J Respir Crit Care Med* 153:650-655, 1996.
14. Marwah O, Sharma O: Bronchiectasis: How to identify, treat and prevent, *Postgrad Med* 97:149-159, 1995.
15. Morrison W, Wilsman N, Fox L et al: Primary ciliary dyskinesia in the dog, *J Vet Int Med* 1:67-74, 1987.
16. Voorhout G, Goedegebuure S, Nap R: Congenital lobar emphysema caused by aplasia of bronchial cartilage in a Pekinese puppy, *Vet Pathol* 23:83-84, 1986.
17. Anderson W, King J, Flint T: Multifocal bullous emphysema with concurrent bronchial hypoplasia in two aged Afghan hounds, *J Comp Path* 100:469-473, 1989.
18. Lobetti R, Leisewitz A, Spencer J: *Pneumocystis carinii* in the miniature dachshund: Case report and literature review, *J Sm Anim Pract* 37:280-285, 1996.
19. Lobetti R: Common variable immunodeficiency in miniature dachshunds affected with *Pneumocystis carinii* pneumonia, *J Vet Diagn Invest* 12:39-45, 2000.
20. LaRue M, Garlick D, Lamb C et al: Bronchial dysgenesis and lobar emphysema in an adult cat, *J Am Vet Med Assoc* 197:886 888, 1990.
21. Roperto F, Brunetti A, Saviano L et al: Morphologic alterations in the cilia of a cat, *Vet Pathol* 33:460-462, 1996.
22. Bradford J, De Camp P: Bronchiectasis, *Surg Clin N Amer* 46:1485-1492, 1966.
23. Nicotra M, Rivera M, Dale A et al: Clinical, pathophysiologic and microbiologic characterization of bronchiectasis in an aging cohort, *Chest* 108:955-961, 1995.
24. Norris CR, Griffey SM, Samii VF et al: Comparison of results of thoracic radiography, cytologic evaluation of bronchoalveolar lavage fluid and histologic evaluation of lung specimens in dogs with respiratory tract disease: 16 Cases (1996-2000), *JAVMA* 218(9)1456-1461, 2001.
25. Myer W, Burt J: Bronchiectasis in the dog: Its radiographic appearance, *J Am Vet Rad* 14:3-11, 1973.
26. Kirchner B, Port C, Magnoc T et al: Spontaneous bronchopneumonia in laboratory dogs infected with untyped *Mycoplasma* spp, *Lab Anim Sci* 40:625-628, 1990.
27. O'Brien J: Chronic bronchitis in the dog, *Vet Annual* 14:125-128, 1973.
28. Padrid P, Hornof W, Kurpershoek C et al: Canine chronic bronchitis, *J Vet Int Med* 4:172-180, 1990.
29. Clercx C, Peeters D, Snaps F et al: Eosinophilic bronchopneumopathy in dogs, *J Vet Intern Med* 14:282-291, 2000.
30. Brownlie S: A retrospective study of diagnosis in 109 cases of canine lower respiratory disease, *J Sm Anim Pract* 31:371-376, 1990.
31. Dye J, McKiernan B, Rozanski E et al: Bronchopulmonary disease in the cat: Historical, physical, radiographic, clinicopathologic and pulmonary functional evaluation of 24 affected and 15 healthy cats, *J Vet Int Med* 10:385-400, 1996.
32. Moise N, Wiedenkeller D, Yeager A et al: Clinical, radiographic, and bronchial cytologic features of cats with bronchial disease: 65 cases (1980-1986), *J Am Vet Med Assoc* 194:1467-1473, 1989.
33. Padrid P, Snook S, Finucane T et al: Persistent airway hyperresponsiveness and histologic alterations after chronic antigen challenge in cats, *Am J Respir Crit Care Med* 151:184-193, 1995.
34. Allan G, Howlett C: Miliary broncholithiasis in a cat, *J Vet Med Assoc* 162:214-216, 1973.
35. Hoover J, Howard-Martin M, Bahr R: Chronic bronchitis, bronchiectasis, bronchiolitis, bronchiolitis obliterans, and bronchopneumonia in a rottweiler with primary ciliary dyskinesia, *J Am Anim Hosp Assoc* 25:297-304, 1989.
36. Douglas S, Hall L: Bronchography in the dog, *Vet Rec* 72:901-903, 1959.
37. Edwards D, Patton C, Bemis D et al: Immotile cilia syndrome in three dogs from a litter, *J Am Vet Med Assoc* 183:667-672, 1983.
38. Bishop E, Medway W, Archibald J: Radiological methods of investigating the thorax of small animals, including a technique for bronchography, *N Am Vet* 36:477-483, 1955.
39. Agasthian T, Deschamps C, Trastek V et al: Surgical management of bronchiectasis, *Ann Thorac Surg* 62:976-980, 1996.

CHAPTER 52

Chronic Bronchitis in Dogs

Ned F. Kuehn

Definition and Etiology

Chronic bronchitis is essentially an incurable disease of insidious onset usually seen in middle age or older dogs of the small breeds. It is characterized clinically by a chronic, persistent cough and characterized pathologically by chronic inflammation of the airways, as well as mucus hypersecretion.[1] The cough is usually productive with gagging, but because dogs do not expectorate, the production of excess mucus may be difficult to recognize. Chronic bronchitis in humans is defined as chronic or recurrent excessive mucus secretion in the bronchial tree, occurring on most days for at least 3 months of the year during at least 2 years. The diagnosis is made in absence of other specific pulmonary diseases such as cancer, pneumonia, and tuberculosis.

Because of their shorter lifespans, the definition is modified somewhat for dogs.[2] Chronic bronchitis in dogs is defined as a condition of chronic or recurrent excessive mucus production in the bronchial tree for at least 2 consecutive months in the preceding year, and manifested clinically by chronic coughing. As in man, the chronic hypersecretion of bronchial mucus is not attributable to other lung disease. Therefore, the diagnosis of chronic bronchitis requires fulfillment of three major criteria:

1. Chronic cough
2. Evidence of excessive mucus or of mucus hypersecretion
3. Exclusion of other chronic cardiorespiratory diseases (e.g., congestive heart failure, chronic bacterial pneumonia, pulmonary neoplasia, parasitism, and fungal pneumonia). In dogs, coexisting diseases (e.g., congestive heart failure and airway collapse) may be present and may complicate the diagnosis and treatment of chronic bronchitis.

The most common functional sequela of chronic bronchitis is chronic airflow obstruction, which is generally referred to as chronic obstructive pulmonary disease (COPD).[3]

Pathophysiology and Pathogenesis

Chronic bronchitis is characterized pathologically by excessive viscid mucus or mucopus (mucopurulent matter) in the tracheobronchial tree.[3] The viscid mucus contains a large number of neutrophils and macrophages admixed with varying amounts of cellular debris and edema fluid. Smaller bronchi are often occluded by thick mucus plugs. The bronchial mucosa is usually hyperemic, thickened, and edematous. Polypoid proliferations often project from the mucosa into the bronchial lumen. Patchy pneumonia is a complicating factor in about one quarter of the dogs. Emphysema is a much less important lesion in the dog than in humans, and is primarily confined to the edges of the lung lobes.

It is generally accepted that the development of chronic bronchitis is the result of a vicious cycle of airway damage and patient response. The airways are protected in health by a set of pulmonary defense mechanisms that includes normal ciliary action, normal quantity and quality of mucus, efficient collateral ventilation, and an efficient cough mechanism.[4] Persistent infection or chronic inhalation of airborne irritants can result in sustained injury to the bronchial epithelium, stimulating metaplastic transformation of the ciliary epithelium, hyperplasia and hypertrophy of mucus-secreting glands and cells, and hyperemia and cellular infiltration of the bronchial mucosa. Chronic saccular dilatation and destruction of the walls of bronchi and bronchioles (bronchiectasis) may result from long-standing airway inflammation.[1] Once bronchiectatic airway changes occur, they are irreversible. Furthermore, because all these changes impede normal defense mechanisms, bacterial colonization of the airways commonly results. The irre-

versible airway changes associated with bronchiectasis cause severe impairment of mucociliary clearance, which allows for mucus accumulation in the airways and predisposes those animals to recurrent bronchopulmonary infections.

Toy breeds of dogs often develop weakness of the cartilaginous rings of the trachea and major bronchi, resulting in tracheobronchial collapse during expiration and during coughing. Collapse of the major airways impedes expiratory airflow and efficient clearance of mucus from the bronchial tree, exacerbating the clinical condition of patients with chronic bronchitis.

Chronic insult to the bronchial epithelium not only contributes to decreased efficiency of normal pulmonary defense mechanisms but also promotes the development of functional obstruction to intrapulmonary gas flow. Airway diameter is reduced in chronic bronchitis by a combination of the following mechanisms:

- Edema and cellular infiltration of airway walls
- Copious quantities of tenacious intraluminal mucus
- Localized endobronchial narrowing associated with fibrosis of the lamina propria and polypoid proliferations of the mucosa
- Spasticity of bronchial smooth muscles causing reactive airway narrowing (may not be as significant in dogs as in humans)
- Collapse of larger bronchi associated with weakening of the bronchial walls subsequent to chronic inflammatory activity
- Plugging of smaller airways by tenacious mucus
- Obliteration of bronchioles as a result of inflammatory activity
- Emphysema develops following flooding of the alveoli with mucus

Chronic obstructive pulmonary disease is an insidious condition characterized by minimally reversible airflow obstruction that cannot be explained by any specific or infiltrative lung disease but that occurs as an end result of chronic bronchitis. The minimal reversibility of COPD differentiates it from asthma, which is a disease of significant reversibility of airflow obstruction. The small peripheral airways are the predominant sites of irreversible airflow obstruction. The persistent airway inflammation associated with chronic bronchitis is responsible for the development of refractory airflow obstruction.

The small airways normally only contribute a small percentage of total airway resistance because the tremendous number of small airways dramatically increases the total cross-sectional area for gas flow. Disease of small airways, therefore, must be diffuse and extensive before airway resistance is enhanced sufficiently to bring about clinical signs. Dogs normally have extensive interconnections between alveoli and adjacent respiratory bronchioles. Collateral ventilation through these channels allows alveoli primarily served by obstructed bronchioles to continue to be ventilated. One can therefore appreciate that small airway disease in the dog must be remarkably extensive before clinical signs of shortness of breath associated with COPD are observed. In humans, the diagnosis of COPD relies upon quantitative documentation of airflow obstruction by pulmonary function testing. Enhanced airway resistance and a decline in maximum expiratory airflow rate are characteristic findings. Because pulmonary function testing is not widely available in veterinary medicine, the diagnosis of COPD is usually determined on the basis of clinical and radiographic findings. Extensive obstruction of small airways primarily manifests clinically as expiratory dyspnea. Gas trapping in COPD occurs with premature closure of the small airways during expiration. In advanced cases of COPD, gas trapping may occur during quiet breathing, resulting in a barrel-chested appearance of some patients. Hyperinflation of the lung fields is seen radiographically.

Patients with advanced chronic bronchitis and COPD develop maldistribution of ventilation in relation to blood flow through the lung. This ventilation-perfusion inequality occurs because ventilation is universally reduced within the lung in relationship to blood flow. Chronic hypoxemia stimulates erythropoiesis, resulting in mild to moderate erythrocytosis (secondary polycythemia). The overall increase in airway resistance associated with advanced chronic bronchitis increases the work of breathing and intensifies the hypoxemic state. Vasoconstriction of the pulmonary arteries occurs in response to hypoxemia. This pulmonary hypoxic vasoconstrictor response causes an increase in pulmonary vascular resistance and pulmonary artery pressure. Chronic pulmonary hypertension may lead to right ventricular heart failure (cor pulmonale).

BOX 52-1
Possible Causes of Chronic Bronchitis in Dogs

Atmospheric Pollution
Passive Smoking
Chronic exposure to smoke in poorly ventilated confined spaces

Respiratory Tract Infections
Chronic fungal infection
Chronic bacterial infection
- *Bordetella bronchiseptica*
- *Mycoplasma spp.*
Viral infection
- Canine distemper virus
- Adenovirus (types 1 and 2)
- Herpesvirus
Parasites
- *Filaroides milksi; Filaroides herthi*
- *Crenosoma vulpis*
- *Capillaria aerophila*
- *Dirofilaria immitis*

Genetic or Acquired Defects
α_1-antitrypsin deficiency
Mucociliary defects
Immunodeficiency

Hypersensitivity (Allergic) Lung Disease

Epidemiology, Risk Factors, and Environmental Influences

The causes of chronic bronchitis are poorly understood in the dog, and usually remain unknown in individual patients. The major difficulty in determining the cause of chronic bronchitis is because the disease is detectable only in its advanced stages. This is largely because chronic bronchitis has an insidious onset and lengthy pathogenesis, and the diagnosis is largely based on a descriptive clinical definition.

The three etiologic factors in man considered most important for the hypersecretion of mucus in the bronchial tree are smoking, atmospheric pollution, and infection. Chronic exposure to sulfur dioxide (SO_2), a common atmospheric pollutant, causes mucus hypersecretion, bronchial mucus gland hypertrophy, bronchiectasis, and emphysema in dogs.[5] Box 52-1 lists several possible causes of chronic bronchitis in dogs.

Historical Findings, Clinical Signs, and Progression

Chronic bronchitis is most commonly seen in middle age to older (age greater than 5 years) smaller breeds of dogs (e.g., terriers, poodles, and cocker spaniels); however, the diagnosis should not be overlooked in large breed

dogs.[6] Clinical signs usually seen in patients with chronic bronchitis include:
- Persistent, intractable, productive cough with gagging and production of sputum, which is typically swallowed and thus difficult to document
- Cough may be unproductive, resonant, harsh, hacking during the day and productive during the evening or early morning hours
- Paroxysmal cough precipitated by exercise or excitement
- Obesity
- Cyanosis, collapse, exhaustion, and exercise intolerance
- Pronounced sinus arrhythmia
- Expiratory dyspnea
- Varying periods of remission followed by exacerbation of coughing (exacerbations may be in association with changes in weather, particularly cold weather)
- Systemic signs of illness may be seen during severe exacerbations or episodes of bronchopneumonia.[7]

The clinical diagnosis of chronic bronchitis requires fulfillment of three major criteria: (1) chronic cough on most days for at least 2 consecutive months during the preceding year; (2) evidence of excessive mucus or mucopus hypersecretion; and (3) exclusion of other chronic respiratory diseases.[8] The first two criteria may easily be established with a thorough and accurate history. The third criterion is established only after an exhaustive examination for other causes of chronic cough and dyspnea.

The most important differential diagnoses that must be ruled out are cardiac diseases (typically chronic mitral regurgitation), chronic bacterial pneumonia, pulmonary neoplasia, foreign body bronchitis, hypersensitivity airway disease, dirofilariasis, pulmonary parasites, fungal pneumonia, dysphagia, and megaesophagus.

The physical examination typically does not contribute significantly to the patient evaluation. Diligent auscultation of the chest is important because cardiac diseases (e.g., chronic mitral regurgitation or cor pulmonale) and pulmonary diseases (e.g., tracheal collapse or pneumonia) are often present as coexisting problems or secondary complications in patients with chronic bronchitis. Lung sounds may be normal or abnormal depending on the degree of airway involvement. Paninspiratory crackles and expiratory wheezes are the most commonly heard adventitious (abnormal) breath sounds. In those dogs with coexisting collapse of the intrathoracic trachea, an end-expiratory snap (click) may be heard during coughing or forced expiratory efforts. Nevertheless, it must be stressed that many dogs with chronic bronchitis have normal auscultation findings.

Dogs with severe obstructive lung disease also may show evidence of hyperinflation (barrel-chested appearance), a pronounced expiratory effort, and a prolonged expiratory phase of respiration. The presence of increased respiratory effort during the expiratory phase of breathing should be considered a significant clinical finding because chronic bronchitis is the only common respiratory disorder in dogs to cause expiratory dyspnea.

Differential Diagnosis

Chronic bronchitis is a diagnosis based on clinical exclusion of other chronic respiratory diseases. The presence of coexisting cardiopulmonary disease may, however, complicate the diagnosis of chronic bronchitis. Chronic respiratory diseases associated with either cough or exercise intolerance, or both, that should be excluded include congestive heart failure, tracheal collapse, hypersensitivity (allergic) lung disease, parasitic lung disease, dirofilariasis, neoplastic lung disease, eosinophilic or lymphomatoid granulomatosis, pneumonia, lung lobe abscess, foreign body, lung lobe torsion, diaphragmatic hernia, pleural space disease (e.g., hemothorax, chylothorax, pneumothorax, neoplasia), neuromuscular diseases with secondary aspiration pneumonia (e.g., megaesophagus, myasthenia gravis), laryngeal paralysis, and mediastinal disease (e.g., pneumomediastinum, neoplasia).

Diagnostic Tests

Since the diagnosis of canine chronic bronchitis is largely based on the history of chronic cough, diagnostic tests are performed to rule out other causes of chronic cough. A complete blood count (CBC), serum biochemical profile, and urinalysis are indicated if systemic disease is suspected. In dogs with respiratory abnormalities only, a CBC can be valuable, although it is often normal. An increased white blood cell count may indicate the presence of bronchopneumonia, whereas eosinophilia may suggest an allergic or parasitic pneumonitis. Arterial blood gas analysis may be indicated in some patients with severe obstructive lung disease. An increased $Paco_2$ due to hypoventilation is a grave finding that denotes the onset of ventilatory failure associated with increased work of breathing. All dogs with chronic cough from heartworm endemic areas should have an antigen test (or similar tests) performed to rule out dirofilariasis. A fecal examination (standard flotation and Baermann) should be performed to rule out the presence of lung parasites, if suspected.

Good quality thoracic radiographs are essential to rule out other causes of chronic cough or to disclose complicating conditions such as pneumonia, bronchiectasis, and cardiac disease. Thoracic radiographs from dogs with nonobstructive chronic bronchitis usually show bronchial wall thickening or generalized increased airway-oriented interstitial density or both (Figure 52-1). Bronchial wall thickening is recognized by "doughnut" shadows and "tram lines," which arise from either end-on or longitudinal projections of thickened bronchial walls, respectively. The existence of alveolar infiltrates may indicate concurrent pneumonia or pulmonary edema. Many dogs, however, have normal appearing lung fields; thus the finding of normal thoracic radiographs should not rule out the diagnosis of chronic bronchitis.

The presence of a mild to moderate peribronchial pattern in the thoracic radiograph of an older dog is significant and should not be dismissed as a change compatible with age. Peribronchial and interstitial densities in thoracic radiographs of older dogs have been shown to correlate with significant histologic abnormalities.[9] Likewise, similar changes in the chest radiograph of an older human would be considered a significant sign of peribronchial pathology.

Dogs with obstructive chronic bronchitis (e.g., chronic bronchitis and chronic obstructive pulmonary disease) have radiographic evidence of pulmonary hyperinflation in addition to bronchial wall thickening and a generalized increase in airway oriented interstitial density. Pulmonary hyperinflation is recognized by hyperlucency and enlargement of the lung fields, and by caudal displacement and flattening of the diaphragm. Bronchopneumonia and bronchiectasis may arise as complications of chronic bronchitis. Superimposed bronchopneumonia is recognized radiographically by patchy alveolar infiltrates. Bronchiectasis is identified by saccular or cylindrical dilation of bronchi.

Bronchoalveolar lavage or tracheal wash to collect material for cytology and microbiology should be considered in all dogs suspected of having chronic bronchitis. It is definitely indicated in any dog with chronic bronchitis that has an acute exacerbation of clinical signs. Bronchopulmonary cytology in dogs with chronic bronchitis typically reveals excess mucus with either normal or hyperplastic bronchial epithelial cells; and increased

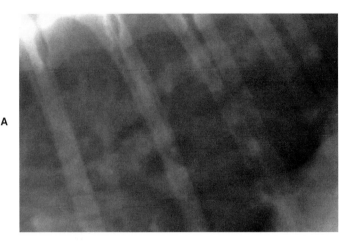

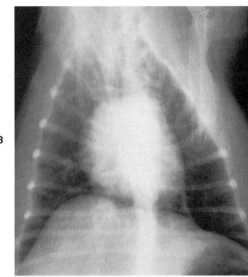

Figure 52-1. A, Close-up view of the dorsocaudal lung lobes on a lateral thoracic radiograph. **B,** Ventrodorsal view of the same thorax. Both views are from a dog with nonobstructive chronic bronchitis and show bronchial wall thickening and a generalized increase in airway-oriented interstitial density.

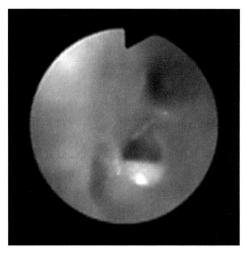

Figure 52-2. Excessive, thick, tenacious mucus may be found in strands or small plaque-like accumulations within the airways. Small airways may be occluded by mucus plugs.

numbers of macrophages, goblet cells, neutrophils, and lymphocytes. Purulent material characterized by increased neutrophils with engulfed bacteria indicates an associated bronchial infection or bronchopneumonia. The presence of large numbers of eosinophils may suggest an underlying hypersensitivity disorder or parasitic disease.

Microbiological culture and sensitivity testing of the fluid obtained during bronchoalveolar lavage or tracheal wash may be indicated to rule out secondary bacterial infection. The airways and lungs of healthy dogs are commonly inhabited by a variety of bacterial flora.[10,11] Growth of small numbers of bacteria on culture does not necessarily imply the presence of infection. In many dogs with chronic bronchitis, bacteria cultured from the airways or lungs merely reflect innocuous colonization rather than infection. Tracheobronchial culture and sensitivity testing

is indicated in newly diagnosed dogs with chronic bronchitis that have radiographic or bronchoscopic evidence of bronchiectasis, and in dogs with an acute exacerbation of previously stable chronic bronchitis. In most of these situations, bronchopulmonary cytology supports the presence of infection based on the findings of intracellular bacteria or the toxic appearance of neutrophils. For the culture results to be meaningful it is essential that sample material for tracheobronchial culture and sensitivity testing is obtained from the lower airways and not the pharynx. The most common isolates are *Bordetella bronchiseptica*, *Streptococcus* spp., *Pasteurella* spp., *Escherichia coli*, *Pseudomonas* spp., and *Klebsiella* spp.

Bronchoscopy may be a useful procedure in helping to establish a clinical diagnosis of chronic bronchitis, especially in dogs lacking the typical radiographic findings of the disease. Bronchoscopy is also valuable in obtaining representative samples from the deeper airways for cytology and culture. The airways of dogs with chronic bronchitis are characterized by erythema and a roughened granular appearance.[3] The mucosa often appears thickened, irregular, and edematous. Occasionally polypoid or nodular proliferations are seen projecting into the bronchial lumen. Excessive thick tenacious mucus may be found in strands or small plaquelike accumulations within the airways. Small airways may be occluded by mucus plugs (Figure 52-2). Collapse of the dorsal tracheal membrane into the lumen of the airway is commonly observed in dogs with chronic bronchitis and indicates the presence of concurrent tracheal collapse. Principal bronchial collapse may be observed in some patients during passive tidal exhalation. These patients typically have a worse prognosis than those without evidence of principal bronchial collapse. Saccular and irregular dilation of secondary or tertiary bronchi indicates the presence of bronchiectasis.

Pathological and Histopathological Findings

Because chronic bronchitis is largely a clinical diagnosis, tissue biopsy is not required for confirmation. Fibrosis; edema; and cellular infiltration of the lamina propria by lymphocytes, plasma cells, macrophages, and neutrophils are seen histopathologically. A significant proportion of the tracheobronchial wall is occupied by mucous glands. There is both an increase in size and number (hypertrophy) of mucous glands, in addition to an overall increase (hyperplasia) in the number of epithelial goblet cells.[12] Focal ulceration, loss of cilia, and squamous metaplasia of the bronchial epithelium is also found. Extremely severe cases may have medial hypertrophy of the small pulmonary arteries and muscularization of the pulmonary arterioles,[13] associated with right ventricular hypertrophy as a result of chronic hypoxic pulmonary hypertension.

Bronchopulmonary cytology of deep lung samples obtained via bronchoalveolar lavage typically reveals excess mucus, with either normal or hyperplastic bronchial epithelial cells; and a preponderance of nondegenerate neutrophils.[14] Increased numbers of macrophages, goblet cells, and lymphocytes may be present. Bronchial casts of airway mucus (Curschmann's spirals) are sporadically recovered in lavage fluid samples. The presence of increased numbers of neutrophils does not necessarily indicate the presence of bacterial infection. Bacterial infection is not a clinical problem in many dogs with chronic bronchitis. The presence of large numbers of degenerate neutrophils or neutrophils with engulfed bacteria supports the presence of secondary bacterial bronchitis or bronchopneumonia.

Occasionally, dogs with chronic bronchitis have increased numbers of eosinophils in lavage fluid; this may indicate concurrent systemic hypersensitivity or parasitism by gastrointestinal parasites or ectoparasites, underlying hypersensitivity lung disease, or the stage of disease. Increased numbers of eosinophils may be recovered from humans with acute exacerbation of chronic bronchitis, signifying that noninfectious irritants, viruses, and *Mycoplasma* spp. should be considered as possible causes of acute inflammation.[15]

Management and Monitoring

The structural alterations in airway anatomy associated with chronic bronchitis are not readily reversible, if at all. Bronchiectasis, tracheobronchial collapse, and emphysema are permanent, irreversible changes that complicate the management of these patients. Because this disease is essentially incurable, client education is very important. There should be an understanding by the client of the natural history of the problem and the goals of therapy.

Therapy is based on an assessment of the nature and severity of the individual animal's problems. Basically, management of patients with chronic bronchitis is divided into five major categories:

1. Avoidance of exacerbating factors and control of body weight
2. Relief of airway obstruction and inflammation
3. Control of cough
4. Control of infection
5. Oxygen therapy

Factors initiating chronic bronchitis are rarely identified. If an offending agent is identified and exposure continues, cure is rarely achieved and control is simply more difficult. In the unusual situation where exposure to the initiating factors can be curtailed, there are reduced airway inflammatory changes and return of the airway anatomy towards normal. It is recommended that dogs with chronic bronchitis be kept in a clean, cool environment. Exposure to inhaled irritants (e.g., oven and household cleaners, dust or smoke, heat, and humidity) should be avoided. If concurrent airway collapse is present, events promoting stress or excitement should be avoided to reduce paroxysmal bouts of coughing. These dogs, as well as those with marked tracheal sensitivity for cough, should be fitted with a harness rather than a collar.

Many dogs with chronic bronchitis are overweight. The excessive accumulation of extrathoracic, intrathoracic, and intraabdominal fat restricts the respiratory system and thereby decreases lung volume.[3] Obesity decreases thoracic wall compliance, increases the work of breathing, and increases intraabdominal pressure on the diaphragm. A low resting lung volume is present, predisposing the animal to small airway closure, which thereby decreases the efficiency of normal pulmonary defense mechanisms and reduces pulmonary ventilation. Weight reduction improves ventilation, promotes increased exercise capability, enhances arterial oxygenation, and reduces stress on the cardiovascular system. In some dogs, a significant improvement in clinical signs is seen with weight loss alone.

Relief of airway obstruction is generally accomplished by patient-specific combinations of three types of therapy: antiinflammatory medications, bronchodilator medications, and treatments that promote removal of accumulated airway secretions.

Antiinflammatory therapy is the most important aspect of treatment of chronic bronchitis. Chronic bronchial inflammation results in mucus hypersecretion, mucosal bronchial wall thickening, and variable degrees of airway smooth muscle constriction. Weeks to months of therapy may be required to achieve a reduction in airway inflammation, and in some instances control of airway inflammation is never attained.

Because most cases of canine chronic bronchitis do not have a defined cause, the primary basis of medical treatment is to control airway inflammation. Glucocorticoids appear to benefit dogs with chronic bronchitis, presumably by alleviating chronic airflow obstruction by reducing airway inflammation and mucus production, and by decreasing cough by diminishing stimulation of airway sensory nerves responsible for initiating cough.[7,14] Glucocorticoids are the most effective drugs and form the basis of chronic therapy for managing dogs with chronic bronchitis. However, glucocorticoids should not be given to patients with secondary bronchopulmonary infection.

Studies to determine the specific bioavailability of the various glucocorticoid preparations for lung tissue have not been established in the dog. In humans, hydrocortisone seems to have the greatest penetrability for lung tissue, followed by methylprednisolone and prednisone. Oral or parenteral glucocorticoid therapy is typically used in dogs. Many adverse side effects can develop with chronic oral or parenteral glucocorticoid therapy. Short-acting glucocorticoids such as prednisone and prednisolone are associated with fewer side effects than the long-acting preparations such as dexamethasone, methylprednisolone, and triamcinolone. Inhaled glucocorticoid therapy is preferred in human medicine because it allows direct absorption of the drug into the lung and diminishes systemic side effects; however, this route of administration is not feasible for many canine patients.

A 10- to 14-day therapeutic trial using oral prednisone or prednisolone at a dosage of 0.5 to 1 mg/kg every 12 hours is initially recommended. If remission of clinical signs is induced, the dosage should be reduced by half every 10 to 14 days. The dosage of medication should gradually be reduced to the absolute minimum required to maintain improvement of clinical signs (i.e., reduction in cough and improved exercise tolerance). Prolonged alternate or every third day therapy is beneficial in some patients. If the sole administration of prednisone or prednisolone does not bring about significant clinical improvement, combination therapy with a bronchodilator such as albuterol should be undertaken. After 2 to 4 months of maintenance therapy, an attempt should be made to gradually stop treatment entirely. Some dogs may not have worsening of clinical signs for months after stopping therapy. Glucocorticoid therapy should be reinstituted using the guidelines above if exacerbation of disease is observed.

The use of nonsteroidal antiinflammatory drugs has not been evaluated in the treatment of dogs with chronic bronchitis. While thromboxane TXA2 and prostacyclines PGF2 and PGD2 cause bronchoconstriction under experimental conditions, they are not considered at this time to play an important role in the pathogenesis of bronchoconstriction in dogs with chronic bronchitis.

Bronchodilators are widely prescribed in humans to relieve bronchoconstriction associated with chronic bronchitis. Their use in dogs with chronic bronchitis is predicated on the assumption that bronchoconstriction is present and is a significant component of airway obstruction. There is evidence to suggest that beta$_2$-agonist therapy can increase expiratory airflow, reduce wheezing, increase exercise tolerance, reduce cough, and partially resolve radiographic changes when given to some dogs with chronic bronchitis.[7] However, it is difficult to confirm the presence and reversibility of bronchoconstriction in a given dog with chronic bronchitis because pulmonary function tests such as tidal breathing flow volume loops are not widely used. Despite this limitation, probably all dogs with chronic bronchitis should be given the benefit of trial therapy with bronchodilators. The efficacy of bronchodilator therapy should be judged in terms of clinical improvement because relatively few dogs with chronic bronchitis have reversible bronchoconstriction. The sole use of bronchodilators is not advised in dogs that demonstrate clinical improvement with bronchodilator therapy. The inflammatory nature of chronic bronchitis is chronic and progressive, so concurrent use of glucocorticoids is advised.

Beta$_2$-agonists (e.g., albuterol and terbutaline) may be the most effective bronchodilator drugs for use in dogs with chronic bronchitis.[7] These drugs also appear to act synergistically with glucocorticoids to control airway inflammation. Therefore, dogs that demonstrate a positive clinical response to beta$_2$-agonist therapy may have control of their clinical signs with a reduced dosage of both drugs when given in combination. Beta$_2$-agonist therapy should be considered in dogs with exercise intolerance, wheezing on chest auscultation, or failure of adequate response to glucocorticoids. Common side effects of beta$_2$-agonists include restlessness and skeletal muscle tremors. These side effects usually resolve within 2 to 5 days of initiating therapy. Albuterol syrup is recommended at a starting dosage of 0.02 mg/kg PO every 12 hours for 5 days. After 5 days, if a positive response to the initial dosage was not appreciated, the dosage may be increased to 0.05 mg/kg PO every 8 to 12 hours providing that the dog is tolerating the medication. If a positive response to therapy is appreciated, the lowest effective dosage of albuterol that minimizes cough and improves exercise tolerance should be found. Should a positive response not be established within 2 weeks of instituting therapy, further bronchodilator treatment will likely not be effective. The effective dosage for terbutaline has not been clearly defined; however, a dosage of approximately 1 mg/kg PO every 12 hours has been recommended.

The methylxanthine derivatives (e.g., theophylline and aminophylline) previously were most commonly used in the management of canine chronic bronchitis.[16] Although the pharmacokinetics of theophylline in the dog are well established,[17] only anecdotal reports address the occasional effectiveness of this drug for dogs with chronic bronchitis. Like beta-agonists, methylxanthine derivatives seem to act synergistically with glucocorticoids to control airway inflammation.[14] Theophylline is reported to cause relaxation of bronchial smooth muscle, increase mucociliary transport rates, stabilize mast cell membranes, decrease bronchovascular leak, and increase contractibility of fatigued diaphragmatic muscle.[14] Adverse side effects of methylxanthines are likely related to adenosine antagonism and include gastrointestinal distress, tachycardia, and hyperexcitability. The preferred theophylline preparations for dogs are long-acting, slow-release tablet formulations (Theo-Dur Tablets [Key Pharmaceuticals], 20 mg/kg PO every 12 hours; Slo-Bid Gyrocaps [Rhone-Poilenc Rorer], 20 to 25 mg/kg PO every 12 hours).

Anticholinergic agents (e.g., atropine and ipratropium bromide) are potent bronchodilators.[14] Anticholinergic drugs relax airway smooth muscle and reduce mucus production through blockage of vagal nerve transmission to airway smooth muscle and submucosal gland and goblet cells. Atropine has not proven to be an effective bronchodilator in dogs with chronic bronchitis because increased vagal tone is only a minor contributing factor to airway narrowing in this disease. Ipratropium bromide is administered only by inhalation and is not at present a practical alternative for dogs.

Some dogs with chronic bronchitis benefit from methods to facilitate removal of accumulated airway secretions. The inhalation of humidified air via steam inhalation or nebulization moistens thick, tenacious bronchial secretions and thereby facilitates their movement from the airways. An ultrasonic nebulizer is best because it produces the very small particles of water needed to penetrate deep in the airways. Aerosol therapy for hospitalized patients may be accomplished by placing a portable nebulizer in an enclosed cage with the animal. A more expensive alternative is the use of an oxygen cage with humidification and temperature controls. Therapy may be attempted at home by compelling the dog to breathe aerosolized vapors from a portable nebulizer. Treatment in either situation requires a minimum of 15- to 30-minute treatments three or four times daily in order to be effective.

Light exercise after aerosol therapy assists in dislodging bronchial mucus and helps open small airways by promoting increased lung volumes associated with a standing posture. Chest physiotherapy is also beneficial following aerosol therapy to aid in dislodging bronchial mucus. Chest percussion (coupage) is achieved by using a cupped hand to generate vibrations on the patient's thoracic wall, and should be performed three or four times daily for 5 to 10 minutes per session. The success of treatment is judged by the induction of a bout of productive coughing following therapy.

Expectorants may be tried to promote removal of bronchial secretions. Theoretically, these drugs enhance the secretion of less viscous bronchial mucus, but their efficacy is questionable. Medications containing a combination of cough suppressants and expectorants should not be used if the cough is productive because an intact cough reflex is desirable to expel bronchial secretions. Mucolytics such as acetylcysteine are drugs capable of breaking the disulfide bonds that are partially responsible for the viscid nature of airway mucus. Unfortunately, aerosolized acetylcysteine is irritating to bronchial epithelium and can trigger bronchoconstriction.[6] Antiinflammatory therapy, maintenance of normal hydration, and aerosol therapy are probably the most beneficial methods to reduce production and viscosity of airway mucoid secretions.

Cough is an important pulmonary defense mechanism. Effective removal of viscid airway secretions is of great importance in patients with chronic bronchitis. Suppression of cough before resolution of inflammation may result in mucus trapping, which may perpetuate airway inflammation. Once clinical signs suggest that inflammation is resolving (e.g., improved exercise tolerance, improved thoracic radiographs, chronic nonproductive cough), cough suppressants may be advantageous to resolve cough because chronic coughing can lead to repeated airway injury and syncope.[6] The use of antitussives should be restricted to those dogs with periods of nonproductive cough, dogs with chronic cough who are unable to sleep, and dogs with chronic cough due to airway collapse. Narcotic antitussives such as hydrocodone bitartrate and butorphanol are much more effective than over-the-counter anti-tussives such as dextromethorphan. In some dogs, however, dextromethorphan may be effective in controlling cough. The primary side effects of the narcotic antitussives are sedation or drowsiness and constipation. Hydrocodone bitartrate may be given at a dosage of 0.22 mg/kg PO every 6 to 12 hours, or butorphanol at a dosage of 0.05 to 1 mg/kg PO every 6 to 12 hours, both as needed without inducing excessive sedation. Long-term therapy may be required in dogs with severe airway collapse. It is important not to indiscriminately suppress coughing, especially if productive cough or bronchopulmonary infection is present. The cause of an acute exacerbation of cough should be found, if possible, before recommending cough suppressants.

Bacterial infection does not usually play a significant role in the cause or exacerbation of clinical signs in dogs with chronic bronchitis.[14] The signs of bronchial disease typically wax and wane in severity and frequency. Reports describing the therapeutic effect of antibiotics in controlling chronic cough were likely consistent with the waxing and waning nature of untreated cases of chronic bronchitis. Likewise, a positive culture does not necessarily imply infection but may be a result of normal airway contaminants. The use of antibiotics should only be based on demonstrated evidence of bronchial infection. Prompt effective treatment of any bacterial bronchial infection is essential in dogs with chronic bronchitis in order to prevent further perpetuation of airway damage and the development of bronchopneumonia. Culture and sensitivity of lavage fluid from the lungs or lower airways should be considered in dogs with documented evidence of bronchiectasis (either via radiographs or bronchoscopy) or those with an acute exacerbation of symptoms associated with mucopurulent nasal discharge, fever, or radiographic signs of lobar consolidation.

Antibiotic choice should be based on sensitivity results when possible. Broad-spectrum antibiotics are indicated due to the diversity of bacteria commonly isolated in the lung. Lipophilic antibiotics should be employed due to the presence of the blood-bronchus barrier, which limits penetration of many antibiotics into bronchial tissue.[6] Antibiotics of choice include chloramphenicol (50 mg/kg PO every 8 hours), doxycycline (2.5 to 5 mg/kg PO every 12 hours), and enrofloxacin (5 to 10 mg/kg PO every 12 hours or 10 to 20 mg/kg PO every 24 hours); or ciprofloxacin (10 to 20 mg/kg PO every 12 hours or 20 to 40 mg/kg PO every 24 hours). Fluoroquinolones such as enrofloxacin inhibit the metabolism of theophylline, and the combination of the two drugs can result in toxic plasma levels of theophylline.[18] A reduction in the dosage of theophylline by at least 30% is advised if fluoroquinolones are required. Chronic or severe infections may involve various organisms and may require a combination of chloramphenicol, trimethoprim-sulfa (15 mg/kg PO every 12 hours), or clindamycin (11 mg/kg PO every 12 hours) with enrofloxacin or ciprofloxacin to facilitate resolution of the infection.

Oxygen therapy can be used for temporary support during treatment of dogs with severe hypoxemia as a result of acute decompensation of disease or the presence of severe bronchopneumonia.[3] The inhaled air should be humidified to help liquify tenacious bronchial secretions and prevent drying of the airways. Periodic suctioning of the airways with a soft rubber catheter (if the dog is intubated and receiving temporary ventilatory support) or chest physiotherapy (if the patient is mobile) should be attempted to remove accumulated secretions. Animals receiving oxygen therapy and suffering severe obstructive disease should be frequently monitored for hypoventilation because their hypoxic drive stimulus for respiration may be removed by the inhalation of oxygen rich air.

Outcome and Prognosis

Chronic bronchitis is a common, progressive, and chronic airway disorder that can often be managed but is essentially incurable. The prognosis is improved when the airway inflammation can be effectively controlled and exposure to environmental respiratory irritants is reduced. Periods of exacerbation, nevertheless, often characterize the chronic, progressive clinical course of disease in these patients. Fortunately, most dogs are only affected by a recurrent cough. All dogs with chronic bronchitis should have periodic examinations to evaluate the effectiveness of any current therapy and to ensure that secondary bronchopulmonary infections are not present.

The major complications associated with chronic bronchitis are the development of COPD, bronchopneumonia, bronchiectasis, and, in severely affected dogs, cor pulmonale. Bronchopulmonary infections should be treated promptly and effectively. Dogs with bronchiectasis should be inspected regularly (every 3 to 6 months) for the development of bronchopneumonia. Cor pulmonale (right heart failure) is a serious consequence of chronically increased pulmonary vascular resistance. This is a direct complication of advanced chronic bronchitis and indicates a grave prognosis for the patient.

REFERENCES

1. Wheeldon EB, Pirie HM, Fischer EW et al: Chronic respiratory disease in the dog, *J Small An Pract* 18:229, 1997.
2. Prueter JC, Sherding RG: Canine chronic bronchitis. In Spaulding GL, editor: Symposium on respiratory diseases, *Vet Clin North Amer* 15: 1085, 1985.
3. Amis TC: Chronic bronchitis in dogs. In Kirk RW, editor: *Current veterinary therapy*, vol 9, Philadelphia, 1986, WB Saunders.
4. Haschek WM: Response of the lung to injury. In Kirk RW, editor: *Current veterinary therapy*, vol 9, Philadelphia, 1986, WB Saunders.
5. Shore SA, Kariya ST, Anderson K et al: Sulfur-dioxide-induced bronchitis in dogs, *Am Rev Respir Dis* 135:840, 1987.
6. Johnson L: CVT update: Canine chronic bronchitis. In Bonagura JD, editor: *Current veterinary therapy*, vol 13, Philadelphia, 2000, WB Saunders.
7. Padrid PA, Hornof W, Kurperchoek C et al: Canine chronic bronchitis: A pathophysiologic evaluation of 18 cases, *J Vet Intern Med* 4:172, 1990.
8. Pirie HM, Wheeldon EB: Chronic bronchitis in the dog, *Adv Vet Sci Comp Med* 20:253, 1976.
9. Reif JS, Rhodes WH: The lungs of aged dogs: A radiographic-morphologic correlation, *J Am Vet Radiol Soc* 7:5, 1996.
10. Lindsey JO, Pierce AK: An examination of the microbiologic flora of normal lung of the dog, *Am Rev Respir Dis* 117:501, 1978.
11. McKiernan BC, Smith AR, Kissil M: Bacteria isolated from the lower trachea of clinically healthy dogs, *J Am Anim Hosp Assoc* 20:139, 1984.
12. Wheeldon EB, Breeze RG, Pirie HM: Animal model: Chronic bronchitis in dogs, *Am J Path* 96(1):355, 1979.
13. Turk JR, Rantanen NW: Chronic bronchitis, cardiomegaly, and medial hypertrophy of small pulmonary arteries in a dog, *J Small Anim Pract* 23:719, 1982.
14. Padrid P: Diagnosis and therapy of canine chronic bronchitis. In Kirk RW, editor: *Current veterinary therapy*, vol 12, Philadelphia, 1995, WB Saunders.
15. Saetta M, DiStefano A, Maesterelli P et al: Airway eosinophilia in chronic bronchitis during exacerbations, *Am J Respir Crit Care Med* 153:1646, 1994.
16. Papich MG, Bronchodilator therapy. In Kirk RW, editor: *Current veterinary therapy*, vol 9, Philadelphia, 1986, WB Saunders.
17. McKiernan BC, Neff-Davis CA, Koritz GD et al: Pharmacokinetic studies of theophylline in dogs, *J Vet Pharmacol Ther* 4:103, 1981.
18. Intorre L, Mengozzi G, Maccheroni M et al: Enrofloxacin-theophylline interaction: Influence of enrofloxacin on theophylline steady-state pharmacokinetics in the beagle dog, *J Vet Pharmacol Ther* 19:352, 1995.

CHAPTER 53

Feline Bronchial Disease/Asthma

Jeff D. Bay • Lynelle R. Johnson

Definition and Etiology

Feline bronchial disease (feline asthma or bronchitis) is one of the most common respiratory diseases in cats. It is recognized clinically by various combinations of cough, wheeze, exercise intolerance, and respiratory distress and is characterized pathologically by inflammation of the lower airways without an obvious identifiable cause. Young- to middle-age cats are most commonly affected. The Siamese breed may be overrepresented, although cats of any breed are susceptible.

Pathophysiology and Pathogenesis

Like asthma in humans, the pathophysiology of feline bronchial disease is not altogether known. However, considerable research has been completed on these syndromes in recent decades, and the disease in cats has been better characterized by the use of an experimental model of antigen-induced inflammatory bronchial disease.[1-5] Clinical signs range from intermittent cough to severe respiratory distress; these are attributable to airway obstruction caused by bronchial inflammation, with subsequent smooth muscle constriction, epithelial edema, and mucous gland hypertrophy and hyperactivity.[6-9] These changes are reversible in some cats that have primarily hyperresponsive, inflamed airways; however, chronic inflammation may lead to permanent pathology in other cats and is evidenced by airway fibrosis or emphysema.[10]

Decreased airflow in the small airways is caused by excessive mucus secretion, airway edema, cellular infiltrates, and smooth muscle hypertrophy and constriction. Following Poiseuille's law, airflow through a bronchus or bronchiole is proportional to the radius of the tube raised to the fourth power.[11] Therefore, a 50% reduction in airway luminal size results in a sixteenfold increase in resistance to airflow, and airway mucus, edema, or bronchoconstriction can reduce airway diameter and diminish airflow significantly. Correspondingly, therapy that leads to small increases in airway lumen diameter can dramatically increase airflow and reduce clinical signs.

Severe lower airway obstruction in cats with asthma can lead to lung hyperinflation because they are unable to exhale completely past the narrowed airways, resulting in air trapping. Lung hyperinflation may cause an enlarged, barrel-chested appearance; or can be appreciated by a flattened, caudally-displaced diaphragm and increased pulmonary radiolucency on thoracic radiographs of cats with bronchial disease. Chronic airway inflammation and obstruction in this manner can induce such dramatic intraluminal pressure for significant periods that permanent airway dilation (bronchiectasis) and loss of pulmonary elastic support structures (emphysema) may result. Bronchiectasis and emphysema have been noted radiographically and histopathologically in some cats with chronic bronchial disease.[6,7,10,12] In contrast, complete obstruction of a mainstem bronchus may cause atelectasis of the corresponding lung lobe because air is unable to enter or exit and residual air is resorbed. For unknown reasons, this process seems to affect the right middle lung lobe in cats with bronchial disease more often than other lobes, as noted in radiographic series of these patients.[7,8]

Coughing may be initiated by a variety of factors in cats, including airway compression; the presence of foreign material, noxious gases, tissue, mucus, or fluid in the tracheobronchial tree; airway inflammation; or airway smooth muscle contraction. Cough in cats with bronchial disease may result from stimulation of irritant receptors due to the presence of excess mucus or inflammatory mediators in inflamed and constricted airways. Cough is seen more commonly in cats with airway disease than in those with pulmonary parenchymal disease or congestive heart failure because cough receptors are located in the airways, but not in the alveoli.[13]

Asthma is characterized by localized accumulation of inflammatory cells in the airway, particularly eosinophils and activated lymphocytes. Eosinophils appear to be primary effector cells in the development of asthmatic airway pathophysiology in cats as well as in humans. Highly charged cationic proteins found within eosinophil granules may be released into airways, causing epithelial disruption and sloughing, and smooth muscle hyperreactivity.[14] Studies in mice have shown that local interleukin-5 (IL-5) secretion from activated T lymphocytes plays a pivotal role in causing migration of activated eosinophils into airways, participating in the pathogenesis of bronchial hyperreactivity and lung damage.[15] These events may also take place in cats with bronchial disease.

Adhesion molecules contribute to selective cellular recruitment responses and permit cell-cell and cell-substratum attachments.[16] Intercellular adhesion molecule-1 (ICAM-1) is found on vascular endothelium and epithelium. Interaction of ICAM-1 with eosinophils is important for cell recruitment to human airways and for the eventual development of bronchial inflammation and hyperresponsiveness.[17] Interactions of intercellular adhesion molecules could be an important target for therapeutic intervention, although the role of these agents in the pathogenesis of feline bronchial disease has not yet been confirmed.

In vitro studies have suggested that serotonin, a primary mediator released from feline mast cells, contributes to airway smooth muscle contraction in the cat.[5] Smooth muscle cell responsiveness of tracheal and bronchial smooth muscle tissue from immune-sensitized cats was examined in the presence and absence of serotonin receptor blockade with cyproheptadine. The strength of contraction was attenuated in the presence of cyproheptadine,[5] implicating a role for serotonin in the bronchoconstriction that occurs in this model of antigen-stimulated airway hyperresponsiveness. Whether serotonin plays a role in naturally occurring disease has not been established. In this same study, prevention of leukotriene production with an inhibitor of 5-lipoxygenase had no effect on contraction of airway smooth muscle *in vitro*, suggesting that leukotriene metabolites might not play a role in feline bronchoconstriction.

Epidemiology and Risk Factors

In human asthma, allergens are risk factors for development and expression of disease, and aeroallergens are also important triggers of the inflammatory process.[18,19] The role of allergens and nonspecific airway irritants in feline bronchial disease is unknown; however, irritants may exacerbate or initiate the inflammation and airway obstruction of asthma. Conditions that might be identified as stimulants of clinical signs in cats with bronchial disease include allergens, air pollution, and aerosolized irritants.

Viral, bacterial, mycoplasmal, or parasitic respiratory tract infections also have the potential to trigger airway inflammation. Viral (e.g., rhinovirus, influenza, and respiratory syncytial virus) respiratory infections are the most common cause of asthma exacerbations in children,[20] and infections early in life may play a role in asthma development.[21] Respiratory infections increase airway hyperresponsiveness, possibly by causing or enhancing bronchial inflammation via stimulation of local cytokine secretion. Some respiratory infections may be protective for the development of asthma in humans, possibly by stimulating a T helper 1 cytokine profile (i.e., gamma interferon) that shifts the balance away

from allergic inflammation.[22] In cats, the relationship between upper respiratory tract infections and asthma remains unclear, although in a recent study, 25% of cats evaluated for signs of asthma had clinical signs consistent with upper respiratory tract infection.[6]

The role of Mycoplasma in initiation or exacerbation of clinical signs associated with feline bronchial disease remains speculative. *Mycoplasma* spp. were isolated from airway washings in 4 of 9 cats with bronchial disease,[7] and *Mycoplasma* spp. have not been recovered from the airways of healthy cats.[23,24] If present within the airway, Mycoplasma could potentially increase bronchoconstriction and airway edema by prolonging the activity of Substance P. In rodent studies, *Mycoplasma* spp. have been reported to degrade neutral endopeptidase, an enzyme responsible for Substance P degradation.[25,26]

Historical Findings and Clinical Signs

Clinical signs most often apparent in cats with bronchial disease include a combination of cough, wheeze, and abnormal or difficult respiration. Decreased airflow is responsible for the clinical signs of cough, wheeze, and lethargy. These signs are often chronic or slowly progressive; however, cats with severe exacerbations may present acutely with open mouth breathing, dyspnea, and cyanosis due to bronchoconstriction. Mildly affected cases may only have occasional and brief episodes of bronchoconstriction and cough separated by long periods without symptoms. Exacerbation or induction of clinical signs may occur in association with exposure to potential allergens or irritants such as new litter (possibly perfumed), cigarette or fireplace smoke, perfumed household items (e.g., carpet cleaners, air fresheners, deodorants, and hair spray), dust associated with remodeling, or seasonal pollens. Clinical signs commonly worsen with stress or exercise. Weight loss may be apparent in cats suffering from chronic bronchial disease; however, cats that have restricted activity due to respiratory disease can be overweight.

Differential Diagnosis

Cough is fairly specific for tracheobronchial disease in the cat because cats with pulmonary edema due to heart disease do not typically cough. Airway foreign bodies are rare but should be ruled out. Pulmonary parasitic infestation with *Paragonimus*, *Aelurostrongylus*, or *Capillaria*, although uncommon, may cause many of the same clinical findings as those present in cats with asthma (e.g., local and peripheral eosinophilic inflammation and bronchoconstriction). Infection with *Bordetella* can lead to upper respiratory tract signs, and occasionally coughing is noted.[27] Parenchymal diseases (e.g., bacterial pneumonia) are relatively uncommon in cats, and cats usually display a less pronounced cough than dogs. Occasionally, cats with chylothorax cough intermittently; however, the cough that occurs with bronchial disease is more frequent. Dyspnea or respiratory distress is common in cats with acute congestive heart failure and is often found in cats with pleural effusion or pneumothorax. Physical examination findings are helpful in distinguishing among these various disorders.

Diagnostic Tests

PHYSICAL EXAMINATION

Many asthmatic cats can appear normal at rest, and thoracic auscultation may be unremarkable. Because bronchial disease is an obstructive disease of the small, lower airways, most affected cats exhibit a prolonged expiratory phase of respiration, and audible wheezes or crackles may be heard with or without the aid of a stethoscope, usually during expiration. Air trapped distal to obstructed airways can lead to diminished thoracic wall compressibility and a barrel-shaped appearance to the chest. Many cats exhibit increased tracheal sensitivity and cough with cervical tracheal palpation.

BLOODWORK

Approximately 20% of cats with bronchial disease have a peripheral eosinophilia,[6-8] and the likelihood of eosinophilia may increase as disease severity worsens.[6] This finding is not specific however because several other possible diagnoses (e.g., lungworm or heartworm infections, gastrointestinal parasitism, or ectoparasites) may also cause peripheral eosinophilia. A stress leukogram may be apparent. Chronic hypoxemia could potentially cause a compensatory increase in hematocrit, although this is relatively uncommon. Biochemical profiles rarely yield information specific to bronchial disease. Some cats have hyperglobulinemia, suggestive of chronic immunological stimulation. Heartworm antibody and antigen serology is recommended for cats that exhibit respiratory symptoms and reside in a heartworm-endemic region.

FECAL EXAMINATION

Airway parasitic infestations with *Paragonimus*, *Aelurostrongylus*, or *Capillaria* can occur. Therefore fecal examination, including a flotation with or without centrifugation (to find *Paragonimus* and *Capillaria* eggs), and a Baermann sedimentation (to detect *Aelurostrongylus* first-stage larvae) is recommended as part of the diagnostic work-up.

RADIOLOGY

Routine thoracic radiographs can be within normal limits in some cats with bronchial disease, and the diagnosis should not be ruled out based solely upon these results. The classic lung pattern in a cat with bronchial disease includes evidence of bronchial wall thickening (doughnuts or railroad tracks) because of airway inflammation (Figure 53-1). Air trapping may also be evident in the peripheral lung fields. Signs suggestive of lung hy-

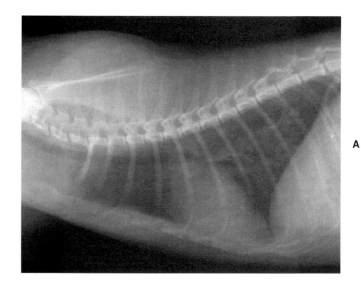

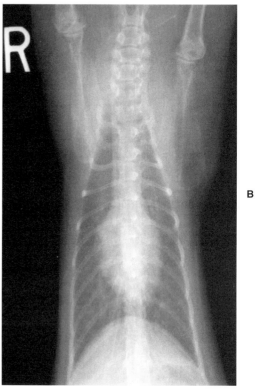

Figure 53-1. A, Lateral and **B,** ventrodorsal thoracic radiographs of a cat with bronchial disease. Notice the prominent bronchiolar radiographic pattern, especially in the caudal lung fields, seen as multiple doughnuts and railroad tracks.

perinflation and air trapping include increased lucency to the lungs and flattening or caudal displacement of the diaphragm (Figure 53-2). A small percentage of cats may have evidence of right middle lung lobe atelectasis, indicated by opacity in this lobe and a right mediastinal shift.[7,8] Rarely, cats with bronchial disease may develop pneumothorax or rib fractures secondary to chronic airway compromise and respiratory distress.[28]

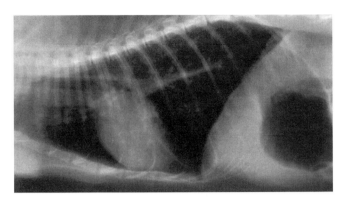

Figure 53-2. *Lateral thoracic radiograph of a cat with bronchial disease. Notice the lung hyperinflation as evidenced by the flattened, caudally-displaced diaphragm. A gas-filled stomach, caused by aerophagia, can be seen on this view. (Courtesy Dr. John D. Bonagura, The Ohio State University, Columbus, Ohio.)*

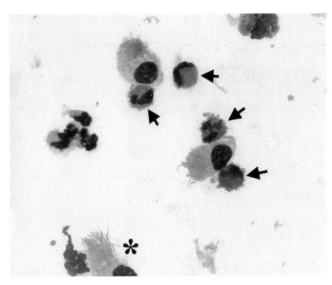

Figure 53-3. *Photomicrograph of transtracheal wash fluid cytology obtained from the cat described in Figure 53-1. Several ciliated, columnar epithelial cells (*) are seen, along with many eosinophils (arrows) (100×). The cytological differential count revealed 45% eosinophils and 40% neutrophils, and no evidence of infectious agents.*

ENDOTRACHEAL WASH (ETW)/ BRONCHOALVEOLAR LAVAGE (BAL)

Cytologic examination of airway samples from asthmatic cats generally provides evidence of airway inflammation, with increased numbers of eosinophils and/or neutrophils (Figure 53-3). A preponderance of eosinophils may be found in tracheobronchial washings from healthy cats,[23,29-31] therefore eosinophilic airway washes are not pathognomonic for asthma or bronchial disease. In a recent study, the number of eosinophils and neutrophils in BAL samples of cats with bronchopulmonary disease correlated well with disease severity.[6]

Despite the fact that a role of infectious agents in the pathogenesis of bronchial disease has not been established, aseptically handled samples of ETW or BAL fluid should be submitted for culture of aerobic bacterial and mycoplasmal organisms and for antibacterial susceptibility testing. A mixed population of aerobic bacteria has been cultured from cats with asthma, but similar bacteria can be cultured from the airways of healthy cats, so the significance of a positive culture is unknown at this point.[6] These bacteria may be colonizing the airways rather than causing true pulmonary infection. A positive culture result could be considered more meaningful if a pure culture with a large number of organisms is grown on primary culture plate media (not enrichment broth), or if intracellular bacterial organisms or a preponderance of one type of bacterium are visualized upon ETW or BAL cytology. Since oropharyngeal bacteria can contaminate samples, cytology should be carefully evaluated for the presence of squamous cells, indicating that oropharyngeal contents have likely been deposited in the sample.

Isolation of *Mycoplasma* spp. is difficult and requires specialized growth media. Therefore, before collection of samples, it is recommended that the laboratory be contacted for information on proper submission of airway specimens. The role of *Mycoplasma* in feline respiratory disease remains unknown; however, these species are potentially important because *Mycoplasma* has been cultured from airways of cats with respiratory disease[7] but not from healthy cats.[23,24]

PULMONARY FUNCTION TESTS

Pulmonary function testing is commonly utilized in human medicine for the evaluation of respiratory disease, including use in the diagnosis and monitoring of therapeutic response in patients with asthma or chronic bronchitis. Parameters such as vital capacity, airway resistance, total lung capacity, and forced expiratory volume can be measured to evaluate airway disorders and to assess response to therapy.[32] Because patient cooperation with pulmonary function tests is limited in veterinary species, identical evaluations cannot be completed; however, some methods have been developed to examine airway mechanics in anesthetized or awake cats. In awake animals, measurement of flow-volume loops during tidal breathing can be used as a noninvasive means of evaluating pulmonary function. The use of tidal breathing flow volume loops has confirmed that cats with bronchial disease have an increased ratio of expiratory time to inspiratory time, decreased area under the expiratory curve, lower expiratory flow rates, decreased tidal breathing expiratory volumes, and increased mean lung resistance.[33] These changes in resistance during the expiratory phase of respiration are compatible with lower airway obstructive disease.

Additional techniques are being investigated that would allow noninvasive measurements of pulmonary mechanics, and use of a whole-body plethysmograph has proven useful in assessing airway reactivity in normal cats.[34] Application of this technique to cats with bronchial disease would allow confirmation of airway hyperresponsiveness and quantification of the response to bronchodilators. Other measures of airway responsiveness and pulmonary mechanics require anesthesia and therefore have not been applied to a wide number of clinical cases. However, one study of cats with bronchial disease showed that lung resistance increased with disease severity, providing an objective means for assessment of disease.[6]

Pathological and Histopathological Findings

Eosinophilic and/or neutrophilic bronchial inflammation with smooth muscle hyperplasia are common histopathological findings in cats with bronchial disease. Hyperplasia and hypertrophy of goblet cells and submucosal glands are also common features, as is subsequent mucus accumulation with inflammatory cellular debris in the bronchial lumen (Figures 53-4 and 53-5). Epithelial erosion can be seen, especially in severe cases. Lobular and bullous emphysema, which may occur as a possible consequence of chronic obstructive airway disease, has been described in a small number of cats with bronchial disease.[10] Similarly, bronchiectasis has been reported in some cats with chronic bronchial disease.[10,12]

Treatment

There is no consistently reported strategy for the treatment of bronchial disease in cats, and very little research has been completed to evaluate specific treatments in cats. An expert panel has determined four components of asthma treatment in humans:

1. Use of objective measurements of lung function to assess asthma severity and to monitor the course of therapy
2. Establishment of environmental control measures to avoid or eliminate factors that precipitate asthma symptoms or exacerbations
3. Utilization of comprehensive pharmacologic therapy for long-term management of disease that is designed to reverse and prevent airway inflammation and to manage asthma exacerbations
4. Employment of patient education that fosters a partnership among the patient, his or her family, and clinicians[35]

A similar approach modified for veterinary patients and clients would be recommended in the treatment of cats with bronchial disease.

EMERGENCY MANAGEMENT

In cats that present with acute, severe respiratory distress (e.g., cyanosis and open mouth breathing), diagnostic tests should be delayed, stress should be minimized, and an oxygen enriched environment (oxygen cage with Fio_2 of at least 40%) should be provided. Initially, bronchodilator therapy (e.g., terbutaline 0.01 mg/kg IV, IM, or SC) should be used to combat acute bronchoconstriction. Inhaled bronchodilator medication (e.g., albuterol) may be used if the equipment is available and if the patient tolerates this method of administration. Visual inspection of respiratory rate and effort

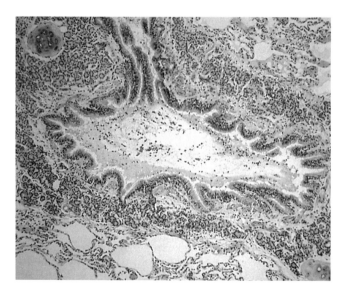

Figure 53-4. Histological section of a bronchus from a cat with bronchial disease. Note accumulation of mucus and inflammatory cells in the lumen, epithelial hyperplasia and folding, smooth muscle hypertrophy, and increased numbers of mucous glands (200×). (Courtesy of Dr. Margaret A. Miller, University of Missouri, Columbia.)

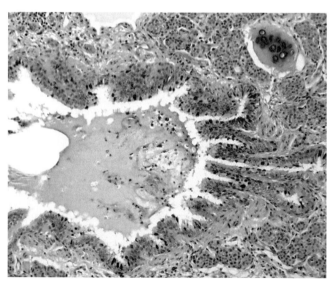

Figure 53-5. Histological section of a bronchus from a cat with bronchial disease. Note accumulation of mucus and inflammatory cells in the lumen, epithelial hyperplasia and folding, smooth muscle hypertrophy, and increased numbers of mucous glands. The Alcian blue/PAS stain (pH 2.5) highlights the numerous epithelial goblet cells (400×). (Courtesy of Dr. Margaret A. Miller, University of Missouri, Columbia.)

during the first hour of therapy will allow assessment of the therapeutic response. A positive response is expected within 30 to 45 minutes, and is indicated by a decrease in respiratory frequency and effort. If the cat does not respond favorably in that time, a repeated dose of bronchodilator medication is warranted and a rapidly acting corticosteroid (e.g., dexamethasone 0.25 to 2 mg/kg IV or IM) should be administered. If no response is seen to this combination of drugs, alternate causes for dyspnea should be investigated. If the cat remains severely dyspneic, intubation and positive pressure ventilation with 100% oxygen may be needed to facilitate diagnostic testing, including radiography, cardiac evaluation, and respiratory tract cytology and bacteriology.

Once the patient is stable, a complete diagnostic evaluation for feline asthma as outlined above is recommended. If corticosteroids have been administered to control respiratory distress, airway cytology may lack the classic inflammatory response and may therefore be of diminished benefit.

Atropine is an effective bronchodilator; however, its anticholinergic effects can cause tachycardia and inspissation of bronchial mucus that might worsen airway obstruction. Epinephrine is also a potent bronchodilator, but it should only be used in cats that are dying or those in which cardiac disease has been ruled out because its alpha and beta-1 agonist activities may cause arrhythmias, vasoconstriction, and systemic hypertension. Aminophylline exhibits weaker bronchodilatory activity than terbutaline and is not recommended as the first choice in emergency situations. Beta-blockers (e.g., propranolol and atenolol) should not be administered to cats in which bronchial disease is a possible cause for respiratory distress. Cats rely heavily on sympathetic tone for bronchodilation, and inhibition of beta-agonist activity may have dire consequences in these patients.

Initiation of emergency medications at home may be recommended in cats with a previous diagnosis of asthma that experience frequent asthma attacks. An injection of terbutaline or a dose of inhaled albuterol can be given by the owner at the onset of acute dyspnea; however, emergency veterinary attention should be sought if no response is seen within 15 to 30 minutes. It is important to stress that proper diagnosis and chronic therapy should be pursued in such cases.

CHRONIC THERAPY

Decrease Allergen/Irritant Exposure

Because environmental allergens and nonspecific irritants may be important risk factors in the initiation and exacerbation of asthma in cats, asthma care may be improved by identification of offending allergens and institution of steps to avoid these in the environment. A therapeutic trial of isolation in one room where allergens are minimized may help determine the degree of effect that allergens play in an individual cat's bronchial disease. Similarly, switching the cat's litter, especially eliminating dust and perfumes, may assist in diminishing clinical signs of asthma.

Corticosteroids

The most consistent, reliable, and effective treatment for feline asthma or bronchitis is high-dose (initially), long-term, oral corticosteroids. Reduction of underlying inflammation is recommended even in relatively asymptomatic cats because human asthmatics often have evidence of chronic airway inflammation even when clinical signs are not present.[36] Inhaled corticosteroids are utilized principally in humans, thereby allowing the topical use of an extremely effective drug without the degree of harmful side effects that systemic corticosteroids can induce. Cats can be treated with inhaled corticosteroids using pediatric spacers and aerosolization chambers, but administration can be expensive, labor-intensive, and may not be well tolerated. Fortunately most cats are relatively resistant to the health-threatening side effects of systemic corticosteroids, which can be used safely in the majority of cats. Oral prednisone or prednisolone (1 to 2 mg/kg PO BID for 7 to 10 days) is recommended, with a slow taper of the dose over 2 to 3 months in cats that respond. No benefit has been reported for the use of longer-acting oral corticosteroids. Long-acting repository glucocorticoids can be used as an alternative when owners are unable to medicate the cat orally. Methylprednisolone acetate (Depo-Medrol®) can be given at a dose of 10 to 20 mg/cat IM or SC every 2 to 4 weeks.

Bronchodilators

Bronchodilators seem to be most useful in human and feline patients during acute exacerbations caused by bronchoconstriction. These agents may also be utilized in chronic management in an attempt to decrease the dose of corticosteroids needed to control clinical signs, especially if corticosteroid-induced side effects (e.g., diabetes mellitus or concurrent infectious diseases) become problematic. The primary goal of therapy, however, should be to control the underlying airway inflammation, and substitution of systemic corticosteroids by inhalant corticosteroids may be more appropriate in these situations. Bronchodilators may also be added to chronic therapy if corticosteroid administration alone does not induce a sufficient decrease in symptoms.

Bronchoconstriction can be reversed using beta-2 adrenergic agonists (e.g., terbutaline 0.625 mg PO BID) in some cats with asthmatic signs that have airway hyperreactivity or increased airway resistance.[6,37] Cats that have airway obstruction due to remodeling of the airways are less likely to show a positive response. Beta-agonists are effective for quick relief of bronchospasm because of their direct action to induce smooth muscle relaxation, and injectable terbutaline is recommended for management of acute exacerbations of asthma. Potential side effects of terbutaline administration include tachycardia, agitation and hypotension due to slight beta-1 agonist activity.

Methylxanthine derivatives (e.g., theophylline and aminophylline) have been used extensively, and may be useful in some cats with bronchopulmonary disease. This class of drug appears to cause bronchodilation via a combination of mechanisms. Theophylline may inhibit a phosphodiesterase isoenzyme, increasing cAMP concentrations and causing bronchodilation; it may inhibit adenosine, a mediator of bronchoconstriction; or it may interfere with intracellular calcium mobilization. Other positive effects on the respiratory tract include inhibition of mast cell degranulation and increased strength of respiratory muscles. Pharmacokinetic studies have established a dose for long-acting oral preparations of theophylline (Theo-Dur® tablets or Slo-Bid® gyrocaps) of 20 to 25 mg/kg PO every 24 hours in the evening.[38,39] These drugs are not currently on the human market, and it is not known whether generic long-acting theophylline products are bioequivalent in the cat. A suggested initial dosage of generic sustained-release theophylline is 10 mg/kg PO once daily in the evening.

Cyproheptadine

In vitro studies have shown that serotonin, a mediator released from mast cells, contributes to airway smooth muscle contraction; and that cyproheptadine, a serotonin antagonist, significantly attenuates this response.[5] Reports have not been published to corroborate this response in the clinical setting; however, it is possible that blockade of serotonin might alleviate clinical signs in vivo. A trial of cyproheptadine (1 to 4 mg/cat PO BID) can be utilized in cats in which high doses of corticosteroids and bronchodilators are not effective in eliminating the clinical signs of cats with bronchial disease. Potential side effects of cyproheptadine are related to its other antiserotonin effects, and include lethargy and increased appetite. Approximately $2\frac{1}{2}$ days are required to reach steady-state drug concentrations, and several more days may be required to appreciate a clinical response.[40]

Cyclosporine

With knowledge of the role activated T cells play in the pathophysiology of asthma, it can be theorized that cyclosporine, a potent inhibitor of T cell activation, may be effective in asthma therapy. In cats with experimentally-induced asthma, cyclosporine therapy diminished structural derangements in airway histopathology and attenuated functional changes in airway reactivity.[3] Cyclosporine therapy might be indicated for those cats with especially severe or end-stage bronchial disease, or for those that are unresponsive to more standard medical management, although no clinical trials have been carried out to date. Based upon studies in experimentally-induced feline asthma,[1,3] the initial recommended dose is 10 mg/kg PO BID (olive oil-based Sandimmune®) or 3 mg/kg PO BID (microemulsion Neoral®); however, cyclosporine blood levels should be checked weekly until a stable, therapeutic dose (500 to 1000 ng/ml whole blood trough level) is achieved, and then evaluated monthly thereafter. Experience with cats receiving renal transplants indicates that lower doses of cyclosporine and whole blood trough levels between 250 and 500 ng/ml may achieve immunosuppression.[41] Continued monitoring of blood levels is important because the oral absorption of cyclosporine is unpredictable. Feeding a high-fat meal at the time of cyclosporine administration may increase its oral bioavailability.

Leukotriene Modifiers

Leukotrienes are inflammatory mediators that may contribute to the pathophysiology of certain forms of asthma in humans and in some animal models by causing airway smooth muscle contraction, increased microvascular permeability, stimulation of mucus secretion, decreased mucociliary clearance, and by acting as eosinophil chemoattractant agents.[42] The role of leukotrienes in the pathogenesis of feline bronchial disease has not been established, and contradictory results have been reported with measurement of urine leukotriene metabolite concentrations in cats with asthma.[43,44] While several clinical studies have shown modest clinical improvement in asthmatic people using leukotriene receptor antagonists[45] or inhibitors of 5-lipoxygenase,[46] an *in vitro* study using feline airways demonstrated no decrease in airway contraction in response to a 5-lipoxygenase inhibitor.[5] Therefore, until more research is completed in cats, these medications cannot be recommended at this time.

Antiinterleukin-5 Antibody

Interleukin-5 (IL-5), a cytokine secreted from activated T cells, appears to participate in asthma pathology by inducing eosinophil migration into the airways and bronchial hyperreactivity.[14] The IL-5 gene of cats has been sequenced[47]; however, the role of this mediator in feline bronchial disease has not yet been elucidated. Preliminary research in cats with experimentally induced asthma treated with a nebulized anti-IL-5 antibody appears promising,[48] but more information is required before its use can be recommended.

Antibiotics

Respiratory bacterial infections are rarely associated with clinical bronchial disease in cats, and bacteria may be cultured from tracheobronchial washes in healthy cats.[6] Therefore, antibiotics are rarely indicated or effective for the treatment of asthma in cats. Exceptions include cats in which a pure, heavy growth of bacteria is grown on the primary culture plate; and those in which Mycoplasma spp. is cultured. Mycoplasma spp. have not been found to colonize the lower respiratory tract of healthy cats[23,24]; therefore, a trial of doxycycline or other anti-mycoplasma antibiotics might be considered pending culture results.

Inhaled Medications

Medications for respiratory conditions given via inhalation offer the advantage of high drug concentrations within the airways while attenuating systemic side effects. Inhaled corticosteroids and bronchodilators are the current standard of care for human asthmatic patients. Controlled clinical trials on the use of inhaled medications in cats have not yet been reported; however, anecdotal recommendations have been presented.[43] The primary disadvantage of utilizing this method of treatment in feline patients is their lack of tolerance of the face mask that is placed over the nose and mouth, especially when symptoms of respiratory distress are present. The use of inhalant medications in cats requires three pieces of equipment:

1. The metered dose inhaler (MDI) that contains the medication
2. A spacer into which the medication is sprayed so that activation of the MDI does not need to be coordinated with inhalation
3. An anesthetic face mask that connects the spacer with the cat's mouth and nose.

This type of apparatus is used to treat infants or children suffering from asthma. The recommended protocol for cats entails fitting the three pieces of equipment together, actuating (spraying) the MDI to fill the spacer with medication, then placing the face mask over the cat's nose and mouth for 7 to 10 inspirations.[43] Recommended inhaled medications include albuterol (Ventolin®, Proventil®), a short-acting beta-2 agonist bronchodilator used for acute worsening of symptoms; salmeterol (Serevent®), a long-acting beta-2 agonist bronchodilator; and/or fluticasone propionate (Flovent®, 110-220 μg/puff), a corticosteroid utilized as chronic therapy.[43] Future clinical reports on the response to inhaled medication will help guide therapy. In general, the type of medication and frequency of administration need to be tailored to each patient's symptoms and concurrent oral medications, and adjusted based upon response.

Monitoring

Evaluation of clinical response to treatment is the usual and most practical means of monitoring cats with bronchial disease. Effective therapy should eliminate or significantly minimize the clinical signs. Repeating thoracic radiographs to compare with those taken prior to therapy provides an objective means to evaluate the response to treatment. The diagnosis of bronchial disease should be questioned if a significant response is not appreciated within 1 to 2 weeks of initiating proper treatment. Ensuring that the owner has been able to medicate the cat at home is imperative in the evaluation of clinical response to therapy. If a cat has not responded to proper therapy and other diseases have been ruled out, a trial of injectable methylprednisolone acetate should be considered. Measurement of lung function, if available, would provide an objective evaluation of both initial disease severity and response to therapy.

Outcome and Prognosis

The majority of cats with bronchial disease respond to appropriate therapy, yet it should be assumed that lifelong treatment may be required. Spontaneous resolution of asthma is relatively common in children that grow out of their asthma as they become adults. Although this scenario has not been documented in cats, some feline patients with bronchial disease can be tapered off their medications with no apparent return of symptoms. A small percentage of cats may succumb to acute, severe bronchoconstriction and subsequent respiratory distress, especially when proper emergency therapy is delayed. Some owners may choose euthanasia for cats that do not quickly respond to chronic therapy, those that do not tolerate the administration of medications, or those that experience severe drug side effects.

Areas for Further Research

No clinical studies have been published comparing different treatment modalities for bronchial disease in cats. Most of the information in this area is extrapolated from research in human patients, and opinions regarding therapy in cats are shared from veterinarian to veterinarian via anecdotal reports. One difficulty causing the shortfall of research is the lack of an easily obtained, readily available, objective method for obtaining a definitive diagnosis.

Asthma appears to be more prevalent in some families, and children that have a close relative with asthma or allergies have a higher incidence of asthma. Identification of genes associated with asthma will allow further understanding of its pathophysiology, and can improve diagnostic capabilities and early therapeutic intervention.

REFERENCES

1. Mitchell RW, Cozzi P, Ndukwu IM et al: Differential effects of cyclosporine A after acute antigen challenge in sensitized cats in vivo and ex vivo, Br J Pharmacol 123:1198-1204, 1998.
2. Mitchell RW, Ndukwu IM, Leff AR et al: Muscarinic hyperresponsiveness of antigen-sensitized feline airway smooth muscle in vitro, Am J Vet Res 58(6):672-676, 1997.
3. Padrid PA, Cozzi P, Leff AR: Cyclosporine A inhibits airway reactivity and remodeling after chronic antigen challenge in cats, Am J Respir Crit Care Med 154:1812-1818, 1996.
4. Padrid P, Snook S, Finucane T et al: Persistent airway hyperresponsiveness and histologic alterations after chronic antigen challenge in cats, Am J Respir Crit Care Med 151:184-193, 1995.
5. Padrid PA, Mitchell RW, Ndukwu IM et al: Cyproheptadine-induced attenuation of type-I immediate-hypersensitivity reactions of airway smooth muscle from immune-sensitized cats, Am J Vet Res 56(1):109-115, 1995.
6. Dye JA, McKiernan BC, Rozanski EA et al: Bronchopulmonary disease in the cat: Historical, physical, radiographic, clinicopathologic, and pulmonary functional evaluation of 24 affected and 15 healthy cats, J Vet Intern Med 10(6):385-400, 1996.
7. Moise NS, Wiedenkeller D, Yeager AE et al: Clinical, radiographic, and bronchial cytologic features of cats with bronchial disease: 65 cases (1980-1986), J Am Vet Med Assoc 194(10):1467-1473, 1989.
8. Corcoran BM, Foster DJ, Luis Fuentes V: Feline asthma syndrome: A retrospective study of the clinical presentation in 29 cats, J Sm Anim Pract 36:481-488, 1995.
9. Greenlee PG, Roszel JF: Feline bronchial cytology: Histologic/cytologic correlation in 22 cats, Vet Pathol 21:308-315, 1984.
10. Howard EB, Ryan CP: Chronic obstructive pulmonary disease in the domestic cat, Calif Vet 6:7-11, 1982.
11. West JB: Mechanics of breathing. In West JB, editor: Respiratory physiology: The essentials, ed 5, Baltimore, 1995, Williams & Wilkins.
12. Norris CR, Samii VF: Clinical, radiographic, and pathologic features of bronchiectasis in cats: 12 cases (1987-1999), J Am Vet Med Assoc 216(4):530-534, 2000.

13. Korpas J, Tomori Z: Cough and other respiratory reflexes. In Herzog H, editor: *Progress in respiration research,* vol 12, Basel, Switzerland, 1979, S. Karger.

14. Weller P: The immunobiology of eosinophils, *N Engl J Med* 324:1110-1118, 1991.

15. Hogan SP, Koskinen A, Matthaei KI et al: Interleukin-5-producing CD4+ T cells play a pivotal role in aeroallergen-induced eosinophilia, bronchial hyperreactivity, and lung damage in mice, *Am J Respir Crit Care Med* 157:210-218, 1998.

16. Albelda SM: Endothelial and epithelial cell adhesion molecules, *Am J Respir Cell Mol Biol* 4:195-203, 1991.

17. Wegener CD, Gundel RH, Reilly P et al: Intercellular adhesion molecule-1 (ICAM-1) in the pathogenesis of asthma, *Science* 247: 456-459, 1990.

18. Sporik R, Holgate ST, Platts-Mills TA et al: Exposure to house-dust mite allergen (Der pl) and the development of asthma in childhood, *N Engl J Med* 323:502-507, 1990.

19. Wills-Karp M: Immunologic basis of antigen-induced airway hyperresponsiveness, *Ann Rev Immunol* 17:255-281, 1999.

20. Johnston SL, Pattemore PK, Sanderson G et al: Community study of role of viral infections in exacerbations of asthma in 9-11 year old children, *BMJ* 310:1225-1228, 1995.

21. Martinez FD, Wright AL, Taussig LM et al: Asthma and wheezing in the first six years of life, *N Engl J Med* 332:133-138, 1995.

22. Shaheen SO, Aaby P, Hale AJ et al: Measles and atopy in Guinea-Bissau, *Lancet* 347:1792-1796, 1996.

23. Padrid PA, Feldman BF, Funk K et al: Cytologic, microbiologic, and biochemical analysis of bronchoalveolar lavage fluid obtained from 24 healthy cats, *Am J Vet Res* 52(8):1300-1307, 1991.

24. Randolph JF, Moise NS, Scarlett JM et al: Prevalence of mycoplasmal and ureoplasmal recovery from tracheobronchial lavages and of mycoplasmal recovery from pharyngeal swab specimens in cats with or without pulmonary disease, *Am J Vet Res* 54(6):897-900, 1993.

25. Borson DB, Brokaw JJ, Sekizawa K et al: Neutral endopeptidase and neurogenic inflammation in rats with respiratory infections, *J Appl Physiol* 66(6):2653-2658, 1989.

26. Tamaoki J, Chiyotani A, Tagaya E et al: Airway hyper-responsiveness to neurokinin A and bradykinin following *Mycoplasma pneumoniae* infection associated with reduced epithelial neutral endopeptidase, *Microbiol* 144(Pt 9):2481-2486, 1998.

27. Welsh RD: *Bordetella bronchiseptica* infections in cats, *J Am Anim Hosp Assoc* 32(2):153-158, 1996.

28. Hardie EM, Ramirez O, Clary EM et al: Abnormalities of the thoracic bellows: Stress fractures of the ribs and hiatal hernia, *J Vet Intern Med* 12(4):279-287, 1998.

29. Hawkins EC et al: Cytologic characterization of bronchoalveolar lavage fluid collected through an endotracheal tube in cats, *Am J Vet Res* 55(6):795-802, 1994.

30. McCarthy G, Quinn PJ: The development of lavage procedures for the upper and lower respiratory tract of the cat, *Irish Vet J* 40:6-9, 1986.

31. McCarthy GM, Quinn PJ: Bronchoalveolar lavage in the cat: Cytological findings, *Can J Vet Res* 53:259-263, 1989.

32. West JB: Tests of pulmonary function. In West JB, editor: *Respiratory Physiology: The essentials,* ed 5, Baltimore, 1995, Williams & Wilkins.

33. McKiernan BC, Dye JA, Rozanski EA: Tidal breathing flow-volume loops in healthy and bronchitic cats, *J Vet Intern Med* 7(6):388-393, 1993.

34. Hoffman AM, Dhupa N, Cimetti L: Airway reactivity measured by barometric whole-body plethysmography in healthy cats, *Am J Vet Res* 60(12):1487-1492, 1999.

35. National Asthma Education and Prevention Program: *Expert Panel report 2: Guidelines for the diagnosis and management of asthma* (National Institutes of Health pub no 97-4051), Bethesda, MD, 1997, NIH.

36. Beasley R, Roche WR, Roberts JA et al: Cellular events in the bronchi in mild asthma and after bronchial provocation, *Am Rev Respir Dis* 139:806-817, 1989.

37. McKiernan BC, Johnson LR: Clinical pulmonary function testing in dogs and cats, *Vet Clin North Am Small Anim Pract* 22(5):1087-1099, 1992.

38. Dye JA, McKiernan BC, Jones SD et al: Sustained-release theophylline pharmacokinetics in the cat, *J Vet Pharmacol Therap* 12:133-140, 1989.

39. Dye JA, McKiernan BC, Neff-Davis CA et al: Chronopharmacokinetics of theophylline in the cat, *J Vet Pharmacol Therap* 13:278-286, 1990.

40. Norris CR, Boothe DM, Esparza T et al: Disposition of cyproheptadine in cats after intravenous or oral administration of a single dose, *Am J Vet Res* 59(1):79-81, 1998.

41. Gregory CR: Immunosuppressive agents. In Bonagura JD, editor: *Kirk's current veterinary therapy: Small animal practice,* vol. 13, Philadelphia, 2000, WB Saunders.

42. Busse WW: Leukotrienes and inflammation, *Am J Respir Crit Care Med* 157:S210-S213, 1998.

43. Padrid P: Feline asthma: Diagnosis and treatment, *Vet Clin North Am Small Anim Pract* 30(6):1279-1293, 2000.

44. Mellema MS, Gershwin LJ, Norris CR: Urinary leukotriene E4 levels in cats with allergic bronchitis [abstract], *Proceedings of the 17th annual forum Am Coll Vet Intern Med* 724, 1999.

45. Lofdahl CG, Reiss TF, Leff JA et al: Randomized, placebo controlled trial of effect of a leukotriene receptor antagonist, montelukast, on tapering inhaled corticosteroids in asthmatic patients, *BMJ* 319:87-90, 1999.

46. Liu MC, Dube LM, Lancaster J: Acute and chronic effects of a 5-lipoxygenase inhibitor in asthma: A 6-month randomized multicenter trial, *J Allergy Clin Immunol* 98:859-871, 1996.

47. Padrid PA, Qin Y, Wells TNC et al: Sequence and structural analysis of feline interleukin-5 cDNA, *Am J Vet Res* 59(10):1263-1269, 1998.

48. Padrid P: CVT update: Feline asthma. In Bonagura JD, editor: *Kirk's current veterinary therapy: Small animal practice,* vol. 13, Philadelphia, 2000, WB Saunders.

CHAPTER 54

Bronchoesophageal Fistulas

Darcy H. Shaw

Definition and Etiology

Bronchoesophageal fistulas (BEF) can be acquired or congenital. They represent an abnormal communication between the bronchial tree and the esophagus, which results in leakage of esophageal contents into airways or movement of air into the esophagus. The embryology of congenital BEF in dogs and cats has not been described. In humans, postulated causes of congenital BEF include incomplete closure of the laryngotracheal furrow,[1] failure of complete separation and persistent attachment between the tracheobronchial tree and the esophagus,[2] bronchopulmonary foregut malformation,[3] and the localized effects of intrauterine infection.[2] The most common cause of acquired BEF in dogs is trauma associated with a bone esophageal foreign body.[4] In humans, acquired BEF can occur secondary to neoplasia, trauma, infectious disease (e.g., tuberculosis), and esophageal diverticuli.[5] Tracheoesophageal[6-10] and gastrobronchial[11] fistulas have also been reported in dogs and cats but are less common than BEF.

Bronchoesophageal fistulas have been reported in 16 dogs[4,12-20] and 2 cats.[21,22] It is difficult to determine precisely how many of these cases had congenital BEF, and how many had acquired lesions. Nine of the 16 dogs had a bone esophageal foreign body at the time of diagnosis, which presumably resulted in an acquired BEF. None of the cats had an esophageal foreign body. The criteria for the diagnosis of a congenital BEF in humans include: (1) the absence of past or present inflammation, (2) the absence of adherent lymph nodes, and (3) the presence of mucosa and a definite muscularis mucosae within the fistula.[2,23] The mucosa of a congenital fistula can be lined with squamous or columnar epithelium and the transition from squamous (esophageal) to columnar (respiratory) epithelium may be an additional criterion.[24] Although histological examination of the fistula was not performed in all of the reported cases, at least 3 dogs (one of which also had a bone esophageal foreign body)[12,17,18] and 1 cat[22] had criteria to support a congenital cause.

In dogs, almost all BEF have occurred in the caudal esophagus and involved bronchi of the right middle or caudal lung lobe. In only 2 dogs the fistula involved the accessory lobe and the left caudal lobe.[16,18] In contrast, the BEF involved the left caudal lung lobe in both cats. This has been attributed to an anatomical difference between the species: the caudal esophagus lies to the left of midline in cats and to the right of midline in dogs.[19]

In humans, four types of congenital BEF have been described: type I, an esophageal diverticulum with a fistula at its tip; type II, a simple fistula; type III, a fistula with a cyst near its end in the pulmonary tissue; and type IV, a fistula into a sequestered area of pulmonary tissue.[25] Type II fistulas are most common in humans.[23] In dogs and cats, although the descriptions are not very detailed in some reports, it appears that type I (10 cases)[4,12,14,17-19] and type II (7 cases)* fistulas are most common.

Clinical Findings

Bronchoesophageal fistulas have been diagnosed in dogs ranging in age from 6 months to 7 years.[12-19] The cats were 2 and 4 years old.[21,22] The mean ages of dogs with esophageal foreign bodies and presumed acquired BEF, and of those without an underlying cause and presumed congenital BEF, were 4.1 and 3.2 years, respectively. There is clearly a considerable overlap in the age range of these groups. Although one would expect congenital BEF to be diagnosed early in life, most cases of congenital BEF in humans are diagnosed in the third decade of life.[24] Possible explanations for the delayed diagnosis include the presence of an occluding membrane over the fistula which subsequently ruptures, limitation of passive leakage due to the orientation of the fistula, or the formation of a one-way flap valve by the mucosa near the fistula on the esophageal side.[23] All dogs with BEF have been small breeds, with terriers and Miniature Poodles predominating. This predisposition may relate to the propensity of small breeds to acquire esophageal foreign bodies.[17] Two thirds of the reported cases in dogs have occurred in females or spayed females.[4,12-19]

Regardless of the cause, all animals with BEF develop chronic or recurring respiratory infections because of contamination of the lower respiratory tract with esophageal contents. Most dogs and cats are presented because of a chronic cough caused by leakage of esophageal contents into the airways and the development of localized pneumonia. Coughing after eating (or especially, drinking) oc-

---

*References 4, 13, 15, 16, 21, and 22.

curs in some animals. Other signs may include lethargy, anorexia, regurgitation, dyspnea, pyrexia, abnormal lung sounds, and weight loss.[4,12-15] The duration of clinical signs in reported cases varied from 3 days to 2 years, with most having signs for weeks to months.[4,12-22]

Diagnosis

An inflammatory leukogram is present in most animals but it is surprisingly absent in others.[4,14] Findings on survey radiographs of the thorax usually reveal a localized alveolar, bronchial, and/or interstitial pattern in the right caudal and/or middle lung lobe in dogs and in the left caudal lung lobe in cats.[4,21,22] Pleural fluid is present in some animals[4] and has been attributed to either pleural inflammation adjacent to the fistula or to severe localized pneumonia. A foreign body may be observed in the caudal esophagus. A transient megaesophagus has also been documented in one dog with BEF caused by an esophageal foreign body.[15]

The results of transtracheal aspiration cytology have been reported in two cases, revealing septic neutrophilic inflammation.[12,15] In one case, the cytologic detection of *Simonsiella* spp., an oral commensal organism, in the transtracheal aspiration fluid suggested contamination of the lower airway with material from the pharynx or upper gastrointestinal tract.[26] The presence of *Simonsiella* spp. is only significant if the transtracheal aspiration was done appropriately with no oral contamination of the catheter or fluid during the procedure. Predictably, bacteria cultured from transtracheal aspiration fluid of animals with BEF reflect their oral and esophageal source and have included *Escherichia coli, Staphylococcus intermedius, Bacteroides fragilis, Actinomyces* spp., *Enterococcus cloacae,* and nonhemolytic streptoccoci.[12,15]

When BEF is suspected, an esophagram utilizing diluted barium (20% to 30% weight/volume) is the diagnostic test of choice.[4] The thin consistency of this barium mixture is better able to identify small fistulas, compared with barium of a thicker consistency or barium mixed with food. Oral iodinated contrast agents should be avoided because they are more irritating to pulmonary tissue.[4] Fluoroscopic examination may be of additional benefit in animals with small fistulas or those with fistulas that do not fill easily due to their orientation. Although fistulas may be visualized endoscopically in the esophagus or bronchi, endoscopy is considered to be less sensitive than an esophagram in humans.[23,24] In dogs, esophagrams have successfully demonstrated BEF and revealed opacification of the right middle and/or caudal bronchus in most cases (Figure 54-1). Esophageal traction diverticuli in the region of the fistula have also been observed in many dogs.[4,12]

Histopathological examination of the fistula usually reveals stratified squamous epithelium and stratified columnar epithelium near the esophageal and bronchial ends, respectively.[12-15,17,18,22] Excised pulmonary tissue reveals varying degrees of atelectasis, suppurative bronchopneumonia, necrosis, and the presence of foreign material in airways and alveoli.[12-15,17-19,22]

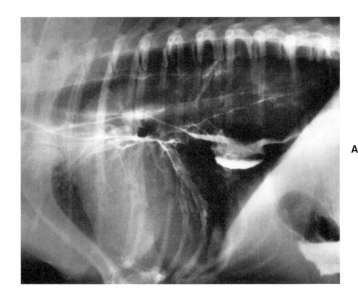

A

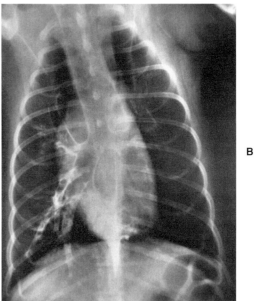

B

Figure 54-1. A, *Lateral and* ***B,*** *ventrodorsal thoracic radiographs of a dog after oral barium administration. A caudal esophageal diverticulum appears to communicate with the right caudal or accessory bronchus resulting in opacification of the right bronchial tree. Megaesophagus is also present. A bronchoesophageal fistula connecting the diverticulum to the right caudal bronchus was identified during surgery. (From Basher AWP, Hogan PM, Hanna PE et al: Surgical treatment of a congenital bronchoesophageal fistula in a dog, J Am Vet Med Assoc 199(4):479-482, 1991.)*

Treatment

Successful treatment requires a thoracotomy and excision of the fistula. Lung lobectomy of the subserved lobe(s) is usually required because of extensive damage from infection and difficulty in exposing and excising the fistula without damage to the vascular supply of the lobe.[27] Removal of an esophageal foreign body may also be required and should be done via esophagotomy. Because of the fistula, anesthetic gases may escape into the esophagus and stomach, and gas accumulation may be exacerbated by the use of positive pressure ventilation. Consequently, special techniques (e.g., endobronchial intubation of the unaffected side, high frequency oscillatory ventilation, or the creation of an escape valve by placement of a gastrostomy tube) may be required.[2]

Prognosis

The prognosis and outcome of animals treated surgically is good. Of the 18 reported cases of BEF in dogs and cats, 12 were treated surgically. Of these 12 animals, 9 had a full recovery and 3 died of postoperative complications. Treatment and outcome were not reported in 5 animals, and one animal was not treated.[4,12-22]

REFERENCES

1. Bekoe S, Magovern GJ, Liebler GA et al: Congenital bronchoesophageal fistula in the adult, *Chest* 66:201-203, 1974.
2. Smith DC: A congenital bronchoesophageal fistula presenting in adult life without pulmonary infection, *Br J Surg* 57:398-400, 1970.
3. Chu W, Mullen JL: Congenital bronchoesophageal fistula in the adult, *J Am Med Assoc* 239:855-856, 1978.
4. Park RD: Bronchoesophageal fistula in the dog: Literature survey, case presentations, and radiographic manifestations, *Comp Cont Ed* 6(7):669-677, 1984.
5. Lazopoulos G, Kotoulas C, Lioulias A: Congenital bronchoesophageal fistula in the adult, *Eur J Cardiothorac Surg* 16:667-669, 1999.
6. Dodman NH, Baker GJ: Tracheoesophageal fistula as a complication of an esophageal foreign body in the dog: A case report, *J Small Anim Pract* 19:291-296, 1978.
7. Beitzel C, Brinker WO: Surgical removal of an esophageal foreign body which had penetrated the trachea, *J Am Vet Med Assoc* 129:241-242, 1956.
8. Schebitz H: Rontgenbefund einer oesophago-trachealfistel nach fremdkorperperforation beim hund, *Tierarztl Umschau* 15:87, 1960.
9. Pearson H: Symposium on conditions of the canine esophagus I: Foreign bodies in the esophagus, *J Small Anim Pract* 7:107-116, 1966.
10. Freeman LM, Rush JE, Schelling SH et al: Tracheoesophageal fistula in two cats, *J Am Anim Hosp Assoc* 29:531-535, 1993.
11. Silverstone AM, Adams WM: Radiographic diagnosis: Gastrobronchial fistula in a dog, *Vet Radiol Ultrasound* 40:477-479, 1999.
12. Basher AWP, Hogan PM, Hanna PE et al: Surgical treatment of a congenital bronchoesophageal fistula in a dog, *J Am Vet Med Assoc* 199(4):479-482, 1991.
13. Fox SM, Allan FJ, Guilford WG et al: Bronchoesophageal fistula in two dogs, *N Zealand Vet J* 43:235-239, 1995.
14. Busch DS, Noxon JO, Merkley DF: Bronchoesophageal fistula in a dog, *Canine Pract* 16(2):25-29, 1991.
15. Van Ee RT, Dodd VM, Pope ER et al: Bronchoesophageal fistula and transient megaesophagus in a dog, *J Am Vet Med Assoc* 188(8):874-876, 1986.
16. Caywood DD, Feeney DA: Acquired esophagobronchial fistula in a dog, *J Am Anim Hosp Assoc* 18:590-594, 1982.
17. Pearson H, Gibbs C, Kelly DF: Esophageal diverticulum formation in the dog, *J Small Anim Pract* 19:341-355, 1978.
18. Foor JC: A congenital bronchoesophageal fistula in a dog, *Minnesota Vet* 14:9-11, 27-28, 1974.
19. Thrall DE: Esophagobronchial fistula in a dog, *J Am Vet Radiol Soc* 14:22-25, 1973.
20. Kleine LJ: Radiologic examination of the esophagus in dogs and cats, *Vet Clin N Am* 4:663, 1974.
21. Reif JS: Solitary pulmonary lesions in small animals, *J Am Vet Med Assoc* 155:717-722, 1969.
22. Muir P, Bjorling DE: Successful surgical treatment of a bronchoesophageal fistula in a cat, *Vet Rec* 134:475-476, 1994.
23. Risher WH, Arensman RM, Ochsner JL: Congenital bronchoesophageal fistula, *Ann Thorac Surg* 49:500-505, 1990.
24. Kim JH, Park KH, Sung SW et al: Congenital bronchoesophageal fistulas in adult patients, *Ann Thorac Surg* 60:151-155, 1995.
25. Braimbridge MV, Keith HI: Esophago-bronchial fistula in the adult, *Thorax* 20:226-233, 1965.
26. Burton SA, Honor DJ, Horney BS et al: What is your diagnosis? (Transtracheal aspiration in a dog with bronchoesophageal fistula), *Vet Clin Path* 21(4):112-113, 1992.
27. Fingeroth JN: Surgical diseases of the esophagus. In Slatter DS, editor: *Textbook of small animal surgery*, ed 2, vol 1, Philadelphia, 1993, WB Saunders.

CHAPTER 55

Bronchopulmonary Dysplasia

John P. Hoover • Michael S. Davis

Definition and Etiology

Dysplasia is defined as abnormal cellular or tissue development. Bronchopulmonary tissues that may become dysplastic include those in the tracheobronchial tree (i.e., cartilage, fibrous connective tissue, elastin, collagen, and smooth muscle), mucosa (i.e., respiratory epithelium and bronchial glands), alveoli, interstitium (i.e., fibrocytes and elastin) and vessels (i.e., endothelium, elastin, and smooth muscle).

In human medicine, the term bronchopulmonary dysplasia (BPD) refers to a specific syndrome in neonates originally described in 1967 as a chronic, noninfectious respiratory insufficiency (i.e., hypoxia, hypercapnia, increased pulmonary resistance, and decreased pulmonary compliance) caused by prematurity, oxygen toxicity, and barotrauma.[1] This condition is a sequela to respiratory distress syndrome (RDS), in which there is abnormally high surface tension within the alveoli, resulting in alveolar collapse and filling with fluid. In some patients with RDS a thickened, glassy, hyaline-like membrane consisting of clotted exudate[2] covers the alveolar walls and respiratory airways, leading to the term hyaline membrane disease (HMD). The formation of hyaline membranes begins within hours in the injured neonate lung.[3]

The term BPD has been associated in human medicine with short-term life-threatening pulmonary disease.[4,5] With increasing survival of patients with BPD, a new definition has evolved to encompass any chronic lung disease (CLD) of neonates resulting from incomplete or inappropriate repair of inflamed and injured lung tissue.[3,4] RDS has been recognized in foals, calves, and piglets,[6] and a clinical syndrome analogous to human neonatal BPD could theoretically follow in the lungs of animals.

Pathogenesis

BPD is multifactorial, but the factors of greatest importance in its development are prematurity, barotrauma, and oxygen toxicity.[3-5] Neonate lungs, especially preterm, are not fully developed at birth.[4,5] In humans, immaturity of pulmonary cell junctions,[7] low levels of protective antioxidant enzymes,[8] decreased surfactant levels,[9] and decreased factors that promote lung differentiation and re-

generation[10] appear to contribute to the development of BPD. Immature lungs in premature neonates are deficient in alveolar surfactant phospholipids, which increases airway surface tension leading to alveolar collapse and development of hyaline membrane disease.[11,12] BPD in humans has been primarily associated with preterm infants that develop respiratory distress and have been treated with high levels of inspired oxygen (Fio_2) and positive pressure ventilation (PPV).[3-5,12,13]

PPV expands collapsed alveoli in the atelectatic surfactant-deficient lung of neonates with severe RDS. However, overdistention of the small terminal airways is a source of ongoing barotrauma, bronchiolar ischemia, and necrosis.[3,14] BPD has also been seen in term human infants that received PPV for pneumonia, aspiration, and patent ductus arteriosus (PDA).[15] Damage to the lung by oxygen free radicals due to oxygen toxicity[3,13] may be more important than barotrauma in producing lung damage in newborn piglets.[16] High inspired oxygen concentrations facilitate increased generation of oxygen free radicals through the hypoxanthine-xanthine oxidase system.[4,17-21] Both surfactant production and function are altered by these reactive oxygen species, making the lungs more vulnerable to injury.[21] Therefore, oxidative stress appears to play a pivotal role in the development of CLD or BPD.[3] Damage by peroxidation can also occur in the absence of oxygen toxicity from oxygen radicals that are produced by activated phagocytes.[22] Regardless of the source, oxygen radicals increase the damage to many different cellular compounds and exacerbate preexisting pulmonary dysfunction.[4]

With pulmonary endothelial damage from inflammation, there is leakage of plasma albumin, as well as leakage and activation of coagulant proteins into the airways, interstitium, and alveoli.[23] Increased hyaluronan and decreased available plasminogen favor fibrin deposition in the damaged pulmonary tissues and airways.

Polymorphonuclear leukocytes (PMNs) play an important part in the development of lung injury.[24-26] Activated PMNs generate oxygen free radicals, release secretory hydrolases[27-30] and elastase,[31,32] partially inactivate the primary pulmonary proteinase inhibitor alpha-1 proteinase,[33,34] and generate arachidonic acid metabolites.[35,36] The resulting inflammation is associated with pulmonary epithelial leakage of albumin and activated coagulant proteins, and may exaggerate the repair process and promote development of pulmonary fibrosis.[22] PMN elastase is the main proteolytic enzyme for pulmonary interstitial, bronchial, and vascular elastin. Elastin is a critical component of the lung interstitium, participates in the maintenance of elastic recoil and stabilization of alveolar volume, and helps to maintain small airway and blood vessel patency during breathing.[37,38] Elastase-proteinase inhibitor imbalance has been associated with destruction of lung connective tissue and fibrosis characteristic of BPD.[39-43]

Other cells (e.g., mast cells and alveolar macrophages) may also play a role in the initiation of oxidative stress and BPD. Tryptase is a serine protein specific to mast cells that has been shown to be a potent fibroblast mitogen.[44] Tryptase-positive mast cell hyperplasia in BPD suggests a role of mast cells, as well as tryptase in the pathogenesis of the disease.[44] Pulmonary alveolar macrophages (PAMs) are potent sources of free radicals.[22,45,46] Endothelin-1 synthesized and secreted by the tracheal epithelial cells and/or PAMs in rabbits has a priming effect on PAMs to produce superoxide anion and may be correlated with the development of BPD.[47] Activated PAMs produce fibronectin, which is a potent chemoattractant, attachment factor and growth factor for fibroblasts.[22] Fibronectin is increased in adults that develop fibrotic lung disease and in the tracheal effluent of infants that develop BPD.[48] Overstimulation of PAMs and increased fibronectin release is associated with pulmonary fibrosis.[22]

Endogenous antioxidant compounds such as vitamins A, C, E, and glutathione normally scavenge free radicals.[49] Vitamin A (retinol) also promotes epithelial regeneration during recovery from lung injury in BPD.[50] Vitamin A deficiency results in lung histopathology similar to BPD.[51] Magnesium deficiency increases the susceptibility of cells and tissues to peroxidation, exacerbates inflammation, decreases the immune response, exaggerates release of catecholamines in stress, and decreases energy metabolism.[52] Many of the chemical compounds vital to the antioxidant systems (e.g., vitamin E and Mg) are transferred from dam to offspring very late in gestation and thus may be deficient in neonates, particularly premature neonates.[3] Maintenance of these compounds is highly dependent on nutrition, and inadequate food intake may make premature neonates more susceptible to lung injury by free radicals.[53]

Polyunsaturated fatty acids (PUFAs) and plasmalogens are the two main substrates for lipid peroxidation in surfactant.[54] Neonatal animals contain triglycerides that are richer in PUFAs than older animals.[55,56] Supplementation with n-3 PUFAs may suppress synthesis of cytokines (e.g., IL-1β and TNF-α) and appears to improve tolerance to oxygen toxicity in animals.[57,58]

Pathology

The pathological lesions of BPD appear to result from disordered growth and repair. The structural immaturity of the neonatal lung is a key component in the development of BPD. Lung maturation occurs late in gestation and progresses through the neonatal period.[59] Elastin production and normal deposition is necessary for the development of alveoli, and elastin metabolism is altered in experimental models of BPD.[37] At term birth, the alveoli are simple saccules that mature to more complex alveolar acini during the first few days to weeks of life.[59] Inflammation during this period can disrupt normal alveolar development, and persistence of the relatively inefficient saccular architecture.[59,60]

BPD consists of an early inflammatory reaction with proliferation and hypercellularity that is followed by variable healing and fibrosis.[22] An abnormal balance between elastin production and breakdown[39,40,43] by elastase from PMNs,[22] along with abnormal distribution and deposition of elastin and collagen in the immature lung, contributes to the abnormal pattern of alveolar growth and differentiation.[61-63]

BPD in humans is currently divided into three phases with different but overlapping pathologic and histologic patterns[5,61,64]: (1) an early inflammatory phase, followed by (2) a subacute or reparative phase, and then (3) a chronic phase with remodeling of airways (Table 55-1).

EARLY INFLAMMATORY PHASE

This phase is characterized by an irregular distribution of hyperinflation and atelectasis. Interstitial edema and inflammation occur, with epithelial necrosis of the small conducting and terminal airways. This is followed by interstitial and bronchiolar fibrosis, and then prominent areas of hyperinflation. Histologically there is resorption of fibrotic tissue without complementary alveolization, which leads to hyperexpanded or oversimplified alveoli.[5,61]

SUBACUTE FIBROPROLIFERATIVE (REPARATIVE) PHASE

This phase is characterized histologically by an irregular pattern of atelectasis and hyperinflation with hyperplasia of type II pneumocytes, hypertrophy of bronchial and bronchiolar smooth muscle, and interstitial and perialveolar fibrosis. During this phase the pulmonary tissues may undergo a repair process[5] involving platelets, PMNs, and alveolar macrophages.[22] Normal saccules and alveoli are interposed between foci of alveoli with thickened overexpanded saccular walls, increased collagen, and myofibroblasts.[5]

CHRONIC FIBROPROLIFERATIVE (REMODELING) PHASE

This phase is characterized by hyperexpansion and cystic-looking lungs with areas of emphysema, thickening and fibrosis of the interstitium, and replacement of type I pneumocytes by type II cells.[12] Airway remodeling may occur histologically[5] and tracheo- and bronchomalacia with airway collapse is a common finding in infants.[65,66]

The changes in developing alveoli and the interstitium are most severe, characterized by areas of atelectasis and hyperinflation that can lead to emphysematous

TABLE 55-1   Progression of Radiographic, Gross, and Histological Findings with Bronchopulmonary Dysplasia (BPD)*

Phases of BPD	Radiographic Findings	Gross Findings	Histological Findings
Acute Inflammatory (Less than 1 week)	Atelectasis Reticulogranularity Air bronchograms Pulmonary interstitial edema	Atelectasis Pulmonary edema	Atelectasis and hyperinflation of alveoli Peribronchial and perivascular edema Interstitial and bronchiolar inflammatory infiltrates
Subacute Fibroproliferative (Reparative) (1 to 3 weeks)	Areas of atelectasis Areas of hyperinflation Increased air bronchograms Alveolar densities	Irregular pattern of atelectasis and emphysema	Hypertrophy of bronchial smooth muscle Interstitial, bronchial and perialveolar fibrosis Hyperplasia of type II pneumocytes and decreased alveoli Airway epithelial necrosis and squamous metaplasia
Chronic Fibroproliferative (Remodeling) (1 month or longer)	Cystic-appearing lungs Hyperexpansion (hyperlucency) Cardiomegaly (in some)	Hyperinflated lungs Bullae and cyst formation Airway collapse	Interstitial thickening and fibrosis Replacement of type I with type II pneumocytes Tracheobronchomalacia

*Modified from reports of human infants with BPD.[5,12,71]

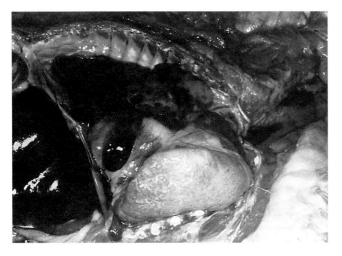

Figure 55-1. *Gross postmortem showing a hyperinflated cranial portion of the left cranial lung lobe with bullae formation projecting to the right side, and atelectasis of the right middle and caudal lung lobes in a 5-month-old chow chow with bronchial cartilage dysplasia. (From Hoover JP, Henry GA, Panciera RJ: Bronchial cartilage dysplasia with multifocal lobar bullous emphysema and lung torsions in a pup, J Am Vet Med Assoc 201(4):600,1992.)*

blebs.[3] Alveolar interstitial support (elastin) is disordered and replaced by fibrosis.[38,39,41,42,63] The alveoli are markedly decreased in number and enlarged[14] due to the failure of normal sacculation postnatally[59] and septal destruction with fibrosis.[14] With septal distraction there may be bullae formation[43] (Figure 55-1).

In the large airways, there is submucosal glandular hypertrophy, increased smooth muscle, squamous metaplasia of the mucosal epithelium, submucosal fibrosis, inflammatory infiltrates, and granulation tissue.[14,67] In severe cases of BPD airway necrosis occurs with intraluminal debris accumulation.[68] The bronchioles have marked smooth muscle hypertrophy, focal mucosal squamous metaplasia, and marked chronic inflammatory infiltrates with fibrosis.[14,67] Peribronchiolar and perivascular edema and fibrosis occur, and commonly, bronchiolar collapse.[65,66]

Muscular hypertrophy of the medial layer and endothelium of the arterioles is accompanied by fibrosis. Irreversible destruction of the capillary bed decreases vascular cross-sectional area[14] and leads to increased pulmonary vascular resistance and cor pulmonale.[3] The collective result is loss of capillary surface area and pulmonary hypertension, and thickening of the airways (smooth muscular hypertrophy and fibrosis) with luminal narrowing.[69]

Pathophysiology

Initially, neonates with RDS have widespread areas of atelectasis. Consequently the overall surface available for gas exchange is reduced and the lung is stiff, resulting in hypoxia and hypercapnia. With PPV, especially with increased FiO_2, the small airways are damaged and areas of hyperinflation and emphysematous blebs develop.[3] Surfactant deficiency results in areas of alveolar collapse and atelectasis, and development of hyaline membrane disease.[11] Oxidative stress can lead to damage to surfactant and membrane phospholipids, resulting in the release of arachidonic acid and eventual production of proinflammatory eicosanoids.[70] Free radicals can inactivate surfactant, causing an increase in the work of breathing, and can impair the nonspecific immune functions of surfactant.[4,21]

In the early inflammatory phase of BPD, mechanical and oxidative stress injury to the respiratory epithelium and vascular endothelium facilitates plasma transudation into the airways, obstructing the lumen and interstitium, and contributing to perivascular, peribronchiolar and interstitial pulmonary edema.[2,14] Atelectasis with increased lung water in the form of interstitial edema further decreases lung compliance, compromises gas diffusion, and promotes extension of the ongoing inflammatory processes in the alveolar interstitium.

BPD progresses into the subacute healing or reparative phase with bronchial gland and smooth muscle hypertrophy, airway epithelial metaplasia and granulation following necrosis, peribronchial and perivascular edema, and intraluminal airway debris. Airway smooth muscle hypertrophy and excess mucus production lead to increased pulmonary resistance, particularly at the level of the small bronchioles,[5] which is complicated by decreased capacity for mucociliary clearance because of the squamous metaplasia of the airway epithelium.[3] Areas of atelectasis and hyperinflation result in decreased lung compliance. Airway narrowing and obstruction results in increased respiratory effort, especially on expiration.

In the chronic remodeling phase of BPD the interstitium in both the atelectatic and overinflated areas is widened and contains undifferentiated mesenchymal cells, myofibroblasts, and relatively fewer cells and more collagen and elastin around expanded and enlarged alveoli,[60,63] resulting in low lung compliance.[71] Hyperreactivity of airway smooth muscle is a common feature of BPD in humans.[3] Therefore, airway resistance is increased in BPD, resulting in greater residual volume (RV) and RV/total lung capacity ratio consistent with air trapping.[5]

Ventilation distribution is abnormal in BPD. Areas of atelectasis (perfused but not ventilated) alternate with areas of hyperinflation (ventilated but not perfused), leading to marked ventilation/perfusion (V/Q) mismatch.[71] V/Q mismatch is the primary reason for the hypoxemia often found in BPD.[3] Hypercapnia is also common because of alveolar hypoventilation, increased functional dead space, and increased V/Q mismatch.[5] A persistent increase in the work of breathing may lead to a compensated respiratory acidosis.[71]

BPD affects the function, growth, and development of the lung and heart because of the fibroproliferative repair of damaged pulmonary and vascular tissues.[72] Chronic hypoxia and periarteriolar thickening[12] may lead to pulmonary hypertension[3,5,12,71,72] and, eventually, right heart failure.[3,5,72]

Incidence/Prevalence

The clinical incidence of classic BPD secondary to oxygen toxicity or barotrauma in animals is unknown but is likely quite low because of the rarity of such management in veterinary medicine. In addition to RDS in horses, calves, and piglets,[6] numerous animal species are used for modeling BPD in humans.[3,73-75] It is clear that many animal species are susceptible to RDS and the development of CLD with neonatal lung inflammation. If the definition of BPD were expanded to include *any* acquired bronchopulmonary dysplasia secondary to the incomplete or inappropriate repair of inflamed and injured tissue, the incidence of heretofore unrecognized BPD in animals would likely become considerably greater. There have been a few reports of BPD-like disease in the veterinary literature.

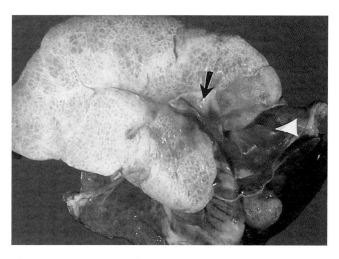

Figure 55-2. *Lungs and heart removed at necropsy from a 5-month-old chow chow with bronchial cartilage dysplasia. Notice the lobar emphysema and 180-degree torsion of the cranial portion of the left cranial lobe, with fibrous adhesion to the atelectic left caudal portion of the left cranial lobe (arrow), and atelectasis of the caudal lung lobe (arrow head). Bullous emphysema with torsion of the right accessory lung lobe is also present.* (From Hoover JP, Henry GA, Panciera RJ: Bronchial cartilage dysplasia with multifocal lobar bullous emphysema and lung torsions in a pup, J Am Vet Med Assoc 201(4):600, 1992.)

In a 1989 report, Freeman and colleagues[76] described lesions consistent with BPD in a foal that had received supplemental oxygen by nasal insufflation. A later correspondence[77] indicated that when tissues from this foal were reanalyzed, they contained equine arteritis virus. They suggested that the viral infection may have played a pivotal role in the development of the foal's clinical disease.

In a 1992 report, Hoover and colleagues[78] described a case of bronchial cartilage dysplasia (BPD-like) in a pup with no history of supplemental oxygen or mechanical ventilation. This animal developed collapse of bronchial lumens, multiple lung lobe torsions, and lobar bullous emphysema (Figure 55-2) secondary to the widespread bronchial cartilage dysplasia. In addition, there was small airway collapse and air trapping in the lung parenchyma (Figure 55-3). The term bullous emphysema was used in this case to be consistent with previous reports.[79-84] In reality, this was a bronchial cyst characterized by septal breakdown, confluence of alveoli, and loss of tethering support of the noncartilaginous airways without the alveolar inflammation associated with true emphysema.[85] No history of any neonatal disease was reported in this patient, so it remains unclear whether the etiology of the lesions in this young dog were congenital or acquired. Retrospectively, the authors suspect that an acquired insult played a major role in the disease.

Collapse of hypoplastic bronchi,[86] bronchogenic cyst,[87] and lung lobe torsion[88] have been associated with BPD in children. Similar conditions have been described in young dogs,[79-81] adult dogs,[82,83] and a cat.[84] Congenital bronchial cartilage aplasia[80] and hypoplasia[82,83] have been associated with lobar emphysema in dogs. Therefore, it appears plausible that analogous conditions

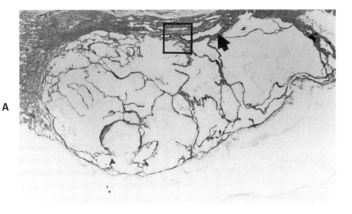

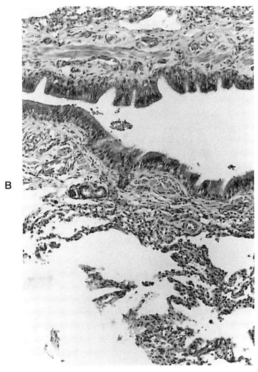

Figure 55-3. *Photomicrograph* **(A)** *H&E stain, bar = 1,100 μm) of a section of the cranial portion of the left cranial lung lobe in the 5-month old Chow Chow. Notice discrete area of emphysema with loss and displacement of alveolar walls, compression of adjacent pulmonic constituents, and a thin walled bronchus (arrow) that contains ciliated pseudostratified columnar epithelium and submucosal glands but lacks cartilage* **(B)** *Inset, bar = 225 μm).* (From Hoover JP, Henry GA, Panciera RJ: Bronchial cartilage dysplasia with multifocal lobar bullous emphysema and lung torsions in a pup, J Am Vet Med Assoc 201(4):601, 1992.)

to BPD of human neonates, or to the chronic lung disease (CLD) of children, may also exist in neonatal and juvenile animals.

Epidemiology and Risk Factors

Known risk factors include prematurity of the lung, RDS, mechanical ventilation injury, and the use of high oxygen concentrations.[3,5,13] Lung defenses and the ability to tolerate hyperoxia, repair, and continued growth can be compromised by undernutrition and deficiencies in micronutrients such as vitamins A and E, copper, zinc, iron, magnesium, selenium, and essential fatty acids.[3,89] Impaired immune function and reduced phospholipids and surfactant may present an additional risk for infection.[89-91]

Acquired infections during the perinatal period may contribute to the development of BPD. Human respiratory syncytial virus has been associated with CLD in humans.[3,92] Nosocomial infections represent an important cause of morbidity and mortality among human infants with BPD. Hyperoxic injury (100% oxygen) of airways and lungs colonized by *Pseudomonas aeruginosa* or a coagulase negative *Staphylococcus epidermitis* resulted in 100% mortality by day 10 in baboons.[93,94] Parainfluenza infection in young rats has been shown to induce airway growth abnormalities associated with persistent pulmonary dysfunction and hyperresponsiveness.[95] These, together with the report of signs consistent with BPD in a foal infected with equine arteritis virus, support the contention that BPD in animals may be associated with some neonatal pulmonary infections.

Recognition of Clinical BPD

Recognition of BPD in veterinary patients depends on a history of bronchopulmonary insult or development of acute RDS with progressive clinical signs, and the general lack of response to treatment. Unfortunately, BPD is difficult to confirm antemortem.

DIFFERENTIAL DIAGNOSIS

The clinical signs of BPD are similar to the diseases that can increase the risk for developing BPD. Therefore the differential diagnosis for BPD could include RDS and HMD in premature neonates; congenital defects such as airway hypoplasia and aplasia in term neonates; and acquired inflammatory conditions such as bronchitis, bronchiolitis, bronchiectasis, bronchopneumonia, and pneumonitis in juveniles.

HISTORY

Patients developing BPD are expected to have a history of lower respiratory tract inflammation, whether it is due to oxygen toxicity, barotrauma, noxious (inhaled or aspirated) or infectious agents. Prematurity and a protracted course of respiratory insult increase the likelihood of BPD.

CLINICAL SIGNS

The clinical signs vary as BPD progresses from the acute inflammatory phase to the chronic fibroproliferative remodeling phase. Respiratory distress, cough, changes in breathing pattern, and auscultation abnormalities may occur. Clinical signs of RDS include increased respiratory rate and effort. As inflammation develops, areas of pulmonary interstitial edema and decreased lung compliance[96] result in a restrictive breathing pattern.[97] As BPD progresses, a breathing pattern more consistent with lower airway obstruction may develop. This pattern features prolonged expiration and low flow rates, caused by compression and collapse of dysplastic lower airways, and eventually leading to air trapping.[97] Because of the hyperinflation, there is often maximal expansion of the thorax and an increased abdominal component to breathing. RDS may become so severe that distress may be characterized by orthopnea.[78] Terminally, ventilation efforts may diminish to apnea. Most veterinary patients will present in the acute inflammatory phase of BPD. The transition from inflammation to dysplasia may be subtle, and in many cases, the first indication that BPD is developing or has developed in an animal with RDS is a lack of continued improvement despite therapy.

Cough is a hallmark sign of lower airway inflammation, but it may not be seen in neonates with early BPD. When a cough develops, it is expected to be productive because of excess mucus transudation and exudation into the airways, and decreased mucociliary clearance.

Initially, breath sounds may be decreased due to atelectasis. As areas of lung inflate and pulmonary edema develops, inspiratory crackles may occur. With chronicity, airway compression and collapse may cause expiratory wheezes and coarse expiratory crackles.

Severe hypoxemia is caused by hypoventilation from airway obstruction, or by increased venous admixture from lung parenchymal disease. The patient may be only partially responsive to increased Fio_2, especially in advanced cases of BPD. This is because of significant right-to-left shunting from regional (lobar) atelectasis and pulmonary hypertension from hypoxia and increased vascular resistance.[3,5,61] Cyanosis of mucous membranes may be seen, although it does not always occur. Animals with BPD can be expected to have decreased Pao_2 (often 75 mm Hg or less) and may have increased $Paco_2$ (45 mm Hg or greater). Intermittent episodes of oxygen desaturation may be associated with apnea, bradycardia, or cyanosis,[3] occurring primarily while the patient is eating or sleeping.[98,99]

Radiography is essential for evaluation of animals with respiratory disease accompanied by a restrictive[100] or obstructive pattern.[101] Radiographs may reveal lower airway obstruction (i.e., airway collapse/compression), or a bronchial, interstitial, vascular, or alveolar pattern. Care must be exercised to stabilize the patient, provide oxygen if necessary, and minimize stress prior to making thoracic radiographs. Compromises in patient positioning may be necessary, and horizontal beam lateral projection should be considered if the animal is in respiratory distress. Other diagnostic procedures may be considered if the animal is stable enough.

Early radiographic signs of BPD in humans may be indistinguishable from other diffuse neonatal lung diseases (see Table 55-1). Initially, the radiographic findings may be indistinguishable from RDS[5] with diffuse atelectasis, reticulogranularity, and air bronchograms. Reticulogranularity represents hyperexpanded alveoli against a background of lung edema, fibrosis, and atelectasis.[71] In the advanced

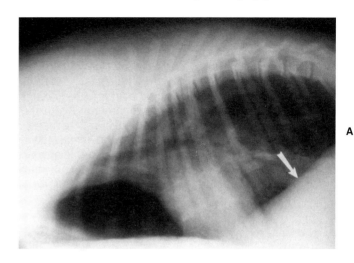

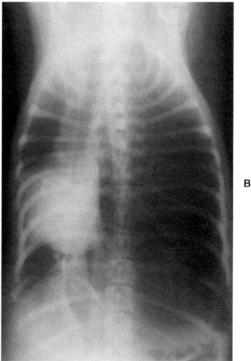

Figure 55-4. *Thoracic radiographs of a 5-month-old chow chow with a history of exercise intolerance, progressive dyspnea, and episodic cough. Hyperinflation of the lungs and flattening of the diaphragm* (arrow) *are evident in a right lateral radiograph* **(A)** *obtained using a horizontal beam. Hyperinflation of the left cranial lung lobe, with displacement of the mediastinum and heart to the right, and atelectasis of the right lung are evident in the dorsoventral view* **(B)**. *(From Hoover JP, Henry GA, Panciera RJ: Bronchial cartilage dysplasia with multifocal lobar bullous emphysema and lung torsions in a pup,* J Am Vet Med Assoc *201(4):601, 1992.)*

stages of BPD, irregularly distributed atelectasis and emphysema may be apparent.

In a canine patient with bronchial cartilage dysplasia, lung hyperlucency with hyperexpansion and flattening of the diaphragm, cystic lungs with bullae or bronchial cyst, and collapse of airways on expiration were all consistent with air trapping (Figure 55-4).

PATHOLOGY

Confirmation of BPD is usually achieved at necropsy and on histopathology. The pup reported by Hoover and colleagues[78] had clinical and radiographic signs, as well as gross necropsy (see Figure 55-1) and histologic findings (see Figure 55-3) consistent with the chronic fibroproliferative phase of BPD and airway remodeling. The foal reported with BPD-like lesions by Freeman and colleagues[76] was more consistent with the radiographic and histologic findings of the late acute inflammatory or early subacute fibroproliferative reparative phase of BPD.

Treatment and Management

The primary pathophysiologic problems are increased work of breathing and decreased efficiency of gas exchange. In BPD, however, often little can be done to alleviate these conditions because of the inherent structural damage that is the hallmark of the disease. Although some respiratory improvement might occur over time in the chronic phase,[61] most veterinary patients will likely succumb during the acute phase.[3] In many respects, management of veterinary BPD cases is not very different from management of human cases.

PREVENTATIVE TREATMENTS IN HUMANS

Therapies intended to prevent BPD in infants include steroids (e.g., antenatal and early postnatal), thyrotropin-releasing hormone to induce antioxidant enzymes, early postnatal surfactant, and antioxidants (e.g., superoxide dismutase and vitamins A and E). Other treatments include inositol and fatty acid supplementation (long-chain n-3 PUFAs).[13] Careful fluid restriction may minimize pulmonary edema and improve lung compliance.[3,13] Whenever ventilation with supplemental oxygen is necessary, high-frequency oscillatory ventilation[13,102] or synchronized (patient-triggered) ventilation[3,13] should be used. Permissive hypercapnea may promote early weaning from mechanical ventilation[13] and thereby reduce barotrauma.

MANAGEMENT OF INFANTS WITH BPD

Therapy includes supplemental oxygen, nutritional support, diuretics, corticosteroids, bronchodilators, and treatment of any infectious agents.[3,13] Other treatments include inhaled nitric oxide (NO) to vasodilate the ventilated areas of the lung, thereby reducing V/Q mismatching and pulmonary hypertension.[103-106] Improvement was reported in some studies of infants with BPD,[107,108] but in other reports infants failed to improve or could not be weaned off the inhaled NO.[103] Several medications (e.g., furosemide, beta-2 agonists, dexamethasone) are being administered to human infants by inhalation; however, variable doses are actually delivered and the mechanism of delivery requires that the patient is ventilated.[13]

PREVENTIVE TREATMENT OF BPD IN ANIMALS

Corticosteroids play important roles in normal prenatal lung maturation,[13] in decreasing inflammation mediated by cells (PMNs and PAMs),[3,13] and in improving the protease-antiprotease ratio.[109] As a result, these drugs are administered before birth in humans to prevent BPD in infants. However, the antenatal use of corticosteroids is controversial because their administration can induce premature parturition in domestic animals. Thus these hormones are not recommended for use in animals unless it is certain that preterm parturition is unavoidable. Proper nutrition of dams during late gestation (especially those with a history of premature births) and avoidance of breeding dams predisposed to premature parturition is recommended. Exercising caution with the use of PPV, avoiding high levels of Fio_2 and neonatal exposure to airway irritants and allergens, and responding quickly to neonatal respiratory infections are all also recommended.

MANAGEMENT OF BPD IN ANIMALS

Treatment is presented in three categories: (1) *supportive*, to maintain the patient and promote homeostasis; (2) *symptomatic*, to relieve clinical signs; and (3) *specific*, to prevent, control or eliminate the definitive cause. If a causal agent can be identified, early treatment may ameliorate this progressive condition. Patients with BPD have impaired pulmonary defense mechanisms and often have a relative inability to clear intraluminal mucus and exudate. Periodic airway suctioning may become necessary, especially if tracheal intubation becomes necessary to ventilate the patient. Any lower respiratory tract infection may exacerbate inflammation[110] and should be treated aggressively.

Antioxidants

Superoxide dismutase (SOD), administered intratracheally in newborn piglets exposed to 100% oxygen for 48 hours, mitigated the inflammatory changes of oxidative lung injury but did not appear to improve surfactant function.[111] Improved oxygenation and pulmonary blood-flow occurred when intratracheal SOD was combined with inhaled NO in a lamb model of persistent pulmonary hypertension.[112] Vitamin A promotes epithelial regeneration[50] and surfactant synthesis in rats,[113] and ventilated preterm human infants,[114] reducing the risk of BPD. Oral or IM administration on alternate days[13] may be worth considering. Human studies suggest that the earlier vitamin A supplementation is started in BPD, the better the response.[115]

Deferoxamine

Deferoxamine, an iron chelator, may protect the neonatal lung from the effects of oxygen exposure. It also appears to allow normal alveolar septation by reducing elastin fiber length and density in hyperoxic neonatal rats[116] and lambs.[63] However, clinical use of deferoxamine in the treatment of BPD in humans or animals has not been established.

Surfactant

In rescue studies where human infants were given exogenous natural surfactant there was reduced mortality and development of BPD.[117] Decreased development of BPD and pulmonary interstitial emphysema was seen using modified bovine surfactant 100 mg/kg IT in baboons[118] and humans.[119] Synthetic protein-free and natural surfactants were compared in a metaanalysis of six human infant studies, revealing clear evidence of the superiority of natural surfactant.[117] Therefore, administration of 100 mg/kg of aerosolized IT natural exogenous surfactant may be considered in animal neonates, especially preterm neonates, with RDS.

Diuretics

Both furosemide and thiazides have been used to treat interstitial pulmonary edema in the early stages of BPD.[13] Diuretics, particularly furosemide, appear to increase lung compliance, decrease airway resistance, and improve V/Q mismatch.[3,13,120,121] There may be an additive effect with theophylline to increase dynamic lung compliance.[122] Improvement in pulmonary function of human infants with BPD given furosemide orally at 1 mg/kg appears to be rapid (less than 1 hour) but lasts less than 6 hours.[123] Furosemide at 2 mg/kg PO daily produced continued improvement in patient oxygenation (pulmonary function) after 1 week of therapy.[124] Inhaled aerosolized furosemide at 1 to 2 mg/kg improved pulmonary function for several hours in preterm neonates without any side effects.[125] Administration of medications by inhalation is problematic in animals, especially when the patient is not intubated. The application, dosages, and routes of administration of these drugs in clinical veterinary patients with BPD are largely unknown. Neonates may respond to and metabolize these medications differently than adults. A suggested guideline for treatment of veterinary patients is summarized in Table 55-2. Clinical veterinary recommendations suggest that furosemide should be administered IV, IM, or PO at 1 to 2 mg/kg, and repeated as needed based on clinical response.

Supportive Treatment

Oxygen supplementation is indicated for hypoxemic patients,[3] but administration should be minimized to avoid increased local oxidative stress.[12,21] The therapeutic goal in human infants is to maintain pulse oximetry readings of 93% to 96%.[3] Maintenance of patient SaO_2 greater than 88% may be difficult using a nasal cannula, and tracheal intubation for PPV may become necessary.[3,13,102,126] When PPV is employed in veterinary patients, either high frequency oscillating ventilation (HFOV)[3,102] or patient syn-chronized ventilation[13] is recommended, using lower TV at peak inspiratory pressures less than 20 cm H_2O initially, and then weaning the patient as response permits.[3,13,102] Permissive hypercapnia may allow earlier weaning of veterinary patients with BPD.[13,127]

Fluid Therapy

Respiratory distress and hypoxia may preclude oral fluid intake and increase insensible fluid losses via the respiratory tract.[128] Adequate colloid osmotic pressure is essential to maintain intravascular fluid volume, but transudation of plasma proteins from the pulmonary vessels and increasing inflammatory proteins within the interstitium in BPD favor edema formation. Excess interstitial water exacerbates BPD, especially during the acute inflammatory phase. Relative fluid restriction of preterm infants at risk for BPD decreased BPD rates and mortality.[129,130] Thus careful restriction of water may be prudent in veterinary patients with RDS and BPD. Colloids should be administered only when needed. Balanced electrolyte crystalloid solutions[128] should be administered IV in sufficient volumes to maintain intracellular water and the minimum plasma volume for organ perfusion while avoiding exacerbation of pulmonary edema.

Nutritional Support

Growth failure is common in infants with severe BPD[3,13] because of increased energy expenditure with decreased intake in RDS. Veterinary neonatal patients with RDS and BPD will likely not nurse, and require nutritional support. Even neonates that are able to eat on their own may tire during feedings, and oxygen supplementation may improve their feeding performance.[3] Nutritional support may best be supplied by alimentary tube feeding using the gastrointestinal tract, but alternatively it can be supplied by parenteral nutrition. Frequent small feedings of a high-calorie, high-lipid diet with supplemental vitamin A, magnesium, and possibly n-3 PUFAs might be considered.

Anti-Tussive Drugs

Airway compression during coughing episodes may cause mechanical irritation to the airways.[131] Centrally acting antitussives may suppress the respiratory control centers as well as the cough. If a productive cough is present, it should not be suppressed because of its vital role in airway clearance. Therefore, centrally acting antitussives should be avoided in neonates, especially if they have BPD. Bronchodilators may act as mild peripheral antitussives by reducing airway compression, thereby avoiding exacerbation of airway inflammation.[131]

Bronchodilators

BPD patients develop airway obstruction due to smooth muscle hypertrophy and airway hyperreactivity.[3,5] Thus bronchodilators and antiinflammatory drugs may be in-

TABLE 55-2   **Suggested Treatments for Bronchopulmonary Dysplasia in Small Animals***

Prevention	Specific Treatments	Supportive Treatments	Symptomatic Treatments
1. Good nutrition for dam: Consider vitamin A and n-3 long-chain fatty acids 2. Avoid breeding dams prone to premature parturition 3. Caution when using O_2 supplementation in neonates (especially when premature): $Fio_2 \leq 60\%$ 4. Antenatal dexamethasone 0.5 mg/kg to dam if premature parturition is imminent	1. Treat any lower airway infections aggressively 2. Administer antioxidants: 　a. Superoxide desmutase (rhSOD): 5 mg/kg IT q 48 hrs ($\leq$7 doses) 　b. Vitamin A: 400-800 U/kg PO q 24-48 hrs 　c. Natural surfactant (Survanta®): 100 mg/kg IT 　d. Furosemide: 1-2 mg/kg PO, IV, IM prn	1. Oxygen supplementation: 　a. Nasal cannula—$Fio_2 \geq 60\%$; if flow rate >0.5 L/min, humidify O_2 with in-line bubbler. Maintain $Sao_2 \geq 88\%$ 　b. Intubation/ventilation: 　　1) Spontaneous 　　2) Assisted: 　　　a) Patient triggered—Tidal volume 6-10 ml/kg, rate 60 bpm 　　　b) Continuous—High frequency oscillatory 　　3) Monitor and maintain $Sao_2 \geq 93\%$; $Pao_2 \geq 100$ mm Hg; $Paco_2$ 45-55 mm Hg 2. Nitric oxide: Tracheal-bronchial catheter 5-80 ppm 3. Fluids—Minimum necessary. Consider reduced sodium isotonic crystalloid maintenance with 2.5% dextrose and KCl (20 mEq/l) $\leq$66 ml/kg/24 hours 4. Nutrition—Stomach tube, naso-esophageal or gastrotomy tube—high calorie, high lipid with vitamin A 400 U/kg $\pm$ n-3 long chain PUFAs	1. Bronchodilators: 　a. Beta-2 agonists: 　　1) Albuterol metered inhalant: 100 µg/activation prn 　　2) Terbutaline: 0.05-0.10 mg/kg PO 　b. Methylxanthines: theophylline 1-2 mg/kg IV q 6-8 hrs 2. Corticosteroids: Dexamethasone 0.5 mg/kg IV or IM q 12-24 hrs and taper off as improves

* Modified from human and animal model studies of bronchopulmonary dysplasia.
IT, Intratracheal; *PUFAs,* polyunsaturated fatty acids.

dicated to decrease the work of breathing. Inhaled beta-2 agonists such as albuterol,[132] metaproterenol,[133] and terbutaline[134] have been shown to increase lung dynamic compliance and reduce pulmonary resistance. Administration is usually by a metered dose inhaler or via jet nebulizer into the inspiratory circuit of a ventilator.[13] Beta-2 and methylxanthine bronchodilators both have some inotropic effect on the diaphragm.[135] Theophylline may have an additive effect with diuretics to improve pulmonary function and patient oxygenation.[123] Concurrent use of antiinflammatory drugs may potentiate bronchodilation by beta-2 agonists and allow reduction in the doses of both.[136,137] Finally, some beta-2 agonists and methylxanthines also have central nervous system stimulatory effects, which might be beneficial for stimulation of respiration in animal neonates that are failing with RDS or BPD. Albuterol can be administered by metered inhalation at 100 µg per activation for intubated veterinary neonates, and terbutaline can be given orally or by injection. Administration should be only as needed, and adjustments in drug dosages should be anticipated because of the immaturity of the neonatal liver.

Antiinflammatory Drugs

Although beta-2 agonists and methylxanthines have some antiinflammatory effects,[138-140] corticosteroids are the mainstay of antiinflammatory therapy. Exogenous steroids improve both pulmonary resistance and lung compliance, decrease oxygen requirements, and may facilitate extubation of ventilator dependent human infants with BPD.[13]

Dexamethasone systemically and by inhalation has been used most commonly for BPD in human medicine. Beclomethasone has also been administered by inhalation with similar effects.[141,142] Studies of inhaled dexamethasone indicated temporary improvement in respiratory function in infants with CLD, and fewer side effects compared with systemic administration.[143] Systemic administration of dexamethasone may be considered in veterinary patients with BPD at 0.5 mg/kg daily, and then tapered if there is continued clinical improvement in respiratory function. Nonsteroidal antiinflammatory drugs have not been effective in reducing the inflammation in the lung with respiratory disease, with the possible exception of heartworm infection.[131,144]

Surgery

In rare instances, surgical intervention may afford some relief from respiratory distress caused by compromised airways or a diseased or torsed lung lobe. Dysplasia of the tracheobronchial cartilage in humans or animals contributes to tracheobronchial chondromalacia. This results in airway collapse and narrowing from lack of structural support during inhalation (extrathoracic airways) and exhalation (intrathoracic airways), and in air trapping in the lung. Tracheal chondrodysplasia seen with BPD in infants has been amenable to surgical stenting.[145] Unfortunately, the primary lesions in BPD are often in the smaller, intrathoracic airways that are not amenable to direct surgical intervention.

Bronchial chondrodysplasia with bronchomalacia can also lead to lung lobe torsion and an acute respiratory crisis, as illustrated in the reported case of canine BPD.[78] The disease was too advanced in this animal to permit surgical intervention. In less severely affected cases with only single lung lobe torsion, a lobectomy might be considered after stabilization of the patient.

Outcome and Prognosis

The likelihood of BPD in animals resolving sufficiently to allow them to have normal activity without respiratory distress appears remote. Recovery from BPD, when it occurs, is a protracted process. In survivors the lung gradually remodels, but the process requires prolonged support and vigilance against additional acquired pulmonary disease. Most human survivors of BPD demonstrate stunted growth, reduced respiratory capacity, and are prone to recurrent infections.[5,71,146] For many veterinary patients, euthanasia because of unresponsive or minimally responsive pulmonary insufficiency is likely to be the predominant outcome.

BPD in its broadest sense may represent a largely unrecognized clinical entity in veterinary medicine. It could be elicited by a variety of severe or prolonged insults that set up a progressive inflammatory condition, resulting in improper lung development of premature neonates and inadequate or inappropriate bronchopulmonary repair.

REFERENCES

1. Northway WH, Rosan RC, Porter DY: Pulmonary disease following respiratory therapy of hyaline membrane disease: Bronchopulmonary dysplasia, *N Engl J Med* 276:357-368, 1967.
2. Weibel ER: *The pathway for oxygen: Structure and function in the mammalian respiratory system,* Cambridge, 1984, Harvard University Press.
3. Farrell PA, Fiascone JM: Bronchopulmonary dysplasia in the 1990s: A review for the pediatrician, *Curr Probl Pediatr* 27:133-163, 1997.
4. Saugstad OD: Chronic lung disease: the role of oxidative stress, *Bio Neonate* 74 (suppl 1):21-28, 1998.
5. Hulsmann AR, van den Anker JN: Evolution and natural history of chronic lung disease of prematurity, *Monaldi Arch Chest Dis* 52(3):272-277, 1997.
6. King AS: *The cardiorespiratory system: Fetal and neonatal circulation and respiration: Neonatal disorders,* Oxford, 1999, Blackwell Science.
7. Merritt TA: Interactions in the immature lung. In Merrit TA, Northway WH, Boynton BR, editors: *Bronchopulmonary dysplasia,* Boston, 1988, Blackwell.
8. Frank L, Sosenko IRS: Development of the lung antioxidant enzyme system in late gestation: Possible implications for the prematurely born infant, *J Pediatr* 110:9-14, 1987.
9. VanGolde LMG, Batenburg JJ, Post M et al: Synthesis of surfactant lipids in developing lung. In Jones CT, Nathaniels PW, editors: *The physiological development of the fetus and newborn,* New York, 1985, Academic Press.
10. Shenai JP, Chytil F, Stahlman MT: Vitamin A status of neonates with bronchopulmonary dysplasia, *Pediatr Res* 19:185-189, 1985.
11. Robertson B: Pathology of neonatal surfactant deficiency, *Perspect Pediatr Pathol* 11:6-46, 1987.
12. Northway WH Jr.: Bronchopulmonary dysplasia: Then and now, *Arch Dis Child* 65:1076-1081, 1990.
13. Barrington KJ, Finer NN: Treatment of bronchopulmonary dysplasia: A review, *Clin Perinatology* 25(1):177-202, 1998.
14. Abman SH, Groothius JR: Pathophysiology and treatment of bronchopulmonary dysplasia, *Pediatr Clin North Am* 41:277-315, 1994.
15. Bancalari E, Gerhardt T: Bronchopulmonary dysplasia, *Pediatr Clin* 33:1-23, 1986.
16. Davis JM, Dickerson B, Metlay L et al: Differential effects of oxygen and barotrauma on the lung injury in the neonatal piglet, *Pediatr Pulmonol* 10:157-163, 1991.
17. Johnson KJ, Fantone JC, Kaplan J et al: In vivo damage of rat lungs by oxygen metabolites, *J Clin Invest* 67:983-993, 1981.
18. Saugstad OD, Hallman M, Abraham J et al: Hypoxanthine and oxygen induced lung injury: A basic mechanism of tissue damage? *Pediatr Res* 18:501-504, 1984.
19. Saugstad OD, Becher G, Grossmann M et al: Acute and chronic effects of xanthine oxidase on lung thorax-compliance in guinea pigs, *Intensive Care Med* 13:30-32, 1987.
20. Russell GAB, Cooke RWL: Randomised controlled trial of allopurinol prophylaxis in very preterm infants, *Arch Dis Child* 73:F27-F31, 1995.
21. Saugstad OD: Bronchopulmonary dysplasia and oxidative stress: Are we closer to an understanding of the pathogenesis of BPD? *Acta Paediatr* 86(12):1227-1282, 1997.
22. Pierce MR, Bancalari E: The role of inflammation in the pathogenesis of bronchopulmonary dysplasia, *Pediatr Pulmonol* 19:371-378, 1995.
23. Groneck P, Gotze-Speer B, Opperman M et al: Association of pulmonary inflammation and increased microvascular permeability during the development of BPD: A sequential analysis of inflammatory mediators in respiratory fluids of high-risk preterm neonates, *Pediatrics* 93:712-718, 1994.
24. Erdmann AJ III, Huttemieir, Landolt C et al: Pure O_2 breathing increases sheep lung microvascular permeability, *Anesthesiology* 58:153-158, 1983.
25. Crapo JD, Barry BE, Foscue HA et al: Structural and biochemical changes in rat lungs occurring during exposure to lethal and adaptive doses of oxygen, *Am Res Respir Dis* 122:521-523, 1980.
26. Crapo JD, Freeman BA, Barry BE et al: Mechanisms of hyperoxic injury to the pulmonary microcirculation, *Physiology* 26:170-176, 1983.
27. Fantone JC, Ward PA: Role of oxygen-derived free radicals and metabolites in leukocyte-dependant inflammatory reactions, *Am J Pathol* 107:170-176, 1982.
28. Weiss SJ, LoBuglio AF: Phagocyte-generated oxygen metabolites and cellular injury, *Lab Invest* 47:5-18, 1982.
29. Klebanoff SJ: Oxygen metabolism and the toxic properties of phagocytes, *Ann Intern Med* 93:380-389, 1980.
30. Newman JH, Loyd JE, English DK et al: Effects of 100% O_2 on lung vascular function in an awake sheep, *J Appl Physiol* 54:1379-1386, 1983.
31. Lee CT, Fein AM, Lippmann M et al: Elastolytic activity in pulmonary lavage fluid from patients with adult respiratory distress syndrome, *N Engl J Med* 304:192-196, 1981.
32. Merritt TA: Oxygen exposure in the newborn guinea pig lung lavage cell populations, chemotactic and elastase response: A possible relationship to neonatal bronchopulmonary dysplasia, *Pediatr Res* 16:798-805, 1982.
33. Ogden BE, Murphy SA, Saunders GC et al: Neonatal lung neutrophil and elastase/proteinase inhibitor imbalance, *Am Rev Respir Dis* 130:817-821, 1984.
34. Gerdes JS, Harris MC, Polin RA: Effect of dexamethasone and indomethacin on elastase, alpha-1-proteinase inhibitor, and fibronectin in bronchoalveolar lavage fluid from neonates, *J Pediatr* 113:727-731, 1988.

35. Fox RB, Holidal JR, Brown DM et al: Pulmonary involvement due to oxygen toxicity: Involvement of chemotactic factors and polymorphonuclear leukocytes, *Am Rev Respir Dis* 123:521-523, 1981.
36. Mirro R, Armestead W, Leffler C: Increased airway leukotriene levels in infants with severe bronchopulmonary dysplasia, *Am J Dis Child* 144:160-161, 1990.
37. Mariani TJ, Sandefur S, Pierce RA: Elastin in lung development, *Exp Lung Res* 23(2):131-145, 1997.
38. Burri PH, Weibel ER: Ultrastructure and morphometry of the developing lung. In Hodson WA, editor: *Development of the lung: Lung biology in health and disease,* vol 6, New York, 1977, Marcel Dekker.
39. Merritt TA, Cochrane CG, Holcomb K et al: Elastase and alpha-1-proteinase inhibitor activity in tracheal aspirates during RDS, *J Clin Invest* 72:656-662, 1983.
40. Bruce MC, Wedig KE, Jentoft N et al: Altered urinary excretion of elastin cross-links in premature infants who develop bronchopulmonary dysplasia, *Am Rev Respir Dis* 131:568-572, 1985.
41. Bruce MC, Schuyler M, Martin RJ et al: Risk factors for the degradation of lung elastic fibers in the ventilated neonate, *Am Rev Respir Dis* 146:294-312, 1992.
42. Fujimura M, Kitajima H, Nakayama M: Increased leukocyte elastase of the tracheal aspirate at birth and neonatal pulmonary emphysema, *Pediatrics* 92:564-569, 1993.
43. Goldstein W, Doring G: Lysosomal enzymes from polymorphonuclear leukocytes and proteinase inhibitors in patients with cystic fibrosis, *Am Rev Respir Dis* 134:49-56, 1986.
44. Lyle RE, Tryka AF, Griffin WS et al: Tryptase immunoreactive mast cell hyperplasia in bronchopulmonary dysplasia, *Pediatr Pulmonol* 19:336-343, 1995.
45. Harrada RN, Bowman CM, Fox RB et al: Alveolar macrophage secretions: Initiators of inflammation in pulmonary oxygen toxicity? *Chest* 81(Suppl):52-53, 1982.
46. Irving LB, Jordana M, O'Brodovich H et al: Alveolar macrophage activation in bronchopulmonary dysplasia, *Am Rev Respir Dis* 133(Suppl):A207, 1986.
47. Kojima T, Hattori K, Hirata Y et al: Endothelin-1 has a priming effect on production of superoxide anion by alveolar macrophages: Its possible correlation with bronchopulmonary dysplasia, *Pediatr Res* 39(1):112-116, 1996.
48. Sinkin RA, Roberts M, LoMonaco MB et al: Fibronectin expression in bronchopulmonary dysplasia, *Pediatr Dev Pathol* 1(6):494-502, 1998.
49. de Zwart LL, Meerman JHN, Meerman JNM et al: Biomarkers of free radical damage applications in experimental animals and in humans, *Free Radical Biology & Medicine* 26(1/2):202-226, 1999.
50. Shenai JP, Mellan BG, Chytil F: Vitamin A status and postnatal dexamethasone treatment in bronchopulmonary dysplasia, *Pediatrics* 106(3):547-553, 2000.
51. Zachman RD: Role of vitamin A in lung development, *J Nutr* 125;6 (suppl):1634S-1638S, 1995.
52. Caddell JL: Evidence for magnesium deficiency in the pathogenesis of bronchopulmonary dysplasia (BPD), *Magnes Res* 9(3):205-216, 1996.
53. Frank L: Effect of oxygen on the newborn, *Fed Proc* 44:2328-2334, 1985.
54. Rudiger M, von Baehr A, Haupt R et al: Preterm infants with high polyunsaturated fatty acid and plasmalogen content in tracheal aspirates develop bronchopulmonary dysplasia less often, *Crit Care Med* 28(5):1572-1577, 2000.
55. Clements JA: Comparative lipid chemistry of lungs, *Arch Intern Med* 127:387-389, 1971.
56. Kehrer JP, Autor AP: Changes in the fatty acid composition of rat lung lipids during development and following age-dependent lipid peroxidation, *Lipids* 12:596-602, 1977.
57. Kehrer JP, Autor AP: The effect of dietary fatty acids on the composition of adult rat lung lipids: relationship to oxygen toxicity, *Toxicol Appl Pharmacol* 44:423-440, 1978.
58. Enderes S, Ghorbani R, Kelley VE: The effect of dietary supplementation with n-3 polyunsaturated fatty acids on the synthesis of interleukin-1 and tumor necrosis factor by mononuclear cells, *N Engl J Med* 320:265-271, 1989.
59. Jobe AJ: The new BPD: An arrest of lung development, *Pediatr Res* 46(4):641-643, 1999.
60. Coalson JJ, Winter V, deLemos RA: Decreased alveolarization in baboon survivors with bronchopulmonary dysplasia, *Am J Crit Care Med* 152(2):640-646, 1995.
61. Hislop AA: Bronchopulmonary dysplasia: Pre- and postnatal influences and outcome, *Pediatr Pulmonol* 23:71-75, 1997.
62. Nerlick AG, Nerlick ML, Muller PK: Patterns of collagen types and molecular structure of collagen in acute post-traumatic pulmonary fibrosis, *Thorax* 42:863-869, 1987.
63. Pierce RA, Albertine KH, Starcher BC et al: Chronic lung injury in preterm lambs, disordered pulmonary elastin deposition, *Am J Physiol* 273(3 Pt 1):L452-460, 1997.
64. Anderson WR: Bronchopulmonary dysplasia: A correlative study by light, scanning, and transmission electron microscopy, *Ultrastruct Pathol* 14:221-232, 1990.
65. Miller RW, Woo P, Kellman RK et al: Tracheobronchial abnormalities in infants with bronchopulmonary dysplasia, *J Pediatr* 111:779-782, 1987.
66. McCubbin M, Frey EE, Wagener JS et al: Large airway collapse in bronchopulmonary dysplasia, *J Pediatr* 114:304-307, 1989.
67. Margraf LR, Tomashefski JF, Bruce MC et al: Morphometric analysis of the lung in bronchopulmonary dysplasia, *Am Rev Resp Dis* 143:391-400, 1991.
68. Binikos DS, Bensch KG: Pathogenesis of bronchopulmonary dysplasia. In Merrit TA, Northway WH, Boynton BR, editors: *Bronchopulmonary dysplasia,* London, 1988, Blackwell Scientific.
69. Coalson JJ, Winter VT, Gerstman DR et al: Pathophysiologic, morphometric, and biochemical studies of the premature baboon with bronchopulmonary dysplasia, *Am Rev Respir Dis* 145:872-881, 1992.
70. Taniguchi H, Taki F, Tagaki K et al: The role of leukotriene B4 in the genesis of oxygen toxicity in the lung, *Am Rev Respir Dis* 133:805-808, 1986.
71. Carey BE, Trotter C: Bronchopulmonary dysplasia, *Neonatal Rad* 15(4):73-77, 1996.
72. Verklan MT: Bronchopulmonary dysplasia: Its effects on the heart and lungs, *Neonatal New* 16(8):5-12, 1997.
73. Frank L, Sonesko IR: Prenatal development of lung antioxidant enzymes in four species, *J Pediatr* 110:106-110, 1987.
74. deLemos RA, Coalson JJ: The contribution of experimental models to our understanding of the pathogenesis and treatment of bronchopulmonary dysplasia, *Clin Perinatol* 19(3):521-539, 1992.
75. Coalson JJ: Experimental models of bronchopulmonary dysplasia, *Biol Neonate* 71(suppl 1):35-38, 1997.
76. Freeman KP, Simmons R, Wilkins PA et al: Recognition of bronchopulmonary dysplasia in a newborn foal, *Equine Vet J* 21(4):292-296, 1989.
77. Wilkins PA, Del Piero F, Lopez J et al: Recognition of bronchopulmonary dysplasia in a newborn foal: Letter to editor, *Equine Vet J* 27(5):398, 1995.
78. Hoover JP, Henry GA, Panciera RJ: Bronchial cartilage dysplasia with multifocal lobar bullous emphysema and lung torsions in a pup, *J Am Vet Med Assoc* 201(4):599-602, 1992.
79. Tennant BJ, Haywood S: Congenital bullous emphysema in a dog: Case report, *J Small Anim Pract* 28:109-116, 1987.
80. Herrtage ME, Clarke DD: Congenital lobar emphysema in two dogs, *J Small Anim Pract* 26:453-464, 1985.
81. Voorhour G, Goedegebure, Nap RC: Congenital lobar emphysema caused by aplasia of bronchial cartilage in a Pekinese puppy, *Vet Pathol* 23:83, 1986.
82. Amis TC, Hager D, Dungworth DL et al: Congenital bronchial cartilage hypoplasia with lobar hyperinflation (congenital lobar empysema) in an adult Pekinese. *J Am Anim Hosp Assoc* 23:321-329, 1987.
83. Anderson WI, King JM, Flint TJ: Multifocal bullous emphysema with concurrent bronchial hypoplasia in two aged afghan hounds, *J Comp Path* 100:469-473, 1989.
84. LaRue MJ, Gerlick DS et al: Bronchial dysgenesis and lobar emphysema in an adult cat, *J Am Vet Med Assoc* 197:886-888, 1990.
85. Mass B, Iheda T, Merange DR et al: Induction of experimental emphysema, *Am Rev Resp Dis* 106:384-391, 1972.
86. Miller KE, Edwards DK, Hilton S et al: Acquired lobar emphysema in premature infants with bronchopulmonary dysplasia: An iatrogenic disease? *Radiology* 138:589-592, 1981.

87. Landing BH, Wells TR: Tracheobronchial anomalies in children, *Perspect Pediatr Pathol* 1:1-32, 1973.

88. Hislop A, Reid L: New pathological findings in emphysema of childhood. Overinflation of a normal lobe, *Thorax* 26:1900-1904, 1971.

89. Frank L, Sosenko IRS: Undernutrition as a major contributing factor in the pathogenesis of bronchopulmonary dysplasia, *Am Rev Resp Dis* 138:725-729, 1988.

90. King RJ, Coalson JJ, deLemos RA et al: Surfactant protein-A deficiency in a primate model of bronchopulmonary dysplasia, *Am J Resp Crit Care* 151(6):1989-1997, 1995.

91. Awasthi S, Coalson JJ, Crouch E et al: Surfactant proteins A and D in premature baboons with chronic lung injury (bronchopulmonary dysplasia): Evidence of inhibition of secretion, *Am J Respir Crit Care Med* 160(3):942-949, 1999.

92. Zambon M: Active and passive immunization against respiratory syncytial virus, *Rev Med Virol* 9(4):227-236, 1999.

93. Coalson JJ, Olsberg CA, Johanson WG Jr et al: The role of infection in the premature baboon with lung injury, *Prog Clin Biol Res* 264:213-221, 1988.

94. Coalson JJ, Gerstmann DR, Winter VT et al: Bacterial colonization and infection studies in the premature baboon with bronchopulmonary dysplasia, *Am Rev Respir Dis* 144:1140-1146, 1991.

95. Uhl EW, Castleman WL, Sorkness RL et al: Parainfluenza virus-induced persistence of airway inflammation, fibrosis, and dysfunction associated with TGF-B$_1$ expression in brown Norway rats, *Am J Respir Crit Care Med* 154:1834-1842, 1996.

96. Arkovitz MS, Garcia VF, Szabo C et al: Decreased pulmonary compliance is an early indication of pulmonary oxygen injury, *J Surg Res* 67(2):193-198, 1997.

97. Turnwald GH, Hoover JP: The initial assessment: identifying abnormal breathing patterns, *Vet Med* 89(2):108-116, 1994.

98. Grag M, Kurzner SI, Bautista DB et al: Clinically unsuspected hypoxia during sleep and feeding in infants with bronchopulmonary dysplasia, *Pediatrics* 81:635-642, 1988.

99. Moyer-Mileur LJ, Nielsen DW, Pfeffer KD et al: Eliminating sleep-associated hypoxemia improves growth in infants with bronchopulmonary dysplasia, *Pediatrics* 98:779-783, 1996.

100. Turnwald GH, Hoover JP: Useful diagnostic test in small animals with a restrictive breathing pattern, *Vet Med* 89(2):130-141, 1994.

101. Turnwald GH, Hoover JP: The diagnostic evaluation of obstructive breathing patterns, *Vet Med* 89(2):117-128, 1994.

102. Claris O, Salle BL: High frequency oscillatory ventilation and the prevention of chronic lung disease, *Pediatr Pulmonol* 16 (suppl):33-34, 1997.

103. Mupanemunda RH, Edwards AD: Treatment of newborn infants with inhaled nitric oxide, *Arch Dis Child* 72:F131-F134, 1995.

104. Frostell C, Fratacci MD, Wain JC et al: Inhaled nitric oxide: A selective pulmonary vasodilator reversing hypoxic pulmonary vasoconstriction, *Circulation* 83:2038-2047, 1991.

105. Rossaint R: Nitric oxide: A new area in intensive care, *Presse Med* 23(18):855-858, 1994.

106. Rossaint R, Falke KJ, Lopez F et al: Inhaled nitric oxide for the adult respiratory distress syndrome, *N Engl J Med* 328:399-405, 1993.

107. Abman SH, Griebel JL, Parker DK et al: Acute effects of inhaled nitric oxide in children with severe hypoxemic respiratory disease, *J Pediatr* 124:881-888, 1994.

108. Banks BA, Seri I, Ischiropoulos H et al: Changes in oxygenation with inhaled nitric oxide in severe bronchopulmonary dysplasia, *Pediatrics* 103(3):610-618, 1999.

109. Yoder MC Jr, Chua R, Tepper R: Effect of dexamethasone on pulmonary inflammation and pulmonary function of ventilator-dependent infants with bronchopulmonary dysplasia, *Am Rev Respir Dis* 143(5 Pt 1):1044-1048, 1991.

110. Hoskins JD, Taboda J: Specific treatment of infectious causes of respiratory disease in dogs and cats, *Vet Medicine* 89(5):443-452, 1994.

111. Davis JM: Superoxide dismutase: A role in the prevention of chronic lung disease, *Biol Neonate* 74(suppl 1):29-34, 1998.

112. Albert G, Davis JM, Robbins CG et al: Superoxide dismutase as an adjunct therapy for inhaled nitric oxide and hyperoxia, *Pediatr Res* 43:272, 1998.

113. Fralson C, Bourbon JR: Retinoids control surfactant phospholipid biosynthesis in fetal rat lung, *Am J Physiol* 266(6 Pt 1):L705-712, 1994.

114. Shenai JL, Kennedy KA, Chytil F et al: Clinical trial of vitamin A supplementation in infants susceptible to bronchopulmonary dysplasia, *J Pediatr* 111:269-277, 1987.

115. Robbins ST, Fletcher AB: Early vs delayed vitamin A supplementation in very-low-birth-weight infants, *J Parenter Enteral Nutr* 17:220-225, 1993.

116. Blanco LN, Frank L: The formation of alveoli in rat lung during the third and fourth postnatal weeks: Effect of hyperoxia, dexamethasone, and deferoxamine, *Pediatr Res* 34(3):334-340, 1993.

117. Halliday HL: Clinical experience with exogenous natural surfactant, *Dev Pharmacol Ther* 13(2-4):173-181, 1989.

118. Maeta H, Raju TN, Vidayasagar D et al: Effects of exogenous surfactant on the development of bronchopulmonary dysplasia in a baboon hyaline membrane disease model, *Crit Care Med* 18(4):403-409, 1990.

119. Hoekstra RE, Jackson JC, Myers TF et al: Improved neonatal survival following multiple doses of bovine surfactant in very premature neonates at risk of respiratory distress syndrome, *Pediatrics* 88(1):10-18, 1991.

120. Ali J, Wood LDH: Pulmonary vascular effects of furosemide on gas exchange in pulmonary edema, *J Appl Physiol* 57:180-167, 1984.

121. Kao LC, Warburton D, Cheng MH et al: Effect of oral diuretic in infants with chronic bronchopulmonary dysplasia: Results of a double-blind crossover sequential trial, *Pediatrics* 74:37-44, 1984.

122. Kao LC, Durand DJ, Phillips BL et al: Oral theophylline and diuretics improve pulmonary mechanics in infants with bronchopulmonary dysplasia, *J Pediatr* 111:439-444, 1987.

123. Kao LC, Warburton D, Sargent CW et al: Furosemide acutely decreases airway resistance in chronic bronchopulmonary dysplasia, *J Pediatr* 103:624-629, 1983.

124. Engelhardt B, Elliot S, Hazinski TA: Short- and long-term effects of furosemide on lung function in infants with bronchopulmonary dysplasia, *J Pediatr* 109:1034, 1986.

125. Pai VB, Nahata MC: Aerosolized furosemide in the treatment of acute respiratory distress and possible bronchopulmonary dysplasia in preterm neonates, *Ann Pharmacother* 34(3):386-392, 2000.

126. Thome U, Kossel H, Lipowski G et al: Randomized comparison of high-frequency ventilation with high-rate intermittent positive pressure ventilation in preterm infants with respiratory failure, *J Pediatr* 135(1):9-11, 1999.

127. Mariani G, Cifuentes J, Carlo WA: Randomized trial of permissive hypercapnia in preterm infants: A pilot study, *Pediatr Res* 41:163A, 1997.

128. Hoover JP: Supportive treatment for dogs and cats with respiratory problems, *Vet Medicine* 89(5):420-431, 1994.

129. Tammela OKT, Koivisto ME: Fluid restriction for preventing bronchopulmonary dysplasia? Reduced fluid intake during the first weeks of life improves the outcome of low-birth-weight infants, *Acta Paediatr* 81:207, 1992.

130. Bell EF, Acarregui MJ: Restricted versus liberal water intake for preventing morbidity and mortality in preterm infants, *Cochrane Database Syst Rev* 2:CD000503, 2000.

131. Hoover JP: Symptomatic treatment of respiratory conditions in dogs and cats, *Vet Med* 89(5):432-442, 1994.

132. Prenninger J, Aebi C: Respiratory response to salbutamol (albuterol) in ventilator-dependant infants with chronic lung disease: Pressurized aerosol delivery versus intravenous injection, *Intens Care Med* 19:251-255, 1993.

133. Kao LC, Durand DJ, Nickerson BG: Effects of inhaled metaproterenol and atropine on the pulmonary mechanics of infants with bronchopulmonary dysplasia, *Pediatr Pulmonol* 6:74-80, 1989.

134. Brudno DS, Parker DH, Slaton G: Response of pulmonary mechanics to terbutaline in patients with bronchopulmonary dysplasia, *Am J Med Sci* 297:166-168, 1989.

135. Howell S, Roussos C: Isoproterenol and aminophylline improve contractility in fatigued canine diaphragm, *Am Rev Respir Dis* 129:118-124, 1984.

136. Padid P, Amis TC: Chronic tracheobronchial disease in the dog, *Vet Clin North Am Small Anim Pract* 22:1203-1229, 1992.

137. Dye JA, Moise NS: Feline bronchial disease. In Kirk RW, Bonagura JD, editors: *Kirk's current veterinary therapy*, vol 11, Philadelphia, 1992, WB Saunders.

138. Boothe DM: Feline respiratory pharmacology, proceeding, *Proc Sheba Feline Med Symp*, Kal-Kan Foods, Vernon, CA, 1990.

139. Boothe DM, McKiernan BC: Respiratory therapeutics, *Vet Clin North Am Small Anim Pract* 22:1231-1258, 1992.

140. McKiernan BC. Current uses and hazards of bronchodilator therapy. In Kirk RW, Bonagura JD, editors: *Kirk's current veterinary therapy*, vol 11, Philadelphia, 1992, WB Saunders.

141. LaForce WR, Brundo DS: Controlled trial of beclomethasone dipropionate by nebulization in oxygen- and ventilatory-dependent infants, *J Pediatr* 122:285-288, 1993.

142. Gei T, Raibble P, Zuerlin T et al: Trial of beclomethasone dipropionate by metered-dose inhaler in ventilator-dependent neonates less than 1500 grams, *Am J Perinatol* 13:5-9, 1996.

143. Lister P, Iles R, Shaw B et al: Inhaled steroids for neonatal chronic lung disease, *Cochrane Database Syst Rev* 3:CD002311, 2000.

144. Raju NV, Bharadwaj RA, Thomas R et al: Ibuprofen use to reduce the incidence and severity of bronchopulmonary dysplasia: A pilot study, *J Perinatol* 20(1):13-16, 2000.

145. Zinman R: Tracheal stenting improves airway mechanics in infants with tracheobronchomalacia, *Pediatr Pulmonol* 19:275-281, 1995.

146. Coates AL: Chronic lung disease in infants: Long-term pulmonary sequelae, *Pediatr Pulmonol* 16(suppl):40-42, 1997.

D. Pulmonary Parenchyma
CHAPTER 56

Bacterial Pneumonia in Dogs and Cats

Colleen A. Brady

Bacterial pneumonia in small animals is characterized by inflammation of the lower airways secondary to bacterial infection. It is a particularly challenging disease for the veterinarian because of the complex host-pathogen interactions, the wide range of clinical manifestations (i.e., from patients with mild, eupneic disease to those with rapidly progressive fatal infections), and the particular challenges of respiratory therapy.

Pneumonia is a leading cause of death in humans in the United States.[1-4] Although similar statistics are unavailable in veterinary medicine, pneumonia is a common diagnosis and is often a complication in hospitalized dogs. Bacterial pneumonia is not well described in cats except for a handful of case series and case reports. This paucity of information makes cats with pneumonia especially difficult to recognize and treat.

Pathogenesis/Pulmonary Defenses

Bacterial bronchopneumonia is characterized by inflammation originating at the bronchioalveolar junction. The bronchiolar alveolar junctions are the sites of greatest vulnerability in the distal respiratory tract, especially to damage by inhaled particles and vapors including droplet nuclei with infectious agents. There are several reasons for this vulnerability to infection. This is a major site of deposition of small particles (0.5 to 3.0 μm in diameter) capable of reaching the deep lung. The bronchiolar epithelium is not protected by the mucous blanket of larger airways or by an effective alveolar macrophage system. Finally, cellular material cleared from the alveolar parenchyma has to exit through the narrow lumen of the parent bronchiole, an easily plugged funnel.[5,6]

The lower airways have an elaborate defense network. Large particles (i.e., greater than 10 μm) are cleared by the nasopharynx, mucociliary clearance, and coughing. Particles smaller than 3 μm are deposited in the alveoli.[6] Bacteria, aerosolized in droplets or conveyed via aspiration, regularly bypass the upper respiratory tract defenses. Thus bacteria are routinely isolated from the lower airways of healthy animals.[7,8] A healthy animal can usually clear bacteria from the lower airways unless sheer numbers, high virulence, or concurrent direct injury overwhelms the pulmonary defenses. In situ alveolar defense mechanisms include surfactant and alveolar macrophages. Surfactant has antibacterial activity against *Staphylococcus* and some gram-negative bacteria.[9] Alveolar macrophages play a key role in the cellular defense of the lung.

The inflammatory response is necessary for effective clearance of most organisms. Complex interactions between macrophages, lymphocytes, and neutrophils regulate the inflammatory and counterinflammatory cascades. As bacteria enter the alveoli, opsonins such as surfactant, immunoglobulins, and fibronectin bind to the bacteria, facilitating macrophage recognition.[10] Alveolar macrophages phagocytize opsonized bacteria and produce the proinflammatory mediators tumor necrosis factor-alpha (TNFα) and interleukin-1 (IL-1).[11,12] Oxidative mechanisms in alveolar macrophages can kill *Staphylococcus,* but not gram-negative organisms.[11] Nonoxidative cellular defense mechanisms include the proteases, lysozymes, and defensins.

Lymphoid tissue in the pulmonary tree enhances the inflammatory response through cytokine activation. Activated T lymphocytes secrete interferons, TNF, and granulocyte-macrophage stimulating factor.[11] Mature B lymphocytes secrete antibodies into the alveoli to activate complement, neutralize pathogens and their toxins, and act as opsonins to enhance macrophage function. The dendritic cells in the interstitium, alveolar walls, and the columnar epithelium of the bronchi are the major antigen-presenting cells in the pulmonary tree.[11]

An influx of neutrophils, in conjunction with alveolar macrophages, creates an effective dual phagocytic defense. Neutrophils are attracted by chemotaxins (e.g., leukotriene-B4 and interleukin-8) that are secreted by activated macrophages.[13,14] The majority of neutrophils in the marginated pool are located within the lung capillaries and must cross into the alveoli for suppurative inflammation to occur. Pulmonary neutrophils adhere to the endothelium, repolarize, pass between the endothelial cells, cross the interstitium, and then pass through the cellular junction between type I alveolar cells into the alveolar space. Neutrophil migration involves interactions between cytokines, endothelial cells, cell adhesion molecules, alveolar epithelial cells, and macrophages.[15]

Once in the alveoli, neutrophils secrete chemokines. These perpetuate the inflammatory response, allowing protein and other mediators to enter the tissue. This inflammatory phase is associated with acute, exudative alveolar injury, and is characterized by necrosis and sloughing of type I pneumocytes. As the injury progresses, cuboidal type II cells proliferate to line the partially denuded alveolar wall. Proliferation of type II cells marks the transition from the exudative to the proliferative phase of inflammation.[6] Once inflammation subsides, type II cells are transformed to type I cells if there is no scarring.[6]

Chronic bronchopneumonia causes destruction of alveolar walls and abscessation due to persistent suppuration. Chronic injury to type II cells can result in metaplasia to squamous, ciliated, or fetal type cells.[6]

Etiology and Risk Factors

Decreased host defenses favor bacterial colonization of the lung. Increased age, organ failure, and poor nutritional status decrease opsonin availability, thus decreasing the efficacy of alveolar macrophages. The mucociliary transport system is directly impaired by bacteria, and through by-products of inflammatory mediators. Many bacterial species affect mucus consistency and volume, impeding normal mucociliary escalator progress.[10, 16]

Many cases of pneumonia in dogs and cats are caused by opportunistic normal airway flora. Environmental conditions that favor proliferation of these bacteria include multi-animal housing; unsanitary conditions; the presence of young, unvaccinated animals; and the presence of animals with upper respiratory disease.[16-19] Secondary bacterial pneumonia is seen following canine distemper virus infection in dogs, and in cats with viral upper respiratory tract infection.[16,20] Underlying conditions that predispose to bacterial pneumonia include other respiratory infections (e.g., viral, bacterial, fungal, or protozoal); poor body condition; metabolic diseases such as diabetes or hyperadrenocorticism; a reduced level of consciousness; neuromuscular diseases; functional or anatomic abnormalities such as ciliary dyskinesia, tracheal hypoplasia, pharyngeal abnormalities, and dysphagia; anesthesia; and surgery.[16,17,20,21]

Hematogenous spread of bacteria is a less common cause of bacterial pneumonia, but is seen in septic patients and secondary to phlebitis.[6,16,20] Bacterial pneumonia is common after aspiration of stomach contents, and is addressed in Chapter 57.

Pathogens

Most bacterial pneumonia is caused by resident microflora in dogs and cats (Table 56-1). Bacterial defenses and offenses are varied and elaborate. Endotoxin has been shown to decrease pulmonary surfactant quantity and quality.[11,16] Exotoxins have direct harmful effects on the pulmonary epithelium. Adhesin proteins facilitate epithelial attachment, and polysaccharide capsules inhibit phagocytosis.[11,16] Gram-negative enteric bacteria are the most commonly isolated bacterial pathogens in dogs with pneumonia.[17,22-25] A recent retrospective study by Angus and colleagues showed that polymicrobial infections may account for up to 43% of dogs with pneumonia.[22]

No comprehensive study of bacterial pneumonia pathogens in cats with pneumonia has been performed. As in dogs, bacteria can be isolated from the lower airways of healthy cats, making interpretation of bacterial cultures difficult.[8,26] However, studies of feline lower respiratory tract disease suggest that polymicrobial infection is common. Common bacterial pathogens in cats include *Pasteurella* spp., *Streptococcus* spp., *Bordetella, E. coli, Pseudomonas,* and *Mycoplasma* spp.[20,21,27] The group eugonic fermenter-4 (EF-4a) bacteria have characteristics similar to *Pasteurella* and have been identified as a cause of suppurative pneumonia in cats.[16,28,29] This group of bacteria has been associated with abscessation in multiple sites including liver, kidney, ear, and the retrobulbar space.

Mycoplasma are normal flora of the oropharynx, and have been recognized as concurrent pathogens in animals with pneumonia. Mycoplasma infections have been demonstrated in dogs and cats,[26,30,31,32] but studies suggest that they may have little clinical significance in dogs.[31] Although mycoplasma have been recovered from the lower airway in healthy dogs, they have not

TABLE 56-1. Common Bacteria Isolated From the Lower Airways and Their Prevalence in Dogs and Cats, Including Special Features of Certain Pathogens[17,20,22,45]

Pathogens	Dog	Cat*	Pathophysiologic Features
Gram Positive			
Staphylococcus Coagulase positive	5%-27%	Unknown +++	Normal flora Exotoxins, polysaccharide capsule
Streptococcus Enterococcus	14%-47%	Unknown ++	Polysaccharide capsule, surface protein A Pneumolysin: exotoxin that inhibits cilia and disrupts the alveolar/blood barrier Associated with hematogenous spread of infection.
Gram Negative	Normal enteric flora include Pseudomonas, E. coli, Klebsiella		
E. coli	17%-43%	Unknown +++	Endotoxin, polysaccharide capsule, adhesins, exotoxin formation.
Pseudomonas	8%-25%	Unknown ++	Adhesins, polysaccharide capsule, alpha hemolysin damages host membranes Antiphagocytic extracellular matrix Exotoxin A causes tissue necrosis Produce fibrinolysin, leukocidin, enterotoxin
Bordetella	3%-23%	Unknown ++	Normal flora of the upper respiratory tract Infectious canine tracheobronchitis Exotoxins inhibit phagocytosis and cause ciliostasis Possible synergistic relationship with Mycoplasma
Pasteurella	26%-45%	Unknown +++	Normal flora of nasopharynx and large airways Endotoxin, adhesions, polysaccharide capsule
Klebsiella	4%-23%	Unknown +	Causes extensive, necrotizing pneumonia
Anaerobic	Note that anaerobic infections usually coexist with either enteric bacteria or staphylococcus infections. A synergistic effect is present when aerobic and anaerobic infections are present.		
Bacteroides	24%	Unknown +	Normal flora Endotoxin, capsule that results in abscess formation, discourages phagocytosis Exotoxin
Clostridium	5%	Unknown +	

*Percentages are not available in the clinical literature so relative frequency is reported as: +++ = High prevalence, ++ = moderate, + = occasional.

been recovered in the lower airway of healthy cats. Therefore, it has been suggested that all mycoplasma infections may have clinical significance in cats and should be treated.[32]

History and Clinical Signs

Historical findings that should prompt consideration of pneumonia include a history of coughing, inadequate vaccination history, exposure to colony situations or unvaccinated animals, or a history of vomiting or anesthesia. Bacterial pneumonia is a well-recognized complication in hospitalized patients, especially in the postoperative period. In one study, 57% of dogs with pneumonia had a concurrent medical problem such as aspiration or immunosuppression, predisposing them to bacterial infection.[31]

The wide range of clinical signs in animals with bacterial pneumonia reflects the wide spectrum of the disease. In dogs, respiratory tract signs may include a moist cough; nasal discharge; tachypnea or dyspnea; and auscultation abnormalities such as crackles, increased bronchovesicular sounds, or wheezes.[16,17,31] Signs of systemic disease are variable and may include fever, anorexia, depression, weight loss, and dehydration. It is important to recognize that many dogs with bacterial pneumonia are not febrile.[17,33]

Cats with bacterial pneumonia often have a concurrent upper respiratory tract infection or a history of nasal discharge.[16,20] Respiratory signs range from no overt abnormalities to severe dyspnea with bilateral crackles on auscultation. Fever is a variable finding. Systemic signs of illness such as anorexia, depression, or vague pain on abdominal palpation may be present.

Diagnosis

The clinical diagnosis of bacterial pneumonia in veterinary medicine is based on a combination of clinical signs, radiographic findings, cytology, and isolation of bacteria in culture. Cats with bacterial pneumonia can be especially difficult to identify. The gold standard for diagnosis in any species is histologic confirmation, although this method is seldom used clinically.[34,35]

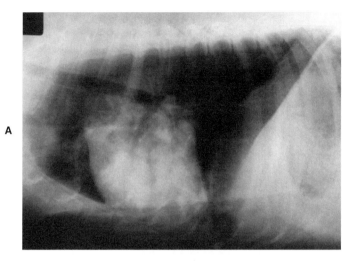

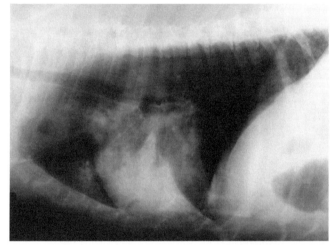

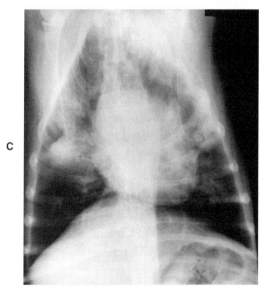

Figure 56-1. A, Right lateral, B, left lateral, and C, ventrodorsal radiographs of a 5-year-old female spayed Rottweiler with bronchopneumonia. A diffuse pulmonary alveolar pattern is evident in the ventral portion of multiple lung lobes (i.e., right cranial, right middle, left cranial, left caudal). Note the lobar separation between the consolidated alveolar pattern in the right middle lung lobe and the aerated right caudal lung lobe (lobar sign).

RADIOGRAPHS

Radiographs are essential for evaluation of patients with pneumonia. Classic radiographic findings of bacterial bronchopneumonia include a cranioventral distribution of alveolar disease (Figure 56-1). It has been suggested that local defense mechanisms are not as effective in the cranial ventral lung lobes. Airway branching is sharper in these areas, and gravity may diminish normal clearance mechanisms.[36] Alveolar consolidation with bronchopneumonia is often more dramatic in the periphery in the early stages and progresses in a central direction. However, a variety of radiographic patterns can be seen with bronchopneumonia, especially in cats (Figures 56-2 and 56-3). For example, bronchopneumonia may present as a diffuse mixed interstitial-bronchial pattern with or without multifocal alveolar patches. Multifocal distribution of patchy alveolar disease can occur in cats with pneumonia, and may not be readily distinguished from metastatic disease on radiographs. Lesions present in the caudal lobes may suggest hematogenous spread or inhaled infection. Small pleural effusions may be observed with severe bacterial pneumonia.[36-38]

Numerous clinical papers have been published debating the relative utility and superiority of the different tests used to diagnose pneumonia in people. Recent studies have shown wide discrepancies among physicians in the interpretation of thoracic radiographs, bronchoalveolar lavage (BAL) analysis, and even histologic samples of affected lungs.[34,39] This is significant because veterinarians often rely exclusively on thoracic radiographs and clinical signs to diagnose pneumonia. It is important to realize the potential limitations of this approach. Although history and clinical signs influence the assessment of alveolar disease, it is critical to identify the cause of alveolar filling. Recognition of an alveolar pattern should prompt exploration of a long list of differential diagnoses, including pulmonary edema, pulmonary thromboembolism, pulmonary hemorrhage, neoplasia, and atelectasis. A recent veterinary review compared the diagnostic utility of the following tests: thoracic radiography, cytology of BAL fluid, and histologic evaluation. The results clearly demonstrated the limitations of using only one diagnostic modality to diagnose respiratory disease.[35]

BACTERIAL ISOLATION

Numerous studies have shown improved morbidity and mortality rates when antimicrobial therapy is based on specific microbial culture results.[17,23,31] Several techniques are employed to bypass the pharynx and larynx and obtain samples for culture from the lower airways. The transtracheal wash is a simple procedure in appropriately selected cases. Endotracheal and bronchoalveolar lavages are also productive but require general anesthesia. Lung aspirates can be very helpful but must be weighed against the risk of pneumothorax.[40]

Cytological evaluation of tracheal/bronchial fluid should be performed; however, interpretation of extracellular bacteria and few to moderate numbers of in-

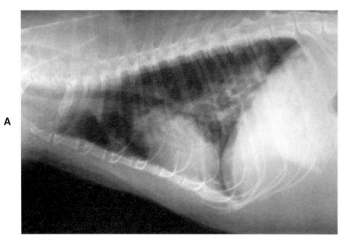

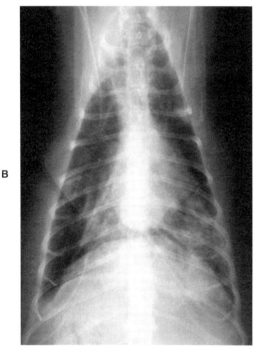

Figure 56-2. **A,** Right lateral and **B,** ventrodorsal radiograph of an 8-year-old castrated male domestic shorthair cat with E. coli pneumonia. An interstitial to alveolar pattern is evident in the right middle, right caudal, and accessory lobes. Note the atypical distribution of disease.

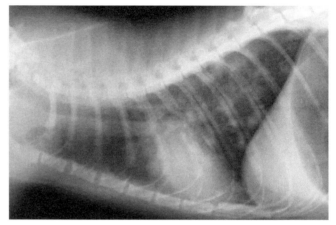

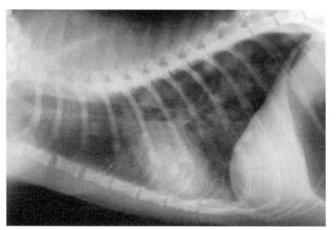

Figure 56-3. **A,** Right lateral and **B,** left lateral thoracic radiograph of a 10-year-old spayed female domestic shorthair cat with bacterial pneumonia confirmed by a postmortem histopathologic examination. A diffuse nodular interstitial pattern is visible.

flammatory cells may be difficult because these are found in healthy dogs and cats.[8,21,24,41] The significance of extracellular bacteria must be correlated with clinical signs and the potential for sample contamination with oral flora. Cytological findings of squamous epithelium or *Simonsiella* bacteria suggest oropharyngeal contamination. Alveolar macrophages are seen in healthy dogs and cats as well as in patients with pneumonia.[8]

The presence of leukocytes with intracellular bacteria confirms active infection (Figure 56-4). A high neutrophil count, especially with degenerate changes, is consistent with active inflammation.[41] Gram-stain evaluation may be considered.[42] Although the presence of bacteria on cytolog-

ical evaluation is supportive of pneumonia, the converse is not true, and the cytological absence of bacteria does not rule out infection. Therefore, it is essential that all samples are cultured for aerobic organisms. Mycoplasma cultures may be indicated. Culturing for anaerobic organisms remains controversial for uncomplicated pneumonia but is indicated in animals with pulmonary abscesses. One study correlating histological evidence of pneumonia with quantitative culture results showed 10^3 or greater colony-forming units (CFU)/ml in samples obtained with a protected sterile brush, 10^4 or greater CFUs/ml in BAL fluid, and 10^5 or greater CFUs/ml in quantitative endotracheal aspiration samples; all are consistent with pneumonia.[8] Another study by Peeters and colleagues suggests that quantitative aerobic cultures greater than 1.7×10^3 CFU/ml are consistent with lower respiratory tract infection in dogs.[25]

Appropriate antibiotic therapy based on bacterial isolation results in increased survival and decreased morbidity.[22] Antibiotic therapy should not be withheld pending sample collection, however. Although it seems intuitive that prior antibiotic use may decrease the yield from cultures taken after antibiotics, this is rarely a clin-

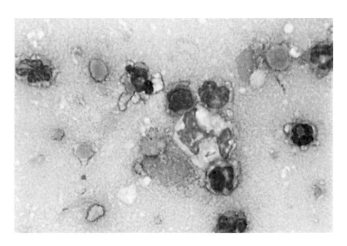

Figure 56-4. A photomicrograph showing intracellular rods within a neutrophil. This is a direct preparation from a fluid sample obtained during endotracheal lavage in a 7-year-old domestic shorthair cat with bronchopneumonia (Wright-Giemsa stain, 400×).

ical problem. Peeters and colleagues found that recent antibiotic therapy did not contribute to negative or minimal quantitative BAL culture results.[25]

HEMATOLOGICAL AND BIOCHEMICAL FINDINGS

Complete blood count (CBC) abnormalities are inconsistently seen in both dogs and cats with bacterial pneumonia.[17,20,22,31] Many animals have a normal leukogram. Moderate to severe cases usually have a leukocytosis with or without a left shift. Very severely affected patients may be leukopenic. A mild anemia is commonly seen in critically ill cats. Biochemical changes are nonspecific. Hypoalbuminemia is common in chronically ill patients and in severe cases, and is due to a shift in hepatic production of albumin to synthesis of acute phase proteins, as well as increased vascular permeability and resultant loss of albumin into the interstitium.

Management and Monitoring

The cornerstones of patient management are comprehensive supportive care and appropriate antibiotic therapy. It is essential to accurately assess respiratory and ventilatory function in patients with lower respiratory disease. A meticulous physical examination, with careful attention to respiratory rate and effort, postural changes, and auscultation abnormalities, is essential to determine the level of care needed. Frequent auscultation by the same individual allows detection of early changes in patient status.

RESPIRATORY MONITORING AND TREATMENT

Pneumonia results in varying degrees of ventilation/perfusion mismatch (V/Q), which may result in hypoxia. Consolidated lung lobes effectively form an intrapul-

monary shunt.[43] Theoretically, hypoxic pulmonary vasoconstriction (HPV) minimizes the volume of blood that is directed to the consolidated area; however, local inflammatory mediators may act as vasodilators and override HPV.[44] Pulse oximetry (SpO_2) is a noninvasive means to help determine if oxygen supplementation is indicated. Arterial blood gas analysis gives an objective measurement of both oxygenation and ventilation. One retrospective study identified significant hypoxemia in 62 dogs with bacterial pneumonia.[45] Most clinically significant hypoxemia is relieved by oxygen supplementation, but hypoxemia caused by a significant intrapulmonary shunt will not be improved by increasing the inspired oxygen concentration.

Oxygen supplementation should be provided if the SpO_2 is less than 94% or if the PaO_2 is less than 80 mm Hg. Methods of administering oxygen include oxygen cages, nasal cannula, flow-by delivery, and oxygen hoods.[46] Oxygen sensors should be used to determine the FiO_2 being provided, when possible. Humidification of oxygen is essential to maintain the health of the mucociliary escalator and facilitate coughing of secretions.

In animals with hypoxia, daily arterial blood gas samples should be analyzed, with serial evaluation of the arterial-alveolar oxygen tension gradient. To ensure accurate comparison from day to day, pulse oximetry readings and daily arterial samples should be obtained while the patient is breathing room air, unless the patient becomes tachypneic or distressed without oxygen supplementation. It is difficult to interpret changes in the alveolar-arterial oxygen tension gradient in animals receiving unknown quantities of supplemental oxygen. An alternative oxygen tension based ratio used commonly in animals receiving oxygen is the $PaO_2:FiO_2$ ratio, which should be greater than 400. Ratios less than 200 are evidence of significant respiratory disease.[6]

Regardless of the means of delivery, the amount of oxygen supplementation should be the minimum required to alleviate respiratory distress. Although oxygen toxicity has not been documented in the veterinary clinical literature, review of the medical literature suggests that it is prudent to avoid oversupplementation.[47,48] Adverse consequences associated with prolonged exposure to high concentrations of oxygen include increased capillary permeability with interstitial and alveolar edema, and denudement of alveolar epithelium and replacement with type II pneumocytes.[48] The degree of absorption atelectasis is linearly related to increases in FiO_2. General guidelines to minimize oxygen toxicity include limiting the FiO_2 to a maximum of 60% if oxygen is needed for longer than 48 hours.[47] Critically ill patients with decreased antioxidant levels may be at increased risk for oxygen toxicity.[11]

Oxygen supplementation may not relieve hypoxemia in severely affected animals. Persistent hypoxemia despite adequate oxygen supplementation, and/or ventilatory muscle fatigue, are indications for mechanical ventilation. Positive pressure ventilation should be considered if the PaO_2 is less than 50 mm Hg while the animal is receiving oxygen supplementation, or if the $PaCO_2$ is greater than 50 mm Hg.[49] If arterial blood gas analysis is not available, severe dyspnea is sufficient indication for ventilation.

FLUID THERAPY

Intravenous fluids are commonly indicated because patients are often adypsic and anorexic. The goals of fluid therapy are twofold: maintain euvolemia, and ensure adequate hydration. The physiologic response to hypoxemia is to increase cardiac output; therefore, an increased fluid volume may be required to maintain euvolemic status.[6] Also, excessive panting and fever may lead to increased water requirements.[50]

Caution must be exercised when administering high doses of intravenous fluids to patients with severe pneumonia because the blood/alveolar barrier is often compromised. Fluid overload can exacerbate compromised lung function, and distinguishing between progression of disease and iatrogenic injury can be difficult.[51,52]

Dehydration may change mucus composition in the respiratory tract, decreasing the efficacy of mucociliary clearance and alveolar emptying. It has been suggested that dehydration may mask alveolar disease because of decreased fluid shift across the alveolar membrane, although this has not been demonstrated convincingly.[53]

ANTIBIOTICS

Traditionally, it was thought to be preferable to obtain samples for culture before starting antibiotics; however, the need to withhold antibiotics before culture is currently controversial. Antibiotics should definitely not be withheld from animals that are hypoxemic or febrile because pneumonia can progress rapidly to a life-threatening condition. Diagnostic samples for culture and sensitivity should be obtained as soon as possible, and treatment with broad-spectrum antibiotics started. Once the pathogen is identified, the antibiotic with the narrowest effective spectrum should be used. Patients that are hemodynamically stable, eating and drinking with no respiratory compromise, may be started on oral antibiotics. All other patients should be hospitalized and treated with intravenous antibiotics.

Initial antibiotics should be selected based on knowledge of individual patients including prior antibiotic therapy, the hospital population, endemic bacterial pathogens, and geographic considerations. Inadequate initial antimicrobial therapy is an independent risk factor for increased mortality in humans with hospital acquired pneumonia.[54] It has been suggested that antibiotic dosages should be increased in leukopenic patients because there is evidence to suggest a direct correlation between decreased circulating leukocytes and decreased alveolar macrophages.[55] Table 56-2 lists broad-spectrum antibiotic choices that may be appropriate for pneumonia.

Nebulization of antibiotics is not recommended by the authors, but has been suggested in specific cases of *Pseudomonas* pneumonia.[56] There are no reports of the efficacy of antibiotic administration in animals with pneumonia, although a series of dogs with *Bordetella* tracheobronchitis (but not pneumonia) were successfully treated with aerosolized gentamicin.[57] Purported benefits of this method of delivery include decreased bacterial counts in airways, lack of systemic absorption of a potentially toxic drug, and more rapid resolution of clinical signs.

Arguments against aerosolized antibiotics include inconsistent drug delivery and airway irritation. It has been suggested that less than 10% to 20% of aerosolized medications in small animals actually reach the bronchi;[58] however, a recent study of aerosolized gentamicin in healthy horses demonstrated high concentrations of gentamicin retrievable in bronchial fluid after aerosolized administration.[59] It has been argued that the respiratory pattern may become more shallow and rapid with progression of disease, thus further decreasing distal delivery of aerosolized particles.[58] Furthermore, there is concern that aerosolized antibiotics may be irritating to inflamed airways, thus exacerbating bronchoconstriction.[59] There is no direct evidence to support or deny the use of this technique, and the controversy is demonstrated in the veterinary or human clinical literature.[58,60]

BRONCHODILATORS

The use of bronchodilators is controversial in animals with pneumonia. Bronchodilators may be inappropriate for animals with primarily alveolar disease and may worsen V/Q mismatch. They may suppress the cough reflex by altering airflow and airway diameter. Arguments supporting the use of beta-agonist bronchodilators include increased airflow and improved mucokinetics as a result of improved ciliary activity, and an increase in the serous component of bronchial secretions. In addition, beta $_2$agonists may have direct antiinflammatory effects by decreasing mucosal edema and down-regulating cytokine release.[58]

Methylxanthine bronchodilators have also been advocated, although the mechanism of action is not well understood. In addition to bronchodilation, potential beneficial effects of methylxanthine use in pneumonia include increased mucociliary transport rates, inhibition of mast cell degranulation, and decreased microvascular leak.[58] Theophylline may increase the strength of diaphragm contractility, which may alleviate ventilatory fatigue.[62] Caffeine infusions are being evaluated in human pediatric ICUs to accomplish the same goal.[63] Theophylline serum concentrations are increased by concurrent use of fluoroquinolones, although the clinical significance of this is unknown.[58]

MUCOLYTICS

Acetylcysteine is sporadically mentioned in the veterinary literature. The mucolytic effects of N-acetylcysteine (NAC) are caused by its effect of breaking down disulfide bonds in thick airway mucus. NAC is a precursor to glutathione, which is a scavenger of free radicals associated with inflammation.[58] Although aerosolized NAC may improve antibiotic delivery,[64] aerosolized NAC can cause reflex bronchoconstriction from its direct irritant effects.[65] Proven benefits of this drug have not been demonstrated in the veterinary clinical literature.

NEBULIZATION AND COUPAGE

Nebulization is the delivery of water droplets to the lower airways to increase hydration of the mucociliary system.

TABLE 56-2. Suggested Antibiotic Regimes in Dogs and Cats with Bacterial Pneumonia

	First Choice (Mild Disease)	Second Choice (Severe Disease)
Dog		
Stable (oral)	Trimethoprim/sulfonamide* 15 mg/kg PO q12h **or** Cephalexin 20 mg/kg PO q8h	Enrofloxacin 5 mg/kg PO q12h **or** Amoxicillin/clavulanate 15 mg/kg PO q12h
Unstable (parenteral)		Ampicillin 22 mg/kg IV q8h **with** Enrofloxacin† 10-15 mg/kg IV q24 **or** Amikacin‡ 15 mg/kg IV q24h **or** 2nd or 3rd generation cephalosporin
Cat		
Stable (oral)	Amoxicillin/clavulanate 15 mg/kg PO q12h	Clindamycin 10 mg/kg PO q12h
Unstable (parenteral)	Cefazolin 10 mg/kg IV q8h **or** Ampicillin 22 mg/kg IV q8h **or** Clindamycin 10 mg/kg IV q12h	Cefoxitin 15 mg/kg IV q4h **or** Ticarcillin/clavulanate 50 mg/kg IV q6h **or** Enrofloxacin** 5 mg/kg IV q24h **or** 3rd generation cephalosporin

*Trimethoprim/sulfonamide is not advised in certain breeds such as Dobermans, rottweilers, and other black and tan dogs, and in dogs with known platelet disorders or keratoconjunctivitis sicca.

†Enrofloxacin should not be used in dogs under 6 months of age. It may be prudent to avoid this drug in giant breed dogs less than 1 year of age.

‡Amikacin should not be used in animals with renal disease or poor renal perfusion. Daily monitoring of urine sediment is advised for early detection of casts.

For effective penetration of the lower airways, water particles must be between 0.5 and 3.0 micrometers. Vaporizers and humidifiers are not effective for this goal.[66]

Coupage of the chest is a form of physical therapy designed to stimulate the cough reflex. Effective coupage of the chest wall with a repeated, firm action effectively mobilizes airway secretions. Atelectasis can exacerbate respiratory insufficiency; therefore, recumbent patients should be turned every 1 to 2 hours and supported in an upright position several times a day. Short walks should be encouraged. Coughing is an important clearance mechanism, and antitussive agents should not be routinely used in patients with pneumonia.

THE REFRACTORY PATIENT

A select population of patients with pneumonia does not respond to conventional therapy. Patients at greater risk include pediatric and geriatric patients and those with concurrent immunosuppression or other significant disease. Although a poor response may be anticipated in severely debilitated animals, it can also occur in patients in seemingly good condition. Negative prognostic markers in people include hypoalbuminemia, leukopenia, thrombocytopenia, and an increased serum creatinine concentration.[3]

Failure to respond to standard treatment may result from antibiotic failure, concurrent viral or fungal pathogens, consolidated lung lobes, lung abscesses, incorrect diagnosis, functional or anatomic defects in pulmonary defenses, and development of sepsis.[54,67] In addition, spontaneous pneumothorax secondary to bacterial pneumonia has been reported in 2 dogs.[68] Antibiotic failure can result from bacterial resistance, inadequate local antibiotic concentrations, anatomic limitations, or the development of superinfection.[70,71] Thoracic ultrasound may help identify a nidus of infection such as a consolidated lung lobe or abscess.[72] A lung lobectomy may be required if there is refractory consolidation of a lung lobe, or for diagnostic evaluation.[73,74] A retrospective study of 59 dogs with bacterial pneumonia showed that over 50% of dogs in the selected population benefited from lung lobectomy in the treatment of pneumonia.[74]

Severe bronchopneumonia can lead to Acute Respiratory Distress Syndrome (ARDS) or septic shock in dogs and cats. Progression of pneumonia to ARDS is associated with increased mortality rates.[67] Identification of risk factors for development of ARDS, such as hypoalbuminemia, is a subject of much research in human medicine.[75] Early recognition of sepsis facilitates aggressive intervention. Persistent pyrexia, tachycardia, hypotension, or worsening dyspnea should alert the clinician to potential sepsis.[76]

Home Management

Patients that are weaned off oxygen and are able to eat and drink should be discharged from the hospital on oral antibiotics. Occasionally, in cases of multi–drug-resistant bacteria, owners may need to administer parenteral antibiotics at home. In dry home environments, humidification of the air may be beneficial in maintaining the water content of the upper airway mucociliary system. Although maintenance of systemic hydration should allow for adequate water saturation of the mucous layer, humidification does seem to be of benefit in certain patients. Underlying predisposing causes of pneumonia must also be addressed and resolved, if possible, for optimal outcome.

Clinical experience suggests that recurrent infections become increasingly more difficult to treat. For this reason, it is essential to maintain antibiotic coverage for an adequate duration to prevent recurrence. Antibiotic therapy should therefore be continued for a minimum of 4 weeks and up to 3 months in severe cases. Serial thoracic radiographs are important to determine the progression of disease and to determine the duration of antibiotic treatment. At a minimum, thoracic radiographs should be obtained at 2 weeks and 6 weeks. Antibiotic therapy is continued for a further 2 weeks after the radiographic changes have completely resolved. Repeat thoracic radiographs should be obtained 2 weeks after discontinuing antibiotic therapy to confirm that pneumonia has not recurred.

Patients that are deteriorating in the face of appropriate therapy need more frequent evaluation. Occasionally radiographic signs of alveolar disease do not resolve. Airway exudate that is not effectively cleared from the alveolar spaces leads to consolidation of lung lobes, which may remain subclinical; may result in persistent chronic clinical signs; and occasionally may abscess and rupture, resulting in pyothorax. Surgical intervention is indicated if appropriate antibiotic therapy has been ineffective and a single lung lobe is persistently affected. However, a retrospective study in dogs showed that lung lobectomy was less successful in resolving infectious pneumonia than other types of pneumonia.[73] Lung lobectomy has been reported for treatment of chronic pneumonia in cats, but bacteria were not identified on histopathological examination of the affected lobes in 3 of the 5 cats in that study.[74]

Pulmonary Abscess

Lobar pneumonia is a rapidly confluent, fulminating bronchopneumonia, in which gross evidence of bronchiolar orientation and spread is not evident. The term is used to indicate very aggressive bronchopneumonia. Pulmonary abscesses may arise from severe bronchopneumonia, foreign bodies, trauma, parasitic infections, or neoplasia. A pulmonary abscess secondary to *Mycoplasma* spp. has been reported in 1 cat.[30] Nodular or cavitary lesions may be visible on thoracic radiographs, and thoracic ultrasound can verify fluid-filled structures.[72] Pulmonary abscess is a surgical condition, and the abscess is prone to rupture with subsequent pyothorax.

REFERENCES

1. Bartlett JG, Mundy LM: Community acquired pneumonia, *N Eng J Med* 333(24):1618-1624, 1995.
2. Farr BM, Sloman AJ, Fisch MJ: Predicting death in patients hospitalized for community acquired pneumonia, *Ann J Intern Med* 115:428-436, 1991.
3. Feldman C, Kallenbach JM, Levy H et al: Community acquired pneumonia of diverse aetiology: Prognostic features in patients admitted to an intensive care unit and a "severity of illness" score, *Int Care Med* 15(5):302-307, 1989.
4. Fine MF, Singer DE, Hanusa BH et al: Validation of a pneumonia prognostic index using the Medis Groups Comparative Hospital Database, *Am J Med* 94:153-159, 1993.
5. Brain JD: Factors influencing deposition of inhaled particles. In *Proceedings of the third veterinary respiratory symposium*, Chicago, 1983.
6. Lumb A: Functional anatomy of the respiratory tract. In *Nunn's applied respiratory physiology*, ed 5, Oxford, 2000, Butterworth-Heineman.
7. Hawkins EC, De Nicola DB, Kuehn NF: Bronchoalveolar lavage in the evaluation of pulmonary disease in the dog and cat, *JVIM* 4:267-274, 1990.
8. Padrid PA, Feldman BF, Funk K et al: Cytologic, microbiologic, and biochemical analysis of bronchoalveolar lavage fluid obtained from 24 healthy cats, *Am J Vet Res* 52(8):1300-1307, 1991.
9. Hamm H, Kroegel C, Holfield J et al: Surfactant: A review of its functions and relevance in adult respiratory disorders, *Respir Med* 90:251-270, 1996.
10. Reynolds HY: Bacterial adherence to respiratory tract mucosa—a dynamic interaction leading to colonization, *Semin Respir Infect* 2:8-19, 1987.
11. Reynolds HJ: Lower airway defense mechanisms. In Bone R, editor: *Pulmonary and critical care medicine*, New York, 1998, Mosby Year-Book.
12. Standiford TJ: Cytokines and pulmonary host defenses, *Current Opinions in Pulmonary Medicine* 3(2):81-88, 1997.
13. Lien DC, Henson PM, Capen RL et al: Neutrophil kinetics in the pulmonary microcirculation during acute inflammation, *Lab Invest* 65(2):145-159, 1991.
14. Sibille Y, Reynolds HY: Macrophages and polymorphonuclear neutrophils in lung defense and injury, *Am Rev Resp Dis* 141(2):471-501, 1990.
15. Hogg JC, Walker BA: PMN leukocyte traffic in lung inflammation, *Thorax* 50:819-820, 1995.
16. Greene CE: Respiratory infections. In Greene CE, editor: *Infectious diseases of the dog and cat*, Philadelphia, 1998, WB Saunders.
17. Thayer GW, Robinson SK: Bacterial bronchopneumonia in the dog: A review of 42 cases, *JAAHA* 20:731-735, 1984.
18. Snyder SB, Fisk SK, Fox JG et al: Respiratory tract disease associated with Bordetella bronchiseptica in cats, *JAVMA* 163:293-294, 1973.
19. Welsh RD: Bordetella bronchiseptica infections in cats, *JAAHA* 32:153-158, 1996.
20. Brady CA, Gardelle O, Van Winkle TJ et al: Bacterial pneumonia in cats: 30 cases (abstract). In *Proceedings of the International Veterinary Emergency and Critical Care Symposium*, Orlando, Florida, 2000.
21. Moise NS, Wiedenkeller D, Yeager A et al: Clinical, radiographic, and bronchial cytologic features of cats with bronchial disease: 65 cases (1980-1986), *JAVMA* 194(10):1467-1473, 1989.
22. Angus JC, Jang SS, Hirsch DC: Microbiological study of transtracheal aspirates from dogs with suspected lower respiratory tract disease: 264 cases (1989-1995), *JAVMA* 210:55-58, 1997.

23. Harpster N: The effectiveness of the cephalosporins in the treatment of bacterial pneumonia in the dog, *JAAHA* 17:766-772, 1981.
24. McKiernan BC, Smith AR, Kissil M: Bacterial isolates from the lower trachea of clinically healthy dogs, *JAAHA* 20:139-142, 1984.
25. Peeters D, McKiernan BD, Weisiger RM et al: Quantitative bacterial cultures and cytological examination of bronchoalveolar lavage specimens in dogs, *JVIM* 14:534-541, 2000.
26. Dye JA, McKiernan BC, Rozanski EA et al: Bronchopulmonary disease in the cat: Historical, physical, radiographic, clinicopathologic, and pulmonary functional evaluation of 24 affected and 15 healthy cats, *JVIM* 10(6):385-400, 1996.
27. Moses BL, Spaulding FL: Chronic bronchial disease of the cat, *Vet Clin North Am* 15(5):929, 1985.
28. Drolet R, Kenefick K, Hakomaki M et al: Isolation of group fermenter-4 bacteria from a cat with multifocal suppurative pneumonia, *JAVMA* 189(3):311-312, 1986.
29. Weyant RS, Burris JA, Nichols DK et al: Epizootic feline pneumonia associated with CDC group EF-4a bacteria, *Lab Animal Sci* 44:180-183, 1994.
30. Crisp M, Birchard S, Lawrence A et al: Pulmonary abscess caused by a *Mycoplasma* spp. in a cat, *JAVMA* 191(3):340-342, 1987.
31. Jameson PH, King LA, Lappin MR et al: Comparison of clinical signs, diagnostic findings, organisms isolated, and clinical outcome in dogs with bacterial pneumonia: 93 cases (1986-1991), *JAVMA* 206(2):206-209, 1995.
32. Randolph JR, Moise NS, Scarlett JM et al: Prevalence of mycoplasmal and ureaplasmal recovery from tracheobronchial lavages and of mycoplasmal recovery from pharyngeal swab specimens in cats with or without pulmonary disease, *Am J Vet Res* 54(6):897-900, 1993.
33. Brownlie SE: A retrospective study of diagnoses in 109 cases of canine lower respiratory disease, *JSAP* 31:371-376, 1990.
34. Corley DE, Kirtland SH, Winterbauer RH et al: Reproducibility of the histologic diagnosis of pneumonia among a panel of four pathologists: Analysis of a gold standard, *Chest* 112(2):458-465, 1997.
35. Norris CR, Griffey SM, Samii V et al: Comparison of results of thoracic radiography, cytologic evaluation of bronchoalveolar lavage fluid, and histologic evaluation of lung specimens in dogs with respiratory tract disease: 16 cases (1996-2000), *JAVMA* 218(9):1456-1461, 2001.
36. Suter PF: Lower airway and pulmonary parenchymal diseases. In Suter PF, editor: *Thoracic radiography*, Weltsil, Switzerland, 1984, PF Suter.
37. Lamb CR: The canine lung. In Thrall DE, editor: *Textbook of veterinary diagnostic radiology*, Philadelphia, 1994, WB Saunders.
38. Texeira LR, Villarino MA: Antibiotic treatment of patients with pneumonia and pleural effusion, *Curr Opin Pulmon Med*, 4(4):230-234, 1998.
39. Albaum MN, Hill LC, Murphy M et al: Interobserver reliability of the chest radiograph in community acquired pneumonia, *Chest* 110(2):343-350, 1996.
40. Teske E, Stokaf A, van den Ingh TSG et al: Transthoracic needle aspiration biopsy of the lung in dogs with pulmonic disease, *JAAHA* 27:289-294, 1991.
41. Hawkins EC, DeNicola DB, Plier ML: Cytological analysis of bronchoalveolar lavage fluid in the diagnosis of spontaneous respiratory tract disease in dogs: A retrospective study, *JVIM* 9(6):386-392, 1995.
42. Papazian L, Antillo-Touati A, Pacal T et al: Diagnosis of ventilator associated pneumonia: An evaluation of direct examination and presence of intracellular organisms, *Anesthesiology* 87(2):268-276, 1997.
43. Hanly P, Light R: Lung mechanics, gas exchange, pulmonary perfusion, and hemodynamics in a canine model of acute Pseudomonas pneumonia, *Lung* 165(5):305-322, 1987.
44. Gea J, Roca J, Torres A et al: Mechanism of abnormal gas exchange in patients with pneumonia, *Anesthesiology* 75:782-789, 1991.
45. Wingfield WE, Matteson VL, Hackett T et al: Arterial blood gases in dogs with bacterial pneumonia, *JVECC* 7(2):75-78, 1997.
46. Camps-Palau M, Marks S, Cornick J: Small animal oxygen therapy, *Comp Contin Ed* 21(7):587-599, 1999.
47. Mensack S, Murtaugh R: Oxygen toxicity, *Compend Cont Ed* 21(4):341-351, 1999.
48. Weibel ER: Oxygen effect on lung cells, *Arch Int Med* 128:54-56, 1971.
49. King LG, Hendricks JC: Use of positive-pressure ventilation in dogs and cats, *JAVMA* 204(7):1045-1052, 1994.
50. Rose BD: Hyperosmolal states: Hypernatremia. In Rose BD, editor: *Clinical physiology of acid-base and electrolyte disorders*, ed 4, New York, 1994, McGraw Hill, Inc.
51. Cooligan T, Light RB, Wood L et al: Plasma volume expansion in canine Pneumococcal pneumonia, *Am Rev Respir Dis* 126:86-91, 1982.
52. Hanly P, Light R: Plasma volume expansion and PEEP in a canine model of acute Pseudomonas pneumonia, *Lung* 167(5):285-299, 1989.
53. Caldwell A, Glauser FL, Smith WR et al: The effects of dehydration and pathologic appearance of experimental canine segmental pneumonia, *Am Rev Resp Dis* 112(5):651-656, 1975.
54. Kollef JH: Inadequate antimicrobial treatment: An important determinant of outcome for hospitalized patients, *Clin Infect Dis* 31(Suppl 4):S131-138, 2000.
55. Calame W, Douwes-Idema A, Barselaar M et al: Contribution of alveolar phagocytes to antibiotic efficacy in an experimental lung infection with Streptococcus pneumoniae, *J Infect* 42(4):235-242, 2001.
56. Court MH, Dodman NH, Seeler DC et al: Inhalation therapy, *Vet Clin North Am* 15:1041-1059, 1985.
57. Bemis D, Appel M: Aerosol, parenteral, and oral antibiotic treatment of Bordetella bronchiseptica infections in dogs, *JAVMA* 170:1082-1086, 1977.
58. Boothe DM: Drug therapy of the respiratory tract, *Comp Contin Ed* Suppl 22(3a):6-17, 2000.
59. McKenzie HC, Murray MJ: Concentrations of gentamicin in serum and bronchial lavage fluid after intravenous and aerosol administration of gentamicin to horses, *AJVR* 61:1185-1190, 2000.
60. Wanner A, Rao A: Clinical indications for and effects of bland, mucolytic, and antimicrobial aerosols, *Am Rev Respir Dis* 122:79-87, 1980.
61. Palmer LB, Smaldone GC, Simon SR et al: Aerosolized antibiotics in mechanically ventilated patients: Delivery and response, *Crit Care Med* 26:31-39, 1998.
62. Viires N, Aubier M, Murciano D et al: Effects of aminophylline on diaphragmatic fatigue during acute respiratory failure, *Am Rev Respir Dis* 129:396-402, 1984.
63. Mazzarelli M, Jaspar N, Zin WA et al: Dose effect of caffeine on control of breathing and respiratory response to CO_2 in cats, *J Appl Phys* 60(1):52-59, 1986.
64. Koch T, Heller S, Heissler S et al: Effects of N-acetylcysteine on bacterial clearance, *Europ J Clin Invest* 26(10):884-892, 1996.
65. Ueno O, Lee L-N, Wagner PD: Effect of N-acetylcysteine on gas exchange after methacholine challenge and isoprenaline inhalation in the dog, *Eur Resp J* 2:238-246, 1989.
66. Hendricks JC, King LG: Airway management. In Kirk RW, editor: *Kirk's current veterinary therapy*, ed 13, Philadelphia, 2000, WB Saunders.
67. Parent C, King LG, Walker L et al: Clinical and clinicopathologic findings in dogs with ARDS, *JAVMA* 208(9):1419-1427, 1996.
68. Schaer M, Gamble D, Spencer C: Spontaneous pneumothorax associated with bacterial pneumonia in the dog, *JAAHA* 17:783-788, 1981.
69. Shure D, Moser K, Konapka R: Transbronchial needle aspiration in the diagnosis of pneumonia in a canine model, *Am Rev Resp Dis* 131(2):290-291, 1985.
70. Hoffman S: Mechanisms of antibiotic resistance, *Comp Contin Ed* 23(5):464-473, 2001.
71. Wunderink RG: Ventilator-associated pneumonia: Failure to respond to antibiotic therapy, *Clin Chest Med* 16(1):173-193, 1995.
72. Reichle J, Wisher E: Noncardiac thoracic ultrasound in 75 feline and canine patients, *Vet Rad & Ultrasound* 41:154-162, 2000.
73. Murphy ST, Ellison GW, McKiernan BC et al: Pulmonary lobectomy in the management of pneumonia in dogs: 59 cases (1972-1994), *JAVMA* 210(2):235-239, 1997.
74. Murphy ST, Mathews KG, Ellison GW et al: Pulmonary lobectomy in the management of pneumonia in five cats, *JSAP* 38:159-162, 1997.
75. Mangialardi RJ, Martin FS, Bernard GR et al: Hypoproteinemia predicts acute respiratory syndrome development, weight gain, and death in patients with sepsis, *Crit Care Med* 28(9):3137-3145, 2000.
76. Brady CA, Otto CM, Van Winkle TJ et al: Severe sepsis in cats: A retrospective study of 29 cases (1986-1998), *JAVMA* 217(4):531-535, 2000.

CHAPTER 57

Aspiration Pneumonia

Linda Barton

Morbidity and mortality secondary to the pulmonary aspiration of gastric contents has been recognized as a clinically significant problem in human medicine for more than 100 years. In 1891, the Section of Therapeutics of the British Medical Association formed a committee to investigate the effects of anesthetics on humans with regard to safety, techniques of administration, and resuscitation.[1] One of the conclusions of the committee was that retching and vomiting were commonly associated with complications and doubtless bore a causal relationship to them. Mendelson, in 1946, published a report describing the development of acute respiratory failure in 66 women caused by pulmonary aspiration of stomach contents during labor.[2]

Since that time several studies of medical and surgical patients have identified aspiration of gastric contents as a major cause of acute respiratory failure in adult patients.[3,4] In a large, prospective, multicenter study, 993 human patients with one or more conditions previously identified as risk factors for the development of acute respiratory failure were studied.[3] These patients were then followed to determine the incidence of respiratory failure in each risk group. The incidence of respiratory failure ranged from 2% to 10% in most categories, but increased to 36% in patients with pulmonary aspiration.[3] There was a 94% mortality rate among patients that developed respiratory failure following aspiration.[3]

Because of the temporary loss of protective airway reflexes, patients undergoing anesthesia are at risk for aspiration, especially during induction and recovery. Several large-scale studies of human anesthetic outcome have been conducted, collectively evaluating more than 1 million anesthetic episodes.[5-10] The incidence of aspiration ranged from 1.4 to 6.5 per 10,000 anesthetics. Although the overall incidence is low, significant morbidity and mortality resulted. Warner and colleagues documented aspiration in 67 patients (1:3216 anesthetics) during a 6-year study.[10] Of the 67 patients, 42 had no clinical signs and required no additional respiratory support. One patient died intra-operatively. The remaining 24 patients developed pulmonary complications; 18 required intensive care or respiratory support. Of these, 13 required mechanical ventilation for more than 6 hours, and 3 died. Similar data are not available for veterinary medicine.

In his original review, Mendelson suggested that there were several mechanisms by which aspirated fluid could produce pulmonary damage.[2] He further investigated this theory by instilling a variety of solutions into the lungs of rabbits (e.g., nonacidic fluid, acidic fluid, liquid vomitus of acid or neutral pH, and vomitus containing undigested food). Mendelson concluded that the acidity of the aspirate was the major determinant of the magnitude of the injury. He observed an initial period of cyanosis and labored respiration in all groups, but the signs resolved without sequelae when the material was nonacidic. Animals treated with acidic fluid had the same initial signs followed by subsequent deterioration and death.

Since Mendelson's original work, studies by a number of investigators have further defined the effects of specific characteristics of the aspirate (e.g., pH, volume, the presence or absence of particulate matter, and osmolality) on the degree of pulmonary injury.[11-17] Using acid solutions of various pH values in rabbits, Teabeaut demonstrated that aspirates with pH less than 1.5 caused severe histologic changes, and that those with pH greater than 2.4 caused little or no damage.[11] The severity of pulmonary damage caused by aspirates with pH values between those two levels varied directly with acidity. Based on a single monkey experiment, Roberts and Shirley reported that human patients with greater than 25 mls (0.4 ml/kg) residual gastric volume were at risk for aspiration and severe pulmonary damage if they were anesthetized.[12,13] From these and similar studies, gastric fluid volumes greater than 0.4 ml/kg with a pH less than 2.5 have been used to define anesthetized human patients at risk of clinically significant lung injury should gastric aspiration occur.

The presence of particulate material in the aspirate can also contribute to the severity of lung injury.[11,16,17] Aspiration of large-particulate debris can cause obstruction of major airways.[18,19] Gastric contents containing small food particles can cause severe pulmonary damage even when the pH of the aspirate is well above 2.5.[11,16,17,20] Aspiration of neutral stomach contents containing small, nonobstructing food particles can produce a prolonged inflammatory response similar to that caused by acid.[11,18] Food particles serve as an excellent nidus for secondary bacterial infection.

These generally accepted criteria for aspiration risk have come under scrutiny.[21-23] Critics suggest less stringent gastric volume criteria, and that the "at risk" value for gastric pH should be increased to less than 3.5. Although exact cut-off values are in question, it is generally accepted that significant morbidity can result from aspiration of:
- Small volumes with very low pH, producing a chemical pneumonitis

- Very large volumes of neutral fluid, producing a "near-drowning" syndrome
- Particulate matter, causing obstruction of small airways as well as an inflammatory response[24]

Diagnosis

The diagnosis of aspiration pneumonia is obvious when aspiration has been witnessed; gastric contents are detected in the airway; or when acute respiratory distress develops within a few hours of known vomiting, regurgitation, or anesthesia. The more common, unwitnessed aspiration case is more difficult to diagnose and requires a high index of suspicion. Acute lung injury secondary to aspiration of gastric contents should be suspected in any patient that develops signs of bronchopneumonia or the acute respiratory distress syndrome (ARDS) during hospitalization, especially if the patient has risk factors that would predispose to aspiration.

Box 57-1 lists conditions predisposing patients to aspiration of gastric contents. Many of these risk factors are found in critically ill, hospitalized patients. Ambulatory patients with underlying laryngeal and esophageal disorders, as well as those that are recumbent or have depressed mentation, are at increased risk. Nasogastric

---

BOX 57-1
Conditions Predisposing to Aspiration of Stomach Contents

Impairment of protective airway reflexes
- Coma
- Head trauma
- Metabolic derangements
- Central depressant medications (sedation, general anesthesia)
- Muscle relaxants
- Seizures
- Airway trauma
- Laryngeal/ pharyngeal dysfunction

Large volumes of intragastric food/fluid
- Delayed gastric emptying
  - Ileus
  - Bowel obstruction
  - Pain
  - Anxiety
  - Opioid medication
  - Peristaltic abnormalities
  - Pregnancy
  - Obesity
- Overfeeding by enteral tube
- Recent meal (before emergency anesthesia/surgery)

Impaired function of gastroesophageal sphincter
- Presence of a nasogastric feeding tube
- Achalasia
- Esophageal obstruction
- Abnormalities of esophageal function
  - Megaesophagus
  - Reflux esophagitis
  - Myasthenia gravis

---

tubes, enteral feeding, and hypomotile gut function also place patients at increased risk of aspiration. The presence of a cuffed endotracheal tube does not exclude the possibility of aspiration.[19,25] Involvement of the dependent lung lobes (i.e., right middle, and left and right cranial) supports the diagnosis of aspiration, but is not pathognomonic.[26] In three large published studies of human patients with severe community-acquired pneumonia requiring hospital admission, the number of those patients diagnosed with aspiration pneumonia ranged from 15% to 23%.[27-29]

Pathophysiology

An understanding of the physiological alterations occurring following aspiration is vital to effective patient management. The clinical presentation, a reflection of the pulmonary pathology, varies depending of the severity of the injury and the time between aspiration and presentation. The injury to the lungs varies with the volume and character of the material aspirated. Aspiration of large particles may rarely cause obstruction of the trachea and acute ventilatory failure. Aspiration during vomiting or regurgitation in a patient with intact upper airway reflexes causes laryngospasm and coughing. Vagal-induced reflexes may lead to bradycardia and, potentially, cardiac arrest. In patients with decreased or absent airway reflexes, vomited or regurgitated material spreads quickly throughout the bronchial tree, causing acute lung injury.

Kennedy and colleagues first demonstrated a biphasic pattern of injury in experimental models of acute acid aspiration.[30] The initial phase is caused by direct chemical burn and by the release of potent neuropeptides from afferent nerves located in the airways. The second phase, an acute inflammatory response, is mediated by recruitment and activation of neutrophils in the lung, and is analogous to the process seen in experimental models of ARDS. Secondary bacterial infection can enhance and prolong the lung injury following aspiration. Table 57-1 characterizes the pathophysiologic derangements and clinical signs associated with each phase of injury.

PHASE 1 (AIRWAY RESPONSE)

The first phase of lung injury occurs immediately following aspiration; it consists of a direct chemical burn and stimulation of sensory nerves located in the airway. The injury is characterized histologically by bronchial epithelial degeneration, pulmonary edema, hemorrhage, areas of atelectasis, and necrosis of type 1 alveolar cells.[18] Damage to the airway epithelium results in bronchoconstriction and increased mucus production. Intact epithelium protects the subepithelial tissues from mediators released by inflammatory cells and mast cells. Munakata and colleagues reported that injury to the epithelium resulted in a thirtyfivefold increase in sensitivity of the airway to histamine.[31] In their rat model of acute acid aspiration-induced injury, Kennedy and col-

TABLE 57-1. Phases of Acid Aspiration Lung Injury

	Pathologic Changes	Clinical Signs
Phase 1: Airway Response	Bronchoconstriction, bronchorrhea, airway edema, $\pm$ alveolar edema, impaired mucociliary action, $\pm$ vascular permeability	Dyspnea, tachypnea, $\pm$ cyanosis, $\uparrow$ sputum production, radiographic evidence of local infiltrate, $\uparrow$Paco$_2$, $\downarrow$Pao$_2$
Phase 2: Lung Inflammation	Neutrophil sequestration, $\uparrow\uparrow\uparrow$ pulmonary vascular permeability, high protein pulmonary edema, pulmonary hypertension, hypovolemia	Continued/increased dyspnea, rhonchi, rales, fever, radiographic evidence of consolidation, $\downarrow$ Pao$_2$, $\downarrow/\uparrow$ Paco$_2$, $\pm$ Blood pressure
Phase 3: Bacterial Infection	Bacterial pneumonia, lung abscess, empyema	Fever, $\uparrow$WBC with left shift and toxic neutrophils, new radiograph densities, $\downarrow$ Pao$_2$, $\downarrow/\uparrow$ Paco$_2$

leagues quantified lung injury by measurement of vascular permeability and histologic changes.[30] Increased capillary permeability was demonstrated 1 hour following acid injury. This alteration in permeability is caused by stimulation of sensory nerves located within the tracheobronchial smooth muscle layer. Stimulation of these nerves causes release of multiple potent neuropeptides of the tachykinin family.[32] This group of peptides, which includes substance P, calcitonin gene-related peptide, neuropeptide K, and many others, causes bronchoconstriction and bronchorrhea. In addition they cause dilation of bronchial vessels and increased capillary permeability, resulting in mucosal and submucosal edema and protein extravasation. Martling and Lundberg demonstrated the effect of these neuropeptides on the acute response to acid injury in a rat model.[32] Pretreatment with high dose capsaicin causes an almost total and long-lasting depletion of this group of neuropeptides. Capsaicin pretreatment decreased protein extravasation by 62% in the trachea and 70% in the bronchi of rats following instillation of acidic gastric juice.

Obstruction of small airways secondary to bronchoconstriction, increased mucus production, and exudation of high protein fluid and small food particles results in collapse of alveoli. Hypoxia develops from hypoventilation and shunting in the areas of alveolar collapse. Lung compliance is reduced as airway edema develops. Aspirated material that reaches the alveoli causes dilution and denaturation of surfactant. The resultant alveolar collapse causes additional atelectasis and V/Q mismatch.[19] Following acid injury, patients are more susceptible to secondary bacterial infections because of decreased production of surface immunoglobulins and loss of the normal mucociliary clearance of particulates, mucin, and bacteria.[19]

PHASE 2 (INFLAMMATORY RESPONSE)

In experimental models, the second phase of lung injury begins 4 to 6 hours following aspiration. It is characterized by an additional significant increase in capillary permeability. This increase temporally parallels a marked infiltration of neutrophils into the alveolar space.[30] The increased permeability leads to extravasation of large amounts of proteinaceous pulmonary edema. Sufficient fluid may be lost from the circulation into the alveoli to deplete intravascular volume and cause hypotension.[18]

Clinically, this inflammatory phase lasts for 1 to 2 days, but inflammation continues much longer if particulate material is aspirated. Inflammatory changes are seen in areas of the lung distant to the tissue in direct contact with the aspirated material. Hypoxia worsens because of progressive atelectasis and increasing shunt fraction, and may progress to pulmonary failure. Within 24 to 36 hours, patients often become febrile. Radiographs may show areas of consolidation.[19]

Increased pulmonary vascular resistance can lead to pulmonary hypertension. The increase in pulmonary vascular tone is caused primarily by hypoxic vasoconstriction. In addition, decreased lung volume, decreased compliance, and decreased functional residual capacity can result in impingement of the pulmonary microvasculature because of mechanical forces. Hemodynamic consequences may follow the acute elevation in pulmonary vascular resistance. The low-pressure right ventricle often cannot adapt to sudden increases in pressure, leading to right ventricular dilation; a decrease in right ventricular ejection fraction; and, potentially, right ventricular failure.[18]

A number of investigators have examined the role of neutrophils in the inflammatory phase of acid-induced lung injury.[33,34] Knight and colleagues demonstrated that rats made neutropenic by a specific antineutrophil antibody had significantly decreased lung injury following acid aspiration when compared with similarly treated rats with normal neutrophil counts, using measurements of vascular permeability and histologic evidence of decreased inflammation.[33] The 6-hour permeability index (PI), a measure of increased capillary permeability, was reduced in the neutropenic rats to the level observed following the acute phase of injury (1-hour postinjury). Lung endothelial permeability can be normalized despite the fact that neutrophil sequestration still occurs.[34] It is not the presence of neutrophils, but rather the products of neutrophil activation that produce lung injury. Activated neutrophils may produce tissue damage by generation of oxygen free radicals or by the release of proteolytic enzymes.

Knight and colleagues studied the effects of both antioxidants and proteolytic enzymes on lung injury following acid aspiration.[33] Lack of protection from lung injury 6 hours following pretreatment with either deferoxamine or catalase argues against a primary role for oxidant injury. In contrast, the elevated levels of serine protease activity in fluid collected via bronchoalveolar lavage 6 hours after injury suggest that the inflammatory phase of pulmonary acid injury may be mediated primarily through the release of neutrophil-derived proteolytic enzymes. Elastase is an enzyme released from the azurophilic granules of activated neutrophils. It has been found to cause endothelial cell injury and to destroy lung surfactant proteins by inducing proteolysis. Kaneko and colleagues demonstrated that blockade of neutrophil elastase function was sufficient to normalize the endothelial permeability and the oxygen defects in rabbits following acid aspiration.[34]

More recent studies have investigated recruitment and activation of neutrophils to better understand the pathogenesis of acid induced lung injury and to identify possible therapeutic strategies to modify the inflammatory response. Aspiration induces the release of proinflammatory cytokines such as tumor necrosis factor-α and interleukin-8 (IL-8).[35,36] IL-8 appears to be the major stimulus for neutrophil recruitment into the lung.[36] Modelska and colleagues demonstrated that acid-induced lung injury in rabbits could be significantly reduced by pretreating with antiinterleukin-8 antibody.[37] To become activated, neutrophils must first adhere to the endothelium before migrating into the lung parenchyma. The process of adhesion and subsequent activation is mediated by glycoprotein receptors on the neutrophil, binding to their counter-receptors on the endothelial cell.[38] Members of this family of receptors that play an important role in neutrophil adhesion include E-, L-, and P-selectins; β₂-integrins; and intracellular adhesion molecules (ICAM-1). The expression of L-selectins and β₂-integrins on neutrophils and ICAM-1 on lung endothelium is increased by proinflammatory cytokines. Goldman and colleagues demonstrated that inhibition of neutrophil adhesion receptor CD18 and ICAM-1 limited the inflammatory response in an animal model of acid aspiration lung injury.[39] In contrast, inhibition of β₂-integrins did not prevent the acid induced influx of neutrophils into the lung.[40] Nagase and colleagues used a monoclonal antibody to ICAM-1 in rats both before and 30 minutes following acid-induced lung injury.[41] Intratracheal administration of anti-ICAM-1 significantly inhibited neutrophil accumulation in the lung. There was improvement in gas exchange and mechanical properties of the lung as well as a reduction in the magnitude of the pulmonary edema. Histologically, there was less lung injury.

PHASE 3 (SECONDARY BACTERIAL INFECTION)

By 72 hours following uncomplicated acid aspiration, inflammation begins to resolve. Histological examination shows regeneration of bronchial epithelium, proliferation of fibroblasts, and decreased acute inflammation. Bacterial superinfection may complicate the course of illness. Aspiration of contaminated material greatly increases the risk of infection. Bacterial pneumonia is seen most commonly; however, lung abscesses and empyema may occur. Development of fever in a previously nor-

mothermic animal, increasing neutrophil count in conjunction with a left shift and increasing neutrophil toxicity, and increased pulmonary densities on radiographs 36 hours or longer after aspiration are suggestive of secondary infection.[26]

Prevention

The simplest and most efficient approach to aspiration of stomach contents is prevention. Adherence to simple practices can prevent aspiration in many cases. When animals are anesthetized, the airway should be protected with a cuffed endotracheal tube. Patients should be awake and have normal laryngeal reflexes before the endotracheal tube is removed.

Because of the effects of gastric pH, volume, and the presence of particulate material on the extent of lung injury following aspiration, many techniques have been employed to manipulate these variables to minimize the risk of aspiration in anesthetized patients. Fasting for a minimum of 6 hours has been a longstanding practice for patients undergoing elective anesthetic procedures. The *nil per os* regimen has recently been reevaluated. Fasting has been shown to clear food particles from the stomach, but the effect on gastric pH and volume is not reliable in humans.[24] Hester and Heath showed no correlation between starvation time and gastric pH or volume,[42] and a number of other investigators have demonstrated that many fasted patients have gastric volume and pH values in the at-risk range.[43-45] Maltby and colleagues performed a series of studies in people to evaluate the gastric volume and acidity after the intake of clear fluids.[43-47] They demonstrated that the consumption of water up to 2 to 3 hours before anesthesia did not significantly increase gastric acidity or volume in healthy human volunteers. Gastric volume was significantly decreased in human patients allowed only clear liquids in several studies.[43,44] There appears to be no comparable data for dogs and cats. Solid food intake should be restricted for at least 6 hours before anesthesia; however, there is a large body of evidence in human patients to recommend liberalization of the intake of clear fluids up to 3 hours before anesthesia.[24]

In addition to fasting guidelines, much attention has been given to pharmacological manipulation of gastric pH and volume to reduce the risk of aspiration. Beginning in the 1970s, oral antacids were prophylactically administered to women in labor and other patients predisposed to aspiration.[1] These drugs effectively increased the pH of the gastric contents but caused an increase in gastric volume, especially after repeated dosing. Other disadvantages of antacids include a variable duration of effect, the potential for vomiting, and incomplete mixing with gastric contents.[24] Nonparticulate antacids such as sodium citrate are preferred to magnesium-containing products because of the concern for potential pulmonary damage if particulate matter is aspirated. Clinical and experimental studies in dogs demonstrated that pulmonary damage following aspiration of a particulate antacid resulted in clinical signs and histopathological changes similar to those seen with acid aspiration.[48,49]

To avoid the disadvantages associated with the use of oral antacids, H_2-antagonists and omeprazole have been used to reduce gastric volume and acidity via inhibition of gastric acid secretion. A variety of doses, dosage schedules, and routes of administration have been examined.[50-54] The regimen that produced the most reliable risk reduction in humans was administration of cimetidine at bedtime, followed by cimetidine and metoclopramide on the morning of surgery.[53] Prokinetics such as metoclopramide and cisapride are added to enhance gastric emptying, but they have no effect on gastric secretion. Metoclopramide has also been shown to increase lower esophageal sphincter tone.[55]

Because of the low incidence of clinically significant aspiration, the routine use of antacids, H_2-antagonists, omeprazole, or metoclopramide is not considered necessary or cost effective in humans. Treatment is recommended in patients considered at high risk for aspiration.[24] Intravenous cimetidine and metoclopramide have been recommended for nonfasted veterinary patients requiring emergency anesthesia.[56]

Aspiration in hospitalized patients can be minimized by attempting to maintain host defenses. Patients unable to protect their airways as a result of sedation or a decreased level of consciousness should be intubated.

Enteral feeding predisposes patients to aspiration. In addition, enterally fed patients are at increased risk of secondary bacterial infection if aspiration does occur. Normally, the fasted stomach maintains sterility as a result of its acid pH. The pH of enteral feeding products ranges from 6.4 to 7.0.[57] Alkalinization of the stomach in patients receiving enteral nutrition causes colonization of the stomach with gram-negative bacteria. Providing nutrition via the gastrointestinal tract is very important in the management of critically ill patients and should not be abandoned because of the increased risk of aspiration. Instead, feeding should be delivered in a manner that minimizes the risk. Patients should be fed in an upright position. It has been demonstrated that the incidence of aspiration and the quantity of the material aspirated were greater in human patients treated in the supine position.[58] Drakulovic and colleagues reported that the incidence of microbiologically confirmed pneumonia in a group of mechanically ventilated ICU patients was reduced from 36% in patients fed in a supine position to 9% in patients fed in a semirecumbent position.[59] Aggressive enteral feeding can cause gastric distension and increased gastric pressure.[60] Gastric residuals should be checked by periodic aspiration of the feeding tube. If large volumes are aspirated, the volume fed should be reduced. Patients are often more tolerant of smaller volume and more frequent feedings. Prokinetic agents (e.g., metoclopramide and cisapride) may be used to facilitate gastric emptying. The presence of a nasogastric feeding tube decreases the function of the lower esophageal sphincter, with the potential for increased gastroesophageal reflux.[59] Feeding tubes that do not traverse the lower esophageal sphincter (e.g., nasoesophageal, gastrotomy, or jejunostomy tubes) will decrease, but not eliminate, the risk of aspiration.

Gastric ulcer prophylaxis with agents that act by reducing gastric acidity may also encourage gastric colonization and predispose to pneumonia with gram-negative organisms.[61] Because of a perceived increase in the risk of nosocomial pneumonia associated with the administration of antacids, the use of sucralfate for stress ulcer prophylaxis has been promoted. Studies in humans to evaluate the potential advantage of sucralfate to antacids and H_2-antagonists have produced disparate results.[62-64] A multi-center, 1200-patient, double-blinded, placebo-controlled, randomized study was conducted by the Canadian Critical Care Trials Group, comparing the incidence of nosocomial pneumonia in patients treated with ranitidine to patients receiving sucralfate.[65] Although there was a trend toward a lower rate of pneumonia in the patients receiving sucralfate (19.1% versus 16.2%), there was no significant difference between the two groups.

When small animal patients present with community-acquired aspiration pneumonia, a complete history and careful physical examination should be done to identify potential underlying causes of aspiration. Prevention of recurrences can be minimized only by identification and correction of risk factors. Investigation of suspected esophageal dysfunction may include chest radiographs, a barium swallow, and/or endoscopy. An oral examination should be done to evaluate swallowing and pharyngeal and laryngeal function. A complete neurologic examination should be performed, including tests of neuromuscular function, if indicated. An acetylcholine receptor antibody test should be performed if the patient is suspected of having myasthenia gravis.[26]

Treatment

The short time lag between the airway response to aspiration and the generalized inflammatory response of the lung provides a potential window for therapeutic intervention to modify the inflammatory response. Several investigators have demonstrated that treatments to block neutrophil recruitment and activation following acid aspiration resulted in a reduction in lung injury in animal models.[36,41] Further investigation is needed to determine the clinical usefulness of such strategies. Currently, treatment is limited to supportive measures. A strategy for treatment immediately following a witnessed or suspected aspiration is outlined in Figure 57-1. The initial management of a witnessed or suspected aspiration should follow the ABCs of emergency care.

AIRWAY

Airway patency should be ensured, by endotracheal intubation if necessary. Rarely, large particulate material can obstruct the large airways. Marked inspiratory effort or stridor should raise suspicion of upper airway obstruction. Radiographs are of limited usefulness because patients are often too unstable for the procedure and soft tissue density foreign material is rarely visible.[26] Because of the uncommon occurrence of tracheal obstruction, dyspneic patients should not be sedated for endoscopic examination without strong evidence of tracheal ob-

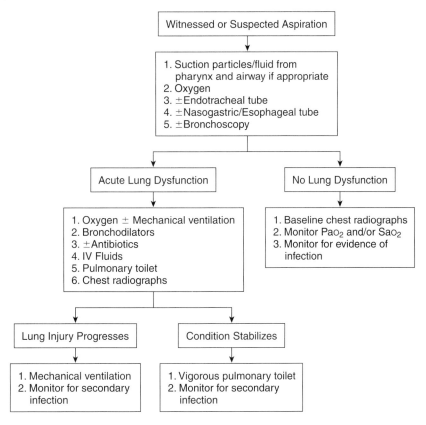

Figure 57-1. *Treatment of witnessed aspiration.*

struction. If necessary, however, examination of the oral cavity, larynx, and proximal trachea can be performed under anesthesia in severely compromised animals. Obstructing material should be removed with alligator forceps, and the mouth and pharynx suctioned. Solid material can be suctioned from the airway of intubated patients immediately following aspiration, but liquid quickly disperses from the large airways into the alveoli. Suctioning stimulates coughing, may remove some of the aspirated material, and can be helpful in confirming the diagnosis.[18] Patients unable to protect their airway should remain intubated. If the patient is at risk for further aspiration because of a fluid-distended esophagus or stomach, a nasoesophageal or nasogastric tube should be placed to remove the accumulated contents.

If aspiration of large particulate material is suspected, and radiographs show evidence of distal airway obstruction, some authors recommend emergency bronchoscopy within the first hour to remove particulate matter and to lavage affected areas.[18,19] If needed, small amounts of saline can be used to clear the airway of secretions or aspirated material. Because acid is quickly neutralized in the lung, bronchoscopy is not recommended unless aspiration of large particles is strongly suspected. Bronchoscopy in a patient in respiratory distress should always be considered a high-risk procedure. Nonbronchoscopic bronchial lavage with large volumes of fluid, and the use of neutral or alkaline solutions for lavage, can be hazardous and are not recommended.[18]

BREATHING

Hypoventilation and intrapulmonary shunt caused by aspiration often result in severe hypoxemia. Humidified oxygen should be delivered by mask, nasal cannula, or oxygen cage as needed to maintain a normal Pao_2. Excessive oxygen administration should be avoided because it has been shown experimentally that hyperoxia increases pulmonary damage after acid aspiration.[66] In this study, rats were exposed to 98% oxygen or room air for 5 hours following acid aspiration. Exposing the acid-injured lung to high levels of oxygen exacerbated the lung injury.

To combat aspiration-induced bronchoconstriction, bronchodilators such as theophylline derivatives (aminophylline) or beta-agonists (terbutaline) are recommended for the first 24 to 48 hours.[18,19,26] Pulmonary edema is a result of increased vascular permeability and not of increased hydrostatic pressure; therefore, diuretic therapy is not indicated. Pulmonary toilet, clearance of secretions from the airways, should be encouraged. Nebulization and coupage are used to humidify secretions and to encourage coughing. Adequate analgesia encourages patients to ambulate and to take deeper breaths, thereby preventing secondary atelectasis.[67]

If Pao_2 or $Paco_2$ cannot be maintained at normal levels, or the work of breathing is felt to be excessive, mechanical ventilation is indicated. Because of the increased shunt fraction, decreased pulmonary compliance, and decreased functional residual capacity, patients with inflammatory lung disease may have high airway pressures and require high levels of positive end expiratory pressure (PEEP) during mechanical ventilation.

CARDIOVASCULAR SUPPORT

Hypoperfusion caused by intravascular volume loss as a result of accumulation of edema fluid in the alveoli may be seen in severely affected patients. Judicious intravenous fluids are required to expand the intravascular volume. Aspiration-induced lung injury produces a high-protein pulmonary edema, caused by increased permeability of the capillary endothelium and not by increased hydrostatic pressure as in cardiogenic edema. The goal of fluid therapy is to deliver the minimum volume required to maintain cardiac output and systemic perfusion. Elevations in capillary hydrostatic pressure above that level will cause increased leakage of fluid into the alveoli through the damaged capillary endothelium. Placement of a pulmonary artery catheter can guide fluid therapy by providing direct measurements of pulmonary capillary wedge pressure and cardiac output. If pulmonary artery catheterization is not available, serial measurement of central venous pressure (CVP) can be used to provide a crude estimate of these values. Both crystalloid and colloid fluids have been recommended for patients with inflammatory lung disease.[26,68] In a dog lung model, there was increased alveolar permeability for albumin and for 150,000-170,000 dalton molecular weight dextran following acid aspiration–induced lung injury.[69] Experimental use of larger molecular weight products such as pentastarch, hetastarch and Oxyglobin® has not been reported.

CORTICOSTEROIDS

Theoretically, the use of corticosteroids should have beneficial effects on noninfectious inflammation. Several published case reports suggested a favorable response to steroid therapy in patients following aspiration of stomach contents containing particulate material.[20] However, one study of particulate aspiration in rabbits showed that corticosteroids interfered with normal healing of the lung following aspiration.[17] Gastric contents containing small food particles were instilled in rabbits, with one group treated with high dose methylprednisolone 1 hour following aspiration and another group of rabbits not receiving steroid therapy. Sections of lung tissue were evaluated histologically 1, 3, 7, and 21 days after instillation. Without steroids, there was a marked inflammatory response. By day 7, well-organized granulomas were seen, often associated with food particles. By day 21, the inflammatory response was resolving. In contrast, there was a reduction in the inflammatory response in the lungs of steroid treated rabbits during the first week following aspiration. On day 21 there was a continuation of the inflammatory response. Many of the remaining granulomas contained large amounts of necrotic debris. The corticosteroids appeared to interfere with the normal housekeeping function of the lung to ingest, eliminate, or isolate foreign material. In a controlled, clinical study of the effect of steroid administration on human patients

following aspiration of gastric contents, there was no significant difference in mortality between the group receiving steroids and group not receiving steroids.[70] However, 7 of 20 patients who received steroids were subsequently diagnosed with gram-negative pneumonia, compared with 0 of the 13 patients not receiving steroid therapy. Because of the lack of proven effectiveness and the potential for harm, corticosteroids are not recommended for the treatment of aspiration pneumonia.

ANTIBIOTICS

Administration of antibiotics immediately following a witnessed aspiration event is controversial. Aspiration of normal stomach contents does not cause infection; however, lungs damaged by aspiration are susceptible to secondary infection. Many human texts recommend that antibiotics be withheld until clinical evidence of infection is seen.[18,19] They argue that prophylactic antibiotics may lead to the development of secondary infections with resistant organisms. It can, however, be difficult to document infection in a patient following aspiration. Fever, leukocytosis, the presence of pulmonary infiltrates, and the production of thick tenacious sputum are nonspecific responses to uncomplicated, sterile chemical pneumonitis.

The risk of bacterial infection is increased if contaminated material is aspirated. Patients that are hospitalized before aspiration are at greater risk for infection. During hospitalization, the oropharynx becomes colonized by gram-negative organisms. Elevated gastric pH secondary to gastric ulcer prophylaxis with antacids and H_2-antagonists or enteral feeding allows bacterial colonization of the stomach and increases the risk for infection following aspiration. Aspiration of esophageal contents (without gastric acid to inhibit the growth of bacteria) places dogs with megaesophagus at increased risk for infection. In a review of 32 dogs diagnosed with aspiration pneumonia and megaesophagus at North Carolina State University, aerobic bacterial cultures of transtracheal wash fluid were positive in 91% (20/22) of the dogs in which the procedure was performed.[26] Food particles act as a nidus for infection, and routine antibiotic therapy is recommended for patients following aspiration of particulate material.[25] Periodontal disease is considered a risk factor for immediate infection in people.[26] In light of the common presence of periodontal disease in small animals, the high incidence of aspiration of contaminated material, and the difficulty documenting infection in patients with pneumonitis, the use of antibiotics may be justified in veterinary patients.

A tracheal wash should be performed to obtain material for cytologic and microbiologic evaluation before initiation of antibiotics. Previous antibiotic therapy is not a contraindication for a tracheal wash. In a study of 395 human patients with community-acquired pneumonia requiring hospital admission, the diagnostic yield was not significantly different in 62 patients who had received antibiotics before admission from those who had not.[71] Positive cultures were found with equal frequency in the two groups. Parenteral broad-spectrum antibiotics should be given empirically pending the results of culture and sensitivity.

Empiric antibiotic selection differs among patient populations. Human patients with community-acquired infections are more likely to have anaerobic infections.[72] Anaerobes were isolated in 88% of human patients with community-acquired infection, compared with 35% of patients with hospital-acquired pneumonia.[72] The role of anaerobes in small animals is not known.[26] In humans with aspiration pneumonia, *Streptococcus pneumoniae*, other *Streptococcus* spp., *Staphylococcus* spp., and gram-negative bacilli are the most common aerobes recovered.[29,72] The incidence of infection with gram-negative organisms is higher in hospital-acquired infections, reflecting colonization of the oropharynx during hospitalization. Gram-negative bacilli were the predominant isolates in 74% of human cases with hospital-acquired infection in one study of aspiration pneumonia.[72]

E. coli, Klebsiella, Pasteurella, and *Streptococcus* spp. are the most common organisms reported in dogs with lower respiratory tract infection.[56,73] The reports do not indicate the cause of the pneumonia or separate community-acquired from hospital-acquired infections. First generation cephalosporins have been recommended for both human and veterinary patients with community-acquired aspiration pneumonia, but many contemporary gram-negative isolates are resistant to these drugs.[56,73,74] or Trimethoprim/sulfonamide, amoxicillin/clavulanate combinations, or chloramphenicol are also recommended.[26,73] In animals with severe hospital-acquired infections, where the chance for resistant gram-negative organisms is increased, an additional agent such as enrofloxacin should be added. Enrofloxacin has excellent penetration through the blood-bronchus barrier, but has minimal activity against anaerobes and should not be used as a single agent.[56] Aminoglycosides have characteristics that may make them less desirable agents for treating pneumonia because they achieve only 30% to 40% of their serum level in endobronchial secretions, and they are not optimally effective at the lower pH levels found in bronchial secretions associated with pneumonia.[60] Most beta lactam drugs only reach 15% to 20% of their serum level in endobronchial secretions.

Antibiotics should be given for a minimum of 3 to 4 weeks. Patients should be treated for 1 week beyond complete resolution of clinical signs and radiographic changes.[26] Changes on radiographs will usually lag behind clinical improvement and therefore are generally not useful in guiding initial therapy.[75] Radiographs should be reevaluated 5 to 7 days after completion of antibiotic therapy.

If aspiration is suspected, but there are no adverse clinical signs, the patient should be carefully observed for the next several hours. Respiratory rate and effort, development of a cough or wheeze, and oxygenation (measured by pulse oximetry or arterial blood gases) should be monitored for the next several hours. Warner reported a study of 67 human patients with witnessed aspiration during anesthetic procedures.[10] Of these, 42 patients with witnessed aspiration developed no clinical signs within 2 hours. None of these patients subsequently required respiratory support or developed pulmonary complications. Twenty-four people developed clinical signs of aspiration; 18 of these patients required

respiratory support and admission to the ICU. Of those, 13 patients required ventilation and 3 patients died.

Persistent localized pulmonary densities, unresolved atelectasis, or recurrent pneumonia in spite of elimination of predisposing causes suggests the possibility of persistent foreign material. Bronchoscopy and/or thoracotomy may be required.[26]

REFERENCES

1. McIntyre JWR: Evolution of Twentieth Century attitudes to prophylaxis of pulmonary aspiration during anesthesia, *Can J Anaesth* 45(10):1024, 1998.
2. Mendelson CL: The aspiration of stomach contents into the lungs during obstetric anesthesia, *Am J Obstet Gynecol* 52:191, 1946.
3. Fowler AA, Hamman RF, Good JT: Adult respiratory distress syndrome: Risk with common predispositions, *Ann Intern Med* 98:593, 1983.
4. Doyle RL, Szaflarski N, Modin GW et al: Identification of patients with acute lung injury, *Am J Respir Crit Care Med* 152:1818, 1995.
5. Olsson GL, Hallen B, Hambraeus JK: Aspiration during anaesthesia: A computer-aided study of 185,358 anaesthetics, *Acta Anaesthesiol Scand* 30:84, 1986.
6. Cohen MM, Duncan PG, Pope WDN et al: A survey of 112,000 anaesthetics at one teaching hospital, *Can Anaesth Soc J* 33:22, 1986.
7. Tiret L, Desmonts JM, Hatton F et al: Complications associated with anaesthesia: A prospective survey in France, *Can Anaesth Soc J* 33:336, 1986.
8. Leigh JM, Tytler JA: Admissions to the intensive care unit after complications of anaesthetic techniques over 10 years, *Anaesthesia* 45:814, 1990.
9. Kaller SK: Aspiration pneumonitis: Fact or fiction? *Probl Anesth* 2:29, 1988.
10. Warner MA, Warner ME, Weber JG: Clinical significance of pulmonary aspiration during the perioperative period, *Anesthesiology* 78(1):56, 1993.
11. Teabeaut JR: Aspiration of gastric contents: An experimental study, *Am J Pathol* 28:51, 1952.
12. Roberts RB, Shirley MA: Antacid therapy in obstetrics, *Anesthesiology* 53:83, 1980.
13. Roberts RB, Shirley MA: Reducing the risk of acid aspiration during cesarean section, *Anesth Analg* 53:859, 1974.
14. Greenfield LJ, Singleton RP et al: Pulmonary effects of experimental graded aspiration of hydrochloric acid, *Ann Surg* 170(1):74, 1969.
15. James CF, Modell JH, Gibbs CP et al: Pulmonary aspiration—effects of pH and volume in the rat, *Anesth Analg* 63:665, 1984.
16. Schwartz DJ, Wynne JW et al: The pulmonary consequences of aspiration of gastric contents at pH values greater than 2.5, *Am Rev Respir Dis* 121:119, 1980.
17. Wynne JW, Reynolds JC et al: Steroid therapy for pneumonitis induced in rabbits by aspiration of foodstuff, *Anesthesiology* 51:11, 1979.
18. Boysen PG: Pulmonary aspiration of stomach contents. In Shoemaker WC, Ayres SM, Grenvik A et al, editors: *Textbook of critical care,* ed 3, Philadelphia,1995, WB Saunders.
19. Britto J, Demling RH: Aspiration lung injury, *New Horizons* 1(3):435, 1993.
20. Coriat P, Labrosse J et al: Diffuse interstitial pneumonitis due to aspiration of gastric contents, *Anaesthesia* 39:703, 1984.
21. Rocke DA, Brock-Utne JG, Rout CC: At risk for aspiration: New critical values of volume and pH? *Anesth Analg* 76:665, 1993.
22. Schreiner MS: Gastric fluid volume: Is it really a risk factor for pulmonary aspiration? *Anesth Analg* 87:754, 1998.
23. Gorback MS: Cut-off values and aspiration risk, *Anesth Analg* 69:407, 1989.
24. Kallar SK, Everett LL: Potential risks and preventive measures for pulmonary aspiration: New concepts in preoperative fasting guidelines, *Anesth Analg* 77:171, 1993.
25. Kluger MT, Short TG: Aspiration during anaesthesia: A review of 133 cases from the Australian Anaesthetic Incident Monitoring Study (AIMS), *Anaesthesia* 54:19, 1999.

26. Hawkins EC: Aspiration pneumonia. In Bonagura JD, editor: *Kirk's current veterinary therapy*, vol 12, Philadelphia, 1995, WB Saunders Co.

27. Torres A, Serra-Batlles JS, Ferrer A et al: Severe community-acquired pneumonia: Epidemiology and prognostic factors, *Am Rev Respir Dis* 144:312, 1991.

28. Leroy O, Santre´ C, Benscart C et al: A five-year study of severe community-acquired pneumonia with emphasis on prognosis in patients admitted to an intensive care unit, *Int Care Med* 21:24, 1995.

29. Leroy O, Vandenbussche C, Coffinier C et al. Community-acquired aspiration pneumonia in intensive care units: Epidemiological and prognosis data, *Am J Respir Crit Care Med* 156:1922, 1997.

30. Kennedy TP, Johnson KJ, Kunkel RG et al: Acute acid aspiration lung injury in the rat: Biphasic pathogenesis, *Anesth Analg* 69:87, 1989.

31. Munakata M, Huang I, Mitzner W et al: Protective role of epithelium in guinea pig airway, *J Appl Physiol* 66;1547, 1989.

32. Martling CR, Lundberg JM: Capsaicin sensitive afferents contribute to acute airway edema following tracheal instillation of hydrochloric acid or gastric juice in the rat, *Anesthesiology* 68:350, 1988.

33. Knight PR, Druskovich G, Tait AR et al: The role of neutrophils, oxidants, and proteases in the pathogenesis of acid pulmonary injury, *Anesthesiology* 77:772, 1992.

34. Kaneko K, Kudoh I, Hattori S et al: Neutrophil elastase inhibitor, ONO-5046, modulates acid-induced lung and systemic injury in rabbits, *Anesthesiology* 87:635, 1997.

35. Goldman GR, Welbourn L, Kobizk CR et al. Tumor necrosis factor-α mediates acid aspiration-induced systemic organ injury, *Ann Surg* 212(4):513, 1990.

36. Folkesson HG, Matthay MA, Hebert CA et al: Acid aspiration induced lung injury in rabbits is mediated by interleukin-8 dependent mechanisms, *J Clin Invest* 96:107, 1995.

37. Modelska K, Pippet JF, Folkesson HG et al. Acid-induced lung injury: Protective effect of anti-interleukin-8 pretreatment on alveolar epithelial barrier function in rabbits, *Am J Respir Crit Care Med* 160:1450, 1999.

38. Hogg JC, Doerschuk CM: Leukocyte traffic in the lung, *Ann Rev Physiol* 57:97, 1995.

39. Goldman GR, Welbourn L, Kobzik L et al: Neutrophil adhesion receptor CD18 mediates remote but not localized acid aspiration injury, *Surgery* 117:83, 1995.

40. Doerschuk CM, Winn RK, Coxson HO et al: CD18-dependent and independent mechanisms of neutrophil migration in the pulmonary and systemic microcirculation of rabbits, *J Immunol* 144:2327, 1990.

41. Nagase T, Ohga E, Sudo E et al: Intercellular adhesion molecule-1 mediated acid aspiration-induced lung injury, *Am J Respir Crit Care Med* 160:1450, 1999.

42. Hester JB, Heath ML: Pulmonary acid aspiration syndrome: Should prophylaxis be routine? *Br J Anaesth* 49:595, 1977.

43. Maltby JR, Sutherland AD, Sale JP et al: Preoperative oral fluids: Is a five-hour fast justified prior to elective surgery? *Anesth Analg* 65:1112, 1986.

44. Sutherland AD, Maltby JR, Sale JP et al: The effect of preoperative oral fluid and ranitidine on gastric fluid volume and pH, *Can J Anaesth* 34:117, 1987.

45. Hutchinson A, Maltby JR, Reid CRG: Gastric fluid volumes and pH in elective inpatients: Part 1, coffee or orange juice versus overnight fast, *Can J Anaesth* 35:12, 1988.

46. Scarr M, Maltby JR, Jani K et al: Volume and acidity of residual gastric fluid after oral fluid ingestion before elective ambulatory surgery, *Can Med Assoc J* 141:1151, 1989.

47. Maltby JR, Lewis P, Martin A et al: Gastric fluid volume and pH in elective patients following unrestricted oral fluid until three hours before surgery, *Can J Anaesth* 38:425, 1991.

48. Bond VK, Stoelting RK, Gupta CD: Pulmonary aspiration after inhalation of gastric fluids containing antacids, *Anesthesiology* 51:452, 1979.

49. Gibbs CP, Schwartz DJ et al: Antacid pulmonary aspiration in the dog, *Anesthesiology* 51(5):380, 1979.

50. Detmer MD, Pandit SK, Cohen PJ: Prophylactic single-dose oral antacid therapy in the preoperative period: Comparison of cimetidine and Maalox®, *Anesthesiology* 51:270, 1979.

51. Gallagher EG, White M, Ward S et al: Prophylaxis against acid aspiration syndrome, *Anaesthesia* 43:1011, 1988.

52. Pandit SK, Kothary SP, Pandit UA et al: Premedication with cimetidine and metoclopramide: Effect on the risk factors of acid aspiration, *Anaesthesia* 41:486, 1986.

53. Manchikanti L, Marrero TC, Roush JR: Preanesthetic cimetidine and metoclopramide for acid aspiration prophylaxis in elective surgery, *Anesthesiology* 61:48, 1984.

54. Atanassoff PG, Alon E, Pasch T: Effects of single-dose intravenous omeprazole and ranitidine on gastric pH during general anesthesia, *Anesth Analg* 75:95, 1992.

55. Cotton BR, Smith G: Single and combined effects of atropine and metoclopramide on lower esophageal sphincter pressure, *Br J Anaesth* 53:869, 1981.

56. Stone SS, Pook H: Lung infections and infestations: Therapeutic considerations. In Spaulding GL, editor: *Problems in veterinary medicine: Respiratory medicine*, Philadelphia, 1992, JB Lippincott.

57. Pingleton SK, Hinthorn DR, Lui C: Enteral nutrition in patients receiving mechanical ventilation: Multiple sources tracheal colonization include the stomach, *Am J Med* 80:827, 1986.

58. Torres A, Serra-Batles J, Ros E et al: Pulmonary aspiration of gastric contents in patients receiving mechanical ventilation: The effect of body position, *Ann Intern Med* 116:540, 1992.

59. Drakulovic MB, Torres A, Bauer TT et al: Supine body position as a risk factor for nosocomial pneumonia in mechanically ventilated patients: A randomized trial, *Lancet* 354:1851, 1999.

60. Fabian TC: Empiric therapy for pneumonia in the surgical intensive care unit, *Am J Surg* 179(Suppl 2A):18S, 2000.

61. DuMoulin GC, Paterson DG, Hedley-Whyte J et al: Aspiration of gastric bacteria in antacid-treated patients: A frequent cause of postoperative colonization of the airway, *Lancet* Jan:242, 1982.

62. Tryba M: Sucralfate versus antacids or H₂-antagonists for stress ulcer prophylaxis: A meta-analysis on efficacy and pneumonia rate, *Crit Care Med* 19:942, 1991.

63. Prodhom G, Leuenberger P, Korfer J et al: Nosocomial pneumonia in mechanically ventilated patients receiving antacid, ranitidine, or sucralfate as prophylaxis for stress ulcer, *Ann Intern Med* 120:653, 1994.

64. Fabian TC, Boucher BA, Croce MA et al: Pneumonia and stress ulceration in severely injured patients: A prospective evaluation of the effects of stress ulcer prophylaxis, *Arch Surg* 128:185, 1993.

65. Cook D, Guyatt G, Marshall J et al: A comparison of sucralfate and ranitidine for the prevention of upper gastrointestinal bleeding in patients requiring mechanical ventilation, *N Engl J Med* 338:791, 1998.

66. Nader-Djalal N, Knight PR, Thusu K et al: Reactive oxygen species contribute to oxygen-related lung injury after acid aspiration, *Anesth Analg* 87:127, 1998.

67. Rowe S, Cheadle WG: Complications of nosocomial pneumonia in the surgical patient, *Am J Surg* 179(Suppl 2A):63S, 2000.

68. Rudloff E, Kirby R: Colloids: Current recommendations. In Bonagura JD, editor: *Kirk's current veterinary therapy*, vol 13, Philadelphia, 2000, WB Saunders.

69. Glauser FL, Millen JE, Falls R: Increased alveolar epithelial permeability with acid aspiration: The effects of high-dose steroids, *Am Rev Respir Dis* 120:1119, 1979.

70. Wolfe JE, Bone RC, Ruth WE: Effects of corticosteroids in the treatment of patients with gastric aspiration, *Am J Med* 63:719, 1977.

71. Ruiz M, Ewig S, Marcos MA et al: Etiology of community-acquired pneumonia: Impact of age, comorbidity, and severity, *Am J Respir Crit Care Med* 160:397, 1999.

72. Lorber B, Swensonm RM: Bacteriology of aspiration pneumonia: A prospective study of community and hospital-acquired cases, *Ann Intern Med* 81:329, 1974.

73. Vaden S, Papich M: Empiric antibiotic therapy. In Bonagura JD, editor: *Kirk's current veterinary therapy*, vol 12, Philadelphia, 1995, WB Saunders.

74. Quenzer R: A perspective of cephalosporins in pneumonia, *Chest* 93(3):531, 1987.

75. Spain D: Pneumonia in the surgical patient: Duration of therapy and does the organism matter? *Am J Surg* 179 (Suppl 2A):36S, 2000.

CHAPTER 58

Viral Pneumonia

Matthew S. Mellema

Definition and Etiology

Acute viral respiratory disease (e.g., the common cold and influenza) is the most common illness in humans. In veterinary medicine, this preeminence has not been established, but viral infection of the upper respiratory tract is certainly a common occurrence in dogs and cats kept under certain conditions.[1] In contrast, viral pneumonia is far less common than upper respiratory tract disease. Viral pneumonia may be defined as inflammation of the alveolar epithelium, pulmonary interstitium, and pulmonary capillary endothelium as a result of a primary viral infection. Commonly, the inflammatory processes in viral pneumonia also involve the terminal airways, and some infections that primarily cause *bronchiolitis* are also termed viral pneumonia.

Many viral infections of the dog and cat more commonly cause upper airway disease (e.g., infectious laryngotracheitis or "kennel cough"). Lower airway and parenchymal disease from these infections is rare unless the case is severe, the patient is immunocompromized, or the infective virus is delivered by an atypical route (e.g., fine aerosol delivery of viral particles in experimental studies). The term viral pneumonia should be reserved for cases in which involvement of the terminal airways and alveolar structures is substantial and predominant. When the bronchioles and parenchyma are largely unaffected, terms that describe the predominant site of injury are more appropriate (e.g., viral laryngotracheitis, bronchitis, or rhinitis). In addition, viral diseases that manifest as focal granulomas when the lung is involved (e.g., feline infectious peritonitis) are referred to as granulomatous pulmonary diseases rather than pneumonia.

The term *pneumonia* may be considered a misnomer when discussing primary viral infections of the pulmonary parenchyma, and many prefer to use the term *pneumonitis*. Pneumonia implies that a significant degree of exudate is to be found within the distal airways, which is seldom the case in uncomplicated viral pneumonia. Viral pneumonia may also be referred to as *atypical pneumonia* because of the relative lack of exudate within the airspaces.

The most prevalent causative agents vary between species and with geographic location. In humans, the principal viral causes of pneumonia also vary with patient age and immune status. These factors may be of similar importance in dogs and cats but have not been widely studied.[2] Viral pneumonia is typically the result of an infection that gained access to the host by the inhaled or oropharyngeal route. Whereas fine aerosols containing viral particles are often generated in experimental studies, in naturally occurring disease the virus is typically spread within larger droplets of excretions and secretions. The lung parenchyma may become affected by direct invasion of respiratory epithelium via the airways. Alternatively, the lung may obtain its viral load secondary to viremia and blood-borne dissemination. Transplacental transmission of some respiratory viral pathogens has been described.[3]

The primary causes of viral pneumonia in dogs are canine distemper virus (CDV), canine adenovirus type-II (CAV-2), and parainfluenza virus type-II (formerly parainfluenza SV5).[4,5] Although reoviruses, coronaviruses, herpesviruses, and parvoviruses have all been recovered from dogs suffering from respiratory disease, their importance as causes of primary viral pneumonia is either limited or uncertain.[4,6-10] In the cat, the predominant causes of primary viral pneumonia include feline herpesvirus (FHV-1), feline calicivirus (FCV), and poxvirus.[11,12] Reoviruses have on occasion been recovered from cats with respiratory disease but are not thought to be a significant cause of pneumonia. Likewise, infection with either feline immunodeficiency virus (FIV) or feline leukemia virus (FeLV) may result in some pulmonary involvement within the context of a systemic disease process, but pneumonia is not thought to be a common manifestation of those viral infections.[13-15] Feline infectious peritonitis (FIP) infection can result in pulmonary granulomas but represents a pathologic process distinct from those of the viral pathogens to be discussed here.[16,17]

Pathophysiology

The response of the lower airways and pulmonary parenchyma to injury is somewhat stereotypic, and in many cases it can be difficult to determine whether a viral or a noninfectious cause underlies observed pulmonary pathology. Epidemiological evidence suggests that the majority of viral infections of the lung in animals produce asymptomatic or subclinical disease. When clinical disease of the lung does occur, many different viruses initiate a similar cascade of events. After gaining access to host tissues via inhalation or the oropharyngeal route, some viruses replicate within the respiratory tract without dissemination (e.g., parainfluenza type-II), whereas others replicate in extrapulmonary sites before spreading to the respiratory epithelium (e.g., canine distemper virus).

The lungs have both innate and acquired immune effector systems, and each plays a role in the defense against and response to viral infection.[18,19] The mucociliary clearance mechanism sweeps viral particles that are trapped in the airway surface fluid layer out of the lung. Immunoglobulins can neutralize virus by preventing attachment and penetration. Secretory IgA and locally synthesized IgG as well as serum-derived IgG and IgM can contribute to this virus-neutralizing activity. The role of surfactant and complement components in nonspecific pulmonary immunity continues to be an active area of research.[18,20] Complement fixation can cause lysis of the larger enveloped viruses.[21] The insertion of the complement membrane attack complex serves to trigger apoptosis of virus infected cells. Another important component of the humoral system of pulmonary antiviral defense is the interferon family of cytokines. The interferons can inhibit viral replication, promote degradation of messenger RNA, and inhibit the initiation of protein synthesis, in addition to their effects on cellular immunity,[22] thereby disrupting viral replication.

In addition to the humoral mechanisms, a host of effector cells also play a role in pulmonary antiviral defense.[19] Lymphocytes are essential to the generation of a maximal antiviral response. Cytotoxic T lymphocytes (CTL) initiate the death of virus-infected host cells when viral antigens presented on the membrane of the infected cells are recognized by T cell receptors. Natural killer (NK) cells also serve a role in eliminating infected cells. The helper T cells of the T_{H1} subset are essential for activation of cytotoxic cells as well as the secretion of cytokines such as interferons. In addition, the helper T cells promote the generation of antibodies by B-lymphocytes.

The alveolar macrophage is a phagocytic cell charged with keeping the alveolar spaces clear of debris and potentially harmful microorganisms. The alveolar epithelium is not ciliated and thus cannot use the mucociliary clearance system to remove foreign material. The alveolar macrophage can ingest foreign matter as well as host cells that have become apoptotic or necrotic. The phagocytic activity of the alveolar macrophage helps to maintain patency of the airspaces, survey the airspaces for foreign antigen, and remove cells and cellular remnants that might serve as media for the growth of microorganisms. In addition to its phagocytic role, the alveolar macrophage is an important source of cytokines and chemokines.

When pulmonary antiviral defenses are inadequate, delayed, or excessively activated, primary viral pneumonia may occur. Common to all forms of viral pneumonia is widespread injury to type I alveolar pneumocytes. Viral pneumonia is often categorized as interstitial pneumonia because the lesions typically are centered in the alveolar walls and the interstitium. However, it is important to understand the course of events of pulmonary viral infection and how the distribution and nature of the lesions change over time. Initially, respiratory viruses injure bronchial, bronchiolar, and alveolar cells, and this initial injury leads to an influx of neutrophils. The direct injury and subsequent inflammatory response lead to the desquamation of epithelial cells, and the lumen of bronchioles and alveoli can become filled with desquamated cells, macrophages, mononuclear cells, and neutrophils. Tissue damage also promotes the leakage of protein-rich fluid into the airspaces. At this early stage the process is better described as a *bronchopneumonia* than as an interstitial pneumonia.

As the disease progresses, the majority of the lesions may be identified in the alveolar walls and interstitium. This transition has prompted some pathologists to use the term *bronchointerstitial pneumonia* to describe the lesions associated with viral infection of the lung parenchyma. As the type I pneumocytes desquamate, the alveolar epithelium is repopulated with hyperplastic type II pneumocytes as long as the alveolar basement membrane remains intact. This shift from type I to type II pneumocytes is initially associated with a thickening of the alveolar epithelium. If the underlying cause resolves, the hyperplastic type II pneumocytes will differentiate into type I pneumocytes with their characteristic flattened profile.

In the acute stage of viral pneumonia, both proliferative and infiltrative lesions are noted. The alveolar septa become thickened and edematous. The septa are typically infiltrated with lymphocytes, histiocytes, and the occasional plasma cell. Neutrophil infiltration also occurs in the acute stage, but neutrophils are seldom the primary cell type seen in later lesions in the absence of secondary bacterial infection. As the disease progresses the alveoli may be free of exudate, but protein-rich fluid in the airspaces may lead to hyaline membrane formation. Hyperplasia of airway and vascular smooth muscle cells may be evident, and microscopic granuloma formation can be seen. Giant cell formation may occur because of virus-induced cell fusion, and capillary thrombosis may be observed. Some viral infections (e.g., herpesvirus, poxvirus, and adenovirus) cause significant cellular necrosis and therefore a more severe acute inflammatory response.

The lesions in viral pneumonia are generally diffuse, in contrast to the cranioventral distribution of lesions typical of bacterial pneumonia. Rather, the lesions may be more pronounced in the dorsocaudal lung fields, although the reason for this distribution is not understood at present. In acute interstitial pneumonia, three distribution patterns have been described: septal perilobular, peribronchiolar, and perialveolar. Each of these patterns may have a viral etiology depending on the agent and the point at which the sample was obtained.

The severity and duration of the illness often depend on the infective dose of virus delivered to the respiratory tract.[23] In cases with a persistent source of alveolar injury, chronic interstitial pneumonia can develop. The hallmark of chronic interstitial pneumonia is pulmonary fibrosis, and there is often a mononuclear cellular infiltrate in the interstitium and persistent hyperplasia of type II pneumocytes.

On gross inspection, the lungs of a patient with viral pneumonia have several significant changes. When the chest is opened the lungs fail to collapse, appear diffusely red to gray, and may be mottled in appearance. Rib impressions may be noted on the visceral pleural surface, and the lungs often feel rubbery to the touch. On the cut surface, the lungs appear meaty and there is minimal visible exudate in the airspaces unless a secondary bacterial pneumonia has developed.

The effects of viral pneumonia on lung function can be significant. Exudate in the airways can cause airway narrowing and decrease airflow. Altered ventilatory patterns and capillary thrombosis can lead to ventilation-perfusion mismatching. In addition, many of the inflammatory cytokines produced in response to viral infection are vasoactive and can alter hypoxic vasoconstriction and further compromise ventilation and perfusion matching.[24] Infiltration of the interstitium and conversion to a type II pneumocyte alveolar epithelium can potentially diminish oxygen diffusion. The edematous and thickened alveolar septa reduce pulmonary compliance and increase the work of breathing.[25] Dyspnea may therefore be observed in the absence of hypoxemia.[26] Extrapulmonary signs of viral pneumonia may manifest if the virus infects tissues other than the lung or if the pulmonary insult results in a systemic inflammatory response.

Long-term sequelae of prior viral pneumonia have not been widely studied in veterinary medicine. Chronic interstitial pneumonia can lead to pulmonary fibrosis. A growing body of evidence in humans suggests that viral respiratory disease may be related to the development and exacerbation of bronchial asthma.[27] Although such an association has not been documented in cats, the author has seen new cases of asthma develop in a closed colony of blood donor cats shortly after an outbreak of calicivirus. Controlled studies investigating a link between viral disease and asthma in cats are lacking at present.

Secondary Bacterial Pneumonia

Uncomplicated viral pneumonia often leads to mild, self-limiting disease. Unfortunately, secondary bacterial invasion is a common complication that can result in significantly increased morbidity and mortality, and can hamper efforts to correctly identify a primary viral pathogen. On thoracic radiographs a cranioventral distribution of pulmonary infiltrates may be noted, which is inconsistent with primary viral pneumonia. Additionally, secondary bacterial pneumonia may result in toxic changes in the leukocytes in a peripheral blood smear, which would be unusual in an uncomplicated viral pneumonia.

Viral and bacterial pathogens may be synergistic in the pneumonic lung, and experimental evidence supports the notion of viral-bacterial synergism in multi-pathogen pneumonia.[28-35] Viral pathogens can significantly impair pulmonary antibacterial defenses, both directly and indirectly. Viral infection can result in loss of ciliated epithelium from the conducting airways and thus compromise mucociliary clearance. Cellular desquamation and protein leakage can produce a suitable medium for bacterial growth in the airways. In addition, consolidated lung represents a relatively hypoxic environment that may indirectly impair bacterial defenses because many immune cells utilize oxygen-derived radicals to kill microbes.[34] Both canine adenovirus type II and parainfluenza have been shown to damage the respiratory epithelium and promote invasion by bacteria and mycoplasma. Several other mechanisms of viral-induced depression of antibacterial defenses have been proposed. Viral infection has been shown to enhance susceptibility to bacterial attachment and colonization,[36] and to diminish surfactant production. Macrophage chemotaxis, bacterial ingestion, and bacterial killing may all be diminished by concurrent viral infection.[33,37]

Viral infection has been experimentally shown to diminish pulmonary antibacterial defenses in a time-dependent fashion.[38] In some models, bacterial defenses abruptly decline at day 7 to day 8 postviral infection, but are reestablished at day 9 to day 10.[38] The extent of depression appears to vary with the viral dose, and the most severe depression of antibacterial defenses appears to correlate with a period of rapidly declining viral titers. Importantly, the experimental results suggest that for synergism to occur the viral infection must precede the bacterial infection.

The immunosuppressive effects of canine distemper virus warrant special mention. Distemper virus replicates within lymphoid cells and causes lympholysis, resulting in profound lymphopenia and thymic atrophy. The suppression of lymphocyte activity can lead to depression of both humoral and cellular immune responses.

Epidemiology

Specific detailed epidemiological data regarding each potential cause of viral pneumonia in dogs and cats is lacking. Moreover, much of the data available is derived from colonies or quarantine facilities and may not be broadly applicable to the pet population.[4,5,9,39,40] In dogs, viral pneumonia is often a disease of young puppies,[2] possibly because of exposure to pathogenic viruses before vaccination or during the period when maternally derived immunity is insufficient to prevent disease yet adequate to prevent full protection from vaccination. Many dogs and cats spend little time in close contact with other members of their species except during early life. Lastly, some viruses capable of causing pneumonia may be passed from carriers to their offspring.

Viral respiratory disease is often seen when many animals are housed together. Crowding, relatively poor ventilation, stress, and increased likelihood of exposure to carriers all can contribute to increased prevalence of respiratory disease. Upper respiratory disease in cats often occurs in catteries, boarding facilities, and shelters. Feline poxvirus pneumonia is more likely to occur in the late summer or early fall,[41] possibly because rodent carrier populations are highest during this period. Most canine viral respiratory disease occurs in shelters, laboratory colonies, quarantine facilities, breeding colonies, and boarding kennels. One study of random-source dogs in a quarantine facility showed that respiratory disease developed in 52% of the dogs during the quarantine period.[5] Of the viral diseases identified in this population, distemper was the most common and most likely to be fatal.

Differential Diagnosis

Differential diagnosis for viral pneumonia includes conditions that can produce an acute, diffuse alveolar injury, as well as those producing an acute interstitial pneumonia independent of a primary injury to the alveolar epithelium (Box 58-1). Noninfectious causes are eliminated first. Next, nonviral infectious agents (e.g., bacteria, mycoplasma, fungi, and protozoa) that might be consistent with the patient's signs are investigated. Finally, viruses that might result in the clinical presentation can be considered.

The differentiation of infectious from noninfectious causes of acute, diffuse, interstitial pulmonary infiltrates can be challenging. History, laboratory data, and extra-

---

BOX 58-1

Differential Diagnosis of Acute Diffuse/ Multifocal Pulmonary Infiltrates

Noninfectious Causes (Both Dogs and Cats)
- Inhaled toxins
  - Smoke inhalation, noxious gases
  - Prolonged oxygen therapy
- Ingested toxins
  - Paraquat
- Adverse drug reactions
- Hypersensitivity pneumonitis
- Endogenous/metabolic toxins
  - Uremic pneumonitis
- Cardiogenic pulmonary edema
  - Congestive heart failure (left-sided)
- Noncardiogenic pulmonary edema
  - Acute Respiratory Distress Syndrome (ARDS)
  - Neurogenic pulmonary edema
  - Upper airway obstruction
- Autoimmune disease
  - Systemic lupus erythematosis
- Unknown (idiopathic)

Infectious Causes
- Bacterial/mycoplasmal/mycobacterial pneumonia
- Mycotic pneumonia
- Protozoal pneumonia
- Viral pneumonia (dogs)
  - Canine distemper virus
  - Canine adenovirus type II
  - Parainfluenza virus type II
- Viral pneumonia (cats)
  - Feline herpesvirus
  - Calicivirus
  - Poxvirus

---

pulmonary clinical signs can often distinguish between the various causes of acute pulmonary injury. In many cases, lung biopsy and diagnostic techniques based on molecular biology may be required for a definitive diagnosis. Determining the agent(s) responsible for an infectious pneumonia relies predominantly on cytology and culture of samples of lung tissue and/or airway lining fluid. In the case of parasitic pneumonia, the examination of stool samples, in some instances, can circumvent the need to obtain samples from the respiratory tract. A history and clinical picture consistent with an infectious pneumonia can suggest a viral etiology when no other form of microorganism can be identified. In many cases, identification of the specific virus responsible for an episode of pneumonia is not necessary because treatment is largely supportive in nature. It is unlikely that virus isolation techniques to distinguish CAV-2 from parainfluenza type II will alter the outcome in an individual case. Distinguishing distemper from the other causes of viral pneumonia in dogs, however, has important prognostic implications, particularly if neurologic signs are evident.

In cats, differentiating between calicivirus and herpesvirus infection can often be based on presentation, oral, ocular, and upper respiratory findings. In severe cases, obtaining a specific viral diagnosis may be of use because some chemotherapeutic options exist to treat herpetic diseases that are ineffective in the treatment of caliciviral infection. Poxvirus can nearly always be distinguished from the other causes of viral pneumonia based on accompanying skin lesions typical of that illness.[12]

The pursuit of a specific viral diagnosis may be of more utility when faced with an outbreak rather than an isolated case. Identifying the virus responsible in such instances may help rational determination of appropriate isolation and prophylactic measures. For example, starting an early intranasal B. bronchiseptica/parainfluenza vaccination program in a breeding kennel is unlikely to alter the spread of an outbreak of distemper in that population. It may also be appropriate to pursue the specific identification of a viral pathogen when atypical signs are noted and one suspects a new strain or species may be responsible. Such investigations have led to the identification of strains with different tropisms, and also help in the formulation of future vaccines. Newer techniques becoming available, such as polymerase chain reaction, are of such high sensitivity that viral components can be isolated from many healthy animals. This underscores the care that must be taken when attributing a given patient's illness to a viral pathogen.

Viral Pneumonia in Dogs

In dogs, viral respiratory infection typically results in large airway disease (e.g., laryngotracheitis or "kennel cough") and primary viral pneumonia is rarely recognized. However, many of the causative agents of kennel cough can result in viral pneumonia in severe cases or in experimental studies in which infective virus is delivered as a fine aerosol. In addition, many cases of kennel cough represent infections with both viral and bacterial pathogens (e.g., parainfluenza virus and *Bordetella bronchiseptica*); therefore viral pneumonia is commonly associated with the development of secondary bacterial pneumonia. However, several viral agents can cause *primary* viral pneumonia in dogs, independent of subsequent bacterial invasion. Whereas a number of viral agents have been implicated in case reports of lower respiratory disease, the bulk of clinically recognized viral pneumonia can be attributed to three viruses: canine distemper, parainfluenza virus, and canine adenovirus (CAV-2).

CANINE DISTEMPER

Canine distemper is the agent most commonly associated with life-threatening or chronically debilitating viral pneumonia in dogs. Carré originally described the disease in 1905. Over the last century, vaccination of dogs for this disease has become standard practice in many parts of the world. Despite extensive vaccination of the at-risk population, significant disease caused by distemper is still seen. The illness likely persists because of the presence of unvaccinated carriers and the exposure of dogs to virus either before vaccination or before protective antibody titers develop. Outbreaks of disease within vaccinated populations have been described.[42,43]

Distemper is caused by a virus related to the human measles virus and is classified as a morbillivirus. The viral genome is in the form of RNA and the entire genome has been sequenced.[44] Exposure is generally thought to occur via aerosol and fine droplets. The virus initially replicates in lymphoid tissues such as the tonsils and bronchial lymph nodes. Following initial viral replication, viremia develops and the virus spreads to more peripheral lymphoid tissues. Another period of viral replication occurs within the peripheral lymphoid tissue. Distemper virus is pantropic and invades a wide range of tissue and cell types. The virus often targets epithelial cells, and many of the clinical signs of the disease reflect viral infection of epithelial surfaces and secondary bacterial invasion. Infection of the central nervous system often leads to the clinical signs of acute encephalitis and may also result in chronic disease.[45,46] Distemper infection is immunosuppressive because of both lympholysis and alteration of cytokine responses.[47-51] Secondary bacterial pneumonia is particularly common following distemper virus infections of the lung.

History and Clinical Signs

The clinical signs of distemper are often sufficient to distinguish it from the other major causes of viral pneumonia in dogs.[52] Patients with distemper are generally much more seriously ill than those suffering from CAV-2 or parainfluenza. The diversity of clinical signs observed reflects both the pantropism of the virus and the profound immunosuppression it can induce. Distemper has been shown in experimental infections to cause a biphasic fever (around day 5 and around day 11 postinoculation), but the initial febrile period may often be missed in clinical disease.[7,53,54] Gastrointestinal signs can include both vomiting and diarrhea. Signs of respiratory involvement may include cough, dyspnea, and a mucopurulent oculonasal discharge. Weight loss and dehydration may be substantial. Neurologic signs are variable and may include myoclonus, seizures, and vision loss. Some of the classic signs of distemper such as hyperkeratosis of the footpads are more chronic manifestations of the disease, and are seldom present at the time pneumonia is most likely to develop. This description of clinical signs is that of a classic distemper case, but distemper can mimic a variety of other diseases and cases seldom fit a textbook picture. Regarding the pulmonary manifestations of distemper, the virus should be high on the differential list if pneumonia is present in the face of lymphopenia, neurologic signs, ocular signs, or a recent history of exposure to a multi-dog environment such as a shelter. Similarly, if an overwhelming infection with a relatively uncommon parasite is diagnosed, concurrent distemper infection should be considered.[55,56]

Diagnostic Testing

The diagnosis of distemper is often made based on history and clinical signs. The chemistry profile, complete blood count, and urinalysis may have few changes, particularly in the acute stages of the disease. Depending on the viral strain involved, a significant lymphopenia may be noted. Thoracic radiographs may initially show a diffuse interstitial pattern that progresses to a diffuse bronchial and alveolar pattern if secondary bacterial bronchopneumonia develops or if pulmonary necrosis is extensive. Eosinophilic viral inclusion bodies in the nucleus or cytoplasm of leukocytes, erythrocytes, or epithelial cells may support the tentative diagnosis (Figure 58-1).[57-59]

Definitive diagnosis may be made using immunohistochemistry (Figure 58-2), viral isolation, or polymerase chain reaction amplification of unique viral sequences of nucleic acid.[60-64] Heparinized blood is considered the best sample on which to attempt viral isolation, but distemper can be a challenging virus to grow in the laboratory. Electron microscopy of tissue samples can identify viral particles but has low sensitivity and is not specific. ELISA-based assays for both distemper-specific antibodies and viral antigen have also been used successfully and offer a more rapid alternative to virus neutralization assays.[65,66] Serum antibody titers may at times be misleading because of the immunosuppression produced by distemper infection and widespread vaccination of dogs for this disease.

Fluorescent antibodies with specificities for distemper antigens may be applied to acetone-fixed conjunctival scrapings, tonsilar swabs, and buffy coat smears; however, these samples may yield false negative results during the acute phase of the disease. Distemper virus and viral antigens often persist longer in the epithelial cells of the lower respiratory tract.[67] Transtracheal aspirates can often yield diagnostic samples when conjunctival scrapings are negative. Although bronchoalveolar lavage (BAL) samples are likely to yield useful information, the

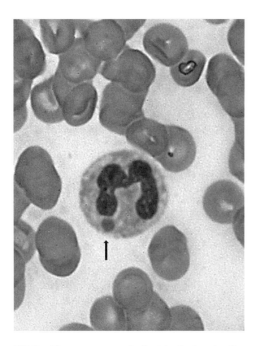

Figure 58-1. *The presence of viral inclusion bodies can increase the index of suspicion for viral illness. However, identifying inclusion bodies seldom allows one to make a definitive diagnosis. In this photograph of a peripheral blood smear an inclusion body resulting from canine distemper virus infection is identified in a neutrophil. (Courtesy Dr. P.J. Dickinson, University of California-Davis).*

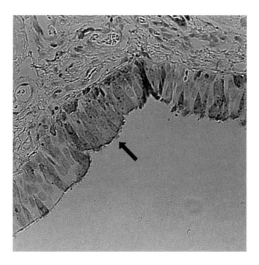

Figure 58-2. *Immunohistochemistry of lung tissue from a dog that died of an infection with canine distemper virus. The airway epithelial cells containing distemper antigen show up as darker and stippled in appearance (arrow) in this photograph. Immunohistochemistry is one method by which a specific viral diagnosis may be made. (Courtesy Dr. P.J. Dickinson, University of California-Davis).*

patients are often quite ill and the risks of anesthesia in this setting warrant careful consideration,[68] and contamination of bronchoscopic and anesthetic equipment may occur. Viral antigens may persist in bladder epithelial cells beyond the acute stage of the disease.[69-71] Fortunately, the attenuated virus of vaccines does not spread to nonlymphoid tissues, and prior vaccination generally does not interfere with fluorescent antibody–based diagnostics.

Pathological and Histopathological Findings

The extrapulmonary gross pathological and histopathological findings in distemper viral infection are well described.[7,53,54,72-74] The lungs have a variable appearance on gross examination (Figure 58-3). Secondary bacterial pneumonia can substantially increase the amount of gross hemorrhage and consolidated or devitalized parenchyma. The lungs are often mottled gray and dark red, and fail to deflate when the chest is opened. Thymic atrophy may be notable in young dogs. Rib impressions may be apparent on the visceral pleural surface. Purulent exudate may be visible in the airways if secondary bacterial pneumonia was present antemortem.

Uncomplicated distemper infection of the lung is typically associated with a diffuse interstitial pneumonia. A necrotizing bronchiolitis and necrosis and desquamation of pneumocytes may be seen. Mild alveolar edema is commonly noted, and the alveolar septa may be thickened, with infiltration of the interstitium with mononu-

clear cells. Hyperplasia of type II pneumocytes is seen. Multinucleated giant cells may be found in the bronchial lining, alveolar septa, and in the alveolar spaces. The formation of fused cells is similar to the giant cell pneumonia also seen in human measles. The alveolar airspaces may contain macrophages and desquamated epithelial cells. The histopathological findings in distemper pneumonia can be modified by secondary bacterial invasion. When secondary bacterial invasion has occurred the lesions are typically those of a purulent bronchopneumonia, with the airways and alveoli filled with neutrophils, cellular remnants, and mucin.

Management and Monitoring

Serial evaluation of respiratory and neurologic status is advised in the management of distemper pneumonia. Respiratory rate and effort should be recorded at regular intervals. Patients with worsening respiratory signs should have oxygenation evaluated by pulse oximetry or arterial blood gas analysis. Repeated thoracic radiographs may be helpful in making an earlier diagnosis of secondary bacterial pneumonia in patients with deteriorating respiratory function. Transtracheal aspirates often provide suitable samples for culture and sensitivity determination and allow appropriate antibiotic selection when secondary bacterial pneumonia is suspected.

The clinical management of distemper pneumonia is largely supportive, and no specific therapy is presently available. Maintaining adequate nutrition and fluid support are central to patient care. Distemper can often result in severe gastrointestinal signs, and dogs intolerant of enteral feeding may require parenteral nutritional support. Because of the profound immunosuppression, ad-

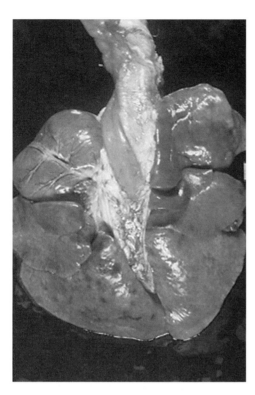

Figure 58-3. The gross appearance of the lungs from a dog that died of an infection with canine distemper virus. The lungs fail to collapse fully, are rubbery to the touch, and have a diffusely mottled appearance. On cut surface the lungs had a meaty appearance and less exudate was noted in the airways than in bacterial pneumonia. (Courtesy Dr. P.J. Dickinson, University of California-Davis).

ministration of broad-spectrum antibiotics is advised. Nebulization and coupage may be helpful. Nebulization followed by gentle removal of accumulations of nasal discharge from the external nares may improve patient comfort. Patients with dyspnea and those with documented hypoxemia should receive supplemental oxygen. In severe cases, respiratory failure may prompt the institution of mechanical ventilatory support.

Distemper is closely related to the human measles virus and some treatments used in the management of measles giant cell pneumonia may be considered. Ribavirin is a nucleoside analogue with broad *in vitro* activity against both RNA and DNA viruses. Aerosolized ribavirin administration has been reported to be effective for treatment of measles pneumonia, and is FDA approved for the treatment of respiratory syncytial virus pneumonia in people.[75,76] Efficacy studies and dosing schemes for this agent in the treatment of distemper pneumonia are lacking at present. Successful outcomes in human patients with giant cell pneumonia, treated with corticosteroids in combination with other drugs, have been reported.[77] Studies have also evaluated the use of steroids in experimental distemper infections.[78] However, the use of a drug that can cause immunosuppression and lympholysis to treat a viral infection associated with the same adverse effects is generally not ad-

vised. No controlled studies of steroid therapy for giant cell pneumonia are available at present.

Vitamin A deficiency has been shown to be a risk factor in the development of measles in humans.[79] The World Health Organization (WHO) advises that children in areas of the world where measles prevalence is high receive vitamin A supplements. Further, it has been shown that the administration of 200,000 IU per day of vitamin A for 2 days to children suffering from measles can reduce overall mortality as well as pneumonia-specific mortality.[80] The use of vitamin A as an adjunct therapy in the treatment of distemper pneumonia bears further investigation.

Prevention of distemper relies on isolation of affected animals and vaccination of unaffected dogs.[81] Vaccination is considered the single most important prevention strategy. In one study, 94% of the cases could be attributed to nonvaccinated patient status.[82] In unvaccinated populations the disease strikes dogs of all ages. Both attenuated live virus and recombinant distemper virus vaccines are available. Distemper vaccines in puppies are generally given starting at 6 to 7 weeks of age and every 3 weeks thereafter until three doses have been given. In adult dogs a single dose of attenuated live virus or multiple doses of recombinant vaccine are administered to generate protective immunity. Additional distemper vaccine is administered on an annual or biennial schedule. Vaccinated animals may remain susceptible to isolated respiratory infection. This observation places distemper among the rule-outs for kennel cough.

Isolation of affected dogs helps to prevent transmission. Distemper virus is relatively labile. Both detergents and disinfectants are suitable for removing viral infectivity.

Prognosis

The prognosis for acute distemper virus infection is fair to guarded. Pneumonia often occurs in more severe cases. Progressive signs of acute encephalitis generally warrant a worse prognosis. The dose of infective virus received often correlates with the length and severity of illness, although viral strain and host factors also play a role.

CANINE ADENOVIRUS TYPE II (CAV-2)

Canine adenovirus type II is another pathogen that can cause kennel cough in dogs. CAV-2 is closely related to CAV-1, the causative agent of infectious canine hepatitis. Canine adenovirus type II infection is common and highly contagious. In severe cases, both bronchiolitis and interstitial pneumonia can develop,[83-86] and studies have implicated adenovirus as the sole pathogen in young kennel-origin dogs with pneumonia.[85,87,88] Co-infection with distemper virus has also been reported.[89,90]

Adenoviral infection is generally acquired by inhalation of aerosol droplets. The virus proliferates within the respiratory tract without dissemination to extrapulmonary sites. The virus is shed in respiratory secretions and can persist within the lung for up to a month in the absence of clinical disease.

History and Clinical Signs

Patients suffering from adenoviral pneumonia often have a history of exposure to other dogs in a kennel or shelter environment within the prior month. Clinical signs include mild fever, oculonasal discharge, coughing, and weight loss (or failure to gain weight in young dogs). Signs are often limited to the upper and lower respiratory tract, and evidence of significant systemic illness is generally lacking. A more pronounced febrile response may correlate with more rapid recovery.

Diagnostic Testing

The diagnosis of adenoviral pneumonia is typically made based on history and clinical signs. The minimum database is often unremarkable unless the patient has concurrent distemper virus infection or secondary bacterial pneumonia. Thoracic radiographs typically reveal a bronchointerstitial pattern. Cranioventral alveolar infiltrates may be seen if bacterial pneumonia develops. Nasal, tonsilar, and ocular swabs/scrapings may provide a specific viral diagnosis, and transtracheal aspirates or BAL can also yield diagnostic samples. Unlike those of distemper virus, the inclusion bodies of CAV-2 are basophilic and nuclear. A definitive diagnosis can be made via viral isolation as well as by fluorescent antibody methodologies. Hemagglutinin testing (HA), complement fixation testing (CF), and observation of a cytopathogenic effect (CPE) in canine cell cultures can indicate the presence of pathogenic viral particles, but specific identification is typically performed via virus neutralization (VN) testing. Each of these techniques has been developed for adenovirus testing but availability may vary. Acute and convalescent titers can be obtained, but in most cases of CAV-2 respiratory disease the patient will be fully recovered before convalescent titers are drawn. However, because the virus can persist in the respiratory tract for weeks after recovery, identification of adenovirus can alter the recommendations for how long an individual dog should be isolated.

Pathological and Histopathological Findings

Adenovirus infection can result in widespread necrosis and exfoliation of bronchiolar and alveolar epithelium. The initial insult leads to a mild infiltration of the alveolar interstitium with neutrophils and lymphocytes. Interstitial edema can be found, with some leakage of protein-rich fluid into the airways. Proliferation of type II pneumocytes is seen. The overall pattern of lesions is one of bronchointerstitial pneumonia with a necrotizing bronchiolitis. If histopathology is performed on samples obtained shortly after the acute illness, the appearance may be that of a proliferative or hyperplastic bronchitis and bronchiolitis.

Management and Monitoring

Patients with adenoviral pneumonia often present much less systemically ill than those with distemper. Dogs that are not overtly dyspneic and are not hypoxemic may be managed as outpatients if they are eating and drinking adequately. Cases with more severe respiratory compromise (e.g., because of the primary viral illness, coinfection with distemper, or secondary bacterial pneumonia) are better managed initially as inpatients. Canine adenovirus type II is highly contagious and the virus is relatively resistant and can persist in the environment for months. For these reasons, it is advisable to hospitalize these patients for the minimum possible time. Isolation of affected animals is essential to the prevention of spread of an outbreak.

The medical management for adenoviral pneumonia is supportive, and no specific therapies are available. The general measures recommended are similar to those described for distemper pneumonia. Ribavirin has *in vitro* activity against adenoviruses, and successful treatment of adenoviral pneumonia in humans with both intravenous and nebulized ribavirin has been reported.[91-93] Reports of ribavirin for treatment of adenoviral pneumonia in dogs are lacking. The mortality rate associated with CAV-2 is low and the use of antiviral agents in typical cases is unwarranted.

The prevention and limitation of outbreaks of CAV-2 depend on both vaccination and prolonged isolation of recovering animals. Attenuated CAV-2 vaccines are available and are given according to the same schedule as distemper vaccines. Maternally derived antibodies can interfere with responses to CAV-2 vaccines in puppies up to 3 to 4 months of age. The ability of CAV-2 to persist for up to 4 weeks in the respiratory tract of recovering animals suggests that animals diagnosed with this viral infection should be isolated for this time.

Thorough cleaning of facilities with bleach or phenolic-based disinfectants (e.g., Lysol) is essential to containing the spread of the disease. Prevention strategies in animal housing facilities include routine cleaning, maintaining adequate ventilation, and ensuring vaccination before admission. Full quarantine of all animals within a facility for several weeks may be required to contain a significant outbreak.

Prognosis

The prognosis for respiratory disease secondary to CAV-2 infection is generally quite favorable. Most dogs will recover fully with minimal in-hospital care. The long-term effects of respiratory adenoviral infection are uncertain. Experimental infection in dogs has led to altered airway responsiveness to later respiratory challenges. The experimental data suggest that adenoviral infection may result in airway hypersensitivity to bronchoconstriction for a time.[94-96] The relevance of these observations to the naturally-occurring disease is uncertain. Treatment with nedocromil sodium appears to alleviate airway dysfunction in experimental infections.[97]

CANINE PARAINFLUENZA VIRUS TYPE II

Canine parainfluenza virus type II (CPIV) was formerly termed parainfluenza SV-5 and is among the viral causes of kennel cough in dogs.[98] CPIV is a paramyxovirus; it is enveloped and contains single stranded RNA. Similar to CAV-2, severe parainfluenza virus infections can lead to the development of pneumonia. Transmission of CPIV is by inhalation of aerosol droplets. The virus replicates within the respiratory tract, is shed in respiratory secretions, and causes localized infection. It does not replicate within macrophages, and this helps to prevent dissemination of infective virus.

History and Clinical Signs

The history and clinical presentation are often identical to that for CAV-2 infection. It is generally diagnosed in young dogs and in those with a recent history of exposure to a kennel or shelter environment. The typical clinical signs are those of rhinitis and tracheobronchitis, with conjunctivitis and bronchopneumonia less commonly seen. Persistent cough is the most common owner complaint. The signs are typically mild unless the patient has secondary infection with either bacterial pathogens or distemper virus.

Diagnostic Testing

Similar to CAV-2, uncomplicated CPIV pneumonia results in minimal changes in the standard database. Thoracic radiographs generally reveal a bronchointerstitial pattern. Canine parainfluenza virus type II causes localized infection of the respiratory tract and conjunctiva. Cytology of BAL or transtracheal aspirates may reveal a lymphocytic, neutrophilic, or mixed inflammatory response. Inclusion bodies, when seen, are typically cytoplasmic. Appropriate samples for viral isolation include nasal and ocular swabs, conjunctival scrapings, transtracheal aspirates, and BAL fluid. Virus isolation may be performed by inoculation of embryonating chicken eggs. CPIV contains a hemagglutinin protein, and hemagglutination inhibition (HI) testing can be used to identify the virus by using specific antiserum. Acute and convalescent serum samples drawn 3 weeks apart may be used for both HI and serum neutralization testing. A fourfold rise in titer is considered significant and indicates recent infection.

Pathological and Histopathological Findings

Within the respiratory tract, CPIV causes diffuse bronchiolitis and mild epithelial necrosis.[98-100] Submucosal edema and infiltration of bronchiolar and alveolar structures with a mixed inflammatory cell infiltrate may be noted. CPIV can cause destruction of ciliated epithelium and allow invasion by bacteria and mycoplasma. Substantial bronchopneumonia occurs rarely in immunocompetent dogs. In tissue culture, parainfluenza virus can induce the formation of multinucleated giant cells, but the giant cell pneumonia of measles or distemper is not seen clinically with CPIV infection.[101]

Management and Monitoring

General management and monitoring of CPIV pneumonia is identical to that for CAV-2 infection. Aerosolized ribavirin has been used in the treatment of parainfluenza pneumonia in humans but controlled studies are lacking.[102] Specific therapies for the treatment of CPIV infection are lacking. Experimentally, it is difficult to produce significant respiratory disease in dogs with CPIV alone. If a patient shows significant respiratory compromise, and CPIV is the only pathogen isolated, a thorough evaluation of the dog's immune status is warranted.

Vaccination is central to the prevention of CPIV infection. Both parenteral and intranasal vaccine preparations are available. Parenteral vaccines include attenuated CPIV in combination with distemper and CAV-2. Intranasal vaccines include avirulent live *B. bronchiseptica* in combination with modified live CPIV. Parenteral vaccine schedules for CPIV follow those for distemper and CAV-2. The intranasal vaccine may be given to puppies as young as 2 weeks old because maternally derived antibodies do not interfere with the generation of a local immune response. Intranasal vaccines may be readministered yearly to maintain the immune response. In addition, many boarding facilities advise intranasal vaccination before admission. In breeding colonies where CPIV, specifically, or kennel cough, in general, is a significant problem, intranasal administration to all puppies at 2 weeks of age is advised.

The disease produced by CPIV is generally mild and seldom warrants hospital admission. The disease is sufficiently contagious that home management of cases is advised whenever possible. When animals with CPIV are hospitalized they should be isolated from other patients to decrease aerosol transmission. Housing facilities should be thoroughly cleaned with bleach.

Prognosis

The prognosis for uncomplicated CPIV is excellent. Secondary bacterial pneumonia can worsen the prognosis if antibiotic resistant bacterial pathogens are identified. CPIV is unlikely to produce significant respiratory disease in the immunocompetent canine, thus the prognosis in dogs with CPIV pneumonia may be determined by an underlying cause of immunosuppression rather than by the viral illness itself.

Viral Pneumonia in Cats

Infectious pneumonia is less commonly seen in the feline species than in dogs. Respiratory compromise from infectious disease in cats is more often seen because of upper respiratory viral infection or pyothorax. As in dogs, many of the viral causes of large airway or upper respiratory tract disease can also cause pneumonia in severe cases. Several different viruses have been isolated from cats with respiratory disease, but most viral pneumonia in cats is caused by feline herpesvirus-1 (FHV-1), feline calicivirus (FCV), or poxvirus.

FELINE HERPESVIRUS-1 (FHV-1)

Infection with FHV-1 in cats is often referred to as rhinopneumonitis or rhinotracheitis. The virus is also referred to as feline rhinotracheitis virus. In addition to respiratory signs, the ocular changes associated with FHV-1 infection are often the most severe manifestation of the disease. Feline herpesvirus-1 is an alpha-herpesvirus with double-stranded DNA. During replication this virus can yield both enveloped and naked particles. There are multiple strains but only one serotype.

Exposure to FHV-1 is by the oronasal or conjunctival route.[103] Direct cat-to-cat transmission is probably typical, although contact with excretions/secretions can also lead to exposure. The virus probably is spread only rarely by aerosol exposure. Chronic carriers that shed intermittently even when not overtly ill expose other cats to the virus. One study estimates that 90% of cats worldwide have been exposed to FHV-1.[104] After primary inoculation of oral, nasal, or conjunctival mucosa the virus undergoes rapid replication within epithelial cells. This period of rapid replication induces cytolysis. Viremia generally does not occur, and viral spread to and replication within the viscera is rare. Following initial infection, latent infection can be lifelong, with virus residing in sensory ganglia. The severity and extent of the disease can be worsened by concurrent infection with FIV or FeLV.[105]

History and Clinical Signs

Feline herpes viral infections may manifest in susceptible cats recently exposed to the virus, or as a recrudescence of the infection in carrier cats. In older carrier cats there may be a history of a stressful event such as travel or boarding, or administration of corticosteroids. Young stray cats and cats adopted from shelters are often afflicted with the disease. In some studies, the prevalence of feline respiratory viruses was greater in rescue catteries than in breeding catteries.[106]

The course of the viral illness is usually self-limiting over a period of 1 to 3 weeks. The predominant clinical signs are typically those of upper respiratory disease and keratoconjunctivitis[107] including fever; lethargy; sneezing; oculonasal discharge; and, occasionally, hypersalivation. Keratitis may manifest as the characteristic linear dendritic ulcers of FHV-1. In young kittens, herpesvirus infection may present as "fading kitten" syndrome. Pneumonia has been reported to develop in some younger patients.[108,109] Although pneumonia is uncommon in FHV-1 infection, it may cause coughing, which is otherwise uncommon in the disease. The primary differentials for upper respiratory tract infection with pulmonary involvement are feline calicivirus, *Bordetella bronchiseptica*, and *Chlamydia psittaci.* Bordetellosis has recently emerged as a feline respiratory tract pathogen of previously under-appreciated importance.[110-113]

Diagnostic Testing

A tentative diagnosis can often be made based on history and clinical signs, particularly if the characteristic dendritic ulcers are present. Changes in the complete blood count, chemistry profile, and urinalysis are usually minimal or nonspecific. Thoracic radiographs may show a diffuse bronchointerstitial pattern. Although

some manifestations of FHV-1 related disease may present a diagnostic challenge, cats with FHV-1 infection of such severity as to present with pneumonia are generally shedding virus in large quantities. Oropharyngeal, nasal, or conjunctival swabs may be submitted for virus isolation.[104,114] Conjunctival scrapings or nasal swabs may be submitted for immunofluorescent antibody based tests to detect viral antigens. Polymerase chain reaction primers and protocols have been used to detect FHV-1 in cases of ocular disease and are easily modified for samples from the respiratory tract.[114-120] Serum neutralization and ELISA titers may be determined from venous blood samples but vary substantially and appear to correlate poorly with the clinical status of the patient.[104]

Pathological and Histopathological Findings

In those cases in which the epithelial cells of the lower respiratory tract are exposed to virulent virus, pneumonia can occur. Exposure of the lung to virus does not necessarily mean pneumonia will develop. Viral replication is optimal in cooler, superficial sites, and thus signs of ocular, oropharyngeal, and nasal disease are far more common. When pneumonia does develop it is an interstitial pneumonia with necrosis of the bronchial, bronchiolar, and alveolar epithelial surfaces. As with other viruses that cause necrosis of the pulmonary epithelia, the influx of neutrophils can be considerable and create an appearance similar to bacterial bronchopneumonia. The airways and alveolar septae may have accumulations of mixed inflammatory cells. Fibrinous, protein-rich exudate in the airways is not atypical. Secondary bacterial pneumonia commonly occurs.

Management and Monitoring

Most cats with FHV-1 infection are managed as outpatients, and FHV-1 pneumonia is generally only seen in severe cases. Patients with severe FHV-1 infections warrant determination of FIV and FeLV status. Mortality in FHV-1 cases is usually caused by dehydration, malnutrition, and secondary bacterial infection. For this reason the primary focus of acute care should be nutritional support, enteral or parenteral fluids, and treatment with broad-spectrum antibiotics. Antibiotic choice initially is biased towards those with activity against *Chlamydia, Mycoplasma,* and *Bordetella* spp. because each of these agents can cause similar clinical signs. The tetracyclines are reasonable first-line antibiotics in this setting. Cats with significant nasal disease seldom eat adequately. Resolving secondary bacterial rhinitis and using humidification therapy to moisten secretions can help an earlier return to voluntary eating. In the interim, nutritional support may be provided through an esophagostomy tube.

Often pneumonia is part of a larger fading kitten syndrome and intensive care and monitoring are required. Kittens with severe FHV-1 infections rarely take in adequate nutrition, and blood glucose measurement should be among the early diagnostics performed. Supplementation of parenteral fluids with dextrose is often required until full nutritional support is provided.

The use of specific antiherpetic antiviral medications (e.g., Acyclovir) to treat FHV-1 infection has been studied, particularly in the context of topical treatment of ocular disease. The efficacy of these agents has not been established in the treatment of the respiratory manifestations of FHV-1 infection. The doses needed to produce effective serum levels of both acyclovir and valacyclovir tend to produce excessive toxic side effects and preclude their systemic usage in all but the most severe cases.[121-123] Newer antiviral agents that are currently in development appear to hold greater promise.

Adjunctive therapies may also be considered in the treatment of FHV-1 pneumonitis. Lysine has been suggested to have an indirect antiviral effect by limiting the availability of arginine. One study suggested that oral lysine may be of use in the treatment of ocular FHV-1 disease, but clinical trials are lacking at present.[124] Such an effect has not been shown in regard to the respiratory epithelium; however, a dose of 250 mg lysine orally twice daily appears to be associated with relatively few side effects and could be used as an adjunct therapy. Similarly, oral administration of interferon-alpha (5 to 25 units per day) has been proposed as a secondary therapy in the treatment of FHV-1 infection.[125] This dose of interferon appears to improve the patient's clinical state but does not alter viral shedding.

Prevention of FHV-1 infection involves routine vaccination and isolation of cats with overt disease.[126,127] Attempts to isolate carriers are probably not worthwhile in most cases. Both modified live and killed virus vaccines are available. A minimum of two doses of vaccine should be administered to kittens, separated by a 3- or 4-week interval. Intranasal vaccine can be administered to promote rapid mucosal immunity in young kittens or cats entering a new multi-cat household, boarding facility, or shelter. Maternal antibodies generally do not interfere with the acquisition of mucosal immunity. In catteries, early intranasal vaccine administration programs can help limit acute disease and the development of chronic rhinitis or rhinosinusitis.

Prognosis

The prognosis for FHV-1 is variable. Young kittens infected with FHV-1 that present as fading kittens have a guarded prognosis. For cats presenting with upper respiratory signs, the mortality rate is low but chronic morbidity is common. Recrudescent disease is common in some settings (e.g., catteries or in cats with comorbid conditions requiring corticosteroid therapy). Pneumonia generally only occurs in more severe cases and suggests a less favorable prognosis.

FELINE CALICIVIRUS (FCV)

Feline calicivirus is another common cause of upper respiratory disease in cats that can, in severe cases, result in pneumonia. It is thought that infection with FCV results in pneumonia more often than FHV-1, but the frequency with which naturally occurring FCV infection results in pneumonia is uncertain. Experimental studies using aerosol delivery of heavy doses of infective virus appear to produce pneumonia with greater frequency than is seen in clinical practice[128-131]; however, most cats probably acquire FCV via direct contact with other cats and not by inhalation of fine aerosols. There is only one serotype but multiple subtypes. Some strains appear to have greater tropism for pneumocytes than other strains.[132]

Feline calicivirus is a single-stranded RNA virus. Exposure is via inhalation or ingestion of saliva, excretions, or secretions from shedding cats. Direct contact is a more important route of exposure than inhalation of fine aerosols. The virus persists long enough in the environment that indirect exposure is likely possible in multi-cat environments. Coinfection with either FIV or FHV increases the severity of the disease.

History and Clinical Signs

Patients with respiratory disease caused by FCV infection often present with historical and clinical findings similar to those seen in FHV-1 infection. The disease is more often noted in kittens than in adult cats, and it is primarily a disease of multi-cat environments such as catteries or shelters.[106] New kittens introduced to homes with adult cats will often manifest signs of upper respiratory disease within days or weeks of arrival. The predominant clinical signs include altered eating patterns because of oral ulceration and pain, sneezing, low-grade fever, oculonasal discharge, rhinitis, and conjunctivitis. Coughing may be noted in cases with pneumonia but generally is not prominent. Dyspnea may be noted and may be the chief complaint in some cases.

Cats with FCV infections generally appear less systemically ill than those suffering from FHV-1. Two important differences between FHV-1 and FCV infection are that FCV does not cause keratitis, and FHV-1 rarely causes oral ulceration. These differences may help to make a tentative diagnosis while awaiting further diagnostics.

Diagnostic Testing

The differences between the clinical signs associated with the two most common causes of viral respiratory disease in cats often allow a tentative diagnosis to be made; further diagnostics may not be pursued in an isolated case. To obtain a definitive viral diagnosis, nasal swabs, oropharyngeal swabs, or conjunctival scrapings may be submitted for virus isolation. Fluorescent or immunohistochemical antibody-based assays can also be applied to conjunctival scrapings as well as tonsillar biopsies.[133] Serology is generally not helpful because of widespread vaccination in many parts of the world. Polymerase chain reaction can be used to identify feline calicivirus nucleic acid sequences.[119]

The minimum clinical database typically has few changes or those of a nonspecific inflammatory illness. Thoracic radiographs may show patchy infiltrates. FIV status should be determined because coinfection with FIV can be associated with more severe disease and has prognostic implications.[134]

Pathological and Histopathological Findings

Some strains of FCV have strong tropism for type I pneumocytes. On gross inspection the lungs appear edematous with sharply demarcated, solid, dark purple lesions near the lung periphery. The infiltrates are often patchy in distribution, and approximately 20% of cats have sharply demarcated bands of lung congestion. The pulmonary lesions of calicivirus infection are those of an acute to subacute interstitial pneumonia.[128] Caliciviral infections typically produce less bronchiolitis than is seen with other viral pneumonias. Necrosis of type I pneumocytes can lead to leakage of protein rich fluid into the airspaces and initiate an influx of neutrophils. Hyaline membranes may form. As the disease progresses, the predominant lesions are proliferation of type II pneumocytes and infiltration with mononuclear inflammatory cells.

Management and Monitoring

Management principles are similar to those for FHV-1 infections. Oral ulceration can make nutritional support challenging. Few cats with painful ulcers will tolerate oral rinses, although these products may speed the healing of painful ulcers. Cats may be tempted to eat by providing appetizing, aromatic foods and administrating small doses of intravenous diazepam before the presentation of a meal. In cases where oral intake of nutrition is inadequate, placement of an esophagostomy tube should be considered. Maintaining adequate hydration and electrolyte balance via parenteral fluids is an important component of any treatment plan. Blood glucose levels should be monitored early in the management of kittens with FCV infections that have not been eating. Supplementation of fluids with dextrose can help maintain blood glucose levels until nutritional status improves.

Caliciviral infections tend to cause less severe systemic signs than those caused by FHV-1, and many cats can be managed as outpatients. Isolation of affected animals is important to prevent the spread to unaffected, susceptible cats. Patients with more severe respiratory compromise should be managed as inpatients. Dyspneic cats should be provided with supplemental oxygen. When pneumonia is present, antibiotics should be administered. As in FHV-1 infection, tetracyclines are an appropriate class of antibiotic to start with until sensitivity results are available. No specific antiviral medications are available for the treatment of caliciviral infections in cats. Ribavirin has *in vitro* activity against calicivirus but *in vivo* produced more severe illness in calicivirus infected cats.[135,136]

The cornerstone of prevention is the routine vaccination of household cats. Several parenteral vaccines (both modified live virus and inactivated adjuvanted virus) are available. Vaccine schedules follow those for FHV-1. Newer vaccines continue to be developed. Intranasal vaccines can be given if a cat is about to enter a high-risk environment such as a boarding facility. However, the intranasal route is more likely to produce side effects such as signs of upper respiratory tract inflammation. In boarding facilities, cats from different households should be housed separately. Physical barriers and a distance of at least a meter should separate cats from different homes. Cats can sneeze macrodroplets of respiratory secretions to a distance of nearly 2 meters. Thorough cleaning of housing as well as food and water bowls is essential.

Prognosis

The prognosis for recovery from caliciviral respiratory disease is generally favorable. Disease is often mild and self-limiting; however, many cats can become lifelong carriers and shed virus fairly constantly. Some animals may develop chronic oropharyngeal disease, but chronic lower respiratory tract disease has not been reported.

FELINE COWPOX

Cowpox infection is an uncommon cause of viral pneumonia in the cat.[12,41,137] It is found only in Europe and Asia where wild rodents serve as reservoir hosts, and hunting reservoir animals typically leads to feline infections. The peak incidence of feline cowpox infection is during late summer and early fall when rodent populations are at their greatest. The initial presenting complaint is typically multifocal skin lesions. The appearance of the lesions is variable; they can be mistaken for cat bite abscesses or eosinophilic granulomas. Samples of the skin lesions can be evaluated microscopically for the presence of eosinophilic cytoplasmic inclusion bodies. Fluorescent antibodies can be applied to samples of the skin lesions to detect cowpox antigens. Material from skin lesions can also be submitted for virus isolation. Serum antibody titers are generally diagnostic because the disease is not widespread in cats and vaccines are not available. When pneumonia or other systemic signs are noted, the prognosis is generally poor. Cowpox can cause extensive pulmonary necrosis and a significant purulent inflammatory response can be noted. Feline cowpox has not been reported in North America. The disease is zoonotic, and owners of infected cats should be advised to consult their physicians.

Conclusion

Viral infections of the upper respiratory tract are common in dogs and cats. Although these viruses can produce pneumonia, they generally only do so in severe cases or when the patient is immunocompromised. Canine distemper is unique in this regard because this virus can itself produce significant immune suppression. For this reason canine distemper is more likely to produce clinically significant viral pneumonia than most other agents. Viral strains vary in their tropism, and those that favor pneumocytes are more likely to produce interstitial pneumonia when they gain access to the lower respiratory tract. Viral infections of the lung typically produce a pattern of lesions termed *bronchointerstitial pneumonia*. Early lesions are predominantly centered on the airways and may be purulent. Over time the primary focus of the lesions becomes alveolar, and interstitial and mononuclear infiltrates are typical. Viral pneumonia in dogs is largely because of canine distemper virus, canine adenovirus type II, and parainfluenza virus type II. In cats, viral pneumonia is typically the result of infection with feline herpesvirus-I or feline calicivirus, although in Western Europe feline cowpox pneumonia has been noted. Viral infection can suppress pulmonary antibacterial defenses, and secondary bacterial pneumonia is common. Treatment of viral pneumonia is generally supportive although a few antiviral agents warrant consideration in the treatment of dogs and cats. The prognosis for viral pneumonia is often good although systemic illness, secondary bacterial infections, and coinfection with other viruses can lead to worsening of the outcome.

REFERENCES

1. Walter JH, Kirchhoff A: Causes of illness in young dogs in necropsy files (1980-1993), *Berl Munch Tierarztl Wochenschr* 108(4):121-126, 1995.
2. Krakowka S, Koestner A: Age-related susceptibility to infection with canine distemper virus in gnotobiotic dogs, *J Infect Dis* 134(6):629-632, 1976.
3. Krakowka S, Hoover EA, Koestner A et al: Experimental and naturally occurring transplacental transmission of canine distemper virus, *Am J Vet Res* 38(7):919-922, 1977.
4. Binn LN, Eddy GA, Lazar EC et al: Viruses recovered from laboratory dogs with respiratory disease, *Proc Soc Exp Biol Med* 126(1):140-145, 1967.
5. Binn LN, Alford JP, Marchwicki RH et al: Studies of respiratory disease in random-source laboratory dogs: Viral infections in unconditioned dogs, *Lab Anim Sci* 29(1):48-52, 1979.
6. Van Rensberg IB, De Clerk J, Groenewald HB et al: An outbreak of African horsesickness in dogs, *J S Afr Vet Assoc* 52(4):323-325, 1981.
7. Appel MJ, Menegus M, Parsonson IM et al: Pathogenesis of canine herpesvirus in specific-pathogen-free dogs: 5- to 12-week-old pups, *Am J Vet Res* 30(12):2067-2073, 1969.
8. Kakuk TJ, Conner GH: Experimental canine herpesvirus in the gnotobiotic dog, *Lab Anim Care* 20(1):69-79, 1970.
9. Binn LN, Lazar EC, Helms J et al: Viral antibody patterns in laboratory dogs with respiratory disease, *Am J Vet Res* 31(4):697-702, 1970.
10. Binn LN, Marchwicki RH, Keenan KP et al: Recovery of reovirus type 2 from an immature dog with respiratory tract disease, *Am J Vet Res* 38(7):927-929, 1977.
11. Kahn DE, Hoover EA: Infectious respiratory diseases of cats, *Vet Clin North Am* 6(3):399-413, 1976.
12. Vestey JP, Yirrell DL, Aldridge RD: Cowpox/catpox infection, *Br J Dermatol* 124(1):74-78, 1991.
13. Bart M, Guscetti F, Zurbriggen A et al: Feline infectious pneumonia: A short literature review and a retrospective immunohistological study on the involvement of Chlamydia spp. and distemper virus, *Vet J* 159(3):220-230, 2000.
14. Hawkins EC, Kennedy-Stoskopf S, Levy JK et al: Effect of FIV infection on lung inflammatory cell populations recovered by bronchoalveolar lavage, *Vet Immunol Immunopathol* 51(1-2):21-28, 1996.
15. Ritchey JW, Levy JK, Bliss SK et al: Constitutive expression of types 1 and 2 cytokines by alveolar macrophages from feline immunodeficiency virus-infected cats, *Vet Immunol Immunopathol* 79(1-2):83-100, 2001.
16. Weiss RC, Scott FW: Pathogenesis of feline infectious peritonitis: Pathologic changes and immunofluorescence, *Am J Vet Res* 42(12):2036-2048, 1981.
17. Montali RJ, Strandberg JD: Extraperitoneal lesions in feline infectious peritonitis, *Vet Pathol* 9(2):109-121, 1972.
18. Welliver RC, Ogra PL: Immunology of respiratory viral infections, *Ann Rev Med* 39:147-162, 1988.
19. Woodland DL, Hogan RJ, Zhong W: Cellular immunity and memory to respiratory virus infections, *Immunol Res* 24(1):53-67, 2001.
20. LeVine AM, Whitsett JA, Hartshorn KL et al: Surfactant protein D enhances clearance of influenza A virus from the lung in vivo, *J Immunol* 167(10):5868-5873, 2001.
21. McSharry JJ, Pickering RJ, Caliguiri LA: Activation of the alternative complement pathway by enveloped viruses containing limited amounts of sialic acid, *Virology* 114(2):507-515, 1981.
22. Sen GC: Viruses and interferons, *Annu Rev Microbiol* 55:255-281, 2001.
23. Shanley JD, Pesanti EL: The relation of viral replication to interstitial pneumonitis in murine cytomegalovirus lung infection, *J Infect Dis* 151(3):454-458, 1985.
24. Liu SF, Dewar A, Crawley DE et al: Effect of tumor necrosis factor on hypoxic pulmonary vasoconstriction, *J Appl Physiol* 72(3):1044-1049, 1992.
25. Freihofer AF, Brooks SM, Loudon RG et al: Functional effects of influenzal pneumonia, *Chest* 66(Suppl):36S-37S, 1974.
26. Manning HL, Mahler DA: Pathophysiology of dyspnea, *Monaldi Arch Chest Dis* 56(4):325-330, 2001.
27. Micillo E, Bianco A, D'Auria D et al: Respiratory infections and asthma, *Allergy* 55(Suppl 61):42-45, 2000.
28. Jakab GJ: Sequential virus infections, bacterial superinfections, and fibrogenesis, *Am Rev Respir Dis* 142(2):374-379, 1990.
29. Jakab GJ: Mechanisms of bacterial superinfections in viral pneumonias, *Schweiz Med Wochenschr* 115(3):75-86, 1985.
30. Jakab GJ, Warr GA: The participation of antiviral immune mechanisms in alveolar macrophage dysfunction during viral pneumonia, *Bull Eur Physiopathol Respir* 19(2):173-178, 1983.
31. Jakab GJ: Viral-bacterial interactions in pulmonary infection, *Adv Vet Sci Comp Med* 26:155-171, 1982.
32. Jakab GJ: Immune impairment of alveolar macrophage phagocytosis during influenza virus pneumonia, *Am Rev Respir Dis* 126(5):778-782, 1982.
33. Jakab GJ, Warr GA, Sannes PL: Alveolar macrophage ingestion and phagosome-lysosome fusion defect associated with virus pneumonia, *Infect Immun* 27(3):960-968, 1980.
34. Jakab GJ, Green GM: Pulmonary defense mechanisms in consolidated and nonconsolidated regions of lungs infected with Sendai virus, *J Infect Dis* 129(3):363-367, 1974.
35. Jakab GJ, Green GM: Immune enhancement of pulmonary bactericidal activity in murine virus pneumonia, *J Clin Invest* 52(11):2878-2884, 1973.
36. Nickerson CL, Jakab GJ: Pulmonary antibacterial defenses during mild and severe influenza virus infection, *Infect Immun* 58(9):2809-2814, 1990.
37. Warr GA, Jakab GJ: Alterations in lung macrophage antimicrobial activity associated with viral pneumonia, *Infect Immun* 26(2):492-497, 1979.
38. Green G: Antimicrob Agents Chemother 1966:26-29.
39. Bjotvedt G, Geib LW, Mann PH: The role of canine distemper in respiratory disease of non-conditioned laboratory dogs, *Lab Anim Care* 19(6):789-794, 1969.
40. McCandlish IA, Thompson H, Cornwell HJ et al: A study of dogs with kennel cough, *Vet Rec* 102(14):293-301, 1978.
41. Bennett M, Gaskell RM, Gaskell CJ et al: Studies on poxvirus infection in cats, *Arch Virol* 104(1-2):19-33, 1989.
42. Ek-Kommonen C, Sihvonen L, Pekkanen K et al: Outbreak of canine distemper in vaccinated dogs in Finland, *Vet Rec* 141(15):380-383, 1997.
43. FitzGerald K: Distemper in vaccinated dogs, *Vet Rec* 115(7):158-159, 1984.
44. Sidhu MS, Husar W, Cook SD et al: Canine distemper terminal and intergenic non-protein coding nucleotide sequences: completion of the entire CDV genome sequence, *Virology* 193(1):66-72, 1993.
45. Raw ME, Pearson GR, Brown PJ et al: Canine distemper infection associated with acute nervous signs in dogs, *Vet Rec* 130(14):291-293, 1992.
46. Vandevelde M, Kristensen B, Braund KG et al: Chronic canine distemper virus encephalitis in mature dogs, *Vet Pathol* 17(1):17-28, 1980.
47. Bencsik A, Malcus C, Akaoka H et al: Selective induction of cytokines in mouse brain infected with canine distemper virus: structural, cellular and temporal expression, *J Neuroimmunol* 65(1):1-9, 1996.

48. Grone A, Frisk AL, Baumgartner W: Cytokine mRNA expression in whole blood samples from dogs with natural canine distemper virus infection, *Vet Immunol Immunopathol* 65(1):11-27, 1998.

49. Iwatsuki K, Okita M, Ochikubo F et al: Immunohistochemical analysis of the lymphoid organs of dogs naturally infected with canine distemper virus, *J Comp Pathol* 113(2):185-190, 1995.

50. Krakowka S, Cockerell G, Koestner A: Effects of canine distemper virus infection on lymphoid function *in vitro* and in vivo, *Infect Immun* 11(5):1069-1078, 1975.

51. Toman M, Svoboda M, Rybnicek J et al: Secondary immunodeficiency in dogs with enteric, dermatologic, infectious or parasitic diseases, *Zentralbl Veterinarmed (B)* 45(6):321-334, 1998.

52. Blixenkrone-Moller M, Svansson V, Have P et al: Studies on manifestations of canine distemper virus infection in an urban dog population, *Vet Microbiol* 37(1-2):163-173, 1993.

53. Appel MJ: Pathogenesis of canine distemper, *Am J Vet Res* 30(7):1167-1182, 1969.

54. Appel MJ: Distemper pathogenesis in dogs, *J Am Vet Med Assoc* 156(12):1681-1684, 1970.

55. Carrasco L, Hervas J, Gomez-Villamandos JC et al: Massive Filaroides hirthi infestation associated with canine distemper in a puppy, *Vet Rec* 140(3):72-73, 1997.

56. Sukura A, Laakkonen J, Rudback E: Occurrence of Pneumocystis carinii in canine distemper, *Acta Vet Scand* 38(2):201-205, 1997.

57. Dobos-Kovacs M: Studies on the diagnostic value of cell inclusions in canine distemper, *Acta Vet Acad Sci Hung* 25(2-3):185-200, 1975.

58. Watson AD, Wright RG: The ultrastructure of cytoplasmic inclusions in circulating lymphocytes in canine distemper, *Res Vet Sci* 17(2):188-192, 1974.

59. Watson AD, Wright RG: The ultrastructure of inclusions in blood cells of dogs with distemper, *J Comp Pathol* 84(3):417-427, 1974.

60. Axthelm MK, Krakowka S: Immunocytochemical methods for demonstrating canine distemper virus antigen in aldehyde-fixed paraffin-embedded tissue, *J Virol Methods* 13(3):215-229, 1986.

61. Frisk AL, Konig M, Moritz A et al: Detection of canine distemper virus nucleoprotein RNA by reverse transcription-PCR using serum, whole blood, and cerebrospinal fluid from dogs with distemper, *J Clin Microbiol* 37(11):3634-3643, 1999.

62. Miry C, Ducatelle R, Thoonen H et al: Immunoperoxidase study of canine distemper virus pneumonia, *Res Vet Sci* 34(2):145-148, 1983.

63. Motohashi T, Nakagawa H, Okada T: Fluorescent antibody technic in diagnosis of canine distemper, *Vet Med Small Anim Clin* 64(12):1057-1060, 1969.

64. Fairchild GA, Steinberg SA, Cohen D: The fluorescent antibody test as a diagnostic test for canine distemper in naturally infected dogs, *Cornell Vet* 61(2):214-223, 1971.

65. von Messling V, Harder TC, Moennig V et al: Rapid and sensitive detection of immunoglobulin M (IgM) and IgG antibodies against canine distemper virus by a new recombinant nucleocapsid protein-based enzyme-linked immunosorbent assay, *J Clin Microbiol* 37(4):1049-1056, 1999.

66. Blixenkrone-Moller M, Pedersen IR, Appel MJ et al: Detection of IgM antibodies against canine distemper virus in dog and mink sera employing enzyme-linked immunosorbent assay (ELISA), *J Vet Diagn Invest* 3(1):3-9, 1991.

67. Fairchild GA, Wyman M, Donovan EF: Fluorescent antibody technique as a diagnostic test for canine distemper infection: detection of viral antigen in epithelial tissues of experimentally infected dogs, *Am J Vet Res* 28(124):761-768, 1967.

68. Connolly MG, Jr., Baughman RP, Dohn MN et al: Recovery of viruses other than cytomegalovirus from bronchoalveolar lavage fluid, *Chest* 105(6):1775-1781, 1994.

69. Bui HD, Tobler LH, Van Pelt LF et al: Canine bladder epithelial cells in culture: Susceptibility to canine distemper and measles viruses, *Am J Vet Res* 43(7):1268-1270, 1982.

70. Dagle GE, Zwicker GM, Adee RR et al: Cytoplasmic inclusions in urinary bladder epithelium of dogs, *Vet Pathol* 16(2):258-259, 1979.

71. Richter WR, Moize SM: Ultrastructural nature of canine distemper inclusions in the urinary bladder, *Pathol Vet* 7(4):346-352, 1970.

72. Deem SL, Spelman LH, Yates RA et al: Canine distemper in terrestrial carnivores: A review, *J Zoo Wildl Med* 31(4):441-451, 2000.

73. Leisewitz AL, Carter A, van Vuuren M et al: Canine distemper infections, with special reference to South Africa, with a review of the literature, *J S Afr Vet Assoc* 72(3):127-136, 2001.

74. Wadman-Taylor WM: Canine distemper, *Vet Rec* 119(2):52, 1986.

75. Gururangan S, Stevens RF, Morris DJ: Ribavirin response in measles pneumonia, *J Infect* 20(3):219-221, 1990.

76. Forni AL, Schluger NW, Roberts RB: Severe measles pneumonitis in adults: Evaluation of clinical characteristics and therapy with intravenous ribavirin, *Clin Infect Dis* 19(3):454-462, 1994.

77. Rupp ME, Schwartz ML, Bechard DE: Measles pneumonia: Treatment of a near-fatal case with corticosteroids and vitamin A, *Chest* 103(5):1625-1626, 1993.

78. Nara PL, Krakowka S, Powers TE: Effects of prednisolone on the development of immune responses to canine distemper virus in beagle pups, *Am J Vet Res* 40(12):1742-1747, 1979.

79. West CE: Vitamin A and measles, *Nutr Rev* 58(2 Pt 2):S46-S54, 2000.

80. D'Souza RM, D'Souza R: Vitamin A for treating measles in children (Cochrane Review), *Cochrane Database Syst Rev* 2, 2001.

81. Chappuis G: Control of canine distemper, *Vet Microbiol* 44(2-4):351-358, 1995.

82. Patronek GJ, Glickman LT, Johnson R et al: Canine distemper infection in pet dogs, II: A case-control study of risk factors during a suspected outbreak in Indiana, *J Am Anim Hosp Assoc* 31(3):230-235, 1995.

83. Castleman WL: Bronchiolitis obliterans and pneumonia induced in young dogs by experimental adenovirus infection, *Am J Pathol* 119(3):495-504, 1985.

84. Ducatelle R, Thoonen H, Coussement W et al: Pathology of natural canine adenovirus pneumonia, *Res Vet Sci* 31(2):207-212, 1981.

85. Ducatelle R, Palmer D, Ossent P et al: Immunoperoxidase study of adenovirus pneumonia in dogs, *Vet Q* 7(4):290-296, 1985.

86. Grad R, Sobonya RE, Witten ML et al: Localization of inflammation and virions in canine adenovirus type 2 bronchiolitis, *Am Rev Respir Dis* 142(3):691-699, 1990.

87. van Rensburg IB, Greenberg M: Adenovirus pneumonia in a puppy, *J S Afr Vet Assoc* 54(4):267-269, 1983.

88. Wright NG, Thompson H, Cornwell HJ: Canine adenovirus pneumonia, *Res Vet Sci* 12(2):162-167, 1971.

89. Ducatelle R, Maenhout D, Coussement W et al: Dual adenovirus and distemper virus pneumonia in a dog, *Vet Q* 4(2):84-88, 1982.

90. Shirota K, Azetaka M, Fujiwara K: A case of canine respiratory adenovirus infection associated with distemper, *Nippon Juigaku Zasshi* 42(2):265-270, 1980.

91. Buchdahl RM, Taylor P, Warner JD: Nebulised ribavirin for adenovirus pneumonia, *Lancet* 2(8463):1070-1071, 1985.

92. Sabroe I, McHale J, Tait DR et al: Treatment of adenoviral pneumonitis with intravenous ribavirin and immunoglobulin, *Thorax* 50(11):1219-1220, 1995.

93. Shetty AK, Gans HA, So S et al: Intravenous ribavirin therapy for adenovirus pneumonia, *Pediatr Pulmonol* 29(1):69-73, 2000.

94. Quan SF, Lemen RJ, Witten ML et al: Changes in lung mechanics and reactivity with age after viral bronchiolitis in beagle puppies, *J Appl Physiol* 69(6):2034-2042, 1990.

95. Quan SF, Witten ML, Grad R et al: Changes in lung mechanics and histamine responsiveness after sequential canine adenovirus 2 and canine parainfluenza 2 virus infection in beagle puppies, *Pediatr Pulmonol* 10(4):236-243, 1991.

96. Quan SF, Witten ML, Grad R et al: Acute canine adenovirus 2 infection increases histamine airway reactivity in beagle puppies, *Am Rev Respir Dis* 141(2):414-420, 1990.

97. Anderson KA, Lemen RJ, Weger NS et al: Nedocromil sodium inhibits canine adenovirus bronchiolitis in beagle puppies, *Toxicol Pathol* 28(2):317-325, 2000.

98. Appel MJ, Percy DH. SV-5-like parainfluenza virus in dogs, *J Am Vet Med Assoc* 156(12):1778-1781, 1970.

99. Lemen RJ, Quan SF, Witten ML et al: Canine parainfluenza type 2 bronchiolitis increases histamine responsiveness in beagle puppies, *Am Rev Respir Dis* 141(1):199-207, 1990.

100. Wagener JS, Minnich L, Sobonya R et al: Parainfluenza type II infection in dogs: A model for viral lower respiratory tract infection in humans, *Am Rev Respir Dis* 127(6):771-775, 1983.

101. Crandell RA, Brumlow WB, Davison VE: Isolation of a parainfluenza virus from sentry dogs with upper respiratory disease, *Am J Vet Res* 29(11):2141-2147, 1968.

102. Wendt CH, Weisdorf DJ, Jordan MC et al: Parainfluenza virus respiratory infection after bone marrow transplantation, *N Engl J Med* 326(14):921-926, 1992.

103. Gaskell RM, Povey RC: Transmission of feline viral rhinotracheitis, *Vet Rec* 111(16):359-362, 1982.

104. Maggs DJ, Lappin MR, Reif JS et al: Evaluation of serologic and viral detection methods for diagnosing feline herpesvirus-1 infection in cats with acute respiratory tract or chronic ocular disease, *J Am Vet Med Assoc* 214(4):502-507, 1999.

105. Kawaguchi Y, Mikami T. Molecular interactions between retroviruses and herpesviruses, *J Vet Med Sci* 57(5):801-811, 1995.

106. Binns SH, Dawson S, Speakman AJ et al: A study of feline upper respiratory tract disease with reference to prevalence and risk factors for infection with feline calicivirus and feline herpesvirus, *J Feline Med Surg* 2(3):123-133, 2000.

107. Stiles J: Feline herpesvirus, *Vet Clin North Am Small Anim Pract* 30(5):1001-1014, 2000.

108. Fulton RW, Cho DY, Downing M et al: Isolation of feline herpesvirus 1 from a young kitten, *Vet Rec* 106(23):479-481, 1980.

109. Feinstein L, Miller GF, Penney BE: Diagnostic exercise: Lethal pneumonia in neonatal kittens, *Lab Anim Sci* 48(2):190-192, 1998.

110. Hoskins JD, Williams J, Roy AF et al: Isolation and characterization of Bordetella bronchiseptica from cats in southern Louisiana, *Vet Immunol Immunopathol* 65(2-4):173-176, 1998.

111. Binns SH, Dawson S, Speakman AJ et al: Prevalence and risk factors for feline Bordetella bronchiseptica infection, *Vet Rec* 144(21):575-580, 1999.

112. Dawson S, Jones D, McCracken CM et al: Bordetella bronchiseptica infection in cats following contact with infected dogs, *Vet Rec* 146(2):46-48, 2000.

113. Jensen AL, Iversen L, Lee MH et al: Seroprevalence of antibodies to Bordetella bronchiseptica in cats in the Copenhagen area of Denmark, *Vet Rec* 143(21):592, 1998.

114. Burgesser KM, Hotaling S, Schiebel A et al: Comparison of PCR, virus isolation, and indirect fluorescent antibody staining in the detection of naturally occurring feline herpesvirus infections, *J Vet Diagn Invest* 11(2):122-126, 1999.

115. Hara M, Fukuyama M, Suzuki Y et al: Detection of feline herpesvirus 1 DNA by the nested polymerase chain reaction, *Vet Microbiol* 48(3-4):345-352, 1996.

116. Reubel GH, Ramos RA, Hickman MA et al: Detection of active and latent feline herpesvirus 1 infections using the polymerase chain reaction, *Arch Virol* 132(3-4):409-420, 1993.

117. Stiles J, McDermott M, Bigsby D et al: Use of nested polymerase chain reaction to identify feline herpesvirus in ocular tissue from clinically normal cats and cats with corneal sequestra or conjunctivitis, *Am J Vet Res* 58(4):338-342, 1997.

118. Suchy A, Bauder B, Gelbmann W et al: Diagnosis of feline herpesvirus infection by immunohistochemistry, polymerase chain reaction, and in situ hybridization, *J Vet Diagn Invest* 12(2):186-191, 2000.

119. Sykes JE, Allen JL, Studdert VP et al: Detection of feline calicivirus, feline herpesvirus 1 and Chlamydia psittaci mucosal swabs by multiplex RT-PCR/PCR, *Vet Microbiol* 81(2):95-108, 2001.

120. Weigler BJ, Babineau CA, Sherry B et al: High sensitivity polymerase chain reaction assay for active and latent feline herpesvirus-1 infections in domestic cats, *Vet Rec* 140(13):335-338, 1997.

121. Nasisse MP, Dorman DC, Jamison KC et al: Effects of valacyclovir in cats infected with feline herpesvirus 1, *Am J Vet Res* 58(10):1141-1144, 1997.

122. Hirschberger J: Administration of acyclovir (virustatic) to cats, *Tierarztl Prax* 16(4):427-430, 1988.

123. Owens JG, Nasisse MP, Tadepalli SM et al: Pharmacokinetics of acyclovir in the cat, *J Vet Pharmacol Ther* 19(6):488-490, 1996.

124. Maggs DJ, Collins BK, Thorne JG et al: Effects of L-lysine and L-arginine on *in vitro* replication of feline herpesvirus type-1, *Am J Vet Res* 61(12):1474-1378, 2000.

125. Hargis AM, Ginn PE: Feline herpesvirus 1-associated facial and nasal dermatitis and stomatitis in domestic cats, *Vet Clin North Am Small Anim Pract* 29(6):1281-1290, 1999.

126. August JR: Feline viral respiratory disease. The carrier state, vaccination, and control, *Vet Clin North Am Small Anim Pract* 14(6):1159-1171, 1984.

127. Chappuis G, Brun A, Precausta P et al: Immunization against respiratory diseases in cats, *Comp Immunol Microbiol Infect Dis* 1(3):221-227, 1979.

128. Hoover EA, Kahn DE: Experimentally induced feline calicivirus infection: Clinical signs and lesions, *J Am Vet Med Assoc* 166(5):463-468, 1975.

129. Langloss JM, Hoover EA, Kahn DE: Diffuse alveolar damage in cats induced by nitrogen dioxide or feline calicivirus, *Am J Pathol* 89(3):637-648, 1977.

130. Langloss JM, Hoover EA, Kahn DE: Ultrastructural morphogenesis of acute viral pneumonia produced by feline calicivirus, *Am J Vet Res* 39(10):1577-1583; 1978.

131. Ormerod E, McCandlish IA, Jarrett O: Diseases produced by feline caliciviruses when administered to cats by aerosol or intranasal instillation, *Vet Rec* 104(4):65-69, 1979.

132. TerWee J, Lauritzen AY, Sabara M et al: Comparison of the primary signs induced by experimental exposure to either a pneumotrophic or a "limping" strain of feline calicivirus, *Vet Microbiol* 56(1-2):33-45, 1997.

133. Dick CP, Johnson RP: Immunohistochemical detection of feline calicivirus in formalin-fixed, paraffin-embedded specimens, *Can J Vet Res* 53(3):331-335, 1989.

134. Reubel GH, George JW, Higgins J et al: Effect of chronic feline immunodeficiency virus infection on experimental feline calicivirus-induced disease, *Vet Microbiol* 39(3-4):335-351, 1994.

135. Povey RC: *In vitro* antiviral efficacy of ribavirin against feline calicivirus, feline viral rhinotracheitis virus, and canine parainfluenza virus, *Am J Vet Res* 39(1):175-178, 1978.

136. Povey RC: Effect of orally administered ribavirin on experimental feline calicivirus infection in cats, *Am J Vet Res* 39(8):1337-1341, 1978.

137. Hinrichs U, van de Poel H, van den Ingh TS: Necrotizing pneumonia in a cat caused by an orthopox virus, *J Comp Pathol* 121(2):191-196, 1999.

CHAPTER 59

Fungal Pneumonia

Carol R. Norris

Mycotic infections of the lung can arise from primary pathogenic fungal organisms such as *Histoplasma capsulatum*, *Blastomyces dermatitidis*, *Coccidioides immitis*, and *Cryptococcus neoformans*. Fungal pneumonia can also be caused by secondary or opportunistic pathogens when defects in host immunocompetence exist.[1] Fungal organisms are distributed widely in the environment, with endemic areas in many regions of North America. Airborne spores, which can subsequently be inhaled by mammals, are part of the reproductive cycle of many fungi.[2] Because the respiratory tract is a common portal of entry, especially for the primary pathogens, localized infection resulting in fungal pneumonia often results. Dissemination to the lungs and other organs from a different portal of entry can also occur (e.g., via the gastrointestinal tract or skin wounds).

Clinical signs of systemic fungal infections reflect the underlying organ involvement. When the lower respiratory tract is affected, coughing, tachypnea, dyspnea, and exercise intolerance are often seen. Hematologic findings are generally nonspecific and do not help with definitive diagnosis of disease. Clinical chemistries may reveal hypoalbuminemia, hyperglobulinemia, and hypercalcemia.[3] Hypercalcemia is speculated to be induced by mediators of bone resorption associated with the granulomatous response to fungal infection.[4] Thoracic radiography may demonstrate interstitial, alveolar, bronchiolar, or mixed patterns; lobar consolidation; discrete nodules or cavitary lesions; hilar lymphadenopathy; pleural effusion or thickening; or pneumothorax. Serology is helpful in establishing the diagnosis of some fungal infections (coccidioidomycosis and cryptococcosis, in particular) and less useful in others. Cytologic specimens obtained from tracheal washes, bronchoalveolar lavage (BAL), fine-needle aspiration of the pulmonary parenchyma, and thoracocentesis can be examined for the presence of intra- or extracellular fungal organisms. Histologic specimens can also be used to identify the fungal agents. Special stains such as periodic acid Schiff (PAS), Gridley's fungal, and Gomori's methenamine silver stain (GMS) are recommended to aid in the identification of organisms. Culture of cytologic or histologic samples can be performed; however, only qualified personnel should handle cultures of fungi with an infectious phase that grows on culture media because of the risk of inadvertent infection. Polymerase chain reaction (PCR), although not commercially available at present, will likely aid in the diagnosis of fungal diseases in the future.

Antifungal Therapy

The ideal antifungal agent must have effective intrinsic antimycotic activity, be able to target the fungal organism in vivo, and be able to selectively kill the fungus without harming the host.[5] Evaluation of the most effective treatment regimens for fungal infections has been hampered by the paucity of prospective studies in the veterinary literature. It is particularly difficult to draw conclusions about the efficacy of these drugs in fungal pneumonia because pneumonia may occur as an isolated infection or be a component of more severe disseminated disease. Patient outcome is obviously influenced by the extent of disease, with dissemination being more difficult to treat and carrying a more guarded prognosis. The major classes of antifungal agents used in fungal pneumonia in dogs and cats include polyene antibiotics (amphotericin B and hamycin); azoles (ketoconazole, itraconazole, and fluconazole); antimetabolites (flucytosine); and chitin synthesis inhibitors (nikkomycin and lufenuron).

Amphotericin B is a polyene antibiotic that is isolated from the aerobic organism *Streptomyces nodosus*. Its mechanism of action involves the irreversible binding of sterols in cell membranes, including ergosterol in fungal membranes and cholesterol in mammalian cell membranes. Affinity for ergosterol is greater than affinity for cholesterol, which accounts for the greater toxicity against fungal organisms.[2] Death of the fungal organism results from alterations in cell membrane permeability. Leakage of sodium, potassium, and hydrogen ions ultimately leads to cell lysis.[3] Amphotericin B has additional immunomodulatory effects by stimulating host macrophages.[3] Amphotericin B is a broad spectrum antifungal, with efficacy against *Blastomyces*, *Histoplasma*, *Cryptococcus*, *Coccidioides*, *Candida*, and *Zygomycetes*. *Aspergillus* is usually resistant.[2] Amphotericin is traditionally formulated as an intravenous deoxycholate preparation. The major side effect is nephrotoxicity, caused by alterations in renal tubular epithelial cell permeability. Changes in permeability allow for increased chloride ion delivery to the distal tubules and subsequent decreased glomerular filtration rates caused by tubuloglomerular feedback.[3] This response is blunted if patients are sodium-loaded; therefore, some protocols call for 0.9% sodium chloride diuresis before amphotericin administration. The recommended dose of regular amphotericin is 0.15 to 0.5 mg/kg intravenously three times a week, with the lower end of the dose range being used in cats. A relatively new lipid-complexed preparation of amphotericin B has been shown to be less nephrotoxic and allows for higher cumulative doses.[6] Decreased nephrotoxicity is caused by rapid uptake of the lipid complexes by cells of the reticuloendothelial system, allowing for decreased renal uptake.[3] Additionally, the lung and other organs with high reticuloendothelial cell activity receive higher doses of amphotericin B, which can enhance killing of fungal organisms. Doses range from 0.5 to 2.2 mg/kg intravenously three times weekly, with the lower end of the dose range being used in cats. Other toxic side effects of amphotericin include vomiting, anorexia, fever, hypokalemia, hypomagnesemia, renal tubular acidosis, and phlebitis. Serial serum creatinine and blood urea nitrogen (BUN) concentrations should be measured, and therapy discontinued if the serum creatinine exceeds 3 mg/dl or the BUN exceeds 60 mg/dl.

Azole antifungal drugs are classified as imidazoles (e.g., ketoconazole) or triazoles (e.g., itraconazole and fluconazole). Their mechanism of action is by inhibition of ergosterol synthesis in fungal cell membranes. Specifically, they inhibit the fungal P450-dependent lanosterol C14-demethylase enzyme. Some also bind to mammalian P450 enzyme systems and block conversion of lanosterol to cholesterol.[5] Ketoconazole and itraconazole are lipid-soluble compounds extensively metabolized by the liver; as a result, they interact with drugs that inhibit or induce P450 enzymes. They are mainly excreted in the bile and, to a lesser extent, in the urine. Both compounds require an acid environment for oral absorption and have improved bioavailability when given with a meal. Ketoconazole has more side effects than the triazoles because of its higher affinity for mammalian P450 enzymes.[5] Side effects of ketoconazole in dogs and cats include vomiting, anorexia, diarrhea, hepatotoxicity, lightening of the hair coat, thrombocytopenia, and adrenal insufficiency. The dose of ketoconazole is 5 to 30 mg/kg PO divided BID. Itraconazole can be associated with gastrointestinal side effects, hepatotoxicity, and cutaneous skin eruptions, and is given at a dose of 5 to 10 mg/kg PO once or twice daily. In comparison to ketoconazole and itraconazole, fluconazole is water-soluble, has minimal hepatic metabolism, and is largely excreted unchanged in the urine. It is administered at a dose of 2.5 to 10 mg/kg PO, SID, or BID. Drug dosage should be adjusted in patients with renal insufficiency. Bioavailability is high, with absorption independent of gastric acidity and food intake. High concentrations are achieved in sputum, and it is thought to penetrate into pulmonary secretions well.[5] Side effects are most commonly gastrointestinal. All azole antifungals are administered orally; fluconazole is also available as an intravenous preparation.

Flucytosine is an antimetabolite that interferes with pyrimidine metabolism. It inhibits DNA, RNA, and protein synthesis. When used as a sole agent, fungal resistance develops rapidly. In practice, it is most commonly used with amphotericin B, and has synergistic effects. Side effects include anorexia, vomiting and diarrhea, bone marrow suppression, and cutaneous eruptions. The dose in dogs ranges from 25 to 175 mg/kg PO divided TID to QID with amphotericin; and in cats, up to 250 mg PO divided BID to QID with amphotericin.

Chitin synthesis inhibitors (e.g., nikkomycin and lufenuron) interfere with the structural and functional integrity of the fungal cell wall.[3] Lufenuron has only been evaluated in a single report of canine coccidioidomycosis,[7] and further studies need to be performed to determine the efficacy of this class of antifungal drug for treatment of mycotic pneumonia.

Histoplasmosis

Histoplasma capsulatum, a dimorphic fungus, exists as a free-living mycelium in the soil and as a yeast in host tissues. It is endemic in the river valleys of the Mississippi, Missouri, and Ohio.[8] Inhalation of the infective microconidia produced by the mycelium allows the organism to convert into the yeast phase at body temperature. The organism is phagocytized by the host's alveolar macrophages and undergoes intracellular replication. The intracytoplasmic yeasts range from 2 to 4 μm in diameter and have a nonstaining clear cell wall and a central basophilic nucleus (Figure 59-1).[9] Infection can be limited to the respiratory tract or may disseminate to other tissues by hematogenous and lymphatic routes. Tissues of the reticuloendothelial system are affected most commonly. *H. capsulatum* most commonly causes subclinical disease.[10-13] Pulmonary and disseminated histoplasmosis occur less often, with either an acute or chronic course. The incubation period is typically about 12 to 16 days.[3] The host's immune response, especially

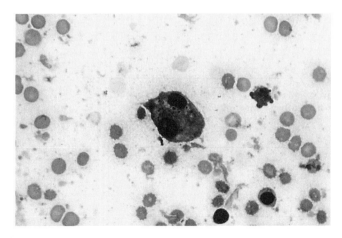

Figure 59-1. *The intracytoplasmic yeast phase of* Histoplasma capsulatum *made from an impression smear of the lung. (150X; Wright's stain)* (Courtesy Dr. Tripp Almy, University of California, Davis.)

cell-mediated immunity, determines the clinical form of disease.[8] Histoplasmosis was formerly thought to primarily affect dogs and to be uncommon in cats[14]; however, this has been refuted.[15]

CANINE PULMONARY HISTOPLASMOSIS

Disseminated histoplasmosis develops in young dogs of either sex[12,13]; no breed predisposition has been reported.[16] Clinical signs relating to the respiratory tract in dogs with histoplasmosis were reported in 17% to 50% of dogs and included coughing and dyspnea.[3,13,16] Hematologic findings are not specific for histoplasmosis, and tend to reflect underlying organ involvement. Histoplasma organisms have been identified in monocytes, neutrophils, and eosinophils in peripheral blood smears.[17,18] Common findings include a normocytic, normochromic, nonregenerative anemia and leukocytosis caused by neutrophilia.[13,16,17] Hypercalcemia in canine histoplasmosis is less commonly reported, in comparison with feline histoplasmosis and canine blastomycosis.[3,19]

Thoracic radiographic findings may be normal even with histologic evidence of discrete pulmonary lesions.[20] This discrepancy is speculated to be caused by the small size of the nodules (often less than 5 mm). Abnormal radiographic findings include interstitial (often nodular), alveolar, and bronchial patterns[16,21,22]; lobar consolidation[9]; hilar lymphadenopathy[22,23]; calcified nodules[21]; and pleural effusion.[9,17] In dogs that have recovered from histoplasmosis, calcified lesions may be present on thoracic radiography.[21,22]

Antibodies against H. capsulatum can be detected using complement fixation (CF) and agar-gel immunodiffusion (AGID) tests, and may support a diagnosis of histoplasmosis. False positive and false negative results are common.[9,16] Cross-reactivity to other fungal organisms can cause false positive results.[13,16] Negative titers can be seen in dogs that are terminal or that have a chronic well localized lesion.[22] Because of these inaccuracies, serology should not be used as the sole diagnostic test for canine histoplasmosis.[3]

Identification of H. capsulatum organisms within mononuclear cells or, less commonly, granulocytes (e.g., neutrophils or eosinophils), provides a definitive diagnosis. Additionally, cytological specimens can be obtained by tracheal wash, bronchoalveolar lavage, fine-needle aspiration of the lung, and thoracocentesis.[9,17,18,24] Identification of organisms on histologic examination with routine hematoxylin and eosin stains is difficult. Instead, special stains including PAS, GMS, or Gridley's fungal stain should be used.[9] To improve diagnostic yield, evaluation of more than one sample is recommended.[13] Culture can be performed on cytological and histological samples, but because the microconidia produced by the mycelial growth are infectious to humans, only qualified personnel should handle these samples. False negative culture results can occur.[13,16,25] An additional drawback of culture is the long time required to grow the organism (i.e., up to 4 weeks).[13]

Hilar lymphadenopathy with secondary airway obstruction occurs in some cases of chronic histoplasmosis.[22,23] Hilar lymphadenopathy may be an extension of pulmonary disease when local immunity has failed, or it may develop from local hypersensitivity to H. capsulatum antigen. Cytological examination of fluid from tracheal washes or bronchoalveolar lavage is recommended to rule out active infection with histoplasmosis. In the absence of active infection, corticosteroids (e.g., prednisone at a dose of 2 to 4 mg/kg/day) have been shown to resolve hilar lymphadenopathy secondary to histoplasmosis.[23]

Pulmonary histoplasmosis in the dog may be self-limiting, and the prognosis is considered to be fair to good.[12] Because of the risk of dissemination, however, antifungal therapy is recommended in patients with clinical histoplasma pneumonia. Disseminated histoplasmosis, which in most cases still involves the pulmonary parenchyma, requires treatment with antifungal agents because most patients die without therapy. Ketoconazole and itraconazole are both reported to be good treatment options, with amphotericin added to the protocol in fulminant cases.[3] Reports comparing the efficacy of these antifungal agents in canine histoplasmosis are lacking. Further studies on the use of lipid-complexed amphotericin B are warranted because of the high concentration of amphotericin attained inside phagocytic cells where histoplasmal organisms reside.

FELINE PULMONARY HISTOPLASMOSIS

Histoplasmosis is the second most commonly reported fungal infection in cats, after cryptococcosis.[26] It appears to affect cats of all ages,[19,25] with a possible predisposition for females in one study.[19] No breeds have been identified to be at increased risk. Clinical signs relating to the respiratory tract (e.g., dyspnea, tachypnea, and cough) were seen in 38% to 93% of cats.[14,19,25,26] The most common clinicopathological abnormalities include anemia, neutrophilia, and lymphopenia.[14,25] Hypercalcemia has also been reported.[19] Many cats have tested negative for FeLV and FIV,[14,15,19] although a more recent review found a 22.9% incidence of concurrent disease, including FeLV infection in 12.5% to 17.9%, with the low end of the range representing the cases in that report, and the high end of the range representing the comparative literature review.[26]

Abnormalities on thoracic radiography were reported in 70% to 93% of cats with histoplasmosis, and consisted mainly of miliary or diffuse interstitial infiltrates.[14,25,26] Nodular, alveolar-interstitial, and alveolar patterns have also been described.[15,21] Cats may have radiographic evidence of interstitial infiltrates without associated clinical signs of respiratory disease.[14]

Serology for antibodies against H. capsulatum appears to have limited utility in the diagnosis of histoplasmosis in cats, but most studies have only evaluated this immunodiagnostic tool in a small number of patients.[14,19] As in dogs, cytological or histological examination provides a definitive diagnosis. Cytology of specimens obtained by tracheal wash, bronchoalveolar lavage, fine-needle aspiration of the lung, and thoracocentesis has demonstrated intracellular histoplasma organisms in cats.[14,19] The organisms may also be found in circulating leukocytes.[14]

Whereas ketoconazole has been used successfully in the treatment of disseminated histoplasmosis, some cats may either be refractory to it or show substantial side effects.[15,19,27] Treatment with amphotericin B may also be associated with substantial adverse effects in cats and has not been particularly effective in the treatment of this disease.[14,28] Itraconazole appears to be better tolerated than ketoconazole or amphotericin B and may be more efficacious.[19] All 8 cats with histoplasmosis in one study were eventually cured with a course of itraconazole (range, 60 to 130 days), although 2 cats had recurrence of disease that required additional treatment with itraconazole (range, 60 to 90 days).[19] Previously the prognosis for feline histoplasmosis was guarded to poor[14]; however, with the availability of itraconazole, the prognosis appears to be substantially improved.

Blastomycosis

Blastomycosis is caused by infection with a dimorphic fungus, *Blastomyces dermatitidis*, which is a free-living saprophyte at temperatures less than 35° C and a yeast in tissues at body temperatures of 37° C or greater.[2,29] It is thought to be a soil saprophyte, although its exact ecological niche is unknown. Geographically, it is restricted to regions near large waterways in North America.[29,30] In infected tissue the organism is a thick-walled yeast, 5 to 20 μm in diameter (Figure 59-2). Usually a single bud is attached by a broad base to a mother cell.[3,29] The wall of the yeast is double contoured and refractile. In culture, mold colonies contain branching septate mycelia (1 to 2 μm in size) that form round or piriform conidia (2 to 10 μm in diameter).[3] Outbreaks of blastomycosis are asso-

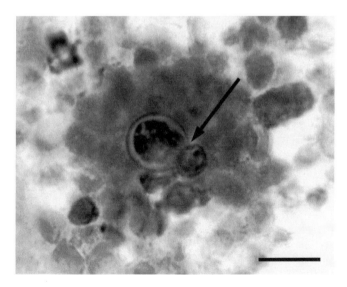

Figure 59-2. Blastomyces dermatitidis: *Impression smears of material collected from a dog living in Wisconsin. The arrow points to broad-based budding, which is characteristic for this type of yeast. (Wright-Giemsa stain. Bar = 10 μm.)* (Courtesy Dr. Patricia McManus, University of Pennsylvania.)

ciated with close proximity to water, sandy and acidic soil or debris, the presence of wildlife and their excreta, and disruption of soil.[30] Infection occurs by inhalation of the aerosolized conidiophores, which are subsequently deposited in the alveoli. Alveolar macrophages phagocytize the conidia, which are then transformed from the mycelial to the yeast phase.[3] Humoral immunity is not considered protective, but cell-mediated immunity may clear infection locally in the lungs. If cell-mediated immunity is inadequate, the yeasts may gain access to the pulmonary interstitium and from there disseminate to the rest of the body by hematogenous and lymphatic routes. Blastomycosis incites intense pyogranulomatous inflammation. Unlike other deep mycotic infections, it is unknown if a subclinical infection occurs. Incubation periods range from 5 to 12 weeks.

CANINE PULMONARY BLASTOMYCOSIS

Blastomycosis is seen more commonly in young male dogs,[31,32] with sporting dogs and hounds (especially bluetick coonhounds, treeing-walker coonhounds, pointers, and weimeraners) being at increased risk for infection.[32] Dogs are considered a sentinel for infection in humans, having a 10 times higher incidence of disease than man.[30] The respiratory tract is often involved in canine blastomycosis, with an incidence of 88% in one study.[29] Not all dogs have clinical signs relating to the respiratory tract, although cough, dyspnea, and exercise intolerance have been reported in 43% to 49% of dogs.[29,33] Laboratory abnormalities include a mild regenerative anemia, neutrophilia, lymphopenia, monocytosis, hyperglobulinemia, hypoalbuminemia, and hypercalcemia.[29,33,34]

Radiographic abnormalities have been described in up to 85% of clinically affected dogs and include a miliary nodular interstitial pattern (with or without a bronchial or alveolar pattern); multifocal, poorly marginated interstitial nodules; hilar or sternal lymphadenopathy; rare cavitary lesions; pleural effusion; pneumothorax; or pneumomediastinum.[29,30,33-37] Hilar lymphadenopathy is believed to be less commonly present in canine blastomycosis than in histoplasmosis or coccidioidomycosis.[2] Thoracic radiographs may also be normal.[29,31,36]

Serology employing the AGID test for antibodies against blastomycosis may be used in conjunction with a compatible history, clinical signs, and radiographic findings to confirm a diagnosis. AGID was previously reported to have a sensitivity of 91% and specificity of 96%[38]; however, a recent report documented the radioimmunoassay (RIA) against the WI-1 antigen of *B. dermatitidis* to be a superior test.[39] The latter study compared the RIA and AGID and found a sensitivity of 92% and 41%, respectively, and 100% specificity for both assays. False negative results with serology may occur early in the course of disease or following disease progression.[3]

Definitive diagnosis of blastomycosis relies on identification of the organism on cytological or histological examination. In dogs with blastomycosis, examination of tracheal wash fluid demonstrated organisms in 3 of 7 dogs, compared with BAL fluid, in which organisms were identified in 5 of 7 dogs.[24] The lower sensitivity of tracheal wash cytology is speculated to be due to the primary interstitial site of this infection.[34] Another report showed the diagnostic yield of lung aspirates to be 47% (7 of 16 dogs); tracheal wash, 30% (3 of 10 dogs); and bronchoalveolar lavage, 25% (1 of 4 dogs).[29] *Blastomyces dermatitidis* was also identified from a direct fecal smear in a dog with acute pulmonary blastomycosis that swallowed his own sputum.[40] Direct fecal examination may represent a simple, noninvasive diagnostic alternative to collection of other pulmonary diagnostic specimens. Histological examination of the lungs is characterized by purulent to pyogranulomatous lesions with broad-based budding yeasts.[3,30] Culture is not recommended in-house because of the potential risk of human exposure to the mycelial form of the organism, and commercial laboratories should be alerted to the possibility of blastomycosis.[34] In one study, only 2 of 17 (12%) dogs had a positive culture result.[29]

Treatment of blastomycosis has been successful in 60% to 75% of cases, although relapses occur in approximately 20% of dogs.* Dogs with more severe lung lesions on thoracic radiography had lower survival rates and higher relapse rates in one study.[35] Ketoconazole appears less effective than itraconazole with a lower response rate and higher relapse rate.[3,35] Itraconazole has been shown to be as effective as treatment with combination ketoconazole and amphotericin B.[29] Fluconazole has not been evaluated in canine blastomycosis to date. The standard preparation of amphotericin, (or amphotericin lipid complex), as a monotherapy has also been used with good success.[6,35]

FELINE PULMONARY BLASTOMYCOSIS

Similar to dogs, blastomycosis most commonly affects young male cats, although in general blastomycosis is rare in cats.[26,41] Earlier studies reported a higher incidence of disease in Siamese cats; but a recent large, retrospective study refuted a predisposition for the Siamese breed and instead found Abyssinians and Havana browns to be at higher risk.[26] The most common clinical signs of blastomycosis in cats are dyspnea and coughing, described in 59% of cases in 1 report.[26] Approximately 10% of cats have positive FeLV tests.[26]

Thoracic radiographic abnormalities appear to be common and may reveal pulmonary nodules, an interstitial pattern, or pleural effusion.[26,42] The AGID test for antibodies to *B. dermatitidis* appears to be less reliable in cats than in dogs,[26,41] although further studies using this test and perhaps the RIA are warranted. Cytologic examination of pleural effusion or BAL fluid specimens may prove to be the most accurate diagnostic method aside from histologic examination.[41,42] Characteristic histologic changes include interstitial granulomas comprised of neutrophils, macrophages, lymphocytes, plasmacytes, and blastomyces organisms.[42,43] Alveoli in affected areas may be filled with fungal organisms, pyogranulomatous infiltrates, fibrin, and blood.[42] Evidence

of pulmonary blastomycosis was seen in 13 of 22 cats necropsied in one report[26] and in 14 of 23 cats by cytologic or histological examination in another.[41]

In the literature, therapy for blastomycosis in cats has been either rarely attempted[26,41] or provided late in the course of disease for severely affected patients.[41,42] This could explain the relatively poor response rate ranging from 0% to 17%.[41,42] Not all of the cats in these studies had pulmonary lesions, so it is difficult to determine the response to therapy in cats with pulmonary blastomycosis. Prognosis, overall, appears to be poor.

Coccidioidomycosis

Coccidioidomycosis is caused by infection with the soil-borne fungus *Coccidioides immitis*, found in the ecological niche known as the lower Sonoran life zone. This region includes parts of California, Arizona, Utah, New Mexico, Nevada, and Texas. The organism exists as a mycelial phase in soil and culture media, and forms multinucleate arthroconidia (2 to 4 μm in diameter and 3 to 10 μm long).[3] The arthroconidia can be dispersed by wind and germinate to form new hyphae, or serve as the infectious form of the organism. Inhalation serves as the major route of infection. Once inhaled, the arthroconidia are converted to immature spherules that subsequently undergo endonuclear division and intracytoplasmic partitioning to form mature spherules containing internal endospores. The mature spherule, measuring 20 to 200 μm in diameter, eventually breaks open, releasing hundreds of endospores.[2] In the body, the endospores mature to become spherules. The incubation period in dogs is 1 to 3 weeks.[3]

The most common form of coccidioidomycosis is an asymptomatic self-limiting respiratory tract infection that is cleared by the host's cell-mediated immunity.[44] The disease can become disseminated in animals with impaired cell-mediated immunity or in those with massive exposure to the organism. Disease is considered disseminated if it progresses past the hilar lymph nodes.[3] Compared with dogs, cats are believed to be relatively refractory to the development of coccidioidomycosis.[45]

CANINE PULMONARY COCCIDIOIDOMYCOSIS

Most cases of canine coccidioidomycosis have been described in young male dogs,[46] with a possible predisposition for boxers and Doberman pinschers.[47,48] Clinical signs of respiratory disease compatible with early nondisseminated pulmonary infection have been reported in 78% of dogs before dissemination.[48] This primary respiratory illness most commonly lasts about 2 weeks and is followed by asymptomatic infection for 3 to 5 months before signs of dissemination became apparent. Hematological changes are nonspecific and include mild nonregenerative anemia; leukocytosis (or less commonly, leukopenia); monocytosis; hyperglobulinemia; and hyperfibrinogenemia.[49] Eosinophilia has been reported but is much less common than in man.[49]

*References 3, 6, 31, 33, 35, and 37.

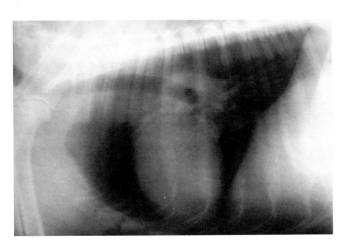

Figure 59-3. Hilar lymphadenopathy in a dog with pulmonary coccidioidomycosis.

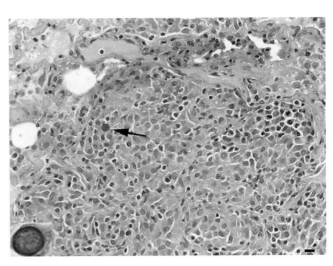

Figure 59-4. Granulomatous inflammation associated with coccidioidomycosis in a dog. The insert shows a spherule with endospores. (PAS stain.) (Courtesy Dr. Stephen M. Griffey, University of California, Davis.)

Abnormalities on thoracic radiography are very common because the main portal of entry of coccidioidomycosis is the lung. One study evaluating radiographic features of canine coccidioidomycosis noted abnormalities in 32 of 38 dogs.[46] In this study, the most common pattern was interstitial, with nodular, linear, or amorphous densities. Other patterns were mixed, with 12 dogs having interstitial-bronchiolar and 5 dogs having interstitial-alveolar patterns. Cavitary lesions, lobar consolidation, pleural effusion or thickening, mediastinal widening (presumptively caused by enlarged cranial mediastinal lymph nodes), and mineralized nodules have also been reported, although rarely.[46,49] Hilar lymphadenopathy was very common, occurring in 28 of these 38 dogs (Figure 59-3).[46]

AGID serology is an important diagnostic and prognostic tool in coccidioidomycosis. The AGID test can pick up precipitin antibodies (IgM) or complement-fixing antibodies (IgG).[44] The precipitin test becomes positive 2 weeks postinfection, then negative after 4 to 5 weeks. It may become positive again if dissemination occurs. A false negative result may occur with infection less than 2 weeks or greater than 5 weeks in duration, or in fulminating infection in immunocompromised patients. The complement-fixing test becomes positive shortly after the precipitin test. The magnitude of the titer reflects the severity of infection. Titers of less than 1:16 may indicate past exposure or infection, localized disease, or chronic infection. Titers greater than 1:32 suggest active disseminated disease.[3] False negative results are also seen with fulminating or early infection. Serial evaluation of complement-fixing titers has been recommended for monitoring clinical improvement, but titers may be elevated for more than a year following therapy.[3] Therapy should not be discontinued until titers are less than 1:16 and clinical signs have been resolved for at least 2 months.

Examination of cytological specimens may reveal the characteristic double-walled spherules containing endospores, although they may not be seen because they are present in low numbers.[3,24] Organisms are more likely to be found on histologic examination (Figure 59-4). Culture should only be performed by qualified personnel because the arthrospores are highly infectious.

Amphotericin B or azoles can be used in the treatment of canine coccidioidomycosis. Results of amphotericin B therapy have been inconsistent and associated with nephrotoxicity.[47,49,50] Long-term therapy (6 to 12 months) with ketoconazole or itraconazole has been successful in clinically affected dogs.[3,47,49] Some of these dogs relapsed when therapy was discontinued and required additional treatment. There are few studies critically evaluating different treatment protocols. A report of the chitin synthesis inhibitor, lufenuron, in dogs with pulmonary coccidioidomycosis demonstrated clinical improvement, although radiographic evidence of disease and complement-fixing titers often remained unchanged.[7] The role of chitin synthesis inhibitors should be evaluated further. Prognosis of pulmonary coccidioidomycosis is good, but is guarded in disseminated disease.[3]

FELINE PULMONARY COCCIDIOIDOMYCOSIS

Cats of any age (range, 1 to 15 years, mean 6.2 years), sex, and breed can be infected with *C. immitus.*[26,45] Compared with dogs, dermatologic lesions are the most common manifestation of coccidioidomycosis in cats, and respiratory signs are seen less often (56% and 25%, respectively, for skin and respiratory signs).[45] Concurrent immunosuppressive disorders were noted in only 7.5% of cases, with the majority of cats being FeLV and FIV negative.[26,45] As with other fungal diseases, hemograms and biochemical profiles are not specific for the diagnosis of coccidioidomycosis. Common abnormalities include a mild nonregenerative anemia, neutrophilic leukocytosis, and hyperglobulinemia.[3,26,45]

Most cats in the veterinary literature did not have thoracic radiographic evaluation, making it difficult to draw conclusions about radiographic patterns in feline coccidioidomycosis. The lack of thoracic radiography is likely caused by the relative rarity of respiratory signs in the cat. Hilar lymphadenopathy and pleural effusion or thickening have been reported.[45]

Serologic testing using AGID is valuable in the diagnosis of feline coccidioidomycosis. In one study, all 39 cats tested using the AGID test for precipitin and complement-fixing antibodies were positive at some time during the course of their disease.[45] Precipitin antibodies were present in 82% of the cats at the time of initial presentation. The cats with negative precipitin antibodies may have had early infection, fulminant disease, or been immunosuppressed.[51] In cats, serial monitoring of complement-fixing titers may not be useful in evaluating the progression or resolution of disease.[45] Culture, cytology, and histopathology have been used successfully in the diagnosis of feline coccidioidomycosis.[26,45]

Little information is available in the veterinary literature about the use of antifungal medication for feline coccidioidomycosis, especially with disseminated disease. Ketoconazole has been the most commonly used antifungal, with uncommon use of itraconazole and fluconazole.[45] The azoles do not appear to be curative because relapses are common after drug withdrawal. In one study of localized (usually cutaneous) or disseminated coccidioidomycosis, 32 of 48 (66.7%) cats responded to therapy, although 11 of these cats relapsed.[45] As in dogs, long-term therapy (up to 43 months) may be required.[45] Amphotericin B (standard preparation or lipid encapsulated) has not been reported to date as therapy for feline coccidioidomycosis.[3]

Cryptococcosis

Cryptococcosis is infection with the saprophytic encapsulated yeast-like organism *Cryptococcus neoformans var neoformans* or *gattii.* The organism has a worldwide distribution and has been isolated predominantly from pigeon excreta, and from bark and leaf litter of certain Eucalyptus trees. It is especially common in the southeast and southwest United States, southern California, and the east coast of Australia.[3] The pigeon is believed to be the most important vector of *C. neoformans,* although the birds do not develop clinical infection, presumptively because of their high body temperature (42° C).[3,52] Most infections are caused by environmental exposure to the yeast-like phase. In infected tissue, the organism is a variably sized yeast (diameter ranging from 3.5 to 7 μm) surrounded by a heteropolysaccharide capsule (diameter ranging from 1 to 30 μm). Reproduction in tissues occurs asexually by budding from a narrow base, forming blastoconidia. The buds may break off when they are different sizes, explaining the variation in size of the organisms in tissue.[53]

The mode of infection in dogs and cats is unknown but is speculated to result from inhalation of airborne organisms. Because of the relatively large size of the yeasts, they mainly impact the upper respiratory passages.[2,54] Smaller dessicated forms of the yeast are also infective and can settle out in the airways and alveoli, leading to mycotic pneumonia.[3,54] Not all animals that have inhaled cryptococcal organisms develop disease; in one study, 14% of asymptomatic dogs and 7% of asymptomatic cats had positive nasal cultures.[55] Immunosuppression is associated with development of cryptococcosis in humans, and is thought to play a role in affected cats.[26,56-58] In dogs, the contribution of immunosuppressive factors leading to cryptococcosis is more controversial.[59-62] The gelatinous capsule contributes to the pathogenicity of the cryptococcal organism by inhibiting phagocytosis, plasma cell function, and leukocyte migration.[3] Lesions may thus be present without a substantial inflammatory response. The host immune response determines the type and severity of disease. Humoral immunity with resultant antibody production is not considered protective. Cell-mediated immunity results in granulomatous inflammation and can lead to prevention of, or recovery from, infection. If the host cannot contain the infection, dissemination by direct extension from a portal of entry or by hematogenous routes can occur. Cryptococcal pneumonia usually occurs as part of disseminated disease.[3,52,53,61,63] There are no reports in the literature describing clinicopathologic findings, results of thoracic radiography, or treatment modalities and outcome in a series of dogs or cats with isolated cryptococcal pneumonia. A lack of uniformity in studies describing infection of the lung with *C. neoformans* makes it difficult to draw conclusions or make recommendations about cryptococcal pneumonia in dogs or cats.

CANINE PULMONARY CRYPTOCOCCOSIS

Affected dogs are usually young (less than 4 years) and large breeds, with a predisposition for Doberman pinschers, Great Danes, and German shepherds.[59,64] Earlier reports of canine cryptococcosis described central nervous system and ocular lesions as being most common[2,3,59]; a more recent report found rhinosinusitis to be the primary site of infection as it is in cats.[64] Pneumonia as the sole manifestation of cryptococcal infection is not typical in dogs and generally implies multisystemic dissemination of the organism.[3,59,63] Inadequate data are present in the veterinary literature to fully characterize the clinical signs and thoracic radiographic findings in dogs with cryptococcal pneumonia; however, isolated reports provide some information about pulmonary involvement. In one review, a dry cough was present in 3 of 28 dogs, but thoracic radiographic or histopathological findings from the lung parenchyma were not consistently available.[53] Another report revealed thoracic radiographic findings of hilar lymphadenopathy and multiple small nodular densities throughout the pulmonary parenchyma that corresponded to cryptococcal granulo-

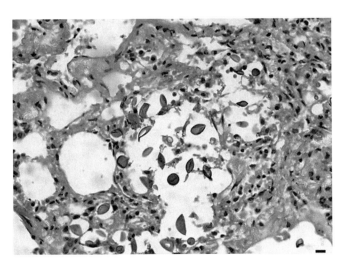

Figure 59-5. *Cryptococcal organisms surrounded by granulomatous inflammation. (PAS stain.)* (Courtesy Dr. Stephen M. Griffey, University of California, Davis.)

mas on histologic examination.[63] Other reports of canine cryptococcosis with evidence of disease on thoracic radiography or lung histology reported secondary bacterial rather than fungal bronchopneumonia.[59,60,65] Canine cryptococcal pneumonia has been rarely diagnosed antemortem, but evidence of respiratory tract (usually pulmonary parenchymal) involvement in disseminated cryptococcosis was reported in up to 50% of cases.[53] Histologic features can include effacement of the pulmonary parenchyma by granulomatous inflammation and budding yeasts of *C. neoformans* (Figure 59-5).[61,63] Granulomas are composed of histiocytes, small mononuclear cells, and fibroblasts.[63] Giant cells have been variably present.[61] Therapy with azoles and amphotericin B with or without flucytosine has been attempted. Because cryptococcal pneumonia is generally seen in disseminated cases, prognosis is guarded to poor.

FELINE PULMONARY CRYPTOCOCCOSIS

Cats of any age can develop cryptococcosis, and the Abyssinian and Siamese breeds are thought to be overrepresented.[26] In most studies, males are predisposed to infection,[52,58,66] although this was disputed in a large retrospective study.[26] Cryptococcosis is the most common deep fungal infection in cats; however, it generally affects the upper respiratory passages, eyes, central nervous system, lymph nodes, and skin. The incidence of pulmonary lesions is variable, being reported in 0% to 67% of cases.[2,52,54,66] Cats with FeLV or FIV infection are thought to be at higher risk for development of cryptococcal infection, are more likely to have advanced or disseminated disease, and have a higher likelihood of treatment failure.[52,56-58,66] Clinicopathologic tests have reported anemia, mature neutrophilia, eosinophilia, and hyperproteinemia.[26]

In one report of cryptococcosis in cats, lesions were identified on thoracic radiography in 27.8% of cases.[26] Thoracic radiography can be normal despite cryptococ-

cal pneumonia, and other diagnostic tests (e.g., tracheal wash or bronchoalveolar lavage) may be indicated.[67] Serology, using a commercial cryptococcal antigen latex agglutination test, is a sensitive, specific, and noninvasive diagnostic test.[68,69] There are few false negative results with the antigen test, but they can occur with localized infection.[68] False positive titers are also uncommon.[3] In comparison, antibody titers are not useful diagnostically because of the high incidence of false negative results in infected animals.[69] Serial monitoring of serum cryptococcal antigen titers is recommended during treatment, and a favorable prognosis is associated with a drop in titer of at least one order of magnitude.[58]

Treatment is generally long term, with continuation of antifungal medication until 1 month after resolution of clinical signs and a decrease in antigen titer by at least two orders of magnitude, preferably until the titer is negative.[58] Azoles or amphotericin B (with or without 5-flucytosine) have been used successfully, albeit long term, in cats with cryptococcosis.* It is not possible to determine from previous reports which antifungal was most effective for cryptococcal pneumonia in cats.

Opportunistic Fungal Pneumonia

Histoplasmosis, blastomycosis, coccidioidomycosis, and cryptococcosis are primary pathogens capable of causing disseminated fungal disease in dogs and cats. Secondary or opportunistic fungal pathogens have inherently low virulence and generally only produce disease when host resistance to infection is impaired.[1] The remainder of the chapter will discuss opportunistic canine and feline fungal pneumonia.

ASPERGILLOSIS

Aspergillus spp. are ubiquitous soil saprophytes that are most commonly described as pathogens causing rhinitis and sinusitis in the dog. *A. terreus, A. deflectus, A. fumigatus,* and other aspergillus species have been associated with pulmonary parenchymal infection in the dog.[1,72-76] *Aspergillus* spp. including *A. fumigatus* have been isolated from the lungs of cats.[77] *A. terreus* belongs to a unique group within the aspergillus species that has the ability to produce aleurospores in infected host tissue, and has additional virulence factors that distinguish it from other nonpathogenic soil isolates.[78] The majority of cases of disseminated aspergillosis in dogs are caused by *A. terreus,* and lack clinical signs or radiographic evidence of respiratory tract involvement.[78] However, in one study, 4 of 10 dogs with disseminated disease had microscopic granulomas confined to vessels within alveolar septa.[74] The portal of entry of aspergillosis in dogs is unknown and is suggested to be the respiratory tract with a primary asymptomatic pulmonary infection; or possibly the gastrointestinal tract, skin, or urinary tract.[78,79] Dissemination likely takes place by hematogenous spread.[79]

*References 3, 26, 58, 66, 70, and 71.

Young German shepherds appear to be at high risk for disseminated aspergillosis.[1,73-75,78] There is speculation about a genetically determined aspergillus-specific immune defect because of the high incidence of disease in this breed.[74,78] Evaluation of some of these dogs for a generalized immunodeficiency with immunoglobulin quantification, serum complement C3 and C4 and total hemolytic complement determination, lymphocyte blastogenesis, and neutrophil function by nitroblue tetrazolium testing was performed.[78] Three of 9 dogs had low serum IgA levels, which were speculated to be associated with a defect in local secretory IgA immunity. The only other abnormality of immune function was a nonspecific elevation in IgG concentrations.

Thoracic radiography in dogs with disseminated aspergillosis is usually normal because of the rarity of macroscopic respiratory tract involvement.[72-74,78] Discospondylitis is much more commonly seen.[72,74] In reports of dogs with respiratory tract disease, radiographic examination demonstrated hilar lymphadenopathy,[73,76] pleural effusion,[74,76] interstitial or alveolar patterns,[72,75,76] lobar consolidation,[75] and a cavitary lesion.[75] Antibody titers appear to have limited use in the diagnosis of disseminated aspergillosis.[1,74,79] A diagnosis of aspergillosis should be made by a positive culture of affected tissue or pleural fluid, or by direct visualization of the organism on cytological or histological examination (Figure 59-6).[74]

Limited information is available regarding treatment of pulmonary or disseminated aspergillosis in dogs. Amphotericin B, hamycin (a polyene antibiotic), and ketoconazole have been used with disappointing results.[73,74,76,79] Itraconazole was used in 4 dogs with disseminated aspergillosis, none of which had pulmonary parenchymal involvement, resulting in long-term survival.[80] Further studies are needed to determine the most effective antifungal regimen in dogs with pulmonary aspergillosis. It is generally agreed that the prognosis in dogs with disseminated aspergillosis is grave.

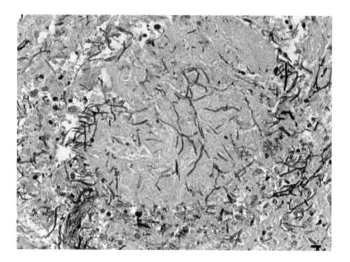

Figure 59-6. *Fungal hyphae within a granuloma from a dog with disseminated aspergillosis. (GMS stain.)* (Courtesy Dr. Stephen M. Griffey, University of California, Davis.)

Feline disseminated aspergillosis has traditionally been described in terminally ill, young (less than 2 years) cats,[77,81] although a more recent retrospective study found the disease in middle age to older cats.[26] A high incidence of predisposing immunosuppression has been reported, including panleukopenia, FIP, FeLV, FIV, endoparasites, recent surgery, or dystocia.[77,81] Diagnosis of feline disseminated aspergillosis has almost always been made postmortem.[26,77,81] Histological lesions included acute necrotizing inflammation with centrally located septate hyphae.[77] These hyphae commonly invaded adjacent blood vessels. Interestingly, in comparison to canine disseminated aspergillosis, feline disseminated aspergillosis commonly had lung involvement (up to 67% of reported cases).[26,77,81] Prognosis for this disease in cats is grave.

SPOROTRICHOSIS

Sporothrix schenckii is a dimorphic fungus that lives as a mycelium in the soil and in culture, and as a yeast at body temperature.[3] The yeast appears as pleomorphic round, oval, or cigar-shaped cells measuring 2 to 3 μm wide and 3 to 10 μm long. Dissemination in the dog is rare, but occurs in 38% to 50% or more of feline cases.[3,26] Young male cats, with a possible predisposition for the Siamese breed, are most commonly affected.[26] The majority of cases are diagnosed by cytological examination, although culture and histological examination have also been useful.[3,26] Itraconazole is currently the treatment of choice,[3] but the prognosis for the disseminated form of disease is guarded. Sporotrichosis is considered highly zoonotic in cats, and to a lesser extent in dogs, and care must be taken when handling patients and exudative material.

CANDIDIASIS

Candida spp., including *C. albicans*, are normal inhabitants of the upper respiratory, gastrointestinal, and genitourinary systems.[3] Immunosuppression or prolonged antibiotic usage may allow proliferation and dissemination of *Candida* spp.[3,72] Disseminated disease, including pulmonary parenchymal involvement, is rare in dogs and cats.[72,81,82] Diagnosis is often made postmortem with culture and histological examination, and the prognosis is grave.

MISCELLANEOUS OPPORTUNISTIC FUNGI

Sporadic cases of zygomycosis[83] and hyalohyphomycosis[84] in the dog, and zygomycosis and penicilliosis in the cat,[26] have been associated with pulmonary involvement. Disease is rare, diagnosis is generally made postmortem, and prognosis is grave.

REFERENCES

1. Watt P, Robins G, Galloway A et al: Disseminated opportunistic fungal disease in dogs: 10 cases (1982-1990), *J Am Vet Med Assoc* 207:67-70, 1995.

2. Roudebush P: Mycotic pneumonias, *Vet Clin North Am Small Anim Pract* 15(5):949-969, 1985.
3. Taboada J: Systemic mycoses. In Greene C, editor: *Infectious diseases of the dog and cat,* Philadelphia, 2000, WB Saunders.
4. Dow SW, Legendre AM, Stiff M et al: Hypercalcemia associated with blastomycosis in dogs, *J Am Vet Med Assoc* 188:706-707, 1986.
5. Heit M, Riviere J: Antifungal therapy: Ketoconazole and other azole derivatives, *Comp Contin Ed* 17(1):21-31, 1995.
6. Krawiec D, McKiernan B, Twardock A et al: Use of an amphotericin B lipid complex for treatment of blastomycosis in dogs, *J Am Vet Med Assoc* 209:2073-2075, 1996.
7. Bartsch R, Greene R: New treatment of coccidioidomycosis, *Vet Forum* 14(4):50-52, 1997.
8. Wolf A: Histoplasmosis. In Greene C, editor: *Infectious diseases of the dog and cat,* Philadelphia, 2000, WB Saunders.
9. Kowalewich N, Hawkins E, Skowronek A et al: Identification of Histoplasma capsulatum organisms in the pleural and peritoneal effusions of a dog, *J Am Vet Med Assoc* 202:423-426, 1993.
10. Rhoades J: Canine histoplasmosis, *Am J Pub Health* 62:1512-1519, 1972.
11. Marx M, Eastin C, Turner C et al: The influence of amphotericin B on histoplasma infection in dogs, *Arch Environ Health* 21:649-655, 1970.
12. Huss B, Collier L, Collins B et al: Polyarthropathy and chorioretinitis with retinal detachment in a dog with systemic histoplasmosis, *J Am Anim Hosp Assoc* 30:217-224, 1994.
13. Clinkenbeard K, Cowell R, Tyler R: Disseminated histoplasmosis in dogs: 12 cases (1981-1986), *J Am Vet Med Assoc* 193:1443-1447, 1988.
14. Wolf A, Belden M: Feline histoplasmosis: A literature review and retrospective study of 20 new cases, *J Am Anim Hosp Assoc* 20:995-998, 1984.
15. Clinkenbeard K, Cowell R, Tyler R: Disseminated histoplasmosis in cats: 12 cases (1981-1986), *J Am Vet Med Assoc* 190:1445-1448, 1987.
16. Mitchell M, Stark D: Disseminated canine histoplasmosis: A clinical survey of 24 cases in Texas, *Can Vet J* 21:95-100, 1980.
17. VanSteenhouse J, DeNovo R: Atypical histoplasma capsulatum infection in a dog, *J Am Vet Med Assoc* 188:527-528, 1986.
18. Clinkenbeard K, Cowell R, Tyler R: Identification of Histoplasma organisms in circulating eosinophils of a dog, *J Am Vet Med Assoc* 192:217-218, 1988.
19. Hodges R, Legendre A, Adams L et al: Itraconazole for the treatment of histoplasmosis in cats, *J Vet Int Med* 8:409-413, 1994.
20. Silva-Ribeiro V, Ferreira-Da-Cruz M, Wanke B et al: Canine histoplasmosis in Rio de Janeiro: Natural and experimental infections, *J Med Vet Mycol* 25:319-322, 1987.
21. Burk R, Corwin L: The radiographic appearance of pulmonary histoplasmosis in the dog and cat: A review of 37 case histories, *J Am Vet Rad Soc* 19:2-7, 1977.
22. Ackerman N, Cornelius L, Halliwell W: Respiratory distress associated with histoplasma-induced tracheobronchial lymphadenopathy in dogs, *J Am Vet Med Assoc* 163:963-967, 1973.
23. Schulman R, McKiernan B, Schaeffer D: Use of corticosteroids for treating dogs with airway obstruction secondary to hilar lymphadenopathy caused by chronic histoplasmosis: 16 cases (1979-1997), *J Am Vet Med Assoc* 214:1345-1348, 1999.
24. Hawkins E, DeNicola D: Cytologic analysis of tracheal wash specimens and bronchoalveolar lavage fluid in the diagnosis of mycotic infections in dogs, *J Am Vet Med Assoc* 197:79-83, 1990.
25. Kabli S, Koschmann J, Roberstad G et al: Endemic canine and feline histoplasmosis in El Paso, Texas, *J Med Vet Mycol* 24:41-50, 1986.
26. Davies C, Troy G: Deep mycotic infections in cats, *J Am Anim Hosp Assoc* 32:380-391, 1996.
27. Noxon J, Digilio K, Schmidt D: Disseminated histoplasmosis in a cat: Successful treatment with ketoconazole, *J Am Vet Med Assoc* 181:817-818, 1982.
28. Breitschwerdt E, Halliwell W, Burk R et al: Feline histoplasmosis, *J Am Anim Hosp Assoc* 13:216-222, 1977.
29. Arceneaux K, Taboada J, Hosgood G: Blastomycosis in dogs: 115 cases (1980-1995), *J Am Vet Med Assoc* 213:658-664, 1998.
30. Cote E, Barr S, Allen C et al: Blastomycosis in six dogs in New York state, *J Am Vet Med Assoc* 210:502-504, 1997.
31. Legendre A, Rohrback B, Toal R et al: Treatment of blastomycosis with itraconazole in 112 dogs, *J Vet Intern Med* 10:365-371, 1996.
32. Rudmann D, Coolman B, Perez C et al: Evaluation of risk factors for blastomycosis in dogs: 857 cases (1980-1990), *J Am Vet Med Assoc* 201:1754-1759, 1992.
33. Legendre A, Walker M, Buyukmihchi N et al: Canine blastomycosis: A review of 47 clinical cases, *J Am Vet Med Assoc* 178:1163-1168, 1981.
34. Legendre A: Blastomycosis. In Greene C, editor: *Infectious diseases of the dog and cat,* Philadelphia, 1990, WB Saunders.
35. Legendre A, Selcer B, Edwards D et al: Treatment of canine blastomycosis with amphotericin B and ketoconazole, *J Am Vet Med Assoc* 184:1249-1254, 1984.
36. Walker M: Thoracic blastomycosis: A review of its radiographic manifestations in 40 dogs, *Vet Radiol* 22:22-26, 1981.
37. Dunbar M, Pyle R, Boring J et al: Treatment of canine blastomycosis with ketoconazole, *J Am Vet Med Assoc* 182:156-157, 1983.
38. Legendre A, Becker P: Evaluation of the agar-gel immunodiffusion test in the diagnosis of canine blastomycosis, *Am J Vet Res* 41:2109-2111, 1980.
39. Klein B, Squires R, Lloyd J et al: Canine antibody response to *Blastomyces dermatitidis* WI-1 antigen, *Am J Vet Res* 61:554-558, 2000.
40. Baumgardner D, Paretsky D: Identification of *Blastomyces dermatitidis* in the stool of a dog with acute pulmonary blastomycosis, *J Med Vet Mycol* 35:419-421, 1997.
41. Miller P, Miller L, Schoster J: Feline blastomycosis: A report of three cases and literature review (1961 to 1988), *J Am Anim Hosp Assoc* 26:417-424, 1990.
42. Brieder M, Walker T, Legendre A et al: Blastomycosis in cats: Five cases (1979-1986), *J Am Vet Med Assoc* 193:570-572, 1988.
43. Sheldon W: Pulmonary blastomycosis in a cat, *Lab Anim Care* 16:280-285, 1966.
44. Barsanti J, Jeffery K: Coccidioidomycosis. In Greene C, editor: *Infectious diseases of the dog and cat,* Philadelphia, 1990, WB Saunders.
45. Greene R, Troy G: Coccidioidomycosis in 48 cats: A retrospective study (1984-1993), *J Vet Int Med* 9:86-91, 1995.
46. Millman T, O'Brien T, Suter P et al: Coccidioidomycosis in the dog: Its radiographic diagnosis, *J Am Vet Radiol Soc* 20:50-65, 1979.
47. Wolf A, Pappagianis D: Canine coccidioidomycosis: Treatment with a new antifungal agent: ketoconazole, *Calif Vet* 35:25-27, 1981.
48. Maddy K: Disseminated coccidioidomycosis of the dog, *J Am Vet Med Assoc* 132:483-489, 1958.
49. Armstrong P, DiBartola S: Canine coccidioidomycosis: A literature review and report of eight cases, *J Am Vet Med Assoc* 19:937-946, 1983.
50. Jackson J, Mauldin R, Bauman D et al: Treatment of canine coccidioidomycosis with ketoconazole: Serological aspects of a case study, *J Amer Anim Hosp Assoc* 21:572-578, 1985.
51. Pappagianis D, Zimmer B: Serology of coccidioidomycosis, *Clin Microbiol Rev* 3:247-268, 1990.
52. Gerds-Grogan S, Dayrell-Hart B: Feline cryptococcosis: A retrospective evaluation, *J Am Anim Hosp Assoc* 33:118-122, 1997.
53. Medleau L, Barsanati J: Cryptococcosis. In Greene C, editor: *Infectious diseases of the dog and cat,* Philadelphia, 1990, WB Saunders.
54. Wilkinson G: Feline cryptococcosis: A review and seven case reports, *J Small Anim Pract* 20:749-768, 1979.
55. Malik R: Asymptomatic carriage of Cryptococcus neoformans in the nasal cavity of dogs and cats, *J Med Vet Mycol* 35:27-32, 1997.
56. Ramos-Vara J, Ferrer L, Visa J: Pathological findings in a cat with cryptococcosis and feline immunodeficiency virus infection, *Histol Histopath* 9:305-308, 1994.
57. Barrs V, Martin P, Nicoll R et al: Pulmonary cryptococcosis and Capillaria aerophila infection in an FIV-positive cat, *Aust Vet J* 78:154-158, 2000.
58. Jacobs G, Medleau L, Calvert C et al: Cryptococcal infection in cats: Factors influencing treatment outcome, and results of sequential serum antigen titers in 35 cats, *J Vet Int Med* 11:1-4, 1997.
59. Sutton R: Cryptococcosis in dogs: A report on 6 cases, *Aust Vet J* 57:558-564, 1981.
60. MacDonald D, Stretch H: Canine cryptococcosis associated with prolonged corticosteroid therapy, *Can Vet J* 23:200-202, 1982.

61. Gelatt K, McGill L, Perman V: Ocular and systemic cryptococcosis in a dog, *J Am Vet Med Assoc* 162:370-375, 1973.
62. Collett M, Doyle A, Reyers F: Fatal disseminated cryptococcosis and concurrent ehrlichiosis in a dog, *J S Afr Vet Med Assoc* 58:197-202, 1987.
63. Carlton W, Feeney D, Zimmerman J: Disseminated cryptococcosis with ocular involvement in a dog, *J Amer Anim Hosp Assoc* 12:53-59, 1976.
64. Malik R, Dill-Macky E, Martin R et al: Cryptococcosis in dogs: A retrospective study of 20 consecutive cases, *J Med Vet Mycology* 33:291-297, 1995.
65. Tiches D, Vite C, Dayrell-Hart B et al: A case of canine central nervous system cryptococcosis: Management with fluconazole, *J Am Anim Hosp Assoc* 34:145-151, 1998.
66. Malik R, Wigney D, Muir D et al: Cryptococcosis in cats: Clinical and mycological assessment of 29 cases and evaluation of treatment using orally administered fluconazole, *J Med Vet Mycol* 30:133-144, 1992.
67. Hamilton T, Hawkins E, DeNicola D: Bronchoalveolar lavage and tracheal wash to determine lung involvement in a cat with cryptococcosis, *J Am Med Vet Assoc* 198:655-656, 1991.
68. Medleau L, Marks A, Brown J et al: Clinical evaluation of a cryptococcal antigen latex agglutination test for diagnosis of cryptococcosis in cats, *J Am Vet Med Assoc* 196:1470-1473, 1990.
69. Flatland B, Greene R, Lappin M: Clinical and serologic evaluation of cats with cryptococcosis, *J Am Vet Med Assoc* 209:1110-1113, 1996.
70. Malik R, Craig A, Wigney D et al: Combination chemotherapy of canine and feline cryptococcosis using subcutaneously administered amphotericin B, *Aust Vet J* 73:124-128, 1996.
71. Medleau L, Jacobs G, Marks M: Itraconazole for the treatment of cryptococcosis in cats, *J Vet Int Med* 9:39-42, 1995.
72. Clercx C, McEntee K, Snaps F et al: Bronchopulmonary and disseminated granulomatous disease associated with Aspergillus fumigatus and Candida species infection in a golden retriever, *J Amer Anim Hosp Assoc* 32:139-145, 1996.
73. Jang S, Dorr T, Biberstein E et al: Aspergillus deflectus in four dogs, *J Med Vet Mycol* 24:95-104, 1986.
74. Neer T: Disseminated aspergillosis, *Comp Contin Ed* 10:465-471, 1988.
75. Guerin S, Walker M, Kelly D: Cavitating mycotic pulmonary infection in a German shepherd dog, *J Sm Anim Pract* 34:36-39, 1993.
76. Kahler J, Leach M, Jang S et al: Disseminated aspergillosis attributable to Aspergillus deflectus in a Springer Spaniel, *J Am Vet Med Assoc* 197:871-874, 1990.
77. Fox J, Murphy J, Shalev M: Systemic fungal infections in cats, *J Am Vet Med Assoc* 173:1191-1195, 1978.
78. Day M, Penhale W, Eger C et al: Disseminated aspergillosis in dogs, *Aust Vet J* 63:55-59, 1986.
79. Kaufman A, Greene C, Selcer B et al: Systemic aspergillosis in a dog and treatment with hamycin, *J Am Anim Hosp Assoc* 30(2):132-136, 1994.
80. Kelly S, Shaw S, Clark W: Long-term survival of four dogs with disseminated Aspergillus terreus infection treated with itraconazole, *Aust Vet J* 72:311-313, 1995.
81. Ossent P: Systemic aspergillosis and mucormycosis in 23 cats, *Vet Rec* 120:330-333, 1987.
82. Greene C, Chandler F: Candidiasis. In Greene C, editor: *Infectious diseases of the dog and cat,* Philadelphia, 1990, WB Saunders.
83. Miller R, Turnwald G: Disseminated basidiobolomycosis in a dog, *Vet Pathol* 21:117-119, 1984.
84. Walker R, Monticello T, Ford R et al: Eumycotic mycetoma caused by Pseudallescheria boydii in the abdominal cavity of a dog, *J Am Vet Med Assoc* 192:67-70, 1988.

CHAPTER 60

Lipid Pneumonia

Carol R. Norris

Introduction

Lipid pneumonia, a type of noninfectious inflammatory or irritant pneumonia, is characterized by intra- or extracellular globules of lipid in the alveolar spaces, often with mixed inflammatory cells and fibrosis. It is triggered by the intraalveolar presence of fatty substances and results in patchy consolidation of the lung.[1-3] Lipid pneumonia can be further classified as exogenous lipid pneumonia (ELP) or endogenous lipid pneumonia (EnLP) based on the source of lipid.[4] Exogenous lipid pneumonia results from inhalation or aspiration of mineral, vegetable, or animal oils, whereas EnLP occurs when cholesterol and other lipids are released into the alveoli following breakdown of pulmonary cell walls.[5] Fatty substances in either form of lipid pneumonia can

be identified by special stains (e.g., Sudan black, Sudan red, and oil-red-O); polarized light; and tissue chromatography.[6,7] In humans, EnLP can also result from fat emboli, pulmonary alveolar proteinosis, and lipid storage disorders.[4]

Both forms of lipid pneumonia have been described in dogs and cats,[1,5,8,9] ELP has been reported in cattle and horses[10,11]; and EnLP has been reported in raccoons, opossums, ferrets, llamas, and rodents.[12-16] In dogs, pulmonary alveolar proteinosis, a related pulmonary disorder associated with the accumulation of endogenous lipids, has also been described.[17-19] It differs from EnLP in that the alveoli become filled with periodic acid-Schiff (PAS) positive lipoproteinaceous material, believed to be caused by a defect in surfactant turnover.[19] Additionally, in pulmonary alveolar proteinosis, pulmonary interstitial architecture is maintained, in comparison with the inflammatory and fibrotic response seen with lipid pneumonia.[17]

Exogenous Lipid Pneumonia

ETIOLOGY AND PATHOGENESIS

Exogenous lipid pneumonia results from the inhalation or aspiration of fatty material of mineral, vegetable, or animal origin that leads to an inflammatory foreign body reaction and fibrosis in the lung.[4] Access of lipid to the airways and pulmonary parenchyma may be enhanced by recumbency, sedation or anesthesia, anatomic defects (e.g., cleft palate), gastrointestinal disorders (e.g., megaesophagus or gastroesophageal reflux), and neurologic deficits.[3,4,7,20] Normal pulmonary defense mechanisms, including the cough reflex, an intact mucociliary apparatus, and an active alveolar macrophage phagocytic response, may fail to provide adequate protection for the lung from the aspirated lipid.

The severity and type of pathologic lesion in the lung is dependent on the origin of the lipid.[3,4] Mineral oil does not irritate the pharyngeal mucosa, and consequently does not elicit a cough reflex when aspirated.[3] Once mineral oil gains access to the tracheobronchial tree, it inhibits the motility of the mucociliary apparatus by altering the viscoelastic properties of airway secretions.[4,7,20] Mineral oil in the alveolar spaces is emulsified (finely subdivided) and ingested by alveolar macrophages. The macrophages are unable to metabolize the chemically inert mineral oil, and after a time they degenerate, releasing the oil back into the alveoli.[20] The lipid initiates a local cell-mediated inflammatory response that eventually leads to fibrosis.[21]

In contrast to mineral oils, highly refined vegetable oils are free of fatty acids and do not emulsify.[3,6,8] Unless they are rancid, they do not trigger an inflammatory response, and are removed from the lung largely by expectoration.[4,6] Lipids of animal origin have a high fatty acid content and are hydrolyzed by pulmonary lipases. In the alveolar spaces, these liberated fatty acids cause a severe mononuclear and giant cell inflammatory reaction.[6] Animal oils have also been described to cause connective tissue proliferation, especially in the alveolar walls, as well as varying degrees of necrosis.[4]

CLINICAL FEATURES AND HISTORICAL FINDINGS

Exogenous lipid pneumonia has rarely been reported in dogs and cats. There is only a single case report in the veterinary literature of lipid pneumonia in the dog, and the authors were unable to definitively determine whether it was the exogenous or endogenous form.[9] In that case, supportive evidence that it was the exogenous form included the presence of muscle fiberlike structures in one bronchoalveolar lavage sample, suggesting the possibility of food aspiration. In cats, chronic forced administration of mineral oil for treatment of constipation and hair balls appears to be the most common cause of

ELP.[8,22] Clinical signs can range from a complete absence of symptoms, to mild tachypnea or cough, to severe respiratory distress.[8,9,22,23] In severe cases, dyspnea, increased abdominal effort, and cyanosis have been observed.[22] Crackles may be present on thoracic auscultation. Body temperatures were either normal or not reported.

DIAGNOSIS

The hemogram can be normal or may reflect the underlying inflammatory process, especially if there is a secondary bacterial infection.[22,23] Thoracic radiographic changes are variable and not specific for ELP.[9] In cats, radiography may show a diffuse nodular interstitial pattern that can mimic neoplastic, fungal, and parasitic diseases.[24] Severe lobar consolidation and hyperinflation corresponding to a histologic diagnosis of emphysema have also been reported in chronic cases of ELP in cats.[8,22] The role of computed tomography (CT), which is instrumental in the diagnosis of ELP in humans,[7] has not been evaluated in dogs or cats to date. In humans, CT scans not only demonstrate abnormalities that may not be visible on survey thoracic radiography but also detect attenuation values of tissue in the fat range.[3,7]

Cytology of fluid obtained from tracheal washes or bronchoalveolar lavages may be normal or demonstrate foamy lipid-laden macrophages, with or without other inflammatory cells.[8,9,21] In humans, special stains such as Sudan black, Sudan red, and oil red-O help with the identification of lipid-laden macrophages.[7] The cytoplasm of the macrophages is typically honeycombed with large fat vacuoles.[6] Culture of lavage fluid may be useful in determining the need for antibiotic therapy for secondary infections. On histologic examination, alveolar spaces are filled with extracellular lipid droplets, and in the phagocytic alveolar macrophages, intracellular lipid droplets.[8] Fibrosis, a key feature of ELP in humans, may also be present.[4,8,20]

TREATMENT

Discontinuation of forced administration of petroleum-based products for treatment of hair balls and constipation is prudent in animals with ELP. Treating secondary bacterial infections, correcting underlying defects that may favor aspiration, and providing supportive care (including oxygen supplementation, if required), are also recommended.[4,23,25] In humans (and presumably in some animals), chronic repeated aspiration of lipids triggers a local cell-mediated immune response important in the development of interstitial fibrosis.[20] In humans, the use of corticosteroids is controversial, but is speculated to diminish active pneumonitis that can lead to permanent fibrosis.[25]

PROGNOSIS

Prognosis depends on the amount of lipid aspirated; the severity of the granulomatous inflammatory response to the lipid; the development of secondary infections; and the chronicity of aspiration, which influences progression to permanent changes in the lung such as fibrosis. Although there are case reports in the literature of cats being administered mineral oil chronically (more than 3 or 4 years) that ultimately died as a result of severe ELP,[8,22] one retrospective study evaluating lipid pneumonia in all cats undergoing necropsy during a 13-year period at a veterinary medical teaching hospital failed to identify any cat with the exogenous form of the disease.[1] In some humans with ELP, malignant transformation to bronchogenic carcinoma has been reported.[4,6] It is unknown if the lipids themselves are carcinogenic, or if the secondary pulmonary inflammation and fibrosis predisposes to cancer.[4] The prognosis for patients with bronchogenic carcinoma and ELP is poor. There are no reports of bronchogenic carcinoma complicating ELP in dogs or cats to date.

Endogenous Lipid Pneumonia

ETIOLOGY AND PATHOGENESIS

Endogenous lipid pneumonia results from damage to pneumocytes, causing degeneration of the cells and subsequent release of cholesterol and cholesterol esters into the alveolar spaces. Injury to type II pneumocytes leads to overproduction of cholesterol-containing surfactant, and a fall in arterial oxygen gas tension with a concomi-

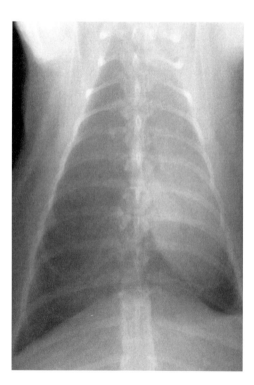

Figure 60-1. A dorsoventral thoracic radiograph of a cat with bronchopulmonary dysplasia. Atelectasis of the left cranial lobe with secondary hyperinflation of the right lung lobes and a leftward mediastinal shift are noted. After lobectomy, histological examination revealed a secondary bronchopneumonia and EnLP. Lobectomy was curative.

tant increase in arterial carbon dioxide gas tension.[26] Lipid in the alveoli incites an inflammatory reaction with subsequent phagocytosis of the lipid by alveolar macrophages. On histological examination, EnLP is characterized by intra- or extracellular cholesterol crystals or clefts, multinucleated giant cells, interstitial fibrosis, and hyperplasia of type II pneumocytes.[1,5]

The etiopathogenesis of EnLP in humans and animals is multifactorial, including obstructive bronchopulmonary disease, inhalation of noxious substances, deranged lipid metabolism, lipid storage disorders, fat emboli, hypophysectomy, and dietary deficiency of pantothenic acid.[3,13,16,27,28] Endogenous lipid pneumonia has also been reported to be idiopathic in humans and cats.[1,6] In the cat, pulmonary diseases (usually accompanied by bronchial obstruction on a microscopic level) associated with the development of EnLP include neoplasia; noninfectious inflammatory disease (e.g., bronchitis, bronchiectasis, necrotizing bronchiolitis, and uremic pneumonitis); pulmonary arterial thrombosis; cryptococcal pneumonia; and bronchial dysgenesis (Figure 60-1).[1,5,29]

Forty-two percent of cats in one study had an underlying obstructive pulmonary disease that was the likely cause of EnLP.[1] In contrast to humans, in whom obstructive pulmonary disease is usually secondary to neoplasia, in cats, noninfectious inflammatory disease and pulmonary arterial thrombosis were most commonly the cause of obstruction. In the remainder of cats, no specific cause of the EnLP was found.

CLINICAL FEATURES AND HISTORICAL FINDINGS

The clinical features of EnLP were retrospectively evaluated in 24 cats with histological confirmation of the disease.[1] Most cats with EnLP had nonspecific clinical signs of lethargy, anorexia, and weight loss. Of those with signs relating to the respiratory system, tachypnea, dyspnea, and cough were most commonly reported. The majority of cats were middle age or older and there was no obvious sex or breed predisposition. In most cases, the physical examination primarily represented findings associated with concurrent or primary disease processes. EnLP often occurred as an incidental finding and as a marker of other more severe disease, rather than a cause of morbidity by itself.

DIAGNOSIS

Clinicopathological abnormalities in cats with EnLP were nonspecific and reflected underlying or concurrent diseases.[1] Abnormalities on thoracic radiography were common but, as in humans, were not pathognomonic for EnLP.[25] Pleural effusion, a diffuse interstitial or bronchointerstitial pattern, multifocal infiltrates with or without confluence in the hilar region, discrete pulmonary nodules, and hyperinflation are examples of thoracic radiographic abnormalities reported in cats with EnLP.[1] Pleural effusions were classified as modified transudates or as chylous effusions and were likely related to the underlying diseases such as neoplasia or cardiac failure.[1] In humans, diffuse interstitial to fine nodular infiltrates are believed to develop as a result of initial alveolar filling followed by movement of lipid-laden macrophages into the interstitium and the resultant edematous, inflammatory, and fibrotic reaction.[18,30] Some cats with EnLP had normal thoracic radiographs[1]; these cats had only mild or microscopic changes of EnLP on histological examination.

Few diagnostic tests specific for the respiratory tract have been performed in cats with documented EnLP, making it difficult to draw conclusions about their utility in the antemortem diagnosis of EnLP. In humans, cytology of sputum samples and bronchoalveolar lavage fluid, as well as advanced imaging (e.g., computed tomography and magnetic resonance), are important in establishing the diagnosis of EnLP.[7] Cytological evaluation may reveal macrophages that stain positive for lipid using special stains.[7] These macrophages have a granular foamy cytoplasm containing fine punctate vacuoles.[6]

In cats, histological lesions of EnLP have been well described.[1] The majority of cats had a multifocal distribution of lesions that were macroscopic in size. These lesions were most commonly subpleural in location, followed by parenchymal and perivascular locations. Obstructive pulmonary disease leads to clearance defects in the lungs, resulting in a subpleural accumulation of macrophages.[28] Concurrent inflammatory infiltrates, including lymphocytes, plasma cells, and neutrophils, were seen in the majority of cats. Inflammation is believed to arise secondary to release of lipid from damaged and degenerating pneumocytes, which acts as a direct irritant.[3] Other histological lesions included cholesterol clefts, multinucleated giant cells, necrosis, fibrosis, and mineralization. Damage to type II pneumocytes results in excessive production of surfactant having a high cholesterol content. This surfactant undergoes phagocytosis by alveolar macrophages, resulting in cholesterol crystals or clefts (Figure 60-2).[1] The cholesterol is released extracellularly when alveolar macrophages degenerate.[18] Cholesterol crystals are irritating and stimulate the formation of multinucleated giant cells.[3]

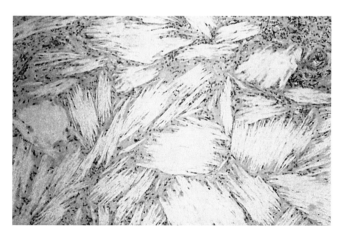

Figure 60-2. *An H&E stained histological specimen from the pulmonary parenchyma of a cat with EnLP showing characteristic cholesterol clefts.* (Courtesy of Dr. Stephen M. Griffey, University of California, Davis.)

TREATMENT

Because most of the available information on EnLP in cats is based on a retrospective study[1] of cats with histologic specimens collected at the time of necropsy, little data is available on treatment of this condition. In humans, focal areas of EnLP and the inciting obstructive lesion are often surgically removed because chronic EnLP has been reported to undergo malignant transformation.[6] It is unknown whether treatment of the underlying disease or removal of an obstructive lesion in cats would resolve the EnLP, or even if chronic EnLP could undergo malignant transformation in this species. Furthermore, cats often have diffuse obstructive pulmonary disease involving most lung lobes, which may not be amenable to focal resection. Idiopathic EnLP in humans may be successfully treated with corticosteroids[25]; this therapy has not been evaluated in cats.

PROGNOSIS

The lesions of EnLP in all cats retrospectively evaluated were believed to be an incidental finding at the time of necropsy.[1] In no cat were lesions severe or extensive enough to be the cause of death; rather, in many cases death was presumed to occur due to severe lesions of concurrent underlying bronchopulmonary disease. The authors speculated that in many cats, EnLP may serve as an indicator of potentially severe underlying obstructive pulmonary disease.

REFERENCES

1. Jones D, Norris C, Samii V et al: Endogenous lipid pneumonia in cats: 24 cases (1985-1998), *J Am Vet Med Assoc* 9:1437-1440, 2000.
2. Robbins S: *Pathologic basis of disease*, Philadelphia, 1989, WB Saunders.
3. Wright B, Jeffrey P: Lipoid pneumonia, *Seminars in Respiratory Infections* 5:314-321, 1990.
4. Spickard A, Hirschmann J: Exogenous lipoid pneumonia, *Arch Intern Med* 154:686-692, 1994.
5. Jerram R, Guyer C, Braniecki A et al: Endogenous lipid (cholesterol) pneumonia associated with bronchogenic carcinoma in a cat, *J Amer An Hosp Assoc* 34:275-280, 1998.
6. Felson B, Ralaisomay G: Carcinoma of the lung complicating lipoid pneumonia, *Am J Radiol* 141:901-907, 1983.
7. Gondouin A, Manzoni P, Ranfaing E et al: Exogenous lipid pneumonia: A retrospective multicentre study of 44 cases in France, *Eur Resp J* 9:1463-1469, 1996.
8. Chalifoux A, Morin M, Lemieux R: Lipid pneumonia and severe pulmonary emphysema in a persian cat, *Feline Prac* 17:6-10, 1987.
9. Corcoran B, Martin M, Darke P et al: Lipoid pneumonia in a rough collie dog, *J Sm Anim Pract* 33:544-548, 1992.
10. Smith B, Alley M, McPherson W: Lipid pneumonia in a cow, *New Zealand Vet J* 16:65-67, 1968.
11. Scarratt W, Moon M, Sponenberg D et al: Inappropriate administration of mineral oil resulting in lipoid pneumonia in 3 horses, *Equine Veterinary Journal* 30:85-88, 1998.
12. Weller W: Alveolar lipoproteinosis. In Jones T, Mohr M, Hunt R, editors: *Monographs on pathology of laboratory animals*, New York, 1985, Springer-Verlag.
13. Emi Y, Higashiguchi R, Konishi Y: Pulmonary lipidosis. In Jones T, Mohr M, Hunt R, editors: *Monographs on pathology of laboratory animals*, New York, 1985, Springer-Verlag.
14. Hamir A, Hanlon C, Rupprecht C: Endogenous lipid pneumonia (multifocal alveolar histiocytosis) in raccoons *(Procyon lotor)*, *J Vet Diagn Invest* 8:267-269, 1996.

15. Fox J: Subpleural histiocytosis. In Fox J, editor: *Biology and diseases of the ferret*, Philadelphia, 1988, Lea & Febiger.
16. Brown C: Endogenous lipid pneumonia in opossums from Louisiana, *J Wildlife Dis* 24:214-219, 1988.
17. Silverstein D, Green C, Gregory C et al: Pulmonary alveolar proteinosis in a dog, *J Vet Intern Med* 14:546-551, 2000.
18. Fisher M, Roggli V, Merten D et al: Coexisting endogenous lipoid pneumonia, cholesterol granulomas, and pulmonary alveolar proteinosis in a pediatric population: A clinical, radiographic and pathologic correlation, *Ped Path* 12:365-383, 1992.
19. Jefferies A, Dunn J, Dennis R: Pulmonary alveolar proteinosis (phospholipoproteinosis) in a dog, *J Sm Anim Pract* 28:203-214, 1987.
20. Lauque D, Dongay G, Levade T et al: Bronchoalveolar lavage in liquid paraffin pneumonitis, *Chest* 98:1149-1155, 1990.
21. Midulla F, Strappini P, Ascoli V et al: Bronchoalveolar lavage cell analysis in a child with chronic lipid pneumonia, *Eur Resp J* 11:239-242, 1998.
22. De Souza H, Dos Santos A, Ferreira A et al: Chronic lipidic pneumonia in a cat, *Feline Prac* 26:16-19, 1998.
23. Hawkins E: Disorders of the pulmonary parenchyma. In Nelson R, Couto C, editors: *Essentials of small animal internal medicine*, St Louis, 1992, Mosby Year-Book.
24. Hawkins E: Diseases of the lower respiratory system. In Ettinger S, Feldman E, editors: *Textbook of veterinary internal medicine*, ed 4, Philadelphia, 1995, WB Saunders.
25. Chin N, Hui K, Sinniah R et al: Idiopathic lipoid pneumonia in an adult treated with prednisolone, *Chest* 105:956-957, 1994.
26. Verbeken E, Demedts M, Vanwing J et al: Pulmonary phospholipid accumulation distal to an obstructed bronchus, *Arch Pathol Lab Med* 113:886-890, 1989.
27. Beaver D, Ashburn L, McDaniel E et al: Lipid deposits in the lungs of germ-free animals, *Arch Pathol* 76:565-570, 1963.
28. Dungworth D: The respiratory system. In Jubb K, Kennedy P, Palmer N, editors: *Pathology of domestic animals*, ed. 4, Orlando, 1993, Academic Press.
29. LaRue M, Garlick D, Lamb C et al: Bronchial dysgenesis and lobar emphysema in an adult cat, *J Am Vet Med Assoc* 197:886-888, 1990.
30. Felson B: *Chest roentgenology*, Philadelphia, 1973, WB Saunders.

CHAPTER 61

Protozoal Pneumonia

Michael R. Lappin

Toxoplasmosis

DEFINITION AND ETIOLOGY

Toxoplasma gondii is a protozoan in the phylum *Apicomplexa*.[1] The coccidian life cycle is completed only in the gastrointestinal tract of cats, and results in the passage of oocysts in feces for about 7 to 14 days after primary infection. Oocysts are passed unsporulated and are not infectious; infectious sporozoites develop into oocysts after 1 to 5 days of exposure to oxygen. Sporulated oocysts are infectious in the environment for months to years. A tissue phase occurs in most mammals, including dogs and cats. Tachyzoites are the rapidly dividing tissue stage (Figure 61-1), and bradyzoites are the slowly dividing tissue phase.[1]

PATHOPHYSIOLOGY

Infection with *T. gondii* occurs following ingestion of any of the three life stages, or transplacentally and during lactation when the host has its primary infection during gestation. Cats are most commonly infected by ingesting *T. gondii* bradyzoites during carnivorous feeding. Dogs are more likely than cats to be coprophagic, therefore ingestion of sporulated oocysts is a possible means of infection for dogs. After primary infection, sporozoites or bradyzoites penetrate the intestinal mucosa and disseminate in the blood and lymph as tachyzoites.[1] Rapid intracellular replication occurs, which destroys the infected cells, causes tissue necrosis, and releases tachyzoites that infect other cells (Figure 61-2). This cycle continues, resulting in severe clinical illness and death unless the immune system attenuates replication, leading to the formation of tissue cysts containing bradyzoites in extraintestinal tissues. It is likely that bradyzoites persist in tissues for the life of the host and can be reactivated during states of immunosuppression, resulting in repeated rapid replication and recurrent clinical illness. Respiratory disease is due to tachyzoite replication.

INCIDENCE/PREVALENCE

Toxoplasma gondii infection is common; the seroprevalence of infection is approximately 30% in cats and humans and approximately 20% in dogs in the United States.[1,2] Although the incidence of disease is unknown, clinical signs are rarely recognized. In the absence of immunosuppression, clinical illness is usually inapparent in dogs and cats.

RISK FACTORS

Respiratory disease from toxoplasmosis is recognized most commonly in transplacentally or lactationally infected animals[3-5] and in animals with reactivated infection caused

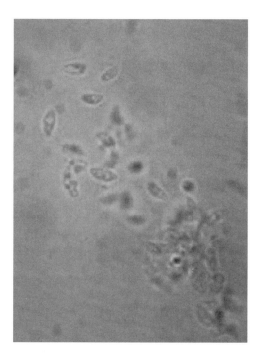

Figure 61-1. *Unstained tachyzoites of* Toxoplasma gondii. *The banana-shaped organisms replicate intracellularly until the host cell is destroyed. This stage of the organism is occasionally detected in BAL fluid.*

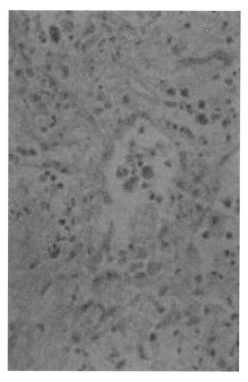

Figure 61-2. *Immunohistochemical stain of lung tissue from an FIV-seropositive cat that died of pneumonic toxoplasmosis.*

by acquired immunodeficiency such as that associated with immunosuppressive therapy,[6] retroviral infection (cats),[7] or canine distemper virus infection (dogs).[8]

CLINICAL FINDINGS

When tissue cysts are fed to cats, approximately 10% to 20% develop self-limiting, small bowel diarrhea. Inflammatory bowel disease is an uncommon manifestation of the intestinal cycle in cats. Fatal extraintestinal toxoplasmosis usually has an acute course; pulmonary, hepatic, central nervous system (CNS), and pancreatic tissues are most commonly involved.[9] Disseminated toxoplasmosis in cats results in depression, anorexia, and fever; this is followed by hypothermia, dyspnea, peritoneal effusion, icterus, and usually death.* If lactational or transplacental infection occurs in kittens, dyspnea is common and usually progresses to death. In one study of fatal toxoplasmosis of cats, *T. gondii* or characteristic lesions were found in the lungs of 84 of 86 cats examined.[9] Acquired immunodeficiency such as that associated with retroviral infection or immunosuppressive drugs can allow bradyzoites in tissue cysts to revert to tachyzoites and disseminate. Dyspnea occurred in some cats with reactivated toxoplasmosis following renal transplantation.[1,6] Chronic clinical syndromes occur in some cats with extraintestinal infection; anterior or posterior uveitis, fever, muscle hyperesthesia, weight loss,

anorexia, seizures, ataxia, icterus, diarrhea, and pancreatitis are most common.[1,2,13]

In dogs, *T. gondii* replication in lungs and other extraintestinal tissues commonly occurs, and occasionally results in clinical disease. When clinical signs occur, fever, dyspnea, vomiting, diarrhea, and icterus are most common.[1,8] Dyspnea or pneumonia was reported in 8 of 13 histologically proven cases.[8] Concurrent canine distemper virus infection was common and likely potentiated clinical toxoplasmosis by inducing immune suppression. Dogs with myositis present with weakness, stiff gait, or muscle wasting; rapid progression to tetraparesis and paralysis with lower motor neuron dysfunction can occur. Ataxia, seizures, tremors, cranial nerve deficits, paresis, and paralysis are the most common manifestations of CNS toxoplasmosis.[1] Ventricular arrhythmias from myocardial infection occur in some dogs. Ocular manifestations (e.g., retinitis, anterior uveitis, iridocyclitis, and optic neuritis) occur in some dogs with toxoplasmosis, but are less common than in the cat. Before 1988, some cases thought to be canine toxoplasmosis were probably *Neospora caninum* because the clinical presentations of the two organisms can be similar and they are difficult to differentiate by light microscopy.

DIAGNOSTIC TESTS

Because disseminated disease commonly occurs with toxoplasmosis, many laboratory abnormalities have been noted. These include nonregenerative anemia; neutrophilic

---

*References 1, 3, 4, 6, 7, and 9-12.

leukocytosis; lymphocytosis; monocytosis; neutropenia; eosinophilia; proteinuria; bilirubinuria; increases in serum protein and bilirubin concentration; and creatinine kinase (CK), alanine aminotransferase, alkaline phosphatase, and lipase activities.[1,2] Diffuse interstitial pattern, diffuse alveolar pattern, or pleural effusion are the most common radiographic abnormalities in dogs and cats with pulmonary involvement.

The antemortem definitive diagnosis of feline or canine toxoplasmosis can be made if the organism is demonstrated. Bradyzoites or tachyzoites are occasionally detected in tissues, effusions, bronchoalveolar lavage fluids, aqueous humor, or cerebrospinal fluid (CSF). Bronchoalveolar lavage cytological findings reveal increased numbers of neutrophils and macrophages.[12,14] Cerebrospinal fluid protein concentrations and cell counts are often higher than normal in dogs and cats with CNS toxoplasmosis; the predominant white blood cells are small, mononuclear cells, but neutrophils also are commonly found. Polymerase chain reaction can be used to detect organismal DNA in aqueous humor, CSF, effusions, bronchoalveolar lavage fluid, or blood. However, detection of T. gondii DNA in blood does not correlate to clinical disease in cats.[15]

Because Toxoplasma gondii–specific antibodies can be detected in the serum of normal cats and dogs, as well as in those with clinical signs of disease, it is impossible to make an antemortem diagnosis of clinical toxoplasmosis based on these tests alone.[1,2] Of the commercially available IgM and IgG serum tests, IgM correlates better with clinical toxoplasmosis because this antibody class is usually not detected in healthy animals. The antemortem diagnosis of clinical toxoplasmosis can be tentatively based on the combination of:

- Demonstration of antibodies in serum which documents exposure to T. gondii
- Demonstration of an IgM titer greater than 1:64 or a fourfold or greater increase in IgG titer which suggests recent or active infection
- Clinical signs of disease referable to toxoplasmosis
- Exclusion of other common causes of the clinical syndrome
- Positive response to appropriate treatment

Some cats and dogs with clinical toxoplasmosis will have reached their maximal IgG titer or will have undergone antibody class shift from IgM to IgG by the time serologic evaluation is performed. Thus the failure to document an increasing IgG titer or a positive IgM titer does not exclude the diagnosis of clinical toxoplasmosis. Because some healthy cats and dogs have extremely high serum antibody titers, and some clinically ill cats and dogs have low serum antibody titers, the magnitude of titer is relatively unimportant in the clinical diagnosis of toxoplasmosis. Because the organism cannot be cleared from the body, most cats and dogs will remain antibody-positive for life, so there is little reason to repeat serum antibody titers after clinical disease has resolved.

On histopathology, the characteristic findings associated with toxoplasmosis are tissue necrosis and pyogranulomatous inflammation.[1,3,8,9] The organism is often but not always noted on histological examination.

Immunohistochemistry and polymerase chain reaction can be used to confirm the presence of the organism in tissues.

MANAGEMENT

Supportive care including fluid and oxygen therapy should be administered as indicated. Drugs with anti-Toxoplasma activity that have been used to treat some affected dogs and cats include clindamycin hydrochloride, potentiated sulfonamides, pyrimethamine, minocycline, azithromycin, and clarithromycin.[1] Clindamycin is usually administered at 12.5 mg/kg, PO, q12h for at least 4 weeks. The drug can also be given parenterally during the acute phase of illness. Trimethoprim sulfa is usually administered at 15 mg/kg, PO, q12-24h for at least 4 weeks. Anti-Toxoplasma doses of the other drugs listed are unknown for dogs and cats. To date, dogs or cats with pulmonary toxoplasmosis from organism replication have generally died in spite of anti-Toxoplasma therapy and extensive supportive care. With uveitis, use topical, oral, or parenteral corticosteroids to avoid secondary damage to the eye induced by inflammation; glaucoma and lens luxations are very common in cats.[1]

To avoid infection, dogs and cats should only be fed processed foods and should not be allowed to hunt.

OUTCOME AND PROGNOSIS

The prognosis is poor for cats and dogs with acute, disseminated toxoplasmosis because of organism replication, particularly if immunodeficiency exists. Chronic toxoplasmosis often responds to therapy. In chronic cases, recurrence of clinical signs may be more common if treatment duration is less than 4 weeks. There is currently no drug that can totally clear the body of the organism, and so recurrences of some syndromes (e.g., uveitis) are common.

Neosporosis

DEFINITION AND ETIOLOGY

Neospora caninum is a coccidian previously confused with T. gondii because of similar morphology.[1,16] The sexual cycle is completed in the gastrointestinal tract of dogs and results in the passage of oocysts in feces.[17-21] Sporozoites develop into oocysts within 24 hours of passage. Tachyzoites (a rapidly-dividing stage) and tissue cysts containing hundreds of bradyzoites (a slowly-dividing stage) are the other two life stages.

PATHOPHYSIOLOGY

Dogs are infected by ingestion of bradyzoites but not tachyzoites. Transplacental infection has been well documented; dams that give birth to infected offspring can repeat transplacental infection during subsequent pregnancies.[21,22] The pathogenesis of the disease is primarily related to intracellular replication of tachyzoites. Although organism replication occurs in many tissues including the lungs, clinical illness is primarily neuromuscular in dogs. Whereas encephalomyelitis and myositis develop in experimentally infected kittens, clinical disease in naturally infected cats has not been reported.[23]

INCIDENCE/PREVALENCE

Canine neosporosis has been reported in many countries around the world. Seroprevalence of infection has varied from 0% to 29%.[21] The incidence of respiratory disease is not known but is likely to be uncommon.

EPIDEMIOLOGY AND RISK FACTORS

Dogs can be infected from the ingestion of infected placental tissues.[20] Whether other intermediate hosts play a role in maintenance of infection is unknown, but white-tailed deer are commonly seropositive.[24] Thus free-roaming dogs may be at increased risk of infection. Because repeated transplacental infections occur, there is increased risk for puppies from a bitch that has previously produced infected puppies.[22] Administration of glucocorticoids may activate bradyzoites in tissue cysts, resulting in clinical illness.

CLINICAL FINDINGS

Clinical disease tends to be most severe in congenitally infected puppies, but dogs as old as 15 years have been clinically affected.[21,25-28] In one dog presented primarily for respiratory disease, cough was the principal sign.[27] Ascending paralysis with hyperextension of the hindlimbs in congenitally infected puppies is the most common clinical manifestation of the disease. Muscle atrophy occurs in many cases. Polymyositis and multifocal CNS disease can occur alone or in combination. Clinical signs can be evident soon after birth or may be delayed for several weeks. Neonatal death is common. Pneumonia, myocarditis, dysphagia, ulcerative dermatitis, and hepatitis occur in some dogs.[16,21] It is unknown whether clinical disease in older dogs is due to acute, primary infection or exacerbation of chronic infection.

DIAGNOSTIC TESTS

Hematological and biochemical findings are nonspecific.[1] Myositis commonly results in increased CK and aspartate aminotransferase (AST) activities. Cerebrospinal fluid abnormalities include increased protein concentration (20 to 50 mg/dl) and a mild, mixed inflammatory cell pleocytosis (10 to 50 cells/dl) consisting of monocytes; lymphocytes; neutrophils; and, rarely, eosinophils. Interstitial and alveolar patterns can be noted on thoracic radiographs.

Definitive diagnosis is based on demonstration of the organism in CSF or tissues. Tachyzoites are rarely identified on cytologic examination of bronchoalveolar lavage, transthoracic aspirate, CSF, or imprints of dermatological lesions. Mixed inflammation with neutrophils, lymphocytes, eosinophils, plasma cells, macrophages, and tachyzoites was noted on transthoracic aspirate of 1 dog with lung disease.[27] The organism can be differentiated from *T. gondii* by electron microscopy, immunohistochemistry, and polymerase chain reaction.

A presumptive diagnosis of neosporosis can be made by combining appropriate clinical signs of disease with positive serology or presence of antibodies in CSF and the exclusion of other etiologies inducing similar clinical syndromes (in particular, *T. gondii*). *Neospora caninum* oocysts can be detected in feces by PCR.[29]

On histopathology, mixed inflammation with lymphocytes, plasma cells, neutrophils, and macrophages was found in the interstitium, alveoli, and pleura of 1 dog that was euthanized because of respiratory disease.[27] Infection of CNS structures causes mononuclear cell infiltrates, which suggests an immune-mediated component to the disease pathogenesis. Intact tissue cysts in neural structures are generally not associated with inflammation, but ruptured tissue cysts induce inflammation.

MANAGEMENT

The untreated disease generally results in death. Although most dogs die, several have survived after treatment with trimethoprim-sulfadiazine combined with pyrimethamine; sequential treatment with clindamycin hydrochloride, trimethoprim-sulfadiazine, and pyrimethamine or clindamycin alone. Administration of trimethoprim-sulfadiazine at 15 mg/kg, PO, BID for 4 weeks with pyrimethamine at 1 mg/kg, PO, SID for 4 weeks or clindamycin at 10 mg/kg, PO, TID, for 4 weeks is currently recommended for the treatment of canine neosporosis.[1,28]

OUTCOME AND PROGNOSIS

The prognosis for dogs presented with severe neurological involvement is grave. Treatment of clinically affected dogs should be initiated before the development of extensor rigidity, if possible. The single reported dog with respiratory disease was euthanized.[27]

Bitches that whelp clinically affected puppies should not be bred. Glucocorticoids should not be administered to seropositive animals, if possible, because a potential exists for activation of infection. Dogs should be housed in yards, should not be allowed to hunt, and should be fed processed foods.

Pneumocystosis

DEFINITION AND ETIOLOGY

Pneumocystis carinii is a saphrophytic organism with worldwide distribution that has characteristics of protozoans, yeasts, and fungi.[30-31]

PATHOPHYSIOLOGY

The organism is found in the alveoli of some normal animals. Disease only occurs in immunosuppressed individuals. Replication of the organism in the alveoli induces infiltrates of lymphocytes, plasma cells, and macrophages;

this produces an alveolar-capillary blockage. Disseminated infection is rare in dogs and people. Disease has been detected in cats given corticosteroids.[32]

INCIDENCE AND RISK FACTORS

Pneumocystosis in animals is extremely rare and is only associated with concurrent immune deficiency. Miniature dachshunds with common variable immunodeficiency syndrome are affected most commonly.[30,31,33]

CLINICAL FINDINGS

Most affected dogs have been less than 1 year of age.[30,31,34,35] Predominant findings are dry cough, dyspnea, and progressive weight loss. Dermatopathies such as demodecosis and pyoderma, which likely reflect the immune deficiency, occur in most cases.

DIAGNOSTIC TESTS

Neutrophilic leukocytosis, polycythemia, eosinophilia, and monocytosis occur in some dogs but are nonspecific findings.[30] Common blood gas abnormalities include hypoxemia, hypocapnia, and an increased arterial-alveolar gradient. On thoracic radiographs, interstitial to alveolar patterns predominate.[30,31,36] Cor pulmonale can develop. Cytologic demonstration of the organism in transthoracic aspirates, transtracheal wash specimens, or lung biopsies is used to make the final diagnosis.[30,31,37] Immune function deficits have been documented in affected dachshunds.[33] Diffuse interstitial pneumonia characterized by free and phagocytosed organisms in the alveolar spaces is found on histopathological examination.[30,31]

MANAGEMENT AND MONITORING

Potentiated sulfonamides at 30 mg/kg, q12hr, PO; or 15 mg/kg, q8hr, PO give the best results.[30,31] Pentamidine, carbutamide, trimetrexate, the combination of clindamycin and primaquine, and the combination of dapsone and trimethoprim have been used to treat pneumocytosis in some dogs. Supportive care including oxygen therapy, bronchodilators, nebulization, and mucolytic agents should be administered as indicated.

OUTCOME AND PROGNOSIS

For most cases, death occurs or euthanasia is chosen within days to months after diagnosis.

REFERENCES

1. Dubey JP, Greene CE, Lappin MR: Toxoplasmosis and neosporosis. In Greene CE, editor: *Infectious diseases of the dog and cat*, ed 2, Philadelphia, 1990, WB Saunders.
2. Lappin MR: Feline toxoplasmosis: Interpretation of diagnostic test results, *Seminars Vet Med Surg* 11:154-160, 1996.
3. Dubey JP, Carpenter JL: Neonatal toxoplasmosis in littermate cats, *J Am Vet Med Assoc* 203:1546-1549, 1993.
4. Dubey JP, Johnstone I: Fatal neonatal toxoplasmosis in cats, *J Am Anim Hosp Assoc* 18:461-467, 1982.
5. Dubey JP, Lappin MR, Thulliez P: Diagnosis of induced toxoplasmosis in neonatal cats, *J Am Vet Med Assoc* 207:179-185, 1995.
6. Bernstein L, Gregory CR, Aronson LR et al: Acute toxoplasmosis following renal transplantation in three cats and a dog, *J Am Vet Med Assoc* 215:1123-1126, 1999.
7. Davidson MG, Rottman JB, English RV et al: Feline immunodeficiency virus predisposes cats to acute generalized toxoplasmosis, *Am J Path* 143:1486-1497, 1993.
8. Dubey JP, Carpenter JL, Topper MJ et al: Fatal toxoplasmosis in dogs, *J Am Anim Hosp Assoc* 25:659-664, 1989.
9. Dubey JP, Carpenter JL: Histologically confirmed clinical toxoplasmosis in cats: 100 cases (1952-1990), *J Am Vet Med Assoc* 203:1556-1566, 1993.
10. Feeney DA, Sautter JH, Lees GE: An unusual case of acute disseminated toxoplasmosis in a cat, *J Am Anim Hosp Assoc* 17:311-314, 1981.
11. Henriksen P, Dietz HH, Henriksen A: Fatal toxoplasmosis in five cats, *Vet Parasitol* 55:15-20, 1994.
12. Brownlee L, Sellon RK: Diagnosis of naturally occurring toxoplasmosis by bronchoalveolar lavage in a cat, *J Am Anim Hosp Assoc* 37:251-255, 2001.
13. Lappin MR, Greene CE, Winston S et al: Clinical feline toxoplasmosis: Serologic diagnosis and therapeutic management of 15 cases, *J Vet Int Med* 3:139-143, 1989.
14. Hawkins EC, Davidson MG, Meuten DJ et al: Cytologic identification of *Toxoplasma gondii* in bronchoalveolar lavage fluid of experimentally infected cats, *J Am Vet Med Assoc* 210:648-650, 1997.
15. Burney DP, Spilker M, McReynolds L et al: Detection of *Toxoplasma gondii* parasitemia in experimentally inoculated cats, *J Parasitol* 5:947-951, 1999.
16. Dubey JP, Carpenter JL, Speer CA et al: Newly recognized fatal protozoan disease of dogs, *J Am Vet Med Assoc* 192:1269-1285, 1988.
17. McAllister MM, Dubey JP, Lindsay DS et al: Dogs are definitive hosts of *Neospora caninum*, *Int J Parasitol* 28:1473-1478, 1998.
18. Lindsay DS, Dubey JP, McAllister M: *Neospora caninum* and the potential for parasite transmission, *Comp Cont Ed Pract Vet* 21:317-321, 1999.
19. Basso W, Venturini L, Venturini MC et al: First isolation of *Neospora caninum* from the feces of a naturally infected dog, *J Parasitol* June (87):612-618, 2001.
20. Dijkstra T, Eysker M, Schares G et al: Dogs shed *Neospora caninum* oocysts after ingestion of naturally infected bovine placenta but not after ingestion of colostrum spiked with *Neospora caninum* tachyzoites, *Int J Parasitol* 31:747-752, 2001.
21. Lindsay DS, Dubey JP: Canine neosporosis, *J Vet Parasitol* 14:1-11, 2000.
22. Dubey JP, Koestner A, Piper RC: Repeated transplacental transmission of *Neospora caninum* in dogs, *J Am Vet Med Assoc* 197:857-860, 1990.
23. Dubey JP, Lindsay DS, Lipscomb TP: Neosporosis in cats, *Vet Pathol* 27:335-339, 1990.
24. Dubey JP, Hollis K, Romand S et al: High prevalence of antibodies to *Neospora caninum* in white-tailed deer *(Odocoileus virginianus)*, *Int J Parasitol* 29:1709-1711, 1999.
25. Barber TS, Trees AJ: Clinical aspects of 27 cases of neosporosis in dogs, *Vet Rec* 139:439-443, 1996.
26. Cuddon P, Lin DS, Bowman DD et al: *Neospora caninum* infection in English Springer spaniel littermates: Diagnostic evaluation and organism isolation, *J Vet Int Med* 6:325-332, 1992.
27. Greig B, Rossow KD, Collins JE et al: *Neospora caninum* pneumonia in an adult dog, *J Am Vet Med Assoc* 206:1000-1001, 1995.
28. Ruehlmann D, Podell M, Oglesbee M et al: Canine neosporosis: A case report and literature review, *J Am Anim Hosp Assoc* 31:174-183, 1995.
29. Hill DE, Liddell S, Jenkins MC et al: Specific detection of *Neospora caninum* oocysts in fecal samples from experimentally-infected dogs using the polymerase chain reaction, *J Parasitol* 87:395-398, 2001.
30. Lobetti RG: *Pneumocystis carinii* infection in miniature dachshunds, *Comp Cont Ed Pract Vet* 23:320-327, 2001.
31. Lobetti RG, Leisewitz AL, Spencer JA: *Pneumocystis carinii* in the miniature dachshund: Case report and literature review, *J Small Anim Pract* 37:280-285, 1996.
32. Shiota T, Shimada Y, Kurimotes H et al: *Pneumocystis carinii* infection in corticosteroid treated cats, *J Parasitol* 76:441-445, 1990.

33. Lobetti R: Common variable immunodeficiency in miniature dachshunds affected with *Pneumonocystis carinii* pneumonia, *J Vet Diag Invest* 12:39-45, 2000.
34. Cabañes FJ, Roura X, Majó N et al: *Pneumocystis carinii* pneumonia in a Yorkshire terrier dog, *Med Mycol* 38:451-453, 2000.
35. Hagiwara Y, Fujiwara S, Takai H et al: *Pneumocystis carinii* pneumonia in a Cavalier King Charles Spaniel, *J Vet Med Sci* 63:349-351, 2001.
36. Kirberger RM, Lobetti RG: Radiographic aspects of *Pneumocytis carinii* pneumonia in the miniature dachshund, *Vet Rad Ultrasonog* 39:313-317, 1998.
37. Sukura A, Saaru S, Jarvinen A et al: *Pneumocystis carinii* pneumonia in dogs: A diagnostic challenge, *J Vet Diagn Invest* 8:124-130, 1996.

CHAPTER 62

Atelectasis

Janet Aldrich

Definition and Etiology

Atelectasis has been used to describe a variety of airless, or partially airless,[1] states of the lung, including:

- A lung that has been mechanically compressed until it collapsed
- A lung that has suffered an airway obstruction with subsequent absorption of trapped gases[2-5]
- A lung in which alveoli have collapsed and subsequently been filled with fluid such that no volume loss has occurred[6]
- A lung in which alveoli repetitively collapse and reexpand during tidal breathing[7]

The term atelectasis is also used to describe the newborn lung that has never expanded. In that setting, atelectasis is one component of the respiratory distress syndrome in premature human infants, which is primarily a deficiency of pulmonary surfactant.[8] To avoid confusing the conditions, some authors prefer the term pulmonary collapse for all states of atelectasis except that of the newborn.[2]

The significance of atelectasis, in addition to the underlying disease it represents, is that it interferes with the balance between ventilation (V) and perfusion (Q), causing V/Q mismatch and intrapulmonary shunting, and can therefore promote venous admixture and hypoxemia.[9] In addition, removal of secretions is impaired in the affected areas, which may predispose to infection.[10,11] Identification of atelectasis is important because it is a potentially reversible cause of severe hypoxemia, and specific management protocols both to decrease its risk and to reexpand the lung are available.

Pathophysiology

An extensive discussion of respiratory terminology is beyond the scope of this chapter, but a few definitions are provided for the sake of clarity. Venous admixture refers to all the ways in which blood passes from the right ventricle to the left ventricle without being properly oxygenated. Airway obstruction causes a reduction in the ventilation of a gas exchange unit that is still being perfused, and therefore the blood leaving that unit is not adequately oxygenated. The ventilation/perfusion ratio (V/Q) of that unit is low. If the lung unit is completely unventilated, the V/Q is zero and that area of the lung constitutes an intrapulmonary shunt. V/Q mismatch contributes to venous admixture when the blood from the underventilated lung units mixes with the end capillary blood from other areas of the lung and dilutes the oxygen content of the mixed blood.[12]

ATELECTASIS CAUSED BY MECHANICAL FORCES AND AIRWAY OBSTRUCTION

Parenchymal and extraparenchymal masses (e.g., neoplasia, granuloma, or abscesses); pleural space disease with accumulation of air or fluid (e.g., transudates, or exudates such as pus, blood, or lymph); or intrusion of abdominal contents all constitute extraluminal forces that can compress airways to the point of collapse. These conditions interfere with lung mechanics. Normally, the thoracic cage elastic forces tend to expand the rib cage during inspiration, whereas the elastic and surface tension forces in the lung tend toward collapse. These opposing forces are linked by negative pressure between the visceral and parietal pleura, which are connected by a thin film of fluid that allows back and forth movement but prevents the pleura from being pulled apart.[13] When air enters the pleural cavity, the seal between the pleura is broken, the rib cage springs outward and the lungs collapse. In experimentally created pneumothorax in dogs, venous admixture increased and tidal volume decreased linearly with progressively increasing volumes of pneumothorax.[14] Loss of integrity of the rib cage (e.g., multiple fractured ribs in flail chest) impairs the tendency of the rib cage to spring outward, allowing the underlying lung to collapse. When airways are compressed, the trapped gases are reabsorbed, resulting in alveolar collapse.

Airways may also be obstructed by mural or intraluminal disease. Mural lesions include loss of structural integrity of the cartilaginous airways, as well as inflammatory, infectious, or neoplastic proliferations that protrude into and eventually obstruct the airway. Intraluminal obstruction may be due to foreign bodies[15] or excessive accumulation of secretions caused by allergic and inflammatory airway diseases.[16] Alveoli and lower airways that lack cartilaginous support are held open by collagenous and elastic fibers; by internal distending forces due to transpulmonary pressure; by the nitrogen skeleton supporting the alveoli; and by the presence of surfactant, which diminishes the surface tension forces that tend to collapse the alveoli. Loss of any of these forces can cause small airway and alveolar collapse.[17] Excessive bronchoconstriction may also impair airway diameter sufficiently to cause obstruction. Lastly, atelectasis may be caused by inability to expand the lung because of weakness of respiratory muscles, pain, or centrally mediated respiratory depression.

ABSORPTION ATELECTASIS

Whatever the cause, gases trapped distal to a closed airway are reabsorbed into the pulmonary circulation. Eventually the alveolus becomes airless and therefore will collapse, a process known as absorption atelectasis. The partial pressure of gases in end-capillary mixed venous blood is lower than in the alveoli, thus a gradient for reabsorption exists. Air contains nitrogen, which is poorly soluble and is absorbed more slowly than the highly soluble oxygen. The slowly absorbed nitrogen provides support, a nitrogen "skeleton," for the alveolus until it too is finally absorbed. In patients breathing enriched oxygen mixtures, alveolar collapse occurs faster because the nitrogen skeleton is diminished or absent.[3] In experimental studies of acute atelectasis in dogs breathing 100% oxygen, airway pressure within the obstructed bronchus began to decrease immediately after obstruction and was at its most negative within 3 minutes.[6] The role of absorption in perioperative pulmonary collapse has been challenged, and compression has been suggested as a more important mechanism.[18]

ATELECTASIS WITHOUT VOLUME LOSS

Atelectasis may be associated with edema or with infiltration of inflammatory cells into the collapsed alveoli and airways, thus creating a condition of airlessness without volume loss. Atelectasis was created by obstruction of a bronchus in experimental dogs, and the gross and histopathological features after 6 to 36 hours of obstruction while breathing air were examined.[19]

After 6 hours, histopathological abnormalities were limited to congestion of the alveolar capillaries of the obstructed lobe. After longer periods of obstruction, fluid containing progressively more leukocytes accumulated in the alveoli, which eventually became fluid filled. At the longest duration of obstruction, a reduction in lung lobe size and alveolar diameter was observed. The authors suggest that congestion, edema, and infiltration with inflammatory cells develops early in airway obstruction, and that volume loss is superimposed on this state, thus explaining the discrepancy between clinical findings of atelectasis and post-mortem observations of pulmonary edema.[19]

However, other studies have described a different progression of atelectasis. In dogs breathing 100% oxygen there was a very slight increase in fluid in the collapsed lobes, but the static pressure-volume relationships were unchanged, indicating that neither edema nor interference with surfactant was sufficient to interfere with lung mechanics. Pleural effusion was observed in 1 dog in which the entire left lung was collapsed.[6] In another study of experimental atelectasis in dogs, atelectasis was not associated with an increase in water content in the affected lobe.[20]

REPETITIVE ALVEOLAR COLLAPSE AND REEXPANSION

Dynamic change in alveolar size during tidal ventilation was directly observed using in vivo microscopy in a pig model of lung injury that caused surfactant deactivation.[7] Some alveoli changed size dramatically, and of these, some totally collapsed at end expiration and reinflated during inspiration, a process termed repetitive alveolar collapse and expansion (RACE). There was histological evidence of leukocyte infiltration in these alveoli. The authors speculate that RACE and alveolar overdistension are involved in ventilator-induced lung injury.[7]

COLLATERAL VENTILATION

Absorption atelectasis may be mitigated by entry of gas from adjacent lobules in a process known as collateral ventilation. Respiratory bronchioles and alveolar ducts anastomose between adjacent lung segments in dogs and are the most likely primary sites of collateral ventilation in that species. Interalveolar pores of Kohn and bronchiole alveolar communications provide additional pathways of collateral ventilation.[21]

The predisposition of certain sublobar segments of the canine lung to atelectasis following airway obstruction has been investigated. Segments of lung with a high ratio of pleural surface to volume may be more prone to atelectasis after airway obstruction. In these segments high resistance to collateral flow limits collateral ventilation. Based on these characteristics, the right middle lung lobe and the left upper lobe were predicted to be more likely to develop atelectasis following airway obstruction.[22]

Risk Factors for Atelectasis

ANESTHESIA

Mechanical Factors

During anesthesia, both reduced chest wall movement and relaxation and anterior displacement of the diaphragm contribute to a reduction in lung volume.[23] The reduction in lung volume (decreased functional residual capacity [FRC]) can cause small airway closure and development of absorption atelectasis in the dependent lung.[24-26] In healthy, spontaneously breathing dogs anesthetized for orthopedic procedures, static respiratory compliance declined progressively.[27] The lack of correlation between development of an intrapulmonary shunt in anesthetized patients and radiographic changes typical of atelectasis may be caused by the lack of sensitivity of radiographs to these changes. In human patients without preexisting respiratory disease, atelectasis in dependent lung regions was identified by computerized tomography (CT) during anesthesia, and atelectasis was proposed as the major cause of shunting in anesthetized, lung-healthy patients.[28] In another study, 95 out of 109 lung-healthy, anesthetized human patients developed pulmonary densities seen on CT and interpreted as atelectasis.[29] In postoperative humans, miliary atelectasis was proposed as a cause of acute onset of reduced V/Q without radiographic changes, which responded to maneuvers to produce some deep breaths (dead space ventilation).[30] The authors proposed that atelectasis in postoperative patients should be defined by a severe reduction in V/Q ratio, occurring along a continuum from small areas of atelectasis to complete collapse.[30]

Effect of Inspired Oxygen Concentration

Atelectasis was avoided in human patients that were administered 30% oxygen in nitrogen instead of 100% oxygen during induction of anesthesia.[31,32] Similarly, lowering the preoxygenation inspired oxygen fraction from 100% to 80% reduced the incidence of atelectasis.[33] In a mathematical model, the time to alveolar collapse was shortest when inspired O_2 was increased.[34] Different inert gases (i.e., N_2 or N_2O) had minimal effect on the time to collapse.[34] Although avoidance of excessive oxygen supplementation is desirable, patients who would benefit from perioperative oxygen supplementation should not be denied this therapy. The effects on atelectasis and pulmonary function of giving 30% or 80% oxygen during and for 2 hours after surgery in lung healthy patients were studied at 24 hours postsurgery. At 24 hours postsurgery, CT-determined atelectasis was still present in both groups (30% and 95% respectively, p = 0.12), but there was a poor correlation between alveolar-arterial oxygen difference and the amount of atelectasis. Approximately 40% of patients in both groups had radiographically detectable atelectasis. In this study of the longer-term effects of postoperative atelectasis, pulmonary gas exchange at 24 hours postsurgery was not clinically significantly impaired, and there was no difference between groups.[35]

Accidental Bronchial Intubation

Accidental bronchial intubation occurs when an endotracheal tube is advanced too far down the trachea and enters a mainstem bronchus, resulting in an absence of ventilation in the contralateral lung (see Figure 62-1). Endotracheal tubes move caudally and cranially with flexion and extension of the head and neck, respectively. Thus an endotracheal tube may move into and out of the mainstem bronchus if it is initially positioned too close to this area.[36]

OTHER RISK FACTORS

Chest physiotherapy with hand clapping or a mechanical percussor in anesthetized, paralyzed, ventilated dogs was seen to cause atelectasis on the lateral lung surface.[37] However, percussion therapy is useful in mobilizing respiratory secretions and, combined with rotating the patient, has been useful in improving or resolving atelectasis.[38]

Thoracic compression by elastic bandaging can reduce lung volume below FRC. When lung volume is reduced, shunting occurs that is reversible on restoration of normal lung volume.[39]

Nonobstructive pulmonary consolidation atelectasis was described in human patients following thoracotomy, and ascribed to a decrease in ipsilateral respiratory excursions, possibly due to a combination of pain and phrenic nerve function impairment.[40]

Massive pulmonary collapse as a complication of asthma has been described but appears to be rare.[41]

Atelectasis secondary to prolonged recumbency in a dog with neurologic disease has been reported.[42] Thus frequent repositioning is an essential part of recumbent patient care.

Improper technique while suctioning an endotracheal tube can promote atelectasis. Suction catheters that are too large and that occlude the endotracheal tube prevent room air from flowing freely alongside the catheter, and thus can cause excessive reduction in airway pressure and small airway and alveolar collapse during suctioning.

Consequences of Atelectasis

HYPOXEMIA

In response to alveolar hypoxemia in underventilated alveoli, small arterioles in the hypoxic region constrict, limiting bloodflow.[43] The success of hypoxic pulmonary vasoconstriction (HPV) in mitigating venous admixture depends on the degree and the extent of vasoconstriction. In one anesthetized, open-chest model of atelectasis in dogs, decreased bloodflow to a collapsed lung lobe was partly caused by HPV and partly caused by mechanical (i.e., kinking of lobe vessels) obstruction to bloodflow.[44] Other investigators found that HPV was the major or the entire determinant of decreased flow, with mechanical forces not measurably affecting it.[45-47] HPV developed within 15 minutes, was maximal by 60 minutes, and was maintained thereafter in a canine experimental model.[48] HPV was demonstrated to be stable for 4 hours in experimental dogs but is decreased by acidosis, increased cardiac output, and severe systemic hypoxemia.[49] Acidosis significantly increased shunting during hemorrhagic shock in experimental dogs by impairing HPV or by increasing vascular resistance in the normal lung.[50] In dogs with experimentally induced atelectasis, the HPV response resulting in redistribution of bloodflow away from the atelectic lobe has been demonstrated, but the strength of this response varies between individuals. The response is reduced by the action of vasodilator prostanoids.[51]

DECREASED CLEARANCE OF RESPIRATORY SECRETIONS

Mucociliary function is essential to move respiratory secretions through the airways. The consequences of impaired clearance include accumulation of secretions that eventually may fill the alveoli, and a reduced ability to clear bacteria from an affected area. In a canine model of atelectasis with induced infection, the obstructed lobes had a greatly increased susceptibility to infection.[11] In a pig model of bacterial pneumonia combined with atelectasis, there was decreased bacterial clearance in the collapsed lobe compared with aerated lobes in spite of preservation of phagocytosis and bactericidal effects by alveolar macrophages. The authors concluded that mucociliary function is vital to bacterial clearance.[10] In samples obtained by bronchoalveolar lavage in dogs with experimentally induced atelectasis, impairment of bronchoalveolar lymphocyte function was demonstrated.[52]

REEXPANSION PULMONARY EDEMA

Pulmonary edema may follow rapid expansion of a lung that has been collapsed for several days, and has been reported to be more likely if negative pressure, rather than underwater seal drainage, has been applied to the pleural drain.[53] Reexpansion pulmonary edema is associated with an increase in cytokines and the inflammatory response, both in the reexpanded and in the contralateral lung.[54]

PROLONGED ATELECTASIS

In experimental dogs, complete obstruction of a bronchus was created for periods ranging from 5 weeks to 10 months, after which the patency of the bronchus was reestablished. Biopsies were obtained at various intervals. The atelectatic lobes were small, with a liverlike appearance and rubbery consistency. Reexpansion of the atelectatic lobe resulted in a nearly normal histologic appearance.[55]

In another study in dogs, atelectatic lobes were grossly shrunken to less than one-quarter normal size, with a color and consistency similar to liver. After 2.5 to 32 weeks of atelectasis, a significant right-to-left shunt persisted but resolved following reexpansion of the affected lung.[56]

Clinical Signs

A ventilatory history supportive of atelectasis would include recent anesthesia, high inspired oxygen concentrations, prolonged recumbency, or the presence of any of the other described risk factors. Clinical signs of atelectasis include dyspnea, cyanosis, and tachypnea. Changes in breathing pattern are not necessarily related to hypoxemia. Increased tidal volume and breathing rate were identified in dogs with atelectasis, and were attributed to withdrawal of slowly adapting stretch receptor activity.[57]

The most notable change in thoracic auscultation associated with airway obstruction is a decrease in breath sound intensity. The presence of wheezes (i.e., musical adventitious lung sounds) indicates a significant flow obstruction, but the correlation between airway obstruction and detectable wheezing is variable. Crackles or dry rales (discontinuous lung sounds) indicate closure of small airways and may also be detected in patients with atelectasis.[58,59]

Fever has been reported to be associated with atelectasis in humans and in experimental dogs,[60] but an association could not be demonstrated in human cardiac surgery patients.[61] Atelectasis probably does not cause fever directly.[62] In a rat model of atelectasis, alveolar macrophages produced increased interleukin-1 (IL-1) and tumor necrosis factor (TNF), and these cytokines were thought to be responsible for fever associated with atelectasis.[63]

Diagnostic Tests

BLOOD GAS ANALYSIS

Atelectasis is one cause of venous admixture and therefore of hypoxemia. In patients with atelectasis, the magnitude of the shunt correlates very well with the degree of atelectasis.[36] Arterial blood gas analysis and pulse oximetry are useful tests for the diagnosis of atelectasis.

RADIOLOGY

A definitive diagnosis of atelectasis can be made based on radiographic changes of mediastinal shift, elevation of the hemidiaphragm, rearrangement of the borders of the inflated lung lobes, separation of the heart from the sternum, and asymmetry of the rib cage (Figures 62-1, 62-2, and 62-3). Most signs of atelectasis are more easily seen in dorsoventral or ventrodorsal projections (Figures 62-2, A and B)[64]; however, some types of atelectasis do not result in radiographically detectable volume loss, either because the area of involvement is too small or because the collapsed alveoli have been infiltrated with fluid. Therefore the absence of evidence of atelectasis on radiographs should not exclude the diagnosis.

The radiolucent appearance of normal lung is caused by air in the alveoli and bronchial tree. With atelectasis, the affected lung is denser than normal because of ex-

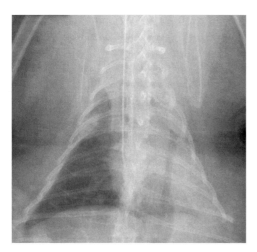

Figure 62-1. *Accidental bronchial intubation. There is evidence of atelectasis of the entire left lung with mediastinal shift to the left. The endotracheal tube is terminating very close to the carina.*

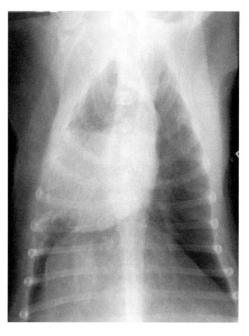

Figure 62-3. *Right middle lung lobe atelectasis during anesthetic recovery. The right middle lung lobe is atelectatic and the heart and mediastinum are shifted to the right.*

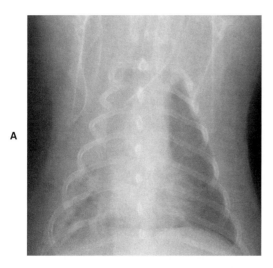

A

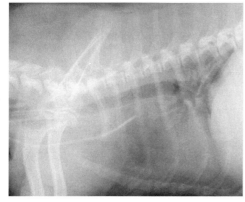

B

Figure 62-2. *Severe atelectasis during anesthetic recovery. Collapse of the right cranial and right middle lung lobes with partial collapse of the right caudal lung lobe, accompanied by mediastinal shift to the right, are evident on the ventrodorsal projection (A). Nearly complete collapse of the right lung lobes is not apparent on the lateral projection (B).*

clusion of air from these areas. The unaffected lobes may be hyperlucent because of compensatory overinflation. Shift of the heart to the affected side and air bronchograms (air-filled bronchus within fluid-filled lung tissue) are noted. The alveolar pulmonary pattern (air bronchograms) is caused by exclusion of air from the alveoli and small peripheral airways because of accumulation of fluid or collapse. If one lobe is affected, the boundary of the alveolar pattern may be identified as the pleural surface of that lobe. There is less air in the lung, and therefore greater lung density during expiration. Radiographs should therefore be taken at peak inspiration to avoid the appearance of an increase in lung density.

The position of the dog or cat while being radiographed is important because diseased lung positioned towards the table in lateral recumbency rapidly collapses.[64] In anesthetized patients, an increase in lung density indicating partial collapse is common, and inflating the lungs a few times before radiographs are taken has been recommended.[65]

The appearance of radiographic changes relative to the development of atelectasis has been reported. In dogs with experimentally induced atelectasis breathing room air, the earliest radiographic changes were observed at 5 hours, whereas in those breathing oxygen the changes were apparent at 1 hour. The early changes consisted only of a mediastinal shift. Depending on the gas present in the alveoli and on the timing of radiographs, a failure to detect atelectasis may occur.[66] Increased density and decreased volume were demonstrated within 1 minute after airway occlusion in a dog breathing 100% oxygen. The authors cautioned that an erroneous diagnosis of pulmonary hemorrhage might be made.[67] In experimental studies of acute atelectasis in dogs breathing 100% oxygen, the affected lobes became opaque radiographically within 5 minutes, but the presence of air bronchograms indicated that the lobe had not yet become completely airless. The volume of the affected lobe decreased by about 25%. Airway pressure within the obstructed bronchus began to decrease immediately after obstruction and was at its most negative within 3 minutes.[6]

COMPUTERIZED TOMOGRAPHY (CT)

The absence of radiographic changes consistent with atelectasis does not rule out the presence of atelectasis, and CT has been reported as a useful imaging modality to identify both the presence and the extent of atelectasis.[68,69]

Differential Diagnosis

An alveolar pattern (air bronchograms) may be caused by the accumulation of a transudate, modified transudate, or exudate in alveoli or by the collapse of the alveoli with resultant exclusion of air. The usual differentials for accumulation of fluid in the alveoli (i.e., water, pus, lymph, and blood) should be considered because these conditions may coexist with atelectasis, and should definitely be considered if there is an alveolar infiltrate with only a slight volume loss.

Treatment

Although high concentrations of inspired oxygen may hasten the development of alveolar collapse, oxygen therapy is an essential part of the treatment for hypoxemia caused by atelectasis. Use of adequate but not excessive concentrations of oxygen is desirable.

If airway obstruction is partial (low V/Q), hypoxemia is responsive to oxygen therapy. If the obstruction is complete (no V/Q), the condition is not responsive to oxygen therapy because the airways are occluded and oxygen cannot reach the alveoli. In that case, positive pressure ventilation may be required to open the closed airways. Positive pressure ventilation provides a hydraulic wedge of air that distends the walls of obstructed airways and allows air passage.[70] A vital capacity (VC) maneuver (i.e., inflation of lungs to 40 cm H_2O for 7 to 8 seconds) reexpanded atelectatic lung in human patients, as detected by CT, and also improved oxygenation.[68] A VC maneuver (i.e., inflating lungs to 40 cm H_2O for 15 seconds every hour) was investigated in anesthetized pigs. No gross, microscopic, or extravascular lung water changes were found.[71] Reexpanded atelectatic lung tissue remained inflated for at least 40 minutes in anesthetized, lung-healthy human patients.[72]

Positive end expiratory pressure (PEEP) of 10 cm H_2O reduced atelectasis in anesthetized, lung-healthy humans.[73] PEEP is used to recruit alveoli, redistribute extravascular lung water, and reduce pulmonary bloodflow through shunt units.[74] PEEP in anesthetized, paralyzed, morbidly obese human patients improved lung volume and respiratory function.[75] The goal of PEEP is to recruit poorly aerated and nonaerated alveoli without overdistending normally aerated alveoli. The success of this maneuver depends in part on the underlying lung disease, with evidence that in patients with acute respiratory distress syndrome (ARDS), it is more effective in inflammatory atelectasis than in mechanical (compression) atelectasis.[69,76]

Treatment of postoperative atelectasis with intravenous aminophylline has been reported to be successful in human patients.[77]

Prompt diagnosis of accidental bronchial intubation is essential. Bilateral auscultation of the thorax should be performed and equality of breath sounds assessed. A decrease in $ETco_2$ (end-tidal carbon dioxide) accompanies the increase in dead space ventilation, but the decrease is transient and not clinically useful.[78]

Outcome and Prognosis

The outcome of patients with atelectasis depends on the underlying disease, if any, and prompt and appropriate intervention to correct life-threatening hypoxemia. Most cases of atelectasis are in patients with known risk factors, especially those associated with anesthesia or prolonged recumbency. These conditions would be expected to respond well to preventive measures and treatment as suggested.

REFERENCES

1. Bendixen HH: Atelectasis and shunting, *Anesth* 25(5):595-596, 1964.
2. Lumb AB: Parenchymal Lung Disease. In Lumb AB, editor: *Nunn's applied respiratory physiology*, Oxford, 2000, Butterworth-Heinemann.
3. West JB: Respiratory system under stress. In West JB, editor: *Respiratory physiology: The essentials*, Philadelphia, 2001, Lippincott Williams & Wilkins.
4. Hasleton PS: Aspiration pneumonia, lung abscess, bronchiectasis, and atelectasis. In Hasleton PS, editor: *Spencer's pathology of the lung*, New York, 1996, McGraw-Hill.
5. Thurlbeck WM, Churg AM: Consequences of aspiration and bronchial obstruction. In Thurlbeck WM, Churg AM, editors: *Pathology of the lung*, New York, 1995, Thieme Medical Publishers.
6. Stein LA, Vidal JJ, Hogg JC et al: Acute lobar collapse in canine lungs, *Invest Rad* 11(6):518-527, 1976.
7. Schiller HJ, McCann UG II, Carny DE et al: Altered alveolar mechanics in the acutely injured lung, *Crit Care Med* 29(5):1049-1055, 2001.
8. Cotran RS, Kumar V, Robbins SL: Diseases of infancy and childhood. In Cotran RS, Kumar V, Robbins SL, editors: *Robbins pathologic basis of disease*, Philadelphia, 1989, WB Saunders.
9. Lumb AB: Distribution of pulmonary ventilation and perfusion. In Lumb AB, editor: *Nunn's applied respiratory physiology*, Oxford, 2000, Butterworth-Heinemann.
10. Drinkwater DC, Wittnich C, Mulder DS et al: Mechanical and cellular bacterial clearance in lung atelectasis, *Ann Thorac Surg* 32(3):235-243, 1981.
11. Shields RT: Pathogenesis of postoperative pulmonary atelectasis, *Arch Surg* 58(4):489-503, 1949.
12. West JB: Gas exchange. In West JB, editor: *Pulmonary pathophysiology*, Philadelphia, 1998, Lippincott Williams & Wilkins.
13. Shapiro BA, Harrison RS, Walton JR: The physiology of external respiration. In Shapiro BA, Harrison RS, Walton JR, editors: *Clinical application of blood gases*, Chicago, 1982, Year Book Medical Publishers.

14. Bennett RA: Cardiopulmonary changes in conscious dogs with induced progressive pneumothorax, *Am J Vet Res* 50(2):280-284, 1989.

15. Buenaventura A, Unger L: Bilateral wheezing from an aspirated vegetable (peanut?) foreign body, *Ann Allergy* January-February: 9-13, 1958.

16. Padrid P, Amis TC: Chronic tracheobronchial disease in the dog, *Vet Clin North Am* 22(5):1203-1229, 1992.

17. Lumb AB: Respiratory system resistance. In Lumb AB, editor: *Nunn's applied respiratory physiology*, Oxford, 2000, Butterworth-Heinemann.

18. Joyce CJ, Baker AB: What is the role of absorption atelectasis in the genesis of perioperative pulmonary collapse? *Anaesth Intensive Care* 23(6):691-696, 1995.

19. Spain DM: Acute non-aeration of lung: pulmonary edema versus atelectasis, *Diseases of the Chest* 25:550-558, 1954.

20. Bradley CA, Arnup ME, Anthonisen NR: Lobar blood flow, blood volume, and water content in atelectasis, *Resp Physiol* 51:333-340, 1983.

21. Robinson NE: Some functional consequences of species differences in lung anatomy, *Adv Vet Sci Comp Med* 26:1-31, 1982.

22. Robinson NE, Milar R: Lobar variations in collateral ventilation in excised dog lungs, *Am Rev Resp Dis* 121:827-834, 1980.

23. Hedenstierna G, Strandberg A, Brismar B et al: Functional residual capacity, thoracoabdominal dimensions, and central blood volume during general anesthesia with muscle paralysis and mechanical ventilation, *Anesthesiology* 62(3):247-254, 1985.

24. Nelin LD, Rickaby DA, Linehan JH et al: Effect of atelectasis and surface tension on pulmonary vascular compliance, *J Appl Physiol* 70(6):2401-2409, 1991.

25. Lumb AB: Elastic forces and lung volume. In Lumb AB, editor: *Nunn's applied respiratory physiology*, Oxford, 2000, Butterworth-Heinemann.

26. Tokics L: V/Q distribution and correlation to atelectasis in anesthetized paralyzed humans, *J Appl Physiol* 81(4):1822-1833, 1996.

27. Corcoran BM, Abercromby RH: Effects of general anaesthesia on static respiratory compliance in dogs, *Vet Rec* 125:450-453, 1989.

28. Hedenstierna F, Tokics L, Strandberg A et al: Correlation of gas exchange impairment to development of atelectasis during anaesthesia and muscle paralysis, *Acta Anaesthesiol Scand* 30:183-191, 1986.

29. Lundquist H, Hedenstierna G, Strandberg A et al: CT-assessment of dependent lung densities in man during general anaesthesia, *Acta Radiol* 36:626-632, 1995.

30. Hamilton WK, McDonald JS, Fischer HW et al: Postoperative respiratory complications, *Anesthesiology* Sep-Oct:607-612, 1964.

31. Rothen HU, Sporre B, Engberg G et al: Atelectasis and pulmonary shunting during induction of general anaesthesia—can they be avoided? *Acta Anaesthesiol Scand* 40(5):524-529, 1996.

32. Rothen HU, Sporre B, Engberg G et al: Prevention of atelectasis during general anaesthesia, *Lancet* 345 (8962):1387-1391, 1995.

33. Hedenstierna G: Time to reconsider the pre-oxygenation during induction of anaesthesia, *Minerva Anesthesiol* 66(5):293-296, 2000.

34. Joyce CJ, Williams AB: Kinetics of absorption atelectasis during anesthesia: A mathematical model, *J Appl Physiol* 86(4):1116-1125, 1999.

35. Akca O, Podolsky A, Eisenhuber E et al: Comparable postoperative pulmonary atelectasis in patients given 30% or 80% oxygen during and 2 hours after colon resection, *Anesthesiology* 91(4):991-998, 1999.

36. Benumof JL: Respiratory physiology and respiratory function during anesthesia. In Miller RD, editor: *Anesthesia*, New York, 2001, Churchill Livingstone.

37. Zidulka A, Chrome JF, Wight DW et al: Clapping or percussion causes atelectasis in dogs and influences gas exchange, *J Appl Physiol* 66(6):2833-2838, 1989.

38. Raoof S, Chowdhrey N, Raoof S et al: Effect of combined kinetic therapy and percussion therapy on the resolution of atelectasis in critically ill patients, *Chest* 115(6):1658-1666, 1999.

39. Nunn JF, Coleman AJ, Sachithanandan R et al: Hypoxaemia and atelectasis produced by forced expiration, *Br J Anaesthesia* 37(3): 3-11, 1965.

40. Culiner MM, Reich SB, Abouav J: Non-obstructive consolidation-atelectasis following thoracotomy, *J Thorac Surg* 372-381, 1959.

41. Aronsohn RB, Pressman JJ: Massive atelectasis in bronchial asthma, *Ann Otol Rhinol* 67(4):1106-1112, 1958.

42. Farrow CS: Postural atelectasis in a dog, *Mod Vet Pract* 65(6):474, 1984.

43. West JB: Blood flow and metabolism. In West JB, editor: *Respiratory physiology*, Philadelphia, 2000, Lippincott Williams & Wilkins.

44. Orchard CH, DeLeon RS, Chakrabarti MK et al: Pulmonary lobe blood flow during ventilation hypoxia and lobar collapse in the dog, *Cardiovasc Res* 19:264-269, 1985.

45. Miller FL, Chen L, Malmkvist G et al: Mechanical factors do not influence blood flow distribution in atelectasis, *Anesthesiology* 70(3):481-488, 1989.

46. Benumof JL: Mechanism of decreased blood flow to atelectatic lung, *J Appl Physiol* 46(6):1047-1048, 1979.

47. Pirlo AF: Atelectic lobe blood flow: Open vs. closed chest, positive pressure vs. spontaneous ventilation, *J Appl Physiol: Respirat Environ Exercise Physiol* 50(5):1022-1026, 1981.

48. Glasser SA, Domino KB, Lindgren L et al: Pulmonary blood pressure and flow during atelectasis in the dog, *Anesthesiology* 58(3):225-231, 1983.

49. Domino KB, Chen L, Alexander CM et al: Time course and responses of sustained hypoxic pulmonary vasoconstriction in the dog, *Anesthesiology* 60:562-566, 1984.

50. Wahrenbrock EA, Carrico CJ, Amundsen DA et al: Increased atelectic pulmonary shunt during hemorrhagic shock in dogs, *J Appl Physiol* 29(5):615-621, 1970.

51. Thomas HM, Garrett RC: Strength of hypoxic vasoconstriction determines shunt fraction in dogs with atelectasis, *J Appl Physiol* 53(1):44-51, 1982.

52. Nguyen DM, Mulder DS, Shennib H: Altered cellular immune function in the atelectatic lung, *Ann Thorac Surg* 51:76-80, 1991.

53. Weissberg D, Refaely Y: Pneumothorax: Experience with 1199 patients, *Chest* 117:1279-1285, 2000.

54. Sakao Y, Kajikawa O, Martin TR et al: Association of IL-8 and MCP-1 with the development of reexpansion pulmonary edema in rabbits, *Ann Thorac Surg* 71(6):1825-1832, 2001.

55. Hinshaw JR, Emerson GL: Histologic studies of the lung during recovery from atelectasis, *Surgical Forum* 9:390-392, 1958.

56. Benfield JR, Harrison RW, Perkins JF Jr. et al: The reversibility of chronic atelectasis, *Surgical Forum* 8:473-478, 1957.

57. Green JF, Kaufman MP: Pulmonary afferent control of breathing as end-expiratory lung volume decreases, *J Appl Physiol* 68(5):2186-2194, 1990.

58. Pasterkamp H, Kraman SS, Wodicka GR: Respiratory sounds: Advances beyond the stethoscope, *Am J Respir Crit Care Med* 156: 974-987, 1997.

59. Kotlikoff MI, Gillespie JR: Lung sounds in veterinary medicine, part I: Terminology and mechanisms of sound production, *Comp Cont Ed Pract Vet* 5(8):634-638, 1983.

60. Lansing AM, Jamieson WJ: Mechanisms of fever in pulmonary atelectasis, *Arch Surg* 87:168-174, 1963.

61. Engoren M: Lack of association between atelectasis and fever, *Chest* 107(1):81-84, 1995.

62. Marik PE: Fever in the ICU, *Chest* 117:855-869, 2000.

63. Kisala JM, Ayala A, Stephan RN et al: A model of pulmonary atelectasis in rats: Activation of alveolar macrophage and cytokine release, *Am J Physiol* 264:R610-R614, 1993.

64. Suter PF: Lower airway and pulmonary parenchymal diseases. In Suter PF, editor: *Thoracic radiography: A text atlas of thoracic diseases of the dog and cat*, Wettswil, 1984, Peter F. Suter.

65. Lord PF: Alveolar lung diseases in small animals and their radiographic diagnosis, *J Sm An Pract* 17:283-303, 1976.

66. Lansing AM: Radiological changes in pulmonary atelectasis, *Arch Surg* 90:52-56, 1965.

67. Fletcher BD, Avery ME: The effects of airway occlusion after oxygen breathing on the lungs of newborn infants, *Radiology* 109:655-657, 1973.

68. Rothen HU, Neumann P, Berglund JE et al: Dynamics of reexpansion of atelectasis during general anaesthesia, *Br J Anaesth* 82(4): 551-556, 1999.

69. Malbouisson LM, Muller J, Constantin J et al: Computed tomography assessment of positive end-expiratory pressure-induced alveolar recruitment in patients with acute respiratory distress syndrome, *Am J Respir Crit Care Med* 163:1444-1450, 2001.

70. Dayman HG, Manning LE: Pulmonary atelectasis: physical factors, *Ann Int Med* 47(3):460-492, 1957.

71. Magnusson L: The safety of one, or repeated, vital capacity maneuvers during general anesthesia, *Anesth Analg* 91(3):702-707, 2000.
72. Rothen HU: Reexpansion of atelectasis during general anaesthesia may have a prolonged effect, *Acta Anaesthesiol Scand* 39(1):118-125, 1995.
73. Neumann P, Rothen HU, Berglund JE et al: Positive end-expiratory pressure prevents atelectasis during general anaesthesia even in the presence of a high inspired oxygen concentration, *Acta Anaesthesiol Scand* 43(3):295-301, 1999.
74. Gattinoni L, Pelosi P, Crotti S et al: Effects of positive end-expiratory pressure on regional distribution of tidal volume and recruitment in adult respiratory distress syndrome, *Am J Respir Crit Care Med* 151: 1807-1814, 1995.
75. Pelosi P: Positive end-expiratory pressure improves respiratory function in obese but not in normal subjects during anesthesia and paralysis, *Anesthesiology* 91(5):1221-1231, 1999.
76. Puybasset L: Regional distribution of gas and tissue in acute respiratory distress syndrome, III. Consequences for the effects of positive end-expiratory pressure, *Intensive Care Med* 26(9):1215-1217, 2000.
77. Robbins JJ, Schonberger SH, Jackson SC et al: Successful treatment of postoperative atelectasis by intravenous injection of aminophylline, *J Thor Card Surg* 49(5):874-880, 1965.
78. Johnson DH, Chang PC, Hurst TS et al: Changes in PETCO$_2$ and pulmonary blood flow after bronchial occlusion in dogs, *Can J Anaesthiology* 39(2):184-191, 1992.

CHAPTER 63

Pulmonary Contusion

C. Bisque Jackson • Kenneth J. Drobatz

Pulmonary contusion (PC) is an anatomic and physiologic lung lesion that occurs secondary to a nonpenetrating, compression-decompression injury to the thoracic wall.[1,2] It has become a major cause of morbidity and mortality in both human and veterinary medicine. In humans, deceleration injuries associated with automobile accidents, blasts (e.g., high energy shock waves produced by an explosion), and high-velocity missiles (e.g., bullets with velocities in excess of 2000 feet per second passing within a few centimeters of the lung)[3] are mechanisms of injury documented to result in severe pulmonary contusion.[2,3] High speed automobile accidents are currently the most common cause of PC in both humans and veterinary patients sustaining severe thoracic trauma. Other injuries such as crush injuries, falls, animal interactions, and human abuse have also been observed in animals; however, any major force acting on the chest wall can result in pulmonary contusion.

In humans, thoracic injury is responsible for approximately 25% of trauma-related deaths,[4-6] and the incidence of lung contusion secondary to blunt chest trauma has been reported to range from 50% to 60%.[7] In dogs, the incidence of thoracic trauma secondary to motor vehicular accidents has been reported at 38.9%.[8] Of all types of thoracic injury, PC has been reported to be the most common, accounting for approximately 50% of all chest injuries in dogs and cats.[8,9]

PC is often associated with other thoracic and extrathoracic injuries.[10,11] The physical forces during trauma may produce a variety of concurrent injuries such as pneumothorax, fractured ribs, head trauma, and various bone fractures.[8-12] Morbidity therefore depends both on the severity of the PC and the number and severity of concurrent injuries. Rapid detection of PC is paramount to the successful management of these patients. Often the lung injury is masked by other more dramatic injuries at which resuscitative measures are aimed. Extensive pulmonary lesions can be rapidly fatal because of progressive hypoxia and acute respiratory failure.[13-15] Many cases, however, are mild and associated with few other injuries. Pulmonary contusion tends to be insidiously progressive during the first 24 to 48 hours.[14,16,17] Animals can present with adequate pulmonary function but then quickly deteriorate. If the animal survives the acute crisis, the pulmonary lesion usually resolves completely within 7 to 10 days after the injury, with few complications. Mortality in humans has been reported to range from 22% to 50%.[18,19] Powell reported a mortality rate of 18% in dogs sustaining PC.[11]

History

The first report of pulmonary trauma without associated chest wall injury was described in 1761, in which a carriage wreck victim sustained a fatal lung injury: *"A 16-year-old boy was injured when a wheel passed over his chest, when he fell while attempting to jump on a moving horse cart. At autopsy, there was no external evidence of chest wall injury, but both lungs were severely contused with small lacerations. Beer was noted in the stomach."*[20] From then, little was written about lung trauma until the beginning of the twentieth century, when high explosives were utilized in warfare. During World War I, fatalities from explosions were thought to be caused by the inhalation of toxic vapors from the blast (e.g., carbon monoxide and phosgene); a sudden vacuum effect in gas-containing parts of the body (i.e., the lungs); or a direct shock effect on the central nervous system.[20,21] An elaborate set of studies performed in the early 1900s demonstrated the hallmark pathophysiologic finding of blast injuries: severe intrapulmonary hemorrhage.[22]

Throughout the "Great War," the Spanish Civil War, and the bombing of Britain, many publications described soldiers that were found dead on the battlefield without any evidence of external injury. These victims had sustained blast injuries that resulted in progressive respiratory dysfunction and death. Autopsies revealed severe pulmonary hemorrhage.[23-26] Various theories surfaced regarding whether these pulmonary lesions were caused by the effect of suction on the lungs (negative pressure wave), excessive distention of the lungs with air (positive pressure wave), or the direct impact of blast on the chest wall. This prompted further studies of blast-induced pulmonary injury. Zuckerman's animal studies during the 1940s demonstrated that the lung injury was caused by the direct impact of the pressure wave from the blast on the chest wall and that the degree of pulmonary hemorrhage directly correlated to the distance from the blast.[27]

Severe lung injuries after battlefield explosions became well recognized during and after World War II. Burford and Burbank described the "wet lung" injury of battlefield victims and found that it *produced more than its normal amount of interstitial and intra-alveolar fluid,* and *". . . in all wounds of the chest the bronchopulmonary tree not only has more fluid to rid itself of, but becomes less capable of doing so."*[28,29] Vigorous intravenous fluid resuscitation in combat hospitals was implicated as the cause for the progressive pulmonary compromise after thoracic trauma in these victims.[28,29]

Before the 1960s, little was written about pulmonary contusion in the nonmilitary setting. Alfano and DeMuth were the first to document the high morbidity and mortality associated with thoracic trauma and pulmonary contusion in victims sustaining motor vehicular accidents.[1,3] Further studies in the 1960s demonstrated that direct damage to the lung, rather than bony injury, was the cause of respiratory dysfunction in these patients.[30] Over the next 10 years, published data from animal studies unraveled the pathophysiological derangements, mechanism of injury, and radiographic findings associated with PC.[1,13,14,30] Vietnam War surgeons further detailed the impact of high-velocity missiles and blasts upon lung tissue using sophisticated laboratory and monitoring techniques.[15,31,32] Much of today's awareness and management of pulmonary contusion is taken from investigative work performed during the 1960s and 1970s.

Pathophysiology

Pulmonary contusion results in structural and physiological changes in the lung parenchyma that, depending on the extent and severity of the injury, can culminate in acute respiratory failure. Ventilation/perfusion mismatch, increased lung water, elevated intrapulmonary shunt, and loss of lung compliance can develop as a result of progressive lung injury[13,33,34] and can subsequently result in hypoxemia, hypercarbia or hypocapnia, and an increased work of breathing.[13,32,35] Reduced surfactant levels 24 to 48 hours postinjury have also been implicated as a contributing factor in the pulmonary derangement.[35]

Hypoxemia that accompanies PC often parallels the severity and extent of parenchymal involvement, as well as the presence of associated pulmonary and systemic injuries.[4] The magnitude, rate, and duration of the applied force, as well as the size and age of the patient, directly modify the biological response.[4,14] The additional forces of acceleration, deceleration, compression, shear, and torsion can indirectly contribute to the severity of the injury.[18] The extent of lung injury can range from mild focal bruising in one lobe to extensive, diffuse hemorrhage in both lungs.

Various animal models of pulmonary contusion have yielded qualitative and conflicting results concerning the pathophysiology of hypoxemia.[2,16,31,35-37] A set of well-controlled experimental studies in dogs, in which blank cartridges were fired against a metal plate taped to the chest wall, demonstrated the histopathological and physiological alterations that occurred following blunt chest trauma.[2,16,37,38] Data from these experiments revealed a progressive pulmonary parenchymal change that occurred over time. The initial damage is caused by disruption of capillaries and small vessels leading to immediate interstitial and alveolar hemorrhage.[16,31,38] Within 1 to 2 hours of injury, marked accumulation of edema and a moderate infiltrate of mononuclear and polymorphonuclear cells occurs within the lung interstitium. The alveolar architecture structure usually remains intact with minimal destruction. Approximately 24 hours after injury, a significant cellular response occurs in which the architecture of the lung becomes obliterated by a massive accumulation of inflammatory cells (primarily mononuclear cells), fibrin, and red blood cells.[16,38,39] Within 48 hours, more fibrin, cell debris, granules from type II alveolar cells, and inflammatory cells can be noted. Lymphatics become dilated and filled with protein. Hemorrhage is most intense in lung tissue surrounding solid structures such as the ribs, liver, heart, vertebral column, and hilar structures.

With the knowledge of the histopathological changes that can occur 24 to 48 hours after injury, it was easier to explain the progressive gas diffusion barrier that occurred during that time.[3,16] Thus the clinical course of patients suffering from chest injuries may deteriorate 24 to 48 hours postinjury.[1,16]

Although the exact mechanism of the production of lung contusion is not clear, direct impact on the lung and indirect forces during deceleration have both been implicated.[18,32] The sudden and direct impact of a portion of the lung on the chest wall can cause disruption of the microvasculature with interstitial extravasation of red cells and plasma causing local flooding of alveoli. The indirect impact results from severe and rapid chest compression and decompression, creating high pressure gradients between vessels and alveoli. This type of event causes diffuse pulmonary interstitial hemorrhage without requiring direct lung trauma.[18,32,40]

Diagnosis

The diagnosis of PC must be suspected in any patient subjected to severe thoracic trauma and is based on physical examination findings and thoracic radiography.[1] Initial evaluation of trauma patients sustaining contusions can be difficult because they may not present with a single injury and the lung changes may not be immediately evident. This can result in a delay in onset of respiratory symptoms, which may lead to errors in diagnosis and serious miscalculation of outcome. If contusions are not apparent immediately after the trauma, manifestation usually occurs within 24 hours.[1] For this reason, continuous observation of a thoracic trauma patient is usually recommended for the first 1 to 2 days after injury.

In humans, pulmonary contusion commonly exists as a single entity without accompanying trauma to the chest wall, especially in young patients with highly elastic chest walls.[1,18,35] It can, however, be associated with other thoracic and nonthoracic injuries. Pulmonary contusion alone has been reported to occur in 50% of dogs sustaining motor vehicular accidents.[8] In dogs, the most commonly associated thoracic injuries included pneumothorax, pleural effusion (hemothorax), rib fractures, pulmonary bulla or hematoma, and pneumomediastinum.[8,11] Nonthoracic injuries associated with PC include pelvic and long bone fractures, head trauma, spinal cord injury, and abdominal trauma.[11] Because of the insidious nature of lung contusion, attention can be diverted to other more dramatic nonthoracic injuries, resulting in a delay in instituting therapy.[1] If rib fractures are present, it is likely that respiratory compromise is caused by underlying contused lung, rather than the mechanical difficulties associated with the fractures.[1] Most human patients with fractured ribs are likely to have localized areas of contusion, whereas patients without rib fractures tend to have diffuse parenchymal damage.[1] In veterinary patients, most severe cases of pulmonary contusion are not associated with concurrent rib fractures or other discontinuity of the chest wall.

Clinical signs vary with the extent of injury. Some animals may have very mild signs of respiratory impairment. Most, however, have initial signs of respiratory compromise consisting of tachypnea, dyspnea, open mouth breathing, and increased bronchovesicular sounds. Signs suggestive of more serious contusion include hemoptysis, crackles on auscultation, and cyanosis.[1,41] Tachycardia is common because of pain, hypoxia, or hemorrhagic shock. Cardiac arrhythmias can occur because of traumatic myocarditis or a hypoxic myocardium.

THORACIC RADIOGRAPHS

Radiographs are one of the most important means of diagnosing pulmonary contusion and associated thoracic injuries; however, they should only be obtained in patients

that are stable enough to tolerate the procedure. The radiographic appearance of PC consists of nonanatomic pulmonary infiltrates with a diffuse or patchy alveolar or interstitial pattern (Figure 63-1).[42] The classic radiographic findings may be evident at presentation or may take 12 to 48 hours to appear.[1,14,17,27,39] Complete resolution of pulmonary infiltrates usually occurs within 7 to 10 days after the injury.[2,42] The disturbance of respiratory function may be quite disproportionate to the extent of anatomical disturbance shown radiographically; thus initial radiographs may fail to indicate the full extent of the injury.[1,14] Additional follow-up radiographs are important in patients with continued pulmonary compromise.

COMPUTERIZED TOMOGRAPHY

Computerized tomography (CT) is the imaging tool considered to be most accurate in assessing the pulmonary

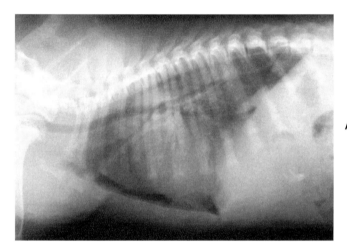

A

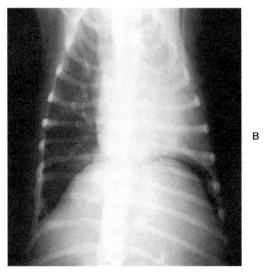

B

Figure 63-1. Right lateral **(A)** and ventrodorsal **(B)** radiographs of a pit bull puppy that sustained pulmonary contusion and a small pneumothorax as a result of abuse. Extensive diffuse alveolar infiltrates are present in the left lung. (Photograph courtesy of Dr. Lori Waddell, School of Veterinary Medicine, University of Pennsylvania, Philadelphia.)

parenchyma and the pleural cavity in humans. As such, it is now recommended as a routine diagnostic test in human patients who sustain blunt chest trauma.[43,44] The CT scan is considered far superior to thoracic radiographs in its ability to detect contused pulmonary parenchyma immediately after trauma.[43,45] It additionally has good sensitivity in estimating the lesion size 6 and 12 hours posttrauma. Schild reported that CT underestimated the extent of the lesion in only 8% of cases, whereas conventional chest radiographs underestimated the lesion size in 56%.[45] Wagner further demonstrated the ability of CT scans to predict the need for ventilatory support by determining the percentage of airspace consolidation; when more than 28% of airspace was involved, all patients required mechanical ventilation.[46] Because of the requirement for anesthesia, CT should be performed only in stable patients.

ARTERIAL BLOOD GASES AND OXYGEN TENSION-BASED INDICES

Oxygenation and ventilation can be accurately assessed with arterial blood gases; this can be extremely useful for monitoring the severity of respiratory compromise and guiding and evaluating therapy.[16,39] Many patients with mild PC will have normal arterial blood gases. In more severely affected patients however, various degrees of hypoxemia, hypocapnia, or hypercapnia can occur. Hypoxemia is determined by measuring the arterial oxygen tension (PaO_2) and is defined as a PaO_2 of less than 60 mm Hg (reference range 80 to 100 mm Hg).[47-49] Patients with PaO_2 values less than 70 mm Hg should receive supplemental oxygen. Patients with PaO_2 values below 60 mm Hg, while breathing supplemental oxygen with an FiO_2 exceeding 0.5 may require mechanical ventilation.[49] A PaO_2 of less than 60 mm Hg can cause tissue hypoxia, metabolic acidosis, and cardiac arrhythmias, further worsening the condition of an already compromised patient.[47-49] Pulse oximetry, which measures arterial saturation of hemoglobin, is an additional rapid and noninvasive method of assessing pulmonary function. An arterial hemoglobin saturation (SpO_2) of 90% approximately equals a PaO_2 of 60 mm Hg.[47]

Arterial blood gases also provide information about the ventilatory status of the patient by measuring the $PaCO_2$ (reference range 30 to 40 mm Hg).[40,41] The hypoxemia associated with PC can centrally stimulate a compensatory ventilatory drive resulting in a low $PaCO_2$. Conversely, the pain associated with fractured ribs or impaired respiratory drive from head trauma can cause patients to hypoventilate, resulting in hypercapnia. Severe pulmonary parenchymal damage can also occasionally result in a high $PaCO_2$.[16,35] Hypercapnia, defined as a partial pressure of carbon dioxide greater than 60 mm Hg, can result in respiratory acidosis, neurologic abnormalities, and increased intracranial pressure.[47-49] Mechanical ventilation is indicated if severe hypoventilation is present (i.e., $PaCO_2$ greater than 50 mm Hg with a pH of 7.25 or less).[49]

The PaO_2:FiO_2 ratio is another indicator of pulmonary injury that can be easily calculated from arterial blood gases obtained while the patient is receiving oxygen supplementation.[47,48] This ratio has been used as a rough estimate of intrapulmonary shunt.[40,50] In humans with pulmonary contusion, an initial PaO_2:FiO_2 ratio of less than 300 was significantly associated with increased mortality and the need for mechanical ventilation.[51] The alveolar-arterial oxygen tension gradient (A–a gradient) is another oxygen tension–based index that provides an estimate of the extent of ventilation/perfusion mismatch. The A–a gradient can be calculated from an arterial blood gas, and a gradient greater than 20 mm Hg indicates that venous admixture is occurring.[41]

Treatment

PC rarely exists as a single entity. Many patients present in shock with concurrent thoracic, abdominal, and head injuries. Therefore, application of the general principles for the management of trauma victims is essential for each patient. A thorough and rapid assessment of the patient is crucial for initial treatment (Box 63-1). Initial assessment should be directed at the respiratory, cardiovascular, and neurological systems.

RESPIRATORY SYSTEM AND OXYGEN THERAPY

A rapid and thorough assessment of airway patency should be performed, consisting of observation of respiratory rate and effort and the character of chest wall excursions, auscultation, and a brief oropharyngeal examination, if it is tolerated by the patient. Coexisting thoracic conditions (e.g., airway obstruction, pneumothorax, hemothorax, flail chest, or diaphragmatic hernia) that can seriously compromise pulmonary function may be detected during this survey. In dogs sustaining PC after motor vehicle accidents, 47% had concurrent pneumothorax, 34% had pleural effusion, and 13% had rib fractures.[11] Such lesions are best managed before the lung contusion reaches its maximum extent because the combination of injuries may be incompatible with life.

Establishing a patent airway is the first priority. Animals with severe PC can have hemoptysis with thick, blood-tinged oral secretions. The oral cavity should be

---

BOX 63-1
Treatment of Pulmonary Contusion

1. Treat associated thoracic and life-threatening nonthoracic injuries
2. Oxygen administration to maintain oxygen saturation >90%
3. Decision for endotracheal intubation or management with spontaneous ventilation
4. Optimize pain control
5. Avoid fluid overload
6. Avoid unnecessary barotrauma
7. Prophylactic antibiotics: ***not indicated***
8. Corticosteroids: ***not indicated*** (exception: severe upper airway obstruction or bronchospasm)

cleared of secretions if they are impeding airflow. If complete airway obstruction is present, immediate intubation, airway suctioning, and ventilatory support is imperative. If endotracheal intubation is impossible because of pharyngeal or laryngeal obstruction, emergency tracheostomy is required. Unconscious patients, or those suffering from severe intracranial trauma, should be intubated and mechanically ventilated.

Pneumothorax should be promptly evacuated via needle thoracocentesis, which may also determine the presence of a hemothorax. Flail chest should be treated with intercostal nerve blocks for pain relief. Stabilization of most flail segments is unnecessary in the emergency setting. Following evacuation of a pneumothorax (and, if necessary, stabilization of the chest wall), ventilatory function should be restored if hypoventilation is a contributing factor to respiratory compromise.[52]

All patients with PC should receive supplemental oxygen because most are hypoxic to some degree and they are commonly in shock. Oxygen supplementation can be provided with a face mask, nasal prongs, nasopharyngeal catheter, or an oxygen cage, as dictated by equipment availability and the severity of respiratory compromise. Intubation and mechanical ventilation are required when oxygen supplementation and thoracocentesis do not restore adequate ventilation and patient stabilization.

CARDIOVASCULAR SYSTEM AND FLUID THERAPY

Assessment of the cardiovascular system is important in all trauma victims. Hypovolemic shock can follow severe blood loss; hypovolemia and inadequate perfusion can be assessed by evaluation of the heart rate, pulse quality, mucous membrane color, and capillary refill time. Many patients with PC lose minimal volumes of blood into the lungs despite severe pulmonary dysfunction. If hypovolemia is present because of hemorrhage in other parts of the body, restoration of adequate tissue perfusion is imperative, although it is sometimes challenging in PC patients with impaired pulmonary vascular integrity.

Fluid therapy has been an area of controversy since Burford and Burbank described "wet lung" in soldiers with chest injuries during World War II.[28] The adverse effects of fluid therapy in PC, and the optimal resuscitative efforts, have been under investigation for decades. Early experimental models of PC demonstrated that vigorous fluid resuscitation, especially with large volumes of rapidly administered crystalloids, predisposed to a more severe and progressive lung lesion with worsening hypoxemia, lung water accumulation, and lesion size.* Although studies in animals have reproduced results suggesting that massive fluid administration has a negative effect after PC, the clinical data to support this concept have been ambiguous. Studies on soldiers injured during the Vietnam War found that the volume of blood transfused correlated with the degree of hypoxemia, but only in soldiers who had sustained chest trauma.[55] Tranbaugh reported that trauma patients sustaining PC

who presented in hypovolemic shock had increased measured lung water content after resuscitation in comparison to trauma patients presenting in shock who had no lung injury.[56] Other studies reviewed the outcomes of mechanically ventilated patients with PC and found no evidence supporting the notion that the use of balanced salt solutions, when given in needed volumes for clinical resuscitation, produced deleterious pulmonary effects.[40] Furthermore, Johnson demonstrated that mortality and the need for ventilatory support did not correlate with the volume of crystalloid infused.[51] Contusion did not appear to be worsened by hemodilution and a lowered plasma oncotic pressure; rather, a compensatory pulmonary mechanism (e.g., increased lymph drainage as demonstrated in hemorrhagic-shock models) was evoked as an explanation for these findings.[51]

It is generally recommended that fluid therapy should be titrated to restore and maintain optimum cardiac output and tissue perfusion. Careful monitoring is essential to avoid overhydration, especially in patients with severe PC, because of the possibility of increased capillary permeability. Conversely, fluid restriction and dehydration should be avoided. The type and volume of fluid required for stabilization is dependent upon the cardiovascular status and associated injuries of the individual patient. Crystalloids, colloids, and blood products are fluids commonly utilized for the resuscitation of patients sustaining PC. Typically, in the hemorrhaging patient with PC, the optimal method of fluid resuscitation would be to use blood products such that the patient only receives what has been lost from the intravascular space. Aggressive and meticulous management in an ICU setting may be necessary for more critical patients, in which central venous pressure, urinary output, arterial blood pressure, and cardiac output should be assessed.

Until recently there have been few alternatives to massive volume resuscitation in the hemorrhaging trauma victim. Many patients suffer blood loss from other injuries and require massive fluid therapy with crystalloids and blood products. Recently, potentially useful resuscitative fluids have been developed that appear to restore perfusion with minimal fluid volume. Hypertonic saline solutions offer many beneficial effects for the resuscitation of patients in shock. Studies have shown effective restoration of tissue perfusion, cardiac output, blood pressure, and splanchic blood flow in animal models with hemorrhagic shock treated with small volumes of hypertonic fluid.[57,58] In animal models of head trauma sustaining hemorrhagic shock, hypertonic saline therapy led to substantially less brain edema and lower intracranial pressures than isotonic crystalloid solution.[59] Hypertonic saline is therefore a potentially useful adjunctive therapy directed at rapidly restoring circulatory function without deleterious pulmonary effects, although currently no data exist on the use of hypertonic saline in patients after thoracic injury.

The recommended dose is a combination of hypertonic saline (5% to 7% solution) with 6% dextran-70 at 4 ml/kg delivered over 5 minutes as a one-time bolus. It is important to closely monitor pulmonary function after hypertonic solution administration because increased

*References 2, 14, 16, 17, 35-37, 53, and 54.

pulmonary capillary permeability could cause the efflux of the solution into the pulmonary interstitium, further worsening fluid influx and edema.

The use of hemoglobin substitutes in the resuscitation of hemorrhagic shock has become another area of investigation. Recently developed solutions appear capable of restoring perfusion with minimal fluid volumes, and thus offer potential benefits in the setting of lung injury with associated hemorrhage.[60] Diaspirin cross-linked hemoglobin is under investigation in experimental animal models as an alternative resuscitative measure.[60,61]

CORTICOSTEROIDS

The use of corticosteroids in the treatment of PC remains controversial, and currently there are few data supporting their use.[2,3,14,38] Theoretically, corticosteroids could help to inhibit the pulmonary inflammatory response and relieve bronchospasm. Indeed, some canine studies have shown a diminution in hypoxemia and lesion size with corticosteroids administered immediately after the injury.[3,62] Svennevig demonstrated that human trauma patients treated immediately after the injury with high dose methylprednisone (30 mg/kg) had reduced pulmonary vascular resistance and mortality.[63-65] Many others, however, have documented little histopathological, physiological, or clinical benefit from corticosteroid use.[2,14,38] In addition, corticosteroid use in patients with PC could be detrimental because pulmonary bacterial clearance may be impeded, predisposing patients to pulmonary infection.[66] Powell reported no difference in duration of oxygen administration or hospitalization between dogs that received glucocorticoids and those that did not.[11] If corticosteroids are indicated (e.g., in patients with concurrent spinal cord injury), early use and monitoring for gastrointestinal ulceration should be implemented.

ANTIBIOTICS

It has been hypothesized that contused lung may be predisposed to bacterial infection.[1,3,38,67] For decades, treatment with prophylactic antibiotics was the standard of care for humans with PC. It was theorized that extravasation of fluid and blood into the alveolar and interstitial spaces provided a culture medium for bacterial growth, especially in debilitated patients. Studies in the 1970s showed that 50% to 70% of people with PC developed pneumonia in the contused segment of lung, and that 35% would go on to develop pulmonary abscess, pneumonitis, or empyema. Many of these patients, however, were mechanically ventilated.[4] Richardson and colleagues documented decreased lung bacterial clearance following fluid therapy in an experimental canine model of PC, suggesting that contused lungs may be more susceptible to bacterial infections.[66] To date, however, no infectious process has yet to be identified as part of the pathogenesis of PC. Powell reported a 1% incidence of bacterial pneumonia in dogs with PC; however, this particular dog was mechanically ventilated.[11] The majority of dogs in that study did not develop pneumonia despite a lack of antibiotic therapy.[11] Currently, antibiotic therapy is not indicated in PC unless bronchopneumonia develops or there is an associated injury (e.g., an open fracture). The prophylactic use of antibiotic therapy should be avoided to reduce the development of bacterial resistance.

DIURETICS

Currently, diuretics are not recommended in the treatment of PC, especially in volume-depleted patients. Diuretic administration in a volume-depleted patient with pulmonary contusion can complicate hypovolemia, thereby further decreasing tissue oxygen delivery. This can precipitate cardiovascular collapse. If clinical evidence of volume overload and pulmonary edema are observed, furosemide can be administered (1 to 2 mg/kg, IV). Strict attention must be paid to volume status and urine output in any patient receiving diuretic therapy.

PAIN CONTROL

Pain management should be considered in any patient encountering blunt chest trauma. The massive force required to generate PC is often associated with significant soft tissue injury of the chest cavity and, possibly, rib fractures. Pain from these injuries can suppress ventilatory efforts and hinder tussive efforts. Pain can cause or worsen respiratory acidosis caused by hypoventilation. In humans, effective analgesia has been shown to improve ventilatory function, decrease morbidity and mortality, and allow patients to be effectively managed without mechanical ventilation.[67,68] Commonly used narcotics in veterinary medicine include butorphanol, buprenorphine, morphine, and hydromorphone. Narcotics should be used with caution in any patient with pulmonary disease because they can centrally suppress ventilatory drive. Rib fractures are commonly treated with intercostal nerve blocks, thereby reducing the required amount of systemically administered opioids, especially if there is concern about respiratory depression. In humans with PC, epidural or intrathecal administration of morphine or fentanyl has replaced intercostal nerve blocks as the standard method of chest wall analgesia because it results in less significant respiratory depression.[68]

MECHANICAL VENTILATION

Before the 1970s, all human patients sustaining severe blunt chest trauma underwent mechanical ventilation. Studies in the 1970s in people, however, demonstrated that morbidity and mortality were not improved with mechanical ventilation, and the complications associated with ventilation, including sepsis and tracheostomy complications, possibly worsened outcome.[69] In 1975, Trinkle implemented a selective intubation protocol for thoracic trauma patients who sustained respiratory compromise because of PC.[70] This protocol represents the most significant therapeutic advance for PC over the last three decades and has significantly reduced mortality (Box 63-2).[71]

BOX 63-2
Criteria Indicating Endotracheal Intubation and Mechanical Ventilation for Patients with Pulmonary Contusion[49,71]

1. Unconscious
2. Upper airway obstruction or evidence of large amounts of blood in the airways
3. Evidence of hypoxemia: Pao_2 <60 mm Hg with an Fio_2 >50%
4. Evidence of hypoventilation: $Paco_2$ >50 mm Hg, despite pain relief
5. Evidence of progressive respiratory deterioration or fatiguing ventilatory drive
6. Severe head trauma or indication of increased intracranial pressure (e.g., altered mentation, anisocoria, or bradycardia with hypertension)

Campbell reported ventilator management and outcome for dogs requiring mechanical ventilation because of severe PC.[72] This study showed that survival rate to discharge was 30% for dogs with PC that needed to be mechanically ventilated, and that dogs weighing more than 25 kg had a better outcome.[72] Pneumonia and acute respiratory distress syndrome (ARDS) were causes for progressive lung injury in dogs that did not survive.[72] Intensive monitoring with aggressive ventilatory care by trained personnel is essential in these patients.

Prognosis/Outcome

The prognosis associated with pulmonary contusion depends largely upon the extent of lung injury, the severity and number of other thoracic and nonthoracic injuries, and the cardiovascular status at the time of presentation.[3] In humans, mortality rates have been reported to range from 25% to 38%,[7,52,68,73,74] of which 50% of deaths occurred within the first few minutes of admission.[19] Powell reported a mortality rate of 18% in dogs with PC.[11] In that study, dogs were either euthanized or died because of financial constraints, severity of concurrent injuries, or progressive pulmonary failure.[11] Of the dogs that died from progressive pulmonary failure, death occurred within the first 4 hours for the majority of the patients. In the remaining dogs, death occurred 48 to 72 hours after admission.[11]

Predictors of mortality in humans include: (1) respiratory rate less than 5, (2) systolic blood pressure less than 100 mm Hg, and (3) older patients. Factors that do not seem to influence mortality include: (1) the mechanism of lung injury, (2) the number of days on a mechanical ventilator, (3) respiratory rate greater than 5 in the trauma room, and (4) amount of blood products infused.[19] Other factors that have been associated with increased mortality include concurrent head trauma and other severe thoracic and extra-thoracic injuries. Craniocerebral trauma, especially when associated with massive hemorrhage, is the most common cause of mor-

tality in humans sustaining PC, with most deaths occurring within the first 24 hours.[19,68,71] The presence of concomitant flail chest has been associated with a greater chance of mechanical ventilation (from 20% to 50%) and mortality (from 16% to 42%).[51,68] Turchin reported no difference in the morbidity between patients with PC and nonthoracic injuries (extremity injuries) to those with PC alone.[75] Patients with spinal fractures and pulmonary contusion, however, had the worst outcomes.[75] In patients with extremity fractures and pulmonary contusion, outcome was related more to the presence of PC than to the fracture and its treatment.[75] Such prognostic criteria have not yet been evaluated in veterinary medicine.

The pulmonary derangements associated with PC improve rapidly in most patients.[3] Clinical improvement and radiographic resolution of the contused lung usually occur within 3 to 5 days.[2,3] Conservative management with supplemental oxygen therapy usually results in a good outcome in the majority of human patients with PC.[71] Currently, controversy exists as to whether associated short- and/or long-term pulmonary complications occur in humans.[76] Pneumonia has been reported in humans as a sequela to PC; however, this has been seen mostly in patients that were mechanically ventilated either for severe pulmonary dysfunction or for surgery.[4] This has also been reported in veterinary medicine.[11,72] Rare reports of hematomas, pseudocysts, pulmonary abscess, and ARDS have additionally been reported to occur in dogs secondary to PC.[11,41,72] In humans, ARDS has been reported to develop in 38% to 50% of human patients sustaining PC.[77]

Long-term respiratory disability in humans is still unknown. Some investigators report that long-term respiratory difficulties are uncommon,[76] whereas others report them as commonplace.[78] Late pulmonary dysfunction may occur secondary to local inflammatory responses in the injured lung, systemic inflammatory responses related to associated injuries, or development of nosocomial pneumonia.[73] Kishikawa reported a decrease in the functional residual capacity and oxygenation in patients following PC that correlated with pulmonary fibrosis on thoracic CT.[78] No comparable reports exist in veterinary medicine; however, it has been suggested that delayed pulmonary fibrosis may occur secondary to PC in dogs.[41]

Conclusion

PC is a common sequela of blunt chest wall trauma. Alveolar and interstitial hemorrhage worsens over 24 to 48 hours and then generally resolves over 5 to 7 days. The diagnosis of PC should be based upon a recent history of thoracic trauma and respiratory dysfunction at admission, in conjunction with thoracic radiographic findings. In humans, a thoracic CT scan is superior to a radiograph in identifying PC and may be helpful in predicting the need for mechanical ventilation. Pulmonary dysfunction can manifest as severe respiratory distress on admission or can develop insidiously. Parenchymal consolidation and edema are maximal 48 to 72 hours after the lung injury. Arterial blood gas monitoring is a useful means of assessing hypoxemia and the progression of lung injury. Clinical and radiographic improvement occurs unless pulmonary infection or ARDS develops. Early recognition of patients with PC is paramount. Management is mostly supportive and includes judicious fluid administration, oxygen supplementation, hemodynamic monitoring, and pain control. Despite current therapeutic interventions, patients sustaining PC still face significant morbidity and mortality.

REFERENCES

1. Alfano G, Hale HW: Pulmonary contusion, *Journal of Trauma* 5:647-658, 1965.
2. Trinkle JK, Furman RW, Hinshaw MA et al: Pulmonary contusion, pathogenesis and effects of various resuscitative measures, *Ann Thoracic Surg* 16:568-573, 1973.
3. DeMuth WE, Smith JM: Pulmonary contusion, *Am J Surg* 109:819-823, 1965.
4. Jones KW: Thoracic trauma, *Surg Clin North Am* 60:957-981, 1980.
5. Dougall AM, Paul ME, Finley RJ et al: Chest trauma: current morbidity and mortality, *J Trauma* 17:547-553, 1977.
6. Lewis FR: Thoracic trauma, *Surg Clin No Am* 62:97-104, 1982.
7. Kirsh MM, Pellegrini RV, Sloan HE: Treatment of blunt chest trauma, *Surgery Annual* 4:51-90, 1972.
8. Spackman CJ, Caywood DD, Feeney DA et al: Thoracic wall and pulmonary trauma in dogs sustaining fractures as a result of motor vehicular accidents, *JAVMA* 185:975-977, 1984.
9. Tamas PM, Paddleford RR, Krahwinkel DJ: Thoracic trauma in dogs and cats presented for limb fractures, *JAAHA* 21:161-166, 1985.
10. Jackimczyk K: Blunt chest trauma, *Emerg Medicine Clinics North Am* 11:81-96, 1993.
11. Powell LL, Rozanski EA, Tidwell AS et al: A retrospective analysis of pulmonary contusion secondary to motor vehicular accidents in 143 dogs: 1994-1997, *JVECC* 9:127-136, 1999.
12. Griffin DJ, Walter PA, Wallace LJ: Thoracic Injuries in cats with traumatic fractures, *VCOT* 7:98-100, 1994.
13. Garzon AA, Seltzer B, Karlson KE: Physiopathology of crushed chest injuries, *Annals Surg* 168:128-136, 1968.
14. Fulton RL, Peter ET, Wilson JN: The pathophysiology and treatment of pulmonary contusions, *J Trauma* 10:719-730, 1970.
15. Lichtmann MW: The problem of contused lungs, *J Trauma* 10:731-739, 1970.
16. Fulton RL, Peter ET: The progressive nature of pulmonary contusion, *Surgery* 67:499-506, 1970.
17. Daniel RA, Cote WR: "Wet lung," an experimental study, *Ann Surg* 127:836-857, 1948.
18. Shin BS, McAslan TC, Hankins JR et al: Management of lung contusion, *American Surgeon* 45:168-175, 1979.
19. Stellin G: Survival in trauma victims with pulmonary contusions, *Am Surg* 57:780-784, 1991.
20. Cohn SM: Pulmonary contusion: Review of the clinical entity, *J Trauma* 42:973-979, 1997.
21. Mott FW: The effects of high explosive upon the central nervous system, *Lancet* 1:331-338, 1916.
22. Hooker DR: Physiological effects of air concussion, *Am J Physiol* 67:219-274, 1924.
23. Lockwood AL: Surgical experiences in the last war, *Br Med J* 1:356-358, 1940.
24. Dean DM, Thomas AR, Alison RS: Effects of high-explosive blast on the lungs, *Lancet* 2:224-226, 1940.
25. Falla ST: Effect of explosion-blast on the lungs, *Br Med J* 1:225-256, 1940.
26. Barcroft J: Lung injuries in air raids, *Br Med J* 1:239-242, 1941.
27. Zuckerman S: Experimental study of blast injuries to the lungs, *Lancet* 2:219-224, 1940.
28. Burford TH, Burbank B: Traumatic wet lung, *J Thoracic Surgery* 14:415-424, 1945.
29. Brewer LA, Burbank B, Samson PC et al: The "wet lung" in war casualties, *Ann Surg* 123:343-362, 1946.
30. Reid JM, Baird WLM: Crushed chest injury: Some physiological disturbances and their correction, *Br Med J* 1:1105-1109, 1965.
31. Mosley RV, Vernick JJ, Doty DB: Response to blunt chest injury: A new experimental model, *J Trauma* 10:673-683, 1970.
32. Ratliff JL, Fletcher JR, Kopriva CJ et al: Pulmonary contusion, a continuing management problem, *J Thoracic Cardio Surgery* 62:638-644, 1971.
33. Oppenheimer L, Craven KD, Forkert L et al: Pathophysiology of pulmonary contusion in dogs, *J Appl Physiol* 47:718-728, 1979.
34. Craven KD, Oppenheimer, Wood LDH: Effects of contusion and flail chest on pulmonary perfusion and oxygen exchange, *J Appl Physiol: Respir, Envir & Exercise Physiol* 47:729-737, 1979.
35. Nichols RT, Pearce HJ, Greenfield LJ: Effects of experimental pulmonary contusion on respiratory exchange and lung mechanics, *Arch Surg* 96:723-730, 1968.
36. Rutherford RB, Valenta J: An experimental study of "traumatic wet lung," *J Trauma* 11:146-166, 1971.
37. Richardson JD, Franz JL, Grover FL et al: Pulmonary contusion and hemorrhage: Crystalloiod versus colloid replacement, *J Surg Res* 16:330-336, 1974.
38. Shepard GH, Ferguson JL, Foster JH: Pulmonary contusion, *Ann Thoracic Surg* 7:110-119, 1969.
39. Erickson DR, Shinozaki T, Beekman E et al: Relationship of arterial blood gases and pulmonary radiographs to the degree of pulmonary damage in experimental pulmonary contusion, *J Trauma* 11:689-694, 1971.
40. Bongard FS, Lewis FR: Crystalloid resuscitation of patients with pulmonary contusion, *Am J Surg* 148:145-151, 1984.
41. Crowe DT: Traumatic pulmonary contusions, hematomas, pseudocysts, and acute respiratory distress syndrome: An update- Part I, *Compendium* 5:396-401, 1983.
42. Crawford WO: Pulmonary injury in thoracic and nonthoracic trauma, *Radiol Clin North Am* 11:527-541, 1973.
43. Wagner RB, Crawford WO, Schimpf PP: Classification of parenchymal injuries of the lung, *Thoracic Radiology* 167:77-82, 1988.
44. Green R: Lung alterations in thoracic trauma, *J Thoracic Imaging* 2:1-11, 1987.
45. Schild HH, Strunk H, Weber W et al: Pulmonary contusion: CT vs plain radiographs, *J Computer Assisted Tomography* 13:417-420, 1989.
46. Wagner RB, Jamieson PM: Pulmonary contusion. Evaluation and classification by computed tomography, *Surg Clin North Am* 69:31-40, 1989.
47. Marino PL: Hypoxemia and hypercapnia. In Marino PL: *The ICU book*, ed 2, Philadelphia, 1997, Williams & Wilkins.
48. Pierce LNB: Practical physiology of the pulmonary system. In Pierce LNB: *Guide to mechanical ventilation and intensive respiratory care*, Philadelphia, 1995, WB Saunders.
49. Pierce LNB: Mechanical ventilation: Indications, basic principles of ventilator performance of the respiratory cycle, and initiation. In Pierce LNB: *Guide to mechanical ventilation and intensive respiratory care*, Philadelphia, 1995, WB Saunders.
50. Lucas CE, Ledgerwood AM: Pulmonary response of massive steroids in seriously injured patients, *Ann Surg* 194:256-261, 1981.
51. Johnson JA, Cogbill TH, Winga ER: Determinants of outcome after pulmonary contusion, *J Trauma* 26:695-697, 1986.
52. Keller JW, Meckstroth CV, Sanzenbacher L et al: Thoracic injuries due to blunt trauma, *J Trauma* 7:541-550, 1967.
53. Fulton RL, Peter ET: Physiologic effects of fluid therapy after pulmonary contusion, *Am J Surg* 126:773-777, 1973.
54. Fulton RL, Peter ET: Compositional and histologic effects of fluid therapy following pulmonary contusion, *J Trauma* 14:783-790, 1974.
55. Collins JA, James PM, Bredenberg CE et al: The relationship between transfusion and hypoxemia in combat casualties, *Annals of Surgery* 188:513-520, 1978.
56. Tranbaugh FS, Elings VB, Christensen J et al: Determinants of pulmonary interstitial fluid accumulation after trauma, *J Trauma* 22:820-826, 1982.
57. Velasco IT, Pontieri V, Rocha M et al: Hyperosmotic NaCl and severe hemorrhagic shock, *Am J Physiol* 239:H664-H673, 1980.
58. Velasco IT, Oliveisa MA: A comparison of hypersomotic and hyperoncotic resuscitation from severe hemorrhagic shock in dogs, *Circ Shock* 21:338-341, 1987.
59. Wisner DH, Schuster L, Quinn C: Hypertonic saline resuscitation of head injury: Effects on cerebral water content, *J Trauma-Inj Infect & Crit Care* 30:75-78, 1990.

60. Cohn SM, Zieg PM, Rosenfield AT et al: Resuscitation of pulmonary contusion: Effects of a red cell substitute, *Crit Care Med* 25:484-491, 1997.
61. Schultz SC, Hamilton IN, Malcolm DS: Use of base deficit to compare resuscitation with lactated Ringer's solution, haemaccel, whole blood, and diaspirin cross-linked hemoglobin following hemorrhage in rats, *J Trauma-Inj Infect & Crit Care* 35:619-625, 1993.
62. Franz JL, Richardson JD, Grover FL et al. Effect of methylprednisolone sodium succinate on experimental pulmonary contusion, *J Thorac & Cardiovasc Surg* 68:842-844, 1974.
63. Svennevig JL, Bugge-Asprheim B, Bjorgo S et al: Methylprednisolone in the treatment of lung contusion following blunt chest trauma, *Scand J Thorac Cardio Surg* 14:301-305, 1980.
64. Svennevig JL, Bugge-Asprheim B, Vaage J et al: Corticosteroids in the treatment of blunt injury of the chest, *Injury* 16:80-94, 1984.
65. Svennevig JL, Bugge-Asprheim B, Geiran O et al: High dose corticosteroids in thoracic trauma, *Acta Chir Scand* 526(Suppl):110-119, 1985.
66. Richardson JD, Woods D, Johanson WG et al: Lung bacterial clearance following pulmonary contusion, *Surgery* 86:730-735, 1979.
67. Freedland M, Wilson RF, Bender JS, et al: The management of flail chest injury: Factors affecting outcome, *J Trauma* 30:1460-1468, 1990.
68. Clark GC, Schecter WP, Trunkey DD: Variables affecting outcome in blunt chest trauma: Flail chest vs. pulmonary contusion, *J Trauma* 28:298-304, 1988.
69. Ransdell HT: Treatment of flail chest injuries with a piston respirator, *J Trauma* 5:412-420, 1965.
70. Trinkle JK, Richardson JD, Franz JL et al: Management of flail chest without mechanical ventilation, *Ann Thorac Surg* 19:355-363, 1975.
71. Richardson JD, Adams L, Flint LM: Selective management of flail chest and pulmonary contusion, *Ann Surg* 196:481-487, 1982.
72. Campbell VL, King LG: Pulmonary function, ventilator management, and outcome of dogs with thoracic trauma and pulmonary contusions: 10 cases (1994-1998), *JAVMA* 217:1505-1509, 2000.
73. Demling RH, Pomfret EA: Blunt chest trauma, *New Horizons* 1:402-421, 1993.
74. Lewis FR, Thomas AN, Schlobohm RM: Control of respiratory therapy in flail chest, *Ann Thorac Surg* 29:170-176, 1975.
75. Turchin DC, Schemitsch EH, McKee MD et al: A comparison of the outcome of patients with pulmonary contusions versus pulmonary contusions and musculoskeletal injuries, *American Academy of Orthopedic Surgeons 1996 Annual Meeting*-Scientific Program: Paper No. 87.
76. Livingston DH, Richardson JD: Pulmonary disability after severe blunt chest trauma, *J Trauma* 30:562-567, 1990.
77. Pepe PE, Potkin RT, Reus DH et al: Clinical predictors of the adult respiratory distress syndrome, *Am J Surg* 144:124-130, 1982.
78. Kishikkawa M, Yoshioka T, Shimazu T et al: Pulmonary contusion causes long-term respiratory dysfunction with decreased functional residual capacity, *J Trauma* 31:1203-1210, 1991.

CHAPTER 64

Smoke Inhalation

Kenneth J. Drobatz

Introduction

Structure fires are a relatively common occurrence in large cities. In 1996 alone, there were 1550 dwelling fires in Philadelphia. Despite this common problem, animals that present with smoke exposure are relatively rare in veterinary emergency medicine. At the University of Pennsylvania, only 27 dogs and 22 cats were admitted to the emergency service with a diagnosis of smoke exposure during a 10-year period.[1,2] During this same period approximately 8000 to 10,000 dogs and cats were examined per year in the emergency service. Smoke exposure therefore represents an extremely small proportion of the population of dogs and cats seen in a large urban veterinary emergency service. Given this infrequent occurrence, it is not surprising that there is a paucity of information regarding this clinical condition in the veterinary literature. Except for a few case reports and review articles, there are only two case series published regarding the clinical manifestation of dogs and cats presenting to a veterinary facility.[1,2] The veterinary clinical information regarding smoke inhalation/exposure presented in this chapter will be largely derived from the information in these studies.

The range of physiological compromise with which these animals are presented can be wide. Most animals have only minor respiratory signs or ocular irritation, whereas others may have severe respiratory and neurologic compromise that can result in death. Hence, despite its rarity, it is important that the veterinary clinician be familiar with the pathophysiology, clinical manifestations, therapeutic rationale, and prognosis of smoke exposure/inhalation in order to provide the best care for these critically ill animals.

Dogs and cats with smoke exposure seen at veterinary clinics tend to be young, with a median age of approximately 3 years.[1,2] The author suspects that these animals are not more likely to suffer smoke inhalation, but are more likely to survive the smoke exposure and make it to the veterinary hospital compared with older animals. Experimental animal models have demonstrated that older dogs tend to do worse than younger ones.[3]

The majority of smoke exposure cases were presented in the colder months of the year. Of 40 instances of smoke exposure, 21 (53%) presented between November and February; 8 (20%) between the months of March and June; and 11 (27%) between July and October.[1,2] This likely reflects the greater incidence of dwelling fires because of space heater accidents, heater malfunctions, and the use of Christmas lights.

Pathogenesis

Three major pathophysiologic insults result from smoke inhalation: tissue hypoxia, thermal damage, and pulmonary irritation. The spectrum of respiratory compromise can range from mild respiratory problems to pulmonary failure. Different components of smoke result in differing physiologic insults. The type of material that is burned, the heat that is generated, and the amount of oxygen available determine the components of smoke during combustion. Although extensive knowledge regarding the individual chemicals that may be present and the resultant damage they can induce in the pulmonary tissue is interesting, it is nearly impossible to know what an individual animal has inhaled.

The clinical signs attributed to tissue hypoxia are primarily associated with the cardiovascular system and the neurological system. No animals in a recent study of smoke exposure manifested severe cardiovascular compromise except for intermittent ventricular arrhythmias, but immediate and delayed neurological abnormalities can develop ranging from mild depression to seizures, stupor, or coma.[1,2]

Tissue hypoxia occurs for a variety of reasons including decreased inspired oxygen concentration, decreased ability to carry oxygen, decreased tissue perfusion, and disruption of the cells' ability to utilize oxygen. It is often reported that dogs and cats are found unconscious at the scene of the fire but quickly regain consciousness once removed from the smoke and allowed to breathe fresh air or oxygen.[1,2] This initial loss of consciousness likely reflects decreased Fio_2 secondary to CO_2 production from combustion, which can lower ambient oxygen concentration to 15%.[4] In addition, tissue hypoxia occurs as a result of inhalation of carbon monoxide and cyanide and production of methemoglobinemia. Carbon monoxide (CO) has 200 to 250 times the affinity for hemoglobin compared with oxygen. The binding of CO to hemoglobin decreases blood oxygen content and therefore decreases tissue oxygen concentration. Carbon monoxide not only decreases blood oxygen content but also shifts the hemoglobin/oxygen saturation curve to the left, preventing release of oxygen to the tissues from the hemoglobin. In addition, CO may have cardiotoxic effects by directly binding myoglobin, and it also poisons the mitochondrial cytochrome oxidase system.[5]

Combustion of wool, plastics, polyurethane, silk, nylon, rubber, paper products, and other materials can produce cyanide. Cyanide binds to the ferric ion on Cytochrome A_3 and also arrests the tricarboxylic acid cycle. As a result, cell production of ATP must rely on less efficient anaerobic glycolysis, a cycle resulting in increased production of lactate. Finally, heat denaturation of hemoglobin, oxidation of nitrogen, and combustion of nitrites can cause methemoglobinemia, further compromising tissue oxygen delivery.[6]

Direct thermal injury to pulmonary tissue also occurs. Because of the efficient heat exchange capacity of the upper airways, most thermal injury is limited to the upper airways, whereas the lower airways are spared. Inhalation of steam, however, can result in direct injury to the lower airways and alveoli. Swelling, inflammation, and edema of the supraglottic area and larynx often occur within the first several hours of injury and can be worsened by aggressive fluid therapy. In a clinical study in dogs, tracheostomy for upper airway injury was necessary between 24 and 72 hours after fire exposure in 2 dogs.[2]

Chemical irritants in smoke include sulfur dioxide, chlorine gas, and acroleins. Irritants cause direct injury by producing acid and alkali burns of the respiratory mucosa, by formation of free radicals, and by protein denaturation (acroleins). They also contribute to respiratory dysfunction by inciting reflex bronchoconstriction and pulmonary inflammation. The clinical result may range from mild tachypnea to life-threatening respiratory distress. The irritants may cause pulmonary injury anywhere along the pulmonary tract. High water-soluble irritants tend to cause upper airway lesions, and low water-soluble irritants can penetrate to the lower airways and alveoli, causing damage there. The irritants may also inactivate surfactant within seconds of the inhalation of smoke, causing atelectasis and decreased compliance.[3]

Particulate materials cause mechanical irritation and reflex bronchoconstriction. Also, superheated particles may contribute to mucosal burn and dissolved irritant gases may cause chemical irritation and injury to the respiratory mucosa.

It is clear that the numerous components of smoke can produce a wide spectrum of effects. Keeping these effects in mind when assessing and treating these patients will provide for a more comprehensive and effective approach to management.

Clinical Signs

The clinical signs of smoke inhalation vary depending upon the intensity and duration of exposure, the heat generated, and the components of smoke. Therefore the range of signs can range from mild to life threatening. The systems most commonly affected are the respiratory, neurological, ophthalmic, and cutaneous. The most common clinical signs in dogs noted at the scene of the fire include stupor or coma (47%), coughing/gagging (35%), and respiratory difficulty (35%).[2] Other less commonly reported signs include weakness/ataxia, foaming from the mouth, and rubbing at the eyes.[2] In cats, difficulty breathing (44%), open mouth breathing (44%), vocalizing (44%), coughing (22%), loss of consciousness

(22%), and lethargy (22%) were the most common clinical signs noted at the fire scene.[1]

Physical Examination

The majority of animals with smoke exposure are relatively stable. Most of the physical manifestations of smoke exposure are a result of tissue hypoxia, thermal damage, and irritation of mucous membranes. The majority of dogs and cats have normal rectal temperature and pulse rates. Respiratory rate is often increased because of pulmonary irritation, bronchoconstriction, and hypoxia. Oral mucous membrane color tends to be normal, although hyperemia is not uncommon. Tissue irritation, increased carbon dioxide concentration, carbon monoxide concentration, or cyanide concentrations may all contribute to the hyperemia.

Conjunctivitis, blepharospasm, rubbing at the eyes, corneal ulceration, and edema caused by chemical, particulate, and thermal irritation are also relatively common in animals exposed to smoke. Skin lesions are relatively rare, and animals most commonly have soot covering their haircoat and a smoky smell. When present, skin burns indicate a close exposure to the fire and possibly greater thermal and smoke exposure for the pulmonary system. Pulmonary effects tend to be worse when smoke inhalation and skin burns occur together, and a more serious prognosis is warranted in those cases.

Loss of consciousness followed by recovery at the fire scene is often reported. At presentation, the majority of dogs and cats are relatively normal neurologically, or mildly depressed. Rarely, an animal will present with severely altered mentation ranging from seizures to stupor or coma. Also uncommonly, a dog or cat that presents with relatively normal mentation or mild depression can progress to severely altered mentation hours or a few days after smoke exposure.

The majority of dogs and cats have an increased respiratory rate. Upper airway sounds may occur as a result of mucosal swelling from irritation and thermal injury. Lower airway abnormalities are relatively common and are manifested as increased bronchovesicular sounds and crackles. Expiratory wheezes may be heard because of small airway narrowing from bronchoconstriction and mucosal edema. Rarely, localized areas of decreased airway sounds may occur because of small airway obstruction from mucosal swelling, mucosal sloughing, and particulate debris.

Diagnostic Evaluation

An emergency database including packed cell volume, total solids, blood glucose, blood urea nitrogen, electrolytes, and blood gas analysis should be evaluated in critically ill patients with smoke exposure. Packed cell volume tends to be higher and blood glucose lower in dogs and cats more severely affected with smoke exposure. A persistent metabolic acidosis may indicate carbon monoxide intoxication, methemoglobinemia, or cyanide

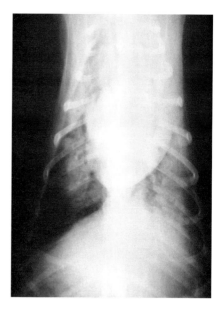

Figure 64-1. Dorsal-ventral thoracic radiograph of a dog with smoke inhalation on the first day of hospitalization. Note the generalized, severe alveolar pattern in most of the lung fields. This is an example of a severely affected smoke inhalation dog.

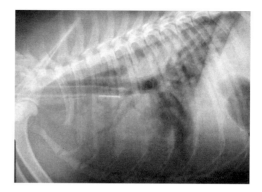

Figure 64-2. A lateral thoracic radiograph of the same animal in Figure 64-1, taken later on the first day of hospitalization. Again, note the severe lung changes. This animal has been intubated and is receiving positive pressure ventilation.

intoxication. Cooximetry would be helpful in determining the cause of the metabolic acidosis in this instance.

Arterial blood gas analysis provides an assessment of lung function and should be serially monitored in animals with evidence of respiratory involvement. If arterial blood gases are drawn during oxygen supplementation, evaluation of the ratio of Pao_2:Fio_2 can provide assessment of the lung's ability to oxygenate the blood. The nadir (lowest value) of this ratio in dogs with smoke inhalation tends to occur between 24 and 48 hours after smoke exposure.[2]

Pulse oximetry provides a noninvasive method of assessing hemoglobin oxygenation, although the presence of carboxyhemoglobin or methemoglobin in smoke inhalation patients can render the pulse oximetry readings inac-

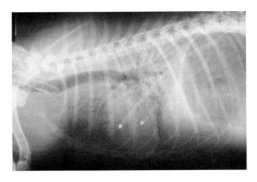

Figure 64-3. *The same animal as in Figures 64-1 and 64-2, but on day 2 of hospitalization. Note that the alveolar pattern is worse and more generalized, consistent with a diagnosis of acute respiratory distress syndrome. This animal is receiving positive pressure ventilation. In addition, note the chest tubes in place. It is not unusual in animals with such severe lung injury to develop pneumothorax when receiving positive pressure ventilation.*

curate. Pulse oximetry readings in these instances tend to overestimate the level of oxygenation of hemoglobin.

Thoracic radiographs also provide another method of assessing lung involvement and its progression. As with many dynamic pulmonary problems, thoracic radiographic changes can lag behind clinical progression. Radiographic changes seen in dogs and cats with smoke inhalation vary, and include bronchiolar, interstitial, and alveolar patterns (Figures 64-1, 64-2, and 64-3). Rarely, a collapsed lung lobe may occur as result of bronchial obstruction from mucosal swelling, sloughing, and debris.

Animals showing ocular irritation should have a thorough examination of the cornea, sclera, conjunctiva, and eyelids. Topical anesthesia will facilitate exploration for foreign bodies of the sclera, conjunctiva, or under the eyelids.

Finally, a complete blood count, chemistry screen, urinalysis, and coagulation parameters should be evaluated in any animal that is critically ill from smoke inhalation.

Treatment

Oxygen supplementation should be provided for any animal showing respiratory or neurological signs. High inspired-oxygen concentrations will improve hemoglobin oxygenation and decrease the half-life of carboxyhemoglobin. There are no specific recommendations for the duration of oxygen therapy, except that high inspired-oxygen concentrations should be administered until the carboxyhemoglobin concentration is less than 10%. Resolution of neurological or respiratory signs is not a clinically useful endpoint because they may not resolve before achieving the target blood concentrations of carboxyhemoglobin. Administering 100% oxygen reduces the half life of carboxyhemoglobin from 4 hours to 30 minutes, but the initial concentration of carboxyhemoglobin is usually unknown. A reasonable clinical goal is probably to administer high concentrations of oxygen (up to 100%) for approximately 2 to 4 hours, and longer in more severely affected patients.

Corticosteroids may decrease inflammation of airways, but studies of different species and different types of corticosteroids have shown mixed results on outcome in smoke inhalation.[2,7,8] At this point, there is no strong evidence supporting the use of corticosteroids in dogs and cats with smoke inhalation.

Prophylactic antibiotics are not warranted in animals with smoke inhalation. Antibiotic therapy should be guided by culture and sensitivity of pulmonary fluid samples, if possible. Animals with smoke inhalation that are intubated and receiving positive pressure ventilation may be particularly susceptible to pulmonary infection and should be monitored accordingly. If pulmonary infection is diagnosed, then broad-spectrum antibiotic administration is warranted.

Chemicals and particulates in smoke can be irritating to pulmonary airways and cause reflex bronchoconstriction. In animals with respiratory signs, bronchodilators such as beta-2 agonists or phosphodiesterase inhibitors may provide some relief.

Nebulization and coupage will help thin and clear pulmonary secretions in more severely affected patients. Rarely, bronchoscopy and suctioning of lower airways may be necessary when debris and secretions obstruct major airways.

Animals with upper airway obstruction may require tracheostomy until the inflammation and swelling of the pharynx and larynx resolves. Mechanical ventilation may be necessary in animals that require a prolonged period of high inspired-oxygen concentration, are fatigued, hypoventilating, or have severe neurologic changes that interfere with ventilation.

Hydration with intravenous balanced electrolyte solution should be maintained to avoid drying and thickening of airway secretions. Pulmonary vascular permeability may be increased, and overhydration should be avoided to minimize accumulation of pulmonary fluid.

Animals with corneal ulceration should be treated with topical broad-spectrum antibiotics. If miosis secondary to ciliary spasm is present, topical atropine should also be administered.

Prognosis

Overall, the survival rate in dogs and cats with smoke exposure (without severe skin burns) that make it to the veterinary hospital alive is approximately 90%. Dogs with minor respiratory signs that do not worsen by the second day tend to do well and are discharged from the hospital after 2 days. Dogs that have severe signs at presentation and worsen by the second day either die within 72 hours or are discharged after 6 or 7 days of hospitalization.[1,2]

REFERENCES

1. Drobatz KJ, Walker L, Hendricks JC: Smoke exposure in cats: 22 cases (1986-1997), *JAVMA* 215:1312-1316, 1999.

2. Drobatz KJ, Walker LM, Hendricks JC: Smoke exposure in dogs: 27 cases (1988-1997), *JAVMA* 215:1306-1311, 1999.
3. Nieman G, Clark W, Wax S et al: The effect of smoke inhalation on pulmonary surfactant, *Ann Surg* 191:171-181, 1980.
4. Dressler DP: Laboratory background on smoke inhalation, *J Trauma* 19:913-915, 1979.
5. Piantadosi CA: Carbon monoxide, oxygen transport, and oxygen metabolism, *J Hyperbaric Med* 2:27-44, 1987.

6. Bizovi KE, Leikin JD: Smoke inhalation among firefighters, *Occup Med* 10:721-733, 1995.
7. Dressler DP, Skornik WA, Kupersmith S: Corticosteroid treatment of experimental smoke inhalation, *Ann Surg* 183:46-52, 1976.
8. Robinson NB, Hudson LD, Riem M et al: Steroid therapy following isolated smoke inhalation injury, *J Trauma* 22:876-879, 1982.

CHAPTER 65

Accidental Drowning and Submersion Injury

Lisa L. Powell

Accidental drowning and submersion injury is a leading cause of morbidity and mortality in humans. Drowning is the third most common cause of accidental death in people less than 44 years old, with 40% of all drowning deaths reported in children less than 5 years of age.[1] Another 15% to 20% of drowning victims are between the ages of 5 and 20 years, and males predominate in all age groups.[1] *Drowning* is defined as death from asphyxia while submerged or within 24 hours of submersion.[2] *Submersion* describes a patient who experiences some water-related distress sufficient to require medical care. Previously, submersion victims were described as *near-drowning* victims. New recommendations by the American Heart Association include the use of the term *submersion victim* instead of *near-drowning victim*.[3] Near-drowning has been reported in veterinary medicine as a case report in a horse.[4] No other reports of this syndrome in animals have been published.

Pathophysiology

Drowning occurs without aspiration of water in about 10% of victims, whereas 90% aspirate fluid into the lungs.[5] All submersion victims experience hypoxemia, either from laryngospasm, in which no aspiration of fluid occurs, or aspiration of fluid, resulting in loss of surfactant causing atelectasis and intrapulmonary shunt. Most (about 85%) submersion victims that survive are thought to have aspirated less than 22 ml/kg of water.[5]

In the 1970s, the medical literature focused on the differences between aspiration of fresh and salt water. It was hypothesized that the hypertonicity of aspirated salt water would result in an osmotic gradient in the lungs, drawing plasma water into the pulmonary interstitial space, resulting in hypernatremia and a decreased circulating blood volume. Aspiration of fresh water was thought to cause a shift of fluid out of the lung and into the circulation, causing hypervolemia and dilution of serum electrolytes, including sodium. Later experimental studies showed that the amount of aspirated water necessary to cause these changes in blood volume was far greater than the amount normally experienced by drowning victims.[6] In one series of 91 people with severe submersion, no serious fluid or electrolyte abnormalities were detected.[7] However, the hypertonicity of sea water may contribute to pulmonary edema through its osmotic effects. The most prominent pathology in victims of both fresh and salt-water submersion injury is the wash-out of surfactant from the alveoli, which results in pulmonary atelectasis and the potential for development of noncardiogenic pulmonary edema.

Other factors important in the morbidity and mortality of submersion victims include the temperature, and potential contaminants within the water. Swimming pools contain few bacteria, but the chlorine can irritate the pulmonary tissues. Fresh water lakes contain bacteria and protozoa. Sea water is contaminated with bacteria, algae, sand, and other particulate matter. Aspiration of this material may predispose to pneumonia in submersion victims that survive the initial hypoxic insult. Particulate matter may obstruct the smaller bronchi and bronchioles, impeding airflow to the associated lung lobes.

Water temperature has an important effect on the survivability of submersion victims. Submersion in ice-cold water (i.e., less than 5° C) increases the chances of survival, in part because of the *diving reflex,* which is present in most mammals. Within seconds of a victim's face contacting cold water, and before unconsciousness, a reflex mediated by the trigeminal nerve sends impulses to the central nervous system, causing bradycardia, hypertension, and preferential shunting of blood to the cerebral and coronary circulations.[1,2] This reflex acts to protect the brain and heart from hypoxia-induced injury. Hypothermia also causes a decrease in metabolic need, protecting the brain from injury. The effects of this response are evidenced by good neurological recovery in victims submerged in icy water, despite the initial presence of coma or other negative neurological prognostic indicators. Hypothermia in patients with submersion injury in warm water, however, is a negative prognostic sign, indicating poor peripheral perfusion and longer submersion times.[1]

Pulmonary edema is commonly seen in submersion victims regardless of the amount of water aspirated.[2] Aspiration of salt water causes fluid shifts from the pulmonary circulation into the alveoli, causing pulmonary edema. Loss of surfactant following both types of aspiration causes pulmonary atelectasis, intrapulmonary shunt, alterations in pulmonary capillary permeability, and resultant noncardiogenic pulmonary edema. Myocardial depression from global hypoxia may also contribute to the development of cardiogenic pulmonary edema. Increased pulmonary resistance due to airway obstruction from laryngospasm, bronchoconstriction, inhaled particulate matter, or inhaled gastric contents may also cause increased pulmonary capillary permeability, contributing to the development of pulmonary edema.[2] Water that is grossly contaminated with large amounts of bacteria and particulate matter may increase the risk of severe pulmonary infection.

Acute, severe cerebral hypoxia is the final common pathway in all drowning victims. In a retrospective review of 96 human submersion victims, all patients presenting to the emergency room that were awake or had only blunted mentation survived.[8] Patients arriving comatose, decorticate, decerebrate, or flaccid had worse outcomes despite aggressive cerebral resuscitation attempts.[8] Hypoxemia results in severe tissue hypoxia, and predisposes to cardiac arrhythmias, myocardial failure, end-organ failure, and severe metabolic acidosis.

Diagnostic Tests and Monitoring

Most submersion victims are pulled from the water and cardiopulmonary resuscitation is attempted at the scene. New recommendations for CPR in submersion victims include immobilization of the cervical and thoracic spine, immediate mouth-to-mouth ventilation, chest compressions if pulseless, and rapid transfer to an emergency room.[3] There is no need to clear the airway of aspirated water, and the Heimlich maneuver should not be performed.

Monitoring of the victim includes continuous electrocardiogram, respiratory rate and effort, lung auscultation, body temperature, mentation and pupil responsive-

ness, arterial blood pressure, serum electrolytes, and arterial blood gas analysis. Continuous pulse oximetry can be used to monitor hemoglobin saturation. Thoracic radiography should be performed when the patient is stable. Serial blood gas analysis should be performed to monitor arterial oxygen tension, carbon dioxide levels, and acid-base status.

Treatment

The goals of treatment include neurologic stabilization, prevention of tissue hypoxia by optimizing arterial blood oxygen tension, and correction of acid-base abnormalities. Hypoxemia, and respiratory and metabolic acidosis should be treated aggressively and early to prevent further neurological and cardiac damage. Oxygen should be administered and, if indicated, the patient should be intubated and artificially ventilated. Guidelines used in human medicine to indicate the need for intubation and assisted ventilation include a Pao_2 of less than 60 mm Hg while on 30% oxygen, with an oxygen saturation of less than 90% or worsening hypercapnia.[1]

Severe pulmonary dysfunction following a submersion episode often progresses to acute respiratory distress syndrome. In most of these cases, oxygen supplementation alone is not sufficient to maintain adequate arterial oxygenation, and the patient must be artificially ventilated. Positive end-expiratory pressure (PEEP) is often needed to decrease intrapulmonary shunt, improve blood oxygenation, and increase lung compliance in atelectatic lung lobes. Artificial surfactant has been used with some success in patients with severe pulmonary dysfunction.[9] Recent experimental therapies include liquid ventilation, inhaled nitric oxide, and intratracheal pulmonary ventilation.[10-12] Submersion victims are at risk for aspiration and should be monitored carefully for development of pneumonia. If the patient was submerged in grossly contaminated water, broad-spectrum antibiotic therapy may be considered. Ideally, a culture should be obtained by tracheal wash or bronchoalveolar lavage prior to antibiotic administration.

Fluid therapy should be guided toward improving tissue perfusion and oxygenation, correcting electrolyte imbalance, and normalizing blood pH; however, excessive fluids must be avoided to prevent worsening of cerebral edema and noncardiogenic pulmonary edema. Central venous pressure, urine output, and arterial blood pressure monitoring can be used to assess fluid requirements and avoid fluid overload. In patients with severe metabolic acidosis and adequate ventilation, sodium bicarbonate should be administered.[5]

Neurological resuscitation is aimed at decreasing cerebral edema and intracranial pressure. Mild hyperventilation (30 mm Hg) has been shown to decrease intracranial pressure by causing constriction of cerebral vessels. However, hyperventilation is not routinely performed because severe vasoconstriction may also decrease cerebral perfusion. Other recommended treatments for suspected increases in intracranial pressure include sedation and head elevation. Current cerebral resuscitation is aimed at preventing secondary neurologic damage caused by on-going hypoxia, acidosis, hypotension, hyperthermia, hyperglycemia, uncontrolled seizure activity, and fluid overload.[1] Evidence exists that hyperglycemia may be associated with secondary brain injury; therefore normoglycemia should be maintained. Hyperthermia and uncontrolled seizure activity both act to increase cerebral oxygen demands and cerebral blood flow. Osmotic diuretics such as mannitol may be used in fluid-resuscitated patients if severe cerebral edema is suspected. Current experimental therapies, including free radical scavengers and lipid peroxidation inhibitors, have failed to improve neurological outcome in patients with postischemic encephalopathy. Glucocorticoid therapy is not recommended because it has not been shown to improve neurological outcome and hyperglycemia may result.[13]

Prognosis

In one study, three factors were associated with 100% mortality in submersion victims younger than 20 years: (1) submersion duration greater than 25 minutes, (2) resuscitation duration greater than 25 minutes, and (3) pulseless cardiac arrest upon arrival at the emergency department.[14] Additional factors associated with a poor prognosis included the presence of ventricular tachycardia or ventricular fibrillation (93% mortality), fixed pupils (89% mortality), severe acidosis (89% mortality), and respiratory arrest in the emergency department (89% mortality).[14] Patients experiencing acute pulmonary edema were found to have mortality rates ranging from 5% to 19%. Level of consciousness and responsiveness also correlated with survival. Deaths occurred only among victims who remained comatose on arrival at the emergency department. No deaths occurred in patients who presented alert or depressed but responsive.[15]

Accidental drowning and submersion injury has not been reported in the small animal literature. Prognosis would depend on the severity of pulmonary injury, the need for mechanical ventilation, and neurological status. Severe hypoxemia and generalized pulmonary infiltrates indicate a poor prognosis, especially if mechanical ventilation is needed. If the patient presents with minimal cerebral injury and mild to moderate lung injury, the prognosis improves.

REFERENCES

1. DeNicola LK, Falk JL, Swanson ME et al: Submersion injuries in children and adults, *Crit Care Clin* 13(3):477-502, 1997.
2. Levin DL, Morris FC, Toro LO et al: Drowning and near-drowning, *Pediatr Clin North Am* 40(2):321-336, 1993.
3. Anonymous: Part 8: Advanced challenges in resuscitation. Section 3: Special challenges in ECC. 3B: Submersion or near-drowning. *Resuscitation* 46(1-3):273-277, 2000.
4. Humber KA: Near drowning of a gelding, *JAVMA* 192(3):377-378, 1988.
5. Modell JH: Drowning, *N Engl J Med* 328(4):253-256, 1993.
6. Modell JH: Serum electrolyte changes in near-drowning victims, *JAMA* 253(4):557, 1985.
7. Modell JH, Graves SA et al: Clinical course of 91 consecutive near-drowning victims, *Chest* 70(2):231-238, 1976.
8. Conn A, Montes J, Barker G: Cerebral salvage in near-drowning following neurologic classification by triage, *Can J Anaesth* 27:201-209, 1980.
9. Norberg WJ, Agnew RF, Brunsvold R et al: Successful resuscitation of a cold water submersion victim with the use of cardiopulmonary bypass, *Crit Care Med* 20:1355-1357, 1992.
10. Moller JC, Schailble TF, Reiss I et al: Treatment of severe non-neonatal ARDS in children with surfactant and nitric oxide in a "pre-ECMO" situation, *Int J Artif Organs* 18:598-602, 1995.
11. Arensman RM, Statter MB, Bastawrous AL et al: Modern treatment modalities for neonatal and pediatric respiratory failure, *Am J Surg* 172:41-47, 1996.
12. Burkhead SR, Lally KP, Bristow F et al: Intratracheal pulmonary ventilation provides effective ventilation in a near-drowning model, *J Pediatr Surg* 31:337-341, 1996.
13. Gabrielli A, Layon AJ: Drowning and near-drowning, *J Fla Med Assoc* 84(7):452-457, 1997.
14. Quan L, Kinder D: Pediatric submersions: Prehospital predictors of outcome, *Pediatrics* 90:909-913, 1992.
15. Quan L, Wentz KR, Gore EJ et al: Outcome and predictors of outcome in pediatric submersion victims receiving prehospital care in King County, Washington, *Pediatrics* 86:586-593, 1990.

CHAPTER 66

Pulmonary Edema

Dez Hughes

Definition

Pulmonary edema is defined as an increase in extravascular lung water (i.e., fluid in the pulmonary parenchyma that is not located in the intravascular space). There are two major pathophysiological forms: high-pressure edema and increased permeability edema. High-pressure edema is caused by elevated pulmonary capillary hydrostatic pressure (usually caused by increased left atrial pressure or fluid overload) and subsequent transudative fluid loss through a largely intact pulmonary microvasculature.[1] Increased permeability edema results from damage to the microvascular barrier or alveolar epithelium and direct leakage of fluid and protein into the interstitium and alveoli.[1] Most causes of high permeability edema have an inflammatory component and are conditions associated with the acute respiratory distress syndrome (ARDS).

Pathophysiology

Understanding the pathophysiology of pulmonary edema requires knowledge of the fluid compartments of the body; of normal and abnormal water, solute, and protein fluxes in the lung; of the processes involved in edema formation; of the defenses that protect against fluid accumulation; and of the mechanisms responsible for clearance of water, solute, and protein from the pulmonary interstitium and alveolar spaces.

There are three major body fluid compartments: the intracellular space, the interstitial space, and the intravascular space. The intravascular and interstitial compartments make up the extracellular space. In part, fluid movement depends upon the permeability of the barrier between compartments and the concentration of molecules within each compartment. The cell membrane is freely permeable to water; water movement across the cell membrane occurs by osmosis, depending upon the relative intracellular and extracellular concentration of molecules. Water will move into the area with the highest concentration of molecules. In addition to water, the microvascular barrier is also freely permeable to small solutes but is relatively impermeable to macromolecules.[2] A protein concentration gradient therefore exists between the intravascular space and the interstitium. The higher concentration of impermeant macromolecules within capillaries exerts an osmotic pressure, the intravascular

colloid osmotic pressure (COP), which acts to retain fluid. Fluid exchange between the intravascular space and the interstitium depends upon the hydrostatic and osmotic pressure gradients between each compartment.[3]

$$\text{Flow} = K_{fc}[(\text{capillary hydrostatic pressure} - \text{interstitial hydrostatic pressure}) + \sigma (\text{capillary COP} - \text{interstitial COP})]$$

The filtration coefficient, K_{fc}, is a measure of how well a specific tissue allows fluid efflux, and is a product of the capillary surface area and hydraulic conductivity. A tissue with a greater microvascular surface area or higher hydraulic conductivity allows more transvascular fluid flow. The reflection coefficient, σ, is a measure of the microvascular barrier permeability to protein. When a membrane is completely impermeable, the full possible colloid osmotic gradient is exerted and the value for the reflection coefficient is 1.0.

In the lung, as in all tissues, the microvascular barrier in small arterioles, capillaries, and small venules is freely permeable to water and electrolytes, and fluid is constantly being extravasated and reabsorbed between the interstitium and blood vessels. At the arterial end of the capillary bed, a hydrostatic pressure gradient in excess of the COP gradient results in transudation of fluid into the interstitium. At the venous end, plasma proteins exert an osmotic force in excess of the hydrostatic pressure gradient, resulting in a net fluid flux into vessels. In all tissues, three mechanisms prevent excessive interstitial fluid accumulation. First, extravasation of fluid into a relatively nondistensible interstitium results in an increased interstitial pressure, thereby opposing further extravasation. Second, following extravasation of low protein fluid, the interstitial COP falls because of dilution and washout of protein, thereby maintaining the COP gradient between the intravascular space and the interstitium. Third, because the perimicrovascular interstitium is not compliant, increased interstitial fluid results in an increased driving pressure for lymphatic drainage.

These alterations in Starling forces, which act to limit interstitial fluid accumulation, have been termed the tissue safety factors.[4,5] Their relative importance varies and depends on the characteristics of the tissue.[6,7] In a distensible tissue that is relatively permeable to protein (e.g., the lungs), the protective effect of COP is less than in other tissues, and increased lymph flow appears a more important safeguard against interstitial edema.[8] This increased permeability to protein is apparent in that the normal protein concentration in lymph from skin or skeletal muscle is about 50% that of plasma, compared with 65% in pulmonary lymph.[9] Because the COP gradient is less important in protecting the lung, the lung is resistant to hypoproteinemia-induced edema formation.[6] Nevertheless, a lower intravascular COP reduces the hydrostatic pressure at which high pressure edema occurs.[10-12]

Pulmonary edema occurs when the rate of interstitial fluid formation overwhelms the protective fluid clearance mechanisms. Because pulmonary gas exchange is vital to maintain life, some specific features of the pulmonary ultrastructure act to protect gaseous diffusion. The alveolar epithelium is impermeable to all blood solutes and is freely permeable to water. This means that there is a huge transepithelial osmotic gradient (in excess of 5000 mm Hg) that prevents fluid accumulation in the alveoli. The length of the diffusion barrier is minimized because alveolar epithelial and capillary endothelial cells are extremely thin and have a fused basement membrane on the gas exchange side of the capillary (Figure 66-1). Because of this fused basement membrane and lack of interstitial tissue, normal interstitial fluid flow occurs on the opposite side of the capillary to gas exchange. The distensibility of the

pulmonary interstitium increases towards the peribronchovascular region, creating an alveolohilar hydrostatic pressure gradient along which interstitial fluid flows.[13,14] Thus excess fluid that is not cleared by the pulmonary lymphatics tends to accumulate in a location where it does not affect gas exchange.

The interstitium was previously thought to play a passive role in edema formation; however, recent evidence suggests that the interstitial matrix may be actively involved in the modulation of interstitial solute flux.[15] The complex, coiled structure of the huge, negatively charged molecules of the interstitial matrix hinders movement of water and solute, thereby contributing to the permeability characteristics of the microvascular barrier. This maze of meshed macromolecules also serves to resist expansion and collapse during conditions of edema and dehydration, respectively. In mild edematogenic states, small increases in volume result in large increases in interstitial hydrostatic pressure that limit extravasation of fluid and that increase lymphatic drainage. In most tissues, as the interstitium becomes gradually more distended it remains noncompliant until a threshold is reached and the interstitial structure abruptly breaks down. This is termed stress relaxation, and it is important because it means that at some point the interstitium will become distensible and edema can rapidly progress. In the lung, the critical point may be that at which cell separation and alveolar flooding occurs. Fluid can then accumulate in the interstitium and alveoli without a corresponding protective rise in interstitial pressure and lymph flow. During increased interstitial fluid flow, interstitial matrix components can be washed out via the lymphatic system, further reducing interstitial resistance to fluid flow. Clinically, this means that as interstitial expansion occurs with edema fluid, and especially once there is communication between the pulmonary interstitium and alveoli, extravascular pulmonary fluid accumulation can greatly increase.

It cannot be overemphasized that hydrostatic pressure is the main determinant of pulmonary fluid extravasation in normal lungs and in both types of pulmonary edema.[1] Hydrostatic pressure modification (e.g., with fluid restriction, diuretics, or vasodilators) is therefore a rational therapy for both increased permeability and high-pressure edema. In severe permeability edema, in which protein can freely cross into the interstitium, hydrostatic pressure reduction may be the only means by which to reduce fluid extravasation.

HIGH PRESSURE EDEMA

As pulmonary capillary pressures increase (usually because of left-sided heart failure or fluid overload), fluid extravasation increases and ultimately overwhelms the lymphatic removal capacity. Fluid then begins to accumulate in the interstitium and flows towards the peribronchovascular interstitium.[13,14] Eventually, edema fluid will distend all parts of the pulmonary interstitium and fluid begins to fill the alveolar space.[16] It appears that, because the alveolar membrane is so impermeable to solutes, alveolar filling does not occur by fluid flow

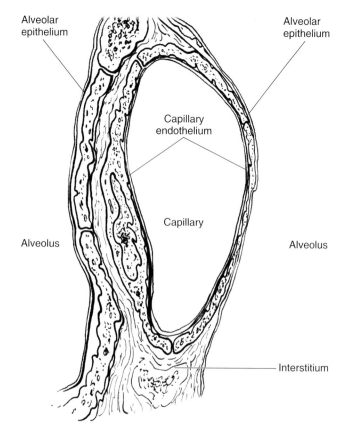

Figure 66-1. *Schematic diagram of the pulmonary ultrastructure. Note the fused basement membranes and lack of interstitial space on the alveolar side of the capillary.*

Alveolar epithelium

Alveolar epithelium

Capillary endothelium

Capillary

Alveolus

Alveolus

Interstitium

through the epithelium; rather, it spills into the airspaces at the junction of the alveolar and airway epithelia.[17] Blood vessel rupture can also occur with hydrostatic edema, as evidenced by the serosanguineous nature of edema fluid seen in some cases of cardiogenic pulmonary edema. Because many forms of left heart failure develop gradually, rises in hydrostatic pressure often occur over a relatively long period, and overt edema can take months to develop depending on the underlying cardiac disease. In contrast, acute increases in hydrostatic pressure (e.g., as occur with chordae tendineae rupture or fluid therapy) can result in a more rapid deterioration. Cardiogenic pulmonary edema occurs at lower hydrostatic pressures when hypoproteinemia is present.[10,11]

INCREASED PERMEABILITY EDEMA

Microvascular barrier injury, either by direct chemical injury or by inflammatory cells and mediators, increases the permeability of the pulmonary microvasculature to protein, which increases fluid extravasation and significantly diminishes the protective effect of colloid osmotic pressure. In addition, the protective fall in interstitial COP (to maintain the intravascular to interstitial COP gradient) that occurs following fluid transudation through an intact barrier is reduced. Consequently, capillary hydrostatic pressure becomes a major determinant of edema formation.[1] Interstitial fluid accumulation can then occur at normal or even low pulmonary hydrostatic pressures, and relatively small rises in capillary hydrostatic pressure result in much greater edema formation. If the alveolar epithelial cells are also damaged, a direct conduit may develop between the intravascular space and the alveoli, and interstitial edema rapidly progresses to alveolar flooding. This explains the greater clinical severity and fulminant course seen in many forms of increased permeability edema compared with hydrostatic edema.

RESOLUTION OF PULMONARY EDEMA

Alveolar fluid clearance occurs by reabsorption into the pulmonary interstitium, followed by clearance into the lymphatics, bronchial vasculature, and pleural space.[18,19] Interestingly, whereas lymphatic drainage is one of the most important mechanisms limiting interstitial fluid accumulation, it is less important in edema resolution.[20] In high-pressure edema, most interstitial edema fluid is cleared via the bronchial circulation[21]; this is probably because of the peribronchovascular pooling of edema fluid. Drainage into, then from the pleural space occurs in both high-pressure and increased permeability edema. Pleural effusion formation and drainage has been demonstrated in animals with increased left atrial pressure,[22] intravascular volume loading,[19] and experimental models of increased permeability edema.[18,23] In fact, pleural effusion formation may be a manifestation of left- and not right-sided congestive heart failure in people and small animals, especially cats,[25] probably because visceral pleural veins drain into the pulmonary veins and, therefore, the left side of the heart.

Absorption of water, solutes, and protein from the alveoli occurs by different mechanisms and at very different rates. Water is reabsorbed rapidly, and protein removal is much slower. Water reabsorption occurs via aquaporins in the cell membrane of type I pneumocytes.[26] Indeed, the osmotic water permeability of type I cells is the highest measured for any mammalian cell membrane.[26] When the alveolar epithelium is intact, alveolar free water (e.g., in fresh water drowning) can be absorbed from the alveoli over the course of minutes. In contrast, reabsorption of sodium-containing alveolar fluid takes a period of hours. It occurs mainly via cyclic AMP-mediated active sodium transport with glucose cotransport through apical sodium channels by type II pneumocytes.[27,28] Fluid absorption occurs against a colloid osmotic gradient, which increases as fluid is reabsorbed and protein remains behind. A rising protein concentration in edema fluid obtained via an endotracheal catheter is a positive prognostic indicator in people with hydrostatic and increased permeability edema.[29]

The mechanism of macromolecule clearance is less well understood, but it occurs at a very slow rate over a period of days.[31,32] Slow macromolecule clearance, the presence of inflammatory cells, and alveolar epithelial and capillary endothelial cell damage or death likely explain the protracted resolution or progression to ARDS often seen with increased permeability edema. Alveolar fluid clearance is slower in humans with ARDS compared with high pressure edema, and impaired alveolar fluid clearance is associated with a higher mortality and longer duration of mechanical ventilation in ARDS patients.[32,33]

PULMONARY EDEMA EFFECTS ON LUNG FUNCTION

There are several deleterious consequences of pulmonary edema in addition to the most serious consequence, which obviously is reduced arterial oxygenation. Edema results in increased airway resistance because of a vagally mediated reflex, airway edema, and vascular engorgement.[34,35] Lung compliance is reduced[34] in affected areas, which reduces total lung volume and causes overdistension of nonedematous regions in artificially ventilated patients, resulting in the potential for barotrauma and volutrauma.

Epidemiology

HIGH-PRESSURE EDEMA

High-pressure edema is usually caused by left-sided heart failure or fluid overload. A relatively small number of common cardiac conditions result in heart failure (e.g., mitral valve disease or dilated cardiomyopathy in dogs; and hypertrophic, thyrotoxic, or restrictive cardiomyopathy or endomyocarditis in cats). Fluid overload has been underemphasized in the veterinary literature, probably because most animals without serious cardiopulmonary disease can tolerate aggressive intravenous fluid rates.[36] Whereas fluid therapy can be tolerated in some animals with pulmonary disease, it can be detrimental in others. Worsening of lung disease caused by pulmonary edema is obviously life threatening, especially if facilities for positive pressure ventilation are not available.

INCREASED PERMEABILITY EDEMA

There are many possible underlying causes of increased permeability edema (Box 66-1). Animals that develop the systemic inflammatory response syndrome (SIRS) or diseases associated with systemic vasculitis or vascular leak are at risk for developing increased permeability pulmonary edema. ARDS is the most refractory and challenging form of increased permeability pulmonary edema. Many conditions categorized as increased permeability and uncertain or mixed etiology edemas can be antecedents of ARDS. As such, ARDS is the end result of an underlying disease process rather than a definitive diagnosis. For example, animals with bacterial, fungal, or protozoal pneumonia can be expected to have some degree of associated pulmonary edema because of parenchymal inflammation. Bacterial pneumonia and other causes of bacterial sepsis are the most common cause of ARDS in dogs.[37] Because ARDS carries such a poor prognosis, the underlying cause should be vigorously pursued and aggressively treated. Only two necropsy-based case series documenting ARDS in dogs have been published[37,38]; therefore, survival rates cannot be determined from the literature. Clinical experience suggests that they are very low.

Toxic lung injury can result from exposure to smoke,[39,40] volatile hydrocarbons, Teflon vapor, paraquat, cis-platinum (cats), and envenomation. Following smoke exposure, cats seem to be less severely affected and have a less complicated clinical course than dogs.[39,40]

Reexpansion edema is a poorly understood phenomenon reported in dogs and cats after acute reexpansion of chronically collapsed lung lobes.[41-43] Suggested mechanisms include decreased surfactant concentration, negative interstitial pressures, and oxygen free radical formation.

In humans, oxygen toxicity has been associated with absorption atelectasis, tracheobronchitis, increased permeability pulmonary edema, and bronchopulmonary dysplasia.[44] Experimental studies in animals have documented marked endothelial cell death, increased permeability edema, reduced airway mucus clearance, and ARDS following prolonged exposure to high inspired oxygen concentrations.[44-46]

Blood transfusion has been associated with increased permeability edema in both humans and dogs.[47,48] Transfusion-related acute lung injury carries a mortality rate of 5% to 14% in people, making it the third leading cause of transfusion-related mortality. The vast majority of cases are caused by HLA (Class I or II) or granulocyte-specific complement activating antibodies.[48]

The clinical relevance of ventilator-induced lung injury has recently been confirmed by the Acute Respiratory Distress Syndrome Network trial. There was a 22% reduction in mortality in ARDS patients with the use of reduced tidal volumes during mechanical ventilation.[49] Experimental observations suggest that excessive tidal volume and/or end-inspiratory lung volume is the main determinant of ventilator-induced lung injury.[49,50] Also implicated in the pathogenesis are inflammatory cells and mediators that may be activated and released either into the alveolar space or systemic circulation following rupture of the alveolar-capillary barrier.[50]

Neurogenic edema is an incompletely understood condition that appears to be caused by increased hydrostatic pressure and increased microvascular permeability.[51,52] The condition is common in dogs but rare in cats, and is usually caused by head trauma or seizures, increased intracranial pressure, upper airway obstruction, or biting an electric cord.[53-55] Most affected dogs are under 1 year of age. In young dogs, the nature of the head trauma or upper airway obstruction can sometimes be trivial (e.g., a slap on the muzzle or a pull on a leash). Older dogs usually have a more serious underlying cause (e.g., seizures or laryngeal paralysis). Signs of dyspnea occur immediately following the incident. The prognosis for full recovery is usually good in young dogs and depends upon the underlying cause in older animals.[53]

Feline endomyocarditis is an intriguing and frustrating condition of as yet undetermined etiology; it is often seen following a stressful episode such as a veterinary visit.[56] Many affected cats are young and present with acute onset of severe dyspnea. Endocardial inflammation and interstitial pneumonia are present in the majority of cases. Clinical experience suggests that the prognosis is poor; however, this is difficult to interpret given the extreme difficulty of establishing a definitive diagnosis before death.

BOX 66-1
Causes of Pulmonary Edema in Dogs and Cats

Increased Permeability Edema

Infectious pneumonia
Pulmonary contusions/
  hemorrhage
SIRS
  Sepsis
  Pancreatitis
  Metastatic neoplasia
  Severe tissue trauma
  Immune mediated
    disease
  Systemic vasculitis
ARDS
Pulmonary
  thromboembolism
Toxic lung injury
Smoke inhalation

Oxygen toxicity
Ventilator-induced lung
  injury
Blood transfusion

High-Pressure Edema

Left-sided heart failure
Fluid overload

Uncertain or Mixed Etiology

Neurogenic edema
Reexpansion edema
High-altitude edema
Feline endomyocarditis

Other

Near drowning

SIRS, Systemic inflammatory response syndrome; *ARDS*, acute respiratory distress syndrome.

Historical Findings and Clinical Signs

Occasionally there are obvious historical indicators of the underlying cause of pulmonary edema (e.g., smoke inhalation, pulmonary contusions, reexpansion pulmonary edema, or previously diagnosed cases of congestive heart disease). In many cases, however, there are more subtle historical findings. Vomiting or regurgitation should raise suspicion of aspiration pneumonia. An older large-breed dog with changes in bark and exercise intolerance may have laryngeal paralysis and concurrent aspiration pneumonia or neurogenic edema. Upper airway obstruction, seizures, head trauma, and electric shock account for almost all cases of neurogenic pulmonary edema. Any potential for anticoagulant rodenticide exposure should prompt coagulation testing because pulmonary and intrapleural hemorrhage is common in animals with anticoagulant rodenticide toxicity.[57,58] Pancreatitis in dogs is usually associated with profuse vomiting, and affected animals may have had a recent diet change or a high-fat meal, or other risk factors such as hyperadrenocorticism, diabetes mellitus, hypothyroidism or epilepsy.[59] A recent stressful episode such as a veterinary visit or travel is noted in many cats with endomyocarditis.[56]

The vast majority of patients with pulmonary edema have moderate to severe tachypnea and dyspnea, the severity of which can sometimes be inversely proportional to the chronicity of disease. For example, some dogs with slowly progressive mitral valve disease can tolerate quite severe edema. Paradoxically, some animals with very severe pulmonary edema may seem to become less dyspneic, potentially because of decreased lung compliance or respiratory muscle fatigue. Animals with neurological disease, sedation, severe hypoperfusion, or respiratory muscle paralysis may not show appropriate signs of respiratory distress relative to the severity of pulmonary alveolar disease.

To assess the severity of dyspnea, one should look for postural manifestations such as an extended neck, abducted elbows, open mouth breathing, an anxious facial expression, and increased or paradoxical abdominal wall movement. Straightening of the neck and open mouth breathing occur in both dogs and cats. Other postural manifestations of more severe dyspnea can vary between species: dogs prefer to stand with abducted elbows, whereas cats tend to sit in sternal recumbency. Constantly changing body position in cats implies a much more severe degree of dyspnea than it does in dogs. Lateral recumbency because of dyspnea is a serious sign in a dog; however, it often means impending respiratory arrest in a cat, especially when combined with marked mydriasis (Figure 66-2).

Most animals with pulmonary edema have harsh lung sounds on auscultation, but crackles may or may not be present. With careful auscultation, the abnormal lung sounds can be localized in some cases (e.g., cranioventral harsh lung sounds or crackles in dogs with aspiration pneumonia, compared with a dorsocaudal distribu-

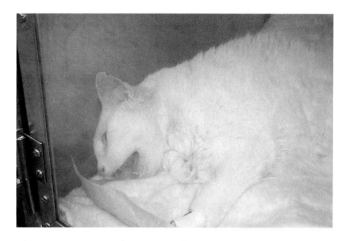

Figure 66-2. Cat with open mouth breathing and impending respiratory arrest. (Courtesy of Dr. Lesley King, University of Pennsylvania, Philadelphia, PA.)

tion in an animal with neurogenic edema). Dogs with cardiogenic edema may have a perihilar distribution of abnormal lung sounds. The majority of dogs in congestive heart failure will also have a systolic heart murmur, a notable exception being some dogs with very low cardiac output cardiomyopathy. Acute and severe decompensation in a dog with relatively stable mitral insufficiency can occur following chordae tendineae rupture. Cats with heart disease usually have harsh lung sounds or crackles and a systolic murmur or gallop rhythm. A concurrent pleural effusion may result in quiet or absent lung sounds in the ventral fields. Palpation of a thyroid nodule in an older cat raises the possibility of hyperthyroidism and thyrotoxic cardiomyopathy.

Initial Management, Monitoring, and Diagnostic Tests

Dogs and cats with pulmonary edema usually present for respiratory distress or become dyspneic during hospitalization. The goals for initial management of patients with respiratory distress are to quantify the severity of the disease process and to stabilize the patient, then to identify the underlying cause. The clinician must remain acutely aware of the fragility of the dyspneic patient. Even a brief physical examination can prove fatal, especially in cats. Consequently, the risks of any manipulation must be cautiously balanced against the potential benefits. If a patient suffers a respiratory arrest, the chance of a successful outcome is greatly reduced. When presented as an emergency, most animals with pulmonary edema will benefit from a short period breathing 100% oxygen before diagnostic testing.

If an animal with suspected pulmonary edema is in severe respiratory distress, empirical therapy may be necessary before diagnostic testing. For example, in the case of a dyspneic cat with diffuse pulmonary crackles and a heart murmur, empirical treatment with furosemide may

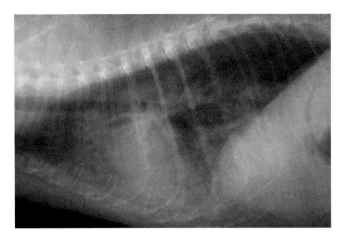

Figure 66-3. Lateral thoracic radiograph of a cat with cardiogenic pulmonary edema. Note the diffuse alveolar/interstitial pattern.

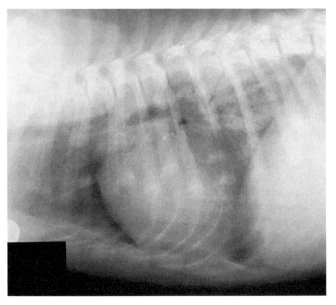

Figure 66-4. Lateral thoracic radiograph of a 5-month-old mixed breed puppy with noncardiogenic pulmonary edema that developed after a transient airway obstruction. Note the classical dorsocaudal distribution of the alveolar pattern. The poor patient positioning and rotation of the radiograph is evidence of severe respiratory distress. This puppy required oxygen supplementation for 24 hours but recovered fully and was discharged from the hospital.

stabilize the cat enough to allow chest radiographs to be safely obtained.

The severity of pulmonary edema is determined primarily by physical examination and by observing the response to oxygen therapy, aided by pulse oximetry or arterial blood gas evaluation. Arterial blood sampling may be too stressful in severe cases, however, and the results may not actually change case management. Hence astute clinical judgment is necessary on an individual case basis.

In a critical patient that presents with dyspnea, more than one cause is not uncommon. The location of the disease in the respiratory tract should be determined as soon as possible. A thorough physical examination should detect most instances of upper airway obstruction, abnormalities of the chest wall and diaphragm, and pleural space disease. If ultrasound is available, confirmation of pleural effusion is simple and almost stress-free. Usually, small airway disease represents feline asthma. Hence localization to the pulmonary parenchyma can be relatively easy in many cases.

Thoracic radiographs are the most clinically useful diagnostic test because they provide information about the whole chest cavity. Unfortunately, they are also potentially the most stressful part of the initial diagnostic evaluation. Whereas dyspneic dogs may tolerate a quick lateral radiograph (often the most useful view), a dorsoventral view with minimal restraint is usually the least stressful in cats. When taking radiographs of dyspneic patients, the equipment should be fully set up before beginning the procedure, and oxygen supplementation should always be available. Short periods without oxygen can be life threatening, especially if the animal struggles during restraint.

Thoracic radiographs usually provide good evidence to distinguish cardiogenic and noncardiogenic components of pulmonary edema on the basis of the lung pattern and the presence or absence of cardiomegaly. Thoracic radiographs are probably most useful in animals with a heart murmur, to determine whether heart disease is likely to be an important factor. In the absence of cardiomegaly, a cardiogenic etiology of pulmonary edema becomes less likely, because with the exception of peracute processes such as chordae tendineae rupture, cardiac enlargement must occur before left atrial pressure can rise. An alveolar pattern, more severe in the perihilar region, is often seen in dogs with cardiogenic edema. Cats with cardiogenic edema occasionally have a perihilar alveolar pattern but usually have diffuse patchy alveolar and interstitial infiltrates (Figure 66-3).

Distended pulmonary veins relative to the corresponding pulmonary artery can be supportive of increased pulmonary venous pressures. A cranioventral alveolar pattern is most compatible with aspiration pneumonia, whereas a dorsocaudal alveolar or interstitial pattern suggests neurogenic pulmonary edema (Figure 66-4). All animals do not have a classic radiographic appearance, and almost all causes of pulmonary edema can cause a diffuse pattern.

A skilled echocardiographer can quickly obtain useful information as to whether there is a cardiac component to pulmonary parenchymal disease. Most dogs with congestive heart failure have mitral valve disease or dilated cardiomyopathy, and cats usually have hypertrophic, restrictive, or intermediate cardiomyopathy or endomyocarditis. The latter is challenging to diagnose in a live animal, but a hyperechoic endocardium is thought to be compatible with the diagnosis. Failure to document left atrial dilation should, in most cases, raise significant doubt that cardiogenic pulmonary edema is occurring. Difficulty positioning a dyspneic animal can limit the echocardiographic interpretation of chamber sizes or wall thickness, however.

Whereas thoracic radiographs provide anatomical information, blood gas analysis and pulse oximetry provide physiological documentation of the severity of the lung disease. Assessment of the severity of dyspnea on physical examination is very useful in documenting changes in pulmonary edema; therefore these tests of lung function are not absolutely essential if they pose a serious risk to the patient. Obtaining a metatarsal arterial blood sample is less stressful than using the femoral artery. Arterial blood gas analysis allows calculation of the alveolar-arterial oxygen tension difference (A–a gradient), which corrects oxygenation for changes in ventilation. The majority of patients with pulmonary edema have an increased A–a gradient, and a diagnosis of serious pulmonary edema is unlikely without an increased A–a gradient. Pulse oximetry is useful providing a meaningful waveform is obtained and the measured heart rate matches that of the animal. An accurate reading may be difficult in cats and also in patients with poor peripheral perfusion, fast heart rates, pigmented skin, or those that are moving.

Arterial blood pressure measurement is of limited diagnostic use; however, because many causes of pulmonary edema can be associated with hypovolemic, cardiogenic, or septic shock, it should be monitored. A metatarsal arterial catheter can be placed percutaneously or by surgical cut down under local anesthesia.[60] Central venous pressure (CVP) measurement can be very helpful in managing patients with pulmonary edema, especially in patients with cardiac dysfunction or oliguria. In the absence of fluid overload, an elevated CVP occurs with right-sided heart failure, pericardial effusion, and right-sided cardiac outflow obstruction. A flow-guided pulmonary arterial catheter can be used to measure pulmonary capillary wedge pressure (an indicator of left atrial pressure), and thermistor-tipped catheters can be used to determine cardiac output. In addition, systemic vascular resistance and oxygen transport and consumption variables can then be calculated, allowing intense scrutiny of cardiopulmonary status. With a special lung water computer, these catheters can also be used to calculate extravascular lung water (EVLW), the fluid content of the lungs excluding fluid within blood vessels. They also have the potential to detect fluid accumulation in the lungs before oxygenation defects.

Many experimental techniques are used to quantitate EVLW, ranging from postmortem wet weight measurement to positron emission tomography. However, the only potentially clinically applicable method is the double indicator dilution technique.[61] Simultaneous boluses of a nondiffusible indicator and a diffusible indicator are injected into the cranial vena cava or right heart. The nondiffusible indicator remains in the intravascular space, and the diffusible indicator equilibrates with the intravascular and extravascular spaces. Indicator concentrations are then determined beyond the left heart. Analysis of the dilution curve of the nondiffusible indicator allows estimation of the pulmonary blood volume. The dilution curve from the diffusible indicator yields the intravascular and extravascular volume. Subtraction of the volume of distribution for the nondiffusible indicator from that of the diffusible indicator allows estimation of extravascular lung water. Clinically applicable techniques use indocyanine green as the nondiffusible indicator and either heat[62] or heavy water[63] as the diffusible indicator. A major disadvantage of the thermodilution technique is that it requires blood sampling from the aorta for accurate measurements. Indocyanine green and heavy water can be analyzed via a central venous line and a peripheral arterial catheter. Double indicator dilution quantitation of EVLW, regardless of the indicators used, has several limitations. Most importantly, results can be seriously affected by poor technique. A nonuniform distribution of lung disease, especially if there are underperfused areas of the pulmonary parenchyma, may render EVLW estimates inaccurate. Another major problem with both techniques is that large blood samples (about 45 ml) are required for generation of the indicator dilution curves.

Using these techniques, an increase in EVLW of 15% to 30% can be detected, and results must differ by more than 15% to 20% to indicate a definite change. Increases of EVLW of 50% to 75% are necessary before alveolar flooding occurs, and gas exchange is not affected until EVLW approximately doubles. Therefore the potential exists to detect subclinical pulmonary edema by EVLW quantitation. Normal EVLW is 6 to 7 ml/kg; it increases to 25 to 35 ml/kg (a 400% to 500% increase) in patients with very severe pulmonary edema. In a study of 101 human patients with pulmonary edema, one group received fluid therapy guided by EVLW measurements, while the other was managed using wedge pressure measurements.[64] The EVLW group had a shorter time on mechanical ventilation (9 compared to 22 days), shorter ICU stays (7 compared to 16 days), and a lower ICU mortality (35% compared to 47%), although because of the small numbers the study failed to achieve statistical significance.[64] There is also evidence that EVLW may be superior to pulmonary capillary wedge pressure in guiding treatment in people with normal wedge pressures and high EVLW because of sepsis or ARDS.[65]

When infectious pneumonia or neoplasia is suspected, specimens should be obtained for cytology and microbiological analysis via transtracheal lavage, endotracheal lavage, or bronchoalveolar lavage. A negative result does not rule out the presence of either disease. The results of bacterial cultures should be weighed against clinical findings, and the likelihood of contamination should be considered. In humans, the protein concentration in edema fluid obtained using a suction catheter has been used to differentiate high-pressure from increased permeability edema.[29,66] In one clinical study in small animals, the average edema fluid protein concentration was lower in those with high-pressure pulmonary edema than in those with increased permeability edema, but the amount of overlap between groups limited diagnostic utility in individual cases.[67] A rising protein concentration in edema fluid obtained via an endotracheal catheter is a positive prognostic indicator in people with hydrostatic and increased permeability edema.[29]

Other ancillary tests to consider in a patient with pulmonary edema depend upon the potential disease processes present. Pulmonary thromboembolism is notoriously difficult to confirm in vivo, and pulmonary angiography, computerized tomographic digital subtraction angiography, or ventilation perfusion scanning may be required. Coagulation testing is often indicated in patients with permeability edema because of the likelihood of disseminated intravascular coagulation associated with many of the underlying disease processes. Abdominal ultrasound can detect conditions such as pancreatitis, intraabdominal neoplasia, or potential septic foci. Blood cultures and fungal, protozoal, or rickettsial titers may be indicated in certain cases. Lastly, in extremely challenging cases, lung biopsy may be necessary to establish a definitive diagnosis.

Treatment

Treatment of pulmonary edema depends upon the underlying cause. In all cases, oxygen must be supplied to ensure adequate tissue oxygenation (i.e., an arterial hemoglobin saturation in excess of 90%, which approximates an arterial partial pressure of oxygen [PaO_2] of 60 mm Hg). When the PaO_2 falls below 60 mm Hg there is a rapid decline in hemoglobin saturation (which is the main determinant of arterial oxygen content) and tissue hypoxia becomes more likely. When the PaO_2 is around 60 mm Hg, any increase in nonessential tissue oxygen consumption can be life threatening. Hypoxemic animals limit their movement and therefore have sufficient tissue oxygen delivery to support major organ systems. However, increased skeletal muscle activity because of agitation or restraint greatly increases skeletal muscle oxygen demand, which can be sufficient to precipitate cardiopulmonary arrest. It is therefore vital to restrict activity and minimize stress in patients with pulmonary edema, especially those with concurrent heart disease. The simplest means to achieve this is to place the animal on cage rest in an oxygen-enriched environment. Opiates such as morphine have been advocated to calm distressed patients; this drug is also a mild venodilator and may therefore actively help in the treatment of pulmonary edema.[68]

Nasal cannulation can be used to provide oxygen supplementation in animals with moderate hypoxemia that will tolerate nasal cannulae or prongs, but placement can be stressful. When placing a nasal cannula after instillation of local anesthetic, full desensitization can take up to 10 minutes. The inspired oxygen concentration achieved using nasal administration depends on the oxygen flow rate relative to the animal's tidal volume, the dead space ventilation, and whether the animal is breathing through its mouth or nose. In a sedated animal breathing solely through its nose, inspired oxygen concentrations can be in excess of 60%.

Positive pressure ventilation (PPV) may be necessary if arterial oxygen saturation cannot be maintained above 90% with noninvasive methods of oxygen supplementation, or in animals with severe hypoventilation or impending respiratory muscle fatigue. Although PPV may be required to sustain oxygenation and ventilation and keep the patient alive, the literature regarding the use of PPV and positive end expiratory pressure (PEEP) to modify the formation and resolution of pulmonary edema is complex. Many factors are involved including the type, duration, and severity of edema; the tidal volume and airway pressures delivered; the mode of ventilation; the timing and amount of PEEP; the effects on cardiac output; and other coexisting disease processes. Thus the scientific evidence is apparently contradictory. With permeability edema, one study showed that PEEP and low tidal volumes reduced EVLW,[69] but other studies documented that increased lung volume and decreased ventilation/perfusion mismatch resulted in improvement in gas exchange but no change in EVLW.[70,71] With high pressure edema, PEEP has been shown to improve oxygenation but may slow edema clearance.[72]

Body position can significantly affect arterial oxygen concentration, and there is a growing body of compelling evidence that prone positioning (sternal recumbency) significantly improves PaO_2 in early ARDS and high-pressure edema; however, it appears to be ineffective in the later fibrotic stages of ARDS.[73-75] In people with acute respiratory failure, repositioning from the supine to the prone position was associated with a mean increase in PaO_2 of 69 mm Hg, which was sufficient to avoid the need for artificial ventilation or to allow a decrease in inspired oxygen concentration and PEEP in ventilated patients.[73] In a pig model of experimentally induced increased permeability edema, the prone position greatly increased oxygenation (mean PaO_2 = 140 ± 112 mm Hg compared with 453 ± 54 mm Hg) and improved the ventilation/perfusion ratio, ventilation/perfusion heterogeneity, and the gravitational ventilation/perfusion gradient.[76] Prone positioning may also improve oxygenation by reducing compression of the dorsal lungs by the heart.[77] Positioning the animal in sternal recumbency is therefore a simple and effective way to improve oxygenation. The differences in oxygenation achieved with changes in body position also mean that extreme caution should be exercised when moving animals out of sternal recumbency. In cases with lateralizing alveolar disease, restraining the animal with the diseased side up can precipitate life-threatening hypoxemia.

Diuretics (usually, furosemide), used to attempt to decrease pulmonary capillary hydrostatic pressure, are an accepted mainstay of treatment in high-pressure edema. In view of the fact that hydrostatic pressure is an important force causing fluid extravasation, diuretic administration is also a logical treatment for increased permeability edema. Furosemide usually increases COP,[78] and it may not reduce plasma volume as much as previously suggested.[79] Furosemide has been shown to decrease lung liquid and shunt fraction in experimental permeability edema in dogs, in the absence of changes in wedge pressure and COP, and even in nephrectomized dogs.[80] It also has beneficial vasoactive effects, and it may increase perfusion to ventilated regions of the lung.[81] Furosemide administration is associated with a large decrease in pulmonary venous resistance, decreased hydrostatic pressure, and decreased transvascular fluid filtration by a nondiuretic mechanism.[82] It appears to cause selective venodilation, especially in the pulmonary veins, by an effect on $Na^+/K^+/Cl^-$ cotransport or chloride-mediated refilling of intracellular calcium stores.[83] Local formation of prostacyclin by vascular tissue has been suggested to mediate its vascular activity.[84] Furosemide reduces lung water accumulation and shunt fraction in dogs with increased permeability edema;[85] however, its effect may be less effective once pulmonary injury is well established.[86]

Some studies have suggested that a constant rate diuretic infusion is more effective in producing diuresis than is bolus administration,[87-89] also resulting in decreased fluctuation in urine output and reduced fluid replacement requirements.[90] Other authors imply that there is no difference with respect to route of administration.[91,92] Importantly, the diuresis induced by bolus administration is more rapid than that achieved by constant rate infusion.[93] Thus intravenous boluses remain the administration route of choice in acute, life-threatening situations.

Vasodilators such as nitroglycerine or nitroprusside are also employed as a means of reducing preload and pulmonary capillary hydrostatic pressure. Nitroglycerin is primarily a venodilator with minimal effects on arterial blood pressure at recommended doses and is usually safe. However, some authorities have questioned its efficacy. Nitroglycerin is available as a transcutaneous paste and is used somewhat empirically at $\frac{1}{4}$ to 2 inches per dog (1 inch contains 15 mg of nitroglycerin). Nitroprusside is a potent arterio- and venodilator that, because of its short half-life, must be given by constant rate infusion. Because its potent arterial dilatory effects can cause severe arterial hypotension, it should only be used with constant monitoring of the electrocardiogram and arterial blood pressure. Used carefully, an arterial dilator may reduce afterload and thereby increase cardiac output without significantly decreasing arterial blood pressure. This effect can be beneficial in dogs with mitral regurgitation and dilated cardiomyopathy. In dogs with decreased myocardial performance, concurrent beta agonism (e.g., with dobutamine) may be necessary. The benefits of vasodilator therapy over furosemide therapy have recently been demonstrated in human clinical trials.[94,95] Intravenous isosorbide dinitrate was a safe and effective treatment for unstable angina and congestive heart failure.[94,95] High-dose intravenous isosorbide dinitrate and low-dose furosemide had significant benefits over a low-dose isosorbide dinitrate, high-dose furosemide protocol.[95] The first regimen resulted in significantly fewer patients requiring artificial ventilation, and a lower incidence of myocardial infarction.

Several interesting new experimental treatments for pulmonary edema may warrant further investigation. Phosphodiesterase inhibitors and beta-2 agonists such as terbutaline and dobutamine facilitate reabsorption of fluid from the alveolar space.[96-98] Nebulized salmeterol can accelerate alveolar liquid clearance, decrease excess lung water, and improve arterial blood gases in experimental models of hydrostatic pulmonary edema.[99] Salmeterol also appears to reduce the risk of high-altitude pulmonary edema.[100] There have also been recent advances exploring the role of growth factors in the lung. The epithelial-specific growth factors are important in lung develop-

ment, inflammation, and repair.[101] Transforming growth factor alpha stimulates in vivo alveolar liquid clearance at a rate similar to beta-adrenergic stimulation by increasing Na^+ uptake by alveolar type II pneumocytes.[102] Vascular endothelial growth factor may play a role in increased permeability edema by increasing microvascular permeability.[103,104] The relevance of these findings in clinical patients remains undetermined, but they raise the possibility of novel treatment modalities (e.g., gene therapy) for pulmonary edema.

Outcome and Prognosis

The prognosis for patients with pulmonary edema obviously depends upon the underlying condition. For hydrostatic edema caused by fluid overload, the prognosis in animals without serious underlying disease is excellent. In contrast, in an old cat with renal insufficiency and thyrotoxic cardiomyopathy, a crystalloid fluid rate of 40 ml/hr could prove fatal. Arguably, the worst mistake in patients with fluid overload is failing to make the diagnosis and assuming that dyspnea is caused by more sinister causes that may lead to euthanasia. The prognosis in patients with cardiogenic edema depends on the severity of underlying cardiac disease. Dogs with mitral insufficiency may live for years, whereas some Doberman pinschers with severe dilated cardiomyopathy fail to survive to hospital discharge. Managing patients with permeability edema can be very challenging. Outcome is likely to be poor in severe cases; however, treatment of mild to moderate disease is often successful. The outcome in animals that require positive pressure ventilation is often poor, and even when advanced intensive care is provided, survival is only around 20%.[105]

REFERENCES

1. Demling RH, LaLonde C, Ikegami K: Pulmonary edema: Pathophysiology, methods of measurement, and clinical importance in acute respiratory failure, *New Horiz* 1:371, 1993.
2. Rippe B, Haraldsson B: Transport of macromolecules across microvascular walls: The two pore theory, *Physiol Rev* 74:163, 1994.
3. Starling EH: On the absorption of fluid from the connective tissue spaces, *J Physiol (Lond)* 19:312, 1896.
4. Guyton AC, Granger HJ, Taylor AE: Interstitial fluid pressure, *Physiol Rev* 51:527-563, 1971.
5. Taylor AE: The lymphatic edema safety factor: The role of edema dependent lymphatic factors (EDLF), *Lymphology* 23:111-123, 1990.
6. Zarins CK, Rice CL, Peters RM et al: Lymph and pulmonary response to isobaric reduction in plasma oncotic pressure in baboons, *Circ Res* 43:925, 1978.
7. Chen HI, Granger HJ, Taylor AE: Interaction of capillary, interstitial, and lymphatic forces in the canine hindpaw, *Circ Res* 39:245-254, 1976.
8. Zarins CK, Rice CL, Smith DE et al: Role of lymphatics in preventing hypooncotic pulmonary edema, *Surg Forum* 27:257-259, 1976.
9. Parker JC, Perry MA, Taylor AE: Permeability of the microvascular barrier. In Staub NC, Taylor AE, editors: *Edema*, New York, 1984, Raven Press.
10. Guyton AC, Lindsay NW: Effect of elevated left atrial pressure and decreased plasma protein concentration on the development of pulmonary edema, *Circ Res* 7:649-657, 1959.

11. Gaar KAJ, Taylor AE, Owens LJ et al: Effect of capillary pressure and plasma protein on development of pulmonary edema, *Am J Physiol* 213:79-82, 1967.

12. Kramer GC, Harms BA, Bodai BI et al: Effects of hypoproteinemia and increased vascular pressure on lung fluid balance in sheep, *J Appl Physiol: Respir Envir Exercise Physiol* 55:1514-1522, 1983.

13. Conhaim RL, Lai-Fook SJ, Staub NC: Sequence of perivascular liquid accumulation in liquid-inflated dog lung lobes, *J Appl Physiol* 60:513, 1986.

14. Bhattacharya J, Gropper MA, Staub, NC: Interstitial fluid pressure gradient measured by micropuncture in excised dog lung, *J Appl Physiol: Respir Envir Exercise Physiol* 56:271, 1984.

15. Aukland K, Reed RK: Interstitial-lymphatic mechanisms in the control of extracellular fluid volume, *Physiol Rev* 73:1, 1993.

16. Staub NC: Alveolar flooding and clearance, *Am Rev Respir Dis* 127:S44-S51, 1983.

17. Conhaim RL: Airway level at which edema liquid enters the air space of isolated dog lungs, *J Appl Physiol* 67(6):2234, 1989.

18. Blomqvist H, Berg B, Frostell C et al: Net fluid leakage (LN) in experimental pulmonary oedema in the dog, *Acta Anaesthesiologica Scandinavica* 34(5):377, 1990.

19. Broaddus VC, Wiener-Kronish JP, Staub NC: Clearance of lung edema into the pleural space of volume-loaded anesthetized sheep, *J Appl Physiol* 68(6):2623, 1990.

20. Mackersie RC, Christensen J, Lewis FR: The role of pulmonary lymphatics in the clearance of hydrostatic pulmonary edema, *J Surg Res* 43:495, 1987.

21. Fukue M, Serikov VB, Jerome EH: Bronchial vascular reabsorption of low-protein interstitial edema liquid in perfused sheep lungs, *J Appl Physiol* 81:810, 1996.

22. Allen S, Gabel J, Drake R: Left atrial hypertension causes pleural effusion formation in unanesthetized sheep, *Am J Physiol* 257 (2 Pt 2):H690-H692, 1989.

23. Wiener-Kronish JP, Matthay MA: Pleural effusions associated with hydrostatic and increased permeability pulmonary edema, *Chest* 93(4):852, 1988.

24. Wiener-Kronish JP, Matthay MA, Callen PW et al: Relationship of pleural effusions to pulmonary hemodynamics in patients with congestive heart failure, *Am Rev Respir Dis* 132(6):1253, 1985;.

25. Kittleson MD: Pathophysiology of heart failure. In Kittleson MD, Kienle RD, editors: *Small animal cardiovascular medicine*, St Louis, 1998, Mosby.

26. Dobbs LG, Gonzalez R, Matthay MA et al: Highly water-permeable type I alveolar epithelial cells confer high water permeability between the airspace and vasculature in rat lung, *Proc Natl Acad Sci USA* 95(6):2991, 1998.

27. Cott GR, Sugahara K, Mason RJ: Stimulation of net active ion transport across alveolar type II cell monolayers, *Am J Physiol* 250(2 Pt 1):C222-C227, 1986.

28. Sakuma T, Okaniwa G, Nakada T et al: Alveolar fluid clearance in the resected human lung, *Am J Respir Crit Care Med* 150:305, 1994.

29. Matthay MA, Wiener-Kronish JP: Intact epithelial barrier function is critical for the resolution of alveolar edema in humans, *Am Rev Respir Dis* 142(6 Pt 1):1250, 1990.

30. Folkesson HG, Matthay MA, Westrom BR et al: Alveolar epithelial clearance of protein, *J Appl Physiol* 80:1431, 1996.

31. Matthay MA, Berthiaume Y, Staub NC: Long-term clearance of liquid and protein from the lungs of unanesthetized sheep, *J Appl Physiol* 59:928, 1985.

32. Verghese GM, Ware LB, Matthay BA et al: Alveolar epithelial fluid transport and the resolution of clinically severe hydrostatic pulmonary edema, *J Appl Physiol* 87(4):1301, 1999.

33. Ware LB, Matthay MA: Alveolar fluid clearance is impaired in the majority of patients with acute lung injury and the acute respiratory distress syndrome, *Am J Respir Crit Care Med* 163(6):1376, 2001.

34. Bernard GR, Pou NA, Coggeshall JW et al: Comparison of the pulmonary dysfunction caused by cardiogenic and noncardiogenic pulmonary edema, *Chest* 108(3):798, 1995.

35. Brown RH, Zerhouni EA, Mitzner W: Visualization of airway obstruction in vivo during pulmonary vascular engorgement and edema, *J Appl Physiol* 78(3):1070, 1995.

36. Cornelius LM, Finco DR, Culver DH: Physiological effects of rapid infusion of Ringer's lactate solution into dogs, *Am J Vet Res* 39:1185, 1978.

37. Parent C, King LG, Walker LM et al: Clinical and clinicopathologic findings in dogs with acute respiratory distress syndrome: 19 cases (1985-1993), *JAVMA* 208:1419, 1996.

38. Turk J, Miller M, Brown T et al: Coliform septicemia and pulmonary disease associated with canine parvoviral enteritis: 88 cases (1987-1988), *JAVMA* 196:771, 1990.

39. Drobatz KJ, Walker LM, Hendricks JC: Smoke exposure in dogs: 27 cases (1988-1997), *JAVMA* 215(9):1306, 1999.

40. Drobatz KJ, Walker LM, Hendricks JC: Smoke exposure in cats: 22 cases (1986-1997), *JAVMA* 215(9):1312, 1999.

41. Stampley AR, Waldron DR: Reexpansion pulmonary edema after surgery to repair a diaphragmatic hernia in a cat, *JAVMA* 203: 1699, 1993.

42. Raptopoulos D, Papazoglou LG, Patsikas MN: Re-expansion pulmonary oedema after pneumothorax in a dog, *Vet Rec* 136:395, 1995.

43. Fossum TW, Evering WN, Miller MW et al: Severe bilateral fibrosing pleuritis associated with chronic chylothorax in five cats and two dogs, *JAVMA* 201:317, 1992.

44. Jenkinson SG: Oxygen toxicity, *New Horizons* 1(4):504, 1993.

45. Wolfe WG, Ebert PA, Sabiston DC Jr.: Effect of high oxygen tension on mucociliary function, *Surgery* 72(2):246, 1972.

46. Laurenzi GA, Yin S, Guarneri JJ: Adverse effect of oxygen on tracheal mucus flow, *N Engl J Med* 279(7):333, 1968.

47. Bennett SH, Geelhoed GW, Aaron RK et al: Pulmonary injury resulting from perfusion with stored bank blood in the baboon and dog, *J Surg Research* 13(6):295, 1972.

48. Popovsky MA: Transfusion and lung injury, *Transfus Clin Biol* 8(3):272, 2001.

49. The Acute Respiratory Distress Syndrome Network: Ventilation with lower tidal volumes as compared with traditional tidal volumes for acute lung injury and the acute respiratory distress syndrome, *N Engl J Med* 342(18):1301, 2000.

50. Ricard JD, Dreyfuss D, Saumon G: Ventilator-induced lung injury, *Curr Opin Crit Care* 8(1):12, 2002.

51. Maron MB: A canine model of neurogenic pulmonary edema, *J Appl Physiol* 59(3):1019, 1985.

52. Maron MB: Analysis of airway fluid protein concentration in neurogenic pulmonary edema, *J Appl Physiol* 62(2):470, 1987.

53. Drobatz KJ, Saunders HM, Pugh CR et al: Non-cardiogenic pulmonary edema in dogs and cats: 26 cases (1987-1993), *JAVMA* 206:1732, 1995.

54. Kerr LY: Pulmonary edema secondary to upper airway obstruction in the dog: A review of nine cases, *JAVMA* (25):207, 1989.

55. Gupta YK, Chugh A, Kacker V et al: Development of neurogenic pulmonary edema at different grades of intracranial pressure in cats, *Ind J Physiol & Pharmacol* 42(1):71, 1998.

56. Stalis IH, Bossbaly MJ, Winkle TJ: Feline endomyocarditis and left ventricular endocardial fibrosis, *Vet Pathol* 32:122, 1995.

57. Sheafor SE, Couto CG: Anticoagulant rodenticide toxicity in 21 dogs, *J Am Anim Hosp Assoc* 35:38, 1999.

58. Berry CR, Gallaway A, Thrall DE et al: Thoracic radiographic features of anticoagulant rodenticide toxicity in 14 dogs, *Vet Radiol Ultrasound* 34:391, 1993.

59. Hess RS, Kass PH, Shofer FS et al: Evaluation of risk factors for fatal acute pancreatitis in dogs, *J Am Vet Med Assoc* 214:46, 1999.

60. Hughes D, Beal MW: Emergency vascular access, *Vet Clin North Am Small Anim Pract* 30(3):491, 2000.

61. Staub NC, Hogg JC: Conference report of a workshop on the measurement of lung water, *Crit Care Med* 8(12):752, 1980.

62. Lewis FR, Elings VB, Hill SL et al: The measurement of extravascular lung water by thermal-green dye indicator dilution, *Ann New York Academy of Sciences* 384:394, 1982.

63. Wallin CJ, Leksell LG: Estimation of extravascular lung water in humans with use of ^2H_2O: Effect of blood flow and central blood volume, *J Appl Physiol* 76(5):1868, 1994.

64. Mitchell JP, Schuller D, Calandrino FS et al: Improved outcome based on fluid management in critically ill patients requiring pulmonary artery catheterization, *Am Rev Resp Dis* 145(5):990-998, 1992.

65. Eisenberg PR, Hansbrough JR, Anderson D et al: A prospective study of lung water measurements during patient management in an intensive care unit, *Am Rev Respir Dis* 136(3):662, 1987.

66. Fein A, Grossman RF, Jones JG et al: The value of edema fluid protein measurement in patients with pulmonary edema, *Am J Med* 67(1):32, 1979.

67. Rozanski EA, Dhupa N, Rush JE et al: Differentiation of the etiology of pulmonary edema by measurement of the protein content, *J Vet Emerg Crit Care* 8:256, 1998.

68. Vismara LA, Leaman DM, Zelis R: The effects of morphine on venous tone in patients with acute pulmonary edema, *Circulation* 54(2):335, 1976.

69. Colmenero-Ruiz M, Fernandez-Mondejar E, Fernandez-Sacristan MA et al: PEEP and low tidal volume ventilation reduce lung water in porcine pulmonary edema, *Am J Respir Crit Care Med* 155(3):964, 1997.

70. Peitzman AB, Corbett WA, Shires GT III et al: The effect of increasing end-expiratory pressure on extravascular lung water, *Surgery* 90(3):439, 1981.

71. Saul GM, Feeley TW, Mihm FG: Effect of graded administration of PEEP on lung water in noncardiogenic pulmonary edema, *Crit Care Med* 10(10):667, 1982.

72. Blomqvist H, Wickerts CJ, Berg B et al: Does PEEP facilitate the resolution of extravascular lung water after experimental hydrostatic pulmonary oedema? *Eur Resp J* 4(9):1053, 1991.

73. Douglas WW, Rehder K, Beynen FM et al: Improved oxygenation in patients with acute respiratory failure: The prone position, *Am Rev Respir Dis* 115(4):559, 1977.

74. Nakos G, Tsangaris I, Kostanti E et al: Effect of the prone position on patients with hydrostatic pulmonary edema compared with patients with acute respiratory distress syndrome and pulmonary fibrosis, *Am J Respir Crit Care Med* 161:360-368, 2000.

75. Lee DL, Chiang HT, Lin SL et al: Prone-position ventilation induces sustained improvement in oxygenation in patients with acute respiratory distress syndrome who have a large shunt, *Crit Care Med* 30(7):1446, 2002.

76. Lamm WJ, Graham MM, Albert RK: Mechanism by which the prone position improves oxygenation in acute lung injury, *Am J Respir Crit Care Med* 150(1):184, 1994.

77. Albert RK, Hubmayr RD: The prone position eliminates compression of the lungs by the heart, *Am J Respir Crit Care Med* 161(5): 1660, 2000.

78. da Luz P, Shubin H, Weil MH et al: Pulmonary edema related to changes in colloid osmotic and pulmonary artery wedge pressure in patients after acute myocardial infarction, *Circulation* 51:350, 1975.

79. Schuster CJ, Weil MH, Besso J et al: Blood volume following diuresis induced by furosemide, *Am J Med* 76:585, 1984.

80. Ali J, Chernicki W, Wood LD: Effect of furosemide in canine low-pressure pulmonary edema, *J Clin Invest* 64(5):1494, 1979.

81. Ali J, Unruh H, Skoog C et al: The effect of lung edema on pulmonary vasoactivity of furosemide, *J Surg Research* 35(5):383, 1983.

82. Demling RH, Will JA: The effect of furosemide on the pulmonary transvascular fluid filtration rate, *Crit Care Med* 6(5):317, 1978.

83. Greenberg S, McGowan C, Xie J et al: Selective pulmonary and venous smooth muscle relaxation by furosemide: A comparison with morphine, *J Pharmacol Exp Ther* 270(3):1077, 1994.

84. Lundergan CF, Fitzpatrick TM, Rose JC et al: Effect of cyclooxygenase inhibition on the pulmonary vasodilator response to furosemide, *J Pharmacol Exp Ther* 246(1):102, 1988.

85. Molloy WD, Lee KY, Girling L et al: Treatment of canine permeability pulmonary edema: Short-term effects of dobutamine, furosemide, and hydralazine, *Circulation* 72(6):1365, 1985.

86. Rusch VW, Artman L, Cheney FW: Effect of furosemide on fully established low pressure pulmonary edema, *J Surg Res* 41(2):141, 1986.

87. Pivac N, Rumboldt Z, Sardelic S et al: Diuretic effects of furosemide infusion versus bolus injection in congestive heart failure, *Int J Clin Pharmacol Res* 18(3):121, 1998.

88. Reiter PD, Makhlouf R, Stiles AD: Comparison of 6-hour infusion versus bolus furosemide in premature infants, *Pharmacotherapy* 18(1):63, 1998.

89. Lahav M, Regev A, Ra'anani P et al: Intermittent administration of furosemide vs. continuous infusion preceded by a loading dose for congestive heart failure, *Chest* 102(3):725, 1992.

90. Luciani GB, Nichani S, Chang AC et al: Continuous versus intermittent furosemide infusion in critically ill infants after open heart operations, *Ann Thorac Surg* 64(4):1133, 1997.

91. Schuller D, Lynch JP, Fine D: Protocol-guided diuretic management: Comparison of furosemide by continuous infusion and intermittent bolus, *Crit Care Med* 25(12):1969, 1997.

92. Reiter PD, Makhlouf R, Stiles AD: Comparison of 6-hour infusion versus bolus furosemide in premature infants, *Pharmacotherapy* 18(1):63, 1998.

93. Copeland JG, Campbell DW, Plachetka JR et al: Diuresis with continuous infusion of furosemide after cardiac surgery, *Am J Surg* 146(6):796, 1983.

94. Cotter G, Faibel H, Barash P et al: High-dose nitrates in the immediate management of unstable angina: Optimal dosage, route of administration, and therapeutic goals, *Am J Emerg Med* 16(3):219, 1998.

95. Cotter G, Metzkor E, Kaluski E et al: Randomised trial of high-dose isosorbide dinitrate plus low-dose furosemide versus high-dose furosemide plus low-dose isosorbide dinitrate in severe pulmonary oedema, *Lancet* 351(9100):389, 1998.

96. Seibert AF, Thomson WJ, Taylor A et al: Reversal of increased microvascular permeability associated with ischemia-reperfusion: Role of cAMP, *J Appl Physiol* 72:389, 1992.

97. Sakuma T, Okaniwa G, Nakada T et al: Alveolar fluid clearance in the resected human lung, *Am J Resp Crit Care Med* 150:305, 1994.

98. Tibayan FA, Chesnutt AN, Folkesson HG et al: Dobutamine increases alveolar liquid clearance in ventilated rats by beta-2 receptor stimulation, *Am J Respir Crit Care Med* 156(2 Pt 1):438, 1997.

99. Frank JA, Wang Y, Osorio O et al: Beta-adrenergic agonist therapy accelerates the resolution of hydrostatic pulmonary edema in sheep and rats, *J Appl Physiol* 89(4):1255, 2000.

100. Sartori C, Allemann Y, Duplain H et al: Salmeterol for the prevention of high-altitude pulmonary edema, *N Engl J Med* 346(21): 1631, 2002.

101. Ware LB, Matthay MA: Keratinocyte and hepatocyte growth factors in the lung: Roles in lung development, inflammation, and repair, *Am J Physiol Lung Cell Mol Physiol* 282(5):L924-L940, 2002.

102. Folkesson HG, Pittet JF, Nitenberg G et al: Transforming growth factor-alpha increases alveolar liquid clearance in anesthetized ventilated rats, *Am J Physiol* 271(2 Pt 1):L236-L244, 1996.

103. Kaner RJ, Ladetto JV, Singh R et al: Lung overexpression of the vascular endothelial growth factor gene induces pulmonary edema, *Am J Respir Crit Care Med* 22(6):657, 2000.

104. Bates DO, Curry FE: Vascular endothelial growth factor increases microvascular permeability via a Ca(2+)-dependent pathway, *Am J Physiol* 273(2 Pt 2):H687-H694, 1997.

105. King LG, Hendricks JC: Use of positive-pressure ventilation in dogs and cats: 41 cases (1990-1992), *J Am Vet Med Assoc* 204(7): 1045-1052, 1994.

CHAPTER 67

Pulmonary Hypertension

Jennifer L. Steele • Rosemary A. Henik

Definition and Etiology

Normal pulmonary artery pressures in small animals, as measured by cardiac catheterization under pentobarbital anesthesia, are 25 ± 5 mm Hg systolic, 10 ± 3 mm Hg diastolic, and mean of 15 ± 5 mm Hg.[1] By definition, pulmonary hypertension (PH) exists when the systolic and/or mean pulmonary artery pressures are elevated to above 30 and 20 mm Hg, respectively.[2,3] PH is further classified as either primary or secondary in etiology. Primary PH is a diagnosis of exclusion because it has no known etiology. Secondary PH develops as a sequela to conditions resulting in impedance of pulmonary venous drainage[4] (usually secondary to increased left atrial pressure[2,3]), pulmonary overcirculation,[2-4] or increased pulmonary vascular resistance.[2-4]

Although canine heartworm disease is considered to be the most well-recognized cause of PH,[2,5] a recent review of 53 dogs with evidence of PH revealed increased pulmonary venous pressure secondary to mitral valve disease as the most common predisposing condition causing PH, accounting for 16 of 53 cases.[5] Other conditions noted in this study, in addition to heartworm disease (5 of 53), included pulmonary thromboembolism (5 of 53), dilated cardiomyopathy (4 of 53), pulmonary fibrosis (3 of 53), and pneumonia (3 of 53).[5] The same review reported 5 dogs in which the pathophysiological mechanism of PH could not be determined,[5] making a diagnosis of primary PH possible in these animals, although this condition has not yet been characterized in veterinary medicine.[2]

Pathophysiology

Recent advances in the understanding of primary PH in humans warrant a discussion of its suspected pathogenesis and proposed risk factors.[3] Findings in humans with the disease indicate that a marked vasoconstrictive tendency is key in the development of primary PH, possibly through the effect of catecholamines,[3] release of the potent vasoconstrictor endothelin by vascular endothelial cells, or decreased production of endothelium-derived relaxation factor (EDRF) from dysfunctional endothelial cells.[3,6] Dysfunctional endothelial cells also produce a local procoagulant environment,[3] and increased production of biologically-active von Willebrand's factor in human patients with primary PH[3,6] may explain the widespread development of thrombosis *in situ* in small pulmonary arteries, resulting in vascular obstruction.[3,7] It is also possible that these microthrombi simply form secondary to stasis of blood within partially occluded vessels.[6] An immune mechanism has also been proposed in humans[6-8] based on the development of primary PH in patients with collagen vascular diseases such as scleroderma, systemic lupus erythematosus, and rheumatoid arthritis.[8] Risk factors have been identified in the development of primary PH in human beings; those which may be pertinent to small animals include systemic hypertension[3]; portal hypertension[3,8,9]; and living at high altitude, usually between 3000 and 5000 m above sea level.[9] However, the low prevalence of primary PH in the human population, estimated at only 2 cases per million,[3] makes the primary form of this disease an unlikely diagnosis in veterinary patients.

A discussion of the normal physiology of the pulmonary circulation is required before describing the abnormalities contributing to secondary PH. When blood flows uninhibited through the pulmonary vascular bed, there is minimal resistance, and a small arteriovenous pressure difference of approximately 2 to 10 mm Hg moves the entire cardiac output with minimal effort by the right heart.[3,10] In comparison, a pressure difference of approximately 90 mm Hg is required to move the same volume of blood across the systemic vascular bed.[3] If cardiac output is increased, resulting in increased flow through the pulmonary circuit (e.g., during exercise), low pulmonary vascular resistance is maintained by increasing the radius of distensible vessels and by recruitment of additional vessels.[3] The relationship between flow, pressure, and resistance is described by the following equation (derived from Poiseuille's law):

$$R = \Delta P/Q = 8\eta l/\pi r^4$$

where R = resistance, ΔP = change in pressure, Q = flow, η = viscosity of fluid, l = length of the vessel, and r = radius of the vessel. Therefore even a small change in the radius of a vessel can have a large impact on resistance within the pulmonary circulation.[3] Other factors influencing vascular resistance in normal and diseased states include total lung tissue mass being perfused (a greater mass decreases resistance), proximal vascular obstruction (e.g., because of pulmonary embolism), and extramural compression of vessels such as by perivascular edema.[3,10]

Three main mechanisms lead to development of secondary PH. First, *impedance of pulmonary venous drainage*[3,10] usually results from structural or functional abnormalities of the left side of the heart, although lesions of the pulmonary veins may also obstruct drainage.[10] Consequently, there is sustained elevation of the pulmonary venous pressure, usually above 25 mm Hg,[3,10] which is transmitted back to the pulmonary arteries.[10] Pulmonary arterial vasoconstriction occurs in response to the passive elevation of pulmonary venous pressure and worsens pulmonary arterial hypertension.[3,10] When this occurs, the arteriovenous pressure gradient rises, although pulmonary bloodflow remains constant or decreases.[3] This impedance of pulmonary venous drainage has been called passive pulmonary hypertension,[3,4] but this term is best applied when there is elevation of pulmonary artery pressure without a significant increase in pulmonary vascular resistance.[3] Conditions that could potentially result in PH by the mechanism of impeded pulmonary venous return include mitral stenosis, mitral regurgitation, cor triatriatum sinister, cardiomyopathies (including hypertrophic, restrictive, and dilated), aortic stenosis,[3,10] congenital pulmonary vein stenosis, pulmonary venoocclusive disease, fibrosing mediastinitis,[10] and systemic hypertension.[3]

The second mechanism of PH involves *increased pulmonary bloodflow,* which most commonly occurs in association with congenital cardiac anomalies such as atrial and ventricular septal defects and patent ductus arteriosus.[2-4] Normally, these defects result in left-to-right shunting of blood because of higher blood pressure in the systemic circulation compared with the pulmonary circulation. When pulmonary bloodflow is doubled, pulmonary vascular resistance decreases in order to maintain pulmonary artery pressure at a constant level.[3] If pulmonary bloodflow is increased four- to six-fold, pulmonary artery pressure rises as the reserve capacity of the pulmonary vascular bed is exceeded.[3] The pulmonary response to increased bloodflow is vasoconstriction, mediated by various endogenous vasoactive substances in an attempt to protect the pulmonary microvasculature.[12] Vascular remodeling occurs in the walls of the small pulmonary arteries because of flow-induced damage[4,12] and prolonged vasoconstriction.[12] Eventually, blood pressure in the pulmonary arterial circulation rises above that of the systemic circulation, reversing shunt bloodflow to right-to-left.[4,12] When the shunted blood (moving left-to-right) enters the right ventricle or pulmonary artery directly, as in a ventricular septal defect or patent ductus arteriosus, there appears to be a higher prevalence of severe and irreversible pulmonary vascular damage.[3] This pathophysiological mechanism is commonly referred to as Eisenmenger's physiology, and describes a collection of abnormalities including increased pulmonary vascular resistance with pulmonary hypertension and reversal of a previously left-to-right shunt.[3,5,13] In small animals, this syndrome has been recognized in association with PDA, aorticopulmonary communication, and ventricular and atrial septal defects.[13]

Although PDA is the most common congenital heart defect in dogs and has been observed in many breeds,[12,13] only a small number of animals actually develop a right-to-left shunt. Left-sided heart failure within the first year of life is more common than pulmonary hypertension.[12] It has also been reported that dogs with early development of pulmonary hypertension have a large-diameter PDA.[12,13] When Eisenmenger's physiology does develop, it usually occurs before the animal is 6 months old,[12,13] and the severity of the vasoreactive and structural vascular changes are at least partially positively correlated to the diameter of the communicating defect.[12] Decreased oxygen tension at high altitudes with associated vasoconstriction might also play a role in the development of Eisenmenger's physiology by exacerbating the pulmonary hypertension that develops with PDA.[12]

The third mechanism by which secondary PH may result is *increased pulmonary vascular resistance.* This category can be further subdivided, based on the etiology of the pulmonary vascular resistance, into conditions resulting in obstruction or obliteration of the pulmonary vasculature or chronic parenchymal diseases of the lung.[2-5,10,14,15] Pulmonary embolization is commonly cited as a cause of PH because of both vascular obstruction and vasoconstriction.[2-4,14] Although pulmonary thromboembolism (PTE) in humans accounts for 300,000 hospitalizations and 50,000 deaths per year in the United States,[14] this condition rarely leads to the development of chronic PH in people.[3] The pathophysiology of this disorder involves both mechanical obstruction of the vessel and reactive vasoconstriction mediated by vasoactive substances.[2,16] Platelets within the clot release histamine, serotonin, and thromboxane A$_2$, and endothelin is released from the endothelium.[16,17] In humans, PH develops when thromboemboli organize and vessels do not recanalize, with incorporation of thromboemboli into the vascular wall. Progression to this stage is reported to be slow, allowing time for right ventricular hypertrophy to develop and compensate for increased vascular resistance. Over time, progressive thrombosis or changes in the uninvolved vascular bed result in worsening of PH.[3] Additionally, acute cor pulmonale has been recognized following acute PTE in humans, with increased pulmonary artery pressure associated with obstruction of greater than 25% of the pulmonary vascular bed.[16] Obstruction of pulmonary vessels with increased vascular resistance can also occur secondary to parasitic diseases such as dirofilariasis[2] and schistosomiasis[4,14]; or embolization of fat, air, amniotic fluid, or tumor cells.[4]

Chronic pulmonary parenchymal diseases may lead to the development of PH. The suspected mechanism is thought to be hypoxia-induced vasoconstriction, although reactive vasoconstriction secondary to tissue acidosis may also contribute.[2,3] Consequently, pulmonary arteries develop muscular (medial) hypertrophy and intimal fibrosis, which sustain the hypertensive state. Lung diseases associated with such changes include chronic bronchitis, emphysema, and pulmonary fibrosis.[2,3,10,18,19] Chronic lung disease may also lead to the development of PH through additional mechanisms; in obstructive lung diseases such as COPD the loss of radial traction around the airways and distortion and rupture of air spaces results in partial destruction of the capillary bed.[18,20] In restrictive pulmonary diseases such as pulmonary fibrosis, radial traction on the airways may be excessive[21] and mechanical distortion may result in compression, destruction, or disordered repair of adjacent vessels.[10,22] Both obstructive and restrictive pulmonary diseases cause a decrease in the cross-sectional area of the pulmonary vascular bed and a rise in pulmonary arterial pressure.[2]

Pulmonary hypertension is considered to be the most important factor contributing to the development of clinical signs in dogs with heartworm disease.[23] In addition to disorders that result in hypoxia-induced vasoconstriction and subsequently increased vascular resistance, conditions such as tracheal collapse and laryngeal paralysis may be associated with intermittent or sustained hypoxia. However, the prevalence of PH in these conditions has not been studied.[2,17] Because dogs have a relatively mild vasoconstrictive response to hypoxia,[2,3,17] PH may only develop in very advanced respiratory disease or when additional factors such as PTE, sepsis, hypercoagulability, or hyperviscosity are present.[17]

Historical Findings and Clinical Signs

PH can affect any age or breed of dog, and a sex predilection has not been identified. Based on published reports of PH in the veterinary literature, the vast majority of cases occur in dogs, but atrial septal defect with associated Eisenmenger's physiology[24] and PDA with PH[25] have been documented in cats. Reported clinical signs vary depending on the underlying disorder and whether the onset was acute or chronic. Most animals exhibit cough, dyspnea, lethargy, exercise intolerance, and cyanosis.[2,17] Cyanosis may be caused by decreased cardiac output with systemic vasoconstriction (peripheral cyanosis) or secondary to ventilation-perfusion mismatch with resultant hypoxemia (central cyanosis).[2] Syncope may occur as a result of decreased left ventricular filling and may be exacerbated by hypoxia.[2,17] Any young animal presenting with a congenital cardiac shunt or an adult animal presenting with heart disease, chronic pulmonary disease, or heartworm disease should be evaluated for evidence of PH.

Physical Examination

Physical examination abnormalities are often related to the underlying disease process, and auscultation of the lungs may reveal significant respiratory pathology. Harsh crackles and wheezes may be heard with chronic bronchitis, and increased end-expiratory effort is a common finding. Fine crackles and tachycardia may be auscultated if the animal has pulmonary edema secondary to heart failure.[2,17] Hyper-resonance within the lungs suggests air trapping, which may occur with emphysema or other chronic obstructive pulmonary diseases.[17]

Abnormalities of heart sounds may suggest PH; a loud pulmonary component of the second heart sound reflects forceful closure of the pulmonic valve with high pulmonary artery pressures. A murmur of tricuspid insuffi-

ciency may occur secondary to right ventricular hypertrophy, or with increased pulmonary artery and right ventricular systolic pressures. If the etiology of pulmonary hypertension is left-sided disease of the heart, other murmurs or gallops may be auscultated. Additional physical examination findings with severe PH include a palpable apex beat on the right side of the thorax, if significant right ventricular hypertrophy exists; and signs of right heart failure including hepatomegaly, ascites, pleural effusion, and jugular venous distension.[2,17]

Diagnostic Testing

CLINICAL PATHOLOGY

Diagnostic investigation of patients at risk for PH requires an organized and thorough evaluation of the underlying disease, and determination of the presence or absence of PH and its consequences.[2,17] Hematological findings may include polycythemia suggestive of chronic hypoxia secondary to high altitude or chronic pulmonary disease, or right-to-left shunt such as in an animal with reversed PDA.[26] Spherocytosis with anemia, thrombocytopenia, or an inflammatory leukogram may be noted with immune-mediated diseases that predispose the animal to PTE and secondary PH. Heartworm disease may result in monocytosis, eosinophilia, and basophilia. If immune-mediated disease is suspected, additional immunologic testing is recommended. Results of antinuclear antibody (ANA) testing must be interpreted with caution, however, because 29% of human patients with PH tested ANA positive, suggesting a possible immunologic basis for PH or exposure to self-antigens secondary to endothelial disruption.[17]

Serum biochemical evaluation may reveal liver enzyme abnormalities because of chronic passive congestion in right heart failure or steroid hepatopathy. Other diseases that predispose animals to PTE and PH may result in characteristic serum biochemical abnormalities including hyperadrenocorticism (increased alkaline phosphatase, alanine transaminase, and cholesterol); nephrotic syndrome (increased cholesterol, decreased albumin, and increased creatinine and blood urea nitrogen in later stages); and sepsis (decreased glucose). An occult heartworm test should be performed to rule out dirofilariasis. Coagulation times and antithrombin III concentrations are indicated to identify animals predisposed to hypercoagulability. Arterial blood gas analysis should be performed whenever possible. Hypoxemia is a characteristic finding in PH, and its severity may indicate the degree of pulmonary dysfunction. Hypercarbia, if present, should be corrected with ventilatory support because it may contribute to PH through acidosis and pulmonary vasoconstriction.[2,17]

RADIOGRAPHIC FINDINGS

A broad spectrum of abnormalities, or none at all, may be seen on thoracic radiographs of animals with PH. Changes most commonly reported include cardiomegaly characterized by right-sided enlargement, pulmonary parenchymal infiltrates, and large, tortuous pulmonary arteries.[2,5,17] Additional radiographic abnormalities may be consistent with pulmonary embolism (abruptly attenuated lobar arteries with contiguous oligemia[27]), right heart failure (pleural effusion and enlarged vena cava[28]), chronic bronchitis or bronchiectasis (thickened bronchial walls with bronchiectasis characterized by dilation of bronchi and the loss of normal bronchial tapering[28]), pulmonary fibrosis, or tracheobronchial collapse.[17] Diseases of the left heart such as mitral valve insufficiency or dilated cardiomyopathy may obscure subtle pulmonary artery and right heart abnormalities.

CARDIOVASCULAR STUDIES

When PH is severe, electrocardiographic findings of deep S waves in leads I, II, III and aVF may suggest right axis deviation.[2,17] In a study of 53 dogs with evidence of PH by echocardiography, electrocardiography was performed in 18 animals.[5] Findings were variable and suggested chamber enlargement associated with the underlying etiology of PH; and arrhythmias, particularly atrial fibrillation and sinus tachycardia.[5]

Typical echocardiographic changes with PH may include right atrial and right ventricular dilation, right ventricular hypertrophy, pulmonary artery dilation (pulmonary artery:aorta >1), and interventricular septal hypertrophy (Figure 67-1, A).[2,17] Left ventricular dimensions may be small and left ventricular shortening fraction may be decreased because of right ventricular volume and pressure overload with resultant paradoxic septal motion.[2] When pulmonary artery pressure is increased, pulmonic valve function is characterized by delayed opening and mid-systolic closure.[17]

Doppler echocardiography provides an excellent noninvasive means of estimating pulmonary artery pressure (PAP) to diagnose PH. Pulmonary hypertension often results in high velocity regurgitation jets across the pulmonic and/or tricuspid valves (Figure 67-1, B).[2,5,17,29] In humans with PH, 80% to 87% of individuals had tricuspid valve regurgitation measurable on continuous wave Doppler echocardiography.[30,31] An invasive or estimated measurement of central venous or right atrial pressure, added to the Doppler-derived systolic trans-tricuspid gradient, is equivalent to the right ventricular and pulmonary artery systolic pressure.[30,31] Pulmonary hypertension is diagnosed when a tricuspid insufficiency jet is greater than 2.8 m/sec in the absence of pulmonic stenosis.[2] Using the modified Bernoulli equation:

$$\Delta P = 4 \times (\text{velocity in m/sec})^2$$

where peak tricuspid regurgitant velocity $\geq$2.8 m/sec estimates a systolic PAP $\geq$32 mm Hg, and a pulmonic insufficiency velocity $\geq$2.2 m/sec estimates a diastolic PAP $\geq$20 mm Hg.[2] Additional Doppler echocardiographic findings in PH include early onset right ventricular ejection followed by a rapid decrease in flow velocity in mid-systole as increased pulmonary artery resistance is encountered, and a shortened time to peak right ventricular ejection velocity.[17,29]

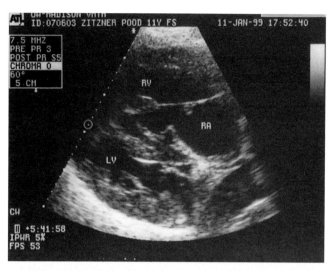

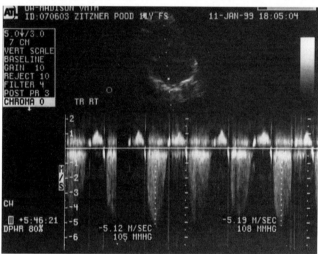

Figure 67-1. A, Two-dimensional echocardiogram obtained from a right parasternal long axis view of the heart in an 11-year-old spayed female toy poodle with pulmonary hypertension of unknown etiology. There is right ventricular and right atrial dilation and right ventricular hypertrophy. **B,** Continuous wave spectral Doppler tracing recorded from the left apex in the dog from Figure 67-1, A. The right ventricular to right atrial systolic gradient is 105 to 108 mm Hg. Because right ventricular systolic pressure is equal to pulmonary artery systolic pressure in the absence of pulmonic stenosis, the pulmonary artery systolic pressure is 105 to 108 mm Hg, documenting severe pulmonary hypertension.

Before Doppler echocardiography, cardiac catheterization of the right heart and pulmonary artery provided definitive diagnosis of PH. A Swan-Ganz balloon-flotation catheter measures central venous, right atrial, right ventricular, pulmonary artery, and pulmonary capillary wedge pressures (PCWP). Measurement of these pressures allows differentiation of the etiology of secondary PH; left-sided cardiac disease results in increased PCWP. Bronchopulmonary or pulmonary vascular diseases result in pulmonary arterial diastolic pressure that is significantly greater than the PCWP.[17] Cardiac catheterization is also helpful in obtaining information regarding response to treatment. Pulmonary artery pressure, cardiac output, and pulmonary vascular resistance may be measured following separate intravenous administration of the bronchodilators aminophylline (10 mg/kg) and terbutaline (0.01 mg/kg).[17] Additional testing with intravenous vasodilators such as hydralazine (1 mg/kg), verapamil (0.05 mg/kg), or nifedipine (<0.1 mg/kg) may also be performed, although close monitoring for systemic hypotension is essential.[17] Evaluation following inhalation of 100% oxygen or nitric oxide (10 to 160 ppm[32,33]) may demonstrate a decrease in PAP secondary to pulmonary vasodilation.[2] Reduced PAP following the above interventions suggests the potential for some reversibility of vascular disease.[2]

SPECIAL STUDIES

Ancillary tests that may assist in the diagnosis of PH include radionuclide angiography to measure right ventricular ejection fraction, and pulmonary angiography to define dilated and/or tortuous pulmonary arteries. Both of these studies may also demonstrate pulmonary perfusion deficits; a mottled perfusion scan may be indicative of generalized lung disease or PH, whereas a segmental distribution of deficits is more characteristic of pulmonary embolic disease.[2,17]

Ventilation/perfusion scintigraphy can diagnose or provide valuable information regarding the severity of PTE, chronic obstructive pulmonary disease (COPD), heartworm disease, and ventilation/perfusion mismatch.[34] Comparison studies of pulmonary angiography, digital subtraction angiography, and ventilation-perfusion scintigraphy of experimental pulmonary emboli (produced by forceful intravenous injection of clotted blood) in dogs revealed that ventilation-perfusion scintigraphy is the best available method to screen dogs with suspected PTE.[35]

Magnetic resonance imaging (MRI) is a valuable technique for diagnosis of PH in people. A study of 17 humans with pulmonary arterial hypertension confirmed by cardiac catheterization revealed good correlation between the measured systolic pulmonary artery pressure and the diameter of the main pulmonary artery.[36] The main pulmonary artery was enlarged in all affected individuals, even those with mild increases in PAP. MRI also provides a direct measurement of right ventricular wall thickness and can detect abnormal intraluminal signal intensity during the cardiac cycle.[36] Spiral computed tomography is another useful diagnostic imaging technique that can detect and differentiate organized mural thrombi and reveal perfusion abnormalities noninvasively in human patients with chronic pulmonary thromboembolism causing PH.[37] Unfortunately, the cost, availability, and the requirement of general anesthesia to perform these tests limits their utility in compromised veterinary patients.

HISTOPATHOLOGY

Histopathological findings from diagnostic lung biopsy or postmortem examination vary depending on the eti-

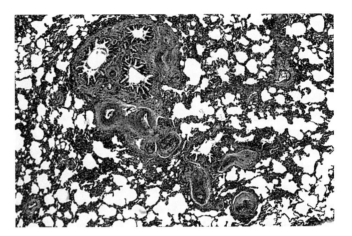

Figure 67-2. Low magnification H & E photomicrograph of a section of canine lung showing tortuous pulmonary arteries with plexiform lesions and medial hyperplasia. In several segments the hyperplastic response is occluding the lumen.

ology of PH. PH caused by impedance of pulmonary venous drainage results in pulmonary capillary remodeling characterized by an increase in extracellular matrix, which develops secondary to a rise in pulmonary venous pressure, as in left heart failure.[11] Diffuse interstitial pulmonary edema, an increase of collagen and elastic fibers in the left atrial endocardium, and multifocal subendocardial nodular fibrosis and mineralization were additional findings in dogs with mitral stenosis.[38]

Pulmonary overcirculation and increased pulmonary vascular resistance result in medial muscular hypertrophy and intimal proliferation,[3,12,14,39-41] which may cause complete obliteration of the vascular lumen.[39] Medial hypertrophy is the first and most common lesion observed in pulmonary hypertension; thickening of the media is actually caused by hyperplasia of smooth muscle cells.[40] Dilatation and plexiform lesions can also be found when vasoconstrictive PH is severe (Figure 67-2).[40,41] Dilatation lesions result from sustained pulmonary arterial hypertension and thinning of the arterial wall. Plexiform lesions arise in smaller branches of muscular pulmonary arteries; the lumen is dilated and contains a plexus of small channels that open at their distal end into a thin-walled, dilated, and patent section of the artery.[40] Plexiform lesions characterize "irreversible" PH, whereas in PH secondary to impedance of pulmonary venous drainage, absence of these lesions correlates with reversibility of PH.[3] Specific histopathological lesions associated with heartworm disease are discussed elsewhere.

Management

Treatment of PH in veterinary patients centers on resolving or alleviating the underlying disease process. Anticoagulant therapy is advisable when PTE is diagnosed in dogs, and heparin[17] or warfarin[3] therapy may be appropriate when PH may result from PTE.[17] Continuous oxygen therapy improves survival in human patients with hypoxic vasoconstriction from various causes[3,17,18] and is a feasible treatment option in small animals with acute-onset or sudden worsening of PH, as in heartworm disease or PTE. Inhalation of nitric oxide (NO), a substance normally produced in vascular endothelial cells, provides selective pulmonary vasodilation without systemic effects.[3,32,42] Nitric oxide is used to treat humans with PH[3,42] and has been shown to decrease mean PAP in newborn foals[32] and dogs[33] with experimentally-induced PH. Clinically, inhaled NO administered at 20 ppm was effective in decreasing mean PAP in a pug with vena cava syndrome secondary to heartworm disease; further decreases in mean PAP were not observed in this dog with higher doses of NO.[33] Nitric oxide is believed to act only on preconstricted vessels, not on those with normal tone, and additional benefits may include oxygen-derived free radical scavenging, decreased development of oxygen toxicosis, decreased platelet and leukocyte aggregation, and attenuation of the inflammatory cascade induced by sequestration of pulmonary leukocytes.[32] Potential harmful effects include prolonged bleeding[32] and pulmonary toxicity caused by accumulation of NO_2, the product of NO oxidation.[33]

Mainstays of chronic treatment of PH include bronchodilators, vasodilators, and diuretics. Theophylline, a bronchodilator, also improves cardiovascular performance in humans with cor pulmonale or COPD and has direct pulmonary vasodilatory effects.[17,18] If diuretics are used to reduce preload, close monitoring of serum potassium concentration is necessary, especially with concurrent use of theophylline or beta-2 agonists such as terbutaline, because these drugs can induce cellular uptake of this electrolyte.[18] Worsening of signs secondary to inspissation of bronchial secretions in COPD may occur with excessive diuretic administration.[17] Vasodilators proven to be effective in either human beings or animals with PH include angiotensin-converting enzyme inhibitors,[17,18] oral calcium-channel blockers,[3,17,18,43,44] hydralazine,[17,18] and intravenous adenosine[3,45] or prostacyclin (epoprostenol).[3,17,46,47] A recent advance in human medicine has been the development of an aerosolized prostacyclin analogue, iloprost.[48] In human studies, milrinone selectively inhibited phosphodiesterase III and decreased PAP and pulmonary vascular resistance; it also had a positive inotropic effect.[49]

Outcome

Information regarding prognosis and survival in animals with PH is lacking.[2,17] In one study of people with PH, those who responded to vasodilator therapy had a 5-year survival rate of 94% compared with 55% in those who did not respond.[44] In human beings with chronic cor pulmonale, survival of 5 to 10 years after the first appearance of peripheral edema is not uncommon.[50] However, at one veterinary institution, most of the animals treated for PH died or were euthanized within 4 months.[17] A greater understanding of conditions that predispose animals to PH, in addition to earlier recognition and treatment of PH, may help to improve survival time and quality of life for affected animals.[2,17]

REFERENCES

1. Thomas WP, Sisson D: Cardiac catheterization and angiography. In Fox PR, Sisson D, Moïse NS, editors: *Textbook of canine and feline cardiology: Principles and clinical practice,* ed 2, Philadelphia, 1999, WB Saunders.
2. Johnson L: Diagnosis of pulmonary hypertension, *Clin Tech Small Anim Pract* 14(4):231-236, 1999.
3. Rich S, Braunwald E, Grossman W: Pulmonary hypertension. In Braunwald E, editor: *Heart disease: A textbook of cardiovascular medicine,* ed 5, vol 1, Philadelphia, 1997, WB Saunders.
4. West JB: Vascular diseases. In West JB: *Pulmonary pathophysiology: The essentials,* ed 5, Baltimore, 1998, Williams & Wilkins.
5. Johnson L, Boon J, Orton EC: Clinical characteristics of 53 dogs with Doppler-derived evidence of pulmonary hypertension: 1992-1996, *J Vet Intern Med* 13:440-447, 1999.
6. Rabinovitch M: Insights into the pathogenesis of primary pulmonary hypertension from animal models. In Rubin LJ, Rich S, editors: *Primary pulmonary hypertension,* New York, 1997, Marcel-Dekker.
7. Burke AP, Virmani R, Farb A: Primary pulmonary hypertension and venoocclusive disease. In Saldana MJ, editor: *Pathology of pulmonary disease,* Philadelphia, 1994, JB Lippincott.
8. Brenot F, Simonneau G: Risk factors for primary pulmonary hypertension. In Rubin LJ, Rich S, editors: *Primary pulmonary hypertension,* New York, 1997, Marcel-Dekker.
9. Moride Y, Abenhaim L, Xu J: Epidemiology of primary pulmonary hypertension. In Rubin LJ, Rich S, editors: *Primary pulmonary hypertension,* New York, 1997, Marcel-Dekker.
10. Farb A, Burke AP, Virmani R: Pulmonary hypertension caused by chronic left heart failure, obstruction of venous return, and parenchymal lung disease. In Saldana MJ, editor: *Pathology of pulmonary disease,* Philadelphia, 1994, JB Lippincott.
11. West JB, Mathieu-Costello O: Vulnerability of pulmonary capillaries in heart disease, *Circulation* 92:622-631, 1995.
12. Oswald GP, Orton CE: Patent ductus arteriosus and pulmonary hypertension in related Pembroke Welsh Corgis, *J Vet Med Assoc* 202(5):761-764, 1993.
13. Bonagura JD, Lehmkuhl LD: Congenital heart disease. In Fox PR, Sisson D, Moïse NS, editors: *Textbook of canine and feline cardiology: Principles and clinical practice,* ed 2, Philadelphia, 1999, WB Saunders.
14. Virmani R, Farb A, Burke AP et al: Thromboembolic pulmonary hypertension, intravenous drug addiction, and rare forms of pulmonary embolization. In Saldana MJ, editor: *Pathology of pulmonary disease,* Philadelphia, 1994, JB Lippincott.
15. Saldana MJ, Arias-Stella J: Pulmonary hypertension and pathology at high altitudes. In Saldana MJ, editor: *Pathology of pulmonary disease,* Philadelphia, 1994, JB Lippincott.
16. Schulman DS, Matthay RA: The right ventricle in pulmonary disease, *Cardiol Clin* 10(1):111-135, 1992.
17. Johnson LR, Hamlin RL: Recognition and treatment of pulmonary hypertension. In Bonagura JD, Kirk RW, editors: *Kirk's current veterinary therapy,* vol 12, Philadelphia, 1995, WB Saunders.
18. Klinger JR, Hill NS: Right ventricular dysfunction in chronic obstructive pulmonary disease: Evaluation and management, *Chest* 99:715-723, 1991.
19. Wright JL, Petty T, Thurlbeck WM: Analysis of the structure of the muscular pulmonary arteries in patients with pulmonary hypertension and COPD: National Institutes of Health nocturnal oxygen therapy trial, *Lung* 170:109-124, 1992.
20. West JB: Obstructive diseases. In West JB: *Pulmonary pathophysiology: The essentials,* ed 5, Baltimore, 1998, Williams & Wilkins.
21. West JB: Restrictive diseases. In West JB: *Pulmonary pathophysiology: The essentials,* ed 5, Baltimore, 1998, Williams & Wilkins.
22. Phan SH: Endothelial cells in pulmonary fibrosis. In Phan SH, Thrall RS, editors: *Pulmonary fibrosis,* New York, 1995, Marcel-Dekker.
23. Hirano Y, Kitagawa H, Sasaki Y: Relationship between pulmonary arterial pressure and pulmonary thromboembolism associated with dead worms in canine heartworm disease, *J Vet Med Sci* 54(5):897-904, 1992.
24. Church DB, Allan GS: Atrial septal defect and Eisenmenger's syndrome in a mature cat, *Aust Vet J* 67:380, 1990.
25. Jeraj K, Ogburn P, Lord PF et al: Patent ductus arteriosus with pulmonary hypertension in a cat, *J Am Vet Med Assoc* 172(12):1432-1436, 1978.

26. Duncan JR, Prasse KW, Mahaffey EA: Erythrocytes. In Duncan JR, Prasse KW, Mahaffey EA: Veterinary laboratory medicine: Clinical pathology, ed 3, Ames, IA, 1994, Iowa State University Press.

27. Sottiaux J, Franck M: Pulmonary embolism and cor pulmonale in a cat, J Small Anim Pract 40:88-91, 1999.

28. Burk RL, Ackerman N: The thorax. In Burk RL, Ackerman N: Small animal radiology and ultrasonography: A diagnostic atlas and text, ed 2, Philadelphia, 1996, WB Saunders.

29. Moïse NS, Fox PR: Echocardiography and Doppler imaging. In Fox PR, Sisson D, Moïse NS, editors: Textbook of canine and feline cardiology: Principles and clinical practice, ed 2, Philadelphia, 1999, WB Saunders.

30. Yock PG, Popp RL: Noninvasive estimation of right ventricular systolic pressure by Doppler ultrasound in patients with tricuspid regurgitation, Circulation 70(4):657-662, 1984.

31. Berger M, Haimowitz A, Van Tosh A et al: Quantitative assessment of pulmonary hypertension in patients with tricuspid regurgitation using continuous wave Doppler ultrasound, J Am Coll Cardiol 6:359-365, 1985.

32. Lester GD, DeMarco VG, Norman WM: Effect of inhaled nitric oxide on experimentally induced pulmonary hypertension in neonatal foals, Am J Vet Res 60(10):1207-1212, 1999.

33. Hirakawa A, Sakamoto H, Misumi K et al: Effects of inhaled nitric oxide on hypoxic pulmonary vasoconstriction in dogs and a case report of vena cava syndrome, J Vet Med Sci 58(6):551-553, 1996.

34. Berry CR, Daniel G, O'Callahan M: Pulmonary scintigraphy. In Berry CR, Daniel GB: Handbook of veterinary nuclear medicine, Raleigh, NC, 1996, North Carolina State University Press.

35. Koblik PD, Hornof W, Harnagel SH et al: A comparison of pulmonary angiography, digital subtraction angiography, and 99mTc-DTPA/MAA ventilation-perfusion scintigraphy for detection of experimental pulmonary emboli in the dog, Vet Radiol 30(3):159-168, 1989.

36. Bouchard A, Higgins CB, Byrd BF et al: Magnetic resonance imaging in pulmonary arterial hypertension, Am J Cardiol 56:938-942, 1985.

37. Roberts HC, Kauczor HU, Schweden F et al: Spiral CT of pulmonary hypertension and chronic thromboembolism, J Thorac Imag 12(2):118-127, 1997.

38. Lehmkuhl LB, Ware WA, Bonagura JD: Mitral stenosis in 15 dogs, J Vet Intern Med 8:2-17, 1994.

39. Pyle RL, Park RD, Alexander AF et al: Patent ductus arteriosus with pulmonary hypertension in the dog, J Am Vet Med Assoc 178(6): 565-571, 1981.

40. Wagenvoort CA, Wagenvoort N: Pulmonary hypertension in cardiac left to right shunts. In Wagenvoort CA, Wagenvoort N: Pathology of pulmonary hypertension, New York, 1977, John Wiley and Sons.

41. Turk JR, Miller JB, Sande RD: Plexogenic pulmonary arteriopathy in a dog with ventricular septal defect and pulmonary hypertension, J Am Anim Hosp Assoc 18:608-612, 1982.

42. Clark RH, Kueser TJ, Walker MW et al: Low-dose nitric oxide therapy for persistent pulmonary hypertension of the newborn, N Engl J Med 342(7):469-474, 2000.

43. Packer M: Therapeutic application of calcium-channel antagonists for pulmonary hypertension, Am J Cardiol 55:196B-201B, 1985.

44. Rich S, Kaufmann E, Levy PS: The effect of high doses of calcium-channel blockers on survival in primary pulmonary hypertension, N Engl J Med 327(2):76-81, 1992.

45. Driessen B, Haskins SC, Pascoe PJ et al: Haemodynamic effects of ATP in dogs during hypoxia-induced pulmonary hypertension, J Vet Pharmacol Therap 22:213-219, 1999.

46. Epoprostenol for primary pulmonary hypertension, The Medical Letter 38(968):14-15, 1996.

47. McLaughlin VV, Genthner DE, Panella MM et al: Reduction in pulmonary vascular resistance with long-term epoprostenol (prostacyclin) therapy in primary pulmonary hypertension, N Engl J Med 338(5):273-277, 1998.

48. Hoeper MM, Schwarze M, Ehlerding S et al: Long-term treatment of primary pulmonary hypertension with aerosolized iloprost, a prostacyclin analogue, N Engl J Med 342(25):1866-1870, 2000.

49. Dent G, Magnussen H, Rabe KF: Cyclic nucleotide phosphodiesterases in the human lung, Lung 172:129-146, 1994.

50. Fishman AP: Pulmonary hypertension and cor pulmonale. In Fishman AP, Elias JA, Fishman JA et al, editors: Fishman's pulmonary diseases and disorders, ed 3, New York, 1998, McGraw-Hill.

CHAPTER 68

Acute Lung Injury and Acute Respiratory Distress Syndrome

Daniel L. Chan • Elizabeth A. Rozanski

Acute (adult) respiratory distress syndrome (ARDS) is a leading cause of respiratory failure in critical care medicine. This syndrome is typified by an exaggerated inflammatory response that develops within the lungs. ARDS was first described in the human literature in the late 1960s.[1] Since that time, acute lung injury (ALI) and the more severe ARDS have been appreciated as common sequelae in patients with systemic inflammation or infection. With advances in critical care techniques and supportive care, many patients with life-threatening diseases are initially resuscitated, only to later succumb to multiple organ dysfunction syndrome (MODS) including respiratory failure (ALI and ARDS).[2,3]

In recent years, veterinary critical care clinicians have recognized a similar syndrome of acute respiratory failure in dogs.[4-10] Other differentials for acute respiratory distress in critically ill dogs include pneumonia, pulmonary thromboembolism, or congestive heart failure/volume overload. It is unclear whether cats develop ARDS in a similar fashion. Whereas critically ill cats certainly develop worsening respiratory distress, this is often caused by volume overload and pleural effusion rather than primary pulmonary pathology. Additionally, many of the common risk factors (e.g., sepsis, pneumonia, and nonfatal thoracic trauma) that occur in people and dogs are far less common in cats.

Definition

In order to advance scientific knowledge, for overall improvement in management of the disease, and to provide universal agreement on its classification, a consensus statement to define ARDS in people was adopted by the American-European Consensus Committee in 1994.[11] ARDS was recognized as a more severe subset of ALI. The actual criteria proposed to define ALI and ARDS are as follows: (1) acute onset of respiratory distress; (2) presence of bilateral pulmonary infiltrates on chest radiographs; and (3) pulmonary artery wedge pressure equal to or lower than 18 mm Hg, or no clinical evidence of left atrial hypertension. Patients with ALI are further defined as having a Pao_2:Fio_2 ratio of 300 or less, whereas the definition of ARDS requires a ratio of 200 or less.[11-13]

In practice, ARDS is widely recognized as the development of respiratory failure, as evidenced by the above criteria, in a patient with a predisposing medical or surgical risk factor. In humans, risk factors for the development of ALI and ARDS may be of pulmonary or extrapulmonary origin. Pulmonary risk factors include those that result in direct injury to the lungs (e.g., pneumonia; pulmonary contusion; and inhalation of noxious gases, including high concentrations of oxygen) and noncardiogenic pulmonary edema (e.g., electrocution).[3] Extrapulmonary risk factors include polytrauma, sepsis, and systemic inflammatory response syndrome (SIRS).[3,12] Logically, the presence of more than one risk factor increases the likelihood of the development of ALI and ARDS. In general, any disease process that warrants admission to an ICU is considered severe enough to predispose the patient to developing ALI. Furthermore, humans with ALI are also highly susceptible and often succumb to MODS characterized by the failure of a variety of organs including the kidneys or liver.[13,14]

Risk factors for ALI and ARDS in dogs are less well defined. In one of the few studies on the subject, 19 dogs were identified with histopathological changes consistent with ARDS.[9] Similarly to people with ARDS, pneumonia and sepsis were identified as the most common risk factors.[10] Despite the recognition that ARDS does occur in dogs, the veterinary literature currently lacks a large-scale review of ARDS in critically ill dogs, as well as a consensus statement defining ALI/ARDS in this patient population.

Mechanism of Lung Injury

The mechanism of lung injury is an area of active research in critical care medicine. Although great strides in understanding the pathogenesis of ALI have been made since the first description in late 1960s, the mortality rate due to ALI/ARDS remains high. In an attempt to hasten the development of effective therapy for ARDS, the Acute Respiratory Distress Syndrome Clinical Network (ARDSnet) was established in 1994 by the National Heart, Lung, and Blood Institute and the National Institutes of Health (www.ardsnet.org). This organization has supported many research trials elucidating the mechanism of lung injury, and has developed many clinical trials aimed at reducing the morbidity and mortality of ARDS.

Although the intricacies of its pathogenesis remain quite complex, it is easiest to think of ALI/ARDS as the development of pulmonary edema resulting from an increase in endothelial permeability, in response to an inflammatory process. As critical injury or illness progresses, the normally resilient pulmonary capillaries and alveoli become very permeable, allowing the leakage of protein-rich serum into the alveolar spaces. The presence of this fluid further incites the inflammatory response and results in circulation of a variety of more intense inflammatory mediators such as cytokines and leukotrienes. Radiographically, this fluid may be appreciated as bilateral alveolar infiltrates (Figure 68-1), and functionally as abnormal gas exchange (hypoxemia) and decreased lung compliance. Relative surfactant deficiencies contribute to alveolar collapse. The inflammatory process represents an overzealous response on the part of both cellular and humoral immune systems.

Cellular mediators of ALI/ARDS include primarily neutrophils and macrophages, although monocytes, lymphocytes, and platelets (platelet aggregation) may also be involved. Humoral mediators include a variety of cytokines with TNF-α, and IL-1, IL-6, and IL-8 considered particularly important.[13,14] Complement and the generation of arachidonic acid metabolites may also contribute to the inflammatory response.[13,14]

Pulmonary arterial hypertension results from increased pulmonary vascular resistance caused by destruction or obstruction of the vascular bed, and from hypoxic pulmonary vasoconstriction.[13] Untreated pulmonary hypertension may result in right-sided cardiac dysfunction.

Stages of Lung Injury

In affected people, histological evaluation of lung samples obtained via biopsy or autopsy may reflect three separate phases of lung injury. In the first phase, which occurs immediately after the development of lung injury, the changes are classified as exudative. Exudative changes

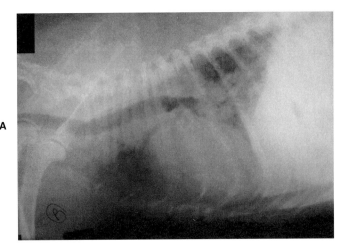

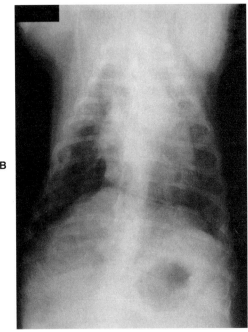

Figure 68-1. A, Right lateral and **B,** ventrodorsal radiographs of a dog with bilateral alveolar infiltrates, commonly seen in patients with ARDS.

reflect the presence of protein-rich edema fluid, hyaline membranes, and white blood cell infiltrates. As ALI/ARDS progresses, histological changes represent the proliferative phase. This phase is characterized by proliferation of type II pneumocytes, which attempt to restore the damaged epithelium. Finally, as the disease resolves, histological examination reflects the fibrotic phase, which is characterized by an influx of fibroblasts. Interestingly, in long-term human ALI/ARDS survivors, minimal pulmonary functional abnormalities are present.

Management Strategies

Management of affected people involves early recognition and treatment of abnormalities and supportive care

until resolution occurs. Supportive care typically includes fluid therapy and management of the underlying disease. As in many conditions, directed therapy is more likely to be beneficial. Although a specific antimicrobial therapy (e.g., an aminoglycoside) may be more effective against bacterial pneumonia in some cases of nosocomial infection, in other cases, particularly when there may be fungal involvement, other therapies are required. Certain conditions also require more aggressive intervention (e.g., surgical drainage of abdominal infection) because unchecked sepsis leads to an increased likelihood of worsening ARDS or MODS.[15] Transfusions of blood products should be limited to patients deemed in critical need of oxygen-carrying support because transfusion-associated lung injury is common in human ARDS patients. Other supportive measures are directed at maintaining vital organ perfusion and function but may present complex problems for patient management. For example, although it is common for people with severe renal dysfunction to undergo hemodialysis, the application of hemodialysis commonly results in transiently decreased oxygen saturation and may significantly impact tissue oxygen delivery.[16]

Since the first description of ARDS, and despite advances in critical care, mortality has remained close to 50%.[13] A variety of pharmacological interventions have been proposed in an attempt to limit some of the devastating changes that accompany ALI/ARDS. Clinical trials have investigated the use of vasopressors, vasodilators, surfactant replacement, nutritional interventions, patient positioning, and global antiinflammatory drugs. Vasopressors are utilized to support blood pressure and/or to improve cardiac output rather than as a specific treatment for the lungs. Fluid therapy and the associated need for vasopressor intervention may reflect the clinical decisions that the clinician has made about fluid balance. For example, if the clinician favors relative hypovolemia as a treatment strategy for ARDS, it may be difficult to maintain adequate blood pressure without using vasopressors in a septic patient. Another dilemma surrounds the use of vasodilators in an attempt to limit pulmonary arterial hypertension, which can be common in ALI/ARDS patients.[14] Although pulmonary arterial hypertension can be alleviated by intravenous vasodilators such as nitroprusside, nitroglycerin, and prostaglandin E_1, their effects are not isolated and can lead to systemic hypotension.[17] Furthermore, nonselective pulmonary vasodilation may increase intrapulmonary shunting and worsen hypoxemia.[17]

More novel approaches include the use of specific agents targeting many of the inflammatory mediators. However, no effective drug has been identified to date.[18] This is perhaps not surprising given the multitude of mediators involved and similar failures in other multifaceted diseases such as sepsis, systemic inflammatory response syndrome, and multiple organ dysfunction syndrome.

Most, if not all, people with ARDS require intermittent positive pressure ventilation for respiratory support. Because of the inflammatory process within the lungs, the lungs become stiff or noncompliant. This is clinically appreciated by the necessity of requiring increasingly higher and higher airway pressures to inflate the lungs to a specific volume. For example, in a normal 20-kg dog, a peak inspiratory pressure of 10 to 15 cm H_2O would result in a inspired tidal volume of 150 to 250 ml of air, whereas a dog with severe ARDS (and poor lung compliance) would require an inspiratory pressure of 40 cm H_2O or more to achieve the same inspiratory tidal volume. As may easily be imagined, an individual patient is not able to consistently maintain that degree of inspiratory effort (work) without the rapid onset of respiratory fatigue because the work (W) of breathing is measured by the product of pressure and volume.

Intermittent positive pressure ventilation (IPPV) permits the delivery of higher concentrations of oxygen and prevents respiratory fatigue and subsequent failure. However, inspired oxygen concentrations of greater than 60% have been associated with oxygen toxicity.[19] Positive end-expiratory pressure (PEEP) is commonly employed in order to recruit additional alveoli that may be collapsed and not participating in ventilation. Additionally, the application of PEEP should permit the maintenance of arterial oxygen saturation at lower concentrations of inspired oxygen. Negative effects of PEEP include decreasing cardiac output because of inhibition of cardiac filling. Additionally, IPPV may also paradoxically worsen lung injury and contribute to ongoing lung abnormalities and increase the likelihood of contracting ventilator-associated pneumonia. To minimize ventilator-related pulmonary injury, lung-protective ventilatory strategies have been developed; these have recently been shown to be quite effective in humans.[20] Ventilating at lower tidal volumes and higher PEEP pressures has been documented to increase survival and to limit ventilator-dependent days in people with ARDS.[21]

Other supportive care measures designed to address the underlying disease processes include intravenous fluid support, antimicrobials, gastric ulcer prophylaxis, and nutritional interventions. In humans, optimal fluid management remains highly controversial in the treatment of ARDS.[22] Many believe that restricting intravenous fluids reduces pulmonary edema and improves gas exchange,[13] whereas others have gone as far as to use diuretics and colloids in the management of ARDS patients.[23] Criticalists continue to debate the advantages and disadvantages of aggressive fluid therapy versus mild dehydration; however, no consensus has been reached at this time.

In dogs, very little is known about optimal therapeutic approaches in the treatment of ALI/ARDS. Certainly, standard supportive measures such as fluid therapy, transfusions, antimicrobials, and nutritional interventions are beneficial in many severe conditions. However, as with other systemic inflammatory diseases, addressing the underlying cause is ideal. As critical care techniques advance, increasing numbers of dogs will receive mechanical ventilation as part of their overall medical management. It is prudent for the clinician to try to distinguish ALI/ARDS from other disease processes for which directed therapies are available. The other common causes of hospital-onset respiratory disease in dogs include pneumonia, pulmonary thromboembolism, and congestive heart failure/volume overload, all of which may be more treatable than advanced ARDS. It is un-

clear how many dogs with ALI/ARDS may be sufficiently supported to allow for return of pulmonary function given that several weeks are required for pulmonary recovery. However, in cases with potentially reversible underlying disease, long-term mechanical ventilation offers the best chance for survival and should be pursued.

REFERENCES

1. Ashbaugh DG, Bigelow DB, Petty TL et al: Acute respiratory distress in adults, *Lancet* 2:319-323, 1967.
2. Navarrete-Navarro P, Rodriguez A, Reynolds N et al: Acute respiratory distress syndrome among trauma patients: Trends in ICU mortality, risk factors, complications and resource utilization, *Int Care Med* 27:1133-1140, 2001.
3. Hudson LD, Milberg JA, Anardi D et al: Clinical risks for development of the acute respiratory distress syndrome, *Am J Resp Crit Care Med* 151:293-301, 1995.
4. Turk J, Miller M, Broen T et al: Coliform septicaemia and pulmonary disease associated with canine parvoviral enteritis: 88 cases (1987-1988), *J Am Vet Med Assoc* 196(5):771-773, 1990.
5. Frevert CW, Warner AE: Respiratory distress resulting from acute lung injury in the veterinary patient, *J Vet Intern Med* 6:154-165, 1992.
6. Orsher AN, Kolata RJ: Acute respiratory distress syndrome case report and literature review, *J Am Anim Hosp Assoc* 1:41-46, 1992.
7. Lopez A, Lane IF, Hanna P: Adult respiratory distress syndrome in a dog with necrotizing pancreatitis, *Can Vet J* 36:240-241, 1995.
8. Jarvinen AK, Saario E, Andresen E et al: Lung injury leading to respiratory distress syndrome in young Dalmatian dogs, *J Vet Intern Med* 9:162-168, 1995.
9. Parent C, King LG, Walker LM et al: Clinical and clinicopathologic findings in dogs with acute respiratory distress syndrome: 19 cases (1985-1993), *J Am Vet Med Assoc* 208:1419-1427, 1996.
10. Parent C, King LG, Van Winkle TJ et al: Respiratory function and treatment in dogs with acute respiratory distress syndrome: 19 cases (1985-1993), *J Am Vet Med Assoc* 208:1428-1433, 1996.
11. Bernard GR, Artigas A, Brigham KL et al: Consensus Committee: The American-European Consensus Conference on ARDS: Definitions, mechanisms, relevant outcomes, and clinical trial coordination, *Am J Respir Crit Care Med* 149:818-824, 1994.
12. TenHoor T, Mannino DM, Moss M: Risk factors for ARDS in the United States: Analysis of the 1993 National Mortality Followback Study, *Chest* 119:1179-1184, 2001.
13. Weinacker AB, Vaszar LT: Acute respiratory distress syndrome: Physiology and new management strategies, *Ann Rev Med* 52:221-237, 2001.
14. Brower RG, Ware LB, Berthiaume Y et al: Treatment of ARDS, *Chest* 120:1347-1367, 2001.
15. Anderson ID, Fearon KC, Grant IS: Laparotomy for abdominal sepsis in the critically ill, *Br J Surg* 83:535-539, 1996.
16. Gilli Y, Binswanger U: Continuous pulse-oxymetry during haemodialysis, *Nephron* 55:368-371, 1990.
17. McIntyre RC, Pulido EJ, Bensard DD et al: Thirty years of clinical trials in acute respiratory distress syndrome, *Crit Care Med* 28(9): 3314-3331, 2000.
18. Tasaka S, Hasegawa N, Ishizaka A: Pharmacology of acute lung injury, *Pulm Pharm Ther* 15:83-95, 2002.
19. Halliwell B, Gutteridge JM: Oxygen toxicity, oxygen radicals, transition metals and disease, *J Biochem* 219:1-14, 1984.
20. Lee WL, Detsky AS, Stewart TE: Lung-protective mechanical ventilation strategies in ARDS, *Int Care Med* 26:1151-1155, 2000.
21. The Acute Respiratory Distress Syndrome Network: Ventilation with lower tidal volumes as compared with traditional tidal volumes for acute lung injury and the acute respiratory distress syndrome, *N Engl J Med* 342:1301-1308, 2000.
22. Schuller D, Mitchell JP, Calandrino FS et al: Fluid balance during pulmonary edema. Is fluid gain a marker or a cause of poor outcome? *Chest* 100:1068-1075, 1991.
23. Martin GS: Fluid balance and colloid osmotic pressure in acute respiratory failure: emerging clinical evidence, *Crit Care* 4(suppl 2):S21-S25, 2000.

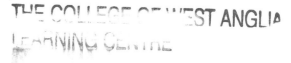

CHAPTER 69

Pulmonary and Bronchial Neoplasia

Jennifer L. Baez • Karin U. Sorenmo

Classification and Etiology

Primary lung tumors in the dog and cat can be described by their site of origin (e.g., bronchial, bronchial gland, or alveolar) and by their pathological appearance (e.g., adenocarcinoma, squamous cell carcinoma, or anaplastic carcinoma).[1,2] Often, it is difficult to classify lung tumors based on location because they tend to be discovered when they are too advanced to identify the site of origin.[2]

There is a strong association between lung cancer and cigarette smoking in humans. An estimated 80% of men and 75% of women that are diagnosed with lung cancer have a history of smoking.[3] More relevant to the situation in dogs and cats, a smaller study showed that 17% of cases of lung cancer among nonsmokers result from passive exposure to smoke during childhood and adolescence.[4] Exposure to other substances such as radon, asbestos, bis(chloromethyl) ether, polycyclic aromatic hydrocarbons, chromium, nickel, and inorganic arsenic compounds has also been associated with increased risk of lung cancer in people.[5,6] Primary lung tumors are rare in dogs and cats, and an etiology in dogs and cats is not as clear. One study found an increased incidence of primary lung tumors in dogs living in urban areas,[7] but an earlier study found no association with urban living.[8] Anatomical conformation may also play a part in susceptibility of dogs, with a report from 1992 showing an increased risk of developing primary lung tumors in brachycephalic dogs exposed to second-hand smoke, compared with dolichocephalic breeds.[9] The assumption that dolichocephalic breeds have a more efficient upper respiratory filtration ability than brachycephalic dogs may explain these differences.

Pathophysiology and Incidence

Lung cancer is the leading cause of cancer death in men and women in the United States, with an incidence exceeding 70 cases per 100,000 men.[10] Although the incidence of primary lung tumors in dogs and cats is reported to be increasing over the last 20 years,[2,11,12] it is still not as common as in humans. Older reports show the incidence of lung cancer in dogs to be 5.6 cases per 100,000 dogs, and only 2.2 cases per 100,000 cats.[13] In general, pulmonary metastatic cancer is more common than primary lung cancer in dogs and cats,[2,14] and patients with multiple lung masses or diffuse pulmonary involvement should be evaluated for a possible nonpulmonary primary tumor.

Geriatric canine and feline animals are the population most commonly diagnosed with primary lung neoplasia. The average age of dogs with primary lung tumors is reported in many studies to be between 9.3 and 10.9 years, with a range of 5 to 12 years.[7,11,15-17] The average age of affected cats is 11 to 12.5 years, with a range of 2 to 18 years.[11,14,17-19]

Historical Findings and Clinical Signs

Clinical signs on presentation depend on the extent of the pulmonary involvement, the presence of metastasis, and associated paraneoplastic syndromes. As many as 25% to 56% of cases are asymptomatic at presentation[7,15,20] and the lung tumor is an incidental finding. In symptomatic cases, the most common (52% to 93%) presenting complaint is a nonproductive cough of several weeks to months duration.[2,7,15,16,21] Less common clinical signs that have been reported include dyspnea associated with hemothorax, pneumothorax, and pleural effusion.[22] Pleural effusions are more commonly associated with primary lung tumors than metastatic lung disease, and effusions are often seen secondary to pleural involvement.[11,18,23] Pleural effusion can result from direct invasion of the pleura or pleural lymphatics by tumor cells.[24] In a study of 210 dogs with primary lung tumors, lethargy and weight loss were seen in 18.1% and 12.4% of the cases, respectively.[7] Other less commonly seen signs were tachypnea, lameness, wheezing, and hemoptysis.[7,15] An uncommon presentation in one report was the appearance of cutaneous flushing associated with two different pulmonary tumors in one dog.[25] Edema of the head and neck from compression of the anterior vena cava (anterior vena cava syndrome) can occur secondary to metastatic spread to mediastinal lymph nodes.[21,23]

Long bones have been reported as the third most common site for metastasis, after lung and thoracic lymph nodes.[15] Lameness can be associated with metastasis to bones, or with the paraneoplastic syndrome, hypertrophic osteopathy (HO).[23,26] Hypertrophic osteopathy is rare in dogs (3% to 17%)[1,7,15,27] but is even more uncommon in cats, with cats according to some reports never exhibiting the syndrome.[18,28-31] The pathogenesis of HO is not fully understood but may be related to increased limb bloodflow, thought to be mediated by a neural afferent component associated with the pulmonary mass.[32] This increased bloodflow leads to a proliferation of connective tissue and periosteum, which is possibly stimulated by prostaglandins or other humoral and neuronal factors.[33,34] One report supporting the suggestion that neuronal factors may be involved in the pathogenesis of HO showed regression of the bony lesions with vagotomy.[35] More recent hypotheses propose the existence of right-to-left shunts, associated with pulmonary neoplasia, that lead to platelet clumps and megakaryocytes circumventing the vasculature of the lungs and migrating to the periphery. Once there, platelets release platelet-derived growth factor (PDGF) that results in increased vascular permeability, which subsequently attracts fibroblasts and inflammatory cells and results in the periosteal reaction seen with HO.[36-41]

Other reported paraneoplastic syndromes include hypercalcemia, which is more commonly associated with lymphosarcoma and anal sac carcinoma. There is one report of hypercalcemia in a dog with epidermoid carcinoma of the lung.[24] In humans, peripheral neuropathy and polymyositis have been associated with lung cancer.[42] Such paraneoplastic syndromes are either not common in the dog or are not recognized, although there is one report of a dog with carcinoma of the lungs presenting with a generalized neuromyopathy.[43]

Clinical signs in cats with primary lung tumors tend to be more variable.[11,12,14,18] In general, clinical signs in cats are referable to disease in the respiratory tract (e.g., tachypnea, dyspnea, and coughing), as well as to metastatic lesions (e.g., lameness caused by skeletal muscle metastasis).[29] Some cats have been reported to present with signs of lameness and pain and no respiratory signs.[44] A recent retrospective study of 86 cats showed that the most common clinical signs in cats with primary lung cancer were weight loss, lameness, and lethargy, in addition to dyspnea and other respiratory signs.[19] The clinical signs with the longest median duration before referral were nonproductive coughing, weight loss, and lameness. Other less commonly reported signs seen in cats include fever and anorexia. Concurrent diseases such as hyperthyroidism, FeLV, and FIV infection are also reported.[1,19]

Biological Behavior

Metastasis of pulmonary neoplasms occurs via the bloodstream or lymphatics, as well as through the airways.[1] It has been reported that more malignant neoplasms spread via lymphatics and blood vessels, whereas less malignant forms spread by direct extension and are limited to the pulmonary parenchyma.[12] In dogs, metastatic lesions tend to occur primarily within the thoracic cavity (e.g., lung, pleura, lymph nodes, heart and pericardium) but other sites include the kidneys, liver, spleen, bone, brain, and skeletal muscles.* There is one case report of metastatic disease to the brainstem of a dog with primary pulmonary adenocarcinoma.[46] An early study reported that in the dog, metastases most often occurred to the lung itself.[15] This may occur because of the lung's central location with respect to the vascular system and lymphatics, through which metastases are distributed.[15]

In contrast to dogs, 71% of 38 cats in one study had extrapulmonary metastasis at sites that included regional lymph nodes, pleura, mediastinum, heart, kidney, axial skeleton, liver, spleen, esophagus, appendicular skeleton, peripheral arteries, skeletal muscle, bladder, pancreas, adrenal glands, and intestines.[14] A similar distribution of metastasis was reported in other studies.[11,19,24] When correlated with the tumor type in cats in this study, the rate of metastasis was 70% of adenocarcinomas (19/27), 83% of bronchioalveolar carcinomas (5/6), and 60% of squamous cell carcinomas (3/5).[14] Another, larger study involving 86 cats reported that 75.6% of the cats had evidence of metastatic disease.[19] Lymph node metastasis was seen in 25 cats, metastasis to the pleural cavity occurred in 26 cats, and 40 cats had evidence of distant metastasis.[19] Spread to lymph nodes may not be detectable radiographically but is often found on biopsy of the lymph node.[29] Several reports describe unusual presentations of metastatic disease of primary pulmonary neoplasia in cats, with one manifestation in particular involving the digits.[44,47-50] The reason for this particular site of metastasis is not fully understood, but one proposed theory suggests that the vasculature of the feline foot, specifically designed to facilitate heat loss, may increase the probability of digital metastasis.[44] Ocular metastasis has been reported in cats, with one reported cat presenting only for ocular signs.[51,52]

Diagnostic Tests

THORACIC RADIOGRAPHY

The most important tool for diagnosis of a pulmonary neoplasm is thoracic radiography.[1,14,15,21,53] According to a report evaluating pulmonary neoplasia in a colony of beagles, most of the dogs were asymptomatic until the masses were 3 cm in diameter or larger on radiographs.[53] Many factors affect the sensitivity of detection of a lung mass. The tissue surrounding the mass itself can obscure a lesion if the opacity of both tissues is similar. In addition, the opacity of the surrounding pulmonary parenchyma depends on how well the lung is aerated when the radiograph is taken.[23] A well-inflated lung, or a radiograph taken at full inspiration, optimizes the visibility of smaller lesions. Nonetheless, it was shown in one study that the lower limit for visualization of pulmonary lesions is 3 to 5 mm.[23] The necessity of taking three views of the thorax (i.e., right lateral, left lateral, and ventrodorsal projections) to better visualize lesions

---

*References 2, 12, 15, 17, 18, and 45.

has also been well documented.[23,54,55] Commonly, small nodules (less than 1 cm) that are not seen in the ventrodorsal view are easily seen in a lateral projection.

Despite following these guidelines, lesions may be obscured for other reasons. One study showed that 24 of 179 radiographs did not show evidence of pulmonary neoplasia despite positive necropsy findings.[23] Possible reasons include the presence of nodules less than 3 mm in size, and lesions hidden in atelectatic lung lobes or pleural effusion. In addition, some nodules up to 10 mm were not detected because of their location; in the subpleural space, hilar area, and caudal lung lobes it can be difficult to identify lesions because of overlying tissues and nearby organs.[23]

In dogs, primary pulmonary neoplasms are most commonly identified as solitary masses from one to several centimeters in diameter (Figures 69-1 and 69-2).[23] Other patterns seen in dogs include multiple nodular lesions (metastatic disease), disseminated mixed alveolar-interstitial and peribronchial patterns, and a homogenous alveolar pattern involving one or several lung lobes or marked lobar consolidation.[17,23] Pulmonary tumors may be found in the right lung as often as in the left lung in both dogs and cats.[14,19] However, a few reports suggest that the right lung is more commonly affected in dogs because of the larger parenchymal area.[12,45] Some authors note a correlation between radiographic appearance and histologic description of pulmonary neoplasia.[14,23] One review of primary lung tumors in the dog and cat found that squamous cell carcinomas were typically located in the perihilar region in the dog, though in cats the more common location appeared to be the middle and peripheral portions of the lung.[18] Adenocarcinomas were mostly found in the lung periphery, whereas bronchioalveolar carcinomas were seen as solitary nodules in the middle and peripheral lung regions. Once again, a difference in presentation was seen in cats, with adenocarcinomas in the feline lung appearing more as an amorphous consolidation of the pulmonary parenchyma. Occasionally, dogs had a mixed alveolar/interstitial pattern or consolidation as in the cat.[18] Conversely, other studies have shown no correlation between radiographic pattern and histological diagnosis.[17]

Radiographically, the appearance of primary lung tumors in cats tends to be more variable.[1,11,14] A study of 20 cats with primary lung tumors did not reveal one characteristic appearance but rather many different presentations including a solitary mass, multiple masses, consolidated lung lobes, a nodular interstitial pattern, pleural effusion, and a normal appearance.[11] Another review examined radiographs from 41 cats with primary lung tumors and found that 56% of the cats had focal

A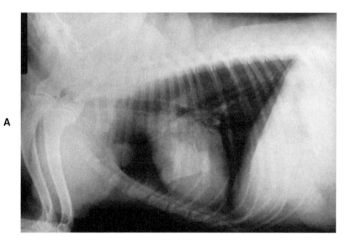

B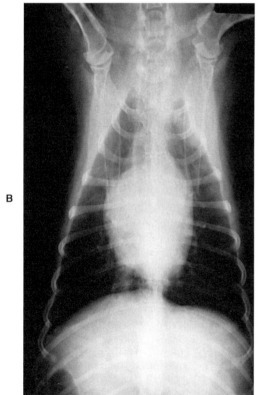

*Figure 69-1. **A**, Lateral and **B**, ventrodorsal radiographs of a 9-year-old dog with a well-circumscribed pulmonary neoplasm in the left cranial lung lobe.*

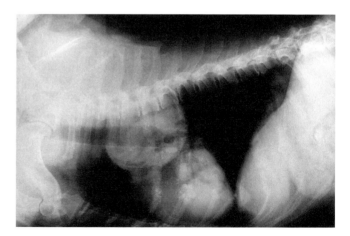

Figure 69-2. Lateral radiograph of a 10-year-old basset hound with a large, well-circumscribed neoplasm in the perihilar region, as well as multiple small pulmonary masses overlying the cardiac silhouette.

abnormalities (including solitary or multiple masses), 20% had a localized pattern, 24% had a diffuse pattern, and 7% of the cats had a normal radiographic appearance.[14] The variety of radiographic patterns makes it difficult to correlate the histological appearance of pulmonary tumors in cats to radiographic appearance. In the series of 41 cases, adenocarcinomas were either seen as well circumscribed, occasionally cavitated lesions in the middle or peripheral portion of the lung lobe; or as lobar alveolar pulmonary infiltrates, often with calcification.[14] Bronchioalveolar carcinomas were seen as multifocal or diffuse opacities in the middle to peripheral portion of affected lobes, and squamous cell carcinomas of the feline lung were too variable to generalize.[14]

ULTRASONOGRAPHY

Ultrasonography, though not a preferred method of diagnosing primary lung tumors, can be used to evaluate certain disease states in the thoracic cavity.[56] Ultrasound cannot penetrate air-filled structures, which limits its usefulness to consolidated lung lobes or to lung lobes displaced by fluid or a mass. In these cases, ultrasound can be used to visualize a mass and to perform ultrasound guided fine needle aspirates or biopsies. If a pleural effusion is present, ultrasonography can be used to estimate the amount of fluid and to distinguish fluid from soft tissue in the pleural cavity. Because fluid is a good medium for transmission of ultrasound images, masses that are obscured by pleural effusion on radiographs may be visualized using ultrasonography.[56] If a pleural effusion is identified, ultrasound can aid thoracocentesis.

CYTOLOGY

Cytological evaluation of pleural effusion may be helpful, though in general is not very specific because many tumors do not exfoliate into pleural fluid.[57,58] Effusions associated with neoplastic processes tend to be modified transudates or exudates, so neoplasia cannot be automatically ruled out even if the fluid is of low cellularity.[21,24] The usefulness of cytology of pleural effusion seems to vary, as is shown in one study of cats with pulmonary neoplasms, where a diagnosis was confirmed based on the cytology of pleural effusion in 12 of 13 cats that had thoracocentesis performed (Figures 69-3 and 69-4).[19] Conversely, in another study that specifically evaluated cats with lung cancer, samples from 8 cats with known pulmonary neoplasia were analyzed. Pleural effusions were primarily modified transudates, and a positive diagnosis of cancer was only obtained from one sample.[29] Another investigator evaluating prognostic factors in dogs with primary lung tumors found that cytological evaluation did not aid in making a diagnosis or change the outcome in 3 of 67 dogs that had pleural effusion analyzed.[59]

Fluids obtained via tracheal wash or bronchoalveolar lavage can also be cytologically analyzed. These techniques provide the most information when there is interstitial or alveolar disease rather than a focal pulmonary lesion.[7,24,60,61] However, marked inflammation may result in significant epithelial hyperplasia, which can be difficult to differentiate from neoplastic epithelial cells.[24,61] The presence of anaplastic epithelial cells without inflammation makes the diagnosis more straightforward. In human oncology, sputum analysis is used to detect any evidence of dysplastic change. Although not a good test for early detection of lung cancer, severe dysplasia may indicate a high risk for its development.[62] When a solitary

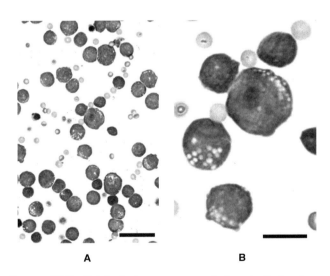

Figure 69-3. Cytological appearance of pleural effusion in an FeLV positive cat with lymphosarcoma. **A,** The neoplastic lymphoblasts are moderately large to large with round nuclei, very fine chromatin, variably sized nucleoli, and a narrow rim of finely vacuolated dark blue cytoplasm. Normal lymphocytes are slightly larger than erythrocytes. Bar = 25 μm. **B,** Higher magnification of A. Bar = 10 μm. (Courtesy Dr. Patricia McManus, University of Pennsylvania, Philadelphia.)

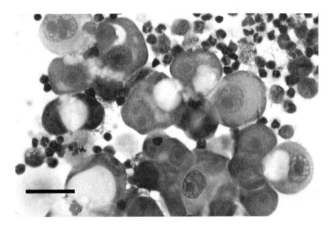

Figure 69-4. Cytological appearance of pleural effusion in a cat with metastatic mammary adenocarcinoma. The neoplastic epithelial cells display classic cytological criteria of malignancy: marked anisocytosis, marked anisokaryosis, large to giant nucleoli, and variable nuclear:cytoplasmic ratios. The cells also display cell to cell adhesion, which helps identify them as epithelial in derivation, although mesotheliomas can also display this trait. The smallest cells in the field are mostly neutrophils and macrophages. Bar = 25 μm. (Courtesy Dr. Patricia McManus, University of Pennsylvania, Philadelphia.)

lung lesion is present, the low yield from tracheal washes or bronchoalveolar lavage may warrant proceeding directly to a biopsy.[59]

OTHER IMAGING MODALITIES

With increased accessibility of imaging modalities such as computed tomography (CT) and magnetic resonance imaging (MRI), identifying pulmonary neoplasia may be possible with yet another type of diagnostic test. In human oncology, CT is used to stage lung cancer when additional information beyond that provided by survey radiographs is needed.[63] CT can also be used to visualize lesions for biopsy in veterinary, as well as in human patients.[64] MRI is thought to be more useful in providing information about the actual size of the tumor and involvement of nearby structures, especially blood vessels.[63,65,66] Ultimately, a biopsy and histopathological diagnosis is still needed for definitive diagnosis, but both CT and MRI can provide useful information for staging and potential treatment of pulmonary tumors.

BIOPSY

Methods to obtain biopsies of pulmonary masses include percutaneous fine-needle aspiration, percutaneous needle core biopsy, transbronchoscopic biopsy, and thoracotomy.[1,21,24,67] Peripherally located lesions may be amenable to transthoracic fine-needle aspiration, although occasionally these tumors have a necrotic center that can preclude a cytological diagnosis.[67] Fine-needle lung aspirates have also been used to diagnose disseminated pulmonary parenchymal disease, and are indicated for patients considered poor candidates for open thoracotomy and biopsy.[68] Contraindications for the procedure include coagulopathy, severe coughing, pulmonary hypertension, pulmonary cysts, and severe bullous emphysema.[68] In general, the complication rate for fine-needle aspirates of the lung in humans is low and includes pneumothorax, pericardial tamponade, pleural effusions, and intrapulmonary hemorrhage with hemoptysis.[69] In one study evaluating transthoracic core needle aspiration biopsy in dogs and cats, pneumothorax occurred in 31% of the cases but required drainage in only 6.2%.[69] However, a diagnosis of malignancy was accurately made in 22 of 27 dogs with pulmonary neoplastic disease.[69] Another smaller study describes the use of fine-needle aspirates of pulmonary masses in 4 dogs, with cytology confirming a neoplastic process in 2 of the dogs.[16] In a similar report reviewing 86 cats with primary lung tumors, a definitive diagnosis was made in 20 of 25 cats by fine-needle aspiration of a mass.[19] In a larger study of 210 dogs, a definitive diagnosis of primary pulmonary neoplasia was made preoperatively in 38.6% of the dogs using a variety of techniques including fine-needle aspiration cytology, which led to a successful diagnosis 79% of the time (52 of 66 attempts).[7] Other techniques to obtain samples for cytological or histopathological analysis include the use of a cutting needle biopsy and transbronchial biopsy via a fiberoptic bronchoscope. Neither of these techniques is routinely used in dogs and cats.[24,68]

If a histopathological or cytological diagnosis cannot be obtained using the methods discussed above, an open lung biopsy may be indicated. Specific indications for thoracotomy and lung biopsy include the presence of a single lesion that has not been successfully diagnosed using less invasive means, the presence of a diffuse process without a concurrent pleural effusion, and the need to specifically treat a solitary pulmonary mass by resecting it.[24] Advantages of this approach include the ability to clearly visualize most structures in the thorax and the opportunity to obtain a large tissue sample or remove the mass under controlled conditions.[24]

Pathological and Histopathological Findings

Neoplasms of the lung can exhibit many different histologic patterns; in general, the neoplasm is named after the most differentiated cell type present.[2] If a tumor is composed entirely of undifferentiated cell types, it is called undifferentiated or anaplastic.[18] Histopathological types of primary pulmonary tumors include adenocarcinomas, squamous cell carcinomas, anaplastic carcinomas, and bronchioalveolar carcinomas. Primary lung tumors of connective tissue origin are less common and include primary hemangiosarcoma,[2] sarcoma,[19] and malignant fibrous histiocytoma.[19] In general, the degree of differentiation correlates with biological behavior. For example, undifferentiated adenocarcinomas, though less common than well-differentiated adenocarcinomas, have a greater tendency to metastasize and are also more invasive.[18] One investigator reported that dogs with a confirmed diagnosis of differentiated adenocarcinoma had a longer survival time than dogs with undifferentiated adenocarcinoma.[7] However, this difference was not statistically significant. In cats, the undifferentiated or poorly differentiated cell type predominates, and one study evaluating 86 cats with primary lung tumors found that the majority of cats (76%) had lung tumors of bronchial origin.[19]

In one study, adenocarcinoma, both differentiated and undifferentiated, was the most prevalent lung tumor type,[2] encompassing 132 of 171 (77%) of all malignant epithelial tumors in dogs and 34 of 47 (72%) in cats. Less commonly occurring cell types included squamous cell carcinomas (in 11 of 171 dogs with malignant epithelial tumors and 2 of 47 cats with malignant epithelial tumors) and bronchial gland carcinomas (in 2 dogs and 6 cats in the same population). Alveolar cell carcinomas also occurred in 26 dogs and 5 cats, and were subclassified into anaplastic small cell, anaplastic large cell, and "adenomatosis."[2] The percentage of adenocarcinomas found in this study is comparable to the reported frequency of 80% in other studies.[13,15,29,53] In another report evaluating 210 dogs with pulmonary tumors, the percentage of dogs with differentiated and undifferentiated adenocarcinoma (74.8%) was similar.[7] Squamous cell carcinoma tends to occur more commonly in humans than in dogs (6%[2] and 1.9%[7]) and cats (4%).[2]

Treatment and Prognosis

The most effective and commonly recommended treatment for pulmonary tumors in dogs and cats is surgical excision.* Additional advantages to performing a thoracotomy include obtaining an accurate diagnosis, accessibility of other lung lobes for evaluation, and staging of the neoplasm by biopsy of the draining lymph nodes. In general, a partial or complete lobectomy is recommended,[18,21,67] and is an excellent option for dogs or cats that have a solitary mass and whose medical status is unaffected by concurrent disease or tumor associated complications.[24] In a group of 15 dogs treated surgically for pulmonary neoplasia, postoperative hospitalization was less than 4 days, and all 15 dogs recovered without major complications.[11,16] Six of these dogs were symptom-free at a mean of 20 months (range 4 to 46 months) following surgery.[16] The remaining nine dogs had died or had been euthanized, and the mean survival time for these dogs treated with surgery alone was 10 months (range 7 to 19 months).[16] All deaths were caused by recurrence of the primary mass or metastatic disease.[16]

In another report of 76 dogs with pulmonary neoplasia treated surgically, 55 of the 76 dogs were in complete remission postoperatively and had a median survival time of 330 days, compared with 28 days for dogs that did not have a complete resection of their tumors.[70] A similar study of 67 dogs with pulmonary neoplasia reported a range of survival from 0 to 1437 days (median 361 days) with hospitalization times from 0 to 12 days (mean 3 days).[59] In a study designed to analyze the incidence of primary lung neoplasia in a beagle colony, survival time in 24 dogs that were not treated after detection of masses was 313 days, with a range of 5 to 1266 days.[53] In 16 of these dogs, however, the masses were small and clinically silent.[53] In another report evaluating 21 cats with primary lung tumors, after surgical resection 18 cats died from metastatic disease with a median survival time of 115 days (range 13 to 1526 days).[71] The cats' survival times were influenced by histological type, with cats more likely to have anaplastic tumors than dogs.[71]

Chemotherapy has not been fully evaluated in the treatment of lung tumors, and information regarding its usefulness or effectiveness in dogs and cats is not available. Chemotherapy is routinely used in human patients with small cell lung cancer, with fourfold to fivefold improvement of survival times over patients not treated with chemotherapy.[72] It may therefore be worth further investigation in dogs and cats with small cell lung cancer. However, small cell lung cancer is rare in dogs and cats, and the response rates seen in human patients with other types of lung cancer treated with chemotherapy are not as impressive. The same trend (response based on histological type) may be seen in companion animals.[72]

Chemotherapeutic agents that have been used as single agents or in combination in dogs with primary pulmonary neoplasia include cyclophosphamide, vincristine, methotrexate, vindesine, and cisplatin.[16] The most favorable response was seen in 2 dogs treated with cisplatin and vindesine, with greater than 50% radiographic reduction of measurable lesions for at least 4 weeks.[16] In a report of 67 dogs with pulmonary masses, additional chemotherapeutics included doxorubicin and mitoxantrone, although the numbers of dogs treated were too small to derive any significant information regarding the impact of these agents on outcome.[59] Patients that might benefit from chemotherapy include those that require palliation for inoperable lesions, or if surgery is contraindicated; animals in which lesions recur after previous surgical excision[11]; or when negative prognostic factors (e.g., histological type and differentiation) or regional lymph node involvement exist (see Figures 69-3 and 69-4). Intracavitary chemotherapy with cisplatin has been shown to have some benefit in patients with malignant pleural effusions.[73]

Radiation therapy is commonly used to treat human patients with certain types of lung cancer, but it is largely untried in veterinary medicine.[67] Complications associated with irradiation of normal lung tissue at doses sufficient to kill neoplastic cells include pneumonitis followed by fibrosis as a later stage.[74] In humans, radiation is used in combination with chemotherapy or alternatively as palliative therapy, and it may be worth investigating in dogs in the future.[21,24]

Prognostic Factors and Outcome

Many prognostic variables have been evaluated in dogs and cats with primary lung tumors. A report of 67 dogs with primary lung neoplasia demonstrated that histologic score, the presence of clinical signs, and regional lymph node involvement affected outcome.[59] When lung tumors were discovered incidentally, the dogs had longer survival times compared with dogs with clinical signs attributable to their tumor (median survival 545 days versus 240 days). Dogs with regional lymph node involvement had shorter disease-free intervals (DFI) (6 days versus 351 days) and median survival times (26 days versus 452 days) than dogs with no lymph node involvement.[59]

The histological type of the tumor may also have prognostic significance. One report noted a correlation between histopathological diagnosis and metastatic rate, with metastasis in 50% of the adenocarcinomas, 100% of the squamous cell carcinomas, and 90% of the anaplastic or anaplastic mixed tumors.[15] In another study, dogs with well-differentiated tumors had longer survival times and DFI (median 790 and 493 days, respectively) than those with moderately (median 251 and 191 days) or poorly (median 5 and 0 days) differentiated tumors.[59] Similar correlation between histological differentiation and outcome was reported in another study: dogs with undifferentiated adenocarcinoma had shorter survival times than dogs with well-differentiated adenocarcinoma.[7] Though not common, dogs with pulmonary tumors diagnosed as squamous cell carcinoma have shorter median survival times (8 months) than dogs with adenocarcinoma (19 months).[16] Dogs with squamous cell carcinoma tend to have more common recurrence and lymph

---

*References 1, 7, 11, 18, 21, and 67.

node metastasis (greater than 90% risk) than those with other histological cell types such as adenocarcinoma (50% risk).[1] A similar correlation between histologic differentiation and prognosis was found in a report of 21 cats with surgical resection of a primary lung tumor.[71] The only prognostic factor identified in those cats was histological differentiation: cats with moderately differentiated lung tumors had a significantly longer survival time (median 698 days, range 19 to 1526 days) than cats with poorly differentiated tumors (median 75 days, range 13 to 634 days).[71]

In addition, the size of the tracheobronchial lymph nodes has prognostic significance: cats without enlarged tracheobronchial lymph nodes at surgery had a median survival time of 412 days, and cats with enlarged nodes had a median survival time of 73 days.[71] However, information about the tracheobronchial lymph node was available in only 12 of 21 cats.[71] A similar result was obtained in a study evaluating 76 cases of dogs with primary lung tumors.[70] Dogs with enlarged lymph nodes had shorter survival times than dogs with normal-sized lymph nodes (median 60 days with enlarged nodes and 345 days with normal-sized nodes).[70] Histological evaluation of the lymph nodes revealed a trend toward longer survival in dogs without histological evidence of metastasis compared with dogs with histological evidence of lymph node metastasis (120 days versus 60 days). However, this difference was not statistically significant.[70] Similar results were found in another study, with a median survival time of 14 months in dogs without lymph node metastasis compared with 10 months in dogs with metastasis. This was not statistically significant, but only small numbers of dogs were involved.[16] The authors concluded that it might be beneficial to remove affected lymph nodes at the time of surgical resection of the lung mass.

The location of the lung tumor may influence survival time.[16] According to a study of 15 dogs, those with tumors located at the base of the lung lobe had a mean survival time of 17.5 months, compared with a mean survival time of 15 months in those with tumors located at the periphery of the lung. Dogs with tumors involving an entire lobe had a median survival time of only 8 months.[16] Finally, size of the lung mass itself may have prognostic significance. In the same report of 15 dogs, 7 dogs with tumors less than 100 cc had mean survival times of 20 months, whereas 5 dogs with tumors that were greater than 100 cc but less than 1000 cc had a mean survival time of only 6.8 months. Other reported prognostic factors in cats include the presence of malignant pleural effusion or presence of metastatic disease, which obviously confers a poor prognosis.[21]

Pulmonary Lymphomatoid Granulomatosis

Pulmonary lymphomatoid granulomatosis (PLG) is a rare disorder seen in humans, dogs, and cats.[75] It has been described in humans as a disease of unknown etiology, with a pleomorphic infiltrate of an atypical lymphoid cell population that primarily centers around and apparently destroys blood vessels.[76] Other cells seen in this disease include small lymphocytes, plasma cells, occasional histiocytes, and eosinophils.[77] A similar cell distribution is seen in young dogs, with infiltrates of the same cells in bronchial lymph nodes and other organs.[17] Although the lesions are composed of lymphoid cells they are quite different from those seen in pulmonary lymphosarcoma.[17] Early reports in the human literature describe the clinical behavior of the disease to be similar to that of lymphoma, and progression of some cases of PLG to a more typical lymphoma was also reported.[76]

There does not appear to be either a breed or gender predilection to PLG.[77] Reported mean and median ages affected range from 2.7 to 8.4 years.[17,77-79] In general, a younger population of animals is affected compared with those with other primary lung tumors.

Clinical signs are similar to those of animals with pulmonary neoplasia (e.g., a nonproductive, dry cough; respiratory distress; anorexia; and weight loss).[17,77-79] Other reported, but less commonly seen symptoms include fever, lameness, peripheral lymphadenopathy, ascites, and vomiting.[17,77-79]

Consistent findings on serum biochemistry panels and urinalysis are not seen. The few reports of PLG describe hemogram abnormalities including leukocytosis, eosinophilia, and basophilia,[77-79] although many of the dogs included in these reports had concurrent or previous heartworm disease.[77,78] In another study of 7 dogs, none of the dogs tested positive for heartworm disease despite having basophilia as a consistent laboratory finding.[79]

Radiographic findings vary from lobar consolidation to large (greater than 5 cm) pulmonary masses.[79] Tracheobronchial lymph nodes were enlarged in 6 out of 7 dogs evaluated.[79] All of the dogs in that report also had a diffuse interstitial pattern, and 5 dogs had small amounts of pleural effusion.[79] Similar findings were reported in another study of 7 dogs with PLG.[77] Two dogs in that report had cranial mediastinal masses as well as sternal lymphadenopathy, and only 1 dog exhibited pleural effusion.[77] Diffuse or multiple nodular densities occurred most often in the diaphragmatic lobes in one study of 8 dogs with PLG.[78] Multiple abnormal pulmonary opacities in a variety of locations were noted in the one cat reported to have PLG,[75] as well as complete alveolar consolidation of the left lung lobes.

The same diagnostic procedures discussed for primary pulmonary neoplasia can be applied to PLG. A definitive diagnosis can only be obtained with histopathology, and in one study, 6 dogs had thoracotomies to obtain diagnostic biopsies.[77] Other procedures pursued in the report of 8 dogs with PLG included bronchoscopy in 2 dogs, and exploratory thoracotomy in 3 of the dogs.[78] In those dogs from which cytologic samples were obtained, the interpretations varied from chronic active inflammation with hemorrhage to other diagnoses (e.g., pyogranulomatous inflammation, eosinophilic granulomatous inflammation, and carcinoma).[78] The samples themselves consisted of erythrocytes, lymphocytes, large numbers of eosinophils, macrophages, and fewer binucleate cells and epithelial cells. This range of cell types seemed to vary depending on when the sample was obtained during the course of the disease; from case to case; and, finally, depending on how the sample was obtained.[78] Ultimately, histopathology is necessary to identify the characteristic angiocentric infiltration of pleomorphic lymphoid cells and the associated vessel destruction, in order to make a diagnosis of pulmonary lymphomatoid granulomatosis.

Metastasis associated with PLG was most commonly seen in the tracheobronchial lymph nodes of affected dogs, and the liver was the most common extrathoracic site of metastasis.[78] Other sites of metastasis were the heart, kidneys, spleen, pancreas, and adrenal gland, each occurring in different dogs.[78] Pleocellular infiltrates were identified at these sites. In humans, the origin of these infiltrates has been analyzed immunohistochemically and identified as T-lymphocytes.[76] In 1996, three cases of cutaneous lymphomatoid granulomatosis in dogs were examined with immunohistochemistry.[80] Two of the 3 dogs demonstrated variable CD3 antigen expression consistent with T-lymphocytes present in the cell population,[80] providing evidence that the disease in companion animals may have similar origins to that of human beings. The etiology of this disorder remains unknown in both animals and humans.

Because PLG is classified as a lymphoproliferative neoplasm, treatment has consisted of chemotherapeutics used in the treatment of lymphoma. In the report of 7 dogs with PLG, 4 were treated with protocols consisting of cyclophosphamide and prednisone; or with combinations of cyclophosphamide, vincristine, cytarabine, and prednisone.[77] Two dogs were treated with prednisone alone. No evidence of improvement was noted radiographically, and the survival time of the 7 dogs ranged from 6 days to 4 years, with a mean of 12.5 months and a median of 3 months.[77] Postorino and colleagues treated 5 dogs with chemotherapy, with some dogs receiving prednisone alone; others receiving prednisone and cyclophosphamide; and still others receiving prednisone, cyclophosphamide, and vincristine.[79] These investigators reported a 60% response rate (3 out of 5 dogs), and they concluded that a combination of cyclophosphamide and prednisone might be the treatment of choice for PLG.

REFERENCES

1. Fox LE, King RR: Cancers of the respiratory system. In Morrison WB, editor: *Cancer in dogs and cats,* Baltimore, 1998, Williams & Wilkins.
2. Moulton JE, von Tscharner C, Schneider R: Classification of lung carcinomas in the dog and cat, *Vet Path* 18:513-528, 1981.
3. Minna JD, Higgins GA, Glatstein EJ: Cancer of the lung. In DeVita VT Jr., Hellman S, Rosenberg SA, editors: *Cancer: Principles and practice of oncology,* ed 3, Philadelphia, 1989, JB Lippincott.
4. Janerich DT, Thompson WD, Varela LR et al: Lung cancer and exposure to tobacco smoke in the household, *N Engl J Med* 323:632, 1990.
5. Fraumeni JF Jr.: Carcinogenesis: An epidemiological appraisal, *J Nat'l Cancer Inst* 55:1039, 1975.
6. Fraumeni JF Jr., Blott WJ: Lung and pleura. In Schottenfeld D, Fraumeni JF Jr., editors: *Cancer epidemiology and prevention,* Philadelphia, 1982, WB Saunders.
7. Ogilvie GK, Haschek WM, Withrow SJ et al: Classification of primary lung tumors in dogs: 210 cases (1975-1985), *J Am Vet Med Assoc* 195:106-112, 1989.
8. Reif JS, Cohen D: The environmental distribution of canine respiratory tract neoplasms, *Arch Environ Health* 22:136-140, 1971.
9. Reif JS, Dunn K, Ogilvie GK et al: Passive smoking and canine lung cancer risk, *Int J Epidemiol* 135:234-239, 1992.
10. Ginsberg RJ, Vokes EE, Raben A: Non-small cell lung cancer. In DeVita VT Jr., Hellman S, Rosenberg SA, editors: *Cancer: Principles and practice of oncology,* ed 5, Philadelphia, 1997, Lippincott-Raven.
11. Melhlaff CJ, Mooney S: Primary pulmonary neoplasia in the dog and cat, *Vet Clin North Am Small Anim Pract* 15:1061-1068, 1985.
12. Moulton JE: Tumors of the respiratory system. In Moulton JE, editor: *Tumors in domestic animals,* Los Angeles, 1990, University of California Press.
13. Dorn CR, Taylor DON, Frye FL et al: Survey of animal neoplasms in Alameda and Contra Costa Counties, California. I. Methodology and description of cases, *J Nat'l Cancer Inst* 40:295-305, 1968.
14. Koblik PD: Radiographic appearance of primary lung tumors in cats. A review of 41 cases, *Vet Radiol* 27:66-73, 1986.
15. Brodey RS, Craig PG: Primary pulmonary neoplasms in the dog: A review of 29 cases, *J Am Vet Med Assoc* 147:1628-1643, 1965.
16. Melhlaff CJ, Leifer CE, Patnaik AM et al: Surgical treatment of primary pulmonary neoplasia in 15 dogs, *J Am Anim Hosp Assoc* 20:799-803, 1984.
17. Barr FJ, Gibbs C, Brown PJ: The radiologic features of primary lung tumours in the dog: A review of 36 cases, *J Small Anim Pract* 27:493-505, 1986.
18. Miles KG: A review of primary lung tumors in the dog and cat, *Vet Radiol* 29:122-128, 1988.
19. Hahn KA, McEntee MF: Primary lung tumors in domestic cats: 86 cases (1979-1994), *J Am Vet Med Assoc* 211:1257-1260, 1997.
20. Nielson SW, Horava A: Primary pulmonary tumors in the dog: A report of 16 cases, *Am J Vet Res* 21:813-830, 1960.
21. Ogilvie GK, Moore AS: Tumors of the respiratory system. In Ogilvie GK, Moore AS: *Managing the veterinary cancer patient: A practice manual,* Trenton, 1995, Veterinary Learning Systems.
22. Dallman MJ, Martin RA, Roth L: Pneumothorax as the primary problem in two cases of bronchioalveolar carcinoma in the dog, *J Am Anim Hosp Assoc* 24:710-714, 1988.
23. Suter PF, Carrig CB, O'Brien TR et al: Radiographic recognition of primary and metastatic pulmonary neoplasms of dogs and cats, *J Am Vet Radiol Soc* 15:3-25, 1974.
24. Stann SE, Bauer TG: Respiratory tract tumors, *Vet Clin North Am Small Anim Pract* 15:535-556, 1985.
25. Miller WH: Cutaneous flushing associated with intrathoracic neoplasia in a dog, *J Am Anim Hosp Assoc* 28:217-219, 1992.
26. Stephens LC, Gleiser CA, Jardine JH: Primary pulmonary fibrosarcoma associated with *Spirocerca lupi* infection in a dog with hypertrophic pulmonary osteopathy, *J Am Vet Med Assoc* 182:496-498, 1983.
27. Brodey RS: Hypertrophic osteoarthropathy in the dog: A clinicopathologic survey of 60 cases, *J Am Vet Med Assoc* 159:1242-1256, 1971.
28. Gram WD, Wheaton LG, Snyder PW et al: Feline hypertrophic osteopathy associated with pulmonary carcinoma, *J Am Anim Hosp Assoc* 26:425-428, 1990.
29. Barr IF, Gruffydd-Jones TJ, Brown PJ et al: Primary lung tumors in the cat, *J Small Anim Pract* 28:1115-1125, 1987.
30. Roberg J: Pulmonary osteoarthropathy, *Feline Pract* 7:6, 18, 20-22, 1977.
31. Nafe LE, Herron AJ, Burk RL: Hypertrophic osteopathy in a cat associated with renal papillary adenoma, *J Am Anim Hosp Assoc* 17:659-662, 1981.
32. Susaneck SJ, Macy DW: Hypertrophic osteopathy, *Compend Contin Educ Pract Vet* 4:689-694, 1982.
33. Lavi Y, Paladuga RK, Benfield JR: Hypertrophic pulmonary osteoarthropathy in experimental canine lung cancer, *J Thorac Cardiovas Surg* 84:373-376, 1982.
34. Morrison WB: Paraneoplastic syndromes of the dog, *J Am Vet Med Assoc* 175:559-561, 1979.
35. Watson ADJ, Porges WL: Regression of hypertrophic osteopathy in a dog following unilateral intrathoracic vagotomy, *Vet Rec* 93:240-243, 1973.
36. Dickinson CJ: The aetiology of clubbing and hypertrophic osteoarthropathy, *Eur J Clin Invest* 23:330-338, 1993.

37. Gladwin AM, Carrier MF, Beesley JE et al: Identification of mRNA for PDGF B-chain in human megakaryocytes isolated using a novel immunomagnetic separation method, *Br J Haematol* 76:333-339, 1990.

38. Huang JS, Huang SS, Kennedy B et al: Platelet-derived growth factor: Specific binding to target cells, *J Biol Chem* 257:8130-8136, 1982.

39. Kaplan KL, Broeckman MF, Chernoff A et al: Platelet alpha-granule proteins: Studies on release and subcellular localization, *Blood* 53:604-618, 1979.

40. Kohler N, Lipton A: Platelets as a source of fibroblast growth-promoting activity, *Exp Cell Res* 87:279-301, 1974.

41. Ross R, Glomset J, Kariya B et al: A platelet-dependent serum factor that stimulates the proliferation of arterial smooth muscle cells *in vitro*, *Proc Nat Acad Sci USA* 71:1207-1210, 1974.

42. Maddeus M, Ginsberg RJ: Diagnosis and staging. In Pearson FG, Cooper JD, Deslauriers J et al, editors: *Thoracic surgery*, New York, 1995, Churchill Livingstone.

43. Sorjonen DC, Braund KG, Joff EJ: Paraplegia and subclinical neuromyopathy associated with a primary lung tumor in a dog, *J Am Vet Med Assoc* 180:1209-1211, 1982.

44. Moore AS, Middleton DJ: Pulmonary adenocarcinoma in three cats with nonrespiratory signs only, *J Small Anim Pract* 23:501-509, 1982.

45. Suter PF, Lord PF: Lower airway and pulmonary parenchymal diseases. In Suter PF, editor: *Thoracic radiography: A text atlas of thoracic diseases of the dog and cat*, Davis, CA, 1984, Stonegate Press.

46. Moore JA, Taylor HW: Primary pulmonary adenocarcinoma with brain stem metastasis in a dog, *J Am Vet Med Assoc* 192:219-221, 1988.

47. Pollack M, Martin RA, Diters RW: Metastatic squamous cell carcinoma in multiple digits of a cat: Case report, *J Am Anim Hosp Assoc* 20:835-839, 1984.

48. May C, Newsholme SJ: Metastasis of feline pulmonary carcinoma presenting as multiple digit swelling, *J Small Anim Pract* 30:302-310, 1989.

49. Scott-Moncrief JC, Elliot GS, Radovsky A et al: Pulmonary squamous cell carcinoma with multiple digital metastases in a cat, *J Small Anim Pract* 30:696-699, 1989.

50. Gottfried SD, Popovitch CA, Goldschmidt MH et al: Metastatic digital carcinoma in the cat: A retrospective study of 36 cats, *J Am Anim Hosp Assoc* 36:501-509, 2000.

51. Gionfriddo JR, Fix AS, Niyo Y et al: Ocular manifestations of a metastatic pulmonary adenocarcinoma in a cat, *J Am Vet Med Assoc* 197:372-374, 1990.

52. Williams LW, Gelatt KN, Gwin RM: Ophthalmic neoplasms in the cat, *J Am Anim Hosp Assoc* 17:999-1008, 1981.

53. Hahn FF, Muggenburg BA, Griffith WC: Primary lung neoplasia in a beagle colony, *Vet Pathol* 33:633-638, 1996.

54. Lang J, Wortman JA, Glickman LT et al: Sensitivity of radiographic detection of lung metastases in the dog, *Vet Radiol* 27:74-78, 1986.

55. Biller DS, Myer CW: Case examples demonstrating the clinical utility of obtaining both right and left lateral thoracic radiographs in small animals, *J Am Anim Hosp Assoc* 23:381-386, 1987.

56. Stowater JL, Lamb CR: Ultrasonography of noncardiac thoracic diseases in small animals, *J Am Vet Med Assoc* 195:514-520, 1989.

57. Gruffydd-Jones TJ, Flecknell PA: The prognosis and treatment related to the gross appearance and laboratory characteristics of pathological thoracic fluids in the cat, *J Small Anim Pract* 19:315-328, 1978.

58. Biery DN: Differentiation of lung diseases of inflammatory or neoplastic origin from lung diseases in heart failure, *Vet Clin North Am Small Anim Pract* 4:711-721, 1974.

59. McNeil EA, Ogilvie GK, Powers BE et al: Evaluation of prognostic factors for dogs with primary lung tumors: 67 cases (1985-1992), *J Am Vet Med Assoc* 211:1422-1427, 1997.

60. Davis GS, Kelley J: Invasive techniques for the diagnosis of respiratory infections, *Clin Lab Med* 2:269-283, 1982.

61. Hawkins EC, Morrison WB, DeNicola DB et al: Cytologic analysis of bronchoalveolar lavage fluid from 47 dogs with multicentric malignant lymphoma, *J Am Vet Med Assoc* 203:1418-1425, 1993.

62. Pilotti S, Ralk EF, Gribaudi D et al: Sputum cytology for the diagnosis of carcinoma of the lung, *Acta Cytol* 26:649, 1982.

63. Gefter WB: Magnetic resonance imaging in the evaluation of lung cancer, *Sem Roentgenology* 25:73-84, 1990.

64. Tidwell AS, Johnson KL: Computed tomography-guided percutaneous biopsy in the dog and cat: Description of technique and preliminary evaluation in 14 patients, *Vet Radiol Ultrasound* 35:445-446, 1994.

65. Casamassima F, Villari N, Fargnoli R et al: Magnetic resonance imaging and high-resolution computed tomography in tumors of the lung and the mediastinum, *Radiother Oncol* 11:21-29, 1988.

66. Kennel SJ, Davis IA, Branning J et al: High resolution computed tomography and MRI for monitoring lung tumor growth in mice undergoing radioimmunotherapy: Correlation with histology, *Med Physics* 27:1101-1107, 2000.

67. Withrow SJ: Lung cancer. In Withrow SJ, MacEwen EG, editors: *Small animal clinical oncology*, ed 3, Philadelphia, 2001, WB Saunders.

68. Roudebush P, Green RA, Diglio KM: Percutaneous fine-needle aspiration biopsy of the lung in disseminated pulmonary disease, *J Am Anim Hosp Assoc* 17:109-116, 1981.

69. Teske E, Stokhof AA, Wolvekamp WTC et al: Transthoracic needle aspiration biopsy of the lung in dogs with pulmonic diseases, *J Am Anim Hosp Assoc* 27:289-294, 1991.

70. Ogilvie GK, Weigel RM, Haschek WM et al: Prognostic factors for tumor remission and survival in dogs after surgery for primary lung tumor: 76 cases (1975-1985), *J Am Vet Med Assoc* 195:109-112, 1989.

71. Hahn KA, McEntee MF: Prognosis for survival in cats after removal of a primary lung tumor: 21 cases (1979-1984), *Vet Surg* 27:307-311, 1998.

72. Ihde DC, Pass HI, Glatstein E: Small cell lung cancer. In DeVita VT, Hellman S, Rosenberg SA, editors: *Cancer: Principles and practice of oncology*, ed 5, Philadelphia, 1997, Lippincott-Raven.

73. Moore AS, Kirk C, Carcona A: Intracavitary cisplatin chemotherapy experience with six dogs, *J Vet Int Med* 5:227-231, 1991.

74. Larue SM, Gillette SM, Poulson JM: Radiation therapy of thoracic and abdominal tumors, *Sem Vet Med and Surg (SA)* 10:190-196, 1995.

75. Valentine BA, Blue JT, Zimmer JF et al: Pulmonary lymphomatoid granulomatosis in a cat, *J Vet Diagn Invest* 12:465-467, 2000.

76. Liebow AA, Carrington CR, Friedman PJ: Lymphomatoid granulomatosis, *Hum Pathol* 3:457-558, 1972.

77. Berry CR, Moore PF, Thomas WP et al: Pulmonary lymphomatoid granulomatosis in seven dogs (1976-1987), *J Vet Int Med* 4:157-166, 1993.

78. Fitzgerald SD, Wolf DC, Carlton WW: Eight cases of canine lymphomatoid granulomatosis, *Vet Pathol* 28:241-245, 1991.

79. Postorino NC, Wheeler SL, Park RD et al: A syndrome resembling lymphomatoid granulomatosis in the dog, *J Vet Int Med* 3:15-19, 1989.

80. Smith KC, Day MJ, Shaw SC et al: Canine lymphomatoid granulomatosis and immunophenotypic analysis of three cases, *J Comp Path* 115:129-138, 1996.

CHAPTER 70

Heartworm Infection

David H. Knight

Definition and Etiology

The heartworm, *Dirofilaria immitis,* is a filarial nematode transmitted between mammalian hosts by vector competent mosquitoes, which also serve as obligatory intermediate hosts in the parasite's life cycle. Domestic and sylvatic canids, domestic cats, and ferrets are the principal definitive hosts of veterinary importance. Though popularly named "heartworm" because some adults are nearly always found in the right ventricle during necropsy dissections of infected animals, in live dogs the worms reside primarily within the lumen of the pulmonary arterial tree. Pulmonary arterial vascular and variable degrees of pulmonary parenchymal disease are consistent distinguishing features of all infections with adult heartworms, but heart, liver and kidney complications also occur commonly in advanced stages of the heartworm disease syndrome.

An appreciation of the heartworm life cycle is central to understanding the pathogenesis of the disease. Embryos, called microfilariae, are released into the blood stream by productive female worms. Ordinarily, microfilariae circulate throughout the body and are ingested from subcutaneous capillaries by female mosquitoes taking a blood meal. Adult worm infections that do not produce a microfilaremia are referred to as being occult. Once ingested by the intermediate host mosquito, the parasite enters the temperature-dependent phase of its life cycle. The microfilariae are transformed into the first larval stage, which migrates from the midgut to the kidney, where they molt twice to the infective third stage, which migrates to the mouth parts of the insect. When the mosquito takes a second blood meal, the infective larvae are deposited in a pool of saliva on the skin, and enter the body of the definitive host through the bite wound. Maturation of infective larvae can occur as rapidly as 7 days at temperatures above 86° F, or take more than 30 days at temperatures below 65° F.[1]

Within the mammalian host, the infective third stage larvae promptly molt to a tissue migratory fourth stage, penetrate the systemic veins within 70 to 90 days postinfection, then begin the adult (fifth) stage of the life cycle. The immature fifth stage adults are embolized to the pulmonary arteries, where they reach maturity at approximately 6.5 months postinfection. This interval from infection to production of microfilariae is the prepatent period. Completion of the life cycle may take an additional month in cats.[2]

Pathophysiology

Most of the disease caused by heartworm infection is attributable to the adult parasites, although microfilariae also contribute to pulmonary interstitial and glomerular nephrotic manifestations in some dogs.[3] At first, heartworm disease in dogs tends to progress insidiously and may take 4 to 5 years before the cumulative effect of repeated infections produces clinically demonstrable signs. Disease tends to be proportional to the severity of infection. Lightly infected dogs, and even many cats, may tolerate live worms without apparent ill effects; however, as worms die, both disease and clinical signs can worsen rapidly. Heavy infections in dogs were commonplace before the increasingly widespread use of chemoprophylaxis during the last 20 years. However, with the greater frequency of heartworm testing now linked to heartworm prevention, most infections are detected before development of serious disease.

Although clinical signs may be slow to develop, pulmonary arterial disease is detectable histologically shortly after arrival of the immature adult worms.[4] These early lesions begin in the small peripheral branches of the pulmonary arteries where the parasites are first deposited, and then progress proximally as the worms grow and additional parasites accumulate with subsequent infections. The early signature histological feature of these heartworm-induced lesions is intimal proliferation accompanied by migration of smooth muscle cells across the internal elastic laminae, and leukocyte infiltration composed primarily of eosinophils. This circumferential obstructive endarteritis at the level of the small- and medium-sized arteries narrows the artery lumen and becomes the major site of increased impedance to bloodflow through the lung. Close contact with the parasite is an important part of the pathogenesis because the lesions are confined to those pulmonary arteries containing adult worms, and the side branches of those vessels. In dogs with systemic arterial aberrant infections, identical lesions also are found in these vessels. Consequently, lesions develop focally in direct proportion to the number and distribution of the worms, accounting for the usual preponderance of disease in the right and to a lesser extent the left caudal lobar pulmonary arteries.

In more heavily infected dogs and cats, the endarteritis becomes continuous with longitudinal ridges of exuberant myo-intimal proliferation in the larger intralobar arteries. These lesions can eventually extend to the main pulmonary artery of the most heavily infected animals, and are grossly visible in necropsy specimens as a roughened and wrinkled appearance of the luminal surface. In the larger branches, smooth muscle proliferation also produces medial hyperplasia. As the lesions evolve, they become less cellular and more fibrotic. However, maturation progresses too rapidly to reflect the age of the lesions, although in general, the more widely they are disbursed the longer worms have been accumulating.

The functional consequence of progressive pulmonary arterial disease in heavily infected dogs is a hemodynamically significant reduction in the cross-sectional area of the vascular bed at the level of the small distributing branches, and loss of distensibility in the large conducting arteries.[3] As pulmonary vascular impedance increases and eventually becomes fixed, pulmonary hypertension develops, especially during exercise-induced increases in bloodflow. The initial narrowing of the small arteries is eventually followed by pressure dilation of the large intra- and extralobar arteries. The right heart is subjected to pressure overloading that, despite compensatory concentric hypertrophy, may eventually lead to right-sided congestive heart failure in cases of chronic cor pulmonale. Unlike dogs, few cats follow this classical progression to congestive heart failure.

In dogs with moderately severe pulmonary hypertension, removal of heartworms by surgical extraction causes a prompt partial reduction in pressure, but the residual pulmonary arterial vascular disease is responsible for most of the impedance to bloodflow.[5] However, after death of the worms, their cuticles soften and worm fragments embolize the peripheral vessels, forming a nidus for thrombosis, which compounds the obstruction because of preexisting structural disease. The greater the underlying pulmonary arterial disease, the more severe the impact of thromboembolism.[6] Despite obstruction of major pulmonary arteries, infarcts are uncommon because of the non-lobulated architecture of dog and cat lungs, which facilitates bronchopulmonary and interpulmonary arterial anastomoses. However, dead worms cause capillary fragility, resulting in pulmonary interstitial edema. Associated with this process, which is not limited to the region of embolization (particularly in cats), is necrosis of type I alveolar epithelial cells and hyperplasia of surfactant-producing cells, similar to the lung injury occurring with acute respiratory distress syndrome (ARDS) in humans.[7] It has been speculated that the prominence of pulmonary intravascular macrophages (PIMs) in cats may contribute to the more diffuse pulmonary manifestations of acute lung injury that characterize heartworm disease in this species, but their role has not been clarified.

Platelet-derived endothelial growth factor is a possible trigger for myo-intimal endovascular disease.[8] Adult heartworms can disrupt the integrity of the endothelial lining, which promotes platelet aggregation at the site of injury. This mechanism appears to be a nonspecific response to injury rather than to the heartworm per se. However, because the pathognomonic proliferative endovascular lesions appear to be covered by intact endothelium, other chronic stimuli may sustain their growth. The presence of heartworm antigen within lung tissue may have pathogenic significance.

Some dogs with occult infections resulting from immune-mediated hypersensitivity to microfilariae develop an interstitial (allergic) pneumonitis caused by the inflammatory response to the microfilariae sequestered by the pulmonary reticuloendothelial system.[9] Phagocytosis of hemoglobin by macrophages of the reticuloendothelial system also contributes to the pulmonary hemosiderosis that speckles the lungs of heavily infected dogs a rusty color. The pathogenesis of this chronic hemolysis is similar to the acute destruction of erythrocytes in caval syndrome dogs.[10] Chronic passive congestion of the liver alters the composition of cholesterol and phospholipids in the erythrocyte membrane, making the cells less elastic and thus more susceptible to trauma as they percolate through entwined masses of worms.

Historically, attention has been focused mostly on the pulmonary arterial structural component of heartworm disease and its resultant functional consequences, but dynamic vasomotor abnormalities have also been recognized.[11,12] For the most part, the importance of vasomotor responses was viewed from the perspective of cardiovascular experimentalists intent on avoiding use of heartworm-infected dogs in protocols investigating vascular control. Because filariasis is a major global disease in humans and dogs, some consideration is now being given to the importance of circulating filarial factors as modulators of vascular responsiveness.

Although heartworms exert experimentally demonstrable alterations in contraction and relaxation of vascular and tracheal smooth muscle, the actual clinical significance remains theoretical. By a yet-to-be definitively determined mechanism, at least partly mediated by cyclooxygenase metabolites, female heartworms and worm products from either patent or occult infections depress acetylcholine-stimulated endothelial-mediated relaxation of pulmonary and femoral arteries.[13] These findings are intriguing because they also quantify a direct relationship between the number of worms and the loss of endothelial-mediated relaxation. Interestingly, heartworm-depressed relaxation was most striking in the spring, though to date this remains an anecdotal observation. Furthermore, the complexity of the influence of heartworm infection on vascular reactivity is evident from the conversion of the normal histamine-induced constriction of pulmonary arteries to endothelial-mediated relaxation. Heartworms or conditioned medium directly increase in vitro constriction of rat tracheal rings, prompting speculation that airway hyperreactivity could contribute to the reported poor racing performance of lightly infected, clinically asymptomatic greyhounds.[14,15] It seems likely that altered vasomotion contributes to the pathogenesis of heartworm disease, but its importance to the clinical manifestations is insufficiently documented to justify revising current medical practices.

Epidemiology and Risk Factors

Heartworm infection is a potential risk to dogs and cats living in temperate to tropical climate zones where vector mosquitoes and microfilaremic hosts coexist. This includes the entire continental United States and Hawaii, but the actual risk varies widely within climatic zones depending on latitude; elevation; seasonal temperature and rainfall; landscape; population densities of both mosquitoes and dogs; use of chemoprophylaxis; and many other variables causing transmission to vary, sometimes substantially, on an annual basis.[16] Even in communities where infection has not been detected, isolation can be broken by the inadvertent importation of a microfilaremic dog. Dogs and peridomestic coyotes are the principal reservoirs, because in cats, microfilaremia, if it occurs, persists for only a few weeks, making them ineffective as a significant source of infection. When the prerequisites are met, infection can be hyperendemic in regions where the duration of infection is limited to only a few summer months.[17] Because environmental temperature controls the maturation rate of infective larvae in vector mosquitoes, transmission has seasonal limits, except in subtropical regions of the country.

Prevalence statistics are relevant only to the conditions existing in a specific geographic area. Furthermore, survey results are influenced by the sample population. In clinic populations in which chemoprophylaxis is commonly administered, the prevalence of infection may be less than 1% to 2%, even if it is a community where most unprotected dogs become infected within a few years. Cats are relatively resistant to infection with adult heartworms. As a rule of thumb, the prevalence of adult heartworm infection in cats is only about 10% of that in dogs living in the same environment. Also, cats are less often bitten by infective mosquitoes because most vector species prefer feeding on dogs. These factors contribute to limiting most cat infections to 4 to 6 worms. The common house mosquito (Culex pipiens) is the principal species that cross-feeds on dogs and cats, and few microfilariae survive to the infective stage in this mosquito.[18] However, based on antibody serological testing, the rate of exposure to transient larval infections in cats is similar to the prevalence of adult heartworm infections in dogs.[19]

Historical Findings

As far as heartworms are concerned, the history is an essential part of the preliminary evaluation preceding initiation or resumption of chemoprophylaxis, and is useful for obtaining diagnostic information about patients that may be infected.

PRETEST HISTORY

The date of birth and age should be part of the patient record. This is particularly important when initiating chemoprophylaxis in puppies because it will determine whether heartworm testing is necessary. If for example, a pup is born after heartworm transmission ceases in the fall, it is unnecessary to test before starting chemoprophylaxis. Similarly, even if a late season infection occurred at the end of October, microfilaria or antigen testing before the end of May would be too soon because the prepatent waiting period would not have expired. The same 7-month interval between suspected date of infection and testing should always be applied to dogs of all ages.

Travel outside the resident community into regions where the risk of infection may be higher and occur at other times of the year should be established and given consideration. When an unexpected positive heartworm test result is obtained, a thorough history of where the dog has been, under what conditions it was living, regularity of prophylaxis administration, dose, and amount of unused medication should be obtained in an effort to make sense of the result, and to understand how and when an infection could have occurred. Test results should always be critiqued and, if suspect, testing should be repeated. For dogs previously receiving chemoprophylaxis, administration since the last evaluation should be recapitulated to ensure instructions were understood and are being followed as prescribed.

DIAGNOSTIC HISTORY

For diagnostic purposes, attention focuses on establishing the frequency, sequence, and timing of events in the development of the clinical signs that prompted the evaluation. With the exception of the acute onset of hemoglobinuria in caval syndrome dogs, physical manifestations of heartworm infection usually develop insidiously. Although clinical signs of heartworm disease may be apparent to a critical observer, they may go unrecognized by pet owners until the disease is quite advanced. The information obtained from the history and physical examination will direct the course of the clinical work-up by providing justification for a methodical selection of diagnostic testing options.

Clinical Signs and Progression

PRECLINICAL INFECTIONS

The most common clinical presentation in dogs, particularly in areas of low endemicity, is a patient in apparent excellent health. In such cases, the infection is usually detected by systematic heartworm antigen testing or by inadvertently finding microfilariae in a blood sample. Asymptomatic, antigen-positive infections can be problematic because other than the antigenemia, there may be no correlative evidence to confirm the diagnosis. In those instances, it is prudent to verify the antigen test result by repeating the test or by running a different antigen test before considering further action. The logical second step is thoracic radiography. In the absence of radiographic evidence consistent with early signs of infection, particularly if there is a reasonably convincing history of chemoprophylaxis and a low level of exposure, the most pragmatic approach may be retesting in 6 months.

COR PULMONALE

The development of classical end-stage clinical signs of heartworm heart disease is invariably preceded by some combination of increased respiratory rate and effort, excessive fatigue during exertion, and increased frequency of coughing. Sometimes the early signs are overlooked or ignored until there is a general loss of body condition and previously disregarded clinical signs worsen. In the late stages of the disease, dogs display obvious disability that may include major weight loss; lethargy; poor stamina, sometimes associated with syncope during abrupt strenuous exertion; heavy breathing; chronic chest cough, occasionally producing blood flecked sputum (or even profuse foaming hemorrhage leading to exsanguination); and abdominal distention with ascites (sometimes accompanied by pleural effusion) in dogs that develop right-sided heart failure. Harsh breath sounds (e.g., crackling inspiratory râles and expiratory wheezes) may be audible, particularly over the caudal dorsal lung lobes. Heart sounds are usually normal, although in severe cor pulmonale cases with pulmonary hypertension, moderately wide and fixed splitting of the second heart sound may be detected. An apical systolic murmur, loudest over the right precordium, develops secondary to tricuspid regurgitation in many dogs with right-sided cardiomegaly and is a consistent finding with caval syndrome. Occasionally, atypical complications such as spontaneous pneumothorax have occurred in cor pulmonale cases, sometimes following adulticide treatment.

Once a dog becomes symptomatic at any time during the clinical course of infection, the etiological diagnosis of heartworm disease is easily confirmed by heartworm antigen testing (cor pulmonale cases are often occult [i.e., microfilaria negative]) combined with thoracic radiography and complemented, in selected cases, with echocardiography. By the time some of the most heavily infected dogs are presented for evaluation, the worms have died and the antigenemia has passed. However, in the aftermath of extensive thromboembolism, the characteristic enlargement of the major pulmonary arteries persists and is easily recognized by thoracic radiography.

ALLERGIC PNEUMONITIS

This is a radiographic clinical diagnosis that may be made in any dog manifesting clinical signs of heartworm disease. Microfilaremia is seldom found in these dogs. Lung sounds are often increased; however, heart murmurs and signs of heart failure are typically absent. The abnormal lung sounds (and radiographic interstitial lung pattern) usually abate after a few days of corticosteroid administration, and respiratory signs improve.

PULMONARY NODULAR EOSINOPHILIC GRANULOMATOSIS

This is an uncommon feature of chronic heartworm infection in dogs, particularly now that late stage infections are themselves relatively infrequent. The clinical signs are nonspecific but typical for symptomatic heartworm-infected dogs, except that fever and peripheral lymphadenopathy are sometimes present. Microfilaremia is usually absent; sometimes, adult heartworms are no longer present, although residual arterial disease attests to prior infection. Like pneumonitis, consideration of this diagnosis is based on radiographic detection. The granulomas may be several centimeters in diameter, and often are multiple and of high radiodensity. Recognition of pulmonary artery enlargement characteristic of heartworm infection is a key observation in connecting these lesions with the infection rather than interpreting them as pulmonary neoplasms.

FELINE HEARTWORM INFECTION

The clinical signs of heartworm infection in cats are less stereotypic than in dogs, and the diagnosis can be easily overlooked if not consciously considered. Most symptomatic cats display variable signs of coughing and difficulty breathing, but anorexia and general malaise manifested by lethargy provide little diagnostic direction.[20] Vomiting, not necessarily associated with eating, is commonly reported, but the nonspecificity and usually benign nature of these events is neither an immediate alert nor an intuitive link to heartworms. Some cats display acute neurological signs including ataxia, seizures, and syncope, but these are uncommon. However, sudden death without prior signs of illness is a common outcome, and it requires a thorough necropsy examination for heartworms, in order to be diagnosed. Because cats are usually lightly infected, caval syndrome and right-sided congestive heart failure occur very infrequently.

There appear to be two vulnerable periods in the course of heartworm infection in cats. The first is associated with the arrival of immature worms in the heart and development of an intense, diffuse pneumonitis. The second occurs when mature adult worms die and produce acute pulmonary embolism. Cats are able to tolerate live heartworms, sometimes for years, and may eventually spontaneously eliminate the infection. The natural life span of heartworms in cats seems to be 2 to 3 years.[21]

Diagnostic Tests

MICROFILARIAE

Microfilariae can be seen in wet blood smears; the buffy coat of microhematocrit tubes; stained blood smears; and occasionally in urine sediment, spinal fluid, or any other body fluid contaminated by blood. However, because they may circulate in low numbers, recovery is facilitated by concentration using either the Knott or millipore filter techniques. Although several filarial parasites infect dogs in the United States, only *D. immitis* and *Dipetalonema reconditum* are detected often enough to be clinically significant, and only *D. immitis* causes disease. For this reason, microfilaria species identification can be important. A microfilaria examination is commonly run to complement serological testing but cannot be relied upon as the primary diagnostic test in dogs and cats. Approximately 25% of all heartworm-infected dogs do not have microfilaremia, and the percentage of occult infections in some syndromes is 100%. Testing before the end of the 6.5-month prepatent period will fail to detect microfilariae, and in the first months of patency, the low number may escape detection if the sample is not concentrated. Light infections often have parasites of only one sex. Particularly when thiacetarsamide was used for adulticide treatment, residual, female unisex infections were common and failed to maintain the microfilaremia. Dogs that develop hypersensitivity to microfilariae (e.g., allergic pneumonitis and some cor pulmonale cases) become permanently occult. Most importantly, chronic monthly administration of all the macrolide endectocides will eventually suppress embryogenesis and eliminate circulating microfilariae.[22,23] If microfilaremia develops in a cat, it persists for only a few weeks, making screening for microfilariae unproductive in this species.

HEARTWORM ANTIGEN SEROLOGY

Antigen testing is the primary method of screening dogs for heartworms and for diagnostic confirmation of infection.[24] Antigenemia is proportional to the number of mature adult female worms and increases transiently when female worms die. ELISA and immunochromatographic heartworm antigen tests are sufficiently sensitive to detect most chronic infections of only one to three female worms. Male unisex infections cannot be detected by antigen serology. Although the percentage of false negative results is highest for light infections, antigen tests also work very well for detecting infected cats having at least one mature female heartworm. Therefore, diagnostic antigen testing of cats suspected of being infected should be performed. However, because infection with mature heartworms is extremely uncommon in clinically healthy cats, it is not cost-effective to use antigen tests for screening this population.

ANTIFILARIAL ANTIBODY SEROLOGY

Because cats are generally lightly infected and may have only male heartworms, testing for heartworm-specific host antibody can be a useful diagnostic method.[25] Because feline immunoglobulin is the target, the commercial antibody tests can be used only in cats. Worms of both sexes can trigger a positive result as early as 2 months postinfection. Most feline infections are spontaneously aborted before maturation; therefore a positive antibody test only documents transient exposure to the parasite, not concurrent infection with adult heartworms. Because heartworm antibody seroprevalence is often 15 to 20 times higher than the adult worm infection rate, and because it is impossible to know whether a larval infection will complete the life cycle, antibody tests in cats do not share the specificity of antigen tests. Therefore antibody screening of cats for heartworm infection is of dubious value other than for risk assessment and justification for chemoprophylaxis. Retesting cats receiving chemoprophylaxis is not helpful because even a

trickle of monthly chemically abbreviated infections can raise a detectable antibody titer.[26]

THORACIC RADIOGRAPHY

Radiography is an extremely valuable tool for establishing a heartworm diagnosis and assessing prognosis. Both attributes derive from the fact that this is a direct approach to detecting organic disease that is often uniquely characteristic and quantifiable. The radiographic signs of heartworm infection parallel the development of pulmonary arterial and parenchymal disease, and fall into a logical sequential pattern that becomes increasingly obvious.[4,27] After history and physical examination, thoracic radiography is the most important preadulticide evaluation of dogs and should be performed whenever clinically significant thromboembolic side effects are anticipated.

Heartworm infection may be detected in survey radiographs as early as 4 to 5 months postinfection. In the early stages, the first signs of pulmonary vascular and periarterial parenchymal disease are found in the periphery of the dorsal wedge of the caudal lung lobes, where the high volume flow to these lobes deposits most of the immature worms. Normally, the vascular pattern in this region is narrow, tapered, and faint. Following infection, the lacy vascular pattern develops into a wider, brighter central linear streak with indistinct margins and a slight peripheral flare. These features are visualized best from the lateral view because in the dorsoventral (DV) or ventrodorsal (VD) views, absorption of x-rays passing through the liver decreases image contrast in this area.

The radiographic features that unmistakably identify heartworm infection in the later stages are enlargement with tortuosity, loss of peripheral taper, and abrupt termination (truncation) of the extra- and intralobar pulmonary arteries (Figure 70-1). These characteristics are particularly evident in the caudal lobes and do not develop in the apical lobes, except when worms accumulate in these arteries in the most heavily infected dogs. The normal dichotomous side branch pattern is rapidly lost beyond the second and third generations as the arteries become progressively dearborized. Coincident to the metamorphosis of the vascular architecture is an increasingly prominent, widespread interstitial lung pattern that is heaviest in the caudal lobes. The pattern radiates peripherally and may be accompanied by variable degrees of focal alveolar consolidation. In the worst cases, the lung disease may obscure proximal segments of the arterial branches, making it difficult to appreciate the characteristic deformities. The main pulmonary artery segment and the right heart silhouette are the last components to enlarge, and do so only after extensive obstruction of the peripheral arterial bed causes chronic pulmonary hypertension. These late changes characterize the cor pulmonale syndrome. Although the pulmonary features will diminish during recovery following adulticide treatment or natural worm death, the enlargement and tortuosity of the major pulmonary arteries persists, as may enlargement of the right side of the heart.

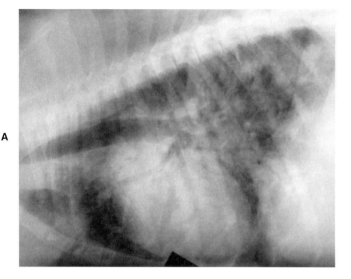

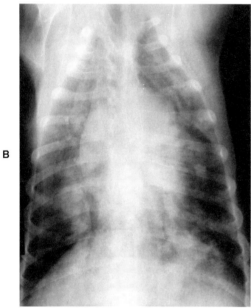

Figure 70-1. *A,* *Lateral and* *B,* *dorsoventral thoracic radiographs of a dog with cor pulmonale caused by chronic heartworm infection. The heavy interstitial, peribronchial, and alveolar lung patterns partially obscure the enlarged, nontapering, truncated peripheral pulmonary arteries in all lung lobes. The trachea is bowed dorsally anterior to the carina by the enlarged main pulmonary segment, which protrudes beyond the cardiac silhouette in the left anterior quadrant of the DV view. The right heart is moderately enlarged.*

The radiographic features of feline heartworm disease differ in subtle ways from those characterizing the disease in dogs.[28] The most common manifestations are variable interstitial lung patterns that may be accompanied by alveolar infiltrates, particularly in the caudal lung lobes. These signs are not specific for heartworm infection, but in the right clinical context support the diagnosis. Unequivocal enlargement of the caudal lobar pulmonary arteries, particularly if unilateral, is distinct evidence, but it is not as common as in chronically infected dogs. Also, tortuosity and truncation are less obvious in survey radiographs than in dogs. The apparent size of these arteries may be exaggerated by periarterial infiltrates, which can fluctuate between one radiographic examination and the next. In cats, the size and shape of the extralobar and peripheral pulmonary arterial branches are visualized more easily in the DV (VD) views. Enlargement of the main pulmonary arterial segment is obscured by the cardiac silhouette, which seldom reveals right-sided cardiomegaly.

PULMONARY ANGIOGRAPHY

Angiography has been used to study the progression of arterial disease in greater detail and is a very useful technique for documenting regional pulmonary arterial obstruction caused by thromboembolism. In the past, angiography provided validation for interpreting survey thoracic radiographs; however, although it is the most vivid method of demonstrating heartworm infection, it is seldom needed today for clinical confirmation.

ULTRASONOGRAPHY

The heartworm cuticle is highly echoic and the body walls create distinctive bright parallel reflections. Where the 2D sector plane intersects the worm's convoluted body, short segmental images resembling "equal" signs are produced. The cavae, chambers of the right heart, main pulmonary artery, and right extralobar branch can be accessed; but in lightly infected dogs, the worms often are restricted to intralobar branches within the lung where they can not be reached by the interrogating sonic beam. Therefore, although heartworms may be a chance finding, echo imaging is not a dependable technique for confirming heartworm infections, except when the infection is heavy. However, ultrasound identification of a worm mass in the tricuspid orifice is the definitive diagnostic test for confirming the caval syndrome. Because heartworms are disproportionately long relative to the length of the pulmonary arteries in cats, there is a greater probability that some portion of the worm can be visualized.[29] Also, because other clinical evidence of heartworm infection in cats may be problematical, ultrasonography may be particularly useful in such instances. Cardiac imaging is only diagnostic for heartworm infection when worms are present in the heart. However, it can provide useful information about cardiac complications secondary to cor pulmonale.

BRONCHIAL LAVAGE

Cytology on endotracheal lung washes is sometimes performed in cats with clinical signs of respiratory disease such as asthma, which is the major condition resembling feline heartworm disease. Eosinophilia is common with both allergic and parasitic diseases but can also be a normal finding in cats. During larval migration through maturation of the heartworm, eosinophils are most numerous in the peripheral blood and bronchial exudate. Lavage is of no differential diagnostic value in distinguishing feline asthma from heartworm infection, and because eosinophilia caused by heartworms is transient, the number of eosinophils relates more to the stage of infection than whether a heartworm infection exists.

HEMATOLOGICAL AND BLOOD CHEMICAL PROFILES

The hematologic and blood chemical testing that is commonly part of the routine medical work-up of heartworm-infected, stable, and healthy animals contributes no essential information for diagnosing heartworm infection. In all instances (heartworm related or otherwise) it should be used selectively to answer clinically relevant questions raised during history taking and physical examination.

Chemoprophylaxis

Because dogs are highly susceptible hosts, it is prudent to protect them during the months of heartworm transmission. There is no winter transmission (December through March) except in the subtropical lower Florida peninsula, and for most of the continental United States the need for prophylaxis begins in late spring and ends mid-fall.[30-32] Owners need to understand when their dogs are at risk because they are the critical link in timely administration of chemoprophylaxis.

Options include daily (diethylcarbamazine) and monthly (ivermectin, milbemycine oxime, and moxidectin) oral, monthly topical (selamectin), and 6-month subcutaneous injectable (sustained release) moxidectin formulations. If dosing conforms to manufacturer's instructions, these products can be used in the most ivermectin-sensitive collies. The monthly and 6-monthly macrolide endectocides provide the highest level of protection and the widest latitude of dosing interval. Each delivers a minimum of 6 weeks retroactive efficacy, which creates a buffer for timing the start of seasonal prophylaxis and inadvertent failure to administer monthly oral and topical doses at precise intervals. Because the monthly macrolides do not convey protection against infections occurring after dose administration, it is important that the last seasonal dose be delayed until transmission has ceased. It is also important that the duration of the sustained release moxidectin formulation encompass the end of the transmission season. Each of the macrolides can be administered to dogs that have patent (microfilaremic) infections, but diethylcarbamazine is specifically contraindicated in such dogs because it may cause fatalities in these circumstances.[4]

Registered ivermectin and milbemycin oxime oral products, and selamectin topical products are available for preventing heartworm infection in cats. Because cats possess some natural resistance to infection and many live more protected lives than dogs, the probability of infection and the risk tolerance of the cat owner deserve consideration before electing heartworm chemoprophylaxis. Cat owners should be advised objectively that cats may become infected and then be allowed to consider

their options. The veterinarian's personal experience with heartworm infection in the community can be a pivotal factor. One thing is certain: any cat given one of these products at the appropriate time of year will not become infected.

Adulticide Treatment

Though nonworking dogs may remain healthy with a light heartworm infection, generally it is preferable to eliminate the parasite. However, pulmonary thromboembolism is an inevitable consequence of destroying heartworms in situ. The severity of this adverse treatment side effect depends on the number of worms and the extent of pulmonary vascular and parenchymal damage already present. The immediate posttreatment and longer-term prognoses can be estimated by staging the patient's clinical status before treatment. It is sufficient to broadly categorize heartworm disease as mild, moderate, and severe (i.e., stages I, II, and III). Caval syndrome is a special category, referred to as stage IV, which is not intended to imply that it is the natural chronological end-stage progression of the disease.

The staging process is based on physical signs and, in particular, radiographic assessment of the arterial and lung disease. Stage I dogs are not symptomatic and have minimal radiographic evidence of early pulmonary arterial vascular disease consistent with heartworm infection. In stage II, clinical signs include sporadic mild cough and possibly increased respiratory effort, associated with moderately enlarged caudal lobar pulmonary arteries on radiographs. By stage III, dogs are definitely symptomatic, and the radiographic signs include extralobar pulmonary arterial enlargement, evidence of extensive interstitial with (or without) alveolar disease, and, possibly, right-sided cardiomegaly.

The most direct method of assessing the number of worms is ultrasonography, but this only provides a relative impression. ELISA antigen tests provide an imprecise measure of heartworm antigenemia reflective of the number of mature female heartworms. Because test reactions tend to saturate rapidly and do not correlate linearly with the amount of antigen, quantitation is of limited value. However, if a stage III dog has a weak ELISA antigen test reaction, it is likely that most if not all of the worms have already died, accounting for the severity of disease. Such cases probably are at little risk of additional pulmonary thromboembolism but also have little to gain from adulticide administration.

Stage I and II dogs usually only suffer mild if any post-adulticide thromboembolic complications and recover uneventfully. The vulnerable period in the convalescence is 7 to 10 days posttreatment, when the worms die and obstruct bloodflow. Exercise limitation during the first month is the most important measure to minimize complications.[33]

Melarsomine dihydrochloride is now the only commercially available adulticide. It is more dependable and efficacious than thiacetarsamide, which it has replaced, and offers the advantages of being nonhepatotoxic; easily administered by deep intramuscular injection, causing only brief soreness and mild swelling; and a split dose schedule for incrementally eliminating the worms. The latter is an advantage in treating stage III infections. The packaged instructions for its use are explicit and should be followed.

Antigen retesting should be repeated 4 to 5 months posttreatment. Complete elimination of the infection will completely seroconvert the antigenemia. If a low antigenemia persists, retesting should be repeated after a few months before electing to repeat the treatment. When clinical improvement in previously symptomatic dogs is satisfactory, retreatment of persistently antigenemic patients may be considered optional.

Adulticide treatment of heartworm-infected cats is generally considered more hazardous than allowing the infection to run its natural course. Therefore, melarsomine is only a treatment of last resort for cats with clinical signs that do not respond satisfactorily to symptomatic treatment with tapered doses of glucocorticosteroids.[25] Melarsomine is tolerated by normal cats, but its use in this species is an off-label application.

Surgical Extraction of Adult Heartworms

Surgical extraction of heartworms via jugular venotomy has been performed successfully in dogs and cats using a variety of forceps, brush, and calculae retrieval devices guided by fluoroscopic visualization. The recovery rate of dogs with stage III infections is better when as many worms as possible are withdrawn before beginning adulticide administration.[34] Extraction is the only effective treatment for the caval syndrome, and given the high rate of complications following adulticide treatment of cats, physically removing worms has potential advantages. A specially designed flexible alligator forceps that permits independent manipulation of the tip and jaws enables recovery of worms from anywhere within the vena cavae, right heart, and pulmonary arteries of dogs. More slender devices are required in traversing the jugular veins of cats, and transvenous retrieval in this species is limited to the cavae, right atrium, and right ventricle.[35] Given the impasse in reaching the pulmonary arteries of cats from peripheral sites, open chest pulmonary arteriotomy may be required. Before electing one of these approaches, the location of worms at accessible sites should be confirmed by ultrasonography.

Microfilariae Elimination

There are no filaricides registered for eliminating circulating microfilariae; however, all the heartworm macrolide endectocides are microfilaricidal at recommended prophylactic dosages, although complete elimination may require several months of administration. Heartworm (not necessarily microfilaria) testing is recommended before initiating chemoprophylaxis in dogs

that may have been infected at least 7 months earlier. This advisory is made to avoid delay in recognizing existing infections and to avoid incorrectly interpreting infections in dogs receiving timely chemoprophylaxis as drug failures. Because no alternative exists, the FDA recognizes the common practice of eliminating microfilariae with one of the macrolides, administered under the supervision of a veterinarian.[36] However, use of concentrated livestock formulations is discouraged because large errors in dose calculation can be fatal. Ordinarily, microfilariae are not specifically targeted until after adulticide therapy is complete. The simplest regime for eliminating potential reservoir dogs (whether adulticide treated or not) is administration of one of the macrolides at the recommended prophylactic dose. If rapid clearance is desired, milbemycin oxime tends to produce the fastest initial rate of decline. When microfilariae are particularly numerous, it is prudent to keep dogs under observation for the first 10 to 12 hours following the first dose of milbemycin oxime because some dogs may develop hypotension and require shock therapy during this interval.[24] Because microfilariae persist for only a few weeks in cats, they require no microfilaricide treatment.

General Medical Support

For most mildly and moderately affected dogs, no medical support other than adulticide treatment is required. Antiinflammatory doses of prednisone in a 10- to 14-day diminishing dose protocol is the most effective treatment for reducing the frequency and severity of heartworm induced coughing. If coughing is heavy before adulticide administration, it is advisable to attempt a partial remission before proceeding because respiratory distress is often temporarily exacerbated by worm emboli. Similarly, dogs that are in right-sided heart failure should be stabilized before adulticide treatment. Cage rest is an essential complement to the judicious use of diuretics. It is important to control the rate at which these patients are dehydrated; this is done by avoiding large doses of diuretics that deplete blood volume before there has been an opportunity for retained fluid to equilibrate from body cavities and tissues. Overzealous diuresis compromises cardiac, renal, and other organ function, and can rapidly transform a weakened patient into one that is completely disabled. Other conventional heart failure drugs (e.g., angiotensin converting enzyme inhibitors and digoxin) are also appropriate.

Pure arteriolar vasodilators such as hydralazine may lower pulmonary blood pressure in some heartworm infected dogs, but the response is unpredictable.[37] Furthermore, this is not a promising adjunctive therapy because the severely sclerotic pulmonary arteries of dogs, which theoretically could benefit from reducing pulmonary hypertension, are probably incapable of dilation. However, inhalation of nitric oxide reduces hypoxic pulmonary vasoconstriction in dogs and has been reported to prevent worsening of pulmonary hypertension during surgical extraction of heartworms in a case of vena cava syndrome.[38] Oxygen and aminophylline may have a small salutary effect on pulmonary hypertension, but the attendant decrease in pulmonary bloodflow attributable to cage rest is more effective in relieving the right ventricular afterload. Aspirin was once recommended for inhibiting release of platelet-derived growth factor and promoting regression of pulmonary arterial endothelial proliferation. However, no clinically apparent benefit has been demonstrated in aspirin-treated dogs,[39] and aspirin actually worsens pulmonary disease in heartworm-infected cats.[40] Furthermore, prolonged bleeding time in aspirin-treated dogs seriously compromises control of hemoptysis, if it occurs.

Clinical Outcome

Heartworm infection in dogs and cats is easily prevented. The key to a successful cure in dogs is detection and treatment in the early stages of disease. Although more pulmonary arterial and lung disease persists as the severity and duration of infection increase, a return to reasonably good health should be expected following adulticide treatment except for the most advanced cases. Survival of heartworm-infected cats is unpredictable.

REFERENCES

1. Slocombe JOD, Surgeoner GA, Srivastava B: Determination of the heartworm transmission period and its use in diagnosis and control. In Otto GF, editor: *Proceedings of the Heartworm Symposium '89*, Washington, DC, 1990, American Heartworm Society.
2. McCall JW, Dzimianski MT, McTier TL et al: Biology of experimental heartworm infection in cats. In Soll MD, editor: *Proceedings of the Heartworm Symposium '92*, Batavia, IL, 1993, American Heartworm Society.
3. Knight DH: Heartworm heart disease. In Simpson CF, editor: *Advances in veterinary science and comparative medicine: Cardiovascular pathophysiology*, New York, 1977, Academic Press.
4. Knight DH: Heartworm infection. In Grieve RB, editor: *The Veterinary clinics of North America: Small animal practice*, vol 17, Philadelphia, 1987, WB Saunders.
5. Kitagawa H, Sasaki Y, Ishihara K et al: Contribution of live heartworms harboring in pulmonary arteries to pulmonary hypertension in dogs with dirofilariasis, *Jpn J Vet Sci* 52(6):1211, 1990.
6. Hirano Y, Kitagawa H, Sasaki Y: Relationship between pulmonary arterial pressure and pulmonary thromboembolism associated with dead worms in canine heartworm disease, *J Vet Med Sci* 54(5):897, 1992.
7. Dillon AR, Warner AE, Molina RM: Pulmonary parenchymal changes in dogs and cats after experimental transplantation of dead *Dirofilaria immitis*. In Soll DM, Knight DH, editors: *Proceedings of the Heartworm Symposium '95*, Batavia, IL, 1996, American Heartworm Society.
8. Schaub RG, Rawlings CA, Keith JC: Platelet adhesion and myointimal proliferation in canine pulmonary arteries, *Am J Pathol* 104:13, 1981.
9. Wong MM: Experimental occult dirofilariasis in dogs with special reference to immunological responses and its relationship to "eosinophilic lung" (tropical eosinophilia) in man, *Asian J Trop Med Public Health* 5:480, 1974.
10. Kitagawa H, Sasaki Y, Matsui A: The half-life of erythrocytes in dogs with pulmonary heartworm disease, *J Vet Med Sc* 54(1):161, 1992.
11. Kaiser L, Tithof PK, Williams JF: Depression of endothelium-dependent relaxation by filarial parasite products, *Am J Physiol* 259:H648, 1990.
12. Mupanomunda M, Williams JF, Mackenzie CD et al: *Dirofilaria immitis:* Heartworm infection alters pulmonary artery endothelial cell behavior, *J Appl Physiol* 82(2):389, 1997.
13. Kaiser L, Williams JF, Meade EA et al: Altered endothelial cell mediated arterial dilation in dogs with *D. immitis* infection, *Am J Physiol* 253:H1325, 1987.
14. Collins JM, Williams JF, Kaiser L: *Dirofilaria immitis:* Heartworm products contract rat trachea *in vitro*, *Exp Parasitology* 78(1):76, 1994.
15. Courtney CF, Sundlof SF, Lane TJ: Impact of filariasis on the racing greyhound, *J Am An Hosp Assoc* 21:421, 185.
16. Walter LL: Risk factors for heartworm infection in northern California. In Soll DM, Knight DH, editors: *Proceedings of the Heartworm Symposium '95*, Batavia, IL, 1996, American Heartworm Society.
17. Stromberg BE, Prouty SM, Averbeck GA et al: Six decades of heartworm in Minnesota. In Soll DM, Knight DH, editors: *Proceedings of the Heartworm Symposium '95*, Batavia, IL, 1996, American Heartworm Society.
18. Genchi G, Di Sacco B, Cancrini G: Epizootiology of canine and feline heartworm infection in northern Italy: Possible mosquito vectors. In Soll MD, editor: *Proceedings of the Heartworm Symposium '92*, Batavia, IL, 1993, American Heartworm Society.
19. Miller MW, Atkins CE, Stemme K et al: Prevalence of exposure to *Dirofilaria immitis* in cats in multiple areas of the United States. In Seward RL, editor: *Recent advances in heartworm disease: Symposium '98*, Batavia, IL, 1999, American Heartworm Society.
20. Atkins CE, DeFrancesco TC, Miller MW et al: Prevalence of heartworm infection in cats with signs of cardiorespiratory abnormalities, *J Am Vet Med Assoc* 212(4):517, 1998.
21. McCall JW, Dzimianski MT, McTier TL et al: Biology of experimental heartworm infections in cats. In Soll MD, editor: *Proceedings of the Heartworm Symposium '92*, Batavia, IL, 1993, American Heartworm Society.
22. Lok JB, Harpaz T, Knight DH: Abnormal patterns of embryogenesis in *Dirofilaria immitis* treated with ivermectin, *J Helminthol* 62:175, 1988.
23. Lok JB, Knight DH, Selavka CM et al: Studies on reproductive competence of male *Dirofilaria immitis* treated with milbemycin oxime, *Trop Med Parasitology* 46(4):235, 1995.
24. Knight DH, Ryan WG, Courtney CH et al: 1999 Guidelines for the diagnosis, prevention and management of heartworm *(Dirofilaria immitis)* infection in dogs. In Seward RL, editor: *Recent advances in heartworm disease: Symposium '98*, Batavia, IL, 1999, American Heartworm Society.
25. Knight DH, Atkins CE, Atwell RB et al: 1999 Guidelines for the diagnosis, treatment and prevention of heartworm *(Dirofilaria immitis)* infection in cats. In Seward RL, editor: *Recent advances in heartworm disease: Symposium '98*, Batavia, IL, 1999, American Heartworm Society.
26. Donoghue A: Effect of prophylaxis on antiheartworm antibody levels in cats receiving trickle experimental infections of *Dirofilaria immitis*. In Seward RL, editor: *Recent advances in heartworm disease: Symposium '98*, Batavia, IL, 1999, American Heartworm Society.
27. Knight DH: Radiographic evaluation of heartworm disease. In Otto GF, editor: *Proceedings of the Heartworm Symposium '86*, Washington, DC, 1986, American Heartworm Society.
28. Selcer BA, Newell SM, Mansour AE et al: Radiographic and 2D echocardiographic findings in 18 cats experimentally exposed to *D. immitis* via mosquito bites, *Vet Rad Ultrasound* 37(1):37, 1996.
29. Venco L, Morini S, Ferrari E et al: Technique for identifying heartworms in cats by 2D echocardiography. In Seward RL, editor: *Recent advances in heartworm disease: Symposium '98*, Batavia, IL, 1999, American Heartworm Society.
30. Watts KJ, Reddy GR, Holmes RA et al: Seasonal prevalence of third stage larvae of *Dirofilaria immitis* in mosquitoes from Florida and Louisiana, *Parasitology* 87(7):322, 2001.
31. Knight DH, Lok JB: Seasonal timing of heartworm chemoprophylaxis in the United States. In Soll DM, Knight DH, editors: *Proceedings of the Heartworm Symposium '95*, Batavia, IL, 1996, American Heartworm Society.
32. Knight DH, Lok JB: Seasonality of heartworm infection and implications for chemoprophylaxis, *Clin Techniques Sm An Pract* 13(2):77, 1998.
33. Hagio M: Influence of exercise on recovery of dogs following heartworm adulticide treatment with melarsomine. In Seward RL, editor: *Recent advances in heartworm disease: Symposium '98*, Batavia, IL, 1999, American Heartworm Society.

34. Moroni S: Surgical removal of heartworms versus melarsomine treatment of naturally treated dogs with high risk of thromboembolism. In Seward RL, editor: *Recent advances in heartworm disease: Symposium '98*, Batavia, IL, 1999, American Heartworm Society.

35. Venco L: Surgical removal of heartworms from naturally infected cats. In Seward RL, editor: *Recent advances in heartworm disease: Symposium '98*, Batavia, IL, 1999, American Heartworm Society.

36. Luddy EA, Sundlof SF: Drugs used in the prevention and treatment of heartworm disease: The regulatory perspective. In Soll DM, Knight DH, editors: *Proceedings of the Heartworm Symposium '95*, Batavia, IL, 1996, American Heartworm Society.

37. Atkins CE, Keene BW, McGuirk SM et al: Acute effect of hydralazine administration on pulmonary arterial hemodynamics in dogs with chronic heartworm disease, *Am J Vet Res* 55(2):262, 1994.

38. Hirakawa A, Sakamoto H, Misumi K et al: Effects of inhaled nitric oxide on hypoxic pulmonary vasoconstriction in dogs and a case report of vena cavae syndrome, *J Vet Med Sc* 58(6):551, 1996.

39. Sasaki Y, Kitagawa H, Ishihara K et al: Improvement in pulmonary arterial lesions after heartworm removal using flexible alligator forceps, *Jpn J Vet Sci* 52(4):743, 1990.

40. Rawlings CA, Farrell RL, Mahood RM: Morphologic changes in the lungs of cats experimentally infected with *Dirofilaria immitis, J Vet Inter Med* 4(6):292-300, 1990.

CHAPTER 71

Pulmonary Thromboembolism

Susan G. Hackner

Pulmonary thromboembolism is the obstruction of a pulmonary vessel, or vessels, by a blood clot. Blood clots may develop locally (primary pulmonary thrombosis) or develop at a distant site and translocate to the pulmonary vasculature (pulmonary embolism). Primary pulmonary thrombosis and pulmonary embolism are difficult to differentiate clinically, and the pathophysiological consequences are similar. As such, the term pulmonary thromboembolism (PTE) is used inclusively to describe these events.

Thromboemboli mechanically obstruct arterial blood-flow, release various humoral factors, and stimulate neurogenic reflexes.[1,2] Subsequent alterations in respiratory and hemodynamic function are responsible for the clinical signs and diagnostic findings in patients with PTE. The condition ranges from incidental, clinically insignificant thromboembolism to massive embolism with sudden death.[3,4] Mortality rates are substantial.[1,5-7]

PTE is extremely underdiagnosed in veterinary patients. Antemortem diagnosis is hindered by a lack of clinical awareness, clinical signs that resemble those of many other disease processes, and the relatively invasive or specialized tests required for definitive diagnosis. In retrospective studies, PTE was suspected antemortem in less than 40% of dogs and in 14% of cats.[8,9]

Incidence

PTE is a significant clinical entity in dogs and cats, but the actual incidence remains unclear. It is probably lower than in humans for several reasons. Deep vein thrombosis (DVT), thrombosis of the deep veins of the pelvis, legs, or arms, is the preceding event to PTE in human patients but does not appear to occur in small animals.[1,10] In addition, humans have multiple inherited hypercoagulabilities that predispose to thromboembolism[11,12] but have not been reported in dogs and cats. It has been estimated that over 20% of human patients with PTE have one or more of these inherited defects.[11]

One study of PTE reported an incidence of 0.9% in the canine necropsy population.[8] Necropsy studies, however, underestimate the incidence of PTE. First, not all patients with PTE die. In addition, thrombi lyse rapidly following death. Experimental data in dogs demonstrates 50% thrombus dissolution within 3 hours.[13] Finally, postmortem identification of thrombi requires careful examination of the pulmonary vasculature. The prevalence of PTE in unselected human autopsies, aimed to identify grossly apparent emboli, was 10%.[14] When particular attention was focused on the vasculature, and microscopic emboli diligently sought, the prevalence exceeded 60%.[14] There are no estimates of the incidence of PTE in cats.

Etiology

Thrombosis depends on three major risk factors: (1) changes in the vessel wall (vascular injury), (2) impairment of bloodflow (stasis), and (3) alterations in the blood constituents (hypercoagulability).[1,10,15,16] This concept, known as Virchow's triad, is fundamental to the understanding and prevention of thromboembolism. Whereas vascular injury and stasis are prothrombotic, true hypercoagulability refers to a quantitative or qualitative defect in the coagulation system. Hypercoagulability can result from platelet hyperaggregability, excessive activation or decreased removal of coagulation factors, deficiencies of natural anticoagulants (e.g., antithrombin III or protein C), or defective fibrinolysis.[12,16,17]

Primary hypercoagulable states are inherited disorders that favor thrombosis.[12,15,16] To date, these have not been reported in dogs and cats. Secondary hypercoagulable states are acquired disorders in patients with underlying systemic disease known to be associated with an increased risk of thrombosis.[12,15,16] In these patients, the pathogenesis is generally multifactorial and complex.

PTE has been shown to be associated with the following conditions in dogs: protein-losing nephropathy; neoplasia; cardiac disease (e.g., dirofilariasis, endocarditis, and cardiomyopathy); necrotizing pancreatitis; immune-mediated hemolytic anemia; hypercortisolism (e.g., naturally-occurring hyperadrenocorticism and corticosteroid therapy); diabetes mellitus; atherosclerosis; sepsis; trauma; and surgical procedures.[4,8,18-30] With the exception of cardiac disease, these conditions are all considered hypercoagulable states: that is, there are hemostatic defects that promote thrombus formation. In retrospective studies of necropsied dogs with PTE, the majority of dogs (59% and 64%) had more than one potentially hypercoagulable condition.[4,8] Dogs with PTE at necropsy were commonly found to have concurrent thrombosis in other organ systems.[8,19,20,24,30]

Although the above conditions are associated with PTE, the actual incidence of thrombosis is variable and unpredictable. It appears that thrombosis is often precipitated by a concomitant hypercoagulable state or prothrombotic situation such as vascular stasis or endothelial injury.

PTE in cats is most commonly associated with cardiac disease (cardiomyopathy) and neoplasia.[31-33] A recent study, however, also reported PTE associated with pancreatitis, immune-mediated hemolytic anemia, protein-losing nephropathy, protein-losing enteropathy, hypercortisolism, and sepsis.[9] In this study, 47% of cats had multiple disease processes that may have predisposed to PTE.

Pathophysiology

The pulmonary vascular bed filters venous blood. As a result, thromboemboli in the venous circulation become trapped in the pulmonary vasculature. In the healthy lung, this vasculature has tremendous reserve capacity; minor occlusions are well tolerated. If occlusion is substantial, however, or if it occurs in a patient with preexisting pulmonary or cardiac compromise, the sequelae are clinically significant.[1,34,35] Such sequelae may be pulmonary and/or hemodynamic.

Pulmonary consequences of PTE have been well defined in experimental canine models and in human pa-

tients. The major consequences include ventilation-perfusion mismatch, bronchoconstriction, hypoxemia, and hyperventilation.[1,28,36-43] Somewhat later, two additional consequences may occur, namely regional loss of surfactant and pulmonary infarction.[44-49]

Total occlusion of a pulmonary arterial vessel results in the absence of bloodflow to the distal lung zone while ventilation continues. That is, by definition, alveolar dead space. Total occlusion, however, is infrequent.[1,36,50] Partial occlusion (either initially, or caused by fibrinolysis in the hours following embolism) results in ventilation-perfusion mismatch with a region of high ventilation-perfusion (high V/Q ratio).[36,39-41] A second immediate consequence of embolism in experimental models is bronchoconstriction in those lung regions with proximal obstruction.[38,43] This results from low levels of carbon dioxide in the alveoli.[38] Teleologically, this should serve to reduce the extent of V/Q mismatch. This bronchoconstriction rarely occurs in patients, however, because they inhale carbon dioxide-rich tracheal "dead space air" into these alveolar zones immediately following the embolic event.[1]

Arterial hypoxemia is a common, although not universal, consequence. Several mechanisms account for its presence and extent.[36,39-41] The variable impact of these mechanisms, together with the common occurrence of hyperventilation, makes it impossible to define an arterial partial pressure of oxygen that excludes the diagnosis of PTE. Ventilation/perfusion differences are a major cause of the hypoxemia.[1,40,41] Blood is diverted from obstructed zones to perfused zones, but the ventilation of these perfused zones may be inadequate to achieve optimum oxygenation. In patients with underlying pulmonary disease, some degree of ventilation/perfusion mismatch may preexist.[1] Furthermore, if a modest degree of diffusion impairment exists in these hyperperfused zones, it may hinder oxygen transfer because of greatly decreased capillary transit times.[1] Reduced cardiac output caused by acute right ventricular decompensation may also contribute to the hypoxemia. As cardiac output decreases, the alveolar-arterial oxygen difference widens. Thus blood returning to the right heart has reduced oxygen saturation. The low mixed venous saturation amplifies the impact of the normal anatomical right-to-left shunt on the arterial oxygen content and magnifies the effect of ventilation/perfusion mismatch.[1]

Hyperventilation generally occurs[1,36,51]; this may ameliorate the hypoxemia and, in the vast majority of patients, lead to variable degrees of hypocapnia. The mechanisms responsible for hyperventilation remain controversial. Stimulation of pulmonary J receptors has been postulated.[51]

Depletion of alveolar surfactant has been demonstrated 24 hours following complete pulmonary arterial occlusion,[45,46] apparently because of failure to deliver components needed for surfactant production to Type II pneumocytes. The resulting edema and atelectasis are generally delayed until the day following embolic occlusion.

Pulmonary infarction is rare because occlusion is rarely complete, and because the lung has an alternate oxygen and nutrient supply via the bronchial arterial circulation.[47-49,52] Where there is concomitant compromise of such supply (e.g., decreased cardiac output or intrinsic pulmonary disease), infarction is more likely.[48]

Hemodynamic consequences of PTE are related to the magnitude of the obstruction and the preexisting status of the cardiovascular and pulmonary systems.[34,53,54] The pulmonary vascular bed has a large reserve capacity, and can compensate for vascular occlusion by recruitment of unused vessels and by capillary dilation.[55] In healthy dogs, greater than 60% of the pulmonary vasculature must be occluded before a significant increase in pulmonary vascular resistance (PVR) and right ventricular afterload occurs.[54] Elevated PVR is a poor prognostic indicator.[1] Increased afterload increases right ventricular oxygen requirements. If these exceed supply, ischemia, arrhythmias, or right ventricular failure ensue.[54,56,57] The resultant decreased venous return to the left ventricle may result in decreased cardiac output and left ventricular failure.[56-58] There is evidence that survival in animals subjected to PTE can be improved by agents that sustain systolic pressure and, therefore, coronary perfusion.[59]

The hemodynamic burden caused by massive PTE is largely caused by mechanical obstruction. Vasoconstriction and the release of humoral substances contribute. An acute and exaggerated increase in PVR beyond what is expected from mechanical obstruction alone has been demonstrated in canine models of PTE.[5,43,60] Postulated mechanisms include the presence of hypoxia-induced vasoconstriction and the release of humoral factors, such as serotonin, from activated platelets on the surface of the thrombus.[61-64]

Pulmonary thromboembolism is a dynamic event. Thrombi can undergo lysis, fragmentation, organization, or growth.[1,50] Pathophysiological consequences reflect such changes, and findings are dependent on the point in time at which they are examined.

Clinical Signs

The severity of clinical signs reflects the magnitude of respiratory and cardiac compromise and the ability of these systems to compensate for the insult. Signs range from mild compromise to profound compromise and death. PTE may also be subclinical.[4,9,65]

Clinical signs are variable and inconsistent and can mimic a multitude of other diseases. The most common signs are dyspnea, tachypnea, and depression.[4,8,9,25-28,66-68] Other signs include coughing, hemoptysis, cyanosis, hypoperfusion, and syncope.[8,9,66] Collapse, shock, and sudden death may result in patients with markedly decreased cardiac output.

Adventitious lung sounds may be auscultated in patients with pulmonary edema, hemorrhage, or bronchoconstriction.[8,66] The presence of pleural effusion is detected as muffled heart and lung sounds. Tachycardia is often present and reflects sympathetic stimulation, hypoxemia, anxiety, or decreased cardiac output.[4,25,27,66] In patients with pulmonary hypertension, a split second heart sound may be auscultated.[25,66] Jugular pulses and peripheral edema are rare findings.[27] Signs of reduced cardiac output may be seen in patients with left heart failure.[27,28,67]

PTE should be suspected in any patient with an acute onset of respiratory signs, particularly if the patient has no prior evidence of respiratory disease. The presence of predisposing conditions or potential hypercoagulable states should increase the index of suspicion.

Differential Diagnosis

PTE should be differentiated from other causes of dyspnea and tachypnea (e.g., pneumonia, pulmonary edema, intrapulmonary hemorrhage, pneumothorax, pleural effusion, and airway obstruction). Where pulmonary hypertension or ventricular dysfunction occur, other causes should be eliminated. These include cardiomyopathy, mitral stenosis, valvular insufficiency, and congenital shunting.

Diagnostic Tests

HEMATOLOGICAL AND BIOCHEMICAL TESTS

These have limited value in the diagnosis of PTE. Abnormal results, when present, generally reflect inflammation, hypoxemia, or stress.[66] Results may be useful, however, in identifying predisposing disease conditions.

THORACIC RADIOGRAPHY

Most dogs with PTE have abnormal thoracic radiographs, but findings are not specific for PTE.[68] Two common radiographic patterns are described in dogs: (1) regional oligemia (hypovascular lung regions), and (2) pulmonary infiltrates.[70] Regional oligemia appears as areas of increased radiolucency and represents reduced vascular filling distal to the thrombotic occlusion. Oligemia is best identified on ventrodorsal and dorsoventral radiographic views. Pulmonary infiltrates are most commonly alveolar but may be either interstitial or mixed alveolar-interstitial.[4,8,69,70] They may be solitary or multiple and may involve more than one lung lobe. They are usually amorphous with indistinct borders. Less commonly, radio-opacity involves an entire lobe, creating distinct lobar borders. Infiltrates are more common in the right and caudal lobes. Rarely, infiltrates may appear as distinct, wedge-shaped densities with the apex toward the pulmonary hilus. Infiltrates represent areas of hemorrhage, atelectasis, or infarction.

Pulmonary vessel changes may be evident, including enlargement of the main pulmonary artery segment and attenuation of a lobar artery or vein.[4,8,70] Pleural effusion and cardiomegaly may also occur.[4,8,70]

Patients with PTE may have normal thoracic radiographs or radiographic findings that are not consistent with the degree of clinical compromise.[4,8,69,70] In canine studies, the percentage of dogs with normal radiographs ranges from 9% to 27%.[4,8,70] In a feline study of PTE, 7% (1/14) had normal thoracic radiographs.[9] Because these are necropsy studies, and thus select for more severely affected patients, the occurrence of normal radiographs in animals with PTE is likely even higher. Thoracic radiographs that underestimate the degree of clinical respiratory compromise are an important clue to the presence of PTE.

ARTERIAL BLOOD GAS ANALYSIS

Arterial blood gas analysis can aid in the diagnosis of PTE, but changes are not pathognomonic. The most common abnormalities are hypoxemia, an increased alveolar-arterial oxygen tension gradient (P[A–a]o_2), decreased oxygen responsiveness, and hypocapnia.[4,8,27,36] Hypercapnia is uncommon but can occur with severe compromise. Blood gas analysis of 15 dogs with PTE showed that 80% were hypoxemic, 100% had an increased alveolar-arterial oxygen gradient, 47% were hypocapnic, and 44% had decreased oxygen responsiveness.[8] These changes, when present, are nonspecific indicators of inefficient gaseous exchange and do not confirm a diagnosis of PTE. Moreover, the presence of normal blood gas values does not exclude PTE. Blood gas abnormalities in cats with PTE have not been reported.

COAGULATION TESTING

The routine coagulogram is not particularly helpful in the diagnosis of thromboembolism; it is commonly normal.[8] If abnormalities are present, they are inconsistent and nonspecific. In a small study of dogs and cats, approximately 50% demonstrated some degree of thrombocytopenia.[9,30] It appears that other changes compatible with consumption (e.g., elevated fibrin degradation products or prolongation of the prothrombin time or activated partial thromboplastin time) are less common.[9,30] There is no known correlation between thrombocytosis or shortened coagulation times and thrombosis. Patients without thrombosis can have shortened coagulation times, but the majority of patients with thrombosis do not have shortened times.

Significant hyperfibrinogenemia may indicate potential hypercoagulability but is not indicative of thromboembolism.[71] Moreover, hyperfibrinogenemia occurs in few of the hypercoagulable states (e.g., some cases of pancreatitis, or with sepsis).

Assay of antithrombin III (ATIII) concentration or activity is more useful but less widely available. A correlation with thrombotic risk has been shown when ATIII deficiency is the primary mechanism for thrombosis (protein-losing nephropathy).[72] Concentration and activity of ATIII may also be decreased as a result of massive thromboembolism. In humans, this is considered a useful adjunctive test for the diagnosis of PTE and DVT, with levels of ATIII often being diminished to a degree compatible with the extent of thrombosis.[72,73] It remains to be evaluated for this use in the dog and cat.

D-dimer is a unique fibrin degradation product that is formed when cross-linked fibrin is proteolyzed by plasmin.[74] Because cross-linkage of fibrin implicates the production of thrombin, elevations in D-dimer concentration imply the presence of both thrombin and circulating plasmin. D-dimer levels are extensively employed as an adjunctive test in human patients with suspected DVT and PTE.[3,73,75-78] The sensitivity of the test has been reported to be 85% to 93%, and the specificity 70% to 77%.[73,75] The overall negative predictive value is high.[75-77] If the clinical suspicion for PTE is low, and the D-dimer test is negative, thrombosis is considered extremely unlikely.[3,75] If the test is positive, further diagnostic tests are indicated. A high D-dimer concentration in human patients has been shown to be correlated with the presence of thrombosis and a higher mortality.[79] Semiquantitative, patient-side latex agglutination tests (e.g., SimpliRED D-dimer test or Agen) appear to be comparable to the standard ELISA assay in human patients.[3,78-80] D-dimer assay is available through several veterinary laboratories, but its utility in the setting of PTE remains to be elucidated.

CARDIAC EVALUATION

Electrocardiographic changes are rarely reported. Sinus tachycardia is likely the most common finding. Changes consistent with right ventricular compromise may be seen (e.g., right axis deviation and cor pulmonale).[66] Myocardial ischemia may result in S-T segment depression or in ventricular premature contractions.[66] These changes are neither sensitive nor specific for PTE.

Elevated pulmonary artery pressure, right ventricular pressure, and central venous pressure occur when vascular obstruction exceeds compensatory limits and pulmonary arterial resistance increases.[26,27,54,81] These changes occur with severe obstruction or with preexisting cardiopulmonary disease. Pulmonary arterial pressure, however, can be deceptive in the evaluation of hemodynamic compromise. As the right ventricle fails and cardiac output decreases, pulmonary arterial pressure falls, despite the presence of an extremely high PVR. Right ventricular hypokinesis is associated with a doubling of the mortality rate in humans.[6] Arterial blood pressure is not a reliable indicator because hypokinesis was present in 40% of human patients with normal systemic arterial blood pressure.[6]

PULMONARY SCINTIGRAPHY

Scintigraphy is commonly used for the diagnosis of PTE in human patients.[3,11,73,82] It has been shown to be sensitive and specific for experimental PTE in dogs and has been successfully utilized clinically in dogs and cats.[28,68,81,83-85] The technique, however, is limited to the few referral facilities with scanning equipment.

The rationale of pulmonary scintigraphy is that occlusion of pulmonary vessels by a thrombus results in areas of the lung that continue to be ventilated despite the absence of perfusion. By radioactive labeling of the pulmonary blood (perfusion scan) and the inspired air (ventilation scan), areas of the lungs with ventilation-perfusion mismatch can be demonstrated via gamma camera (scintigraphy).

Perfusion scans are performed using technetium 99m macroaggregated albumin, which is injected into a central vein.[83,84] A normal perfusion scan virtually excludes a diagnosis of PTE. An abnormal perfusion scan, however, is not specific for PTE: perfusion defects can result from numerous nonthrombotic conditions including pneumonia, edema, contusions, obstructive pulmonary disease, and atelectasis. These conditions are associated with decreased regional ventilation. For this reason, an abnormal perfusion scan should be followed by a ventilation scan. In the patient with PTE, a ventilation scan should be normal.

Ventilation scans are performed by having the patient breathe a nontoxic radioactive gas (e.g., xenon 133 or technetium 99m DTPA radioaerosol).[83,84] These scans can be difficult to perform in dyspneic or stressed dogs. In such situations, a presumption of normal ventilation may be based on the absence of abnormal radiographic densities in the region of abnormal perfusion.[75]

PULMONARY ANGIOGRAPHY

Selective pulmonary angiography remains the gold standard for the diagnosis of PTE.[3,11,69,82,86] It is indicated for the definitive diagnosis or exclusion of PTE when scintigraphy is unavailable or inconclusive. Iodinated contrast medium is rapidly injected via a large-bore catheter into the pulmonary arterial tree. The pulmonary arterial system can then be visualized via thoracic radiography. Intraluminal filling defects, abrupt termination of pulmonary arteries, and the complete absence of arterial branches are diagnostic for PTE (Figure 71-1).[69,86,87] A regional loss of vascularity, asymmetric bloodflow, tortuous pulmonary arteries, and abrupt tapering of peripheral vessels support a diagnosis of PTE but are nonspecific.[86,87] A negative selective arteriogram essentially excludes clinically significant PTE. Because the procedure requires general anesthesia and is invasive, it constitutes a significant risk in the compromised patient. This limits the utility of this technique in clinical veterinary practice.

Nonselective pulmonary angiography is easier and safer than selective techniques. General anesthesia and specialized equipment are typically not required. Contrast medium is injected via a large-bore catheter into the right side of the heart or the jugular vein. The radiographic study, however, is less sensitive and more difficult to interpret than selective angiography because of dilution of the contrast medium by venous blood and the superimposition of vascular structures (Figure 71-2).[69,87] It is indicated in the unstable patient, where the risk of selective angiography is deemed excessive.

SPIRAL COMPUTED TOMOGRAPHIC ANGIOGRAPHY

Spiral computed tomographic (CT) angiography has been evaluated for use in the diagnosis of PTE in humans.[73,75] The technique allows precise visualization of the pulmonary vasculature and is not invasive. Reported sensitivity for the diagnosis of PTE is as high as 95.5%, with a specificity of 97.6%.[73,75] Sensitivity is substantially lower, however, when PTE is confined to subsegmental pulmonary arteries.[73,75] The technique has not yet been described in dogs and cats.

TESTING FOR ASSOCIATED CONDITIONS

The diagnosis or suspicion of PTE should prompt a thorough investigation for conditions that may be associated with hypercoagulation and thromboembolism. Although the presence of such a condition does not confirm PTE, it may provide further support where definitive diagnosis is impossible, and it is essential in clinical management.

Treatment

Treatment of patients with PTE should include: (1) support of the respiratory and cardiovascular systems; (2) the prevention of TE propagation and recurrence; and, possibly, (3) thrombolysis.

It appears that a relatively small percentage of PTEs are immediately fatal.[7,88] In the normal dog, thrombi begin to lyse spontaneously within hours.[13,86] Therefore, if the patient can be supported through the respiratory and

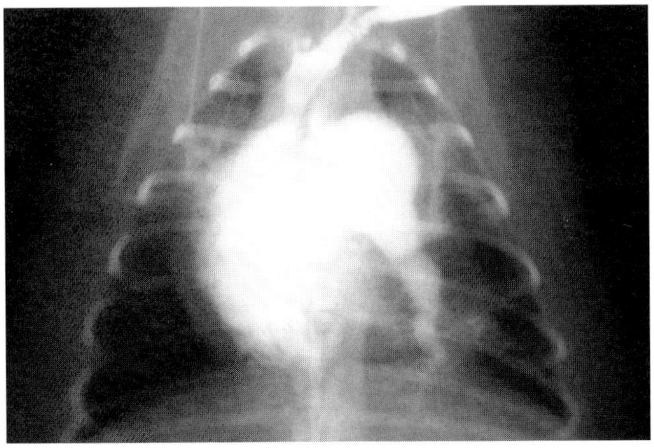

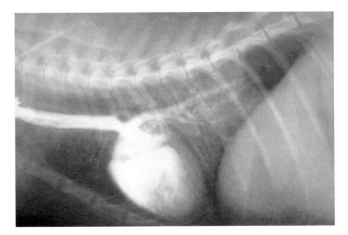

Figure 71-1. *Selective angiogram in a dog with hyperadrenocorticism and acute onset of dyspnea. The ventrodorsal radiographic projection shows abrupt termination of the pulmonary artery.*

Figure 71-2. *Nonselective angiogram in a cat with dirofilariasis. The lateral radiographic projection shows decreased perfusion of the caudal lung field.*

cardiovascular compromise, and further exacerbations can be prevented, survival is possible. In some cases, however, patient compromise may be so extreme that survival is unlikely even if rapid lysis occurs. Moreover, many of these patients have disturbed fibrinolysis, preventing rapid thrombus dissolution. In such cases, pharmacologic thrombolysis may be considered.

RESPIRATORY AND CARDIOVASCULAR SUPPORT

Support of respiratory and cardiovascular function is essential in the patient with clinical PTE. Oxygen supplementation is indicated when dyspnea is evident and/or when arterial partial pressure of oxygen (PaO_2) decreases below 70 mm Hg. In addition to relieving hypoxemia, oxygen supplementation has been shown to dilate pulmonary vessels, improve hemodynamics, reduce pulmonary hypertension, and improve right ventricular function. If appropriate oxygen supplementation is inadequate to correct the hypoxemia, mechanical ventilation is indicated.

Perfusion should be optimized in any patient with hypoxemia. In these patients, arterial oxygen content is deficient, and any decrease in perfusion will further exacerbate the already reduced tissue oxygen delivery. In addition, optimizing perfusion reverses the prothrombotic effects of vascular stasis and hypoxia-induced vascular injury.

Theoretically, bronchodilators may be of benefit. Methylxanthine bronchodilators such as theophylline have small positive inotropic effects and produce sustained pulmonary vasodilation. Theophylline improves diaphragmatic contractility in dogs and reduces respiratory muscle fatigue. These effects may be beneficial in extremely dyspneic or tachypneic patients in whom muscle fatigue may result in respiratory failure.

Positive inotropes such as dobutamine or digoxin may be considered if decreased cardiac contractility and cardiac failure occur, but these are not without risk. Increased cardiac output results in increased pulmonary artery pressures. In addition, hypoxemia and acidosis can increase susceptibility to inotrope-induced arrhythmias.

Vasodilators have been recommended for patients with pulmonary hypertension. Selected patients respond to hydralazine, calcium channel blockers, or angiotensin-converting enzyme inhibitors. Significant side effects can occur, however, because of systemic hypotension. Because there are no clinical data to predict response to these agents, use should be guided by therapeutic trials using cardiac catheterization. Because this is seldom practical in veterinary patients with acute PTE, vasodilator therapy cannot be recommended for these patients.

PREVENTION OF PROPAGATION AND RECURRENCE OF THROMBI

Thrombi tend to propagate, especially in the prothrombotic and hypofibrinolytic patient, and this can result in further compromise. The patient with PTE has proved that it is prothrombotic and, therefore, at risk for additional TE episodes. When death occurs beyond the first few hours following PTE, it is usually caused by a recurrent embolic event.[1,89] Management, therefore, should be focused to prevent such occurrences. Prevention should address all aspects of Virchow's triad including (1) minimizing vascular stasis via the maintenance of adequate perfusion and the prevention of prolonged immobility; (2) minimizing vascular injury via the appropriate use and handling of venous catheters; and (3) altering the hemostatic system via the appropriate use of anticoagulants. In general, these drugs do not lyse existing thrombi; they are indicated to inhibit propagation and prevent recurrent thrombosis. They are most useful in preventing venous thrombosis. Because PTE is primarily a venous event, anticoagulants are indicated in all cases of PTE.

Unfractionated Heparin

Heparin is the most commonly used anticoagulant for the treatment of acute PTE.[3,11,90] Although the use of heparin in patients with disseminated intravascular coagulation may be controversial, its efficacy in preventing thromboembolism is well established.[91-94] Heparin therapy is standard-of-care in human patients with PTE.[90,91]

Unfractionated heparin is composed of naturally occurring mucopolysaccharides of varying molecular weights.[91,95,96] The primary mechanism of action is the potentiation of ATIII activity, leading to the inactivation of a number of coagulation enzymes including thrombin (factor IIa) and factors Xa, IXa, XIa, and XIIa.[90,95,96] Of these, thrombin and factor Xa are the most responsive to inhibition.[90,95,96] The relative effect of heparin on these coagulation factors is dependent on its molecular size. Smaller heparin molecules (i.e., less than 18 saccharide units) are unable to simultaneously bind ATIII and thrombin and are therefore unable to catalyze thrombin inhibition. These molecules, however, are effective in catalyzing factor Xa inhibition. Heparin also catalyzes the inactivation of thrombin by plasma/heparin cofactor II (which acts independently of ATIII).[90,95] Other effects of heparin include decreased blood viscosity, decreased platelet function, increased vascular permeability, and enhanced fibrinolysis via increased tissue plasminogen activator (t-PA).[90,95,97-100] These effects contribute to the hemorrhagic risk.

The anticoagulant effects of a standard dose of heparin vary widely among patients.[90,101] Unfractionated heparin may be poorly absorbed from subcutaneous sites, especially at lower doses.[102] The plasma clearance of heparin depends on a rapid, dose-related saturable cellular mechanism; and a slower, non–dose-related renal clearance.[103] As such, the intensity and duration of effect increase disproportionately with increasing dose.[103] Higher-molecular-weight species are cleared more rapidly than lower-molecular-weight species, resulting in varied anticoagulant activity over time.[90] Binding of heparin to plasma proteins, endothelial cells, and platelets contributes to the unpredictable response.[104] In addition, some patients appear to have heparin resistance, requiring larger doses to achieve a therapeutic effect.[11,90,105-107]

Heparin resistance has been associated with ATIII deficiency, increased heparin clearance, and elevations in heparin binding proteins.[90,106,107]

It has been shown in human patients that, unless a prescriptive heparin nomogram is used, many patients receive inadequate heparinization in the initial 24 to 48 hours of therapy, resulting in an increased incidence of recurrent TE.[91,101,102,108-112] The therapeutic range of heparin has been based on experimental studies in animals and on subgroup analysis of the results of various studies in humans.[102,109,110,113,114] These studies demonstrated that the prevention of thrombus growth required doses of heparin that prolonged the PTT to approximately 1.5 to 2.5 times that of controls. These doses were equivalent to a heparin concentration of 0.2 to 0.4 U/ml by protamine sulfate titration, and 0.3 to 0.7 U/ml by antifactor Xa assay.[11,90,91,106,113] The risk of TE recurrence is increased if the PTT is less than 1.5 times the mean of the normal range.[109,110] Successful heparin therapy, therefore, necessitates monitoring the anticoagulant response using the PTT and/or heparin levels, and titrating the dose to the individual patient. There are, however, limitations in the use of PTT to monitor heparin therapy. Firstly, the PTT is not directly correlated with anticoagulant effect and clinical efficacy.[90] This may be largely because of the fact that the PTT effect of heparin reflects primarily its antifactor IIa activity.[90] Secondly, there is significant variation in PTT sensitivity to heparin using different coagulometers.[11,90] It is recommended that a curve should be established for each machine based on the PTT and associated blood heparin concentrations for 20 to 30 patients.[11,111] Thereafter, monitoring heparin concentrations in individual patients is generally considered unnecessary.

Heparinization guidelines for human patients are established. For patients with suspected or confirmed TE, heparin is generally given as an intravenous bolus followed by continuous-rate infusion.[91,101,108] The American Association of Chest Physicians Consensus Conference on Antithrombotic Therapy established a protocol for intravenous heparinization of PTE patients (Table 71-1).[91] This has been used in dogs but remains to be fully evaluated. Subcutaneous administration of heparin is used less commonly for the treatment of PTE in human patients. An intravenous bolus dose is generally followed by subcutaneous administration every 8 to 12 hours.[90,95,101,102] This protocol has been shown to be adequate, provided that the APTT is prolonged into the therapeutic range; but it is less effective in achieving such a range in a rapid manner.[91,102,115]

Published doses of heparin in dogs vary enormously, ranging from 50 U/kg to 250 U/kg subcutaneously every 6 to 12 hours, to intravenous infusion of 5 to 20 U/kg/hr.[8,26,27,81,116] These are largely anecdotal. One study in healthy beagles demonstrated that subcutaneous heparin doses of 200 U/kg every 6 hours were required to maintain therapeutic levels based on PTT.[117] Another study demonstrated excessive anticoagulation, based on plasma heparin concentrations, using 500 U/kg subcutaneously every 12 hours.[118] Both studies showed marked individual variability in response, emphasizing the importance of monitoring. Moreover, it has been shown

TABLE 71-1. Weight-Based Nomogram for the Intravenous Infusion of Heparin

An intravenous bolus administration of heparin of 80 U/kg is administered, followed by a continuous rate infusion of 18 U/kg/hr.

A PTT is evaluated 6 hours after initiation of therapy. Adjustments are as follows:

PTT	Dose Change (U/kg/hr)	Additional Action	Next PTT
<1.2 × mean normal	+4	Rebolus with 80 U/kg	6 hours
1.2 to 1.5 × mean normal	+2	Rebolus with 40 U/kg	6 hours
1.5 to 2.3 × mean normal	0	0	6 hours for first 24 hours, then daily
2.3 to 3.0 × mean normal	−2	0	6 hours
>3.0 × mean normal	−3	Stop infusion 1 hour	6 hours

From AACP Consensus Committee on Pulmonary Embolism: Opinions regarding the diagnosis and management of venous thromboembolic disease, *Chest* 113(2):499, 1998.

that heparin metabolism may be increased in experimental dogs and in human patients with thromboembolism, such that larger doses may be required compared with healthy subjects.[105]

A study in cats showed marked variation in pharmacokinetics with subcutaneous heparin therapy.[33] Doses needed to achieve apparent therapeutic levels ranged from 175 U/kg to 475 U/kg subcutaneously every 8 hours, and PTT results did not correlate well with plasma heparin concentrations. An effective means of heparinization in small animal patients remains to be established. It would appear prudent to utilize protocols established in human patients and in animal models, and to closely monitor PTT values and/or heparin concentrations.

The most significant adverse effect of heparin therapy is bleeding.[119] The risk increases with dose, recent surgery, trauma, concomitant hemostatic defects, and thrombolytic therapy.[90,119] Studies in humans have demonstrated an increased risk of bleeding with intermittent intravenous administration compared with continuous infusion.[120,121] No difference in major bleeding was detected between continuous intravenous infusion and subcutaneous administration.[115,122] In the event of uncontrolled hemorrhage, treatment with protamine sulfate is indicated.[11,116] If administered within minutes of the last heparin dose, a full neutralizing dose of protamine is 1 mg per 100 U of heparin, given via slow intravenous injection. If 1 hour has elapsed, 50% of the full dose should be administered; if 2 hours have elapsed, 25% of the dose should be administered.

Low Molecular Weight Heparin

The use of low molecular weight heparin (LMWH) is rapidly replacing that of unfractionated heparin in human patients for both the treatment and prevention of PTE. These drugs are manufactured from unfractionated heparin using chemical or enzymatic techniques.[90] They differ from unfractionated heparin in several important respects, including superior bioavailablility (i.e., greater than 90% after subcutaneous injection); a prolonged half-life and predictable renal clearance, enabling once or twice daily dosing; and predictable antithrombotic responses, permitting treatment based on body weight without laboratory monitoring.[90,123-127] Other advantages are their ability to inhibit platelet-bound factor Xa, resistance to inhibition by platelet factor 4, and their decreased effect on platelet function and vascular permeability.[127,128] These characteristics possibly account for the occurrence of fewer hemorrhagic effects at comparable antithrombotic dosages.[128,129]

Small molecular weight fractions lose anti-IIa activity and cannot be monitored with an APTT.[90,127] The drugs can be monitored with an anti-Xa assay, but favorable dose-response characteristics make monitoring unnecessary in most patients, except those in renal failure.[11,90]

In human clinical trials, subcutaneous LMWHs have generally shown similar or superior efficacy when compared with intravenous unfractionated heparin with regard to recurrent venous TE, mortality, and major hemorrhage.[123-125,130,131] Although these drugs are more expensive than unfractionated heparin, the decreased risk and decreased need for monitoring contribute to greater cost-effectiveness.[91] Commercially available LMWHs include dalteparin, enoxaparin, and tinzaparin. There are currently no published reports of their use in veterinary patients.

Warfarin

Warfarin remains the drug of choice for long-term outpatient treatment and prevention of PTE.[11,91,132] Contraindications to therapy include owner noncompliance, significant hepatic disease, and recent surgery of the central nervous system or eye.[133]

Warfarin is an oral vitamin K antagonist, thus inhibiting the activation of vitamin K-dependent factors II, VII, IX, X, and proteins C and S.[132,133] Because of the half-lives of these factors, the anticoagulant effect of warfarin is not immediate. During the first 24 to 48 hours after initiating therapy, only factor VII and protein C are significantly affected.[3,132,133] Inhibition of protein C alone is prothrombotic, thus potentially leading to thrombosis, especially during the first 24 to 48 hours of therapy, before other factors are inhibited. Although inactivation of factor VII will result in PT prolongation, effective anticoagulation does not occur until factor II is inactivated (approximately 48 hours).[3,132] For these reasons, heparin therapy should overlap warfarin therapy for at least the first 2 days, and until therapeutic levels of warfarin are achieved.[3,132,133]

Warfarin therapy is initiated at a dose of 0.05 to 0.1 mg/kg orally once daily in the dog and the cat.[116,134,135] A therapeutic range is generally achieved within 5 to 7 days.[134,135] A study in healthy dogs demonstrated that a loading dose of 6 mg could be safely administered to

dogs weighing 25 to 30 kg (approximately 0.2 mg/kg), to achieve therapeutic levels within 2 days.[136]

Warfarin therapy should be monitored by use of the prothrombin time (PT) and the calculated international normalization ratio (INR). Initial recommendations were to adjust warfarin therapy to achieve a PT of 1.5 times baseline. However, because of the variability of thromboplastins used in the PT assay, current recommendations are to standardize the PT using the international normalization ratio (INR).[11,101,114,132,133] The INR is calculated as follows:

$$INR = (patient\ PT/control\ PT) \times ISI.$$

The ISI, which is provided by the manufacturer, is the international standardization index, and is a measure of the responsiveness of a specific thromboplastin compared to the reference preparation. The therapeutic range for warfarin is an INR of 2.0 to 3.0.* Concomitant administration of unfractionated heparin usually prolongs the INR by an additional 0.5.[3] The INR should be assessed daily until a therapeutic range is achieved. Heparin is then discontinued.[133,137] Gradual weaning of heparin has been recommended in the veterinary literature, although there is little evidence to support this practice. The theory is that weaning may prevent a possible rebound hypercoagulability in patients that are not anticoagulated with warfarin.

The dose-response relationship of warfarin is influenced by drug interactions and other pharmacodynamic factors. Clearance is inhibited by phenylbutazone, metronidazole, trimethoprim-sulfa antibiotics, and amiodarone, resulting in potentiation of effect.[138-142] Cimetidine and omeprazole inhibit clearance to a lesser extent.[132,142,143] Erythromycin and some anabolic steroids potentiate the effects of warfarin via unknown mechanisms.[132,144] Acetaminophen has been reported to augment the effects of warfarin, although this contention has been challenged.[132,142,145,146] In contrast, drugs such as barbiturates, rifampin, and carbamazepine increase metabolic clearance, thus attenuating the anticoagulant effect.[140,145] Increased dietary intake of vitamin K can also decrease the anticoagulant effects of warfarin.[142,145] Hepatic dysfunction and hypermetabolic states, produced by fever or hyperthyroidism, potentiate the effects of warfarin.[132,146]

Because of the risk of hemorrhage, and the influence of diet, comorbidity, and various drugs, continued monitoring of warfarin therapy on an outpatient basis is essential. Initially, recheck twice weekly for 1 to 2 weeks is recommended, then less frequently depending on the stability of the results.[137] If the INR is within therapeutic range, recheck every 4 to 6 weeks is indicated.[133,137] If the INR is below or above range, the dose is increased or decreased, respectively, by 5% to 20% depending on the degree of abnormality, and the INR is reevaluated in 1 to 2 weeks.[133] If the INR is above 5.0, warfarin therapy should be discontinued; when the INR falls below 3.0, therapy can be reinitiated with a dose reduction of 20% to 50%.[133] In the event of warfarin-induced uncontrollable hemorrhage,

---

*References 3, 11, 101, 114, 132, and 133.

therapy should be discontinued and plasma or fresh blood administered.[11,133] Vitamin K can be administered, but the onset of effect is delayed 12 to 24 hours, and it renders the patient refractory to further warfarin therapy for up to 2 weeks.[116,133]

The optimum duration of warfarin therapy in veterinary patients is unclear. In human patients, therapy is recommended for 4 to 12 weeks for a first episode of PTE if there is a reversible risk factor for thrombosis, and for up to 6 months if there is continuing risk.[114,147] Indefinite therapy is recommended in patients with congenital hypercoagulable states, recurrent thromboembolism, or thromboembolism complicating malignancy.[3,114,132,147]

THROMBOLYSIS

Thrombolytic agents are effective, to some degree, in almost all instances of thrombosis. Recent thrombi and arterial thrombi lyse more readily.[148] In human patients, there appears to be a 14-day window for effective administration in cases of PTE.[149] Recognized advantages of thrombolytic therapy include rapid clot lysis, improved pulmonary perfusion, accelerated reversal of right heart failure, and improved hemodynamic stability.[88,150-153] The efficacy of streptokinase (SK), urokinase (UK), and tissue plasminogen activator (t-PA) has been demonstrated in multiple human trials and in canine models.[148,151,153-155] These potential benefits must be weighed, however, against the risk of massive hemorrhage, which is not uncommon.[11,88,101,156] Hemorrhage may be less common when smaller doses are administered directly at the site of the thrombus.[157] Unfortunately, this is often difficult owing to the invasiveness of the procedure and the clinical status of the patient. The introduction of newer, fibrin-specific agents theoretically allows intravenous administration with reduced risk. Additional potential risks of thrombolytic therapy are reperfusion injury and hyperkalemia.[31,156,158] Allopurinol and deferoxamine have been recommended in an attempt to attenuate this effect.[159,160]

In humans, thrombolysis is generally reserved for patients who are hemodynamically unstable or who have echocardiographic evidence of right ventricular dysfunction.[11,88] Studies show that timely intervention with thrombolysis can reduce mortality associated with PTE in these patients.[88,161,162] Limited veterinary experience with these drugs, together with associated risks, make recommendations for their use extremely difficult. Nevertheless, they may be considered if respiratory and cardiovascular compromise is severe or persistent. Contraindications for fibrinolysis therapy include active internal bleeding, hypertension, recent (i.e., within 10 days) surgery or organ biopsy, and severe gastrointestinal bleeding.[11,163]

Streptokinase

Streptokinase (SK) is isolated from the broth of beta-hemolytic streptococci cultures.[164] It binds and activates circulating plasminogen.[148,165] In humans and in cats, the SK-plasmin complex can activate the systemic conversion of plasminogen to plasmin.[166,167] Free plasmin can circulate and induce a lytic state. In the dog, the SK-

plasmin complex is inactivated by alpha$_2$-antiplasmin.[166] SK is therefore more thrombus-specific in the dog. Because of the potential for preexisting anti-SK antibodies, a loading dose is generally recommended.[164]

The use of intravenous streptokinase has been reported in 4 dogs with nonpulmonary TE (3 ileofemoral and 1 cardiac).[160] Doses and protocols varied enormously. Loading doses of 5200 U/kg to 18,000 U/kg were administered over 30 minutes either once or three times (on separate days). Maintenance doses ranged from 2083 U/kg/hr to 9000 U/kg/hr, infused for 3 to 10 hours per day. All dogs showed resolution of the thrombus after 1 to 4 days of therapy. Three dogs demonstrated only minor hemorrhage. Although this study shows that SK can be used safely and efficaciously in dogs, dosage protocols and efficacy in a greater number of patients need to be clarified.

Streptokinase use has been reported in cats with experimental and naturally-occurring aortic TE.[158,167,168] All reports utilized a loading dose of 90,000 U over 20 to 30 minutes, followed by a maintenance dose of 45,000 U/kg/hr for 3 or more hours. Results were disappointing. In experimental cats, few demonstrated thrombolysis at 3 hours.[167] Mortality was high in feline patients (50% to 100%).[158,168] Cats died as a result of bleeding, reperfusion, hyperkalemia, infarction, or presumptive anaphylaxis. It is unclear whether the differences in results in the canine and feline reports are caused by differences in the clot-specificity of SK in these species, to other inherent species differences, to differences in treatment protocols, or to the small numbers of cases involved.

Urokinase

Urokinase (UK), found in urine, is a naturally occurring plasminogen activator, converting plasminogen directly into plasmin.[148,169] It can be produced from fetal cells in culture. UK has shown superior effects compared with SK in humans, and is commonly used both intravenously and locally.[148,155,169] UK is not clot-specific and can lead to a fibrinolytic state. Modified, clot-specific UK compounds (e.g., Pro-UK and PEG-UK) have been developed; these compounds are not activated until they are absorbed onto fibrin.[148,170,171] Dosing regimens for these agents have been evaluated in experimental dogs, but clinical use in small animals has not been reported.[172,173]

Tissue-Type Plasminogen Activator

Tissue plasminogen activator (t-PA) is the major physiologic activator of plasminogen. It is relatively clot-specific in that it has a low affinity for circulating plasminogen. It has a high affinity for fibrin, and plasminogen activation occurs on the surface of fibrin.[174,175] As the clot lyses, plasmin remains bound to the clot. Free plasmin is immediately bound by alpha$_2$-antiplasmin. In humans, t-PA has shown higher success rates and more rapid thrombolysis compared with SK and UK, fewer adverse effects, and is reported to be more effective in the lysis of aged thrombi.[11,176,177] The half-life of t-PA in dogs is 2 to 3 minutes, but thrombolytic effects persist beyond this time.[178] Multiple, small-dose, bolus injections appear to be more effective than a single large-dose bolus, or continuous infusion.

The clinical use of t-PA for PTE in dogs and cats has not been reported. Successful thrombolysis was reported in a dog with aortic thrombosis.[159] The drug was administered at a dose of 1 mg/kg as an IV bolus every 60 minutes for a total of 10 doses. Studies in dogs with experimental PTE have shown that a bolus of 1 mg/kg infused over 15 minutes resulted in rapid thrombolysis without significant hemorrhage.[173,179] Thrombolysis using this regimen was greater than that using UK.[173] Further studies are required to determine the efficacy, safety, and optimal dosing for t-PA in canine patients.

Reports of thrombolytic therapy using t-PA in cats with cardiomyopathy and aortic TE demonstrated rapid fibrinolysis, with 43% of cats regaining limb function within 2 days.[31] Approximately 50% of the cats died acutely, however, because of hyperkalemia, heart failure, or cardiac embolization. The risk-to-benefit ratio of this protocol makes it difficult to recommend.

Prevention

The mortality rate of PTE is substantial, with many deaths occurring rapidly before the diagnosis can be confirmed and effective treatment implemented.[11] Moreover, diagnosis is difficult and treatment of established PTE is not universally successful.[3] This makes prevention imperative in the patient at risk for TE.

Prevention should address all aspects of Virchow's triad. This includes: (1) minimizing vascular stasis by maintaining adequate perfusion and prevention of prolonged immobility; (2) minimizing vascular injury by appropriate use and handling of venous catheters; and (3) altering the hemostatic system via the appropriate use of drugs. Drugs are indicated when there is considered to be significant risk for TE.

ASSESSMENT OF THROMBOEMBOLIC RISK

There are, unfortunately, no objective methods for determining thromboembolic risk in veterinary patients. The incidence of PTE in specific diseases is unknown, and we have few or no laboratory tools to confirm hypercoagulability. In addition, the efficacy of prophylactic measures has not been determined. It is impossible, therefore, to give evidence-based recommendations for the use of prophylactic anticoagulants in small animals. Assessment of risk remains largely subjective. Understanding the risk factors in patient groups and in individual patients forms the basis for such assessment.

In many medical patients, multiple risk factors are present, and the risks are cumulative.[180] That is, a patient with a hypercoagulable state may not develop TE until precipitated by another hypercoagulable state or prothrombotic condition such as catheterization, surgery, hypoperfusion, or glucocorticoid therapy. Such a situation should prompt consideration of anticoagulant therapy.

Undoubtedly, the single most convincing evidence of risk is a prior TE episode. Prophylactic drugs are indicated until the cause is reversed. Cats with cardiomyopathy and evidence of atrial thrombus formation on echocardiogram are candidates for long-term prophylaxis. The author considers sepsis, severe acute pancreatitis, or severe immune-mediated hemolytic anemia (IMHA) to be indications for anticoagulant therapy. Risk stratification, however, is subjective and based on the severity of disease and concomitant risk factors. A study in dogs with IMHA attempted to identify clinical findings associated with a higher incidence of PTE.[26] A high serum bilirubin concentration, multiple intravenous catheterizations, and a higher number of blood transfusions were found to be associated. These clinical findings indicate a more severe hemolytic crisis.

Nephrotic syndrome is a significant risk factor for both venous and arterial thromboembolism. Determination of ATIII concentration or activity might assist in risk assessment and determining the need for aggressive prophylaxis. The risk is reported to be moderate when ATIII concentrations are between 50% and 75% of normal, and marked when ATIII concentrations are less than 50% of normal.[181] Results of human trials, however, are equivocal.[182,183] Risk may also be estimated by the severity of renal protein loss, the existence of potentially contributing factors, and any history of prior thromboembolic events.

Patients with hyperadrenocorticism or diabetes mellitus appear to have a low incidence of thromboembolism, and the need for prophylactic drugs in these patients is doubtful. The risk may increase, however, when another prothrombotic condition is applied (e.g., pancreatitis or surgery). In human patients with hyperadrenocorticism, thromboembolic risk is highly correlated with systemic hypertension. It is the author's opinion that this is true in dogs. That is, whereas anticoagulants are not generally indicated in the dog with uncomplicated Cushing's disease, the patient with hyperadrenocorticism undergoing adrenalectomy is certainly a candidate for anticoagulation, particularly if he/she has hypertension or protein-losing nephropathy. In these patients, prophylactic anticoagulants are generally initiated 1 to 3 days before surgery.

PHARMACOLOGICAL PROPHYLAXIS

Anticoagulants are indicated for the prevention of venous thromboembolism. As such, they form the cornerstone of PTE prevention.[180] Antiplatelet drugs may be considered together with, but not in lieu of, anticoagulants.[180]

Anticoagulants

Anticoagulant prophylaxis is initiated with low-dose, subcutaneous unfractionated heparin. In human patients, fixed doses of 5000 units are administered subcutaneously two or three times daily. This protocol does not require laboratory monitoring and has been shown to reduce the rate of fatal PTE by two thirds.[184-187] Abundant data demonstrate either no increase or small increases in the rates of major hemorrhage.[90,180,184] Wound hematomas are seen more commonly but do not warrant avoidance of heparin.[180,184] Recommended doses of heparin for prophylaxis in small animal patients are largely anecdotal and range from 50 to 200 U/kg subcutaneously two or three times daily. These doses do not appear to result in hemorrhage. Efficacy rates have yet to be assessed.

In human medicine, the use of LMWH has largely replaced that of unfractionated heparin for the prevention of venous TE. In multiple studies, LMWHs have proved to be comparable or superior to unfractionated heparin with respect to prevention.[180,188,189] A meta-analysis of randomized trials showed LMWHs to be associated with a 52% lower incidence of bleeding.[189] There are as yet no reports of the use of LMWHs in small animal patients.

Heparin should be continued until the risk of thromboembolism is considered to be sufficiently decreased. In patients with reversible causes (e.g., pancreatitis or postadrenalectomy), the author continues twice daily heparin for 1 week following clinical recovery. Long-term prophylaxis is indicated where risk continues (e.g., the cat with evidence of cardiac thrombosis, or the dog with recurrent thromboembolism during therapy for IMHA). In such cases, warfarin therapy should be considered. Warfarin is initiated during heparin therapy, and heparin is discontinued when a therapeutic level of warfarin is achieved.

Antiplatelet Drugs

Antiplatelet drugs inhibit platelet adhesion and aggregation, thereby preventing the formation and organization of the primary platelet plug.[190] They are most useful for the prevention of arterial thrombosis (e.g., aortic or cerebrovascular).[190] Although PTE is almost exclusively a venous event in humans, this does not appear to be true in small animals. Moreover, conditions that lead to PTE may also result in arterial thrombosis. In necropsy studies, a significant percentage of animals had thrombosis in multiple organ systems.[8,19,20,24,30] Recent studies in human patients have established that aspirin therapy is effective in preventing venous thromboembolism following surgery.[191] Although it was not as effective as anticoagulant therapy, combined therapy with aspirin was more effective than heparin alone. There is a rationale, therefore, for antiplatelet drugs as adjunctive agents in the prevention of PTE.

Aspirin is the only antiplatelet drug that has been used with any frequency in veterinary patients. Newer antiplatelet drugs appear promising, but veterinary experience with these agents is limited. Aspirin is a cyclooxygenase inhibitor. It irreversibly acetylates the cyclooxygenase enzymes COX-1 and COX-2, thus preventing the formation of various prostaglandins, including thromboxane A_2 (TXA_2) and prostacyclin (PGI_2).[190,192] TXA_2, which is produced by platelets, is largely a COX-1 derived product and induces platelet aggregation.[193,194] PGI_2, which is produced by vascular endothelial cells, is derived from both COX-1 and COX-2 and inhibits platelet aggregation.[193,194] Aspirin is approximately fiftyfold more potent in inhibiting COX-1 than COX-2.[190] Effective antiplatelet therapy with aspirin, therefore, requires small doses that inhibit TXA_2 production while sparing prostacyclin production. The clinical

advantages of such doses have been demonstrated in human patients.[195] Higher doses increase the risk of gastrointestinal toxicity and can decrease the antiplatelet effect.[196] The platelet-inhibitory effect of aspirin persists for the entire lifespan of the platelet (7 to 10 days).[192] Because 10% of circulating platelets are replaced daily, approximately 50% of platelets function normally 5 days following aspirin ingestion.[190,197]

In the dog, an aspirin dose of 0.5 mg/kg orally every 12 hours has been shown to effectively decrease platelet aggregation.[198] Higher doses were less effective and led to increased platelet aggregability after 5 days.[198] In the cat, an aspirin dose of 25 mg/kg twice weekly has been shown to effectively inhibit platelet aggregation.[199] The effect on prostacyclin is unknown. It is possible that ultra-low doses given more frequently may prove to be superior.

Aspirin is a relatively weak antiplatelet drug[190]: it only slightly attenuates platelet aggregability responses to ADP and collagen. The incidence of thromboembolism in human patients on aspirin therapy remains substantial.

The thienopyridines (i.e., ticlopidine and clopidogrel) achieve moderate levels of platelet inhibition.[200] They selectively inhibit ADP-induced platelet aggregation and interfere with the binding of von Willebrand's factor to platelet receptors.[200,201] These agents have no effect on cyclooxygenase, suggesting a synergistic effect with aspirin.[201]

Ticlopidine and clopidogrel have been shown to significantly reduce the risk of arterial thrombosis in humans when compared with placebo and with aspirin therapy.[202,203] Combined therapy with aspirin was shown to be superior to either therapy alone. Significant antiplatelet effects are achieved after 2 to 3 days of therapy, and maximal effects do not occur for 5 to 7 days.[201] Effects persist for 7 to 10 days after cessation, corresponding to the lifespan of the platelet.[201] Ticlopidine has been shown to effectively inhibit platelet aggregation and decrease pulmonary lesions in heartworm-infected dogs.[204] The use of clopidogrel has not been reported in small animals.

Calcium channel blockers have been shown to inhibit platelet aggregation induced by mediators such as ADP, collagen, and epinephrine.[205] This effect may be of value in the treatment of feline hypertrophic cardiomyopathy and other conditions associated with thrombogenesis. A study comparing the antithrombotic effects of aspirin and diltiazem in cats found no significant difference between cats treated with diltiazem alone or in combination with aspirin.[206]

Amrinone has been shown to inhibit platelet activation and to protect against coronary artery thrombosis in experimental dogs.[207] Because other inotropic agents (e.g., catecholamines with alpha$_2$-adrenergic activity) may potentiate thrombosis, amrinone may be advantageous as an inotropic agent in patients with a thrombotic tendency.

Outcome and Prognosis

The prognosis for patients with PTE depends on the severity of respiratory and cardiovascular compromise. Right ventricular hypokinesis is a poor prognostic indicator and is associated with a doubling of the mortality rate in humans.[6] Overall mortality rates for veterinary patients remain unknown but appear to be substantial. Acute, severe compromise and death is not unusual. With appropriate treatment and supportive care, however, many patients survive.

Complete resolution in healthy dogs with experimental PE can occur within days.[13] Resolution may be delayed, however, in patients with defective fibrinolysis. Because some degree of hypofibrinolysis appears to occur in all the hypercoagulable states, delayed resolution is common. Resolution of clinical signs may take days to weeks.

Rates of recurrence have not been reported in dogs and cats. In human patients, these range from 4 to 17%, with most occurring within the first week.[7,162,163] In most patients, standard anticoagulant therapy alone was associated with infrequent recurrences and deaths.[7,131]

Chronic thromboembolic pulmonary hypertension (CTPH) develops in a small number of cases that survive PTE.[1,208,209] Patients present with increasing dyspnea, which inexorably progresses from dyspnea only with exertion to constant dyspnea. Diagnosis is suspected after excluding other causes of dyspnea. Echocardiography is useful to identify pulmonary hypertension. Scintigraphy or angiography usually shows multiple large defects.

REFERENCES

1. Moser KM: Venous thromboembolism, *Am Rev Respir Dis* 141(1):235, 1990.
2. Halmagyi DFJ, Colebatch HJH: Cardiorespiratory effects of experimental lung embolism, *J Clin Invest* 40(12):1785, 1961.
3. Goldhaber SZ: Pulmonary embolism, *N Eng J Med* 339(2):93, 1998.
4. LaRue MJ, Murtaugh RJ: Pulmonary thromboembolism in dogs: 47 cases (1986-1987), *JAVMA* 197(10):1368, 1990.
5. Nelson JR, Smith JR: The pathologic physiology of pulmonary embolism: A physiologic discussion of the vascular reactions following pulmonary arterial obstruction by emboli of varying size, *Am Heart J* 98(6):916, 1959.
6. Goldhaber SZ, De Rosa M, Visani L: International cooperative pulmonary embolism registry detects high mortality rate, *Circulation* 96(Suppl 1):1, 1997.
7. Carson JL, Kelley MA, Duff A et al: The clinical course of pulmonary embolism, *N Eng J Med* 326(19):1240, 1992.
8. Johnson LR, Lappin MR, Baker DC: Pulmonary thromboembolism in 29 dogs: 1985-1995, *J Vet Intern Med* 13(3):338, 1999.
9. Norris CR, Griffey SM, Samii VF: Pulmonary thromboembolism in cats: 29 cases (1987-1997), *J Am Vet Med Assoc* 215(11):1650, 1999.
10. Breddin HK: Thrombosis and Virchow's triad: What is established? *Semin Thomb Hemost* 15(3):237, 1989.
11. Hyers TM: Venous thromboembolism, *Am J Resp Crit Care Med* 159(1):1, 1999.
12. Bick RL, Kaplan H: Syndromes of thrombosis and hypercoagulability: Congenital and acquired causes of thrombosis, *Med Clin N Am* 82(3):409, 1998.
13. Moser KM, Guisan M, Bartimmo EE et al: In vivo and postmortem dissolution rates of pulmonary emboli and venous thrombi in the dog, *Circulation* 48(1):170, 1973.
14. Freiman DG, Suyemoto J: Frequency of pulmonary thromboembolism in man, *N Engl J Med* 272(9):1278, 1965.
15. Joist JH: Hypercoagulability: Introduction and perspective, *Semin Thromb Hemost* 16(2):151, 1990.
16. Schafer AI: The hypercoagulable states, *Ann Intern Med* 102(6):814, 1985.
17. Dahl OE: Mechanisms of hypercoagulability, *Thromb Haemost* 82:902, 1999.
18. Dillon R: Dirofilariasis in dogs and cats. In Ettinger SJ, Feldman EC, editors: *Textbook of veterinary internal medicine*, ed 5, vol 2, Philadelphia, 2000, WB Saunders.
19. Van Winkle TJ, Bruce E: Thrombosis of the portal vein in 11 dogs, *Vet Path* 30(1):28, 1993.
20. Hardie EM, Spaulding K, Malarkey DE: Splenic infarction in 16 dogs: A retrospective study, *J Vet Intern Med* 9(3):141, 1995.
21. Slauson DO, Gribble DH: Thrombosis complicating renal amyloidosis in dogs, *Vet Path* 8(3):352, 1971.
22. Green RA, Kabel AL: Hypercoagulable state in three dogs with nephrotic syndrome, *J Am Vet Med Assoc* 181(9):914, 1982.
23. Keith JC, Rawlings CA, Scharb RG: Pulmonary thromboembolism during therapy of dirofilariasis with thiacetarsamide: Modification with aspirin or prednisone, *Am J Vet Res* 44(4):1278, 1983.
24. Palmer KG, King LG, Van Winkle TJ: Clinical manifestations and associated disease syndromes in dogs with cranial vena cava thrombosis: 17 cases (1989-1996), *JAVMA* 213(2):220, 1998.
25. DiBartola SP, Meuten DJ: Renal amyloidosis in two dogs presented for thromboembolic phenomena, *J Am Anim Hosp Assoc* 16(1):129, 1980.
26. Klein MK, Dow SW, Rosychuk RAW: Pulmonary thromboembolism associated with immune-mediated hemolytic anemia in dogs: Ten cases (1982-1987), *JAVMA* 195(2):246, 1989.
27. Burns MG, Kelly AB, Hornof WJ et al: Pulmonary artery thrombosis in three dogs with hyperadrenocorticism, *JAVMA* 178(4):388, 1981.
28. King RR, Mauderly JL, Hahn FF et al: Pulmonary function studies in a dog with pulmonary thromboembolism associated with Cushing's disease, *J Am Anim Hosp Assoc* 21(4):555, 1985.
29. Hargis AM, Stephens LC, Benjamin SA et al: Relationship of hypothyroidism to diabetes mellitus, renal amyloidosis, and thrombosis in purebred beagles, *Am J Vet Res* 42(9):1077, 1981.
30. Van Winkle TJ, Hackner SG, Liu SM: Clinical and pathologic features of aortic thromboembolism in 36 dogs, *J Vet Emerg Crit Care* 3(1):13, 1994.
31. Pion P: Feline aortic thromboemboli and the potential utility of thrombolytic therapy with tissue plasminogen activator, *Vet Clin North Am Small Anim Practice* 18(1):79, 1988.
32. Laste N, Harpster N: A retrospective study of 100 cases of feline distal aortic thromboembolism: 1977-1993, *J Am Anim Hosp Assoc* 31(4):492, 1995.
33. Smith SA, Lewis DC, Kellerman DL: Adjustment of intermittent subcutaneous heparin therapy based on chromogenic heparin assay in 9 cats with thromboembolism (Abstract), *Proceedings 16th ACVIM forum*, 1998: abstract #9.
34. Sasahara AA: Pulmonary vascular responses to thromboembolism, *Mod Concepts Cardiovasc Dis* 36(10):55, 1967.
35. McIntyre KM, Sasahara AA: Determinants of the hemodynamic response to pulmonary embolism, *Clin Res* 17(3):254, 1969.
36. Dantzker DR, Wagner PD, Tornabene VW et al: Gas exchange after pulmonary thromboembolization in dogs, *Circ Res* 42(1):92, 1978.
37. Burki NK: The dead space to tidal volume ratio in the diagnosis of pulmonary embolism, *Am Rev Respir Dis* 133(5):679, 1986.
38. Severinghaus JW, Swensen EW, Finley TN et al: Unilateral hypoventilation produced in dogs by occluding one pulmonary artery, *J Appl Physiol* 16(1):53, 1961.
39. Stein M, Forkner CE, Robin ED et al: Gas exchange after autologous pulmonary embolism in dogs, *J Appl Physiol* 16(5):488, 1961.
40. D'Alanzo GE, Bower JS, DeHart P et al: The mechanisms of abnormal gas exchange in massive pulmonary embolism, *Am Rev Respir Dis* 128(1):170, 1983.
41. Levy SE, Simmons DH: Mechanism of arterial hypoxemia following pulmonary thromboembolism in dogs, *J Appl Physiol* 39(1):41, 1975.
42. Thomas D, Stein M, Tanabe G et al: Mechanisms of bronchoconstriction caused by thromboemboli in dogs, *Am J Physiol* 206(9):1207, 1964.
43. Gurewich V, Thomas D, Stein M et al: Bronchoconstriction in the presence of pulmonary embolism, *Circ* 27(2):339, 1963.
44. Giammona ST, Mandelbaum I, Foy J et al: Effects of pulmonary artery ligation on pulmonary surfactant and pressure-volume characteristics of the dog lung, *Circ Res* 18(6):683, 1966.
45. Chernick V, Hodson WA, Greenfield LJ: Effects of chronic pulmonary artery ligation on pulmonary mechanics and surfactant, *J Appl Physiol* 21(4):1315, 1966.

46. Finley TH, Swensen EW, Clements JA et al: Changes in mechanical properties, appearance, and surface activity of extracts of one lung following occlusion of its pulmonary artery in the dog, *Physiologist* 3(1):56, 1960.

47. Tsao MS, Schraufnagel D, Wong NS: Pathogenesis of pulmonary infarction, *Am J Med* 72(4):599, 1982.

48. Parker BM, Smith JR: Pulmonary embolism and infarction, *Am J Med* 24(3):402, 1958.

49. Parker BM, Smith JR: Studies of experimental pulmonary embolism and infarction and the development of collateral circulation in the affected lung lobe, *J Lab Clin Med* 49(6):850, 1957.

50. James WS, Minh VD, Monteer MA et al: Rapid resolution of a pulmonary embolus, *West J Med* 128(1):60, 1978.

51. Widdicombe JG: Reflex mechanisms in pulmonary thromboembolism. In Moser KM, Stein M, editors: *Pulmonary thromboembolism*, Chicago, 1973, Yearbook Publishers.

52. Dalen JE, Haffajee CI, Alpert JS et al: Pulmonary embolism, pulmonary hemorrhage, and pulmonary infarction, *N Engl J Med* 296(25):1431, 1977.

53. McIntyre KM, Sasahara AA: Determinants of right ventricular function and hemodynamics after pulmonary embolism, *Chest* 65(5):534, 1974.

54. Ebert PA, Allgood RJ, Jones HW III et al: Hemodynamics during pulmonary artery occlusion, *Surgery* 62(1):18, 1967.

55. West JB: Blood flow and metabolism. In West JB, editor: *Respiratory physiology: The essentials*, ed 5, Baltimore, 1995, Williams & Wilkins.

56. Vlahakes GJ, Turley K, Hoffman JIE: The pathophysiology of failure in acute right ventricular hypertension: Hemodynamic and biochemical correlations, *Circulation* 63(1):87, 1981.

57. Dalen JE, Haynes FW, Hopper FG Jr. et al: Cardiovascular responses to experimental pulmonary embolism, *Am J Cardiol* 200(1):3, 1967.

58. Dennis JS: The pathophysiologic sequelae of pulmonary thromboembolism, *Comp Contin Educ Pract Vet* 13(12):1811, 1991.

59. Molloy WD, Lee KY, Girling L et al: Treatment of shock in a canine model of pulmonary embolism, *Am Rev Respir Dis* 130(5):870, 1984.

60. Elliot CG: Pulmonary physiology during pulmonary embolism, *Chest* 101(Suppl):163S, 1992.

61. Williams MH: Mechanical versus reflex effects of diffuse pulmonary embolism in anesthetized dogs, *Circ Res* 4(5):325, 1956.

62. Thomas DP, Gurewich V, Ashford TP: Platelet adherence to thromboemboli in relation to the pathogenesis and treatment of pulmonary embolism, *N Engl J Med* 274(17):953, 1966.

63. McGoon MD, VanHoutte PM: Aggregating platelets contract isolated canine pulmonary arteries by releasing 5-hydroxytryptamine, *J Clin Invest* 74(3):828, 1984.

64. Rickaby DA, Dawson CA, Mevion MB: Pulmonary inactivation of serotonin and site of serotonin pulmonary vasoconstriction, *J Appl Physiol* 48(4):606, 1980.

65. Ryu JH, Olson EJ, Pellikka MD: Clinical recognition of pulmonary embolism: Problem of unrecognized and asymptomatic cases, *Mayo Clin Proc* 73(9):873, 1998.

66. Dennis JS: Clinical features of pulmonary thromboembolism, *Comp Contin Educ Pract Vet* 15(12):1595, 1993.

67. Adams EW, Hodges DR: Fatal occlusive pulmonary embolism in the dog: A case report, *JAVMA* 134(4):467, 1959.

68. Bunch SE, Metcalf MR, Crane SW et al: Idiopathic pleural effusion and pulmonary thromboembolism in a dog with autoimmune hemolytic anemia, *JAVMA* 195(12):1748, 1989.

69. Suter PF: Lower airway and pulmonary parenchymal disease. In Suter PF, editor: *Thoracic radiography: A text atlas of thoracic diseases of the dog and cat*, Basel, Switzerland, 1984, PF Suter.

70. Fluckiger MA, Gomez JA: Radiographic findings in dogs with spontaneous pulmonary thrombosis or embolism, *Vet Radiol* 25(3):124, 1984.

71. Chooi CC, Gallus AS: Acute phase reaction, fibrinogen level and thrombus size, *Thromb Res Suppl* 53(5):493, 1989.

72. Bick RF: Clinical relevance of antithrombin III, *Semin Thromb Haemost* 8(4):276, 1982.

73. Baker WF: Diagnosis of deep venous thrombosis and pulmonary embolism, *Med Clin N Am* 82(3):459, 1998.

74. Bauer KA, Rosenberg RD: The pathophysiology of the prethrombotic state in humans: Insights gained from studies using markers of hemostatic activation, *Blood* 70(2):343, 1987.

75. AACP Consensus Committee on Pulmonary Embolism: Opinions regarding the diagnosis and management of venous thromboembolic disease, *Chest* 113(2):499, 1998.

76. Bounameaux H, Cirafici P, DeMoerloose P: Measurement of D-dimer in plasma as a diagnostic aid in suspected pulmonary embolism, *Lancet* 337(2):196, 1991.

77. Becker DM, Philbrick JT, Bachhuber TL et al: D-dimer testing and acute venous thromboembolism, *Arch Intern Med* 156(7):939, 1996.

78. De Moerloose P, Minazio P, Reber G et al: D-dimer determination to exclude pulmonary embolism: A two-step approach using latex assay as a screening tool, *Thromb Haemost* 72(1):89, 1994.

79. Kollef MH, Eisenberg PR, Shannon W: A rapid assay for the detection of circulating D-dimer is associated with clinical outcomes among critically ill patients, *Crit Care Med* 26(6):1054, 1998.

80. John MA, Elms MJ, O'Reilly EJ et al: The SimpliRED D-dimer test: A novel assay for the detection of crosslinked fibrin degradation products in whole blood, *Thromb Res Suppl* 58(3):273, 1990.

81. Cornelissen JMM, Wolvekamp WThC, Stokhof AA et al: Primary occlusive pulmonary vascular disease in a dog diagnosed by a lung perfusion scintigram, *J Am Anim Hosp Assoc* 21(3):293, 1985.

82. PIOPED investigators: Value of the ventilation/perfusion scan in acute pulmonary embolism: Results of the prospective investigation of pulmonary embolic diagnosis (PIOPED), *JAMA* 263(12):2753, 1990.

83. Alderson PO, Doppman JL, Diamond SS et al: Ventilation-perfusion lung imaging and selective pulmonary angiography in dogs with experimental pulmonary embolism, *J Nucl Med* 9(1):164, 1978.

84. Koblik PD, Hornof W, Harnagel SH et al: A comparison of pulmonary angiography, digital subtraction angiography, and 99m Tc-DTCPA/MMA ventilation-perfusion scintigraphy for detection of experimental pulmonary emboli in the dog, *Vet Radiol* 30(2):159, 1989.

85. Pouchelon JL, Chetboul V, Devauchelle P et al: Diagnosis of pulmonary thromboembolism in a cat using echocardiography and pulmonary scintigraphy, *J Small Anim Pract* 38(7):306, 1997.

86. Dalen JE, Mathur VS, Evans H et al: Pulmonary angiography in experimental pulmonary embolism, *Am Heart J* 72(4):509, 1996.

87. Newman GE: Pulmonary angiography in pulmonary embolic disease, *J Thorac Imaging* 4(4):28, 1989.

88. Thorpe PE: The role of thrombolytic therapy in pulmonary embolism, *Tech Vasc Interv Radiol* 1(4):199, 1998.

89. Wessler S, Freiman RG, Ballon JA et al: Experimental pulmonary embolism with serum-induced thrombi, *Am J Pathol* 38(1):89, 1961.

90. Hirsh J, Warkentin TE, Shaunessy SG et al: Heparin and low-molecular-weight heparin: Mechanisms of action, pharmacokinetics, dosing, monitoring, efficacy, and safety (Sixth ACCP consensus conference on antithrombotic therapy), *Chest* 119(1 Suppl):65S, 2001.

91. Hyers TM, Agnelli G, Hull RD et al: Antithrombotic therapy for venous thromboembolic disease (Sixth ACCP consensus conference on antithrombotic therapy), *Chest* 119(1 Suppl):176S, 2001.

92. Barritt DW, Jordan SC: Anticoagulant drugs in the treatment of pulmonary embolism: A controlled clinical trial, *Lancet* 1(11):1309, 1960.

93. Kanis JA: Heparin in the treatment of pulmonary thromboembolism, *Thromb Diath Haemorrh* 32(2):519, 1974.

94. Alpert JS, Smith R, Carlson J et al: Mortality in patients treated for pulmonary embolism, *JAMA* 236(12):1477, 1976.

95. Hirsh J: Heparin, *N Engl J Med* 324(12):1565, 1991.

96. Beguin S, Lindhout T, Hemker HC: The mode of action of heparin in plasma, *Thromb Haemost* 60(3):457, 1988.

97. Sobel M, McNeill PM, Carlson PL et al: Heparin inhibition of von Willebrand factor-dependent platelet function *in vitro* and in vivo, *J Clin Invest* 87(5):1787, 1991.

98. Fernandez F, Nguyen P, Van Ryn J et al: Hemorrhagic doses of heparin and other glycosaminoglycans induce a platelet defect, *Thromb Res* 43(4):491, 1986.

99. Barzu T, Molho P, Tobelem G et al: Binding and endocytosis of heparin by human endothelial cells in culture, *Biochem Biophys Acta* 845(2):196, 1985.

100. Blajchman MA, Young E, Ofosu FA: Effects of unfractionated heparin, dermatan sulfate, and low molecular weight heparin on vessel wall permeability in rabbits, *Ann NY Acad Sci* 556(3):245, 1989.

101. Haas SK: Treatment of deep venous thrombosis and pulmonary embolism: Current recommendations, *Med Clin N Am* 82(3):495, 1998.
102. Hull RD, Raskob GE, Hirsh J et al: Continuous intravenous heparin compared with intermittent subcutaneous heparin in the initial treatment of deep vein thrombosis, *N Engl J Med* 315(18):1109, 1986.
103. Olsson P, Lagergren H, Ek S: The elimination from plasma of intravenous heparin: An experimental study on dogs and humans, *Acta Med Scand* 173(5):619, 1963.
104. Hirsh J, van Aken WG, Gallus AS et al: Heparin kinetics in venous thrombosis and pulmonary embolism, *Circulation* 53(4):691, 1976.
105. Simon TL, Hyers TM, Gaston JP et al: Heparin pharmacokinetics: Increased requirements in pulmonary embolism, *Br J Hematol* 39(1):111-120, 1978.
106. Levine M, Hirsh J, Gent M et al: A randomized trial comparing activated thromboplastin time with heparin assay in patients with acute venous thrombosis requiring large daily doses of heparin, *Arch Intern Med* 154(1):49, 1994.
107. Marci CD, Prager D: A review of the clinical indications for the plasma heparin assay, *Am J Clin Pathol* 99(5):546, 1993.
108. Raschke RA, Reilly BM, Fontana JR et al: The weight-based heparin dosing normogram compared with a "standard care" nomogram: A randomized controlled trial, *Ann Intern Med* 119(9):874, 1993.
109. Anand SS, Bates S, Ginsberg JS et al: Recurrent venous thrombosis and heparin therapy: An evaluation of the importance of early activated partial thromboplastin times, *Arch Intern Med* 159(17):2029, 1999.
110. Basu D, Gallus A, Hirsh J et al: A prospective study of the value of monitoring heparin treatment with the activated partial thromboplastin time, *N Engl J Med* 287(7):324, 1972.
111. Brill-Edwards P, Ginsberg JS, Johnston M et al: Establishing a therapeutic range for heparin therapy, *Ann Intern Med* 119(1):104-109, 1993.
112. Hull RD, Raskob GE, Brandt RF et al: Relation between the time to achieve the lower limit of the aPTT therapeutic range and recurrent venous thromboembolism during heparin treatment for deep vein thrombosis, *Arch Intern Med* 157(22):2562, 1997.
113. Chui HM, Hirsh J, Yung WL et al: Relationship between the anticoagulant and antithrombotic effects of heparin in experimental venous thrombosis, *Blood* 49(2):171, 1977.
114. Hirsh J, Hoak J: Management of deep vein thrombosis and pulmonary embolism: A statement for healthcare professionals, *Circulation* 93(12):2212, 1996.
115. Pini M, Pattachini C, Quintavalla R et al: Subcutaneous vs. intravenous heparin in the treatment of deep vein thrombosis—a randomized clinical trial, *Thromb Haemost* 64(2):222, 1990.
116. Rackear DG: Drugs that alter the hemostatic mechanism, *Vet Clin North Am Small Anim Pract* 18(1):67, 1988.
117. Hellebrekers LJ, Slappendal RJ, van den Brom WE: Effect of sodium heparin and antithrombin III concentration on activated partial thromboplastin time in the dog, *Am J Vet Res* 46(12):1460, 1985.
118. Mischke RH, Schuttert C, Grebe SI: Anticoagulant effects of repeated subcutaneous injections of high doses of unfractionated heparin in healthy dogs, *Am J Vet Res* 62(12):1887, 2001.
119. Levine MN, Raskob G, Landefeld S et al: Hemorrhagic complications of anticoagulant treatment (Sixth ACCP consensus conference on antithrombotic therapy), *Chest* 119(1 Suppl):108S, 2001.
120. Glazier RL, Crowell EB: Randomized, prospective trial of continuous versus intermittent heparin therapy, *JAMA* 236(12):1365, 1976.
121. Mant MJ, O'Brien BD, Thong KI et al: Hemorrhagic complications of heparin therapy, *Lancet* 1(8022):1133, 1977.
122. Doyle DJ, Turpie AGG, Hirsh J et al: Adjusted subcutaneous heparin or continuous intravenous heparin in patients with acute deep vein thrombosis: A randomized trial, *Ann Intern Med* 107(4):441, 1987.
123. Levine M, Gent M, Hirsh J et al: A comparison of low-molecular-weight heparin administered primarily at home with unfractionated heparin administered in the hospital for proximal deep-vein thrombosis, *N Engl J Med* 334(11):677, 1996.
124. The Columbus Investigators: Low-molecular-weight heparin in the treatment of patients with venous thromboembolism, *N Engl J Med* 337(10):657, 1997.
125. Simonneau G, Sors H, Charbonnier B: A comparison of low-molecular-weight heparin with unfractionated heparin for acute pulmonary embolism: The THESEE study group, *N Engl J Med* 337(10):663, 1997.
126. Hull RD, Raskob GE, Brandt RF et al: Low-molecular-weight heparin vs. heparin in the treatment of patients with pulmonary embolism, *Arch Intern Med* 160(2):229, 2000.
127. Turpie AGG: Pharmacology of the low-molecular-weight heparins, *Am Heart J* 135(6 Pt 3 Su):S329, 1998.
128. Verstraete M: Pharmacotherapeutic aspects of unfractionated and low-molecular-weight heparin, *Drugs* 40(4):498-530, 1990.
129. Carter CJ, Kelton JG, Hirsh J et al: The relationship between the hemorrhagic and antithrombotic properties of low molecular weight heparins in rabbits, *Blood* 59(6):1239, 1982.
130. Siragusa S, Cosmi B, Piovella F et al: Low-molecular-weight heparins and unfractionated heparin in the treatment of patients with acute venous thromboembolism: Results of a meta-analysis, *Am J Med* 100(3):269, 1996.
131. Gould MK, Dembitzer AD, Doyle RL et al: Low-molecular weight heparins compared with unfractionated heparin for the treatment of acute deep vein thrombosis: A meta-analysis of randomized, controlled trials, *Ann Intern Med* 130(10):800, 1999.
132. Hirsh J, Dalen JE, Anderson DR et al: Oral anticoagulants: Mechanism of action, clinical effectiveness, and optimal therapeutic range (Sixth AACP consensus conference on antithrombotic therapy), *Chest* 119(1 Suppl):8S, 2001.
133. Triplett DA: Current recommendations for warfarin therapy: Use and monitoring, *Med Clin North Am* 82(3):601, 1998.
134. Harpster NK, Baty CJ: Warfarin therapy for the cat at risk for thromboembolism. In Bonagura JD, Kirk RW, editors: *Current veterinary therapy*, vol 12, Philadelphia, 1995, WB Saunders Co.
135. Neff-Davis CA, Davis LE, Gillette EL: Warfarin in the dog: Pharmacokinetics as related to clinical response, *J Vet Pharmacol Ther* 4(2):135, 1981.
136. Monnet E, Morgan MR: Effect of three loading doses of warfarin on the international normalized ratio for dogs, *Am J Vet Res* 61(1):48, 2000.
137. Ansell J, Hirsh J, Dalen J et al: Managing oral anticoagulant therapy (Sixth AACP consensus conference on antithrombotic therapy), *Chest* 119(1 Suppl):22S, 2001.
138. Lewis RJ, Trager WF, Chan KK et al: Warfarin: Stereochemical aspects of its metabolism and the interaction of phenylbutazone, *J Clin Invest* 53(6):1607, 1974.
139. O'Reilly RA: The stereoselective interaction of warfarin and metronidazole in man, *N Engl J Med* 295(7):354, 1976.
140. O'Reilly RA: Stereoselective interaction of trimethoprim-sulfamethoxazole with the separated enantiomorphs of racemic warfarin in man, *N Engl J Med* 302(1):33, 1980.
141. O'Reilly RA, Trager WF, Rattie AE et al: Interaction of amiodarone with racemic warfarin and its separated enantiomorphs in humans, *Clin Pharmacol Ther* 42(3):290, 1987.
142. O'Reilly RA, Rytand D: Resistance to warfarin due to unrecognized vitamin K supplementation, *N Engl J Med* 303(3):160, 1980.
143. O'Reilly RA: Studies on the optical enantiomorphs of warfarin in man, *Clin Pharmacol Ther* 16(2):348, 1974.
144. Weibert RT, Lorentz SM, Townsend RJ et al: Effect of erythromycin in patients receiving long-term warfarin therapy, *Clin Pharmacol* 8(3):210, 1989.
145. Wells PS, Holbrook AM, Crowther NR et al: Interactions of warfarin with drugs and food. A critical review of the literature, *Ann Intern Med* 121(9):676, 1994.
146. Richards RK: Influence of fever upon the action of 3,3-methylene bis-4-hydroxycoumarin, *Science* 97(4):313, 1943.
147. Levine M, Hirsh J, Gent M et al: Optimal duration for oral anticoagulant therapy: A randomized trial comparing 4 weeks with 3 months of warfarin in patients with proximal deep vein thrombosis, *N Engl J Med* 74(2):606, 1995.
148. Marder VJ, Sherry S: Thrombolytic therapy: Current status (1), *N Engl J Med* 318(23):1512, 1988.
149. Daniels LB, Parker JA, Patel SR et al: Relation of duration of symptoms with response to thrombolytic therapy in pulmonary embolism, *Am J Cardiol* 80(2):184, 1997.
150. Goldhaber SZ, Haire WD, Feldstein M et al: Alteplase versus heparin in acute pulmonary embolism: A randomized trial assessing right-ventricular function and pulmonary perfusion, *Lancet* 341(8844):507, 1993.

151. Konstantinides S, Geibel A, Olschewski M et al: Association between thrombolytic treatment and the prognosis of hemodynamically stable patients with major pulmonary embolism: Results of a multicenter registry, *Circulation* 96(3):882, 1997.

152. Dalen JE, Vanes JS, Brooks HL et al: Resolution rate of pulmonary embolism in man, *N Engl J Med* 280(22):1194, 1969.

153. Miller GAH, Sutton GC, Kerr IH: Comparison of streptokinase and heparin in the treatment of isolated acute massive pulmonary embolism, *Br Med J* 2(763):681, 1971.

154. Sasahara AA, Hyers TM, Cole CM et al: The urokinase pulmonary embolism trial (UPET): A national cooperative study, *Circulation* 47(Suppl 2):1, 1973.

155. Sasahara AA, Bell WR, Simon TL: The phase II urokinase–streptokinase pulmonary embolism trial, *Thromb Diath Haemorrh* 33(3):464, 1975.

156. Califf RM, Fortin DF, Tenaglia AN et al: Clinical risks of thrombolytic therapy, *Am J Cardiol* 69(2):12A, 1992.

157. Tapson VF: Rapid thrombolysis of massive pulmonary emboli without systemic fibrinogenolysis: Intra-embolic infusion of thrombolytic therapy, *Am Rev Respir Dis* 145:A719, 1992.

158. Ramsey CC, Riepe RD, Macintyre DK et al: Streptokinase: A practical clotbuster? *Proceedings IVECCS* 225, 1996.

159. Clare AC, Kraje BJ: Use of recombinant tissue-plasminogen activator for aortic thrombolysis in a hypoproteinemic dog, *JAVMA* 212(4):539, 1998.

160. Ramsey CC, Burney DP et al: Use of streptokinase in four dogs with thrombosis, *JAVMA* 209(4):780, 1996.

161. Urokinase pulmonary embolism trial. Phase 1 results, *JAMA* 214(12):2163, 1970.

162. Urokinase-streptokinase pulmonary embolism trial. Phase 2 results, *JAMA* 229(12):1606, 1974.

163. Shafer KE, Santoro SA, Sobel BE et al: Monitoring activity of fibrinolytic agents: A therapeutic challenge, *Am J Med* 76(5):879, 1984.

164. Brogden RN, Speight TM, Avery GS et al: Streptokinase: A review of its clinical pharmacology, mechanism of action, and therapeutic uses, *Drugs* 5(5):357, 1973.

165. McClointock DK, Bell PH: The mechanism of action of human plasminogen by streptokinase, *Biochem Biophys Res Commun* 43(3):694, 1971.

166. Reddy KN, Cercek B, Lew AS et al: Interaction of SK-human plasmin, SK-dog plasmin complexes with alpha$_2$-antiplasmin and alpha$_2$-macroglobulin, *Thromb Res Suppl* 41(5):671, 1986.

167. Killingsworth CR, Eyster GE, Adams T et al: Streptokinase treatment of cats with experimentally-induced aortic thrombosis, *Am J Vet Res* 47(6):1351, 1986.

168. Moore K, Dhupa N, Rush J et al: Clinical experience with streptokinase administration in 27 cats (Abstract), *Proceedings IVECCS* 839, 1998.

169. Sasahara AA: Urokinase: past, present, and future, *Tech Vasc Interv Radiol* 1(3):170, 1998.

170. Zamarron C, Lijnen HR, Van Hef B et al: Biological and thrombolytic properties of proenzyme and active forms of human urokinase obtained from human urine or by recombinant DNA technology, *Thromb Haemost* 52(1):19, 1984.

171. Burke SE, Lubbers NL et al: Comparison of dose regimens for the administration of recombinant pro-urokinase in a canine thrombosis model, *Thromb Haemost* 77(5):1025, 1997.

172. Badylak SF, Voytik S, Klabunde RE et al: Bolus dose response characteristics of single chain urokinase plasminogen activator and tissue plasminogen activator in a dog model of arterial thrombosis, *Thromb Res Suppl* 52(4):295, 1988.

173. Prewitt RM, Hoy C, Kong A et al: Thrombolytic therapy in canine pulmonary embolism. Comparative effects of urokinase and recombinant tissue plasminogen activator, *Am Rev Respir Dis* 141(2):290, 1990.

174. Bachman F, Kruithof KO: Tissue plasminogen activator: Chemical and physiological aspects, *Semin Thromb Haemost* 10(1):6, 1984.

175. Hoylaerts M, Rijken DC, Lijnen HR et al: Kinetics of the activation of plasminogen by human tissue plasminogen activator: Role of fibrin, *J Biol Chem* 257(6):2912, 1982.

176. Goldhaber SZ, Kessler CM, Heit J et al: Randomized controlled trial of recombinant tissue plasminogen activator versus urokinase in the treatment of acute pulmonary embolism, *Lancet* 2(8606):293, 1988.

177. White HD: Comparative safety of thrombolytic agents, *Am J Cardiol* 69(Suppl A):12A, 1992.

178. Eisenberg PR, Sherman LA, Tiefenbrunn AJ et al: Sustained fibrinolysis after administration of t-PA despite its short half-life in the circulation, *Thromb Haemost* 57(1):35, 1987.

179. Shiffman F, Ducas J, Hollett P et al: Treatment of canine embolic pulmonary hypertension with recombinant tissue plasminogen activator: Efficacy of dosing regimens, *Circulation* 78(1):214, 1988.

180. Geerts WH, Heit JA, Clagett GP et al: Prevention of venous thromboembolism (Sixth ACCP consensus conference on antithrombotic therapy), *Chest* 119(1 Suppl):132S, 2001.

181. McGann MA, Triplett DA: Interpretation of antithrombin III activity, *Lab Med* 13(6):742, 1982.

182. Shafer AI: The hypercoagulable states, *Ann Intern Med* 102(6):814, 1985.

183. Gram J, Jespersen J: On the significance of antithrombin III, alpha-2-macroglobulin, alpha-2-antiplasmin, histadine-rich glycoprotein, and protein C in patients with acute myocardial infarction and deep vein thrombosis, *Thromb Haemost* 54(3):505, 1985.

184. Collins R, Scrimgeour A, Yusuf S et al: Reduction in fatal pulmonary embolism and venous thrombosis by perioperative administration of subcutaneous heparin: Overview of results of randomized trials in general, orthopedic, and urologic surgery, *N Engl J Med* 318(8):1162, 1998.

185. Belch JJ, Lowe GDO, Ward AJ et al: Prevention of deep vein thrombosis in medical patients by low-dose heparin, *Scott Med J* 26(2):115, 1981.

186. Cade JF: High-risk of the critically ill for venous thromboembolism, *Crit Care Med* 10(7):448, 1982.

187. Kupfer Y, Anwar J, Senenviratne C et al: Prophylaxis with subcutaneous heparin significantly reduces the incidence of deep vein thrombophlebitis in the critically ill (Abstract), *Am J Respir Crit Care Med* 159(Suppl A):A519, 1999.

188. Mismetti P, LaPorta-Simitsidis S, Tardy B et al: Prevention of venous thromboembolism in internal medicine with unfractionated or low-molecular-weight heparins: A meta-analysis of randomized clinical trials, *Throm Haemost* 83(1):14, 2000.

189. Lederle FA: Heparin prophylaxis for medical patients? *Ann Intern Med* 128(9):768, 1998.

190. Patrono C, Coller B, Dalen JE et al: Platelet-active drugs: the relationships among dose, effectiveness, and side effects (Sixth ACCP consensus conference on antithrombotic therapy), *Chest* 119(1 Suppl):39S, 2001.

191. Pulmonary Embolism Prevention (PEP) Trial Collaborative Group: Prevention of pulmonary embolism and deep vein thrombosis with low dose aspirin: Pulmonary embolism prevention (PEP) trial, *Lancet* 355(10):1295, 2000.

192. Roth GJ, Majerus PW: The mechanisms of the effects of aspirin on human platelets. I. Acetylation of a particulate fraction protein, *J Clin Invest* 56(5):624, 1975.

193. Majerus PW: Arachidonate metabolites in vascular disorders, *J Clin Invest* 72(5):1521, 1983.

194. Patrono C, Ciabattoni G, Patrignani P et al: Clinical pharmacology of platelet cyclooxygenase inhibition, *Circulation* 72(6):1177, 1985.

195. Taylor DW, Barnett HJM, Haynes RB et al: Low-dose and high-dose acetylsalicylic acid for patients undergoing carotid endarterectomy: A randomized controlled trial. ACE trial collaborators, *Lancet* 353(9171):2179, 1999.

196. Roderick PJ, Wilkes HC, Meade TW: The gastrointestinal toxicity of aspirin: An overview of randomized controlled trials, *B J Clin Pharmacol* 35(3):219, 1993.

197. O'Brien JR: Effects of salicylates on human platelets, *Lancet* 1(7546):779, 1968.

198. Rackear D, Feldman B, Farver T et al: The effect of three different dosages of acetylsalicylic acid on canine platelet aggregation, *J Am Anim Hosp Assoc* 24(1):23, 1988.

199. Green C: Effects of aspirin and propanolol on feline platelet aggregation, *Am J Vet Res* 46(12):1820, 1985.

200. Sharis PJ, Cannon CP, Loscalzo J: The antiplatelet effects of ticlopidine and clopidogrel, *Ann Int Med* 129(5):394, 1998.

201. Quinn MJ, Fitzgerald DJ: Ticlopidine and clopidogrel, *Circulation* 100(15):1667, 1999.

202. Haas SK, Easton JD, Adams HP et al: A randomized trial comparing ticlopidine hydrochloride with aspirin for the prevention of stroke in high-risk patients. Ticlopidine aspirin study group, *N Engl J Med* 321(8):501, 1989.

203. CAPRIE Steering Committee: A randomized, blinded, trial of clopidogrel versus aspirin in patients at risk of ischemic events (CAPRIE), *Lancet* 348(10):1329, 1996.
204. Boudreaux MK, Dillon AR, Sartin EA et al: Effects of treatments with ticlopidine in heartworm-negative, heartworm-infected, and embolized heartworm-infected dogs, *Am J Vet Res* 52(12):2000, 1991.
205. Cooke KL, Snyder PS: Calcium channel blockers in veterinary medicine, *J Vet Intern Med* 12(3):123, 1998.
206. Behrend EN, Grauer GF, Greco DS et al: Comparison of the effects of diltiazem and aspirin on platelet aggregation in cats, *J Am Anim Hosp Assoc* 32(1):11, 1996.
207. Sill JC, Bertha B, Berger I et al: Human platelet Ca^{2+} mobilization, glycoprotein IIb/IIIa activation, and experimental coronary thrombosis *in vivo* in dogs are all inhibited by the inotropic agent amrinone, *Circulation* 96(5):1647, 1997.
208. Hawkins EC: Pulmonary parenchymal diseases. In Ettinger SJ, Feldman EC, editors: *Textbook of veterinary internal medicine*, ed 5, vol 2, Philadelphia, 2000, WB Saunders.
209. Rubin LJ: Approach to the diagnosis and treatment of pulmonary hypertension, *Chest* 76(3):659, 1989.

CHAPTER 72

Eosinophilic Pneumonia

Carol R. Norris • Matthew S. Mellema

Eosinophilic pneumonias are a diverse group of infiltrative pulmonary disorders. In many cases the only clear link shared by these diseases is the presence of increased numbers of eosinophils within the tissues of the respiratory tract. Only a few series of eosinophilic pneumonia cases have been published in the veterinary literature, and our understanding of these diseases remains limited.[1,2] Eosinophilic pneumonia disorders can be life-threatening when acute respiratory failure ensues, but they often respond rapidly and completely to corticosteroid therapy, with a relatively minor long-term impact on pulmonary function. The eosinophilic pneumonias are unique among the interstitial lung diseases (ILD) in this regard. In part, the lack of available information on these forms of respiratory disease is caused by this generally favorable prognosis. The pursuit of additional information in the form of lung biopsies and pulmonary function tests is seldom either desired by the owners or needed in the management of these cases. Thus much of what is known about eosinophilic pneumonia in veterinary medicine is either extrapolated from similar disease states in human medicine or based on thoracic radiography, peripheral blood eosinophil counts, and bronchoalveolar lavage cytology rather than histopathology.

Eosinophilic pneumonia can be idiopathic (i.e., primary, of undetermined origin) or be secondary to a known cause. In dogs and cats, eosinophilic lung diseases have been grouped under the umbrella term "pulmonary infiltrates with eosinophils" (PIE), which does not reflect the heterogeneity of these disorders. The term PIE was first coined by Reeder and Goodrich in 1952 and remains widely used in both human and veterinary medicine.[3] Several attempts have been made to introduce and revise categorization schemes for eosinophilic pneumonia, but to date no definitely accepted method of classification exists. The major reason to attempt to classify eosinophilic pneumonia disorders in dogs and cats is to learn more about their etiology, pathogenesis, response to therapy, and prognosis.

Eosinophilic pneumonias in humans are characterized by a predominant eosinophilic infiltrate in the interstitial structures of the lung, including the bronchioles, alveoli, and blood vessels.[4] In the veterinary literature, PIE syndromes include eosinophilic airway disease (eosinophilic bronchitis or asthma) along with eosinophilic pneumonias.[1,5-8] In this chapter, they will be considered as separate disease entities.

Eosinophils

Eosinophils are bone marrow–derived polymorphonuclear granular leukocytes. In contrast to some other types of leukocytes, the eosinophil largely resides within the tissues, and it has been estimated that only 1% of a human's eosinophils are to be found in the blood.[9] The term eosinophil was first employed by Ehrlich in 1879 to describe a subset of granular leukocytes.[10] Since that initial description a number of theories have been proposed regarding their function. Their importance in allergy and immunity to helminth parasites has been recognized for nearly a century, but the exact role of the eosinophil in inflammation remains unclear. The eosinophil has been characterized as beneficial in defense against parasites, but detrimental to host tissues in allergic conditions.

The last two decades have seen an explosion in knowledge of eosinophil biology. These advances have largely been fueled by two factors: (1) the recognition of the eosinophil as an important cell in the pathophysiology of bronchial asthma, and (2) the development of technology to produce animals with specific gene silencing (knockouts). Because bronchial asthma is estimated to affect nearly 10% of the human population of many developed nations, considerable resources have been allocated to asthma research. Unfortunately, in the case of eosinophilic pneumonia, an allergic etiology is not always proven or likely, and research into eosinophil biology outside the context of allergy is more limited.

Knockout mice and the tools of molecular biology have allowed more precise dissection of the factors responsible for the generation of an eosinophilic inflammatory response within the pulmonary tissue. Eosinophils are derived in the bone marrow from a progenitor cell (i.e., the CFU-Eo, or colony-forming unit-eosinophil). One of the major breakthroughs in the understanding of eosinophil biology in the last decade has been the discovery that eosinophils are largely under the influence of helper T lymphocyte (Th2)-derived cytokines. Activated, sensitized Th2 cells release cytokines that lead to expansion of the eosinophil pool; migration of these new cells to the site of inflammation; and, ultimately, activation of eosinophils within the tissues. The production of eosinophils from precursors is regulated by a number of different cytokines including interleukin (IL)-3, IL-5, and granulocyte/macrophage colony stimulating factor (GM-CSF).[11] Once formed, eosinophils migrate through the bone marrow sinus endothelium into the bloodstream under the influence of IL-5 and eotaxin.[12] Eosinophils circulate for less than 24 hours before entering the tissues. In the allergic lung, IL-4 and IL-13 have been shown to control the transmigration of eosinophils across the pulmonary vasculature into the pulmonary tissues.[13,14] Eotaxin and IL-5 also act locally within the lung to promote eosinophil accumulation.[15]

The mature eosinophils of mammals contain at least four types of granules. These have been termed primary granules, specific granules, small dense granules, and microgranules. Although the shape, morphology, size, and abundance of each of these granules may vary with species, they all contain proteins that are potent cytotoxins. Among the component proteins identified are major basic protein (MBP), eosinophil peroxidase (EPO), eosinophil cationic protein (ECP), and eosinophil-derived neurotoxin (EDN). The release of these cytotoxins is thought to be responsible for many of the effector mechanisms of the eosinophils (e.g., killing of helminth parasites, tissue damage in allergic responses, and tumor cell killing). In addition to these cytotoxic proteins, eosinophils can also synthesize and release cytokines, lipid mediators, and derivatives of arachidonic acid (e.g., prostaglandins and leukotrienes). The discovery that eosinophils produce and release these products has led to revision of the concept that these cells are merely transporters for cytotoxins. Instead, it appears that these cells can coordinate and control the inflammatory response in some settings. Further, eosinophils have been shown to be phagocytic and can present antigen to lymphocytes as well, thus contributing to cellular immunity.

The arrival of eosinophils within tissues does not always lead to subsequent activation and degranulation. One of the flaws in some mouse models of asthma is that, whereas eosinophils can be made to accumulate within murine airways in response to aerosolized antigen, they may not release their granular contents upon arrival.[16] Known stimuli for eosinophil activation and degranulation include secretory IgA (sIgA), IL-5, GM-CSF, and IL-3.[17] Recent evidence suggests that in mice and humans IgE is unlikely to have an important role in eosinophil activation.[18,19] The role of IgE in terms of eosinophil activation may be to activate mast cells, which produce TNF-α and IL-1α leading to eotaxin release from epithelial and endothelial cells.[20]

The accumulation of eosinophils within the pulmonary parenchyma can result in decreased pulmonary compliance as well as reduced gas diffusion capacity. This reduction in pulmonary function and increase in the work of breathing can be further exacerbated by the development of noncardiogenic edema as a result of eosinophil degranulation. Patients with eosinophilic pneumonia may exhibit restrictive or obstructive breathing patterns. In humans, hypoxemia is typically more severe in acute eosinophilic pneumonia than in the chronic forms.[4] On thoracic radiographs the infiltrates may appear diffusely alveolar and interstitial, or may take on a more nodular appearance (Figures 72-1 and 72-2). Despite the remarkable cytotoxicity of eosinophil granule proteins, the lungs of human patients show surprisingly little compromise following resolution of eosinophilic pneumonia. Most patients have normal thoracic radiographs following disease resolution.[21]

Classification of Eosinophilic Pneumonia

There is presently no definitely accepted scheme for the classification or categorization of eosinophilic pneumonia in humans or animals. A classification scheme based on "pulmonary versus systemic involvement" and "known cause versus idiopathic origin" will be utilized as a framework here (Box 72-1).[4]

Idiopathic Eosinophilic Pneumonia

In humans, one classification scheme of idiopathic eosinophilic lung disease is based on infiltration of eosinophils into either the pulmonary parenchyma alone, or into multiple organs including the pulmonary parenchyma. Chronic eosinophilic pneumonia (CEP), acute eosinophilic pneumonia (AEP), and some cases of simple pulmonary eosinophilia (Loffler's syndrome) are examples of idiopathic eosinophilic disease that remains localized to the pulmonary parenchyma. Idiopathic hypereosinophilic syndrome and Churg-Strauss syndrome

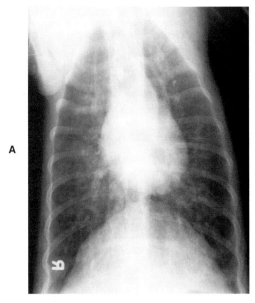

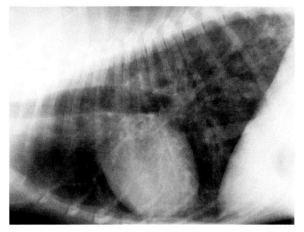

Figure 72-1. A, *Ventrodorsal and* **B,** *lateral thoracic radiographs of a dog with diffuse bilaterally symmetrical interstitial infiltrates caused by eosinophilic pneumonia.* **C,** *Lateral thoracic radiograph of the same dog following therapy with corticosteroids. (Courtesy of Dr. Val Samii, The Ohio State University.)*

are examples of eosinophilic pneumonias that are also associated with infiltration of eosinophils into other tissues.

CHRONIC EOSINOPHILIC PNEUMONIA (CEP)

The features of CEP in humans include an insidious onset of nonspecific respiratory and systemic symptoms, thoracic radiographic or computed tomographic evidence of peripheral alveolar infiltrates, increased percentage of BAL eosinophils, and a dramatic clinical response to oral corticosteroids.[4,22,23] Relapse after discontinuation of corticosteroids is common, especially if tapering is rapid (i.e., less than 6 months).[23] Characteristic histological features include eosinophilic and lymphocytic infiltration in the alveoli and interstitium, with thickened alveolar walls and variable interstitial fibrosis.[23] Bronchiolitis; bronchiolitis obliterans; and mild, nonnecrotizing vasculitis have also been reported.

In dogs, CEP has not been definitively described, although there are multiple reports of chronic idiopathic eosinophilic lung disease described as "pulmonary infiltrates with eosinophils" or "eosinophilic pulmonary gran-

ulomatosis" (EPG) that may represent cases of CEP.[1,24-26] Hilar lymphadenopathy, a feature of EPG in the dog, has been described in humans with CEP.[22] Because of the lack of routine antemortem histological examination before treatment, and the lack of standard criteria for CEP in small animals, this syndrome may go unrecognized or be confused with other types of eosinophilic lung disease.

ACUTE EOSINOPHILIC PNEUMONIA (AEP)

In contrast to CEP, AEP in humans is associated with an acute onset of symptoms (less than 5 to 7 days in duration), severe hypoxemia leading to respiratory failure, diffuse alveolar or mixed alveolar-interstitial infiltrates on imaging, a high percentage of BAL eosinophils, and a dramatic response to corticosteroids.[4,23] Histological examination demonstrates a mixture of eosinophils and edema within the alveoli, bronchi, and interstitium. Vasculitis is not a feature of this disease. Relapses after corticosteroid withdrawal have not been reported.[23] To the authors' knowledge, AEP has not been described in dogs or cats to date.

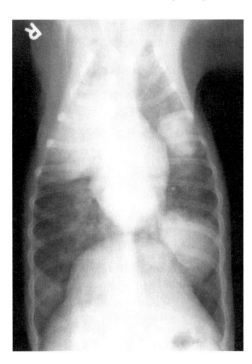

Figure 72-2. *Ventrodorsal thoracic radiograph of a dog with eosinophilic pneumonia. In contrast to the patient described in Figure 72-1, the infiltrates in this case took on a nodular appearance.* (Courtesy of Dr. Val Samii, The Ohio State University.)

<table>
</table>

> **BOX 72-1**
> ## Classification of Eosinophilic Pneumonia
>
> ### Idiopathic Eosinophilic Pneumonia
> Pulmonary involvement only
> - Chronic eosinophilic pneumonia
> - Acute eosinophilic pneumonia
>
> Systemic disease with pulmonary involvement
> - Churg-Strauss syndrome
> - Idiopathic hypereosinophilic syndrome
>
> ### Eosinophilic Pneumonia of Known Cause
> Parasitic infection
> Fungal infection
> Other infectious causes
> Drug-induced
>
> ### Other Pulmonary Syndromes That may Present With Eosinophilia
> Asthma
> Idiopathic pulmonary fibrosis (IPF)
> Langerhans' cell granulomatosis
> Neoplasia
> Bronchiolitis obliterans organizing pneumonia

SIMPLE PULMONARY EOSINOPHILIA (LOFFLER'S SYNDROME)

Simple or transient pulmonary eosinophilia is associated with mild clinical signs, migrating alveolar infiltrates on thoracic radiography, and spontaneous recovery without treatment.[2,23] Parasitic and drug hypersensitivity have been implicated as underlying etiologies, although up to one-third of patients have no identifiable cause.[23]

IDIOPATHIC HYPEREOSINOPHILIC SYNDROME (HES)

Hypereosinophilic syndrome is characterized by a marked, persistent peripheral eosinophilia, orderly and mature eosinophilopoiesis of the bone marrow, and eosinophilic infiltration of multiple organs, of unknown etiology.[27-30] Although rare, this syndrome has been well described in the cat and reported in the dog.[27,31,32] Female cats appear to be affected more often than male cats, and middle age domestic shorthair cats are most commonly reported.[27,31] It has been suggested that rottweilers may be more prone to disorders resulting in eosinophilia, and a report of 3 dogs of this breed with idiopathic hypereosinophilia has been published.[33,34]

Common clinical signs in cats include weight loss, anorexia, vomiting, and diarrhea. Peripheral eosinophil counts may exceed 100,000 cells/μl.[31] Diagnosis depends on ruling out other causes of eosinophilia and on confirming organ infiltration by histologic examination. HES must also be differentiated from eosinophilic leukemia, which is characterized by a disproportionate number of immature eosinophils. In humans, primary eosinophilic leukemia is based on finding more than 5% blast forms on a bone marrow aspirate.[31] Treatment in cats most commonly consists of immunosuppressive doses of glucocorticoids, although hydroxyurea has also been tried.[30,35,36] Prognosis in cats is poor, with a mean survival time from diagnosis to death of 7.5 weeks.[29] Death generally results from tissue infiltration, with eosinophils causing multisystemic organ dysfunction.

CHURG-STRAUSS SYNDROME

The hallmark of Churg-Strauss syndrome, also called allergic angiitis and granulomatosis, is a necrotizing inflammatory vasculitis with granulomatous eosinophilic extravascular tissue infiltration.[4] The typical course of the disease in humans consists of an insidious onset of allergic disease (e.g., asthma with or without allergic rhinitis); development of a peripheral eosinophilia; and then, months to years later, systemic vasculitis.[23] Thoracic radiography may reveal patchy infiltrates, pleural effusion, and hilar lymphadenopathy. Bronchoalveolar lavage and pleural effusion cytologies contain high numbers of eosinophils.[4,23] Although a retrospective study of dogs and cats with eosinophilic pleural and peritoneal effusions has been performed, in the idiopathic cases, histology of organs was not included.[37] It is unknown if any of these animals had systemic vasculitis or granulomas characteristic of this syndrome. The authors are not aware of any reports in the veterinary literature describing Churg-Strauss syndrome in dogs or cats, although there is a reference to an unpublished series of cases of allergic angiitis and granulomatosis in one book.[8]

Eosinophilic Pneumonia of Determined Origin

In contrast to idiopathic eosinophilic pneumonia, a spectrum of eosinophilic lung diseases in which a cause has been determined has been recognized in dogs and cats. Specific details of the diagnosis and treatment of the underlying disorders can be found elsewhere in this text. The goal of therapy is targeted at eliminating the underlying trigger of the pulmonary hypersensitivity. Additionally, prednisone at a dose of 1 to 4 mg/kg (usually divided BID PO) has been commonly used as an adjunct therapy to suppress the hypersensitivity response.[7,38-40]

EOSINOPHILIC PNEUMONIA OF PARASITIC ORIGIN

Dirofilaria immitis infection in dogs and cats has been associated with radiographic evidence of nodular interstitial or alveolar infiltrates and eosinophilic airway lavage fluid.[7,41-46] The pathogenesis of induction of eosinophilic pneumonia in animals with occult heartworm disease involves an excess of antimicrofilarial antibodies that entrap microfilariae within pulmonary capillaries.[38,41,42] This results in hypersensitivity pneumonitis characterized by eosinophilic and neutrophilic infiltration into pulmonary tissue.[7,43] Tests useful in the diagnosis of *D. immitis* include thoracic radiography, Knotts test for microfilaria, heartworm antigen test, heartworm antibody test (cats), and echocardiography.[39,47] A protocol for administration of adulticides (e.g., melarsomine or thiacetarsamide) and microfilaricides (e.g., ivermectin, milbemycin, levamisole, and fenthion) has been reviewed elsewhere.[39] Prednisone has been recommended for treatment of eosinophilic pneumonitis and pulmonary thromboembolism associated with heartworm disease in dogs and cats.[7,38] Other immunosuppressive agents, including cyclophosphamide and azathioprine, have also been used in severe pulmonary eosinophilic pneumonia (pulmonary eosinophilic granulomatosis) presumptively associated with a hypersensitivity to heartworms in dogs.[38] In some regions of the world, the heartworm *Angiostrongylus vasorum* can also cause an eosinophilic pneumonitis in dogs.[48] Ivermectin, fenbendazole, mebendazole, and levamisole have been used in the treatment of *A. vasorum* infection.[48]

Other parasites implicated in eosinophilic pneumonia in dogs and cats include *Aelurostrongylus abstrusus, Capillaria aerophila, Oslerus osleri, Filaroides hirthi and milksi, Crenosoma vulpis, Paragonimus kellicotti, Strongyloides stercoralis, Toxocara* spp., and *Anyclostoma* spp.* A course of an appropriate anthelminthic (e.g., fenbendazole, albendazole, thiabendazole, or levamisole) should be used to eliminate the parasite initially. If signs are severe or fail to completely resolve with anthelminthic therapy, prednisone can be used to suppress the hypersensitivity reaction.

---

*References 2, 6-8, 24, 45, 49, and 50.

EOSINOPHILIC PNEUMONIA OF OTHER INFECTIOUS CAUSES

In humans, infections with *Coccidioides immitus, Pneumocystis carinii, Corynebacterium* spp., *Mycobacterium* spp., and chronic brucellosis have been associated with eosinophilic pneumonia.[4] Additionally, allergic bronchopulmonary aspergillosis (ABPA), a type III hypersensitivity reaction to aspergillus antigens growing in mucous plugs in the airways of asthmatics and distinct from invasive pulmonary aspergillosis, is also associated with eosinophilic pneumonia.[4] In the veterinary literature, chronic bacterial or fungal infections have been purported to cause eosinophilic pneumonia.[7,45,51] However, most reports of dogs or cats with pulmonary coccidioidomycosis, blastomycosis, histoplasmosis, saprophytic fungi, pneumocystosis, and mycobacteriosis have not been associated with eosinophilic pneumonia. Antibiotic or antifungal therapy, ideally based on culture and sensitivity, should be administered to affected patients. Corticosteroids at immunosuppressive doses may result in acceleration or dissemination of infection and should be used with caution.[23]

MISCELLANEOUS PULMONARY DISORDERS WITH EOSINOPHILS

In humans, other pulmonary disorders can be associated with a peripheral eosinophilia or with variable numbers of eosinophils on histologic examination of the lung.[4] Examples include bronchiolitis obliterans with organizing pneumonia (BOOP), asthma/eosinophilic bronchitis, idiopathic pulmonary fibrosis, Langerhans cell granulomatosis, malignancies, and drugs. Bronchiolitis obliterans with organizing pneumonia has been reported in a solitary case report in the dog, and was not associated with eosinophilic infiltration.[52] In dogs and cats, asthma and eosinophilic bronchitis are both associated with eosinophilic infiltration of the airways, sometimes with a peripheral eosinophilia.[5,6,53] Interstitial pulmonary fibrosis (also termed cryptogenic fibrosing alveolitis in humans) has been described in West Highland white terriers, although none of the cases had a peripheral or pulmonary eosinophilia.[54] Langerhans cell granulomatosis (e.g., histiocytosis X or eosinophilic granuloma) was presumptively identified in a dog with dyspnea that had suggestive histological features of the disease; numerous eosinophils were found in the lung.[55] Lymphoma and mast cell neoplasia in particular have been associated with pulmonary eosinophilia in small animals.[8,56]

Drug-induced eosinophilic pneumonia has not been definitively documented in dogs or cats to date. However, if a patient develops eosinophilic pneumonia following the institution of a drug, treatment should be discontinued and either substituted or cautiously reintroduced once the pulmonary lesions have resolved. Drugs commonly used in veterinary practice that have been suggested to cause eosinophilic infiltrates in the lung in humans are listed in Box 72-2. Several illegal drugs, notably cocaine and heroin, have also been associated with eosinophilic pneumonia.[78-80] A particularly

BOX 72-2
Drugs Associated with Eosinophilic Pneumonia in Humans

Aspirin[57]	Methotrexate[69]
Amiodarone[58]	Metronidazole[70]
Ampicillin[59]	Penicillamine[71]
Captopril[60]	Penicillins[72]
Cephalosporins[61]	Phenylbutazone[73]
Chlorpromazine[62]	Piroxicam[74]
Dapsone[63]	Propranolol[66]
Erythromycin[64]	Sulphasalazine[75]
GM-CSF[65]	Tetracycline[76]
Gold salts[66]	Trimethoprim-
Ibuprofen[67]	Sulphamethoxazole[77]
Iodinated contrast medium[68]	

careful history may be required to determine if exposure of the pet to such agents is possible.

Future Directions

The recent advances in molecular biology that have enhanced our understanding of the mechanisms by which eosinophils are recruited to the lung have also led to the discovery of potential new drug targets. Many of the cytokines and chemokines that are involved in eosinophil recruitment signal through a common receptor, CCR3. Compounds that interfere with CCR3 signaling are currently under development and testing, and may offer an alternative to corticosteroids in the future. In addition, antibodies to IL-5 have been investigated and seem to have sufficiently prolonged effects (i.e., weeks to months) to warrant further investigation. In patients that are not able to tolerate systemic steroid administration, the use of inhaled steroids continues to be evaluated. However, given the remarkable efficacy of oral corticosteroids in the treatment of eosinophilic pneumonia, future therapies will need to be rigorously proven to be superior before a change in standard practice would likely be advised.

Conclusion

Eosinophilic pneumonias are a diverse group of pulmonary disorders that share the common feature of increased numbers of eosinophils within the pulmonary parenchyma and alveolar airspaces. The diagnosis typically involves finding diffuse or nodular alveolar-interstitial infiltrates on thoracic radiographs, and *either* elevated eosinophil counts in the peripheral blood or elevated eosinophil percentages in BAL samples. Once the tentative diagnosis has been made, a thorough drug and travel history should be reviewed, followed by investigation to rule out parasitic, fungal, and neoplastic causes. In many cases of eosinophilic pneumonia an underlying cause cannot be identified. Among the known causes, heartworm disease is the

most important in many regions. When an offending organism can be identified, appropriate anthelminthics or antifungals should be administered. Oral corticosteroids remain the mainstay of therapy for all other causes. Prognosis is generally favorable in nonneoplastic cases, although acute eosinophilic pneumonia can cause life-threatening respiratory failure requiring mechanical ventilatory support for a period of days.

REFERENCES

1. Corcoran B, Thoday K, Henfrey J et al: Pulmonary infiltration with eosinophils in 14 dogs, *J Sm Anim Pract* 32:494-502, 1991.
2. Lord P, Schaer M, Tilley L: Pulmonary infiltrates with eosinophilia in the dog, *J Am Vet Radiol Soc* 16:115-120, 1975.
3. Reeder W, Goodrich B: Pulmonary infiltration with eosinophilia (PIE syndrome), *Ann Intern Med* 36:1217-1240, 1952.
4. Cordier J: Eosinophilic pneumonias. In Schwarz M, King T, editors: *Interstitial lung disease*, ed 3, Hamilton, Ontario, 1998, BC Decker.
5. Clercx C, Peeters D, Snaps F et al: Eosinophilic bronchopneumopathy in dogs, *J Vet Intern Med* 14(3):282-291, 2000.
6. Brownlie S: A retrospective study of diagnosis in 109 cases of canine lower respiratory disease, *J Sm Anim Pract* 31:371-376, 1990.
7. Noone K: Pulmonary hypersensitivities, *Current veterinary therapy*, vol 9, Philadelphia, 1986, WB Saunders.
8. Bauer T: Pulmonary hypersensitivity disorders, *Current veterinary therapy*, vol 10, Philadelphia 1989, WB Saunders.
9. Spry C: Eosinophils: *A comprehensive review and guide to the scientific and medical literature*, Oxford, 1988, Oxford University Press.
10. Ehrlich P: Beitrage zur Kenntniss der granulirten Bindegewebszellen und der eosinophilen Leukocythen, *Arch Anat Physiol* 3:166-182, 1879.
11. Nishinakamura R, Miyajima A, Mee P et al: Hematopoesis in mice lacking the entire granulocyte-macrophage colony-stimulating factor/interleukin-3/interleukin-5 functions, *Blood* 88:2458-2464, 1996.
12. Palframan R, Collins P, Williams T et al: Eotaxin induces a rapid release of eosinophils and their progenitors from the bone marrow, *Blood* 91:2240-2248, 1998.
13. Grunig G, Warnock M, Wakil AE et al: Requirement for IL-13 independently of IL-4 in experimental asthma, *Science* 282(5397):2261-2263, 1998.
14. Wills-Karp M, Luyimbazi J, Xu X et al: Interleukin-13: Central mediator of allergic asthma, *Science* 282(5397):2258-2261, 1998.
15. Mould AW, Ramsay AJ, Matthaei KI et al: The effect of IL-5 and eotaxin expression in the lung on eosinophil trafficking and degranulation and the induction of bronchial hyperreactivity, *J Immunol* 164(4):2142-2150, 2000.
16. Malm-Erjefalt M, Persson CG, Erjefalt JS: Degranulation status of airway tissue eosinophils in mouse models of allergic airway inflammation, *Am J Respir Cell Mol Biol* 24(3):352-359, 2001.
17. Kita H, Adolphson C, Gleich G: Biology of eosinophils. In Middleton E, Reed C, Ellis E et al, editors: *Allergy: Principles and practice*, ed 5, St Louis, 1998, Mosby.
18. Kita H, Kaneko M, Bartemes KR et al: Does IgE bind to and activate eosinophils from patients with allergy? *J Immunol* 162(11):6901-6911, 1999.
19. de Andres B, Rakasz E, Hagen M et al: Lack of Fc-epsilon receptors on murine eosinophils: Implications for the functional significance of elevated IgE and eosinophils in parasitic infections, *Blood* 89(10):3826-3836, 1997.
20. Gleich GJ: Mechanisms of eosinophil-associated inflammation, *J Allergy Clin Immunol* 105(4):651-663, 2000.
21. Marchand E, Reynaud-Gaubert M, Lauque D et al: Chronic eosinophilic pneumonia (CEP). A clinical and follow-up study of 61 cases, *Am J Respir Crit Care Med* 155:A329, 1997.
22. Marchand E, Reynaud-Gaubert M, Lauque D et al: Idiopathic chronic eosinophilic pneumonia: A clinical and follow-up study of 62 cases, *Medicine (Baltimore)* 77(5):299-312, 1998.
23. Allen J, Davis W. State of the art: Eosinophilic lung diseases, *Am J Respir Crit Care Med* 150:1423-1438, 1994.
24. Moon M: Pulmonary infiltrates with eosinophilia, *J Sm Anim Pract* 33:19-23, 1992.

25. Yoshikawa K, Hirota Y, Goitsuka R et al: Pulmonary infiltrates with eosinophilia syndrome in a dog, *Jpn J Vet Sci* 49:1160-1161, 1987.

26. von Rotz A, Suter MM, Mettler F et al: Eosinophilic granulomatous pneumonia in a dog, *Vet Rec* 118(23):631-632, 1986.

27. Huibregtse B, Turner J: Hypereosinophilic syndrome and eosinophilic leukemia: A comparison of 22 hypereosinophilic cats, *J Amer Anim Hosp Assoc* 30:591-599, 1994.

28. McEwen SA, Valli VE, Hulland TJ: Hypereosinophilic syndrome in cats: A report of three cases, *Can J Comp Med* 49(3):248-253, 1985.

29. Wilson SC, Thomson-Kerr K, Houston DM: Hypereosinophilic syndrome in a cat, *Can Vet J* 37(11):679-680, 1996.

30. Scott D, Randolph J, Walsh K: Hypereosinophilic syndrome in a cat, *Feline Practice* 15(1):22-28, 1985.

31. Neer T: Hypereosinophilic syndrome in cats, *Compend Cont Ed* 13(4):549-555, 1991.

32. Goto N, Kawamura M, Inoue M et al: Pathology of two cases of canine disseminated hypereosinophilic disease, *Jpn J Vet Sci* 45(3):305-312, 1983.

33. Sykes JE, Weiss DJ, Buoen LC et al: Idiopathic hypereosinophilic syndrome in 3 rottweilers, *J Vet Intern Med* 15(2):162-166, 2001.

34. Lilliehook I, Gunnarsson L, Zakrisson G et al: Diseases associated with pronounced eosinophilia: A study of 105 dogs in Sweden, *J Small Anim Pract* 41(6):248-253, 2000.

35. Harvey R: Feline hypereosinophilia with cutaneous lesions, *J Small Anim Pract* 31:453-456, 1990.

36. Muir P, Gruffydd-Jones TJ, Brown PJ: Hypereosinophilic syndrome in a cat, *Vet Rec* 132(14):358-359, 1993.

37. Fossum T, Wellman M, Relford R et al: Eosinophilic pleural or peritoneal effusions in dogs and cats: 14 cases (1986-1992), *JAVMA* 202(11):1873-1876, 1993.

38. Calvert C, Mahaffey M, Lappin M et al: Pulmonary and disseminated eosinophilic granulomatosis in dogs, *J Amer Anim Hosp Assoc* 24:311-320, 1987.

39. Dillon R: Dirofilariasis in dogs and cats. In Ettinger S, Feldman E, editors: *Textbook of veterinary internal medicine*, ed 5, vol 1, Philadelphia, 2000, WB Saunders.

40. Neer T, Waldron D, Miller R: Eosinophilic pulmonary granulomatosis in two dogs and literature review, *J Amer An Hosp Assoc* 22:593-599, 1986.

41. Calvert CA, Rawlings CA: Pulmonary manifestations of heartworm disease, *Vet Clin North Am Small Anim Pract* 15(5):991-1009, 1985.

42. Calvert C, Losonsky J: Pneumonitis associated with occult heartworm disease in dogs, *JAVMA* 186:1097-1098, 1985.

43. Confer AW, Qualls CW Jr., MacWilliams PS et al: Four cases of pulmonary nodular eosinophilic granulomatosis in dogs, *Cornell Vet* 73(1):41-51, 1983.

44. King R, Zeng Q: Further observations on the characterization of the alveolitis in cats with eosinophilic pneumonitis, *J Vet Int Med* (Abstract) 3:131, 1989.

45. Taboada J: Pulmonary diseases of potential allergic origin, *Sem in Vet Med and Surg (Sm Anim)* 6(4):278-285, 1991.

46. Wong M: Experimental occult dirofilariasis in dogs with reference to immunological responses and its relationship to tropical eosinophilia in man, *SE Asian J Trop Med Pub Health* 5:480-486, 1974.

47. Snyder P, Levy J, Salute M et al: Performance of serologic tests used to detect heartworm infection in cats, *JAVMA* 216(5):693-700, 2000.

48. Martin M, Ashton G, Simpson V et al: Angiostrongylosis in Cornwall: Clinical presentations of eight cases, *J Sm Anim Pract* 34:20-25, 1993.

49. Hayden D, Kruiningen H: Eosinophilic gastroenteritis in German shepherd dogs and its relationship to visceral larva migrans, *JAVMA* 162:379-384, 1973.

50. Hayden D, Kruiningen H: Experimentally induced canine toxocariasis: Laboratory examinations and pathologic changes, with emphasis on the gastrointestinal tract, *Am J Vet Res* 36:1605-1614, 1975.

51. Hamilton T, Hawkins E, DeNicola D: Bronchoalveolar lavage and tracheal wash to determine lung involvement in a cat with cryptococcosis, *JAVMA* 198:655-656, 1991.

52. Phillips S, Barr S, Dykes N et al: Bronchiolitis obliterans with organizing pneumonia, *J Vet Intern Med* 14:204-207, 2000.

53. Dye J, McKiernan B, Rozanski E et al: Bronchopulmonary disease in the cat: Historical, physical, radiographic, clinicopathologic, and pulmonary functional evaluation of 24 affected and 15 healthy cats, *J Vet Int Med* 10(6):385-400, 1996.

54. Corcoran B, Cobb M, Martin M et al: Chronic pulmonary disease in West Highland white terriers, *Vet Record* 144:611-616, 1999.

55. Carroll J, Simon J: Eosinophilic granuloma in a dog, *JAVMA* 150:526-528, 1967.

56. Hawkins E: Pulmonary parenchymal diseases. In Ettinger S, Feldman E, editors: *Textbook of veterinary internal medicine*, ed 5, vol 1, Philadelphia, 2000, WB Saunders.

57. Schatz M, Wasserman S, Patterson R: Eosinophils and immunologic lung disease, *Med Clin North Am* 65(5):1055-1071, 1981.

58. Darmanata JI, van Zandwijk N, Duren DR et al: Amiodarone pneumonitis: Three further cases with a review of published reports, *Thorax* 39(1):57-64, 1984.

59. Poe RH, Condemi JJ, Weinstein SS et al: Adult respiratory distress syndrome related to ampicillin sensitivity, *Chest* 77(3):449-451, 1980.

60. Schatz PL, Mesologites D, Hyun J et al: Captopril-induced hypersensitivity lung disease: An immune-complex-mediated phenomenon, *Chest* 95(3):685-687, 1989.

61. Felman RH, Sutherland DB, Conklin JL et al: Eosinophilic cholecystitis, appendiceal inflammation, pericarditis, and cephalosporin-associated eosinophilia, *Dig Dis Sci* 39(2):418-422, 1994.

62. Shear MK: Chlorpromazine-induced PIE syndrome, *Am J Psychiatry* 135(4):492-493, 1978.

63. Jaffuel D, Lebel B, Hillaire-Buys D et al: Eosinophilic pneumonia induced by dapsone, *BMJ* 317(7152):181, 1998.

64. Abramov LA, Yust IC, Fierstater EM et al: Acute respiratory distress caused by erythromycin hypersensitivity, *Arch Intern Med* 138(7):1156-1158, 1978.

65. Seebach J, Speich R, Fehr J et al: GM-CSF-induced acute eosinophilic pneumonia, *Br J Haematol* 90(4):963-965, 1995.

66. Akoun GM, Cadranel JL, Milleron BJ et al: Bronchoalveolar lavage cell data in 19 patients with drug-associated pneumonitis (except amiodarone), *Chest* 99(1):98-104, 1991.

67. Goodwin SD, Glenny RW: Nonsteroidal antiinflammatory drug-associated pulmonary infiltrates with eosinophilia: Review of the literature and Food and Drug Administration Adverse Drug Reaction reports, *Arch Intern Med* 152(7):1521-1524, 1992.

68. Jennings CA, Deveikis J, Azumi N et al: Eosinophilic pneumonia associated with reaction to radiographic contrast medium, *South Med J* 84(1):92-95, 1991.

69. White DA, Rankin JA, Stover DE et al: Methotrexate pneumonitis. Bronchoalveolar lavage findings suggest an immunologic disorder, *Am Rev Respir Dis* 139(1):18-21, 1989.

70. Kristenson M, Fryden A: Pneumonitis caused by metronidazole, *JAMA* 260(2):184, 1988.

71. Davies D, Jones JK: Pulmonary eosinophilia caused by penicillamine, *Thorax* 35(12):957-958, 1980.

72. Reichlin S, Loveless M, Kane E: Loeffler's syndrome following penicillin therapy, *Ann Intern Med* 38:113-120, 1953.

73. Thuston J, Marks P, Trapnell D: Lung changes associated with phenylbutazone treatment, *BMJ* 1422-1423, 1976.

74. Pfitzenmeyer P, Meier M, Zuck P et al: Piroxicam-induced pulmonary infiltrates and eosinophilia, *J Rheumatol* 21(8):1573-1577, 1994.

75. Wang KK, Bowyer BA, Fleming CR et al: Pulmonary infiltrates and eosinophilia associated with sulfasalazine, *Mayo Clin Proc* 59(5):343-346, 1984.

76. Ho D, Tashkin DP, Bein ME et al: Pulmonary infiltrates with eosinophilia associated with tetracycline, *Chest* 76(1):33-36, 1979.

77. Guerin JC, Chevalier JP, Kofmann J et al: Drug induced interstitial lung diseases after treatment with cotrimoxazole: 2 cases, *Nouv Presse Med* 9(33):2347, 1980.

78. Nadeem S, Nasir N, Israel RH: Loffler's syndrome secondary to crack cocaine, *Chest* 105(5):1599-6000, 1994.

79. Oh PI, Balter MS: Cocaine-induced eosinophilic lung disease, *Thorax* 47(6):478-479, 1992.

80. Brander PE, Tukiainen P: Acute eosinophilic pneumonia in a heroin smoker, *Eur Respir J* 6(5):750-752, 1993.

CHAPTER 73

Parasites of the Lung

Robert G. Sherding

Bronchopulmonary parasites in dogs and cats include nematodes, trematodes, arthropods, and protozoa. This chapter will focus on nematode and trematode infections of the lung. Most respiratory parasite infections are caused by metastrongyloid nematodes. This family includes three parasites formerly grouped together in the genus Filaroides but now considered to be taxonomically separate: *Oslerus (Filaroides) osleri, Filaroides hirthi,* and *Andersonstrongylus (Filaroides) milksi.* The metastrongyloid family also includes *Crenosoma vulpis* and the primary feline lungworm, *Aelurostrongylus abstrusus.* The other lungworm in dogs and cats, *Capillaria aerophila,* also known as *Eucoleus aerophilus,* is not a metastongyloid parasite. The primary trematode lung fluke in dogs and cats is *Paragonimus kellicotti.* Protozoal infections are discussed in Chapter 61, and the pulmonary manifestations of heartworm disease are discussed in Chapter 70.

Lung worm and lung fluke infections are relatively uncommon in domestic dogs and cats. Young animals are most susceptible. Many infections are inapparent or subclinical; however, the most common clinical sign is chronic cough. Severe infections can occasionally cause dyspnea or be complicated by secondary bacterial pneumonia. Thoracic radiography is usually abnormal in animals with overt clinical signs. Respiratory parasites sometimes stimulate increased circulating eosinophils on routine hematology, but this is not consistent. Definitive diagnosis of bronchopulmonary parasitism requires identification of parasite ova or larvae in feces or in airway cytology specimens.

Oslerus (Filaroides) Osleri

This metastrongyloid nematode lives in granulomatous nodules located on the mucosal surface of the distal trachea, tracheal bifurcation, and first-division bronchi in domestic dogs (usually puppies and young dogs less than 1 year of age) and many wild canid species.[1-11]

LIFE CYCLE

Oslerus osleri has a direct life cycle that does not require an intermediate host; thus larvae that are coughed up, swallowed, and passed in the feces can be transmitted directly to another animal.[3,11] In addition, larvae that are expelled from the trachea with respiratory secretions can be transmitted through saliva from dam to puppy during grooming behavior and regurgitative feeding.[4,12] The

prepatent period ranges from 10 to 18 weeks.[3] Oslerus osleri infection is prevalent in North American coyote populations; thus coyotes may be a natural reservoir of infection.[13-16] Similarly, dingos may be a reservoir for this infection in Australia.

CLINICAL SIGNS

The primary clinical sign of *Oslerus osleri* infection is chronic cough.[3,11] Progressively enlarging granulomatous nodules or a series of confluent nodules may obstruct airflow and cause signs such as exercise intolerance, dyspnea, or even death. Spontaneous pneumothorax has been reported in 1 dog.[17]

DIAGNOSIS

The distinctive tracheobronchial nodules can occasionally be detected radiographically as large, space-occupying masses protruding into the lumen near the bifurcation (Figure 73-1). Bronchoscopic visualization is the best way to detect these granulomatous mucosal nodules (Figure 73-2). The most reliable way to definitively diagnose *Oslerus osleri* is to bronchoscopically identify parasitic nodules, accompanied by larvated ova (80 μm) and larvae (230 μm with kinked tail) in airway washings (Figure 73-3) and bronchoscopic biopsies (Figures 73-4 and 73-5).[11] Feces can also be examined for larvae, but this is less rewarding than airway specimens. Zinc sulfate centrifugation-flotation is preferred over the Baermann procedure for detection of *Oslerus osleri* larvae in feces; however, a negative fecal examination by either method is inconclusive, because fecal examination routinely detects no more than a third of active infections.[4,11] This may be attributable to the presence of few larvae, and an intermittent pattern of larval shedding.[18]

TREATMENT

Information concerning treatment of *Oslerus (Filaroides) osleri* is limited mostly to individual case reports. Apparently successful treatment has been reported with fenbendazole,[19] albendazole,[20] oxfendazole,[19,21] ivermectin,[22,23] thiabendazole,[24-26] and levamisole.[27,28] In a prospective trial, fenbendazole and ivermectin were effective in treating gray foxes infected with *O. osleri.*[29] Overall, the treatment of choice for *Oslerus osleri* is either an extended course of fenbendazole (Panacur, 50 mg/kg q24h PO for 10 to 14 days) or ivermectin (Ivomec, 0.4 mg/kg

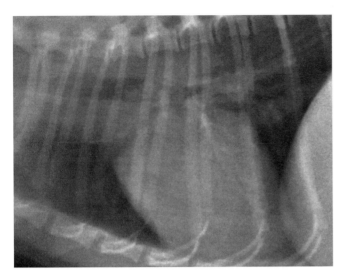

Figure 73-1. *Lateral thoracic radiograph from a young dog with chronic cough and exercise intolerance. A soft-tissue mass is seen within the lumen of the distal trachea that represents a large granulomatous mucosal nodule associated with* Oslerus (Filaroides) osleri *infection.*

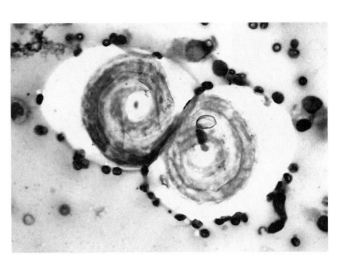

Figure 73-3. *Bronchial cytology from the dog in Figures 73-1 and 73-2 depicts two thin-walled, larvated, metastrongyloid ova typical of* Oslerus (Filaroides) osleri.

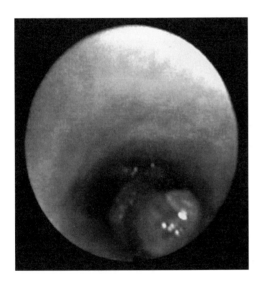

Figure 73-2. *Bronchoscopic appearance of the granulomatous tracheal mass seen in Figure 73-1.*

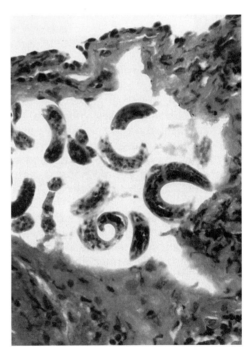

Figure 73-4. *Biopsy of the tracheal nodule in Figures 73-1 and 73-2 reveals numerous larvae of* Oslerus (Filaroides) osleri *embedded in granulomatous inflammatory tissue.*

SC once; do not use in collies).[18] Albendazole has been associated with serious bone marrow toxicity and should be avoided or used very cautiously. In rare cases, severe airway obstruction may necessitate surgical or bronchoscopic removal of the obstructing parasitic nodules.[17]

Filaroides Hirthi

Filaroides hirthi are small metastrongyloid nematodes that live deep in the lung parenchyma (alveoli and terminal airways) of dogs.[11,30-32] *Filaroides hirthi* causes diffuse multifocal interstitial pneumonitis that can be predominantly eosinophilic, mononuclear, or granulomatous.

LIFE CYCLE

Filaroides hirthi has a direct life cycle with a prepatent period of 32 to 35 days.[11] First-stage larvae that are coughed up, swallowed, and passed in the feces are immediately infective and can cause direct horizontal, fecal-oral transmission through coprophagia.[33-37] This mode of transmission has been shown to occur rapidly when infected and unin-

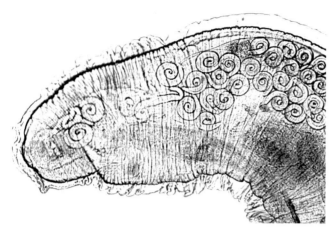

Figure 73-5. *Bronchoscopic mucosal biopsy of a granulomatous tracheal lesion revealed this adult female* Oslerus (Filaroides) osleri *nematode containing numerous ova.*

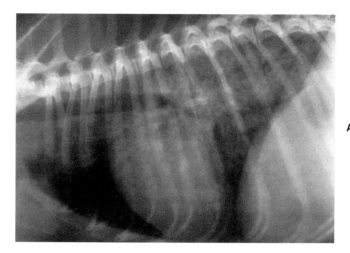

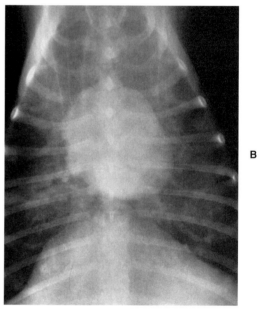

Figure 73-6. A, *Lateral and* **B,** *ventodorsal thoracic radiographs from a 2-year-old female miniature schnauzer infected with* Filaroides hirthi, *showing diffuse interstitial and alveolar infiltrates most severe in the dorsal aspect of the caudal lung lobes.*

fected puppies are kenneled together.[36] In endemically-infected breeding colonies, dam-to-puppy transmission is common and can result in patent infections in puppies less than 3 months of age.[36] Because first-stage larvae are immediately infective, autoinfection can lead to massive overwhelming hyperinfections that cause severe clinical disease and death in severely stressed or immunocompromised dogs.[38-43]

CLINICAL SIGNS

Filaroides hirthi usually causes subclinical interstitial pneumonia but infected dogs occasionally are presented with acute or chronic, progressive signs of cough and dyspnea.[44,45] Fatalities have been reported in severe infections, especially in hyperinfections in immunosuppressed or corticosteroid-treated dogs and in toy breed dogs.[11,18,38,39,41-43]

Filaroides hirthi was originally identified in a laboratory colony of beagles.[30] It was subsequently found to be an endemic problem in other breeding colonies of research dogs, with infection rates approaching 100% in some colonies.[46,47] Dogs from such colonies generally show no clinical signs; however, the parasite produces significant inflammatory lung lesions that can ruin their usefulness in research.[30,47]

DIAGNOSIS

Animals with clinical signs generally have diffuse broncho-interstitial infiltrates on thoracic radiographs (Figure 73-6).[48] Alveolar infiltrates are seen less commonly. These changes may persist for several weeks. A peripheral eosinophilia may be seen, but most cases have no hematological abnormalities. The definitive diagnosis is based on finding ova or first-stage larvae in airway cytology specimens (e.g., aspirates or washings) or feces (Figure 73-7). The most reliable method for examining feces for *Filaroides hirthi* larvae is with zinc sulfate centrifugation-flotation (Figure 73-8). Zinc sulfate flota-tion is 100 times more efficient than the Baermann procedure for concentrating *Filaroides hirthi* larvae from feces.[35]

TREATMENT

Filaroides hirthi can be treated with fenbendazole (Panacur, 50 mg/kg q24h PO for 10 to 14 days)[44,45]; albendazole (Valbazen, 25 to 50 mg/kg q12h for 5 days; repeated in 2 weeks)[49]; or ivermectin (Ivomec, 0.4 mg/kg IV once; do not use in collies). Albendazole has been associated with serious bone marrow toxicity and should be avoided or used very cautiously. Dead and dying worms can elicit a multifocal granulomatous inflammatory response; thus clinical signs and radiographic changes may initially worsen after treatment.[48] If severe, this can be controlled with antiinflammatory doses of corticosteroids for 2 to 3 weeks.

Figure 73-7. *Airway cytology obtained by transtracheal aspiration from the dog in Figure 73-6, depicting a typical larvated metastrongyloid ovum of* Filaroides hirthi *(168×).*

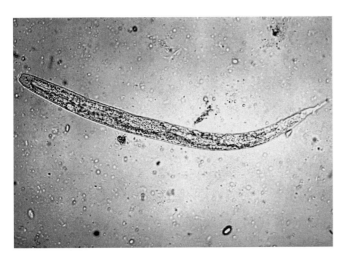

Figure 73-8. *Zinc sulfate centrifugation-flotation (unstained) from the dog in Figures 73-6 and 73-7, showing a* Filaroides hirthi *larva.*

Control of *Filaroides hirthi* infection in kennels and breeding colonies of research dogs can be challenging because of infection rates approaching 100% and direct transmission from dam to puppies.[11] The use of isolation procedures and albendazole treatment substantially reduced the incidence of infection in two breeding colonies,[46] and high-dose ivermectin treatment (1 mg/kg SC, once or twice) controlled the infection rate in another endemically-infected colony.[50]

Andersonstrongylus (Filaroides) Milksi

Andersonstrongylus milksi, also known as *Filaroides milksi, is* a rare metastrongyloid nematode of dogs that has many similarities to *Filaroides hirthi.* There is consid-

erable confusion and some disagreement regarding the taxonomic classification of this parasite.[11] Some of the early reports of this parasite in dogs[10,51-53] are now considered to be misidentifications of *Filaroides hirthi.*[11,18,54] As in other *Filaroides* spp., this lung worm has a direct life cycle. Clinical findings, diagnosis, and treatment are thought to be similar to those of *Filaroides hirthi.*

Aelurostrongylus Abstrusus

Aelurostrongylus abstrusus is a metastrongyloid nematode that primarily infects cats.[11,55,56] This lung worm infection is found worldwide and is most prevalent in feral, stray, and outdoor cats that eat prey. During a 6-month period, 20 of 108 (18.5%) mature stray cats evaluated in an Alabama shelter were infected with Aelurostrongylus.[57] The prevalence in 125 cats in Scotland was 9.6%.[58] In a diverse population of 327 feral adult cats in Australia, the prevalence was 14%,[59] and another study found a prevalence of 39% in 86 feral cats.[60]

LIFE CYCLE AND PATHOGENESIS

The life cycle and pathogenesis of *Aelurostrongylus* have been well described.[55,56,61-68] The adult nematodes live in the terminal bronchioles and alveolar ducts causing bronchiolitis, interstitial and alveolar pneumonia, and muscular thickening of the pulmonary arteries.[61,68-70] The adult female worms are 9 to 10 mm in length and the males are 4 to 6 mm. Eggs produced by the adult nematodes develop within the lung into first-stage larvae that are coughed up, swallowed, and passed in the feces. The indirect life cycle requires a molluscan intermediate host such as a terrestrial snail or slug. Cats can be infected either by ingesting infected snails and slugs; or by eating paratenic transport and storage hosts that feed on snails and slugs, especially prey such as rodents and birds.

In experimentally-infected cats, excretion of larvae begins at 4 to 6 weeks postinfection, peaks at 3 months, and continues for up to 6 to 9 months.[65,68] Larvae remain viable under natural conditions in the soil for at least 1 month, and then within the infected snail intermediate host for 2 years.[63] The third stage larvae can encyst in the viscera of storage hosts such as mice and remain infectious to cats for at least 3 months.[56]

CLINICAL SIGNS

Most *Aelurostrongylus* infections are asymptomatic; however, severe infections can cause chronic cough, dyspnea, and debilitation. Pleural effusion occurs rarely, but one cat with an eosinophilic pleural exudate has been reported.[71] Studies in experimentally infected kittens have shown that the severity of pulmonary disease and clinical signs are related to the infective dose of larvae.[62] A single snail may contain 400 to 600 viable larvae. Mild multifocal pulmonary lesions were evident with an infective dose as small as 50 larvae, but clinical signs were absent. With an infective dose of 100 to 400 larvae, the lung lesions were moderate and the clinical signs were mild. An infective dose of 800 larvae produced progressive pulmonary disease characterized by a dense, mixed inflammatory cell response with signs of cough and exercise intolerance. Higher infective doses (1600 to 3200 larvae) produced severe diffuse pulmonary disease characterized by progressive clinical signs of cough, dyspnea, inappetence, debilitation, and possible death.

Except in severely infected cats, the clinical signs and pulmonary lesions are usually self-limiting within 6 to 9 months[68]; however, the muscular hypertrophy and hyperplasia of the pulmonary artery walls, which can increase in thickness up to 12 times normal and occlude the vessels, may persist for 2 years or more.[68] Although this might be expected to cause pulmonary hypertension, evidence of pulmonary hypertension or right ventricular hypertrophy was not found in cats studied up to 1 year after infection.[72]

DIAGNOSIS

Aelurostrongylus infection should be suspected in cats with bronchopulmonary disease that hunt birds and rodents and that have radiographic findings of diffuse broncho-interstitial and patchy alveolar pulmonary infiltrates (Figure 73-9).[73,74] These radiographic patterns correlate with the dense inflammatory infiltration of lymphocytes, macrophages, and eosinophils around multifocal collections of eggs and larvae. Some cats have a prominent bronchial or miliary nodular pattern. In experimentally infected cats, the alveolar pattern was most pronounced from 5 to 21 weeks after infection, and as the alveolar component resolved, bronchial and miliary interstitial nodular patterns became apparent at 17 to 40 weeks.[73,74] Eosinophilia is an inconsistent hematologic finding in cats with aelurostrongylosis.[57,73] One study concluded that evaluation of serum proteins by electrophoresis is not a useful test in this infection.[75]

Confirmation of *Aelurostrongylus* infection is based on identification of first-stage larvae in airway cytology specimens or in feces using either a Baermann fecal examination or zinc sulfate centrifugation-flotation. Larvae are 0.4 mm in length with a notched tail and configured in a coil or J shape.[56] One study found the Baermann to be a more sensitive clinical diagnostic test than hematology, radiography, or necropsy.[57] However, larvae are shed intermittently in feces in small numbers; thus evaluation of respiratory cytology specimens for larvae can also be very helpful (Figure 73-10).

TREATMENT

Mild *Aelurostrongylus* infections are generally self-limiting without treatment. Cats with significant clinical pulmonary disease are most effectively treated with either fenbendazole (Panacur, 50 mg/kg q24h PO for 10 to 20 days)[76-78] or ivermectin (Ivomec, 0.4 mg/kg SC once).[79] When using fenbendazole it is important to use an extended duration of treatment, because the standard 3-day regimen of fenbendazole was not sufficient to eliminate the infection.[80] Nonspecific adjunctive therapy can include corticosteroids and bronchodilators.

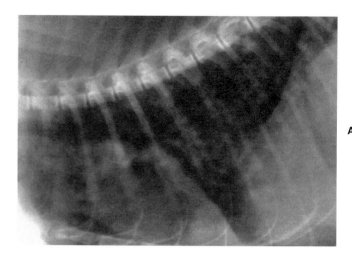

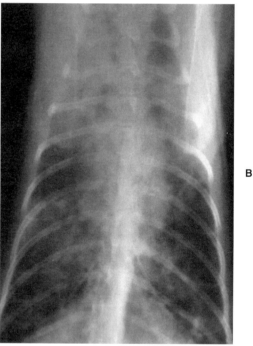

Figure 73-9. **A,** *Lateral and* **B,** *ventrodorsal thoracic radiographs from a young cat infected with* Aelurostrongylus abstrusus, *showing severe diffuse broncho-interstitial infiltrates.*

OTHER PARASITES RELATED TO AELUROSTRONGYLUS

Bronchostrongylus spp. and *Troglostrongylus* spp. may rarely cause lungworm disease similar to aelurostrongylosis in domestic cats. These metastrongyloid nematodes are related to *Aelurostrongylus abstrusus* and primarily infect exotic felid species in Africa.

Crenosoma Vulpis

Crenosoma vulpis is a metastrongyloid nematode parasite found primarily in wild canids (e.g., wolves and

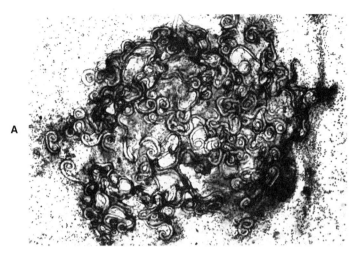

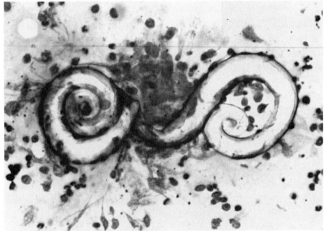

Figure 73-10. *A,* Low *(42×) and* **B**, *high (104× magnifications of broncho-alveolar lavage cytology (stain) from the cat in Figure 73-9, showing the diagnostic appearance of* Aelurostrongylus abstrusus *larvae surrounded by inflammatory cells and mucus.*

foxes) and raccoons in North America and Europe. This lungworm can also occasionally infect dogs, causing chronic bronchopulmonary disease and a productive cough.[11,81-86] In North America, infection is widespread in the wild fox population, and is endemic in red foxes in the northeastern United States and Atlantic provinces of Canada.[85] The prevalence is over 50% in red foxes of Nova Scotia, New Brunswick, and Prince Edward Island (PEI).[84] The general prevalence in 310 dogs from PEI was 3.2%, but in 55 dogs with chronic cough the prevalence was 27.3%.[85] Thus *Crenosoma* can be a significant cause of respiratory disease in dogs residing in rural or urbanized areas populated with foxes.

LIFE CYCLE

The life cycle of *Crenosoma vulpis* involves terrestrial snails and slugs as intermediate hosts and small prey as paratenic hosts, similar to *Aelurostrongylus abstrusus* in cats.[70,83,84] The adult nematodes (females 12 to 16 mm in length and males 4 to 8 mm) live in the bronchi and bronchioles where they cause chronic bronchitis and bronchiolitis. They produce larvated eggs that develop into first-stage larvae that are coughed up, swallowed, and passed in the feces. The indirect life cycle requires terrestrial snails or slugs as intermediate hosts. Dogs are infected primarily by ingesting infected snails and slugs, although ingestion of paratenic transport hosts that feed on snails and slugs may also occur. The prepatent period is 17 to 21 days.

CLINICAL SIGNS

The predominant clinical sign of *Crenosoma vulpis* infection is chronic productive cough. Systemic signs such as fever, inappetence, or weight loss are usually absent.

DIAGNOSIS

On thoracic radiographs, most dogs have a diffuse bronchial or broncho-interstitial pattern that may be indistinguishable from other forms of chronic bronchitis. Alveolar infiltrates are found less commonly. Hematological evaluation often reveals a peripheral eosinophilia.[84,86] Basophilia and monocytosis may also be seen.[86]

Bronchoscopic findings in 9 dogs varied from mild bronchial erythema to severe bronchitis with mucus accumulation and hyperplastic mucosal nodules.[86] One dog had bronchial hemorrhage, and adult worms were visualized in 2 dogs. Tracheobronchial or bronchoalveolar lavage cytology specimens usually show increased mucus, high cellularity, and predominantly eosinophilic inflammation.[84,86,87] First-stage larvae are often observed on cytology.

Definitive diagnosis of *Crenosoma vulpis* infection depends on identification of first-stage larvae in airway cytology specimens, or in feces using either a Baermann procedure or zinc sulfate centrifugation-flotation. The larvae of *Crenosoma* are approximately 300 μm in length with a blunt anterior end and a smooth, tapering tail without notching or kinks. In a report of 10 clinical cases, *Crenosoma* larvae were identified by bronchoalveolar lavage in only 5 of the dogs, whereas the Baermann fecal examination was a more sensitive diagnostic test with positive results in all 10 dogs.[86] Overall, based on the case reports cited here, respiratory cytology positively identifies first-stage larvae in only 50% to 75% of cases confirmed by fecal evaluation. In diagnosing *Crenosoma*, the Baermann procedure was found to be more a reliable fecal test than the zinc sulfate centrifugation-flotation.[85]

TREATMENT

Crenosoma vulpis responds rapidly to treatment with fenbendazole (Panacur, 50 mg/kg q24h PO for 3 to 7 days).[84,85,87,88] Clinical signs and radiographic abnormalities generally improve within 1 week and fecal larvae are absent within 2 to 4 weeks. Other successful treatments for *Crenosoma* have included febantel,[82] levamisole, and diethylcarbamazine.[89] Infected foxes have been treated with ivermectin.[85]

Capillaria Aerophila

Capillaria aerophila, also known as *Eucoleus aerophilus*, is a nematode parasite with worldwide distribution that lives in the tracheobronchial mucosa of dogs, cats, and foxes.[11,90-96] *Capillaria* is classified as a trichuroid nematode. Fecal surveys for *Capillaria* spp. in animals from Columbus, Ohio, found prevalence rates of 1.3% in 1000 humane shelter cats[97] and 1% in 500 stray dogs.[98] In Illinois, the prevalence was 4% in 217 cats from labs, shelters, and homes.[99] The prevalence in Australian cats is 3% to 5%.[95] In a German epidemiological study, *Capillaria* was found in 10% of 70 litters of kittens raised in a farm environment, compared with no infections found in 30 litters of kittens from an indoor environment.[100]

LIFE CYCLE

The adult female worms are 20 to 38 mm in length, and the males are 12 to 25 mm. These parasites occur as white, coiled masses deeply embedded in the mucosa of the trachea and large bronchi, surrounded by collections of ova.[11,18] This results in chronic bronchitis. The direct life cycle involves ingestion of eggs from an infected host that are passed in the feces after being coughed up and swallowed.[11,18] Earthworms may serve as transport paratenic hosts. Excreted eggs embryonate and become infective in about 40 days, remaining viable in the soil for extended periods of up to a year. The prepatent period is 3 to 5 weeks.[18]

CLINICAL SIGNS

Most *Capillaria aerophila* infections are asymptomatic, but this parasite occasionally causes chronic bronchitis with persistent cough.[18,93,95] In severe cases, dyspnea, loss of weight, poor body condition, or complicating bacterial bronchopneumonia may occur, especially in young animals.

DIAGNOSIS

In animals showing clinical signs, thoracic radiographs may reveal a mixed pattern of diffuse peribronchial, interstitial, and alveolar infiltrates (Figure 73-11). Some cases may have a marked peripheral eosinophilia. Airway cytology specimens may show increased mucus, eosinophilic exudates, and the presence of *Capillaria* ova.[93]

The diagnosis is based on identification of double-operculated, yellow-brown ova in fecal flotation or airway cytology specimens (Figure 73-12). *Capillaria* ova must be differentiated from the similar-appearing ova of the intestinal whipworm *Trichuris vulpis* and the nasal nematode *Eucoleus boehmi*.[101] *Capillaria* ova are smaller (less than 70 μm) than *Trichuris* ova, and they have asymmetric bipolar plugs that produce a lopsided appearance.

TREATMENT

The suggested treatment for *Capillaria* is fenbendazole (Panacur, 50 mg/kg q24h PO for 10 to 14 days). It is un-

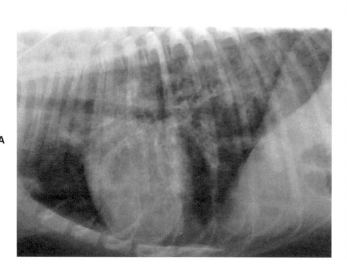
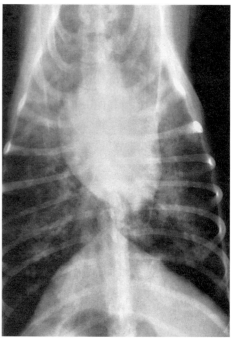

Figure 73-11. A, Lateral and **B**, ventrodorsal thoracic radiographs from a 1-year-old mixed breed dog infected with Capillaria aerophila, showing severe diffuse broncho-interstitial and alveolar infiltrates. This dog presented for cough and mild dyspnea. A CBC revealed a total WBC of 48,200/μl with severe eosinophilia (25,064/μl) and basophilia (1928/μl).

clear from some of the reported cases whether fenben-dazole kills the adult nematodes or merely disrupts egg shedding by a sterilizing effect on female worms.[18] Ivermectin (0.2 to 0.3 mg/kg SC, one or two doses) appears to have successfully treated a cat with pulmonary capillariasis[95] and a dog with nasal capillariasis.[102] Levamisole has also been reported as an effective treatment.[93,96,103] A combination of febantel and praziquantel was not effective for treating *Capillaria* in cats.[104]

Paragonimus Kellicotti

Paragonimus kellicotti is a trematode lung parasite (i.e., lung fluke) that infects wild carnivores and occasionally dogs and cats, especially in the Great Lakes and Gulf of Mexico regions of the United States.[11,105,106]

LIFE CYCLE

The life cycle and pathogenesis of *Paragonimus* have been well studied in experimentally infected cats.[107-110] The lung fluke requires two intermediate hosts: the aquatic snail and the crayfish. Dogs and cats become infected by ingesting infected crayfish or by eating another animal that has recently ingested crayfish. Within 4 to 5 weeks after infection, the flukes are well established in characteristic, radiographically-visible pulmonary cysts, and they begin producing ova that appear in the feces. These cysts are most prevalent in the caudal lung lobes, especially on the right side.[108,110] This distribution may be explained by the migration route of the flukes through the diaphragm. The adult flukes live in pairs within fibrous subpleural cysts that communicate directly with the bronchial system (Figure 73-13). This allows eggs to be readily expelled into the airway where they are coughed up, then swallowed and passed in the feces to complete the life cycle.

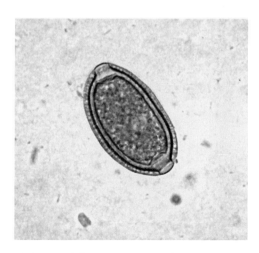

Figure 73-12. *Fecal flotation (unstained) showing the typical bioperculated* Capillaria aerophila *egg. Note the slightly lopsided appearance from asymmetry of the bipolar plugs.*

CLINICAL SIGNS

The typical clinical signs of paragonimiasis are chronic cough, exercise intolerance, and weight loss.[106,111] Hemoptysis is sometimes observed. In some cases, sudden or recurrent episodes of dyspnea can be caused by spontaneous pneumothorax from cyst rupture.[108,112] Experimentally infected cats often have no clinical signs; thus animals with natural *Paragonimus* infection may be asymptomatic and go unrecognized.

DIAGNOSIS

The diagnosis of *Paragonimus* infection is usually suspected from radiographic findings of multiloculated thin-walled pulmonary cysts in dogs (Figure 73-14): and thick-walled cysts and large, ill-defined nodular

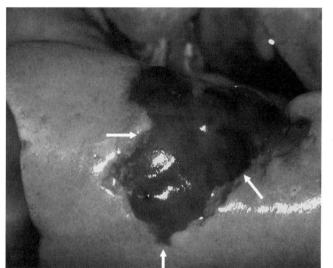

A

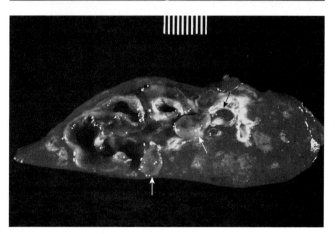

B

Figure 73-13. A, *A large cystic lesion in the right caudal lung lobe caused by* Paragonimus kellicotti. **B,** *Cross-section through the right caudal lung lobe shows a large cavitated lung cyst containing two adult* Paragonimus *flukes (white arrows). Note the cyst communicates with a large bronchus (black arrow). (***B** *used with permission from Pechman RD: The radiographic features of pulmonary paragonimiasis in the dog and cat,* J Am Vet Radiol Society *27:182-191, 1976.)*

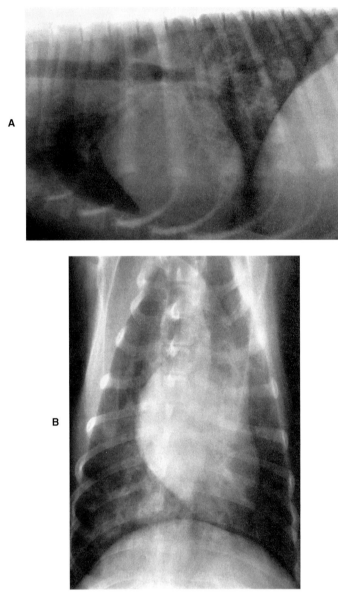

Figure 73-14. A, Lateral and **B,** ventrodorsal thoracic radiographs from a 5-month-old male German shepherd dog infected with Paragonimus kellicotti, showing at least 3 cystic lung lesions—one cranial to the heart (lateral view) in the right cranial lobe, one dorsal to the trachea just cranial to the bifurcation (lateral view), and a large coalescing cavitation in the right caudal lung lobe. The caudal lobe cyst is also associated with mixed pulmonary infiltration.

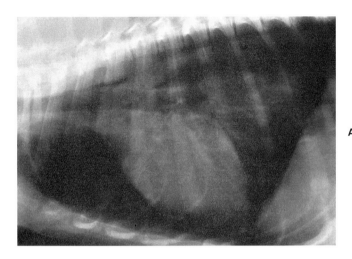

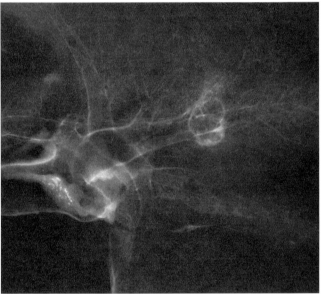

Figure 73-15. A, Lateral thoracic radiograph from a dog infected with Paragonimus kellicotti that presented for acute spontaneous pneumothorax. **B,** Radiograph of the affected lobe after removed postmortem shows a well-delineated thin-walled cyst in the caudal lung lobe that communicates with the lobar bronchus. (**B** reprinted with permission from Pechman RD: The radiographic features of pulmonary paragonimiasis in the dog and cat, J Am Vet Radiol Soc 27:182-191, 1976.)

densities (granulomas) in cats.[106,112] Some animals have radiographic evidence of spontaneous pneumothorax (Figure 73-15). Nonspecific peribronchial and linear interstitial infiltrates are common. Routine laboratory evaluations are unremarkable except for mild eosinophilia in some cases.[108] Definitive diagnosis is based on identification of large yellow-brown, single-operculated ova in feces (using fecal sedimentation or zinc sulfate centrifugation-flotation) or in airway cytology specimens (Figure 73-16).

TREATMENT

Treatment with either praziquantel (Droncit, 25 mg/kg q8h PO for 3 days)[111,113] or fenbendazole (Panacur, 50 mg/kg q24h PO for 10 to 14 days)[114] is highly effective for treating *Paragonimus kellicotti.* Albendazole (25 mg/kg q12h PO for 10 days) is also effective,[115,116] but has a greater risk of serious side effects (e.g., bone marrow toxicity). In one study, within 11 days after praziquantel, the radiographic lung lesions were nearly resolved and eggs were absent from the feces.[113]

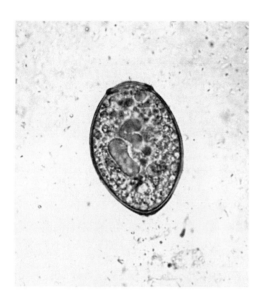

Figure 73-16. *Fecal flotation (104×, unstained) of* Paragonimus kellicotti *ovum from a dog.*

Cuterebra

Cuterebra spp. larvae are the larval forms (bots) of numerous species of arthropod flies that infect mostly rabbits and rodents. Cuterebra can occasionally infect outdoor dogs and cats in spring and summer, especially migrating in the subcutis of the face, head, and neck region. Rarely, Cuterebra can cause respiratory disease when they migrate in the nasopharynx, causing sneezing and unilateral bloody nasal discharge, or in the wall of the cervical trachea, causing clinical signs of cough and dyspnea.[117,118] The diagnosis is made by direct endoscopic visualization of the Cuterebra larvae embedded in the nasopharyngeal or upper airway mucosa. Airway Cuterebra can be treated by endoscopic extraction or by administering ivermectin (0.3 mg/kg subcutaneously once). Corticosteroids (prednisone, 1 mg/kg PO q12h for 2 weeks) may help to reduce the local inflammatory reaction to the parasite.

REFERENCES

1. Barr SC, Lavelle RB, Harrigan KE et al: *Oslerus (Filaroides) osleri* in a dog, *Aust Vet J* 63:334-337, 1986.
2. Bennett D: The diagnosis and treatment of Filaroides osleri in the dog. In Hill CSGGaFWG, editor: *Veterinary annual*, Bristol, UK, 1975, Wright.
3. Clayton HC, Lindsay EF: *Filaroides osleri* infection in the dog, *J Small Anim Pract* 20:773-782, 1979.
4. Dorrington JE: Studies on *Filaroides osleri* infestation in dogs, *Onderstepoort J Vet Res* 35(1):225-286, 1968.
5. Dunsmore JD, Spratt DM: The life history of *Filaroides osleri* in wild and domestic canids in Australia, *Vet Parasitol* 5:275-286, 1979.
6. Schuster R, Hamann F: A case of an *Oslerus osleri* infection (nematoda) in a dog, *Appl Parasitol* 34:125-130, 1993.
7. Jones BR, Clark WT, Collins GH et al: *Filaroides osleri* in a dog, *New Zealand Vet J* 25:103-104, 1977.
8. Kotani T, Horie M, Yamaguchi S et al: Lungworm, *Filaroides osleri*, infection in a dog in Japan, *J Vet Med Sci* 57(3):573-576, 1995.
9. Mills JHL: Filaroidiasis in the dog: A review, *J Small Anim Pract* 8:37-43, 1967.
10. Mills JHL, Nielsen SW: Canine *Filaroides osleri* and *Filaroides milksi* infection, *JAVMA* 149:56-63, 1966.
11. Georgi JR: Parasites of the respiratory tract, *Vet Clin North Am Small Anim Pract* 17:1421-1442, 1987.
12. Polley L, Creighton SR: Experimental direct transmission of the lungworm *Filaroides osleri* in dogs, *Vet Rec* 100:136-137, 1977.
13. Carlson BL, Nielsen SW: Prevalence of *Oslerus osleri* (Cobbold, 1879) in coyotes *(Canis latrans Say)* from Connecticut, *J Wildl Dis* 21:64-65, 1985.
14. Foreyt WJ, Foreyt KM: Attempted transmission of *Oslerus (Oslerus) osleri (Filaroides osleri)* from coyotes to domestic dogs and coyotes, *J Parasitol* 67:284-286, 1981.
15. Morrison EE, Gier HT: Lungworms in coyotes on the Great Plains, *J Wildl Dis* 14:314-316, 1978.
16. Morrison EE, Gier HT: Parasitic infection of *Filaroides osleri*, *Capillaria aerophila* and *Spirocera lupi* in coyotes from the Southwestern United States, *J Wildl Dis* 15:557-559, 1979.
17. Burrows CF, O'Brien JA, Biery DN: Pneumothorax due to *Filaroides osleri* infestation in the dog, *J Small Anim Pract* 3:613-618, 1972.
18. Reinemeyer CR: Parasites of the respiratory system. In Bonagura JD, editor: *Kirk's current veterinary therapy*, vol 12, Philadelphia, 1995, WB Saunders.
19. Bourdoiseau G, Cadore JL, Fournier C et al: Oslerosis of the dog: Diagnostic and therapeutic status, *Parasite* 1:369-378, 1994.
20. van Heerden J, Petrick SW: The treatment of *Filaroides osleri* infestation with albendazole, *J S Afr Vet Assoc* 51:281, 1980.
21. Kelly PJ, Mason PR: Successful treatment of *Filaroides osleri* infection with oxfendazole, *Vet Rec* 116:445-446, 1985.
22. Boersema JH, Baas JJ, Schaeffer F: A persistent case of kennel cough caused by *Filaroides osleri*, *Tijdschr Diergeneeskd* 114:10-13, 1989.
23. Outerbridge CA, Taylor SM: *Oslerus osleri* tracheobronchitis: Treatment with ivermectin in 4 dogs, *Can Vet J* 39:238-240, 1998.
24. Bennett D: Treatment of *Filaroides osleri* infestation in a 16-month-old male Yorkshire terrier with thiabendazole, *Vet Rec* 93(8):226-227, 1973.
25. Hill BL, McChesney AE: Thiabendazole treatment of a dog with *Filaroides osleri*, *J Am Anim Hosp Assoc* 12:487-489, 1976.
26. Levitan DM, Matz ME, Findlen CS et al: Treatment of *Oslerus osleri* infestation in a dog: Case report and literature review, *J Am Anim Hosp Assoc* 32:435-438, 1996.
27. Darke PGG: Use of levamisole in the treatment of parasitic tracheobronchitis in the dog, *Vet Rec* 99:293-294, 1976.
28. Randolph JF, Rendano JVT: Treatment of *Filaroides osleri* infestation in a dog with thiabendazole and levamisole, *J Am Anim Hosp Assoc* 20:795-798, 1984.
29. Blagburn BL, Swango LJ, Hendrix CM et al: Comparative efficacies of ivermectin, febantel, fenbendazole, and mebendazole against helminth parasites of gray foxes, *JAVMA* 189:1084-1085, 1986.
30. Hirth RS, Hottendorf GH: Lesions produced by a new lungworm in beagle dogs, *Vet Path* 10:385-407, 1973.
31. Georgi JR, Anderson RC: Filaroides hirthi sp. n. (Nematoda: Metastrongyloidea) from the lung of the dog, *J Parasitol* 61:337-339, 1975.
32. Beveridge I, Dunsmore JD, Harrigan KE et al: Filaroides hirthi in dogs, *Aust Vet J* 60:59, 1983.
33. Georgi JR: *Filaroides hirthi:* Experimental transmission among beagle dogs through ingestion of first-stage larvae, *Science, New Series* 194:735, 1976.
34. Georgi JR, Fleming WJ, Hirth RS et al: Preliminary investigation of the life history of *Filaroides hirthi Georgi and Anderson, Cornell Vet* 66:309-323, 1976.
35. Georgi JR, Georgi ME, Cleveland DJ: Patency and transmission of *Filaroides hirthi* infection, *Parasitology* 75:251-257, 1977.
36. Georgi JR, Georgi ME: Transmission and control of *Filaroides hirthi* lungworm infection in dogs, *Am J Vet Res* 40:829-831, 1979.
37. Georgi JR, Fahnestock GR, Bohm MF et al: The migration and development of *Filaroides hirthi* larvae in dogs, *Parasitology* 79:39-47, 1979.
38. Craig TM, Brown TW, Shefstad DK et al: Fatal *Filaroidis hirthi* infection in a dog, *JAVMA* 172:1096-1098, 1978.
39. August JR, Powers RD, Bailey WS: *Filaroides hirthi* in a dog: Fatal hyperinfection suggestive of autoinfection, *JAVMA* 176:331-334, 1980.

40. Genta RM, Schad GA: *Filaroides hirthi:* Hyperinfective lungworm infection in immunosuppressed dogs, *Vet Pathol* 21:349-354, 1984.

41. Spencer A, Rushton B, Munro H: *Filaroides hirthi* in a British bred beagle dog, *Vet Rec* 117:8-10, 1985.

42. Valentine BA, Georgi ME: *Filaroides hirthi* hyperinfection associated with adrenal cortical carcinoma in a dog, *J Comp Pathol* 97:221-225, 1987.

43. Carrasco L, Hervas J, Gomez-Villamandos JC et al: Massive *Filaroides hirthi* infestation associated with canine distemper in a puppy, *Vet Rec* 140:72-73, 1997.

44. Rubash JM: *Filaroides hirthi* infection in a dog, *JAVMA* 189:213, 1986.

45. Pinckney RD, Studer AD, Genta RM: *Filaroides hirthi* infection in two related dogs, *JAVMA* 193:1287-1288, 1988.

46. Erb HN, Georgi JR: Control of *Filaroides hirthi* in commercially reared beagle dogs, *Lab Anim Sci* 32:394-396, 1982.

47. Bahnemann R, Bauer C: Lungworm infection in a beagle colony: *Filaroides hirthi,* a common but not well-known companion, *Exp Toxicol Pathol* 46:55-62, 1994.

48. Rendano JVT, Georgi JR, Fahnestock GR et al: *Filaroides hirthi* lungworm infection in dogs: Its radiographic appearance, *J Am Vet Radiol Soc* 20:1-9, 1979.

49. Georgi JR, Slauson DO, Theodorides VJ: Anthelmintic activity of albendazole against *Filaroides hirthi* lungworms in dogs, *Am J Vet Res* 39:803-806, 1978.

50. Bauer C, Bahnemann R: Control of *Filaroides hirthi* infections in beagle dogs by ivermectin, *Vet Parasitol* 65:269-273, 1996.

51. Greenway JA, Stockdale PHG: A case tentatively diagnosed as *Filaroides milksi* in a dog, *Can Vet J* 11:203-204, 1970.

52. Corwin RM, Legendre AM, Dade AW: Lungworm *(Filaroides milksi)* infection in a dog, *JAVMA* 165:180-182, 1974.

53. Cremers HJ, Gruys E, Stokhof AA: An infection with the lungworm *Filaroides milksi* Whitlock, 1956 (Nematoda: Metastrongyloidea) in a dog from Belgium, *Tijdschr Diergeneeskd* 103:85-90, 1978.

54. Webster WA: *Andersonstrongylus milksi* (Whitlock, 1956) n. comb. (Metastongyloidea: Angiostrongylidae) with a discussion of related species in North American canids and mustelids, *Proc Helminth Soc Wash* 48:154-158, 1981.

55. Scott DW: Current knowledge of aelurostrongylosis in the cat, *Cornell Vet* 63:483-500, 1972.

56. Schalm OW, Ling GV, Smith JB: Lungworm infection in cats, *Feline Practice* 41-45, 1974.

57. Willard MD, Roberts MS, Allison N et al: Diagnosis of *Aelurostrongylus abstrusus* and *Dirofilaria immitis* infections in cats from a humane shelter, *JAVMA* 192:913-916, 1988.

58. Hamilton JM: *Aelurostrongylus abstrusus* infestation of the cat, *Vet Rec* 75:417-422, 1963.

59. Coman BJ, Jones EH, Driesen MA: Helminth parasites and arthropods of feral cats, *Aust Vet J* 57:324-327, 1981.

60. Gregory GG, Munday BL: Internal parasites of feral cats from the Tasmanian Midlands and King Island, *Aust Vet J* 52:317-320, 1976.

61. Hamilton JM: Experimental lungworm disease of the cat, *J Comp Pathol* 76:147-157, 1966.

62. Hamilton JM: The number of *Aelurostrongylus abstrusus* larvae required to produce pulmonary disease in the cat, *J Comp Path* 77:343-346, 1967.

63. Hamilton JM, McCaw AW: An investigation into the longevity of first stage larvae of *Aelurostrongylus abstrusus, J Helminthol* 41:313-320, 1967.

64. Hamilton JM, McCaw AW: The role of the mouse in the life cycle of *Aelurostrongylus abstrusus, J Helminthol* 41:309-312, 1967.

65. Hamilton JM: Studies on re-infestation of the cat with *Aelurostrongylus abstrusus, J Comp Path* 78:69-72, 1968.

66. Hamilton JM, McCaw AW: The output of first stage larvae by cats infested with *Aelurostrongylus abstrusus, J Helminthol* 42:295-298, 1968.

67. Hamilton JM: Parenteral infection of the cat by larvae of *Aelurostrongylus abstrusus, J Helminthol* 43:31-34, 1969.

68. Hamilton JM: The influence of infestation by *Aelurostrongylus abstrusus* on the pulmonary vasculature of the cat, *Brit Vet J* 126:202-209, 1970.

69. Dubey JP, Crane WAJ: Lung changes and *Aelurostrongylus abstrusus* infestation in English cats, *Vet Rec* 83:191-194, 1968.

70. Stockdale PH: The pathogenesis of the lesions elicited by *Aelurostrongylus abstrusus* during its prepatent period, *Pathol Vet* 7:102-115, 1970.

71. Miller BH, Roudebush P, Ward HG: Pleural effusion as a sequela to aelurostrongylosis in a cat, *JAVMA* 185:556-557, 1984.

72. Rawlings CA, Losonsky JM, Lewis RE et al: Response of the feline heart to *Aelurostrongylus abstrusus, J Am Anim Hosp Assoc* 16:573-578, 1980.

73. Losonsky JM, Smith FG, Lewis RE: Radiographic findings of *Aelurostrongylus abstrusus* infection in cats, *J Am Anim Hosp Assoc* 14:348-355, 1978.

74. Losonsky JM, Thrall DE, Prestwod AK: Radiographic evaluation of pulmonary abnormalities after *Aelurostrongylus abstrusus* inoculation in cats, *Am J Vet Res* 44:478-482, 1983.

75. Barsanti JA, Hubbell J: Serum proteins in normal cats and cats infected with *Aelurostrongylus abstrusus, Am J Vet Res* 41:775-778, 1980.

76. Smith RE: Feline lungworm infection, *Vet Rec* 107:256, 1980.

77. Hamilton JM, Weatherley A, Chapman AJ: Treatment of lungworm disease in the cat with fenbendazole, *Vet Rec* 114:40-41, 1984.

78. Vig MM, Murray PA: Successful treatment of *Aelurostrongylus abstrusus* with fenbendazole, *Compend Continuing Educ Sm Anim Pract* 8:214-222, 1986.

79. Kirkpatrick CE, Megella BA: Use of ivermectin in treatment of *Aelurostrongylus abstrusus* and *Toxocara cati* infections in a cat, *JAVMA* 190:1309-1310, 1987.

80. Roberson EL, Burke TM: Evaluation of granulated fenbendazole (22.2%) against induced and naturally occurring helminth infections in cats, *Am J Vet Res* 41:1499-1502, 1980.

81. Stockdale PH, Hulland TJ: The pathogenesis, route of migration, and development of *Crenosoma vulpis* in the dog, *Pathol Vet* 7:28-42, 1970.

82. Cobb MA, Fisher MA: *Crenosoma vulpis* infection in a dog, *Vet Rec* 130:452, 1992.

83. McGarry JW, Martin M, Cheeseman MT et al: *Crenosoma vulpis,* the fox lungworm, in dogs, *Vet Rec* 137:271-272, 1995.

84. Shaw DH, Conboy GA, Hogan PM et al: Eosinophilic bronchitis caused by *Crenosoma vulpis* infection in dogs, *Can Vet J* 37:361-363, 1996.

85. Bihr T, Conboy GA: Lungworm *(Crenosoma vulpis)* infection in dogs on Prince Edward Island, *Can Vet J* 40:555-559, 1999.

86. Unterer S, Deplazes P, Arnold P et al: Spontaneous Crenosoma vulpis infection in 10 dogs: Laboratory, radiographic and endoscopic findings, *Schweiz Arch Tierheilkd* 144:174-179, 2002.

87. Peterson EN, Barr SC, Gould WJ III et al: Use of fenbendazole for treatment of *Crenosoma vulpis* infection in a dog, *JAVMA* 202:1483-1484, 1993.

88. Reilly GA, McGarry JW, Martin M et al: *Crenosoma vulpis,* the fox lungworm, in a dog in Ireland, *Vet Rec* 146:764-765, 2000.

89. Stockdale PH, Smart ME: Treatment of crenosomiasis in dogs, *Res Vet Sci* 18:178-181, 1975.

90. Cox DD, Mullee MT: The fox lungworm *(Capillaria aerophila)* in a native cat in eastern Kansas, *Vet Med Small Anim Clin* 62:969-971, 1967.

91. Herman LH: *Capillaria aerophila* infection in a cat, *Vet Med Small Anim Clin* 62:466-468, 1967.

92. Holmes PR, Kelly JD: *Capillaria aerophila* in the domestic cat in Australia, *Aust Vet J* 49:472-473, 1973.

93. Greenlee PG, Noone KE: Pulmonary capillariasis in a dog, *J Am Anim Hosp Assoc* 20:983-985, 1984.

94. Campbell BG: Trichuris and other trichinelloid nematodes of dogs and cats in the United States, *Compend Continuing Educ Sm Anim Pract* 13:769, 1991.

95. Barrs VR, Martin P, Nicoll RG et al: Pulmonary cryptococcosis and *Capillaria aerophila* infection in an FIV-positive cat, *Aust Vet J* 78:154-158, 2000.

96. Norsworthy G: Feline lungworm treatment case report, *Feline Practice* 5:14, 1975.

97. Christie E, Dubey JP, Pappas PW: Prevalence of *Sarcocystis* infection and other intestinal parasitisms in cats from a humane shelter in Ohio, *JAVMA* 168:421-422, 1976.

98. Streitel RH, Dubey JP: Prevalence of *Sarcocystis* infection and other intestinal parasitisms in dogs from a humane shelter in Ohio, *JAVMA* 168:423-424, 1976.

99. Guterbock WM, Levine ND: Coccidia and intestinal nematodes of east central Illinois cats, *JAVMA* 170:1411-1413, 1977.
100. Beelitz P, Gobel E, Gothe R: Fauna and incidence of endoparasites in kittens and their mothers from different husbandry situations in south Germany, *Tierarztl Prax* 20:297-300, 1992.
101. Campbell BG, Little MD: Identification of the eggs of a nematode (*Eucoleus boehmi*) from the nasal mucosa of North American dogs, *JAVMA* 198:1520-1523, 1991.
102. Evinger JV, Kazacos KR, Cantwell HD: Ivermectin for treatment of nasal capillariasis in a dog, *JAVMA* 186:174-175, 1985.
103. Endres WA: Levamisole in treatment of *Capillaria aerophilla* in a cat (a case report), *Vet Med Small Anim Clin* 71:1553, 1976.
104. Corwin RM, Pratt SE, McCurdy HD: Anthelmintic effect of febantel/praziquantel paste in dogs and cats, *Am J Vet Res* 45:154-155, 1984.
105. Herman LH, Helland DR: Paragonimiasis in a cat, *JAVMA* 149:753-757, 1966.
106. Pechman RD Jr.: Pulmonary paragonimiasis in dogs and cats: A review, *J Small Anim Pract* 21:87-95, 1980.
107. Hoover EA, Dubey JP: Pathogenesis of experimental pulmonary paragonimiasis in cats, *Am J Vet Res* 39:1827-1832, 1978.
108. Dubey JP, Stromberg PC, Toussant MJ et al: Induced paragonimiasis in cats: Clinical signs and diagnosis, *JAVMA* 173:734-742, 1978.
109. Stromberg PC, Dubey JP: The life cycle of *Paragonimus kellicotti* in cats, *J Parasitol* 64:998-1002, 1978.
110. Weina PJ, England DM: The American lung fluke, *Paragonimus kellicotti*, in a cat model, *J Parasitol* 76:568-572, 1990.
111. Kirkpatrick CE, Shelly EA: Paragonimiasis in a dog: Treatment with praziquantel, *JAVMA* 187:75-76, 1985.
112. Pechman RD: The radiographic features of pulmonary paragonimiasis in the dog and cat, *J Am Vet Radiol Soc* (17):182-191, 1976.
113. Bowman DD, Frongillo MK, Johnson RC et al: Evaluation of praziquantel for treatment of experimentally induced paragonimiasis in dogs and cats, *Am J Vet Res* 52:68-71, 1991.
114. Dubey JP, Miller TB, Sharma SP: Fenbendazole for treatment of *Paragonimus kellicotti* infection in dogs, *JAVMA* 174:835-837, 1979.
115. Dubey JP, Hoover EA, Stromberg PC et al: Albendazole therapy for experimentally induced Paragonimus kellicotti infection in cats, *Am J Vet Res* 39:1027-1031, 1978.
116. Johnson KE, Kazacos KR, Blevins WE et al: Albendazole for treatment of *Paragonimus kellicotti* infection in two cats, *JAVMA* 178:483-485, 1981.
117. Kazacos KR, Bright RM, Johnson KE et al: *Cuterebra* spp. as a cause of pharyngeal myiasis in cats, *J Am Anim Hosp Assoc* 16:773-776, 1980.
118. Wolf AM: Cuterebra larva in the nasal passage of a kitten, *Feline Practice* 9:25-26, 1979.

CHAPTER 74

Lung Lobe Torsion

Prudence J. Neath

Definition

Lung lobe torsion is a rare condition; details of only 47 dogs [1-12] and 7 cats [13-15] have been reported in the veterinary literature. The torsion occurs when the lung lobe rotates about its bronchovascular pedicle and is unable to return to its normal position. The thin-walled vein collapses easily, whereas the more muscular arterial wall continues to allow bloodflow into the lung. Severe congestion occurs, and consolidation develops as fluid moves into the interstitial tissue and airways. Eventually pleural effusion almost always occurs as fluid moves into the pleural cavity, although rare patients without pleural effusion have been anecdotally seen.

Etiology

The cause of lung lobe torsion in humans and animals has been the subject of debate. The primary event associated with pulmonary torsion in humans is reported to be surgical trauma: a recent literature review found that 36 cases occurred following thoracic surgery, whereas 5 cases followed blunt trauma and 4 cases occurred spontaneously.[16] It has been proposed that deflation of the lung and division of the pulmonary ligaments during surgery may predispose to the development of lung lobe torsion in humans.[17-19] The situation in dogs and cats is less clear. It has been proposed that a combination of lung consolidation or atelectasis (caused by pleural effusion, pneumothorax, trauma, pneumonia, or manipulation during surgery), with increased air or fluid around the lobe, may predispose it to rotate about its axis.[2,3,6,7] However, presumed spontaneous lung lobe torsion has been identified in dogs and cats in which no predisposing factors were discovered.[2,8,12,13] Pleural effusion associated with the spontaneous cases may be a manifestation of the vascular and lymphatic obstruction rather than a predisposing factor.[8,12]

Historical Findings and Clinical Signs

Lung lobe torsion occurs more commonly in large, deep-chested dogs, particularly Afghan hounds.[1-12] Afghan hounds are reported to be 133 times more likely to develop lung lobe torsion than other breeds.[12] Occurrence in cats and small breeds of dog has been reported less often.[2,12-15] Clinical history usually includes progressive dyspnea; coughing; depression; and, in some instances, anorexia, vomiting, and diarrhea.[1-15] There may be a previous history of respiratory disease or trauma.[1-7,9-15] On physical examination, the predominant abnormalities are respiratory signs with dyspnea, coughing, and dull cardiopulmonary sounds on thoracic auscultation. Pyrexia, depression, vomiting, or cardiovascular instability are noted in some instances.[1-15]

Differential Diagnosis

Atelectasis, pneumonia, neoplasia, pulmonary contusion, pulmonary thromboembolism, diaphragmatic hernia, hemothorax, and pyothorax should also be considered in animals with these signs.

Diagnostic Tests

Thoracocentesis is performed to relieve dyspnea and allow fluid analysis. The fluid is often hemorrhagic, but may be clear; serosanguineous; or chylous, with a milky-white appearance with a triglyceride content greater than that of serum. Cytological examination typically reveals an inflammatory cell population with high numbers of neutrophils, lymphocytes, and often erythrocytes and a few modified mesothelial cells.[12] The fluid analysis can become more complicated if an underlying disease is also present. Bacteria are occasionally cultured from the pleural effusion, but pyothorax is rare.[2,6,12,13] Bacteria identified include *Pseudomonas* spp., *Enterococcus* spp., *Proteus* spp., *Staphylococcus* spp., *Enterobacter* spp., and *Serratia* spp.[12] The complete blood count often reveals neutrophilia and, occasionally, anemia; biochemistry results reveal inconsistent changes that may be caused by the underlying disease process rather than the effects of lung lobe torsion.[7,8,10,11-15]

Details of thoracic radiographs are often obscured by pleural effusion; removal of the fluid by thoracocentesis will reveal one or more consolidated lung lobes.[1-15] The finding of severe consolidation of one particular lung lobe, with relative normality of the other lung lobes, should raise suspicion of a lung lobe torsion. Horizontal beam radiographs may allow the lung lobes to be seen more clearly.[2] Radiographic changes are variable depending on the duration of the torsion, the volume of pleural fluid, and whether underlying disease is present. Air bronchograms or air alveolograms are often seen within the affected lobe, but this air usually disperses within a few days as it is replaced by blood or fluid.[2,6,8,11,12] Abnormal bronchial positioning consistent with torsion is sometimes seen (Figure 74-1).[6,12,13]

Positive-contrast bronchography has been used to demonstrate the obstructed orifice of the twisted bronchus.[2] Fiberoptic bronchoscopy may also demonstrate bronchial occlusion; the bronchial mucosa at the site of the obstruction may appear edematous.[5] Thoracic

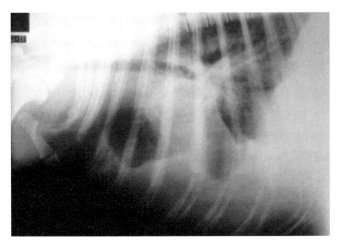

Figure 74-1. Lateral thoracic radiograph of a dog with torsion of the right middle lung lobe, following thoracocentesis to remove the pleural effusion. Note the consolidated lung lobe and abnormal path of the bronchus.

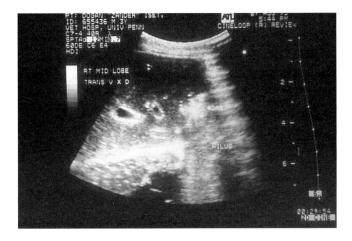

Figure 74-2. Thoracic ultrasound showing obstructed hilus of a torsed lung lobe, filled with fluid.

ultrasound has been used more often in recent years to confirm consolidation of the lung lobe/s and may illustrate filling of the bronchi with fluid (Figure 74-2).[12]

The most commonly affected lobe is the thin, narrow, right middle lung lobe, but the left cranial lobe is affected almost as often.[1-15] Although the left cranial lung lobe is larger than the right middle lobe, neither of these lobes has extensive attachments to the surrounding structures and this may predispose them to torsion. Torsion of any other lung lobe is also possible.

Management and Monitoring

MEDICAL STABILIZATION

Surgical excision of the affected lobe is required, but stabilizing treatment is often needed before surgery. Pleural effusion should be removed by needle thoracocentesis to

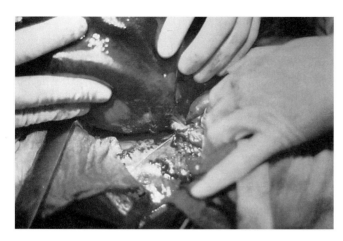

Figure 74-3. *Intraoperative appearance of lung lobe torsion. Note the dark, consolidated lung lobe and twisted hilus.*

alleviate dyspnea. Placement of chest tube/s may be required if the effusion rapidly recurs. Oxygen therapy should be provided via a mask, nasal catheter, or oxygen cage. Fluid resuscitation is required in many cases, and fluid therapy should be provided throughout surgery. Appropriate intravenous antibiotics should be administered, especially if there is evidence of concurrent pneumonia or bacteria in the pleural effusion.

SURGICAL TREATMENT

Exploration of the thorax is performed via a lateral thoracotomy at the fifth intercostal space on the affected side. Care should be taken when entering the thorax because adhesions may have formed between the lung and the thoracic wall. Most twisted lung lobes appear dark, consolidated, friable, and may be necrotic (Figure 74-3). The bronchovascular pedicle should be carefully clamped to prevent release of cytokines into the circulation if the lobe is untwisted during removal. The lobe should always be removed, even if reinflation seems possible. The bronchovascular pedicle can be ligated and divided either by hand or by use of a stapling device. Identification of vascular structures during manual ligation may be aided by de-rotation of the lung lobe, but this is rarely required when a stapling device is used. Biopsies of any abnormal tissue should be obtained (e.g., a mediastinal mass or a mass in the affected lung lobe). If chylothorax is present at the time of surgery, thoracic duct ligation and pericardiectomy should be performed at the time of the initial lung lobe resection. This is particularly important in the case of Afghan hounds, in which the chylothorax is likely to persist following lung lobectomy alone. The position and inflation of the remaining lung lobes should be assessed, and a chest tube placed before closing the thorax.

POSTOPERATIVE CARE

Oxygen therapy may be required postoperatively and can be administered by mask, by nasal catheter, or by place-

ment in an oxygen cage. Appropriate antibiotics should be continued postoperatively until results of bacterial cultures have returned. Analgesia should be provided; parenteral administration of opioids can be supplemented by administration of intrapleural bupivacaine. Drainage of chest tubes should be continued at regular intervals until less than 5 ml/kg/day of fluid is being produced. Fluid intake and output should be monitored, and fluid therapy administered as needed.

Histopathological Findings

A small sample of the resected lung lobe should be submitted for bacterial culture, and the remainder of the lobe submitted for histopathological examination. Histological abnormalities caused by lung lobe torsion usually include hemorrhagic fluid within the bronchi, thrombosis of venous channels, infiltration by plasma cells and lymphocytes, and necrosis.[1,12,18] Histopathological examination may also reveal underlying disease that may have precipitated the lung lobe torsion (e.g., neoplasia or pneumonia).[2,9,12,15]

Outcome and Prognosis

Prognosis for animals with lung lobe torsion is fair to poor depending on whether there is underlying disease and what breed is affected.[1-15] If the pleural effusion has been caused by neoplasia, the long-term prognosis is guarded, depending on the type of neoplasm.[12,13] The majority of animals with spontaneous uncomplicated lung lobe torsion will have a successful outcome.* Hemorrhagic effusion that is not associated with underlying thoracic disease will usually resolve within 3 to 7 days postoperatively. Death of these patients, if it occurs, is often related to systemic inflammation as a result of cytokine release from necrotic lung tissue, which may result in the acute respiratory distress syndrome or cardiovascular collapse.

Chylothorax has often been reported in association with lung lobe torsion, and it is unclear whether it is a cause or a consequence of the torsion.† Chylothorax is thought to develop after disruption or impedance of the thoracic duct or thoracic lymphatics, resulting in lymphangiectasia.[20] Inciting causes include trauma, neoplasia, fungal infection, heartworm disease, and diaphragmatic hernia, but in many cases chylothorax is idiopathic.[20-22] Chylothorax has been diagnosed at the same time as lung lobe torsion,[7,10,12,14] but has also been reported to develop following surgery to correct lung lobe torsion.[2,6,12] Chylothorax resolves within 7 days of lung lobe resection in most cases, without any requirement to perform a thoracic duct ligation or pericardiectomy.[2,12] Persistent chylothorax that fails to resolve after lung lobe resection is a particular problem in Afghan

---

*References 1, 5, 8, 12, 13, and 15.
†References 2, 6, 7, 10, 12, and 14.

hounds; 92% (all but one) of the persistent canine cases in the literature were Afghan hounds.[2,6,7,10,12]

Because Afghan hounds are overrepresented in reports of chylothorax secondary to lymphangiectasia,[20] it has been proposed that their thoracic lymphatic system has a lower tolerance for insults of any kind, increasing their likelihood of developing chylothorax in association with lung lobe torsion.[12] Eight of 14 Afghan hounds in the literature developed chylothorax in association with their lung lobe torsion.[2,6,7,10,12] The prognosis for chylothorax in that breed is poor, with only 17% of dogs surviving to 6 months.[20] Chylothorax associated with lung lobe torsion has only been reported in 1 cat.[14] Although the prognosis for cats with chylothorax is poor, this feline case had a successful outcome following thoracic duct ligation.[14,23]

REFERENCES

1. Rawlings CA, Lebel JL, Mitchum G: Torsion of the left apical and cardiac pulmonary lobes in a dog, *JAVMA* 156:726-733, 1970.
2. Lord PF, Greiner TP, Greene RW et al: Lung lobe torsion in the dog, *J Am Anim Hosp Assoc* 9:473-482, 1973.
3. Alexander JW, Hoffer RE, Bolton GR: Torsion of the diaphragmatic lobe of the lung following surgical correction of a patent ductus arteriosus, *Vet Med Small Anim Clin* 69:595-597, 1974.
4. Critchley KL: Torsion of a lung lobe in the dog, *J Sm Anim Prac* 17:391-394, 1976.
5. Moses BL: Fiberoptic bronchoscopy for diagnosis of lung lobe torsion in a dog, *JAVMA* 176:44-47, 1980.
6. Johnston GR, Feeney DA, O'Brien TD et al: Recurring lung lobe torsion in three Afghan hounds, *JAVMA* 184:842-845, 1984.
7. Williams JH, Duncan NM: Chylothorax with concurrent right cardiac lung lobe torsion in an Afghan hound, *J S Afr Vet Assoc* 57:35-37, 1986.
8. Bretin L, DiFruscia R, Olivieri M: Successive torsion of the right middle and left cranial lung lobes in a dog, *Can Vet J* 10:386-388, 1986.
9. Hoover JP, Henry GA, Panciera RJ: Bronchial cartilage dysplasia with multifocal lobar bullous emphysema and lung torsions in a pup, *JAVMA* 201:599-602, 1992.
10. Gelzer ARM, Downs MO, Newell SM et al: Accessory lung lobe torsion and chylothorax in an Afghan hound, *J Am Anim Hosp Assoc* 33:171-176, 1997.
11. Siems JJ, Jakovlheic S, Van Alstine W: Radiographic diagnosis: Lung lobe torsion, *Vet Radiol & Ultrasound* 39:418-420, 1998.
12. Neath PJ, Brockman DJ, King LG: Lung lobe torsion in the dog: a retrospective study of 22 cases (1981-1999), *JAVMA* 217(7):1041-1044, 2000.
13. Brown NO, Zontine WJ: Lung lobe torsion in the cat, *Am Vet Radiol Soc* 17:219-223, 1976.
14. Kerpsack SJ, McLoughlin MA, Graves TK: Chylothorax associated with lung lobe torsion and a peritoneopericardial diaphragmatic hernia in a cat, *J Am Anim Hosp Assoc* 30:351-354, 1994.
15. Dye TL, Teague HD, Poundstone ML: Lung lobe torsion in a cat with chronic feline asthma, *J Am Anim Hosp Assoc* 34:493-495, 1998.
16. Schamaun M: Postoperative pulmonary torsion: report of a case and survey of the literature including spontaneous and posttraumatic torsion, *Thorac Cardiovasc Surgeon* 42:116-121, 1994.
17. Felson B: Lung torsion: Radiographic findings in nine cases, *Radiology* 162:631-638, 1987.
18. Fisher CF, Ammar T, Silvay G: Whole lung torsion after a thoracoabdominal esophagogastrectomy, *Anesthesiology* 87:162-164, 1997.
19. Goskowicz R, Harrell JH, Roth DM: Intraoperative diagnosis of torsion of the left lung after repair of a disruption of the descending thoracic aorta, *Anesthesiology* 87:164-166, 1997.
20. Fossum TW, Birchard SJ, Jacobs RM: Chylothorax in 34 dogs, *JAVMA* 188:1315-1318, 1986.
21. Willard MD, Conroy JD: Chylothorax associated with blastomycosis in a dog, *JAVMA* 186:72-73, 1985.
22. Myers NC III, Engler SI, Jakowski RM: Chylothorax and chylous ascites in a dog with mediastinal lymphosarcoma, *J Am Anim Hosp Assoc* 32:263-269, 1996.
23. Fossum T, Forrester S, Swenson C et al: Chylothorax in cats: 37 cases (1969-1989), *JAVMA* 198:672-678, 1991.

CHAPTER 75

Respiratory Toxicology

Lori S. Waddell • Robert Poppenga

Toxicant-induced damage to the respiratory tract can occur via inhalation of a toxicant or, in many cases, via the blood following oral, intravenous, or dermal exposure. The respiratory system can be the primary target of a toxicant or can be affected secondarily because of dysfunction of another organ system such as the nervous, cardiovascular, or hematopoietic systems.

Each step of the respiratory process can be affected by toxicants. Toxicants can affect respiratory drive by directly suppressing or stimulating the respiratory center, by altering the response of chemoreceptors to changes in P_{CO_2}, or by increasing metabolic demands because of agitation or fever.[1] For example, opioids depress respiration by decreasing responsiveness of chemoreceptors to CO_2

and by direct suppression of respiratory centers. Hypoventilation can occur as a result of a decrease in either the respiratory rate or tidal volume. Toxicants that cause muscle weakness or muscle rigidity (e.g., botulinum toxin, cholinesterase-inhibiting insecticides, or neuromuscular blocking agents) impair the ability of an animal to expand its chest wall, thus decreasing tidal volume. Airway patency can be compromised in several ways. Toxicant-induced emesis can result in aspiration of stomach contents. Alternatively, obstruction may result from increased secretions (e.g., cholinesterase-inhibiting insecticides) or upper airway edema (e.g., exposure to insoluble oxalate containing plants such as *Philodendron* spp. or *Dieffenbachia* spp.). Toxicant-induced aspiration (e.g., inhalation of volatile petroleum hydrocarbons) can result in severe ventilation-perfusion mismatch and subsequent hypoxia.

Severe local or diffuse lung injury from a variety of toxicants including paraquat and zinc phosphide can result in noncardiogenic pulmonary edema. Cardiogenic pulmonary edema can also be induced by a variety of toxicants; respiratory system involvement is secondary to a primary cardiovascular insult. Examples of toxicants that can cause cardiogenic pulmonary edema include cardiac glycosides, beta-adrenergic antagonists, and ionophores. Disorders of hemoglobin oxygen content and hemoglobin-oxygen interactions, resulting in cellular hypoxia, can occur following toxicant exposure. Cats exposed to acetaminophen present in severe respiratory distress because of the formation of methemoglobin and a concomitant decrease in oxygen delivery to cells. In addition, toxicants causing acute hemolytic anemias (e.g., zinc or *Allium* spp.) or blood loss (e.g., anticoagulant rodenticides) can result in significant respiratory signs. Lastly, there are a number of relatively nontoxic gases (e.g., carbon dioxide, methane, and propane) that, when exposure occurs in a closed environment, can replace oxygen and cause severe hypoxia. These gases are termed chemical asphyxiants and will not be discussed in this chapter.

The following discussion focuses on two intoxications that are associated with significant respiratory signs. Table 75-1 can be consulted for other toxicants that potentially cause either primary or secondary respiratory impairment.

Anticoagulant Rodenticides

Intoxication caused by ingestion of anticoagulant rodenticides is one of the more common toxicoses encountered in small animal practice. It occurs much more commonly in dogs than in cats, perhaps because of the less discriminating eating habits and higher toxicity of anticoagulant rodenticides in dogs. Many distinct but chemically related anticoagulant rodenticides have been developed since the commercial introduction of warfarin in the early 1950s. Warfarin was the first synthetic chemical available for use as an anticoagulant rodenticide. It was derived from the naturally occurring anticoagulant compound called dicoumarol, which is produced on

Penicillium spp. infested sweet clover (*Melilotus* spp.). Dicoumarol was the toxin responsible for a bleeding disorder of livestock, first recognized in the 1920s and associated with the ingestion of improperly cured, moldy, sweet clover hay.

The emergence of warfarin-resistant rodents led to the development of newer, more toxic, "second generation" or "single-dose" anticoagulant rodenticides (e.g., brodifacoum, bromodiolone, coumafuryl, coumatetralyl, chlorophacinone, difenacoum, difethialone, diphacinone, and valone). Of these, brodifacoum is the most widely available and is responsible for most intoxications. Because of the decline in use of warfarin, it is currently uncommon to encounter a case of warfarin intoxication. Thus if a specific anticoagulant cannot be identified, it should be assumed that the animal has been exposed to one of the newer, more biologically persistent chemicals requiring prolonged antidotal treatment.

FORMULATIONS AND TOXICITY

Anticoagulant rodenticides are available in a variety of palatable formulations including treated seed, pellets, paraffin blocks, water-soluble preparations, and tracking powders. Most available formulations contain active ingredient at 0.005% to 0.25% (i.e., 50 to 2500 mg/kg or ppm). Whenever possible, it is important to determine the concentration of active ingredient in the formulation in order to estimate an amount ingested to compare with available toxicity information. Unfortunately, toxicity data are not available for dogs and cats for all anticoagulants. The toxic single oral dose of warfarin in both dogs and cats is reported to be 20 to 300 mg/kg and 5 to 30 mg/kg, respectively.[2] The reported single, oral LD_{50} of brodifacoum for dogs and cats is 0.20 to 4.0 mg/kg and 25 mg/kg, respectively.[2] For diphacinone, the reported single, oral LD_{50} for dogs and cats is 0.9 mg/kg and 15 mg/kg, respectively.[2] Obviously, a potentially toxic dose is substantially less than an LD_{50} dose. Given the relatively long half-lives of many anticoagulants, repeated ingestion over several days of amounts much lower than those reported for single dose toxicity can cause intoxication.

EXPOSURE

Anticoagulant rodenticides are widely available and used extensively. Most exposures result either from access of dogs or cats to improperly placed bait packets or from malicious poisoning. The palatability of the formulations results in ready consumption of the bait if available. The use of bait stations minimizes the chance of access to the baits, but may not prevent access by all animals.

MECHANISM OF TOXIC ACTION

All anticoagulant rodenticides have a common mechanism of toxic action: they inhibit vitamin K 2,3-epoxide reductase and vitamin K quinone reductase in the liver.[2] This inhibition prevents reduction of inactive vitamin K_1 2,3-epoxide to active vitamin K_1 (vitamin K quinol). The resulting lack of active vitamin K_1 in turn

TABLE 75-1. Additional Toxicants with Effects on the Respiratory System

Toxicant	Use/Source	Mechanism of Toxic Action	Respiratory Involvement	Treatment
Zinc phosphide; aluminum phosphide	Rodenticide; fumigant	Release of phosphine gas in stomach and hypothesized direct damage to blood vessels and erythrocytes	Pulmonary edema	Decontamination (initial dilution with milk or bicarbonate solution); S&S care
Organophosphate or carbamate insecticides	Insecticides	Cholinesterase inhibition with resultant cholinergic overstimulation	↑ Respiratory secretions; depolarizing blockade of respiratory muscles	Atropine, pralidoxime are antidotal; decontamination; S&S care
Volatile petroleum hydrocarbons (e.g., gasoline, kerosene, and mineral spirits)	Multiple	Aspiration following ingestion; aspiration potential ↑ with a ↓ viscosity and surface tension and ↑ volatility	Chemical destruction of surfactant in alveoli and distal airways, capillary damage allowing leakage of fluid and blood into alveoli; chemical pneumonitis	Controversy regarding decontamination procedures; provide supplemental oxygen, intubate, provide ventilatory assistance; S&S care
Acetaminophen (Cats)	Analgesic	Methemoglobin formation	Cell hypoxia	Decontamination; N-acetylcysteine is antidotal; S&S care
Botulinum toxin	Elaborated by *Clostridium botulinum;* elaborated from contaminated wound or ingestion of preformed toxin	Failure of cholinergic transmission and autonomic function	Respiratory muscle depression	Antitoxin, ventilatory assistance, S&S care
Opioids	Overdose of legal drug or ingestion of illegal drugs	μ_2 Receptor agonism primarily responsible	Respiratory depression	Decontamination; ventilatory assistance, administration of naloxone
Cyanide	Many laboratory and industrial uses, cyanogenic glycosides found in many plants	Binding of mitochondrial cytochrome oxidase enzyme	Cells cannot utilize O_2, resulting in cell hypoxia	Sodium nitrite and sodium thiosulfate are antidotal; decontamination; administer O_2, S&S care
Ammonia and chlorine gases	Water soluble gases (household, recreational, agricultural and industrial uses)	Local pulmonary damage because of direct cell irritation	Respiratory distress characterized by stridor, wheezing and tachypnea; bronchospasm and edema	Remove from source; external decontamination (e.g., eyes, skin and hair); ventilatory assistance, administer O_2, consider nebulized beta-2 agonists for bronchospasm; S&S care
Zinc	Galvanized metal; pennies minted in 1983 and later	Oxidative damage to red blood cell membranes	Hemolytic anemia	Remove zinc objects; consider chelation; S&S care
Carbon monoxide	Combustion sources (e.g., motor vehicles, heaters or appliances that use carbon-based fuels)	Avidly binds to hemoglobin forming carboxyhemoglobin, shift of O_2 saturation curve to the left making O_2 less available to cells	Cellular hypoxia and anoxia	Remove from source and immediately provide O_2 supplementation

S&S, Symptomatic and supportive.

prevents carboxylation of clotting factors II, VII, IX, and X, which are required for normal clot formation. Depletion of activated clotting factors results in uncontrolled hemorrhage. Respective circulating half-lives of factors II, VII, IX, and X in the dog are 41, 6.2, 13.9, and 16.5 hours, respectively. Factor VII, with the shortest half-life, is depleted first, thus affecting the extrinsic clotting pathway and causing a prolonged one-stage prothrombin time (OSPT). As additional clotting factors are depleted, other coagulation tests such as activated partial thromboplastin time (APTT) and activated clotting time (ACT) become prolonged.

CLINICAL SIGNS

The clinical signs of anticoagulant rodenticide ingestion are variable and include nonspecific signs of illness, respiratory signs, and obvious signs of hemorrhagic shock. Signs include anorexia, lethargy, dyspnea, coughing/hemoptysis, pallor, weakness, fever, lameness, and subcutaneous swellings. Signs of external hemorrhage (e.g., melena, hematochezia, epistaxis, hematemesis, hematuria, gingival bleeding, and bleeding from wounds) may be seen; or internal hemorrhage may be present, resulting in scleral or conjunctival hemorrhage, pain, dyspnea, hypovolemic shock, or neurological signs.[3-5] The clinical signs depend on the site and degree of spontaneous hemorrhage. Respiratory signs are very common; in a retrospective study of 21 dogs that had confirmed anticoagulant rodenticide toxicity, 57% had presenting complaints of dyspnea, whereas 30% presented with coughing/hemoptysis.[6]

CLINICAL DIAGNOSTIC TESTING

Patients that present with respiratory compromise secondary to suspected anticoagulant rodenticide intoxication should receive a clinical work-up including an initial packed cell volume, total solids, and serum dextrose concentration; coagulation parameters; a complete blood count (CBC); chemistry screen; and thoracic radiographs, if the patient is able to tolerate radiography. Coagulation parameters should include testing OSPT, APTT, and a platelet count. If access to a clinical laboratory is not available, an activated clotting time (ACT) and blood smear should be performed. Abnormalities seen on the coagulation screen depend on the length of time from ingestion of the anticoagulant rodenticide. The earliest abnormality is prolongation of the OSPT because of the short half-life of factor VII. As coagulation factors II, IX, and X become depleted, prolongation of the ACT and APTT occurs. Secondary thrombocytopenia, sometimes severe, can be seen and is probably caused by consumption of platelets because of massive, uncontrolled bleeding.[7]

If further coagulation testing is performed, additional abnormalities may include elevated plasma concentrations of fibrin degradation products (FDPs), increased thrombin clotting time, and increased plasma fibrinogen concentration. Although it was once thought that FDP values only increased in patients with disseminated intravascular coagulation, it has been shown that dogs with anticoagulant rodenticide intoxication can also have abnormal values.[6] A clinical test to detect proteins induced by vitamin K antagonism (PIVKA) was developed to potentially distinguish cases of anticoagulant rodenticide intoxication from other severe coagulopathies. Unfortunately, the PIVKA test was documented to be no more reliable than a standard OSPT in these patients.[8]

The CBC may be normal if hemorrhage is acute, or it may reveal anemia if blood loss has been ongoing. If present, anemia may be regenerative or nonregenerative depending on the duration of blood loss. Thrombocytopenia is common, with the severity dependent on the amount of hemorrhage that has occurred. Serum chemistries are usually normal except for decreased globulin and albumin secondary to blood loss, although increases in liver and kidney values may occur if perfusion is severely compromised by hypovolemia.

Thoracic radiographs should be taken if the patient is showing signs of respiratory compromise and is stable enough to tolerate radiography. Common radiographic abnormalities in animals with hemorrhage secondary to anticoagulant rodenticide ingestion include any combination of increased mediastinal soft tissue opacity, extra- and intra-tracheal narrowing, pleural effusion, or a generalized patchy interstitial or alveolar pattern (Figure 75-1).[9,10] These radiographic changes tend to resolve over several days with appropriate care. Abdominal radiographs may show a loss of abdominal serosal detail, or loss of detail and distention in the retroperitoneal space consistent with an effusion. Abdominal ultrasound can confirm the presence of an echogenic abdominal or retroperitoneal effusion.

Comprehensive anticoagulant rodenticide screens are available through many state veterinary diagnostic laboratories. Samples of choice for analysis are whole blood and liver, although anticoagulants may be detected in other tissues. Detection of a specific anticoagulant is useful to guide the duration of vitamin K_1 therapy and to identify exposure sources, which may be important if litigation is being contemplated. However, test results are generally not available quickly enough to influence initial case management.

Gross postmortem examination of animals dying suddenly often reveals massive hemorrhage into a body cavity (e.g., hemothorax, hemomediastinum, or hemopericardium). Substantial intrapulmonary hemorrhage can occur. Most hemorrhages are ecchymotic or suffusive in nature and are not petechial. In general, histopathology does not add much to the gross postmortem findings. Centrilobular hepatic necrosis can result from anemia, poor perfusion, and secondary tissue hypoxia.

MANAGEMENT

Initial stabilization of a patient that presents in respiratory distress secondary to anticoagulant rodenticide ingestion is the same as for any other animal with respiratory distress. Oxygen supplementation is the first step in stabilization while a physical examination is performed. If it is possible to obtain vascular access without too much stress for the patient, an intravenous (IV) catheter should be placed to allow administration of fluids, blood products, and medications and for crisis management in the event of cardiopulmonary arrest. If there are clinical signs of hypovolemic shock (e.g., pale mucous membranes, tachycardia, and poor peripheral pulses), IV fluids and/or blood products should be administered for volume expansion.

Auscultation of the lungs may reveal harsh lung sounds or crackles created by blood within the small airways and alveoli. Auscultation may also reveal dull or decreased lung sounds created by bleeding into the thoracic

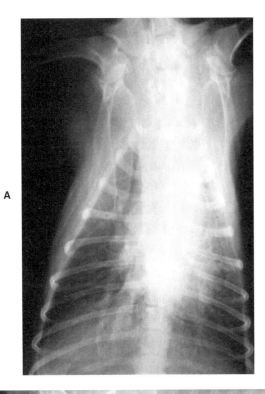

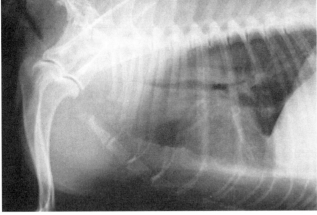

Figure 75-1. **A,** *Ventrodorsal and* **B,** *lateral thoracic radiographs of a 10-year-old female spayed mix breed dog that presented in severe respiratory distress with upper airway stridor and a temperature of 106.5° F. She had a history of brodifacoum ingestion 1 week before presentation. Her initial ACT was greater than 5 minutes. The radiographs show pleural effusion, widening of the cranial mediastinum, tracheal compression, and a diffuse alveolar pattern. She recovered after treatment with fresh frozen plasma, vitamin K₁, and oxygen supplementation.*

cavity. When dull lung sounds are ausculted in an animal with significant respiratory distress, thoracocentesis is indicated to remove the fluid or air, allowing for better lung expansion. However, in the case of a hemothorax secondary to a severe coagulopathy, thoracocentesis may be contraindicated until clotting factors have been provided, to prevent catastrophic bleeding from occurring in the event of tissue trauma during thoracocentesis.

In the acutely bleeding patient with respiratory distress from anticoagulant rodenticide intoxication, active clotting factors are needed immediately. Fresh frozen plasma (FFP) or fresh whole blood should be administered at a dose of 15 to 20 ml/kg or as needed to replace lost blood volume and return the clotting times to normal. Vitamin K₁ should be administered at an initial dose of 5 mg/kg subcutaneously. Intravenous administration is not recommended because of the high frequency of anaphylaxis. Vitamin K₁ should then be administered at 2.5 mg/kg orally twice daily if the patient tolerates oral medications. Oral absorption of vitamin K₁ is superior to subcutaneous administration, especially if given with a meal that has a high fat content. If the patient is unable to tolerate oral medication, the vitamin K₁ should be continued subcutaneously.

If FFP is used to provide active coagulation factors, packed red blood cells (pRBC) may be needed in addition to treat the blood loss anemia. Oxygen supplementation should be provided as long as the patient has significant respiratory compromise from pulmonary or airway bleeding. Intubation and positive pressure ventilation may be required if there is severe respiratory compromise, particularly if the tracheal lumen is narrowed by mediastinal or tracheal wall hemorrhage. If a hemothorax is present and contributing significantly to the patient's respiratory distress, thoracocentesis may be necessary, but should be delayed until active clotting factors have been provided with blood product therapy whenever possible. Pericardial bleeding can also be seen in patients with anticoagulant rodenticide ingestion, and pericardiocentesis may be indicated if tamponade is occurring. As with thoracocentesis, pericardiocentesis should ideally be delayed until active clotting factors have been provided.

Because of the delayed onset of action (3 to 5 days) of anticoagulant rodenticides, there is no need for decontamination procedures when patients present with active bleeding. If an asymptomatic dog or cat presents immediately after witnessed or suspected ingestion of an anticoagulant rodenticide, vomiting should be induced or gastric lavage should be performed. Additionally, the patient should be given activated charcoal and a cathartic, such as magnesium sulfate or sorbitol, and either started on vitamin K₁ at 2.5 mg/kg orally twice daily for 4 weeks or returned for a OSPT in 48 hours to see if enough rodenticide was ingested to create a coagulopathy. If the OSPT is prolonged, the patient should be treated with vitamin K₁ as listed above.

PROGNOSIS

The prognosis for a dog or cat that ingests an anticoagulant rodenticide is excellent if the patient presents immediately after ingestion and decontamination procedures are followed, or if the patient is treated with an appropriate dose of vitamin K₁. For patients that present with clinical signs from bleeding, the prognosis is still very good, unless hypovolemic shock or the degree of dyspnea is severe. Even when an animal presents with severe bleeding, the prognosis remains fair to good because a full recovery is a reasonable expectation with supportive care, blood product therapy, and vitamin K_1.

Paraquat

Paraquat (1,1'-dimethyl-4,4'-bipyridylium dichloride) is a restricted use, highly toxic, quaternary nitrogen herbicide widely used for broadleaf weed control. It has been used for killing marijuana, as a crop dessicant and defoliant, and as an aquatic herbicide. Diquat (1,1'-ethylene-2,2'-dipyridylium dibromide) is a chemically-related compound which is also highly toxic although, unlike paraquat, does not possess significant respiratory toxicity.

FORMULATIONS AND TOXICITY

In the United States, paraquat (as paraquat dichloride) is available as a 37% or 43.8% w/v aqueous formulation. Diquat is formulated as a 36.4% diquat cation liquid. Other formulations can be encountered outside the United States.[11] Paraquat is a blue-green liquid, whereas diquat is brown; this may be a useful clue to possible exposure if residues remain on the skin or hair. Ingested paraquat is quite toxic, with reported LD_{50} values of 110 to 150 mg/kg in rats, 50 mg/kg in monkeys, and 48 mg/kg in cats. Paraquat is also moderately toxic following dermal exposure, with a dermal LD_{50} in rabbits of 236 to 325 mg/kg. In human medicine, paraquat poisoning can be divided into three different categories depending on the amount ingested.[11] Doses of paraquat ion greater than 40 mg/kg body weight results in a rapidly progressing, multi-organ system failure. Moderate intoxication occurs with ingested doses of 20 to 40 mg/kg. Exposures of this magnitude generally result in death because of development of pulmonary fibrosis days to weeks after presentation. Mild toxicity follows ingestion of doses less than 20 mg/kg. Such exposures generally result in full recovery.

EXPOSURE

In humans, most clinically significant exposures to paraquat result from intentional ingestion. In small animals, the most likely intoxication scenario is ingestion associated with malicious poisoning attempts. Skin exposure is generally not regarded as significant unless there is prolonged contact with a concentrated formulation. Inhalation of paraquat used in an agricultural setting does not cause systemic disease because droplet size does not allow penetration of the material deep into the lungs.

MECHANISM OF TOXIC ACTION

Paraquat undergoes cyclic reduction/oxidation in conjunction with NADPH and oxygen, which results in formation of a superoxide radical.[11] The redox cycle involving paraquat, oxygen, and NADPH, along with generation of hydroxyl free radicals, results in cell damage by a number of mechanisms including depletion of NADPH, lipid peroxidation, and DNA and protein destruction. Paraquat and diquat are caustic and produce injury similar to alkaline corrosives on contact with skin, eyes, and mucous membranes. Multisystemic organ damage occurs as a result of free radical formation. Major target organs for paraquat are the gastrointestinal tract, kidneys, and lungs. Paraquat, but not diquat, is actively taken up by Type I and Type II pneumocytes, resulting in alveolar epithelial damage. In humans, a critical plasma threshold is needed for pulmonary uptake to occur.

A biphasic injury pattern occurs in the lungs following toxic exposure to paraquat.[11] An initial destructive phase damages alveolar epithelial cells, resulting in exudative pulmonary edema. A subsequent proliferative phase occurs in which the epithelial layer is replaced by fibrous tissue resulting in severe pulmonary fibrosis, hypoxemia, and death.

CLINICAL SIGNS

The clinical signs of paraquat ingestion include vomiting, diarrhea, lethargy, anorexia, dyspnea, oral ulcerations, oliguria, mucosal irritation, hyperexcitability, incoordination, and convulsions. Paraquat ingestion can result in renal failure, hepatic dysfunction, myocardial necrosis, and acute respiratory distress syndrome (ARDS). Acute signs after ingestion of paraquat include vomiting, hyperexcitability, anorexia, and lethargy. Respiratory signs such as dyspnea and tachypnea usually do not occur until several days after exposure.[12,13] The vagueness of the initial signs makes diagnosis and treatment of paraquat toxicity difficult; the only truly effective treatment for paraquat toxicity is decontamination to prevent absorption. Once the paraquat is absorbed and the patient is showing clinical signs, treatment is supportive only and commonly does not prevent death.

INITIAL STABILIZATION

If an animal is known to have just ingested paraquat, the goal is removal of as much of the toxin from the stomach as possible to prevent absorption. Emesis should be induced or gastric lavage should be performed. Activated charcoal or Fuller's earth should be administered immediately and continued every 4 to 6 hours for 3 to 7 days following ingestion. Intravenous fluids and furosemide should be administered to create a forced diuresis, increasing the rate of excretion of paraquat via the kidneys. Diuresis is most useful in the first 72 hours after ingestion because blood levels of paraquat quickly become very low because of initial rapid excretion in the urine. Hemodialysis is another useful modality in the treatment of paraquat ingestion, but also must be performed within the first 72 hours.[14] The lack of availability of hemodialysis to most veterinarians makes this treatment option more theoretical than practical. Interestingly, oxygen therapy is not recommended as part of the initial stabilization or treatment of paraquat ingestion because oxygen increases the amount of superoxide ions (O_2^-) formed, and superoxideion formation is one of the main mechanisms of action of paraquat toxicity, causing direct tissue damage in the lungs.[13,15] Once an animal presents with clinical signs of respiratory distress, treatment is limited to supportive care.

CLINICAL DIAGNOSTIC TESTING

Thoracic radiographs are indicated in patients with suspected paraquat ingestion that are in respiratory distress. Pulmonary infiltrative changes are most commonly reported, with mixed interstitial and alveolar patterns (Figure 75-2).[12,14,15] The pulmonary changes are consistent with ARDS, and animals given paraquat have been used as a research model for ARDS. Acutely, these patients have pulmonary edema, but pulmonary changes eventually progress to fibrosis. Pneumomediastinum is found in roughly 25% of cases, but the cause of the pneumomediastinum is unknown.[12,14,15] Arterial blood gas analysis can be used to document hypoxemia. The degree of ventilation/perfusion mismatch and intrapulmonary shunting occurring in the lungs can be calculated using the alveolar-arterial oxygen gradient (A–a gradient). If pulmonary mechanics can be measured, restriction of lung volumes and decreased compliance are seen as the lungs progressively become more fibrotic.[13]

Complete blood count and serum chemistry findings are often unremarkable initially after ingestion. Mild changes may be seen secondary to dehydration, resulting in hemoconcentration and mild pre-renal azotemia. More severe abnormalities such as severe azotemia and liver enzyme elevation also occur. Dogs are more predisposed to development of acute renal failure secondary to proximal tubular necrosis than other species, and liver enzymes may be elevated from focal hepatic necrosis. Leukocytosis consisting of a neutrophilia and monocytosis may also occur. An electrocardiogram is indicated if arrhythmias or pulse deficits, secondary to myocardial necrosis, are detected on physical examination.

Detection of paraquat confirms exposure. In humans, plasma concentrations can be used prognostically if the time of ingestion is known, but the applicability of human data to dogs and cats has not been investigated. Few veterinary laboratories offer paraquat analysis; at the present time only the University of Wyoming Veterinary Diagnostic Laboratory offers such testing. Alternatively, testing may be available by contacting the manufacturer, Zeneca Ag Products, through its Emergency Information Network at 1-800-327-8633.

MANAGEMENT

Treatment of dogs or cats suffering from dyspnea caused by paraquat toxicity is mostly limited to supportive therapy. Although supplemental oxygen therapy is not recommended, severely affected patients may require intubation and positive pressure ventilation. The length of time that these patients may require ventilation often makes this option cost-prohibitive. Many additional therapies have been recommended in the treatment of paraquat toxicity, and are either immunosuppressive, an-

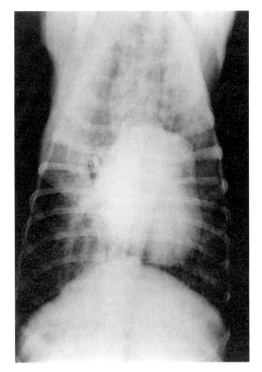

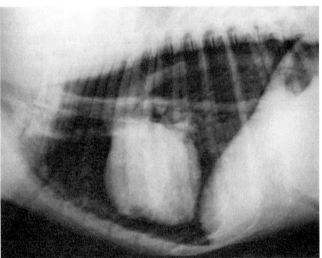

Figure 75-2. *Thoracic radiographs of a dog that presented in respiratory distress following ingestion of paraquat. The radiographs show a diffuse patchy alveolar pattern and pneumomediastinum.* (Radiographs courtesy of Dr. Hester McAllister at the Faculty of Veterinary Medicine, University College Dublin, Ireland.)

tiinflammatory, or aimed at preventing the severe fibrotic changes that occur in the lungs. These include cyclophosphamide, dexamethasone, deferoxamine, superoxide dismutase, acetylcysteine, and nicotinamide.[15] Human studies and experimental animal studies show conflicting data in regards to the usefulness of these additional therapies, with the majority not recommending the use of corticosteroids and cyclophosphamide.

PROGNOSIS

The respiratory effects of paraquat toxicity are progressive and have little response to conventional therapy. Unfortunately, there is no antidote, and the prognosis is extremely guarded because fibrosis and pulmonary failure eventually occur in most cases of paraquat ingestion. Death usually occurs from 3 to 17 days post-ingestion. There have been rare reports of recovery, with at least 1 dog surviving after developing severe respiratory signs.[15]

REFERENCES

1. Hoffman RS: Respiratory principles. In Goldfrank LR, Flomenbaum NE, Lewin NA et al, editors: *Goldfrank's toxicologic emergencies,* ed 6, Stamford, CT, 1998, Appleton & Lange.
2. Felice LJ, Murphy MJ: CVT update: anticoagulant rodenticides. In Bonagura JD, editor: *Kirk's current veterinary therapy,* vol 12, *Small animal practice,* Philadelphia, 1995, WB Saunders.
3. Woody BJ, Murphy MJ, Ray AC et al: Coagulopathic effects and therapy of brodifacoum toxicosis in dogs, *JVIM* 6(1):23-28, 1992.
4. Mount ME: Diagnosis and therapy of anticoagulant rodenticide intoxications, *Vet Clin North Am Small Anim Pract* 18(1):115-129, 1988.
5. DuVall MD, Murphy MJ, Ray AC et al: Case studies on second-generation anticoagulant rodenticide toxicities in non-target species, *J Vet Diag Invest* 1:66-68, 1989.
6. Sheafor SE, Couto CG: Anticoagulant rodenticide toxicity in 21 dogs, *JAAHA* 35:38-46, 1999.
7. Lewis DC, Bruyette DS, Kellerman DL et al: Thrombocytopenia in dogs with anticoagulant rodenticide-induced hemorrhage: Eight cases (1990-1995), *JAAHA* 33:417-422, 1997.
8. Rozanski EA, Drobatz KJ, Hughes D et al: Thrombotest (PIVKA) test results in 25 dogs with acquired and hereditary coagulopathies, *JVECC* 9:73-78, 1999.
9. Berry CR, Gallaway A, Thrall DE et al: Thoracic radiographic features of anticoagulant rodenticide toxicity in 14 dogs, *Vet Rad & Ultrasound* 34:391-396, 1993.
10. Blocker TL, Roberts BK: Acute tracheal obstruction associated with anticoagulant rodenticide intoxication in a dog, *J Small Anim Pract* 40:577-580, 1999.
11. Ekins BR, Geller RJ: Paraquat and diquat. In Ford MD, Delaney KA, Ling LJ et al, editors: *Clinical toxicology,* ed 1, Philadelphia, 2001, WB Saunders.
12. Darke PGG, Gibbs C, Kelly DF et al: Acute respiratory distress in the dog associated with paraquat poisoning, *Vet Rec* 100:275-277, 1977.
13. Gee BR, Farrow CS, White RJ et al: Paraquat toxicity resulting in respiratory distress syndrome in the dog, *JAAHA* 14:256-263, 1978.
14. Bischoff K, Brizzee-Buxton B, Gatto N et al: Malicious paraquat poisoning in Oklahoma dogs, *Vet Human Toxicol* 40:151-153, 1998.
15. O'Sullivan SP: Paraquat poisoning in the dog, *J Sm An Pract* 30:361-364, 1989.

CHAPTER 76

Thoracic Mineralization

Clifford R. Berry • A. Reid Tyson

Interpretation of thoracic radiographs includes evaluation of the extrathoracic structures, the pleural space, the pulmonary parenchyma, and the mediastinum. The reviewer must know and understand normal radiographic anatomy and normal variation, must have a systematic approach to interpretation of the radiograph, and must have an understanding of how pathological processes impact each structure. The basic changes in radiographic anatomy include alterations in number, size, shape, position/location, contours/margins, and opacity. Each of these changes can indicate a pathologic process within the thorax. This chapter will review areas of abnormal mineralization or ossification (change in opacity) within structures that are expected to be soft tissue, fat, or air opacity or alterations in the normal bone structures making up the axial and appendicular skeleton visible on thoracic radiographs.

Three basic pathophysiological processes may result in normal soft tissues becoming calcified or mineralized. The physiology of calcium or phosphorus metabolism has been reviewed elsewhere.[1-4] The three basic mechanisms include dystrophic mineralization, metastatic mineralization, and idiopathic mineralization.[2,5] In the case of dystrophic mineralization, deposition of calcium salts occurs in previously injured, degenerating, or necrotic soft tissues with normal plasma levels of calcium and phosphorus, and in the absence of derangements of calcium metabolism. The most common cause of dystrophic mineralization in small animals is previous inflammation, degeneration, or infection. Another form of dystrophic mineralization occurs in neoplastic tissue and results in a change in radio-opacity within the tumor mass. Tumors that routinely mineralize include adrenal, pulmonary, and prostatic carcinomas.

Metastatic mineralization occurs when calcium salts are deposited in normal soft tissues in the presence of abnormal plasma calcium and phosphorus concentrations.[2] When the product of the calcium and phosphorus plasma concentrations exceeds the solubility product of 70, deposition of mineral in normal soft tissues can ensue. Causes of hypercalcemia can include hyperparathyroidism (primary or secondary), vitamin D toxicity, increased bone catabolism associated with disseminated bone tumors (multiple myeloma), and chronic renal failure with hyperphosphatemia. Metastatic mineralization primarily affects the interstitial tissues of the vasculature (tunica media), kidneys, lungs, and gastric mucosa. The most common causes of metastatic mineralization in small animals are parathyroid-related protein, associated with paraneoplastic syndromes: and chronic renal insufficiency.[4]

In both dystrophic and metastatic mineralization, the calcium deposits can be calcium salts (i.e., noncrystalline amorphous deposits) or calcium-phosphorus apatite crystals that are similar to hydroxyapatite found within the inorganic matrix of bone. Over time these crystals may initiate heterotopic bone formation or osseous metaplasia. This process of mineralization has two distinct processes: initiation and propagation. Calcium deposits are concentrated either intracellularly within the mitochondria of dying cells or in the extracellular space in membrane-bound vesicles.[2] Dystrophic and metastatic mineralization can both occur within the intra and/or extracellular space.

The final type of mineralization is idiopathic mineralization, in which an underlying pathologic cause within the mineralized tissue or abnormalities of serum calcium or phosphorus cannot be determined.[5] The most common instance of idiopathic mineralization in small animals is calcinosis circumscripta.[5] Idiopathic mineralization is also seen in areas of suspected high bloodflow such as the aortic sinus/bulb, although the underlying pathogenesis remains unproven.[6]

In some instances the differences between dystrophic and metastatic mineralization can be difficult to discern. For example, in uremic gastritis, there is an underlying inflammatory change within the gastric mucosa as well as an altered plasma calcium and phosphorus solubility product, both of which are presumed to result in mucosal mineralization of the stomach. The various types of mineralization affecting the extrathoracic structures, pleural space, pulmonary parenchyma, and mediastinum are summarized in Boxes 76-1, 76-2, 76-3 and 76-4.

Extrathoracic Mineralization

Dystrophic mineralization in the extrathoracic structures can be an incidental finding or may require further investigation. Abnormal new bone formation associated with any bony structure, particularly in the presence of other aggressive bone abnormalities, always warrants additional radiographic views or other diagnostic tests. Osteolytic or osteoproliferative lesions associated with the ribs can create the impression of mineral opacities within the pulmonary parenchyma. Spiculated periosteal new bone formation along the diaphyses of the long bones (typically humeri seen on thoracic radiographs) is usually secondary to hypertrophic osteopathy. Evaluation for other thoracic and abdominal masses helps rule out any specific causes of the periosteal reaction. The possibilities of diaphyseal infection secondary to fungal or

---

BOX 76-1
Extrathoracic Mineralizations on Thoracic Radiographs

Dystrophic Mineralization
- Adrenal gland neoplasia (adenoma or adenocarcinoma)
- Amorphous soft tissue mineralization secondary to primary or secondary bone tumors originating in the rib, sternum, pectoral limb, or vertebrae
- Amorphous or spiculated new bone formation along the caudal sternum secondary to *Actinomyces* or *Nocardia* infection
- Spiculated periosteal new bone formation along the long bones secondary to hypertrophic osteopathy
- Degeneration and dehydration of the nucleus pulposus of the intervertebral or intersternebral disk spaces
- Spondylosis deformans of the sternebrae or vertebrae
- Costal cartilage ossification and excessive costochondral junction degenerative changes resulting in pleural indentations or mistaken "pulmonary nodules"
- Focal hepatic mineralizations (intraparenchymal or biliary)
- Egg shell calcification of the gall bladder wall—cholecystitis
- Cholelithiasis
- Calcinosis cutis—Cushing's Syndrome
- Rib callus and repair from previous fracture

Metastatic Mineralization
- Intercostal and abdominal vessel mineralizations—renal failure, primary or secondary hyperparathyroidism
- Gastric wall mucosa—chronic renal failure

Idiopathic Mineralization
- Adrenal gland mineralization in the aged cat
- Pansteatitis in cats
- Cholesterol clefts in the peritoneal space of cats
- Calcinosis circumscripta

---

bacterial infection, or of metastatic disease from distant neoplasia, should also be considered.

Incidental findings associated with new mineral deposition or new bone formation can include degeneration and dehydration of the nucleus pulposus of the intervertebral or intersternebral disks. Spondylosis deformans of the sternebrae or vertebrae is commonly seen in older dogs. Periarticular changes of the scapulohumeral joints and costal cartilage ossification with excessive costochondral junction degenerative changes can result in pleural indentations and should not be mistaken for "pulmonary nodules." These changes are commonly seen in chondrodystrophic breeds such as the dachshund or bassett hound.

Excessive rib callus can occur following repair of previous rib fractures. Usually the margins are smooth, with bony reaction seen along all sides of the rib, and the lesion does not have an aggressive appearance. A malunion is typically present, and rib cortical alignment is not anatomic. A rib-related hypertrophic osteopathic-

BOX 76-2
Pleural Mineralizations That Might Be Seen on Thoracic Radiographs

Dystrophic Mineralization
- Pleural (visceral) osteomas (osseous metaplasia)

Metastatic Mineralization
- Chronic renal failure

Idiopathic Mineralization
- Pleural osseous metaplasia associated with an effusion or constrictive pericarditis

BOX 76-3
Pulmonary Mineralization Seen on Thoracic Radiographs

Dystrophic Mineralization
- Cushing's Disease (acquired or iatrogenic)*
- Aged lungs—bronchial wall mineralization and pleural/pulmonary osteomas (osseous metaplasia)
- Bronchial and tracheal cartilage mineralization
- Linear mineralization of the bronchial walls
- Pulmonary arteries from previous thrombosis and resultant inflammation (postadulticide heartworm treatment is the most common)
- Primary lung neoplasia
- Metastatic disease from osteosarcoma
- Post-fungal infection (histoplasmosis)
- Bronchial wall outlined by barium sulfate aspiration
- Tracheal or bronchial mineralization within luminal neoplasms (chondrosarcoma)

Metastatic Mineralization
- Interstitial and alveolar mineralization secondary to chronic uremia
- Cholecalciferol rodenticide toxicity with associated hypercalcemia and extensive pulmonary mineralization

Idiopathic Mineralization
- Pulmonary alveolar microlithiasis
- Alveolar deposits of barium sulfate from previous aspiration pneumonia

*May not be apparent on the gross pathology as seen on a thoracic radiograph, but can be seen histologically.

BOX 76-4
Mediastinal Mineralizations Seen on Thoracic Radiographs

Dystrophic Mineralization
- Vasculature (e.g., aorta, aortic root, or leaflets)—arteriosclerosis, hypothyroidism
- Coronary artery calcifications—arteriosclerosis
- Lymph node post-fungal infection (histoplasmosis)
- Myocardium—muscular dystrophy, subaortic stenosis, cardiomyopathy*
- Myocardium—chronic renal failure
- Aortic or mitral valve mineralization—endocarditis
- Mineralization of the esophagus in an area of *Spirocerca lupi* infection with malignant transformation to an osteosarcoma
- Esophageal foreign bodies (bones—not true dystrophic mineralization of the esophagus)
- Vascular ring anomalies with partial megaesophagus—retention of mineral material from food in the cranial esophageal lumen
- Megaesophagus—retention of mineral material from food in the esophageal lumen

Metastatic Mineralization
- Vasculature (e.g., aorta, aortic root, or leaflets)—chronic renal failure
- Hypercalcemia resulting in soft tissue mineralization (primary or secondary hyperparathyroidism, paraneoplastic disorders)

Idiopathic Mineralization
- Vasculature (e.g., aorta, aortic root, or leaflets)—hypertension
- Barium mineralization in the sternal lymph nodes secondary to barium leakage into the peritoneal space
- Tracheobronchial lymph node mineralization post barium sulfate aspiration
- Pericardium and pleural osseous metaplasia

*May not be apparent on the gross pathology as seen on a thoracic radiograph, but can be seen routinely histologically.

type of reaction has been reported in dogs with mesothelioma,[7] and with pleural metastatic disease from a pulmonary carcinoma (Figure 76-1).

Evaluation of the cranial abdomen may reveal mineralization of the cranial abdominal viscera. Mineralization in the dorsal and cranial retroperitoneal space in a dog should raise the suspicion of adrenal cortical neoplasia.[8] Adenomas and adenocarcinomas have an equal incidence of dystrophic mineralization, which is presumed to result from areas of secondary ischemia and necrosis.[8] Idiopathic mineralization can be seen in the adrenal gland of the aged cat.[9] This is typically an incidental finding and not associated with adrenocortical tumors, as seen in dogs.

Focal mineralization within the borders of the hepatic silhouette should be further evaluated. Small, pinpoint, generalized mineralizations may occur following infection (histoplasmosis) or parasitic migration (visceral larval migrans).[10] Multifocal choleliths or dystrophic mineralization of the biliary tract can occur secondary to inflammation.[10] If hepatic mineralization is focal and in the right ventral region of the hepatic silhouette, a cholelith is most likely (Figure 76-2). "Egg shell" calcification of the gall bladder wall has also been reported secondary to severe, chronic lymphoplasmacytic cholecystitis and cystic mucinous hyperplasia.[10] Pansteatitis in cats can also cause diffuse mineralization of the mesenteric and falciform fat. These changes may be associated with a history of previous pancreatitis. Additionally, focal areas of nodular fat

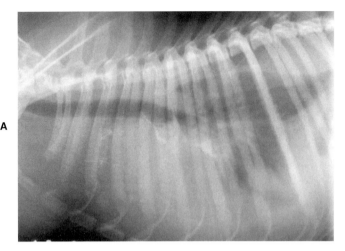

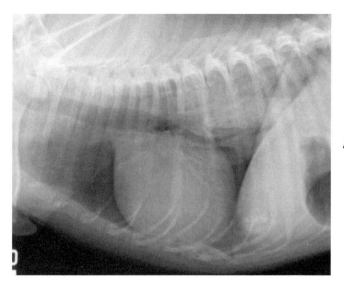

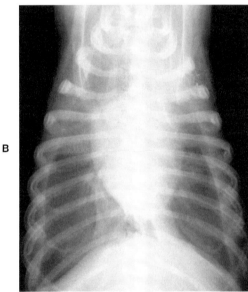

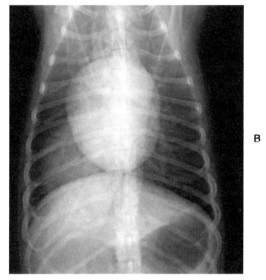

Figure 76-1. A, *Right lateral and* **B,** *ventrodosal radiographs from a 10-year-old mixed breed dog that had a previous left cranial lung lobectomy. The histological diagnosis was a bronchiolar carcinoma. The dog presented with dyspnea and muffled heart sounds. Thoracic radiographs documented a bilateral pleural effusion and irregular, smooth periosteal reactions associated with all ribs. Thoracocentesis revealed carcinoma cells in the pleural fluid.* (Courtesy of Dr. John Graham, College of Veterinary Medicine, University of Florida, Gainesville, Fla.)

Figure 76-2. A, *Left lateral and* **B,** *ventrodosal radiographs of a dog with multiple small mineral opacities within the region of the gall bladder, which were confirmed to be choleliths on ultrasound. The dog presented for clinical signs related to the caudal lung lobe mass.*

necrosis can be found. These are considered to be incidental findings and are not fixed in position within the abdomen. They have been shown to represent mineralization of cholesterol.[11]

Calcinosis cutis may result from iatrogenic or endogenous hyperadrenocorticism, and is presumed to represent degenerative changes in subcutaneous tissue proteins with subsequent dystrophic mineralization.[10,12-15] Other metastatic mineralizations of extrathoracic structures are typically secondary to renal failure, or to primary or secondary hyperparathyroidism.[15] Mineralized structures can include extrathoracic and intrathoracic vessels, renal silhouettes (cortical nephrocalcinosis), and the gastric mucosa. Vascular mineralization of the intercostal vessels has been seen in dogs with hypothyroidism,[15] presumably as a result of hypercholesterolemia and atherosclerosis.[16-19] Calcinosis circumscripta has been reported in the caudal cervical region. These lesions typically appear as finely spiculated mineralized masses that, if excessively large, may impact other organs such as the extrathoracic esophagus or trachea.

Pleural Mineralization

Dystrophic mineralization of the pleural space includes osseous metaplasia (osteomas) of the visceral pleural

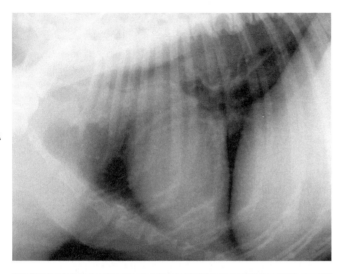

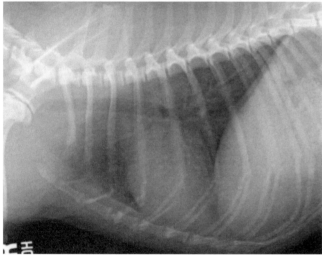

*Figure 76-3. **A, B,** Right lateral radiographs from two dogs with multiple small 2- to 4-mm mineralized nodules throughout the ventral lung fields consistent with pleural/pulmonary osteomas.*

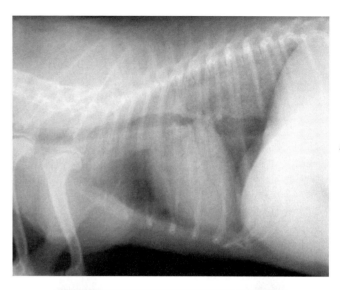

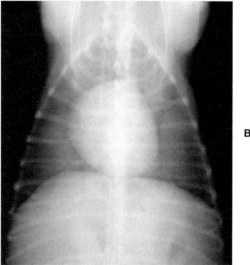

*Figure 76-4. **A,** Right lateral and **B,** ventrodosal radiographs from a 12-year-old, male neutered dog. Generalized interstitial dystrophic mineralization is present. The dog was documented to have pituitary-dependent hyperadrenocorticism. (Courtesy Dr. John Graham, College of Veterinary Medicine, University of Florida, Gainesville, Fla.)*

and sub-pleural surface of the lungs (Figure 76-3). These focal areas of mineralization can extend deeper into the underlying pulmonary parenchyma.[20-22] Typically, osteomas are multifocal and 2 to 4 mm in diameter. They are usually seen in the ventral thorax, and in the author's experience are more common in shelties, collies, and rottweilers. They are usually away from pulmonary vessels and should not be mistaken for pulmonary metastasis. Pulmonary nodules that are truly soft tissue and not mineralized typically cannot be visualized until they are at least 5 to 7 mm in size. Osteomas are more readily identified on the lateral radiographs than on the ventrodorsal or dorsoventral radiographs.

Dystrophic mineralization of the parietal and visceral pleural surface could develop in dogs or cats with chronic inflammatory diseases (e.g., previous chylothorax or pyothorax). Metastatic mineralization of the pleural

space and intercostal musculature can occur in extreme cases of chronic renal failure or other causes of metastatic mineralization.

Pulmonary Mineralization

Dystrophic mineralization of the pulmonary parenchyma can be seen in extreme cases of dogs with iatrogenic or endogenous hyperadrenocorticism.[12,14,23,24] The pulmonary mineralization is typically interstitial in location (Figure 76-4) and can be confused with an unstructured interstitial lung pattern as might be seen with early cardiogenic or noncardiogenic edema.[25] In a prospective study, 2 of 21 dogs with Cushing's syndrome had positive

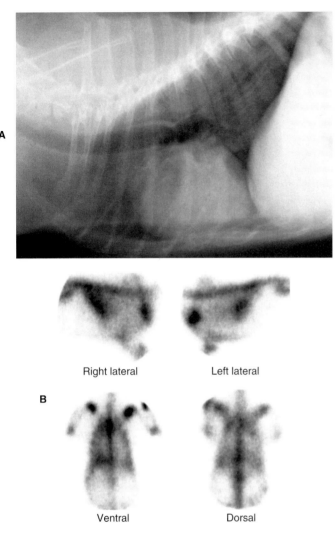

Figure 76-5. A, Right lateral radiograph from a dog with pituitary-dependent hyperadrenocorticism. There is a generalized interstitial pulmonary pattern, corresponding to interstitial dystrophic mineralization. **B,** On ^{99m}Tc-methylene diphosphonate delayed (3-hour postintravenous injection) static images there is generalized pulmonary uptake of the radiopharmaceutical consistent with pulmonary mineralization. (Courtesy Dr. Gregory B. Daniel, College of Veterinary Medicine, University of Tennessee, Knoxville.)

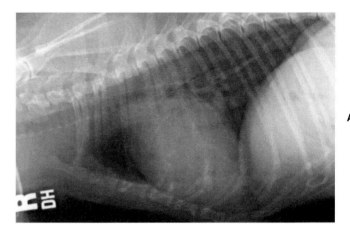

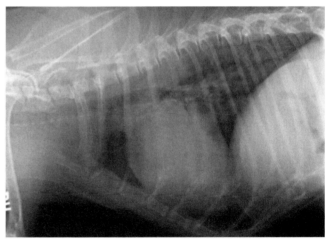

Figure 76-6. A, Right lateral and **B,** left lateral radiographs from a 12-year-old mixed breed dog. There is dystrophic mineralization of the tracheal rings and central airway walls. These changes were considered a geriatric change and not of clinical significance in this dog.

bone scans with a lung uptake pattern consistent with generalized mineralization (Figure 76-5).[24] In necropsies of dogs with Cushing's syndrome, the frequency of pulmonary bronchial and interstitial mineralization has been shown to be as high as 90%.[15]

In older dogs, the bronchial walls can become mineralized, particularly near the trachea and carina.[20,22] Bronchial wall mineralization typically appears as fine linear mineral opacities that correlate with the location of the major airways (Figure 76-6). Mineralization can also be seen within the cartilaginous rings of the bronchi and trachea.

Visceral pleural and pulmonary osteomas can be felt as small 2 to 4 mm nodules along the surface of the lung on gross pathology, and can also extend into the pulmonary parenchyma, typically with a ventral distribution. Some osteoma nodules can be 5 to 7 mm in size when they undergo ectopic ossification or secondary osseous metaplasia.[20,22]

Curvilinear mineralization in the caudodorsal lung fields on the lateral radiograph is consistent with mineralization of the pulmonary arteries (Figures 76-7 and 76-8). Most commonly, these changes are caused by previous thrombosis and the resultant inflammation after a dog has been treated with an adulticide for heartworms.[26] Mineralized pulmonary arteries have also been described in a cat with arteriosclerosis.[5]

Primary lung neoplasia in the cat has been shown to have a high incidence of pulmonary mineralization, particularly when metastatic pulmonary spread of a bronchogenic carcinoma has taken place (Figure 76-9).[27] Intrapulmonary metastatic disease can occur as a result of local invasion, lymphatic spread, bronchial wall invasion, and spread by the hematogenous venous return from the bronchoesophageal vessels into the right heart and pulmonary circulation. In one study of metastatic

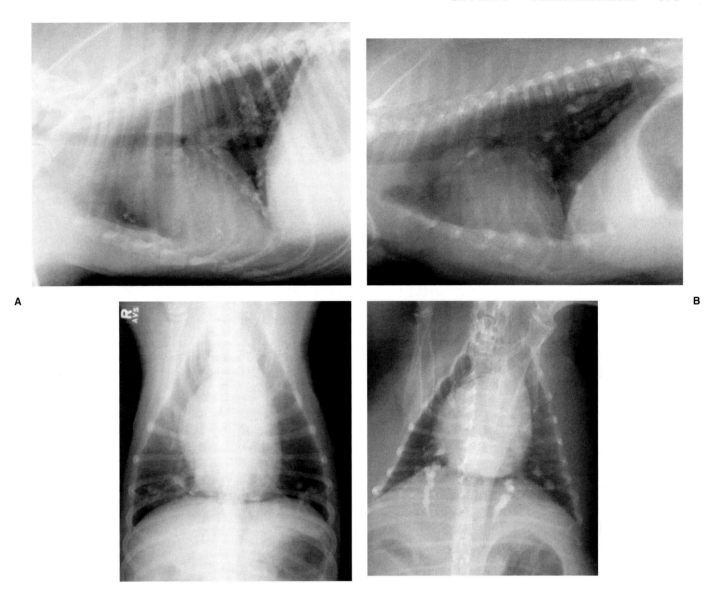

Figure 76-7. **A,** *Right lateral and ventrodosal radiographs and* **B,** *right lateral and dorsoventral radiographs from two dogs with heartworm disease. Both dogs had histories of previous heartworm adulticide therapy. Curvilinear mineral opacities are noted in the ventral and caudal lung fields in both dogs.*

patterns for the cat, however, mineralization was not reported.[28]

Pulmonary metastatic disease from primary bone tumors such as osteosarcoma can undergo mineralization associated with aberrant osteoid deposition (Figure 76-10). Generalized multi-focal mineralized nodules have been described in the dog and cat after histoplasmosis infection.[29,30] These nodules are usually small (less than 5 mm) and do not have associated inflammatory changes around the mineralization (Figure 76-11). These changes are usually seen after the active inflammatory disease has resolved, and the mineralization is presumed to occur during the healing phases of the granulomatous reaction.[29,30]

Intraluminal neoplasms within the trachea or principal bronchi can undergo mineralization, particularly if the tumor is originating from the cartilage of these upper airways (e.g., a chondrosarcoma).[31] Mineralization is usually limited to the neoplasm within the airway. Roentgen findings with these tumors include changes in the normal luminal radio-opacity and alterations in the mucosal margins of the trachea or bronchi.

Metastatic mineralization of the pulmonary parenchyma typically occurs in instances of chronic uremia and hypercalcemia.[15,25] Interstitial pulmonary parenchymal mineralization is composed of either calcium carbonate salts or hydroxyapatite crystals. In the latter instance, the crystals will bind [99m]Technetium-methylene diphosphonate (a radiopharmaceutical that binds to the inorganic matrix of bone).

Metastatic mineralization has also been reported in a cat that had extensive pulmonary mineralization and

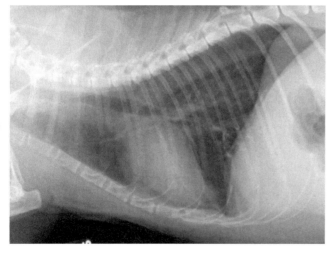

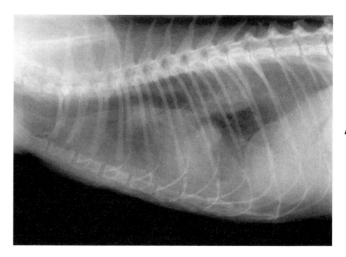

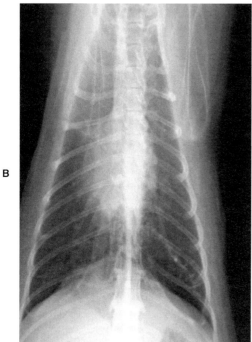

Figure 76-8. A, Right lateral and **B,** ventrodosal radiographs from a cat that had been heartworm antigen positive for 1 year before radiography. The curvilinear mineralized pulmonary arteries are consistent with previous heartworm thromboembolism.

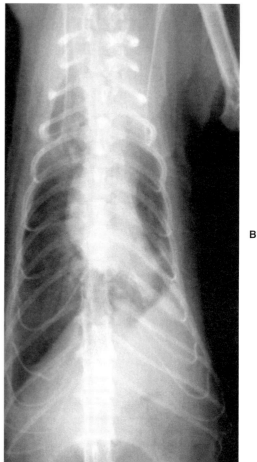

Figure 76-9. A, Right lateral and **B,** ventrodosal radiographs from a 14-year-old cat that presented for cough and tachypnea of recent onset. There is a large mass in the right caudal lung lobe with focal areas of dystrophic mineralization. The histologic diagnosis was a bronchoalveolar carcinoma.

hypercalcemia, presumed to be secondary to cholecalciferol rodenticide toxicity.[32]

Idiopathic mineralization has been described in people and dogs and is termed pulmonary alveolar microlithiasis.[33-35] In these cases, the dogs had focal areas of osseous metaplasia and heterotopic new bone within the alveoli of all lung fields on histologic sections. Radiographically, small, mineralized nodules were present throughout the lung fields. The etiology for this condition is not known. A single case report has been described in a cat where microlithiasis was associated with a bronchopneumonia.[36]

Alveolar deposits of barium sulfate from aspiration pneumonia during or after an upper gastrointestinal series (Figure 76-12) can be seen on sequential radiographs.

Initially, the barium sulfate will outline the major bronchi of the lung lobes in which the barium was aspirated. If the barium sulfate is compartmentalized within the alveoli, the metal opacity will remain over time and even over the life of the animal. If the barium sulfate is phagocytized by

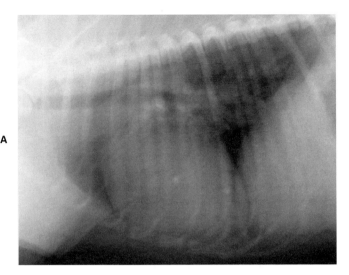

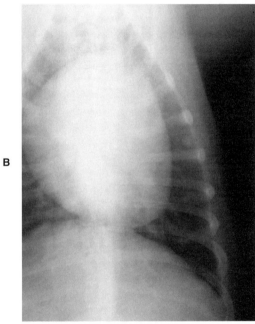

Figure 76-10. A, Right lateral and **B,** collimated ventrodosal radiographs from a dog with previously diagnosed primary osteosarcoma of a long bone. The pulmonary and tracheobronchial metastatic lesions show evidence of mineralization. On histology, these areas were found to be osteoblastic osteosarcoma with osteogenesis and osteoid formation.

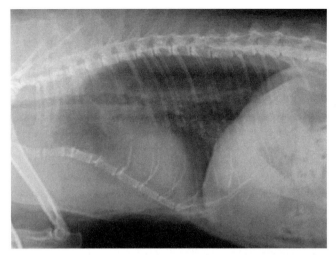

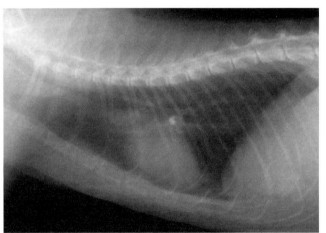

Figure 76-11. A, Right lateral radiograph documenting dystrophic mineralization in the accessory lung lobe of a 9-year-old domestic shorthair cat 1 year after diagnosis of histoplasmosis. The pulmonary mineralization present in the accessory lung lobe remained static in appearance for several years on serial thoracic radiographs. **B,** Right lateral radiograph documenting dystrophic mineralization in the tracheobronchial lymph nodes from a 7-year-old domestic shorthair cat with a similar clinical history.

alveolar macrophages, the barium can be identified within the regional lymph nodes such as the right, central, or left tracheobronchial lymph nodes.

Mediastinal Mineralization

Dystrophic mineralization of the vasculature (e.g., major arterial vessels including the aorta, brachiocephalic trunk, and left subclavian) has been described in animals with hypercholesterolemia, arteriosclerosis, and hypothyroidism.[15,21] These vascular mineralizations can extend out into the intercostal and abdominal arteries.

Coronary artery calcifications are seen in humans with coronary artery disease and atherosclerosis. Coronary artery calcification is rare in the dog, but has been described as an incidental finding.[37] The underlying pathogenesis has not been determined.

The tracheobronchial lymph nodes can remain mineralized after a fungal infection such as histoplasmosis.[28,29] Metal opacity within the tracheobronchial lymph nodes can be seen as a sequel to aspiration of barium sulfate, phagocytosis of barium, and migration of macrophages to the tracheobronchial lymph nodes.

Dystrophic mineralization of the myocardium has been described in a number of conditions in dogs and cats (e.g., muscular dystrophy, subaortic stenosis, and cardiomyopathy).[38,39] These changes are often detectable on gross and especially on histologic examination but may not be apparent radiographically. Myocardial mineralization can also occur associated with other inflammatory

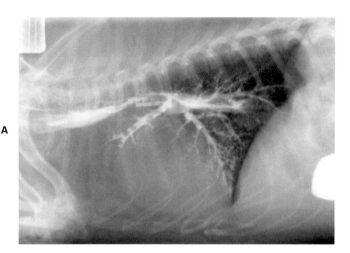

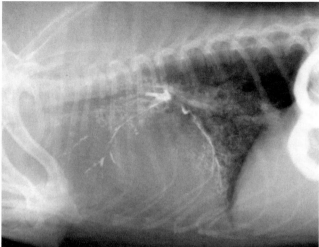

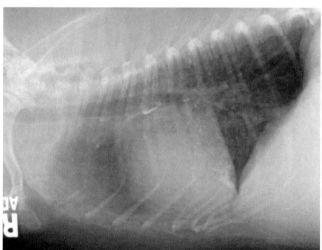

Figure 76-12. *Right lateral radiographs from a dog that underwent an upper gastrointestinal examination.* **A,** *Initial radiograph documents aspiration of barium sulfate (metal opacity) throughout the trachea, major airways and caudal alveolar lung.* **B,** *Right lateral radiograph taken 30 minutes after the initial radiograph documents clearing of the barium sulfate from the trachea and airways.* **C,** *Right lateral radiograph obtained 6 months after the initial gastrointestinal examination and aspiration. Barium is identified in the cranial mediastinal and tracheobronchial lymph nodes. Alveolarization of the barium within the accessory lung lobe is also present.*

conditions such as with parvovirus, toxoplasmosis or leishmania myocarditis.

Aortic or mitral valve endocarditis mineralization can occur as a postinflammatory change associated with granulomatous reactions on the valve leaflets. However, on radiographs, the mineral opacity is not seen as a discrete structure because of the motion associated with the valve leaflets and the timing of the radiographic exposure relative to the cardiac cycle.

Lesions of the esophagus can also result in focal areas of mineralization.[40] Dystrophic mineralization of the esophagus in areas of *Spirocerca lupi* infection can result from granulomatous inflammation or with malignant transformation of the parasitic granuloma to an osteosarcoma. These lesions typically are seen in the caudal esophagus and are best visualized on the lateral radiograph. Esophageal foreign bodies such as bones are not true dystrophic mineralization but can present in typical sites including the thoracic inlet, heart base area, or the lower esophageal sphincter.

Other esophageal mineral opacities may be associated with generalized megaesophagus or vascular ring anomalies with a partial megaesophagus. Vascular ring anomalies result in retention of mineral food material in the cranial esophageal lumen, whereas in generalized megaesophagus, retention of mineral food material can be anywhere within the esophageal lumen.

Metastatic mineralization of the myocardium and primary arterial vasculature (e.g., aorta, aortic root, and leaflets) has been reported in animals with chronic renal failure.[12] Extensive areas of mineralization of the vessels can occasionally be seen (Figure 76-13). Differentials should include hypercalcemia resulting in soft tissue mineralization from other causes.

Tumor mineralization within the pericardium has been reported in a dog with pericardial chondrosarcoma.[41] Idiopathic mineralization of several other mediastinal structures has been reported. Dystrophic mineralization of the pericardium as a cause of effusive-constrictive pericarditis has been described in a 1-year-old rottweiler.[42] Osseous metaplasia of the pericardium and pleural space was evident on histologic evaluation of the pericardium and of pleural samples postthoracotomy and partial pericardectomy. A specific etiology for the osseous metaplasia was not determined.

Mineralization of the primary systemic arterial vasculature including the aorta, aortic root, and primary branches of the aortic root has been seen in cats with

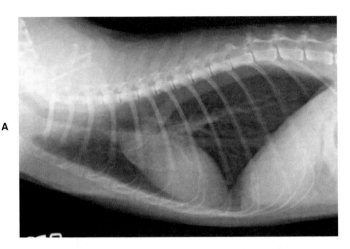

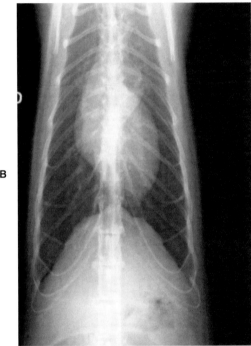

Figure 76-13. A, Right lateral and B, ventrodorsal radiographs from a 14-year-old domestic shorthair cat with a history of chronic renal failure. Extensive aortic and great vessel mineralization is identified consistent with metastatic mineralization of the vessels.

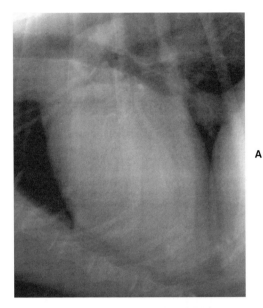

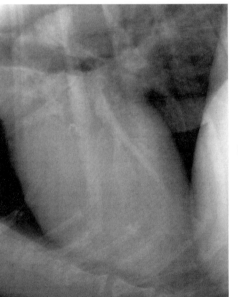

Figure 76-14. A, Right lateral and B, left lateral radiographs from an 8-year-old Greyhound that presented for evaluation of a nasal discharge. On lateral thoracic radiographs, a focal area of curvilinear mineralization was present in the region of the aortic root. This mineralization could not be seen on the ventrodorsal radiograph because of superimposition of other structures. The etiology of this mineralization has not been determined.

systemic hypertension. Additionally, mineralization of the aortic root was reported in 20 dogs without clinical evidence of plasma calcium or phosphorus abnormalities.[6] These changes histologically are similar to Mönckenburg's arteriosclerosis or calcification in humans, although the exact etiopathogenesis has not been determined (Figure 76-14).[6]

Barium localization in the sternal and tracheobronchial lymph nodes (secondary to barium leakage into the peritoneal space or aspiration of barium) has been seen following phagocytosis of the barium and migration of macrophages to the respective regional lymph nodes (see Figure 76-12). Changes within the lymph nodes can be apparent within 24 to 48 hours of barium administration.

Evaluation Using Alternate Imaging Techniques

Extra and intrathoracic mineralization can be evaluated using a number of alternate imaging techniques including special radiographic procedures, echocardiography or thoracic ultrasound, computed tomography, and nuclear scintigraphy. Computed tomography (CT) can be used to evaluate all areas within the thorax, and high resolution CT can be used to evaluate the pulmonary parenchyma.

A generalized area of the lung can be evaluated for mineralization using ^{99m}Tc-methylene diphosphonate (MDP) scintigraphy, for example in dogs with hyperadrenocorticism (see Figure 76-5). These studies are a quick, noninvasive way to evaluate interstitial mineralization within the pulmonary parenchyma, dependent upon the presence of apatite or hydroxyapatite crystals for MDP binding. Uremic interstitial pneumonitis has been associated with calcium hydroxide salts or magnesium salts that will not bind MDP. Additionally, myocardial uptake of ^{99m}Tc-pyrophosphate has been used for imaging acute myocardial necrosis with associated calcium deposition.

Mineralization within the thorax requires careful examination and review to determine the clinical significance of abnormalities identified on the thoracic radiographs. By categorizing the location of the thoracic mineralization, as well as trying to differentiate the types of mineralization (e.g., dystrophic, metastatic, or idiopathic), one can arrive at a reasonable differential diagnosis for the abnormalities identified.

REFERENCES

1. Ganong WF: *Review of medical physiology,* ed 20, New York, 1999, Lange Medical Books/McGraw-Hill.
2. Cotran RS, Kumar V, Robbins SL: *Robbin's pathologic basis of disease,* ed 5, Philadelphia, 1994, WB Saunders.
3. Kurosky LK: Abnormalities of magnesium, calcium and chloride. In Ettinger SJ, Feldman EC, editors: *Textbook of veterinary internal medicine,* ed 5, Philadelphia, 2000, WB Saunders.
4. Nelson RW, Couto CG: *Small animal internal medicine,* ed 2, St Louis, 1998, Mosby.
5. Lefbom BK, Adams WH, Weddle DL: Mineralized arteriosclerosis in a cat, *Vet Radiol Ultrasound* 37(6):420-423, 1996.
6. Douglass JP, Berry CR, Thrall DE et al: Radiographic features of aortic bulb/valve mineralization in 20 dogs, *Vet Radiol Ultrasound* 44(1):20-27, 2003.
7. Craig JA, Helman RG, Walker M: Costal bone changes similar to hypertrophic osteopathy associated with pulmonary and abdominal mesothelioma in a dog, *JAVMA* 186(10):1100-1101, 1985.
8. Penninck DG, Feldman EC, Nyland TG: Radiographic features of canine hyperadrenocorticism caused by autonomously functioning adrenocortical tumors: 23 cases (1978-1986), *JAVMA* 192(11):1604-1608, 1988.
9. Burk RL, Ackerman N: *Small animal radiology and ultrasound: A diagnostic atlas and text,* ed 2, Philadelphia, 1996, WB Saunders.
10. Lamb CR, Kleine LJ, McMillan MC: Diagnosis of calcification on abdominal radiographs, *Vet Radiol* 32(5):211-220, 1991.
11. Schwarz T, Morandi F, Gnudi G et al: Nodular fat necrosis in the feline and canine abdomen, *Vet Radiol Ultrasound* 41(4):335-339, 2000.
12. Lamb CR: Non-skeletal distribution of bone-seeking radiopharmaceuticals, *Vet Radiol* 31(5):246-253, 1990.
13. Huntley K, Frazer J, Gibbs C et al: The radiological features of canine Cushing's syndrome: A review of 48 cases, *J Small Animal Pract* 23:369-380, 1982.
14. Crawford MA, Robertson S, Miller R: Pulmonary complications of Cushing's syndrome: Metastatic mineralization in a dog with high-dose chronic corticosteroid therapy, *J Am Anim Hosp Assoc* 23(1):85-87, 1987.
15. Capen CC: The endocrine glands. In Jubb KVF, Kennedy PC, Palmer N, editors: *Pathology of domestic animals,* ed 3, vol 3, Orlando, 1985, Academic Press.
16. Robinson M: Generalised atherosclerosis in a dog, *J Small Anim Pract* 17(1):1745-1750, 1976.
17. Zeiss CJ, Waddle G: Hypothyroidism and atherosclerosis in the dog, *Compend Contin Educ Pract Vet* 17:1117-1128, 1995.
18. Kagawa Y, Hirayama K, Uchida E et al: Systemic atherosclerosis in dogs: Histopathologic and immunohistochemic studies of atherosclerotic lesions, *J Comp Path* 118:195-206, 1998.
19. Liu S, Tilley LP, Tappe JP et al: Clinical and pathologic findings in dogs with atherosclerosis, *JAVMA* 189:227-232, 1986.
20. Reif JS, Rhodes WH: The lungs of aged dogs: A radiographic-morphologic correlation, *J Am Vet Radiol Soc* 7:5-11, 1966.
21. Suter PF, Lord PF: *Thoracic radiography: A text atlas of thoracic diseases of the dog and cat,* Switzerland, 1988, PF Suter.
22. Meyer W: Radiographic review: The interstitial pattern of pulmonary disease, *Vet Radiol* 21(1):18-23, 1980.
23. Berry CR, Hawkins EC, Hurley KJ et al: Frequency of pulmonary mineralization and hypoxemia in 21 dogs with pituitary-dependent hyperadrenocorticism, *J Vet Intern Med* 14(2):151-156, 2000.
24. Berry CR, Ackerman N, Monce K: Pulmonary mineralization in four dogs with Cushing's syndrome, *Vet Radiol Ultrasound* 35(1):10-16, 1994.
25. Firoozniq H, Pudlowski R, Colimbu C et al: Diffuse interstitial calcification of the lungs in chronic renal failure mimicking pulmonary edema, *Am J Roent* 129:1103-1105, 1977.
26. Ackerman N: Radiographic aspects of heartworm disease, *Seminars in Veterinary Medicine and Surgery (Small Animal)* 2(1):15-27, 1987.
27. Koblik PD: Radiographic appearance of primary lung tumors in cats: A review of 41 cases, *Vet Radiol* 27(3):66-73, 1986.
28. Forrest LJ, Graybush CA: Radiographic patterns of pulmonary metastasis in 25 cats, *Vet Radiol Ultrasound* 39(1):4-8, 1998.
29. Clinkenbeard KD, Wolf AM, Cowell RL et al: Canine disseminated histoplasmosis, *Comp Cont Ed* 11(11):1347-1351, 1989.
30. Schulman RL, McKiernan, Schaeffer DJ: Use of corticosteroids for treating dogs with airway obstruction secondary to hilar lymphadenopathy caused by chronic histoplasmosis: 16 cases (1979-1997), *JAVMA* 214(9):1345-1348, 1999.
31. Carlilse CH, Biery DN, Thrall DE: Tracheal and laryngeal tumors in the dog and cat: Literature review and 13 additional patients, *Vet Radiol* 32(5):229-235, 1991.
32. Peterson EN, Kirby R, Sommer M et al: Cholecalciferol rodenticide intoxication in a cat, *JAVMA* 199(7):904-906, 1991.
33. Thrall DE, Goldschmidt MH, Clement RJ et al: Generalized extensive idiopathic pulmonary ossification in a dog: A case report, *Vet Radiol* 21(3):104-107, 1980.
34. Lui S-K, Suter PF, Ettinger SJ: Pulmonary alveolar microlithiasis with ruptured chordae tendinae in mitral and tricuspid valves in a dog, *JAVMA* 155:1692-1703, 1969.
35. Lord PF: Alveolar lung diseases in small animals and their radiographic diagnosis, *J Small Animal Pract* 17:283-303, 1976.
36. Brummer DG, French TW, Cline M: Microlithiasis associated with chronic bronchopneumonia in a cat, *JAVMA* 194(8):1061-1064, 1989.
37. Schwarz T, Stoerk CK, Renwick M et al: Mineralization of the coronary arteries in the dog (abstract), *Vet Radiol Ultrasound* 40(6):676, 1999.
38. Berry CR, Gashen FP, Ackerman N: Radiographic and ultrasonographic features of hypertrophic feline muscular dystrophy in two cats, *Vet Radiol Ultrasound* 33(6):357-364, 1992.
39. Gaschen L, Lang J, Line S et al: Cardiomyopathy in dystrophin-deficient hypertrophic feline muscular dystrophy, *J Vet Intern Med* 13(4):346-356, 1999.
40. Dvir E, Kirberger RM, Malleczek D: Radiographic and computed tomographic changes and clinical presentation of spirocercosis in the dog, *Vet Radiol Ultrasound* 42(2):119-129, 2001.
41. LaRock RG, Ginn PE, Burrows CF et al: Primary mesenchymal chondrosarcoma in the pericardium of a dog, *J Vet Diagn Invest* 9(4):410-413, 1997.
42. Wright KN, DeNovo RC, Patton CS et al: Effusive-constrictive pericardial disease secondary to osseous metaplasia of the pericardium in the dog, *JAVMA* 209:2091-2095, 1996.

CHAPTER 77

Idiopathic Pulmonary Fibrosis

Brendan M. Corcoran

Definition and Etiology

Pulmonary fibrosis is a pathological end-result of lung parenchymal inflammation. In humans, pulmonary fibrosis is a potential consequence of a wide range of clinical conditions including primary lung disorders (e.g., bronchopneumonia, eosinophilic pneumonia, or acute respiratory distress syndrome); connective tissue diseases (e.g., rheumatoid arthritis); inorganic and organic environmental or occupational pollutants (e.g., silicosis or farmer's lung); drug toxicity (e.g., bleomycin or amiodarone); and idiopathic fibrotic disorders (e.g., idiopathic pulmonary fibrosis or autoimmune pulmonary fibrosis).[1] The extent to which conditions such as the connective tissue disorders and autoimmune diseases result in lung fibrosis in the dog and cat is unknown.

There are specific conditions in both humans and animals in which lung fibrosis is an inevitable pathological consequence of the disease. In humans, this group of diseases is dominated by the occupational/environmental lung diseases and the poorly classified conditions that are grouped under the term idiopathic pulmonary fibrosis (cryptogenic fibrosing alveolitis).[2,3] Information on IPF in the dog and cat is sparse. Recently, lung fibrosis conditions (e.g., chronic pulmonary disease in West Highland white terriers) that are believed to be analogous to idiopathic pulmonary fibrosis in humans have been recognized and partially reported in both the dog[4,5] and cat.[6] In addition, lung fibrosis has been recognized for many years in association with paraquat poisoning in dogs[7,8] and as a complication of Cushing's syndrome[9]; more recently, it was recognized in a case of naturally-occurring bronchiolitis obliterans with organizing pneumonia (BOOP) in a dog.[10] Previously, anecdotal references to a chronic fibrosing condition have appeared periodically in the veterinary literature,[11,12] and two older papers probably described the same clinical entity as IPF.[13,14]

Idiopathic pulmonary fibrosis (IPF) (known as cryptogenic fibrosing alveolitis [CFA] in the United Kingdom and Europe) is a diagnosis of pathological exclusion, where there is no alternative explanation for the cause of lung fibrosis and the lung pathology has clearly identifiable pathological changes. In humans, IPF is a disease of middle to old age, but there is a familial form, believed to involve an autosomal recessive trait with variable penetrance, seen predominantly in the 20- to 40-year age group.

Although there is extensive understanding of the etiology of the diseases that secondarily cause lung fibrosis, little is known of the possible causes of IPF. However, the potential involvement of environmental pollutants cannot be discounted.[15] In humans, the disorder appears to occur in susceptible individuals, and there is evidence that viral, immunologic, and genetic factors play a role in the etiopathogenesis of the disease.[3] IPF in the dog appears to be breed-prevalent, occurs most commonly in the West Highland white terrier (which is prone to allergic skin disease), and Giant cells (epithelial syncytia) reminiscent of viral infection have been noted in lung histopathological sections from affected dogs.[4,13] Anecdotal reports of human patients dating the onset of their symptoms from a flu-like illness have increased speculation that a viral etiology might be implicated.[3] There is an increasing body of evidence associating Epstein-Barr virus (EBV) infection and, to a lesser extent, adenovirus infection with IPF in some human patients.[16-18] Whereas EBV replication is known to occur in the type II alveolar epithelial cells, the exact role of EBV in the pathogenesis of IPF is unknown. It has been suggested EBV acts as an immune trigger or contributes directly to lung injury.[16] Following infection the virus becomes latent, but can continue to promote chronic inflammation and repair, leading to fibrosis.[17] It is recognized that latent viruses can maintain the inflammation and tissue damage caused by other types of injury such as environmental pollutants,[17] and it is possible that a complex interaction between genes, viruses, and environment might be the trigger for IPF. Intriguing preliminary findings from the North West Lung Centre, Wythenshawe Hospital, Manchester, UK, have tentatively identified a clinical improvement in IPF patients treated with antigammaherpes drugs, but the completed data from these studies are not yet available.

Pathophysiology and Pathogenesis

The underlying pathological mechanisms of fibrosis, either in the lung or in any other organ system, are complex and incompletely understood.[18] End-stage lung fibrosis represents an aberrant remodelling process in response to injury.[3,19] The reason for scar formation rather than return to normal structure and function is unknown, but the key to the fibrotic response appears to be the up-regulation of gene expression for a range of cytokines. In particular there is mounting evidence that the transforming growth factor β family (TGF-β) is one of the most important groups of cytokines affecting the function and response of fibroblasts and Type II pneumocytes in the lung fibrosis response.[20] The identification of specific intracellular signals and associated gene expression offers new potential drug therapies for the fibrotic lung diseases.

Further upstream in the pathogenesis of lung fibrosis, a number of other mechanisms have the potential for drug targeting. Both acute and chronic inflammatory mechanisms are implicated in the induction and maintenance of fibrosis. A wide range of inflammatory mediators (e.g., eicosanoids, destructive tissue enzymes, and cytokines such as interleukin-1 [IL-1] and tumor necrosis factor-α [TNF-α]) prime resident tissue cells to increase production of both matrix proteins and additional cytokines such as IL-6, IL-8, and TGF-β.[19-21] Tissue fibroblasts are stimulated to differentiate and proliferate, and to increase production of collagen and other extracellular matrix proteins. The overall process is dynamic with multiple interactions between inflammatory cells and the fibroblast/fibrocyte system; thus the end result of the response to injury cannot be predicted. In lung fibrosis the capacity to arrest aberrant scar formation appears to be overwhelmed, resulting in loss of functional lung, altered lung physiology, and severe clinical signs.

Incidence, Prevalence, and Epidemiology

The incidence of IPF in the dog and cat is unknown, but the condition appears to be prevalent in the terrier breeds and in the West Highland white terrier in particular.[4,5,13] Reports of the incidence of IPF in humans vary greatly and in part reflect the difficulty in diagnosis. The prevalence in the United Kingdom is approximately 6 per 100,000, but closer to 30 per 100,000 in the United States.[22] The overall incidence of human IPF is rising, which probably reflects improvement in diagnosis, and a similar trend may be expected in veterinary medicine as we become more aware of the disease. A gender bias towards males has also been reported for IPF in humans, with males twice as likely to be affected.[22] In one study of West Highland white terriers, 17 were male and 12 were female, giving an approximate ratio of 60% to 40%.[4] The identification of a true male gender bias for IPF in the dog will rely on identification of a much larger number of cases. IPF has a median age of onset of approximately 9 years in the West Highland white terrier.[4]

The incidence of paraquat poisoning is low and sporadic and has become less common over the years because of its reduced use as a herbicide and because of safer handling and storage. Paraquat intoxication does not appear to have an age prevalence, although in one

report the majority of dogs were under 5 years of age.[7] Recently a single case of lung fibrosis, similar to interstitial pneumonia in humans, has been reported in a cat, but the condition appears to be rare in this species.[6]

Risk Factors and Environmental Influences

The question of whether or not environmental industrial airborne pollutants are implicated in canine lung fibrosis is problematic. Obviously, occupational hazard is very important in the genesis of human lung fibrosis.[2] It has been speculated that a single case of BOOP in a dog with attendant lung fibrosis could have been caused by exposure to airborne toxins in the owner's workshop.[10] The author has seen one case of suspected lung fibrosis in a springer spaniel that had ready access to a pottery workshop where the workers used protective face masks, and speculated that the lung disease might have been caused by inhaled particulate material present in the workshop environment. However, beyond such occasional anecdotal reports there is no direct evidence that environmental pollutants are implicated in canine lung fibrosis.

Historical Findings, Clinical Signs, and Progression

Apart from breed predisposition, the only other specific historical features of IPF in the dog are the slow onset and progression of the disease. In the author's experience, coughing occurs late in the disease process and may be the prime reason the owner seeks veterinary advice. The owner may have noted exercise intolerance, dyspnea, and tachypnea, but attributed these signs to advancing age rather than primary respiratory disease.[4] Approximately 30% of cases are presented because of dyspnea. Additional clinical features include intermittent cyanosis and presyncope or syncope. Because the majority of affected dogs are over 9 years of age, concurrent medical problems (e.g., musculoskeletal disorders, endocrinopathies such as hypothyroidism[5] and hyperadrenocorticism, and obesity) may complicate the clinical picture. Additional respiratory conditions can also be present, particularly tracheal collapse and chronic bronchitis, further complicating the clinical presentation. Apart from these presenting signs the dogs are often bright, alert and responsive, and have normal appetite. Despite the respiratory impairment the owners are usually content with the dogs' overall quality of life.

Humans with IPF have a similar clinical presentation, with coughing and breathlessness occurring in equal numbers of patients, and bilateral basilar crackles audible on auscultation in most cases. Finger clubbing is seen in approximately half of the patients.[22] In one report, 30% of human patients had evidence of a concurrent immunological disorder (e.g., polyarthritis, chronic active hepatitis, and Sjögren's syndrome) with the remainder having "lone" CFA.[23] Although there is a single case report of a dog with lung fibrosis and polyarthritis that might have been an early report of IPF,[14] the incidence of concurrent immunological disorders with IPF in the dog is unknown. In the author's experience, concurrent immunological disease appears to be unusual.

The main finding on physical examination in dogs is diffuse pulmonary crackles on thoracic auscultation. Wheezes and rhonchi can also be auscultated in many cases. The intensity of the crackles can be sufficient to make auscultation of the heart difficult.[4,5] Varying degrees of dyspnea, tachypnea, and cyanosis can also be noted.

Specific information on disease progression of canine IPF is not readily available, but it appears to be a slowly progressive disease, and deterioration is inevitable irrespective of treatment. Eventually respiratory failure develops and euthanasia is performed. The expected survival time from the onset of clinical signs varies widely. A range of 3 to 41 months has been reported in the West Highland white terrier, with a median survival of 15.5 months.[4] In human IPF, the median survival can be up to 12 years for desquamative interstitial pneumonitis (DIP), but is only 5 years for the more common usual interstitial pneumonitis (UIP) form. End-stage pulmonary fibrosis in humans results in extreme respiratory distress and total incapacity, followed by death caused by intractable hypoxemia and respiratory failure.[2]

Differential Diagnosis

The major differential consideration in dogs with IPF is chronic bronchitis.[4] Chronic bronchitis is also a disease of small terrier breeds, has a similar clinical presentation and course to IPF, and diffuse pulmonary crackles can be heard on chest auscultation.[24-26] In contrast to IPF, dogs with chronic bronchitis often have minimal radiographic changes and have bronchoscopic evidence of the disease.[25,27] Diffuse pulmonary crackles are also a cardinal sign of pulmonary edema, and conditions causing congestive heart failure and noncardiogenic pulmonary edema must be considered. As IPF results in nonspecific diffuse interstitial radiographic changes, a wide range of interstitial lung diseases (e.g., respiratory infections, pulmonary infiltration with eosinophils, and infiltrative neoplasms) should be considered differential diagnoses for IPF.[4]

In humans, the main differential considerations are the occupational/environmental lung disorders and the connective tissue disorders. An exhaustive list of unclassified (primary) disorders resulting in interstitial disease must also be considered, including sarcoidosis, eosinophilic pneumonia, and acute respiratory distress syndrome.[1]

Diagnostic Tests

Thoracic radiography is important in the diagnosis of IPF in the dog because collection of diagnostic biopsy material is unlikely. The radiographic changes can vary but tend to reflect the severity of the clinical presentation with varying degrees of a diffuse interstitial pattern and right-sided cardiomegaly (Figures 77-1, A and B)[4,5,13] The sensi-

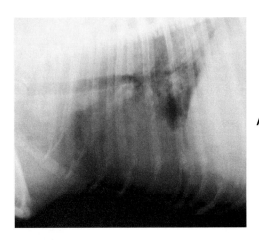

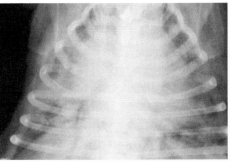

Figure 77-1. A, Lateral and **B,** ventro-dorsal radiographs of the thorax of a dog with histopathologically confirmed idiopathic pulmonary fibrosis, showing a marked diffusely increased interstitial pattern.

tivity and specificity of radiography in the diagnosis of IPF in the dog is unknown. In human IPF the sensitivity and specificity of radiography is very poor, and there is a very poor correlation with severity of disease, unless honeycombing (advanced disease) is present.[3] The radiographic changes in humans can have a more patchy distribution compared with the dog, with an interstitial pattern usually described as reticular or reticulonodular.

Open lung biopsy is the main method for definitive diagnosis of lung fibrosis and the other interstitial lung diseases in humans,[28] but has not been widely adopted in veterinary patients. Although biopsy is necessary for confirmation of lung fibrosis, in a British Thoracic Society study, diagnosis of CFA in humans was still made on the basis of clinical findings in 60% of cases.[29] These clinical findings included breathlessness, finger clubbing and bilateral basilar crackles, typical chest radiographic features, and evidence of impaired gas transfer on lung function tests. Similarly, in dogs with IPF a strong tentative diagnosis can be made on the basis of the clinical presentation of chronic-onset coughing and dyspnea, diffuse pulmonary crackles, and radiographic changes, without necessarily undertaking invasive diagnostic procedures.[4,5] The utility of blood gas analysis in the diagnosis of IPF in dogs is not known, but severely affected individuals have hypoxia with normo- or hypocapnia and alveolar-arterial oxygen gradients typical of ventilation-perfusion mismatch.[4] In human IPF,

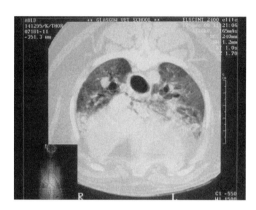

Figure 77-2. *High-resolution computed tomography image of a dog with suspected idiopathic pulmonary fibrosis at a level slightly caudal to the tracheal bifurcation. Notice the generalized ground-glass lung opacity and additional areas of consolidation in the lung periphery. (Courtesy Dr. T. Schwarz, University of Glasgow.)*

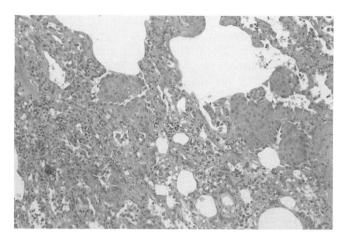

Figure 77-3. *H & E stained section of lung from a dog with idiopathic pulmonary fibrosis. The section illustrates the marked destruction of normal lung architecture, with squamous metaplasia, alveolar fibrosis, and diffuse inflammation.*

pulmonary function tests (e.g., measurement of total lung capacity, single breath carbon monoxide diffusing capacity, and oxygen desaturation on exercise) are also used for the initial diagnosis and assessment, and for monitoring progression and response to therapy.[1,30,31]

In humans, imaging modalities such as high resolution computed tomography (HRCT) can improve diagnostic accuracy by identifying active inflammation, thereby improving the diagnosis, treatment, and management of patients with IPF.[22] Some limited information on HRCT for IPF in the dog is available (Figure 77-2). Video-assisted thoracoscopic lung biopsy has been found to be comparable to open-chest lung biopsy in terms of morbidity and mortality in humans, but has distinct advantages in terms of postoperative care and complications.[32] This technique may prove to be useful for diagnosis of IPF in dogs in the future.

Bronchoscopy and bronchoalveolar lavage (BAL) may be useful tests in canine IPF because they may allow exclusion of chronic bronchitis, which is the major differential diagnosis.[4,5] The limited data on BAL fluid cytology in affected dogs makes assessment of the utility of this diagnostic test difficult. In the majority of cases of canine IPF the BAL samples are normal or have low to moderate mixed populations of inflammatory cells.[4] In human IPF, BAL lymphocytosis is documented in a proportion of patients, and there have been reports that such individuals respond better to therapy.[22,28,33,34] The prognosis further improves if the patient has HRCT results suggestive of an active inflammatory process.

Pathological and Histopathological Findings

The pathological characteristics of paraquat poisoning in dogs are well described but there is little information on the pathology of IPF. Paraquat poisoning results in pro-

gressive and irreversible lung fibrosis, which appears to be preceded by alveolar epithelial detachment and alveolar macrophage activation and recruitment, followed by extensive fibroblast proliferation and laying down of excess collagen.[7,35]

Information on the pathology of canine and feline IPF is sparse. The changes are nonspecific and therefore easily ascribed to a number of etiological factors, particularly viral infections and toxicoses.[13] On gross pathology, the lungs tend to be firm, heavy, and noncollapsable.[5,6,13] Associated right ventricular changes have also been noted (e.g., right ventricular hypertrophy and dilatation). In the limited histopathology reports of IPF in the dog and cat to date, the major finding has been extensive but patchy alveolar fibrosis (Figure 77-3).[4-6,13,14] Additional findings include epithelial cell hyperplasia, localized areas of squamous metaplasia, variable degrees of chronic interstitial inflammation predominantly involving lymphocytes and macrophages, and localized areas of emphysema and peri-arterial fibrosis.[4-6,14] Giant cells, similar to epithelial syncytia, have been reported in three cases, but no viral inclusion bodies have yet been identified.[5,13]

IPF/CFA in humans is divided into two broad histopathological categories.[22] The less common form is known as desquamative interstitial pneumonitis (DIP), and has close similarities to the recent report of feline CFA.[6] DIP mainly involves a lymphocytic cellular reaction with minimal fibrosis and is believed to be either an early form of IPF or a distinct and separate clinical entity. It is also the most amenable to therapy with glucocorticosteroids. Usual interstitial pneumonitis (UIP) is the most common form of IPF/CFA in humans and consists of a mixed inflammatory and fibrosis pattern with a distinctive peripheral distribution.[22] UIP is comparable to the form of IPF reported in the dog.[4,5] The locally extensive nature of the lung pathology, as opposed to widespread diffuse disease, is also comparable between human and canine patients.[4,36]

Management and Monitoring

Often decisions are made not to treat humans with IPF because of the unpredictability of progression of the disease and the poor response to current therapeutic regimes.[37,38] However, some authors question this approach, suggesting that it impedes progress in the diagnosis, management, and treatment of IPF.[28]

The medical treatment of IPF in the dog relies on glucocorticoids (prednisolone) and bronchodilators.[4] There is anecdotal clinical evidence that this drug combination may be beneficial in some cases, but exact figures or data from controlled studies are not available.[4] In human IPF prednisolone is widely used and appears to be beneficial in a number of cases. DIP patients are more responsive to glucocorticoids, reflecting the active inflammatory nature of the condition.[28] Up to 60% of DIP patients respond favorably to such treatment.[39] In the more common UIP where there is extensive fibrosis, glucocorticoids are less effective, which is not surprising because these drugs do not have any effects on the mechanisms of fibrosis.[28] Additional approaches to drug therapy in human patients include immunosuppressive and cytotoxic drugs (e.g., azathioprine and cyclophosphamide). However, convincing data that their use in combination with prednisolone results in a better outcome compared to prednisolone alone are lacking.[28,40,41] Of the two (azathioprine or cyclophosphamide), adjunctive therapy with azathioprine appears to give a marginal improvement over prednisolone therapy alone.[41]

Theoretically, drugs such as colchicine that have antifibrotic activity should be of benefit in IPF. Some studies in human IPF suggested that colchicine was at least as beneficial as prednisolone therapy in terms of clinical improvement and survival, but is a much more benign drug with minimal side effects.[38,42] A more recent study, however, suggests colchicine has no appreciable effect on survival compared to no therapy, and low dose prednisolone therapy gives the best survival outcome.[43] Colchicine inhibits fibroblast proliferation and thereby decreases the rate of collagen synthesis rather than affecting collagen gene transcription.[44] It also has weak inhibitory effects on the release of profibrotic cytokines (e.g., IL-6, TNF-α, IL-1, PDGF, and TGF-β) from inflammatory cells and suppresses production of macrophage-derived growth factor and fibronectin.[44] Through these various mechanisms colchicine should theoretically slow the rate of progression of fibrosis but will not reverse it. The author has no experience in the use of colchicine in IPF dogs, but it may have future applications in this condition.

There is also increasing interest in the development of antifibrotic drugs that either directly affect fibroblast proliferation and function or interfere with the production or activity of profibrotic cytokines. These drugs include cytokine-specific antibodies (e.g., anti-TNF-α), interferon-γ, niacin, taurine, pirfenidone, platelet activating factor antagonists, hydroxyproline analogs, and relaxin,[21,38,45] but clinical trial data on their efficacy in the treatment of IPF are not yet available. Lastly, single lung transplantation is an option in human patients with life-threatening illness.[46,47]

Outcome and Prognosis

With the limited data available it is difficult to provide accurate outcome information and prognosis guidelines for IPF in the dog. In one study of IPF in 29 West Highland white terriers, the median age of onset of clinical signs was 9 years, with a median survival of 15.5 months and a range of 3 to 41 months.[4] The effect of therapy could not be evaluated. Because some dogs survived up to or greater than 3 years, considering the late age of onset (diagnosis), some dogs might live close to their expected life-span. This compares with IPF in humans where the mean age of presentation in one study was 54 years, with a median survival of approximately 5 years.[23] Survival times in humans are best in young patients, especially if they are female,[23] whereas the presence of right-sided cardiomegaly and right axis deviation, suggestive of cor pulmonale, are poor prognostic indicators.[23] Fourteen of 29 cases of IPF in the dog had radiographic evidence of cor pulmonale, but its relationship to survival was not reported.[4]

Human patients with DIP have a much better outcome, with median survival up to 12 years.[28,39] In 20% of DIP patients spontaneous resolution can occur, and this again raises the possibility that DIP may be a separate clinical entity. Outcome in human patients might also be a function of level of care in that IPF patients referred to a specialist interstitial lung clinic have a median survival time significantly greater than those referred to a general respiratory clinic.[47] However, this difference is not seen with patients over 60 years of age. Whether or not specialist intervention in canine IPF would improve survival is not known. Because of the late age onset of clinical signs and the slow progression of the disease, many owners delay presenting their dogs until the disease is well advanced. It is conceivable that more rapid intervention and diagnosis might improve outcome and survival in dogs with IPF.

REFERENCES

1. Schwartz DA, Van Fossen DS, Davis CS et al: Determinants of progression in idiopathic pulmonary fibrosis, *Am J Respir Crit Care Med* 149:444-449, 1994.
2. Hasleton PS: Fibrosing alveolitis. In Hasleton PS, editor: *Spencer's pathology of the lung,* ed 5, New York, 1996, McGraw-Hill.
3. King TE, Cherniak RM, Schwarz MI: Idiopathic pulmonary fibrosis and other interstitial diseases of unknown etiology. In Murray JF, Nadel JA, editors: *Textbook of respiratory medicine,* ed 2, Philadelphia, 1994, WB Saunders.
4. Corcoran BM, Cobb M, Martin MWS et al: Chronic pulmonary disease in West Highland white terriers, *Vet Rec* 144:611-616, 1999.
5. Corcoran BM, Dukes-McEwan J, Rhind S et al: Idiopathic pulmonary fibrosis in a Staffordshire bull terrier with hypothyroidism, *J Small Anim Pract* 40:185-188, 1999.
6. Rhind SM and Gunn-Moore, DA: Desquamative form of cryptogenic fibrosing alveolitis in a cat, *J Compar Pathol* 123:226-229, 2000.
7. Darke PGG, Gibbs C, Kelly DF et al: Acute respiratory distress in the dog associated with paraquat poisoning, *Vet Rec* 100:275-277, 1977.

8. O'Sullivan SP: Paraquat poisoning in the dog, *J Small Anim Pract* 30:361-364, 1989.

9. Crawford MA, Robertson S, Miller R: Pulmonary complications of Cushing's syndrome: Metastatic mineralization in a dog with high-dose chronic corticosteroid therapy, *J Am Anim Hosp Assoc* 23:85-87, 1987.

10. Phillips S, Barr S, Dykes N et al: Bronchiolitis obliterans with organizing pneumonia in a dog, *J Vet Intern Med* 14:204-207, 2000.

11. Bonagura JD, Hamlin RL, Gaber CE: Chronic respiratory disease in the dog. In Kirk RW, Bonagura JD, editors: *Kirk's current veterinary therapy,* ed 10, Philadelphia, 1989, WB Saunders.

12. Martin MWS, Corcoran BM: Diseases of the lung parenchyma. In Price CJ, Sutton JB, editors: *Cardiorespiratory diseases of the dog and cat,* Oxford, 1997, Blackwell Scientific.

13. Cogan DC, Carpenter JL: Diffuse alveolar injury in two dogs, *JAVMA* 194:527-530, 1989.

14. Schiefer B, Hurov L, Seer G: Pulmonary emphysema and fibrosis associated with polyarthritis in a dog, *JAVMA* 164:408-413, 1974.

15. Scott J, Johnston I, Britton J: What causes cryptogenic fibrosing alveolitis? A case control study of environmental exposure to dust, *British Med J* 310:1015-1017, 1990.

16. Egan JJ, Stewart JP, Hasleton PS et al: Epstein-Barr virus replication within pulmonary epithelial cells in cryptogenic fibrosing alveolitis, *Thorax* 50:1234-1239, 1995.

17. Egan JJ, Woodcock AA, Stewart JP: Viruses and idiopathic pulmonary fibrosis, *Europ Resp J* 10:1433-1437, 1997.

18. Stewart JP, Egan JJ, Ross AJ et al: The detection of Epstein-Barr virus DNA in lung tissue from patients with idiopathic pulmonary fibrosis, *Am J Respir Crit Care Med* 159:1336-1341, 1999.

19. Rodeman HP, Binder A, Guven N et al: The underlying cellular mechanism of fibrosis, *Kidney International* 49(Suppl 54):S32-S36, 1996.

20. Martinet Y, Menard O, Valliant P et al: Cytokines in human lung fibrosis, *Arch Toxicol* (Suppl 18):127-139, 1996.

21. Zhang K, Gharaee-Kermani M, McGarry B et al: TNF-α-mediated lung cytokine networking and eosinophil recruitment in pulmonary fibrosis, *J Immunol* 158:954-959, 1997.

22. Chan-Yeung M, Muller NL: Cryptogenic fibrosing alveolitis, *Lancet* 350:651-656, 1997.

23. Turner-Warwick M, Burrows B, Johnson A: Cryptogenic fibrosing alveolitis: Clinical features and their influence on survival, *Thorax* 35:171-180, 1980.

24. Corcoran BM, Luis-Fuentes V, Clarke CJ: Chronic tracheobronchial syndrome in 8 dogs, *Vet Rec* 130:485-487, 1992.

25. Padrid PA, Hornof WJ, Kurpershoek CJ et al: Canine chronic bronchitis: A pathophysiological evaluation of 18 cases, *J Vet Intern Med* 4:172-180, 1990.

26. Wheeldon EB, Pirie HM, Fisher EW et al: Chronic bronchitis in the dog, *Vet Rec* 94:466-471, 1974.

27. Brownlie SE: A retrospective study of diagnosis of 109 cases of canine lower respiratory disease, *J Small Anim Pract* 31:371-376, 1990.

28. Egan JJ, Woodcock AA: Does the treatment of cryptogenic fibrosing alveolitis influence prognosis? *Resp Med* 90:127-130, 1996.

29. Johnston IDA, Prescott RJ, Chalmers JC et al: British Thoracic Society study of cryptogenic fibrosing alveolitis: Current presentation and initial management, *Thorax* 52:38-44, 1997.

30. Agusti C, Xaubet A, Agusti AGN et al: Clinical and functional assessment of patients with idiopathic pulmonary fibrosis: Results of a 3-year follow-up, *Eur Resp J* 7:643-650, 1994.

31. Wells AU, DuBois RM: Prediction of disease progression in idiopathic pulmonary fibrosis, *Eur Resp J* 7:637-639, 1994.

32. Mouroux J, Clary-Meinesz C, Padovani B et al: Efficacy and safety of videothoracoscopic lung biopsy in the diagnosis of interstitial lung disease, *Eur J Cardio-Thoracic Surg* 11:22-26, 1997.

33. Watters LC, Schwarz MI, Cherniack RM et al: Idiopathic pulmonary fibrosis: Pretreatment bronchoalveolar lavage cellular constituents and their relationships with lung histopathology and clinical response to therapy, *Am Rev Respir Dis* 135:696-704, 1987.

34. Haslam PL, Turton CWG, Lukoszek A et al: Bronchoalveolar lavage fluid cell counts in cryptogenic fibrosing alveolitis and their relation to therapy, *Thorax* 35:328-339, 1980.

35. Hampson ECGM, Pond SM: Ultrastructure of canine lung during the proliferative phase of paraquat toxicity, *Brit J Exper Pathol* 69:57-68, 1988.

36. Wallace WAH, Lamb D: Cryptogenic fibrosing alveolitis: A clinico-pathological entity, *Curr Diag Pathol* 3:27, 1996.

37. Meier-Sydow J, Weiss SM, Buhl R et al: Idiopathic pulmonary fibrosis: Current clinical concepts and challenges in management, *Semin Resp Crit Care Med* 15:77-96, 1994.

38. Raghu G: Idiopathic pulmonary fibrosis: A need for treatment with drugs other than corticosteroids-a role for antifibrotic agents? *Mayo Clinic Proceedings* 72:285-287, 1997.

39. Carrington CB, Gaensler EA, Coutu RE et al: Natural history and treated course of usual and desquamative interstitial pneumonia, *New Eng J Med* 298:801-809, 1978.

40. Johnson MA, Kwan S, Snell NJC et al: Randomized controlled trial comparing prednisolone alone with cyclophosphamide and low dose prednisolone in combination in cryptogenic fibrosing alveolitis, *Thorax* 44:280-288, 1989.

41. Raghu G, Depaso WJ, Cain K et al: Azathioprine combined with prednisolone in the treatment of idiopathic pulmonary fibrosis: A prospective double-blind, randomized, placebo controlled clinical trial, *Am Rev Resp Dis* 144:291-296, 1991.

42. Douglas WW, Ryu JH, Bjoraker JA et al: Colchicine versus prednisone as treatment of usual interstitial pneumonia, *Mayo Clinic Proceedings* 72:201-209, 1997.

43. Douglas WW, Ryu JH, Schroeder DR: Idiopathic pulmonary fibrosis: Impact of oxygen and colchicine, prednisone, or no therapy on survival, *Am J Respir Crit Care Med* 161:1172-1178, 2000.

44. Entzian P, Schlaak M, Seitzer U et al: Anti-inflammatory and antifibrotic properties of colchicine: Implications for idiopathic pulmonary fibrosis, *Lung* 175:41-51, 1997.

45. Nicod LP: Recognition and treatment of idiopathic pulmonary fibrosis, *Drugs* 55:555-562, 1998.

46. Egan JJ, Hasleton PS: Cryptogenic fibrosing alveolitis: Diagnosis and treatment, *Hosp Med* 59:364-368, 1998.

47. Lok SS: Interstitial lung disease clinics for the management of idiopathic pulmonary fibrosis: A potential advantage to patients, *J Heart Lung Transplant* 18:884-890, 1999.

E. Pleura, Diaphragm, and Chest Wall

CHAPTER 78

Pleural Transudates and Modified Transudates

Nancy A. Sanders • Meg Sleeper

The pleural space is the area between the parietal and visceral pleural linings of the thoracic cavity. It is often referred to as a "potential space" because it is *almost* devoid of volume-expanding substances under normal circumstances. Approximately 1.5 to 4.0 ml of pleural fluid exists in normal dogs and cats.[1-3] It serves to lubricate and smooth the movements of the thoracic organs during respiration, cardiac contractions, and bodily motion. The pleural space expands to accommodate large volumes of fluid in disease (pleural effusion).

Pleural effusion is not a specific diagnosis; rather, it is the result of various pathological processes. Types of fluid that can accumulate in the pleural space include blood, sterile and septic exudates, chyle, neoplastic effusions, moderately cellular transudates (modified transudates), and pure transudates. This chapter is limited to the discussion of transudates and modified transudates.

A transudate is a minimally cellular, low protein fluid. It has a total protein (TP) concentration less than 2.5 g/dl, and a nucleated cell count less than 1000 cells/µl. A modified transudate has a TP between 2.5 and 3.5 g/dl and a nucleated cell count between 500 and 10,000 cells/µl. The predominant types of nucleated cells in transudates and modified transudates are monocytes, small lymphocytes, and mesothelial cells. Normal or degenerate neutrophils may also be present in varying numbers depending upon the degree of inflammation. Bacteria are generally absent from transudates and modified transudates. In patients with chronic effusions, transudates may transform into modified transudates. Fluid can irritate the pleural lining, thus causing inflammation over time. The inflammatory cells release cytokines that attract even more inflammatory cells (chemotaxis). Furthermore, free water is absorbed over time into the vascular and lymphatic systems, resulting in a fluid that is more concentrated in cells and protein. Thus some overlap between categories of effusion exists (Table 78-1).

	Total Protein (g/dl) Specific Gravity	Nucleated Cell Count (cells/µl)	Possible Cell Types
Transudate	<2.5	<1000	Monocytes Small lymphocytes Mesothelial cells Nondegenerate neutrophils Neoplastic cells
Modified transudate	2.5-3.5	500-10,000	Eosinophils Monocytes Small lymphocytes Mesothelial cells Nondegenerate neutrophils Neoplastic cells
Exudate	>3.0	>5000	Activated macrophages Degenerate neutrophils Bacteria Eosinophils Mesothelial cells Mixed lymphocytes Neoplastic cells

TABLE 78-1. **Classification of Pleural Effusions**

Physiology

Normal fluid production into and removal from the pleural space is dynamic and governed by Starling's forces. Fluid moves into the pleural space from the pulmonary vessels and interstitium as a result of positive hydrostatic pressure in the pulmonary vascular system. Negative atmospheric pressure in the pleural space further influences movement in this direction. The oncotic pressure within the vascular system restricts excessive movement of fluid into the pleural space. The fluid formed is relatively protein free and cell free in comparison to whole blood because of restriction of protein and whole cell movement into the pleural space by the vascular and pleural endothelial linings. Finally, fluid in the pleural space is continuously removed by the lymphatic system. In humans, 5 to 10 liters of fluid pass through the pleural space per day.[1]

Pathophysiology

Abnormal accumulation of fluid in the pleural space occurs for many reasons, and is also explained by Starling's forces. There are two major causes of pleural effusion that, in turn, have various subcategories. The first major etiology is increased fluid flux into the pleural space. For pleural fluid to accumulate, influx must exceed the lymphatic system's capacity to drain the fluid. The subcategories of increased influx include increased hydrostatic pressure, decreased oncotic pressure, and increased vascular permeability (vasculitis). Congestive heart failure, vascular obstruction, and systemic hypertension cause increased vascular hydrostatic pressure. Decreased oncotic pressure results from a decrease in blood protein. Albumin has the most profound effect on oncotic pressure among all of the blood proteins, and hypoalbuminemia is the most common cause of decreased oncotic pressure. Hypoalbuminemia almost always causes the accumulation of pure transudates. Lastly, vasculitis is caused by inflammation of the vascular system. Vasculitis typically allows leakage of whole blood cells and serum into the pleural space, therefore causing the formation of modified transudates and exudates.

The second major etiology of pleural effusion is decreased fluid removal from the pleural space by the lymphatic system, which can lead to effusion even in the absence of increased fluid influx. Decreased lymphatic drainage can result from increased lymphatic pressure (e.g., from congestive heart failure, cardiac tamponade, lymphatic obstruction/stasis, or voluminous abdominal effusions) and leakage of lymph from the lymphatic system (e.g., caused by lymphatic inflammation [lymphangitis], lymphatic dilation [lymphangiectasia], lymphatic neoplasia, or lymphatic duct rupture).

Any pathological process can be complicated by multiple factors; therefore overlap of diseases and fluid categories is common. Furthermore, chronic effusions can change in character over time. As a general rule, disease processes cause pleural transudates and modified transudates by increased vascular hydrostatic pressure or decreased vascular oncotic pressure. Disorders of the lymphatic system typically cause chylous effusions, but modified transudates can also occur.

Etiology

Table 78-2 provides a comprehensive list of diseases that are associated with transudates and modified transudates.

INCREASED HYDROSTATIC PRESSURE

Increased hydrostatic pressure is caused primarily by congestive heart failure, cardiac tamponade, and vascular obstruction. In addition to pleural effusion, peritoneal effusion may also occur. In dogs, any form of heart disease that causes right-sided congestive heart failure, including pericardial effusion, could theoretically cause pleural effusion; however, cardiogenic pleural effusions are most commonly secondary to combined left and right heart failure. Congestive heart failure typically causes both peritoneal and pleural effusions in dogs. Pleural effusion has also been reported in a dog with the cardiopulmonary form of parvovirus infection.[4] In cats, left heart failure can cause pleural effusion, and the most common underlying disease is hypertrophic cardiomyopathy, although other forms of cardiomyopathy are also possible. Diseases that cause biventricular failure are less common, and right heart failure is rare.

Venous obstruction in the cranial vena cava or cranial part of the caudal vena cava can cause pleural effusion, peritoneal effusion, or both. Septic and neoplastic emboli can obstruct great vessels. Thrombi and thromboemboli in systemic and pulmonary vessels are potential serious complications of vasculitis, hypercoagulable states, and long-term indwelling venous catheters. Diseases associated with hypercoagulable states include hyperadrenocorticism, immune-mediated hemolytic anemia (IMHA), pancreatitis, congenital anticlotting factor deficiencies, and protein-losing nephropathies (PLN). These diseases often result in pulmonary thromboembolism (PTE).[5-7] PTE can also result from heartworm infestation.[8] Other causes of pulmonary venous obstruction include solid pulmonary neoplasms and lung lobe torsion (Figure 78-1).[9] Diaphragmatic hernias can cause obstruction of abdominal visceral vasculature entrapped in the diaphragm or thorax, as well as fluid leakage from strangulated organs, lymphatics, and the omentum.

DECREASED ONCOTIC PRESSURE

Diseases that cause low serum TP include primary and secondary hepatopathies, PLNs, protein-losing enteropathies (PLEs), and hemorrhage (e.g., chronic gastrointestinal tract bleeding). As a general rule, effusions occur when the serum albumin concentration is below 1.5 g/dl or when the serum total protein is below 3.5 g/dl.[3] However, diseases that cause protein loss are often multifactorial and may have associated inflammatory components. Thus vasculitis is a potential complication of systemic inflammation, which can

Transudate	Modified Transudate
Increased Hydrostatic Pressure	***Chronic Transudate Vasculitis***
Congestive heart failure	Systemic inflammation/infection
Pericardial effusion	• Sepsis
Heartworm infestation	• Rickettsial infection
Pulmonary thromboembolism	Pancreatitis
Lung lobe torsion	Local lung infection/abscess
Caval syndrome	Immune-mediated disease
	• IMHA
Decreased Oncotic Pressure (Hypoproteinemia)	• ITP
PLE/maldigestion/malabsorption	• SLE
• Inflammatory bowel disease	• Rickettsial infection
• Exocrine pancreatic insufficiency	Allergic/anaphylactic reaction
• Intestinal bacterial overgrowth	• Snake envenomation
• Lymphangiectasia	• Bee sting
• Gastrointestinal lymphoma	• Drug reaction
• Gastrointestinal fungal infection	• Mast cell disease
Liver failure	
• Toxic insult	***Increased Hydrostatic Pressure***
• Drug reaction	Lung lobe torsion
• Chronic active hepatitis	Pulmonary thromboembolism
• Cholangiohepatitis	Diaphragmatic hernia
• Lymphoma/neoplasia	Neoplasia
• Cirrhosis/fibrosis	
• End stage liver disease	***Neoplastic Effusion***
Systemic disease	Mesothelioma
• Protein-losing nephropathy	Lymphoma
• Chronic infection/inflammation	Thymoma
• Amyloidosis	Primary or metastatic lung tumor
• Fanconi syndrome	Carcinomatosis
• Renal lymphoma	
• Rickettsial infection	***Translocation of Abdominal Effusion***
• Heartworm disease	Any abdominal transudate or modified transudate
• Lyme nephritis	
• Systemic lupus erythematosus	
Translocation of Abdominal Transudate	
• Hepatic hydrothorax	
• Peritoneal dialysis	
• Any abdominal transudate	

TABLE 78-2. **Differential Diagnoses for Pleural Transudates and Modified Transudates**

cause pleural effusion at a higher than predicted total protein level.

INCREASED VASCULAR PERMEABILITY

Increased vascular permeability allows leakage of cells and protein through the vascular and pleural endothelial linings into the pleural space, resulting in the formation of modified transudates and exudates. Diseases associated with vasculitis and pleural effusion include pancreatitis, systemic inflammation and infections, allergic reactions, and cancers such as mast cell tumors. Profound hypoproteinemia from vasculitis or peritonitis contributes to effusion formation. Inflammation in the abdomen can also extend directly into the thoracic cavity. For instance, pancreatitis can cause a local peritonitis, and the inflammation can extend through the diaphragm into the thorax. Pancreatitis also causes systemic inflammation by release of pancreatic enzymes and vasoactive substances into the circulatory system, which in turn exacerbates pleural effusion.[10-12]

Tick-borne diseases (especially Rocky Mountain spotted fever and canine ehrlichiosis), and systemic allergic reactions (e.g., overwhelming bee-stings or snake envenomation) can cause vasculitis, systemic inflammation, and subsequent pleural effusion.[13-14] Fluid may leak into any body cavity or the interstitium. Just as with

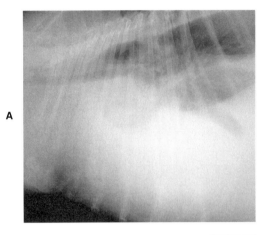

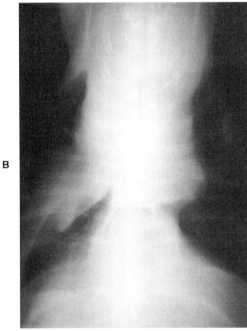

*Figure 78-1. **A,** Lateral and **B,** dorsoventral thoracic radiographs of a dog with a lung lobe torsion pleural effusion.*

other causes of systemic inflammation, the resultant hypoalbuminemia further compounds fluid leakage.

INCREASED LYMPHATIC PRESSURE AND LYMPHATIC LEAKAGE

Increased lymphatic pressure is caused primarily by cardiac disease (e.g., increased right atrial pressures), vascular and lymphatic vessel aberrations (e.g., arteriovenous fistulas), and lymphatic obstruction. Causes of lymphatic obstruction and leakage include lymphatic neoplasia (e.g., lymphangiosarcoma and lymphangioma), lymphatic blockage from extra-lymphatic masses, inflammation of the lymphatic system (e.g., lymphangitis), and lymphangiectasia. Usually, these disease processes cause chylous effusions, but modified transudates can occur, particularly when the patient is anorectic or consumes a low-fat diet.

VOLUME OVERLOAD OF THE LYMPHATIC SYSTEM

Abdominal effusions can overflow into the pleural space indirectly through the lymphatic system. It is theorized that abdominal effusions drained by subdiaphragmatic lymphatics subsequently leak into the thorax. This process has been reported in a dog with bile peritonitis[15] and in dogs with hepatic failure and portal hypertension (hepatic hydrothorax).[16] Pleural effusion has also been reported as a complication of peritoneal dialysis.[17] In the reported case, it was theorized that abdominal fluid overflowed into the thoracic cavity through natural spaces in the diaphragm, such as through the hiatal openings around the esophagus and great vessels. This direct flow of fluid was suggested because analysis of the pleural fluid and dialysate was similar. Contrast studies could not document this communication, however.[17]

Epidemiology

Because pleural effusion is the result of so many different diseases, it is difficult to associate specific breeds of cats and dogs with pleural effusion. Theoretically, breeds predisposed to specific diseases associated with pleural effusion may be more likely to develop pleural effusion. For example, English bulldogs and boxers are predisposed to single, anomalous, right coronary artery and pulmonic stenosis. Mastiffs, samoyeds, miniature schnauzers, and West Highland white terriers also have an increased prevalence of pulmonic stenosis. Labrador retrievers have an increased prevalence of tricuspid valve dysplasia. Such congenital cardiac anomalies could lead to right-sided heart failure and resultant pleural effusion. Ventricular septal defects (VSDs) are a common congenital disease in the cat, but are more likely to result in left-sided congestive heart failure (pulmonary edema). However, even cats with primarily left-sided heart disease can present with pleural effusion.

Golden and Labrador retrievers have an increased incidence of PLN as a result of Lyme nephritis and nonspecific forms of GN in general.[18-20] Wheaten terriers, English cocker spaniels, and Bernese mountain dogs can have a familial form of glomerulonephritis.[21-24] These breeds may, therefore, be more likely to develop pleural effusion secondary to hypoproteinemia. Animals in heartworm endemic areas are naturally more likely to develop pleural effusion as a result of caval syndrome. Older animals and certain breeds such as golden retrievers and boxers are predisposed to neoplasia.[25] These animals may consequently be more likely to get cancer-associated pleural effusion. Afghan hounds have an increased incidence of lung lobe torsion, which often results in pleural effusions (usually chylothorax, but sometimes modified transudates).[26]

The point is that many breeds have breed-associated diseases, some of which may have pleural effusion as a complication. However, to the authors' knowledge, there is no published data of specific breeds, ages, or sex of either dogs or cats with increased incidence of pleural effusion.

Clinical Findings

HISTORY

Animals with pleural effusion have a variety of historical complaints, and symptoms depend upon the underlying disease. Signs most specifically related to pleural effusion include increased respiratory rate and effort, tachypnea, dyspnea, exercise intolerance, and open mouth breathing. The astute pet owner may also notice cyanosis in the severely compromised pet. In dogs, coughing is another common complaint, which may result from pleural irritation. Clients also commonly report that the pet is restless or uncomfortable. Pets are often reluctant to lie down, or they may behave as if it is painful to do so, likely because of discomfort in relation to increased pressure on the diaphragm from the pleural fluid. The restless behavior reflects the pet's attempt to find the most comfortable position that both minimizes diaphragmatic pressure and affords the most lung expansion.

Note that these symptoms are not specific to pleural effusion, and they overlap with signs of primary respiratory and cardiac disease. For example, coughing may also be the result of related or unrelated diseases such as primary lung disease, pulmonary edema, or bronchial compression secondary to cardiac enlargement.

Less specific signs of systemic illness including inappetence, weight loss, lethargy, and depression are common. Weight loss may be more pronounced in patients with diseases such as cardiac failure; cancer; protein-losing diseases (e.g., PLN, PLE, liver disease); and organ failure (e.g., kidney or liver). Gastrointestinal (GI) symptoms, although not specific, may be an indication of primary GI pathology. Polyuria is also common and may result from renal failure, liver failure, or hypercalcemia of malignancy. Polydipsia may also ensue as a result of decreased vascular volume (either from effusion or polyuria) and consequent aldosterone release and activation of the renin-angiotensin system.

The duration and progression of clinical signs depends upon the underlying pathology. In general, any disease causing pleural effusion is progressive without medical and/or surgical intervention. The rapidity of progression depends on the natural course of the underlying disease and on the response to therapy.

PHYSICAL EXAMINATION

Patients with pleural effusion typically, but not always, have physical examination findings attributable to pleural disease. Abnormal physical examination findings include dull lung sounds in the ventral thorax (the dorsal extent depends upon the amount of pleural fluid); and detection of a fluid/air interface via thoracic percussion, tachypnea, and dyspnea. Cats and dogs often sit in sternal recumbency with their elbows abducted. The larger the volume of pleural fluid, the more severe the degree of lung compromise and respiratory signs. The rate at which fluid accumulates also affects the severity of signs. At the same volume, a patient with slowly accumulating pleural fluid may be significantly less compro-

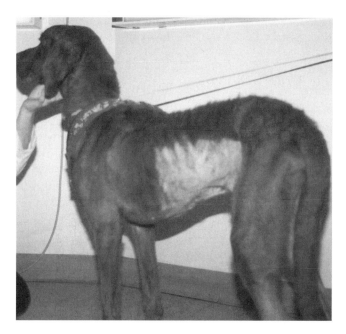

Figure 78-2. Cachectic dog with a protein-losing enteropathy.

mised than an animal that has a rapidly forming effusion because the former patient will have more time to adjust to and compensate for the changes in lung volume. Animals with severe effusion may be dyspneic and/or cyanotic, and as the volume of pleural effusion increases, paradoxical chest movements and abdominal breathing may also occur. The severity of respiratory symptoms is also influenced by other factors such as the patient's packed red cell volume, the presence of underlying lung disease, heart function, acid-base status, and strength. For example, a patient that is anemic or has concurrent primary pulmonary parenchymal disease may have more severe respiratory embarrassment in spite of a lower volume of effusion.

Other abnormal physical examination findings depend upon the underlying disease. Patients with heart disease usually have concurrent signs attributable to heart disease (e.g., murmurs, tachycardia, gallop rhythms, arrhythmias, weak pulses, cardiac cachexia, ascites, subcutaneous edema, jugular pulses, or generalized venous engorgement). Additionally, signs of poor perfusion (e.g., pale mucous membranes and slow capillary refill time) may be present. Pericardial effusion patients typically have muffled heart sounds, pale mucous membranes, and weak pulses. They may also have paradoxical pulses, which is pathognomonic for pericardial effusion. In addition to pleural effusion, animals with hypoproteinemia may have concurrent signs attributable to decreased oncotic pressure including ascites and dependent edema. Extreme muscle wasting may be noted in animals with protein-losing disease, cancer, and cardiac disease (Figure 78-2). Patients with venous obstructive disease may have ascites or asymmetrical limb or dependent edema. Cancer patients may have palpable masses or lymphadenomegaly, PLE patients may have melena upon rectal examination, and patients in liver failure may have altered mentation secondary to hepatoencephalopathy. Uremic breath or melena may be detected in PLN patients in renal failure.

Diagnostics

A full medical work-up to determine the underlying cause is warranted in patients with pleural effusion. One of the most important tests is pleural fluid analysis. At the very least, fluid should be analyzed for protein content, nucleated and red cell counts, and cytological context. Characterization of the fluid is essential to nar- rowing the spectrum of differential diagnoses. The de- termination is not always simple, however, and more elaborate tests such as fibronectin and adenosine deaminase concentrations may be useful. These tests are not specific, however, and do have limitations.[27-29] Bacterial cultures are unlikely to be helpful in transu- dates and modified transudates because these effusions are almost exclusively sterile. However, cases that re- quire frequent thoracocentesis, or that have implants (e.g., chest tubes, pleuro-venous shunts) may develop secondary infections.

The volume of pleural effusion and the degree of res- piratory compromise should dictate how much fluid to remove. If the patient is not dyspneic, then a small sam- ple for diagnostic purposes may be all that is required. If the patient is compromised, then as much fluid as pos- sible should be removed while obtaining the sample for analysis.

A thorough medical work-up should include, at a minimum, lateral and ventrodorsal (VD) thoracic radi- ographs (ideally, before and after thoracocentesis); com- plete blood count (CBC); serum chemistry analysis (CS); urinalysis (UA); and abdominal ultrasound. A VD tho- racic radiograph is preferred over the dorsoventral (DV) view when small volume effusions are present because of the greater magnification of the fluid.[3] In other words, a VD view will more likely detect a small volume of pleural fluid (Figure 78-3). A patient's life should not be threatened to obtain a VD view, however. Special radio- graphic views such as horizontal beam standing laterals may also be helpful in documenting effusion and tho- racic masses. Horizontal beam views are also more ac- commodating to patients with severe respiratory com- promise. If pulmonary or thoracic masses are suspected, thoracic ultrasonography is often very helpful. Ideally, thoracic ultrasound is performed while some of the pleural fluid remains to optimize visualization of in- trathoracic/extrapulmonary structures (Figure 78-4).[30-31]

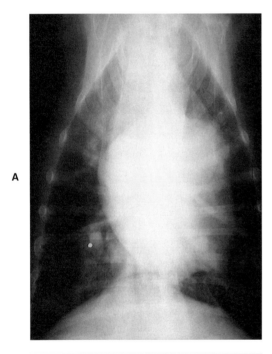

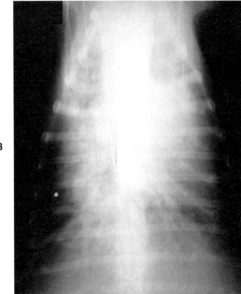

Figure 78-3. A, Dorsoventral compared with **B,** ventrodorsal view of a dog with pleural effusion. Note the enhancement of imaging of the pleural effusion in the ventrodorsal view.

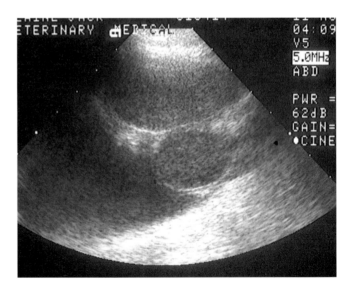

Figure 78-4. Ultrasound image of a thoracic mass surrounded by pleural fluid.

CARDIAC DISEASE

Physical examination findings or thoracic radiographs suggestive of cardiac disease warrant further investigation with an electrocardiogram (EKG), echocardiogram, and heartworm testing. If studies suggest cardiac disease, then evaluation by a cardiologist is ideal (Figure 78-5). More detailed tests such as vascular studies or angiography may be required for specific diagnosis of cardiac disease, especially in the case of complex congenital heart defects.

NEOPLASIA

Intrathoracic neoplasia can cause pleural effusion by vascular compression, and any cancer can cause thromboemboli. Neoplasia can also involve the pleural lining directly. Diagnosis from cytology alone can often be made from cancers that exfoliate easily. Effusions from these cancers are classified as neoplastic effusions, but often fall under the broad category of modified transudates. Lymphosarcoma and mesothelioma are examples of such neoplasms. Careful interpretation is necessary to avoid overdiagnosis of cancer, however, because reactive mesothelial cells are commonly present in chronic effusions with inflammation. Similarly, reactive or increased numbers of lymphocytes are seen with lymphatic leakage. Adenocarcinomas rarely exfoliate cells, except when carcinomatosis is present. When neoplasms do not exfoliate readily, tissue samples for histopathology are required for a definitive diagnosis. Tissue samples can often be obtained by ultrasound-guided aspirate or biopsy if a large intrathoracic or pulmonary mass is present; however, thoracoscopy or exploratory thoracotomy may be necessary for diagnostic samples.

PROTEIN-LOSING ENTEROPATHY

Biochemical and historical implications of PLEs include panhypoproteinemia and gastrointestinal symptoms. Gastrointestinal hemorrhage is suggested by a history of melena or hematemesis, normochromic/normocytic or microcytic/hypochromic anemia, thrombocytosis, increased blood urea nitrogen (BUN):creatinine ratio, panhypoproteinemia, and a positive fecal occult blood test. Further diagnostics to support a diagnosis of PLE include abdominal ultrasound, intestinal biopsies (surgical or endoscopic), serum trypsin-like immunoassay, cobalamin, and folate determination.

HEPATIC DISEASE

If initial medical screening suggests that liver disease is the underlying cause, then further diagnostics to determine the extent and cause of liver disease should be pursued. Chemistry results suggestive of decreased liver function include decreased serum albumin, glucose, and BUN; increased bilirubin; and increased or decreased cholesterol. Commonly, liver enzymes are elevated. More specific tests of liver function include prothrombin (PT) and partial thromboplastin (PTT) times, blood ammonia concentration, and serum bile acids. Abdominal radiographs are useful for evaluating hepatic size. Abdominal ultrasound is also helpful for evaluation of hepatic echogenicity and identification of liver masses. Ultimately, a liver biopsy may be indicated. A liver biopsy should be submitted for histopathology and aerobic and anaerobic culture, if indicated. A full coagulation profile (i.e., PT, PTT, fibrinogen, fibrin degradation products, and manual platelet count) is not only performed as an assessment of liver function but also in anticipation of liver biopsy. It can also be indicative of disseminated intravascular coagulation (DIC), a common complication of fulminant liver failure. Lastly, a coagulation profile will determine if blood products such as fresh frozen plasma or whole blood transfusions are indicated.

PROTEIN-LOSING NEPHROPATHY

Biochemical abnormalities suggestive of a PLN include proteinuria; hypoalbuminemia; hypercholesterolemia; and, at times, azotemia. If a PLN is suspected, further work-up should include a urine culture/sensitivity, an abdominal ultrasound, and a urine protein:creatinine ratio. A variety of diseases, including bacterial and rickettsial infections, chronic inflammation, immune-mediated/autoimmune, heartworm disease, and neoplasia can cause PLNs. Tests to rule out these problems include, but are not limited to, tick serology; thoracic radiographs; antinuclear antibody titer; Coomb's test; heartworm antigen testing; abdominal ultrasound; and ultimately, kidney biopsy. Hypercoagulable states, thromboembolic disease, and hypertension are common complications of PLNs. Therefore, a coagulation profile, antithrombin III quantification, and blood pressure measurement should also be performed in order to help guide therapy.

LYMPHATIC DISEASE

A lymphangiogram is necessary to document lymphatic obstruction and leakage. Once obstruction or leakage is identified, additional diagnostics to determine the cause may include surgical exploration and biopsies.

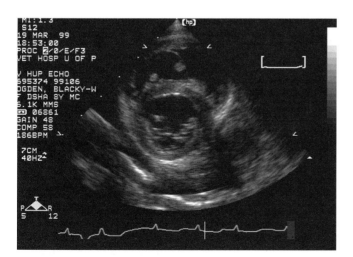

Figure 78-5. *Ultrasound short axis parasternal view of the heart from the right side. Note the pleural effusion surrounding the heart (anechoic space). This cat was diagnosed with restrictive cardiomyopathy and congestive heart failure.*

IDIOPATHIC PLEURAL EFFUSION

Occasionally, an underlying cause of pleural effusion is not found. Lack of diagnosis does not mean the effusion is idiopathic, however: it simply means the cause has not been identified. In such a case, serial pleural fluid analysis and repeat medical work-up should be done until a definitive diagnosis is ascertained.

Management

EMERGENCY MANAGEMENT

Initial emergency stabilization of the dyspneic patient takes priority over diagnostics. Therapeutic thoracocentesis is the most important and helpful procedure, and is life saving in many instances. Oxygen, diuretics, transfusions, and other treatments that do not increase the space into which the lung can expand are futile unless they are done in conjunction with thoracocentesis. Thoracic ultrasound is helpful in guiding thoracocentesis if the fluid is loculated or isolated in pockets.

Other emergency procedures for short-term patient relief may be necessary while pursuit of a definitive diagnosis ensues. If there is primary lung disease, oxygen therapy may be required, even after pleural effusion is evacuated. Oxygen can be delivered by mask, nasal insufflation, oxygen cage, or even mechanical ventilation, depending on the circumstances. Animals in heart failure may need oxygen, diuretics, vasodilators, or antiarrhythmic medications. Hypoproteinemic animals may need colloid support via synthetic colloids, plasma, or albumin transfusions. If the underlying disease is not addressed, however, colloids and oxygen will only be of temporary benefit. It is difficult, impractical, and cost-prohibitive to provide these therapies indefinitely.

MEDICAL THERAPY

Once the patient is stabilized by thoracocentesis and other emergency treatments, a full medical work-up is paramount to definitive diagnosis. It cannot be emphasized enough that pleural effusion itself is not a primary problem: it is always caused by an underlying disease. Symptomatic treatment of pleural effusion alone is futile because pleural fluid will continuously re-form unless the underlying disease is addressed. Definitive treatment will depend on the etiologic diagnosis.

Cardiac Therapy

Specific therapy should be chosen depending on the results of the physical examination and cardiology diagnostics. Congestive heart failure should be addressed with furosemide therapy; however, it is inappropriate to begin treating a patient with significant pleural effusion with diuretics without physically removing the effusion via thoracocentesis first. If furosemide therapy is not successful alone for controlling congestive heart failure, triple diuretic therapy can be initiated with the addition of hydrochlorothiazide and spironolactone. The specific underlying heart disease should be addressed as well.

For example, if the patient is a cat with hypertrophic cardiomyopathy, a beta-blocker (atenolol) or calcium channel blocker (diltiazem) should be added. If there is evidence of myocardial failure (e.g., a dog with dilated cardiomyopathy), a positive inotropic agent such as digoxin should be added. Angiotensin converting enzyme inhibition is warranted to reduce the activity of the renin-angiotensin-aldosterone hormone axis in animals with congestive heart failure. Symptomatic ventricular tachyarrhythmias can be addressed with procainamide or mexilitine (class I antiarrhythmics), sotalol (combined class 2 and 3 antiarrhythmic), or other antiarrhythmic agents. Supraventricular tachyarrhythmias should be addressed by controlling congestive heart failure, and medical management with digoxin, beta blockade, or a calcium channel blocker.

Thyrotoxicosis can result in pleural effusion alone or, more often, in conjunction with underlying primary heart disease. Elevated circulating thyroid hormone results in tachycardia, cardiac hypertrophy, and increased contractility. Although the heart is hyperkinetic at rest, there is less cardiac reserve capacity available and the total cardiac workload increases. Thus hyperthyroidism, especially in the patient with preexisting heart disease, may result in congestive heart failure with or without pleural effusion. Patients at risk of thyrotoxicosis (e.g., cats older than 7 years of age) or with signs suggestive of hyperthyroidism (e.g., weight loss or polyphagia) should be screened for the endocrinopathy. Many of the clinical manifestations of thyrotoxicosis are reversible once a euthyroid state is restored via surgery, medical management, or radioiodine therapy. Until thyrotoxicosis is addressed, a beta-blocker such as atenolol is warranted to protect the heart from elevated circulating thyroid hormone levels.

Cancer Therapy

Thoracic or systemic neoplasia is treated with the appropriate drug or other modality based upon a histological diagnosis. Treatment may require systemic chemotherapeutic agents, radiation therapy, surgical removal or debulking, steroids, intralesional or intracavitary chemotherapeutics, or any combination of the above.

Therapy for Protein-Losing Enteropathy

Protein-losing enteropathies are caused by numerous diseases; therefore, specific treatment depends upon the definitive diagnosis. Causes of PLEs include lymphangiectasia, inflammatory bowel disease (IBD), gastrointestinal lymphoma, infections, immune-mediated diseases, and many other disorders. Treatment often includes special diets formulated from highly digestible and/or novel proteins; steroids for antiinflammatory and antineoplastic purposes; other immunosuppressive drugs (e.g., azathioprine and chlorambucil for immune-mediated disease); and anticancer chemotherapeutics.

Therapy for Hepatic Disease

Treatment of liver disease is both symptomatic and specific. Definitive treatments depend upon the particular hepatopathy. Symptomatic therapy may include fluid therapy, lactulose, nutritional support, antibiotics, vitamin and mineral supplementation (e.g., vitamin K and zinc supplementation), steroids, and S-adenylmethionine.

Therapy for Protein-Losing Nephropathy

The primary cause of a PLN is particularly difficult to identify in most cases. If identified, the primary disease should be treated. Urinary tract and systemic bacterial infections are treated with the appropriate antibiotics based upon a culture and sensitivity. Tick-borne infections are treated with an appropriate anti-rickettsial agent such as doxycycline. Inflammatory foci are treated medically and/or surgically. Cancer is addressed with the appropriate protocol. Nonspecific therapy is also used in conjunction with definitive treatment and is focused on decreasing glomerular protein loss, slowing progression of renal damage, and for symptomatic relief. Moderately restricted protein diets are used to decrease glomerular sclerosis and progression of renal damage. Omega-3 fatty acids can be added as a supplement and are included in some renal diets because their antiinflammatory effects can decrease renal damage from proteases.

Angiotensin converting enzyme inhibitors are used to decrease renal protein loss by selectively vasodilating the efferent glomerular arterioles. They are also beneficial for decreasing systemic arterial blood pressure (systemic hypertension is a common sequela of PLN). Low-dose aspirin is used to block cyclooxygenase and platelet activating factor activities, enzyme pathways theorized to potentiate glomerular damage. Care must be used in animals with overt renal failure or uremic gastritis because aspirin can exacerbate these problems. Gastric protectants such as famotidine, sucralfate, or misoprostol are indicated in the face of GI complications. If anorexia and azotemia are present, then periodic fluid therapy is used to maintain hydration. Steroids are generally not recommended and often have detrimental side effects in patients with PLN. The exception is PLN secondary to systemic lupus erythematosus. Unfortunately, many PLNs are deemed idiopathic, and only nonspecific therapy can be used.

Treatment of Lymphatic Disease

Lymphatic obstruction caused by mass lesions is treated surgically. Lymphangioma/sarcoma is treated with appropriate chemotherapy. Lymphangitis and lymphangiectasia are medically treated with antiinflammatory drugs and low-fat diets with highly digestible proteins. The use of medium-chain triglycerides to supply lipids not carried by the lymphatic system is controversial. Rutin, although also controversial, may decrease leakage of lymphatic fluid into body cavities and the interstitium.

SYMPTOMATIC THERAPY

In many cases, pleural fluid continuously forms despite definitive treatment. The goal of disease-specific therapy is to bring about a cure. Realistically, therapy should decrease the volume of pleural fluid as well as the rate at which it is formed. In most cases, nonspecific therapy is needed in addition to specific medical treatment.

Symptomatic medical therapy includes periodic thoracocentesis and administration of low doses of diuretics. The goal of diuretic therapy is to decrease the frequency and volume of fluid formation in order to decrease the need for repeated emergency room visits for thoracocentesis. Diuretics are used to decrease hydrostatic pressure, and therefore the amount and rate of fluid influx into the pleural space; they are used at the lowest effective dose. In congestive heart failure, furosemide is effective by reducing cardiac preload. Furosemide treatment should be started at the lower end of the dose and gradually increased to effect. Hydration status of the patient should be monitored frequently because dehydration can cause or exacerbate azotemia and worsen clinical signs. If an effusion caused by heart disease is refractory to furosemide therapy, then combination diuretic therapy may be tried.

Diuretics do not remove pleural fluid once it has formed; therefore, thoracocentesis must be performed if significant fluid is present. Complications of thoracocentesis are rare, but they become more likely with frequent thoracocentesis. Complications include pleural scarring and thickening (pleural fibrosis), pneumothorax, iatrogenic infections, cardiac puncture, hemorrhage, and the inherent risks of repetitive sedation.

SURGICAL MANAGEMENT

Surgical management of pleural effusion is indicated when a surgical condition is found or when medical therapy alone is ineffective. Surgical conditions include mediastinal (excluding lymphoma) and solitary lung masses, lung lobe torsions, congenital heart malformations, and diaphragmatic hernias. Surgery is occasionally required to obtain tissue samples for histopathologic diagnosis. If surgery is not curative, then follow-up medical management (e.g., chemotherapy or diuretics) or palliative procedures are necessary.

The goal of nonspecific surgical treatment is to either remove pleural fluid from the thoracic cavity or to decrease fluid production. A nonspecific surgical approach implies that the surgery does not target the underlying cause and, therefore, it is not curative (just as nonspecific medical management does not treat a specific disease and is, therefore, not curative). Chest tubes, thoracic shunts, thoracic omentalization, and pleurodesis are all examples of nonspecific surgical treatment.

Chest Tubes

Chest tubes are occasionally needed for temporary pleural drainage to decrease the frequency of thoracocentesis and its associated risks. They are also used postoperatively when fluid accumulation is expected to continue for a finite period. Chest tubes do not address the underlying cause, however; they are strictly therapeutic and, therefore, should only be used when absolutely necessary and while attempts are made to address the underlying problem. Chest tubes are not feasible for long-term management for several reasons: they cannot be managed at home, they can leak air into the chest if the tubes and connections become worn or disconnect, they can become secondarily infected (especially with nosocomial bacteria), and prolonged implantation in the chest causes irritation that exacerbates effusion.

Palliative Procedures

Several palliative surgical treatment options are available if surgical correction and definitive or nonspecific medical therapy alone are not adequate to control pleural effusion. Palliative procedures are reserved for refractory cases with pleural effusion that persists despite all medical and surgical therapies. Palliative surgical treatments provide additional thoracic fluid drainage or decreased pleural effusion production by various methods.

Pleuro-peritoneal and pleuro-venous shunts and diaphragmatic meshes shift fluid from the chest to the abdomen or venous system.[32] Pleural fluid can be life threatening because it decreases tidal volume and ventilation. Shunting the fluid from the thoracic to the abdominal cavity or venous system shifts the fluid to a space that is less critical to survival. It also provides a larger surface for the fluid to be absorbed into the systemic circulation. Such surgeries do not solve the underlying problem nor are they curative. The goal as with other nonspecific treatments, is to decrease the frequency with which thoracocentesis is performed. Unfortunately, shunts and meshes are not fail-proof. They often malfunction and become obstructed with fibrin. Therefore, thoracocentesis is still occasionally necessary, and multiple surgeries may be necessary to replace or unclog shunts.

Transdiaphragmatic omentalization has been described in the dog and cat for treatment of refractory chylothorax.[33] Insertion of omentum into the thorax works similarly to shunting the fluid into the abdomen. Omentalization increases the absorptive surface for the effusion. Theoretically, this method should prove even more helpful with transudates and modified transudates than with chylous effusions.

Pleurodesis is used to halt or reduce pleural fluid formation by causing fibrosis of the fluid-producing pleural lining. Chemical irritants are instilled into the thoracic cavity to cause adhesions between the visceral and parietal pleura. Some human studies and some experimental studies in animals have shown good success with such procedures.[34] Other studies have been less promising, however.[35,36] Agents used for pleurodesis include tetracycline and quincocrine hydrochloride, nitrogen mustard, bleomycin, 5-fluorouracil, doxorubicin, thiotepa, and talc. Tetracycline hydrochloride appears to be the preferred agent in dogs.[33]

Outcome and Prognosis

There is a large gray zone with respect to outcome and prognosis of pleural effusion, ranging from complete cure to rapid deterioration and death. This is not surprising given the numerous causes of pleural effusion. In general, serious and systemic diseases cause pleural effusions. In the short term, the prognosis is often guarded to grave because it is a life-threatening acute condition and there is a high probability of a serious un-

derlying disease. The long-term prognosis depends upon the diagnosis and the patient's ability to survive the initial crisis.

Effusions secondary to systemic inflammation and infection, and those caused by surgically correctable problems, can completely resolve if the underlying disease is successfully treated. For example, pancreatitis, vasculitis, systemic inflammation and infections, and allergic reactions are potentially reversible. Patients occasionally survive PTE if the underlying cause is successfully treated. Surgically curable diseases such as benign thoracic masses, diaphragmatic hernias, and lung lobe torsions carry a good long-term prognosis provided the patient survives the surgery, anesthesia, and immediate postoperative period. Surgically correctable but not curable diseases such as solitary malignant lung or thoracic tumors also carry a fair to good long-term prognosis. For example, patients with solitary pulmonary adenocarcinoma can survive 1 to 2 years before recurrence of disease.[37] Mesotheliomas can be successfully treated with intracavitary cisplatin for 1 to 2.5 years, and the patients can enjoy good quality lives.[38] Diseases that cannot be cured or that are refractory to medical management carry a worse prognosis (e.g., refractory liver disease, IBD, neoplasia, and PLN).

The prognosis for patients with congestive heart failure depends on the underlying heart disease and interrelated factors (e.g., thyroid status). For example, some dogs with dilated cardiomyopathy, congestive heart failure, and concurrent arrhythmias may live less than a month, whereas dogs with chronic valve disease and congestive heart failure occasionally may live longer than 2 years with appropriate therapy. Animals with dual cavity or eosinophilic effusions are more likely to have cancer, and consequently have a worse prognosis.[10,39]

In general, animals with curable disease should have complete resolution of pleural effusion as well as symptoms if definitive treatment is successful. Patients with diseases that are manageable should, at least, have prolonged periods of remission (symptom-free) or improved quality of life if treatment is pursued. Pleural effusion secondary to refractory or untreatable disease carries a grave short and long-term prognosis.

REFERENCES

1. Forrester D, Troy G, Fossum T: Pleural effusions: Pathophysiology and diagnostic consideration, *Compend Contin Educ Pract Vet* 10:121-136, 1988.
2. Fossum TW: Pleural and extrapleural diseases. In Ettinger SJ, Feldman EC, editors: *Textbook of veterinary internal medicine*, Philadelphia, 2000, WB Saunders.
3. Padrid P: Canine and feline pleural disease, *Vet Clin North Am Small Anim Pract* 30:1295-1307, 2000.
4. Yates RW, Weller RE: Have you seen the cardiopulmonary form of parvovirus infection? *Vet Med* 83(4):380, 382, 384, 386, 1988.
5. LaRue JM, Murtaugh RJ: Pulmonary thromboembolism in dogs: 47 cases (1986-1987), *JAVMA* 197:1368-1372, 1990.
6. Nichols R: Complications and concurrent disease associated with canine hyperadrenocorticism, *Vet Clin North Am Small Anim Pract* 27:309-320, 1997.
7. Dennis JS: The pathophysiologic sequelae of pulmonary thromboembolism, *Compend Contin Educ Pract Vet* 13:1811-1818, 1991.

8. Carr AP, Johnson GS: A review of hemostatic abnormalities in dogs and cats, *J Am Anim Hosp Assoc* 30:475-481, 1994.
9. Dye TL, Teague HD, Pounderstone ML: Lung lobe torsion in a cat with chronic feline asthma, *J Am Anim Hosp Assoc* 34:493-495, 1998.
10. Steyn PF, Wittum TE: Radiographic, epidemiologic, and clinical aspects of simultaneous pleural and peritoneal effusions in dogs and cats: 48 cases (1982-1991), *JAVMA* 202:307-312, 1993.
11. Schaer M: Acute pancreatitis in dogs, *Compend Contin Educ Pract Vet* 13:1771-1780, 1991.
12. Simpson KW: Current concepts of the pathogenesis and pathophysiology of acute pancreatitis in the dog and cat, *Compend Contin Educ Pract Vet* 15:247-251, 1993.
13. Halkin A, Jaffe R, Mevorach D et al: Thoracic complications following snake envenomation, *Am J Med* 102:585-587, 1997.
14. Frendin J, Obel N: Catheter drainage of pleural fluid collections and pneumothorax, *J Small Anim Pract* 38:237-242, 1997.
15. Barnhart MD, Rasmussen LM: Pleural effusion as a complication of extrahepatic biliary tract rupture in a dog, *J Am Anim Hosp Assoc* 32:409-412, 1996.
16. Center SA: Pathophysiology of liver disease: Normal and abnormal function. In Guilford WG et al, editors: *Strombeck's small animal gastroenterology*, Philadelphia, 1996, WB Saunders.
17. Carter LJ, Wingfield WE, Allen TA: Clinical experience with peritoneal dialysis in small animals, *Compend Contin Educ Pract Vet* 11:1335-1338, 1340, 1342-1343, 1989.
18. Dambach DM, Smith CA, Lewis RM et al: Morphological, immunohistochemical, and ultrastructural characterization of a distinctive renal lesion in dogs putatively associated with *Borrelia burgdorferi* infection: 49 cases (1987-1992), *Vet Pathol* 34:85-96, 1997.
19. Cook AK, Cowgill LD: Clinical and pathological features of protein-losing glomerular disease in the dog: A review of 137 cases (1985-1992), *J Am Anim Hosp Assoc* 32:313-322, 1996.
20. Sanders NA: Canine "Lyme nephritis," *Proceedings of the 18th Annual ACVIM Veterinary Medical Forum* 627-628, 2000.
21. Littman MP, Dambach DM, Vaden SL et al: Familial protein-losing enteropathy and protein-losing nephropathy in soft-coated wheaten terriers: 222 Cases (1983-19970), *J Vet Intern Med* 14:68-80, 2000.
22. Lees GE, Helman RG, Homco LD et al: Early diagnosis of familial nephropathy in English cocker spaniels, *J Am Anim Hosp Assoc* 34:189-195, 1998.
23. Reusch C, Hoerauf A, Lechner M et al: A new familial glomerulonephropathy in Bernese mountain dogs, *Vet Rec* 134:411-415, 1994.
24. Minkus G, Brever W, Wanke R et al: Familial nephropathy in Bernese mountain dogs, *Vet Pathol* 31:421-428, 1994.
25. Craig L: Causes of death in dogs according to breed: A necropsy survey of five breeds, *J Am Anim Hosp Assoc* 37:438-443, 2001.
26. Neath PJ, Brockman DJ, King LG: Lung lobe torsion in dogs: 22 cases (1981-1999), *JAVMA* 21:1041-1044, 2001.
27. Hirschenberger J, Pusch S: Fibronectin concentrations in pleural and abdominal effusions in dogs and cats, *J Vet Intern Med* 10:321-325, 1996.
28. Hirschberger J, Pusch S, Loewsch U et al: Validation of commercial human fibronectin assay for use in dogs and cats, *Aust Vet J* 73:196-197, 1996.
29. Hirschberger J, Koch S: Validation of the determination of activity of adenosine deaminase in the body effusions of cats, *Res Vet Sci* 59:226-229, 1995.
30. Stowater JL, Lamb CR: Ultrasonography of noncardiac thoracic disease in small animals, *JAVMA* 195:514-520, 1989.
31. Tidwell AS: Ultrasonography of the thorax (excluding the heart), *Vet Clin North Am Small Anim Pract* 28:993-1015, 1998.
32. Smeak DD, Gallagher L, Birchard SJ et al: Management of intractable pleural effusion in a dog with a pleuroperitoneal shunt, *Vet Surg* 16:212-216, 1987.
33. Lafond E, Weirech WE, Salisbury SK: Omentalization of the thorax for treatment of idiopathic chylothorax with constrictive pleuritis in a cat, *J Am Anim Hosp Assoc* 38:74-78, 2002.
34. Gallagher LA, Birchard SJ, Wiesbrode SE: Effects of tetracycline hydrochloride on pleurae in dogs with induced pleural effusion, *Am J Vet Res* 51:1682-1687, 1990.
35. Gallagher LA, Birchard SJ: Tetracycline hydrochloride pleurodesis: An experimental study in a canine effusion model, *Vet Surg* 17(1):33, 1988.
36. Hawkins E, Fossum T: Medical and surgical management of pleural effusion. In Bonagura J, editor: *Kirk's current veterinary therapy*, vol 13, Philadelphia, 2000, WB Saunders.
37. Shapiro W, Turrell J: Management of pleural effusion secondary to metastatic adenocarcinoma in a dog, *JAVMA* 192:530-532, 1988.
38. Moore AS, Kirk C, Cardona A: Intracavitary cisplatin chemotherapy experience with six dogs, *J Vet Intern Med* 5:227-231, 1991.
39. Fossum TW, Wellman M, Redford RL et al: Eosinophilic pleural or peritoneal effusions in dogs and cats: 14 cases (1986-1992), *JAVMA* 202:1873-1876, 1993.

CHAPTER 79

Chylothorax

Theresa W. Fossum

Management of animals with chylothorax has been greatly refined since the initial report of its surgical treatment in 3 dogs and 1 cat in 1958.[1] However, our ability to effectively treat many affected animals has been hindered by a lack of understanding of the etiology of this devastating disease. Appropriate treatment of affected animals depends foremost on confirming the diagnosis and defining the cause. Once the diagnosis has been made and concurrent diseases ruled out, the value of medical versus surgical treatment must be considered.

Thus a review of the diagnosis of chylothorax and the various underlying conditions associated with it is warranted. This will be followed by a discussion of medical and surgical management of this disease in dogs and cats.

Causes and Associated Diseases

Chylothorax was previously thought to be caused by thoracic duct rupture secondary to trauma; however, this is now known to be a relatively rare cause of chylothorax in animals. Although traumatic rupture of the thoracic duct may occur, the thoracic duct spontaneously heals in most of these animals and clinical signs associated with chylothorax are not recognized.[2,3] More commonly recognized causes include mediastinal lymphosarcoma,[4] cardiomyopathy[5] (particularly secondary to hyperthyroidism), pericardial disease,[6,7] congenital cardiac abnormalities, heartworm infection,[8,9] fungal granulomas, cranial vena cava thrombi, lung lobe torsion, and congenital abnormalities of the thoracic duct.[10] Unfortunately, despite extensive diagnostic work-up, the underlying etiology is undetermined (idiopathic chylothorax) in a majority of animals.[11,12] Because treatment of this disease varies considerably depending on the underlying etiology, it is imperative that clinicians identify concurrent disease processes before instituting definitive therapy.

Any disease that results in high venous pressures may cause chylothorax; cardiomyopathy, pericardial effusion, congenital cardiac abnormalities, and heartworm disease have been associated with chylothorax. Thus a complete cardiac work-up is warranted in any animal with confirmed chylothorax. Treatment of animals with cardiomyopathy and chylothorax should be based primarily on palliation (including thoracocentesis when necessary), and improving cardiac output and decreasing venous pressures with appropriate drug therapy. If pericardial effusion is diagnosed, the underlying etiology should be determined and pericardiectomy performed, if indicated. Although heartworm infection is uncommon in cats, experimental infection with *Dirofilaria immitis* has been shown to result in chylothorax in a small number of cases.[8] Naturally occurring heartworm disease has also been associated with chylothorax in a cat.[9] Therefore it is recommended that animals with chylothorax be screened for heartworm infection.

If an anterior mediastinal mass is identified, a fine-needle aspirate may be performed to determine the tumor or tissue type. Specific therapy (e.g., radiation therapy, chemotherapy, antifungal therapy, or surgery) should then be instituted according to findings. In these animals, the chylous effusion is probably secondary to compression of the cranial vena cava by the mass, and shrinkage of the mass may result in resolution of the pleural fluid. For prognostic purposes, it is prudent to assess FeLV and FIV status in affected cats.

When no obvious underlying disorder can be found, the term "idiopathic" chylothorax is used. Unfortunately, management of animals with idiopathic chylothorax is difficult because no highly effective treatment exists. Until the etiology of chylothorax in these animals is understood, therapy will remain palliative and less than optimal in many instances. One possibility is that these animals have increased volumes of lymph being transported through the thoracic duct. This increased flow may occur secondary to abnormal right-sided venous pressures that cause much of the lymph that would normally be transported from the liver into the venous system to be shunted into the lymphatic system. Minimally elevated venous pressures, in association with other unknown factors, may possibly be sufficient to substantially elevate lymphatic flows through the thoracic duct.

Fibrosing pleuritis is a condition that occurs occasionally in cats with chronic chylothorax. It consists of thickening and fibrosis of the pleura, resulting in gradually progressive compression atelectasis of lung lobes. In addition to chylothorax, pyothorax, feline infectious peritonitis, hemothorax, and tuberculosis have been associated with the development of fibrosing pleuritis in animals. Although the cause of the fibrosis is unknown, it apparently can develop subsequent to any prolonged exudative or blood-stained effusion. Exudates are characterized by a high rate of fibrin formation and degradation. Fibrin formation probably increases because chronic inflammatory exudates, such as chylothorax and pyothorax, induce changes in mesothelial cell morphologic features, resulting in increased permeability, mesothelial cell desquamation, and triggering of both pathways of the coagulation cascade. These desquamated mesothelial cells have also been shown to produce type III collagen in cell culture, promoting fibrosis. Additionally, the chronic presence of pleural fluid might lead to an impairment in the mechanism of fibrin degradation. Fibrinolysis may decrease because direct injury to mesothelial cells may reduce inherent fibrinolytic activity of the cells, and/or the increased fluid volume may dilute local plasminogen activator. Plasminogen activator converts the precursor plasminogen to its active form, plasmin. Fibrinolytic activity in mammals is attributable primarily to this serine protease. In animals with fibrosis, the pleura is thickened by diffuse fibrous tissue that restricts normal pulmonary expansion. Pulmonary function testing in human patients with fibrosing pleuritis has shown a decrease in vital capacity and static compliance, necessitating greater negative intrapleural pressures for any given change in lung volume when compared with healthy patients.

Diagnosis

SIGNALMENT

Any breed of dog or cat may be affected; however, a breed predisposition has been suspected in the Afghan hound for a number of years. Recently, it has been suggested that the Shiba Inu breed may also be predisposed to this disease. Among cats, Oriental breeds such as the Siamese and Himalayan appear to have an increased prevalence. Chylothorax may affect animals of any age;

however, in one study older cats were more likely to develop chylothorax than were young cats.[12] This finding was believed to indicate an association between chylothorax and neoplasia. Although Afghan hounds appear to develop this disease during middle age, affected Shiba Inus have been less than 1 year old. A sex predisposition has not been identified.

HISTORY

Coughing is often the first (and occasionally the only) abnormality noted by owners until the animal becomes dyspneic. Many owners report that they first noticed coughing months before presenting the animal for veterinary care; therefore animals that cough and do not respond to standard treatment of nonspecific respiratory problems should be evaluated for chylothorax. Coughing may be a result of irritation caused by the effusion or may be related to the underlying disease process (e.g., cardiomyopathy or thoracic neoplasia).

PHYSICAL EXAMINATION FINDINGS

Most animals with chylothorax present with a normal body temperature unless extremely excited or severely depressed. Additional findings in patients with chylothorax may include dyspnea, muffled heart and lung sounds, depression, anorexia, weight loss, pale or cyanotic mucous membranes, arrhythmias, murmurs, and pericardial effusion.

RADIOGRAPHY/ULTRASONOGRAPHY

Animals with idiopathic chylothorax have classical radiographic and ultrasonographic signs of a pleural effusion. Other radiographic findings may provide evidence of the underlying cause of chylothorax; for example, a cranial mediastinal mass or cardiomegaly may be evident following removal of the pleural effusion. Animals that have collapsed lung lobes that do not appear to re-expand following removal of chyle or other pleural fluid should be suspected of having underlying pulmonary parenchymal or pleural disease such as fibrosing pleuritis (Figure 79-1). Diagnosis of fibrosing pleuritis is difficult: the atelectatic lobes can have a nodular appearance in the region of the hilus, and they may be confused with metastatic or primary pulmonary neoplasia, lung lobe torsion, or hilar lymphadenopathy (Figure 79-2). Radiographic evidence of pulmonary parenchyma that fails to reexpand after removal of pleural fluid, or lung lobes that have an irregular or scalloped outline, should be considered suggestive of atelectasis with associated pleural fibrosis. Fibrosing pleuritis should also be considered in animals with persistent dyspnea in the face of minimal pleural fluid.

LABORATORY FINDINGS

Fluid recovered by thoracocentesis should be placed in an EDTA tube for cytologic examination. Placing the fluid in an EDTA tube rather than allowing it to clot will permit cell counts to be performed. Although chylous effusions are routinely classified as exudates, the physical characteristics of the fluid may be consistent with a modified transudate. The color varies depending on dietary fat content and the presence of concurrent hemorrhage. The protein content is variable, and measurements are often inaccurate because of interference with the refractive index by the high lipid content of the fluid. The total nucleated cell count is usually less than 10,000/µl and consists primarily of small lymphocytes or neutrophils, with lesser numbers of lipid-laden macrophages.

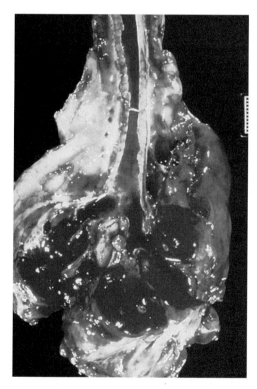

Figure 79-1. Photomicrograph of the lungs of a cat with fibrosing pleuritis associated with chylothorax. Notice the thickened pleura and the rounded appearance of the lung lobes.

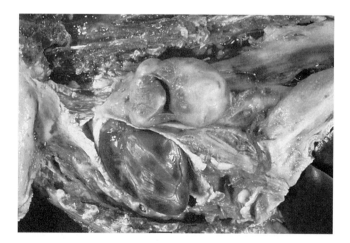

Figure 79-2. Lateral view of lungs of a dog with chronic chylothorax and fibrosing pleuritis. Notice the severe atelectasis and rounded appearance of the cranial lung lobes.

Chronic chylous effusions may contain low numbers of small lymphocytes because of the inability of the body to compensate for continued lymphocyte loss. Nondegenerative neutrophils may predominate if there has been prolonged loss of lymphocytes or if multiple therapeutic thoracocenteses have induced inflammation. Degenerative neutrophils and sepsis are uncommon findings because of the bacteriostatic effect of fatty acids, but can occur iatrogenically if repeated aspirations have been performed. To help determine if a pleural effusion is truly chylous, several tests can be performed including comparison of fluid and serum triglyceride levels, Sudan III stain for lipid droplets, and the ether clearance test. The most diagnostic test is comparison of serum and fluid triglyceride levels. If the effusion is truly chylous it will contain a higher concentration of triglycerides than simultaneously collected serum.

Pseudochylous effusion is a term that has been misused in the veterinary literature to describe effusions that look like chyle, but in which a ruptured thoracic duct is not found. Given the known causes of chylothorax in dogs and cats, this term should be reserved for effusions in which the pleural fluid cholesterol is greater than the serum cholesterol concentration and the pleural fluid triglyceride is less than or equal to the serum triglyceride. Pseudochylous effusions are extremely rare in veterinary patients but may be associated with tuberculosis.

Medical Management

If an underlying disease is diagnosed, it should be treated and the chylous effusion should be managed by intermittent thoracocentesis. If the underlying disease is effectively treated, the effusion often resolves; however, complete resolution may take several months. Surgical intervention should be considered only in animals with idiopathic chylothorax, or in those that do not respond to medical management. Chest tubes should only be placed in animals with suspected chylothorax secondary to trauma (very rare), or when rapid fluid accumulation necessitates that thoracocentesis be performed several times a week to prevent dyspnea, or after surgery. Electrolytes should be monitored because hyponatremia and hyperkalemia have been documented in dogs with chylothorax undergoing multiple thoracocentesis.[13] Clients should be informed that with the idiopathic form of this disease there is no effective treatment that will stop the effusion in all animals. However, the condition may spontaneously resolve in some animals after several weeks or months.

A low-fat diet may decrease the amount of fat in the effusion, which may improve the animal's ability to reabsorb fluid from the thoracic cavity. Commercial low-fat diets are preferable to homemade diets; however, if commercial diets are refused, homemade diets are a reasonable alternative (Boxes 79-1 and 79-2 describe diets with a fat content of about 6% on a dry basis). Care must be taken to ensure adequate calorie intake, despite a low-fat diet, in animals with poor body condition.

BOX 79-1
Canine Homemade Low-Fat Diet*

Ingredient	Amount
Cooked white rice	2⅔ cups
Stewed chicken	⅓ lb
Dicalcium phosphate†	1¼ tsp
GNC Ca-Mg (250 mg Ca, 155 Mg/tab)‡	2 tab
Morton Lite Salt	1 tsp
Zinc (50 mg zinc/tab)§	½ tab
Pet Tab	1 tab
Radiant Valley Natural Selenium (100 mcg Se/tab)§	1 tab
GNC Copper (2 mg copper/tab)‡	1 tab

Directions: Cook the rice without salt. Boil chicken and skim off fat. Crush tablets to a fine powder. Combine all ingredients and mix well. Refrigerate unused portions.

*Calculations based on average published nutrient content of each ingredient indicate this diet meets or exceeds the nutrient requirements for maintenance of adult dogs published by the Associate of American Feed Control Officials. This recipe makes about 1½ lbs. of food that contains 910 kcals of metabolizable energy.
†Dicalcium phosphate 18.5% phosphorus, 22% to 24% calcium, available at farm supply and feed stores.
‡General Nutrition Corp., Pittsburgh PA; available at GNC Nutrition Centers.
§Available at many supermarkets or health food stores.

Medium-chain triglycerides, once thought to bypass the thoracic duct and be absorbed directly into the portal system, are actually transported via the thoracic duct of dogs. Thus they may be less useful than previously believed. It is unlikely that dietary therapy will cure this disease, but it may help in the management of animals with chronic chylothorax.

Benzopyrone drugs have been used for the treatment of lymphedema in humans for years. Whether these drugs might be effective in decreasing pleural effusion in animals with chylothorax is unknown; however, preliminary findings suggest that some animals treated with Rutin (50 to 100 mg/kg, PO, TID) have experienced complete resolution of their effusions.[14] Whether the effusion resolves spontaneously in these animals, or improvement is associated with the drug therapy, requires further study.

Surgical Treatment

Surgical intervention is warranted in animals that do not have underlying disease and in whom medical management becomes impractical. Medical management becomes impractical when thoracocentesis is required more often than once a week, or when repeat thoracocentesis fails to relieve the dyspnea. Surgical options in cases uncomplicated by severe fibrosing pleuritis include mesenteric lymphangiography and thoracic duct (TD) ligation,[11,12,15] subtotal pericardiectomy, omentalization,[16]

BOX 79-2
Feline Homemade Low-Fat Diet*

Ingredient	Amount
Cooked white rice	3⅔ cups
Stewed chicken	½ lb
Dicalcium phosphate†	1½ tsp
GNC Ca-Mg (600 mg Ca/tab)‡	1½ tab
Morton Lite Salt	1 tsp
Taurine tablets (500 mg taurine/tab)§	3 tabs
Zinc (50 mg zinc/tab)¶	½ tab
Feline Pet Tab	3 tabs
Radiant Valley Natural Selenium¶	½ tab
Nature Made Balanced B-50 Complex¶	½ tab
GNC Choline (250 mg choline/tab)‡	1 tab

Directions: Cook the rice without salt. Boil chicken and skim off fat. Crush tablets to a fine powder. Combine all ingredients and mix well. Refrigerate unused portions.

*Calculations based on average published nutrient content of each ingredient indicate this diet meets or exceeds the nutrient requirements for adult maintenance cats published by the Associate of American Feed Control Officials. This recipe makes about 2¼ lbs. of food that contains 1293 kcals of metabolizable energy.
†Dicalcium phosphate 18.5% phosphorus, 22% to 24% calcium, available at farm supply and feed stores.
‡General Nutrition Corp., Pittsburgh PA, available at GNC Nutrition Centers
§Taurine tablets can be purchased at most health food stores and cooperatives as 500 mg and 1000 mg tablets.
¶Available at many supermarkets or health food stores.

passive pleuroperitoneal shunting,[17] active pleuroperitoneal or pleurovenous shunting,[18,19] and pleurodesis.[20,21] Of these, only TD ligation and pericardiectomy are recommended by the author as first line therapies.

THORACIC DUCT LIGATION WITH MESENTERIC LYMPHANGIOGRAPHY

Thoracic duct ligation is performed in cats from a left lateral intercostal thoracotomy or transdiaphragmatically. In dogs the procedure is performed from the right side. The mechanism by which thoracic duct ligation is purported to work is that following thoracic duct ligation, abdominal lymphaticovenous anastomoses form for the transport of chyle to the venous system. Therefore, chyle bypasses the thoracic duct and the effusion resolves. Unfortunately, thoracic duct ligation results in complete resolution of pleural effusion in only 50% of dogs operated[11,22]; in cats the success rate may be even lower (40% or less).[12,23] The advantage of thoracic duct ligation is that if it is successful, it results in complete resolution of pleural fluid, compared with the palliative procedures described below. In addition, it may prevent fibrosing pleuritis from developing. The disadvantages include a long operative time (which is problematic in debilitated animals); a high inci-

dence of continued or recurrent chylous or nonchylous (from pulmonary lymphatics) effusion; and the fact that mesenteric lymphangiography is often difficult to perform, particularly in cats. Without mesenteric lymphangiography, complete ligation of the thoracic duct cannot be ensured. However, an experimental paper assessing lymphangiography in cats suggested that even this technique might not be uniformly successful in verifying complete ligation of the thoracic duct.[24] Additionally, some animals may form collateral lymphatics past the site of the ligature and thus reestablish thoracic duct flow. If chyle flow is directed into the diaphragmatic lymphatics, chylothorax may continue or recur.

For lymphangiography, food is withheld 12 hours before surgery. Either the right side (left side in cats) of the thorax and abdomen, or just the abdomen (if a midline celiotomy is being performed) is prepared for aseptic surgery. If a thoracic approach to the thoracic duct is being used, a right sided (left side in cats) paracostal incision is made in order to exteriorize the cecum. Once the cecum has been exteriorized, a lymph node adjacent to the cecum is located. A small volume (0.1 to 1 ml) of methylene blue (USP 1%, American Quinine, Shirley, NY) is injected into the lymph node to increase visualization of lymphatics. Repeated doses of methylene blue should be avoided because of the risk of inducing a Heinz body anemia or renal failure.[25] Careful dissection of the mesentery near this node allows large lymphatic vessels to be visualized and cannulated with a 22-gauge over-the-needle catheter.[26] Cannulation of this lymphatic is more difficult in the cat than in the dog because cats have more fat in their mesentery and their lymphatics are significantly smaller. Two sutures (3-0 silk) are placed in the mesentery and used to secure in place the catheter and an attached piece of extension tubing. The ends of the suture can be looped over the hub of the extension tubing. An additional suture may be placed around the extension tubing and through a segment of intestine to prevent dislodgement of the catheter. A three-way stopcock is attached to the end of the extension tubing, and a water-soluble contrast agent is injected at a dosage of 1 ml/kg diluted with 0.5 ml/kg of saline. A lateral thoracic radiograph is taken while the last milliliter is being injected. This lymphangiogram can be used to help identify the number and location of branches of the thoracic duct that need to be ligated. It can be repeated following ligation to help determine the extent of lymphangiectasia present in the cranial thorax (Figure 79-3).

The thoracic duct is typically approached in the dog (cat) through a right (left) caudal intercostal thoracotomy (eighth, ninth, or tenth intercostal space); or via an incision in the left diaphragm. Once the duct has been located, hemostatic clips can be used to ligate it. The advantage of using hemoclips (Edward Weck and Co. Inc., Research Triangle Park, NC) is that they can be used as a reference point on subsequent radiographs if further ligation is necessary. However, the author prefers to also place a nonabsorbable suture (e.g., silk) on the duct. Visualization of the thoracic duct can be aided by injecting methylene blue into the lymphatic catheter

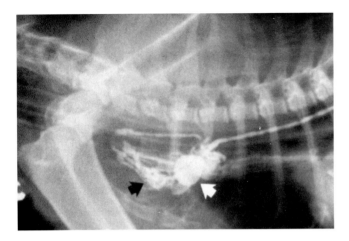

Figure 79-3. Lymphangiogram performed in a cat with chylothorax and thoracic lymphangiectasia. Note the multiple, dilated lymphatics near the entrance of the thoracic duct (arrow) into the venous system.

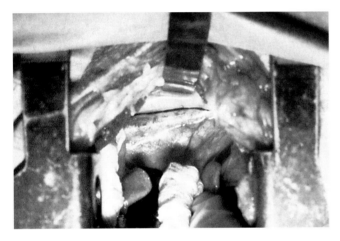

Figure 79-4. Identification of the thoracic duct can be aided by injecting methylene blue either into the lymphatic catheter or directly into a mesenteric lymph node.

(Figure 79-4). If a catheter was not placed, the dye can be injected into a mesenteric lymph node.

PERICARDIECTOMY

In some animals with chylothorax, the pericardium is thickened. This thickening is thought to be a result of chronic irritation by chyle. The thickened pericardium might elevate systemic venous pressures, which in turn might act to impede drainage of chyle into the cranial vena cava while increasing lymphatic flow through the TD. Between May 1998 and October 2000 the author performed pericardiectomy alone or in conjunction with TD ligation in 7 animals with either chylothorax (4 dogs, 2 cats) or serosanguineous pleural fluid after TD ligation that had been performed elsewhere (1 dog). Echocardiography was normal in all of these animals, with the exception of pericardial effusion in 1 dog and a subjectively thickened pericardium in 2 additional dogs. In 1 dog, TD ligation and pericardiectomy were performed at the same time; in 3 dogs and 1 cat, pericardiectomy was performed 2 to 9 months after TD ligation had failed to resolve the pleural effusion; and in 1 dog and 1 cat (each with chylothorax), pericardiectomy alone without concurrent or previous TD ligation was performed. Histopathologic examination of the pericardium showed mild to marked lymphoplasmocytic infiltration of the pericardium in all animals. Clinical signs of pleural fluid resolved in all animals after the pericardiectomy. One dog was lost to follow-up at 6 months but had no evidence of pleural effusion at that time. One additional dog underwent thoracocentesis 4 months after pericardiectomy was performed; further chest taps have not been performed in the past 14 months in that animal. The remaining 5 animals did not require thoracocentesis after the immediate postoperative period and have had no clinical evidence of pleural effusion for a mean of 17 months (range, 5 to 33 months) as of March 2001. The author recommends pericardiectomy in any animal where a serosanguineous effusion continues after TD ligation or where there is echocardiographic evidence of pericardial thickening or pericardial effusion. Additionally, if the pericardium appears thickened at surgery, it should be removed. Further studies are warranted to determine which animals will benefit from pericardiectomy either as sole therapy or in conjunction with TD ligation.

ACTIVE PLEUROPERITONEAL OR PLEUROVENOUS SHUNTING

Active pleuroperitoneal or pleurovenous shunting (Denver double valve pleural effusion shunt, Denver Biomaterials Inc., Evergreen, CO) has been recommended for the treatment of chylothorax in dogs and cats and may be a reasonable consideration in animals in which all other therapies have failed.[18,19,27] Commercially made shunt catheters are available and can be used to pump fluid from the thorax to the abdomen. The catheter is placed under general anesthesia. A vertical incision is made over the middle of the fifth, sixth, and seventh ribs. A purse-string suture is placed in the skin at this site and following the placement of fenestrations in the venous end of the shunt catheter; the catheter is bluntly inserted into the pleural space. A tunnel is created by blunt dissection under the external abdominal oblique muscle, and the pump chamber is pulled through the tunnel. The efferent end of the catheter is then placed into the abdominal cavity through a preplaced purse-string suture and incision located just caudal to the costal arch. The shunt must be placed with the pump chamber directly overlying a rib so that the chamber can be effectively compressed (Figure 79-5). Complications associated with pleuroperitoneal or pleurovenous shunts include: (1) the shunts are expensive; (2) they may easily occlude with fibrin; (3) some animals will not tolerate compression of the pump chamber; and (4) they require a high degree of owner compliance and dedication. Additionally, thrombosis, venous occlusion, sepsis, and

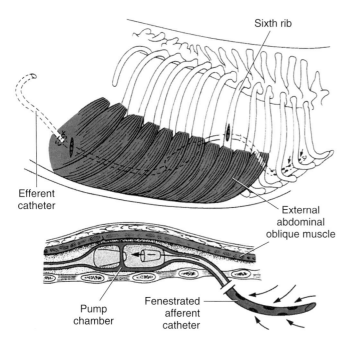

Figure 79-5. *Diagram depicting placement of a pleuroperitoneal shunt. The pump chamber should be positioned over a rib so that it can be manually compressed.* (From Fossum TW, editor: *Small animal surgery,* St Louis, 2002, Mosby.)

electrolyte abnormalities have been reported in human beings.[28-31]

OMENTALIZATION

Omentalization has been reported as a technique to treat animals with chylothorax when other surgical treatments are either not successful or deemed impossible.[16] A fifth or sixth space intercostal thoracotomy is made to provide access to the cranial thorax. A paracostal incision is then made so that a dorsal omental pedicle flap can be raised. The omental flap is brought through an incision in the pars costalis of the diaphragm. Care should be taken to avoid rotation of or excessive tension on the omental pedicle. The omentum is spread out within the thorax to provide a large surface area. An omentopexy is performed by using synthetic absorbable suture to anchor the omentum to the mediastinum in the region of the lymphaticovenous anastomoses between the thoracic duct and the cranial vena cava. Sutures should be placed so that they do not interfere with the blood supply of the omentum. The success of this technique is unproven at this time.

OTHER TREATMENTS

Passive pleuroperitoneal shunting has been recommended as treatment of chylothorax in cats, but this technique is no longer recommended by the author. The goal of placing a fenestrated silastic sheet in the diaphragm was to allow drainage of the chylous fluid into the abdomen where the fluid could be reabsorbed by visceral and peritoneal lymphatics, thereby alleviating the respiratory distress and need for subsequent thoracentesis.[17] The author has not found this technique to be effective, and chronic irritation of the sheeting may be associated with neoplastic transformation of tissues.

Pleurodesis is the formation of generalized adhesions between the visceral and parietal pleura. Adhesions may occur spontaneously in association with pleural effusion, or in some species they can be induced following instillation of an irritating substance into the pleural cavity.[32,33] This technique has been recommended for the treatment of chylothorax in dogs and cats but is not recommended by the author. In order for pleurodesis to occur, the lungs must be able to contact the body wall; however, many animals with chronic chylothorax have some thickening of their visceral pleura, which prohibits normal lung expansion (see the section on fibrosing pleuritis above). Neither mechanical (surgical) pleurodesis or talc administration resulted in pleurodesis in experimental dogs; however, thickening of the pleura did occur in some animals.[33] Chemical or surgical pleurodesis is unlikely to be successful in cats with chylothorax.

MANAGEMENT OF FIBROSING PLEURITIS

The only effective treatment for fibrosing pleuritis is decortication. Decortication gives the best functional result when the pleuritis is of short duration and pulmonary parenchymal disease is minimal. In most cases the thickened pleura is not firmly adherent to the underlying parenchyma and can be removed without severely damaging the underlying lung; however, pneumothorax is a common sequela and usually requires tube thoracentesis. Decortication in human beings carries a good prognosis if only one or two lobes are involved; however, when the fibrosis is diffuse, as occurs in many animals with chylothorax, even with effective decortication a guarded prognosis is warranted. When more than one lung lobe is decorticated, reexpansion pulmonary edema may occur and is often fatal. If decortication is successful, lung expansion and pulmonary function may improve over a 2 to 3 month period. Corticosteroids may be beneficial initially and for 2 to 4 weeks after decortication.

Conclusion

Chylothorax is a complex disease with many identified underlying causes including cardiac disease, mediastinal masses, heartworm disease, and trauma. Management of this disease should be directed at identifying the cause and, if possible, treating the underlying disorder. In cats with idiopathic chylothorax, medical management is initially recommended because the condition may spontaneously resolve. Owners should be aware of the potential development of fibrosing pleuritis in affected cats. When medical management is impractical or unsuccessful, surgical intervention should be considered. Surgical options include mesenteric lymphangiography and thoracic duct ligation, pericardiectomy, omentalization, passive pleuroperitoneal shunting, active pleuroperitoneal or pleurovenous shunting, and pleurodesis. Of these, only TD ligation and pericardiectomy are preferred by the author because if they are successful, the result is complete resolution of the chylothorax, thereby reducing the risk of developing fibrosing pleuritis. Omentalization may be beneficial in some animals as adjuvant therapy, but this procedure may still allow fibrosing pleuritis to occur. Until the etiology of the effusion in animals with idiopathic chylothorax is understood, the treatment success rate will be less than ideal. Future research needs to be directed at determining the pathophysiologic mechanisms underlying this disease.

REFERENCES

1. Patterson DF, Munson TO: Traumatic chylothorax in small animals treated by ligation of the thoracic duct, *JAVMA* 1:452-458, 1958.
2. Hodges CC, Fossum TW, Komkov A et al: Lymphoscintigraphy in healthy dogs and dogs with experimentally created thoracic duct abnormalities, *Am J Vet Res* 53:1048-1053, 1992.
3. Hodges CC, Fossum TW, Evering W: Evaluation of thoracic duct healing after experimental laceration and transection, *Vet Surg* 22:431-435, 1993.
4. Forrester SD, Fossum TW, Rogers KS: Diagnosis and treatment of chylothorax associated with lymphoblastic lymphosarcoma in four cats, *JAVMA* 198:291-294, 1991.
5. Birchard SJ, Ware WA, Fossum TW et al: Chylothorax associated with congestive cardiomyopathy in a cat, *JAVMA* 189:1462-1464, 1986.
6. Fossum TW, Miller MW, Rogers KS et al: Chylothorax associated with right-sided heart failure in 5 cats, *JAVMA* 204:84-89, 1994.
7. Campbell SL, Forrester SD, Johnston SA et al: Chylothorax associated with constrictive pericarditis in a dog, *JAVMA* 206:1561-1564, 1995.
8. Donahoe JM, Kneller SK, Thompson PE: Chylothorax subsequent to infection of cats with Dirofilaria immitis, *JAVMA* 11:1107-1110, 1974.
9. Birchard SJ, Bilbrey SA: Chylothorax associated with dirofilariasis in a cat, *JAVMA* 197:507-509, 1990.
10. Suter PF, Greene RW: Chylothorax in a dog with abnormal termination of the thoracic duct, *JAVMA* 159:302-308, 1971.
11. Fossum TW, Birchard SJ, Jacobs RM: Chylothorax in 34 dogs, *JAVMA* 188:1315-1318, 1986.
12. Fossum TW, Forrester SD, Swenson CL et al: Chylothorax in cats: 37 cases (1969-1989), *JAVMA* 198:672-678, 1991.
13. Willard MD, Fossum TW, Torrance A et al: Hyponatremia and hyperkalemia associated with idiopathic or experimentally induced chylothorax in four dogs, *JAVMA* 199:353-358, 1991.
14. Thompson MS, Cohn LS, Jordan RC: Use of Rutin for medical management of idiopathic chylothorax in four cats, *JAVMA* 215:345-348, 1999.
15. Kerpsack SJ, McLoughlin MA, Birchard SJ et al: Evaluation of mesenteric lymphangiography and thoracic duct ligation in cats with chylothorax: 19 cases (1987-1992), *JAVMA* 205:711-715, 1994.
16. Williams JM, Niles JD: Use of omentum as a physiologic drain for treatment of chylothorax in a dog, *Vet Surg* 28:61-65, 1999.
17. Peterson SL, Pion PD, Breznock EM: Passive pleuroperitoneal drainage for management of chylothorax in two cats, *J Am Anim Hosp Assoc* 25:569-572, 1989.
18. Donner GS: Use of the pleuroperitoneal shunt for the management of persistent chylothorax in a cat, *J Am Anim Hosp Assoc* 252:619-622, 1989.
19. Smeak DD, Gallagher L, Birchard SJ et al: Management of intractable pleural effusion in a dog with a pleuroperitoneal shunt, *Vet Surg* 16:212-216, 1987.
20. Birchard SJ, Fossum TW, Gallagher L: Pleurodesis. In Kirk RW, editor: *Current veterinary therapy*, vol 10, Philadelphia, 1989, WB Saunders.
21. Laing EJ, Norris AM: Pleurodesis as a treatment for pleural effusion in the dog, *J Am Anim Hosp Assoc* 22:193-196, 1986.
22. Birchard SJ, Smeak DD, Fossum TW: Results of thoracic duct ligation in dogs with chylothorax, *JAVMA* 193:68-71, 1988.
23. Harpster NK: Chylothorax. In Kirk RW, editor: *Current veterinary therapy*, vol 9, Philadelphia, 1986, WB Saunders.
24. Martin RA, Leighton D, Richards S et al: Transdiaphragmatic approach to thoracic duct ligation in the cat, *Vet Surg* 17:22-26, 1988.
25. Osuna DJ, Armstrong PJ, Duncan DE et al: Acute renal failure after methylene blue infusion in a dog, *J Am Anim Hosp Assoc* 26:410-412, 1990.
26. Kagan KG, Breznock EM: Variations in the canine thoracic duct system and the effects of surgical occlusion demonstrated by rapid aqueous lymphography, using an intestinal lymphatic trunk, *Am J Vet Res* 40:948-958, 1979.
27. Willauer CC, Breznock EM: Pleurovenous shunting technique for treatment of chylothorax in three dogs, *JAVMA* 191:1106-1109, 1987.
28. Fildes J, Narvaez GP, Baig KA et al: Pulmonary tumor embolization after peritoneovenous shunting for malignant ascites, *Cancer* 61:1973-1976, 1988.
29. Holm A, Rutsky EA, Aldrete JS: Short- and long-term effectiveness, morbidity, and mortality of peritoneovenous shunt inserted to treat massive refractory ascites of nephrogenic origin: Analysis of 14 cases, *Am Surg* 55:645-652, 1989.
30. Smith RE, Nostrant TT, Eckhauser FE et al: Patient selection and survival after peritoneovenous shunting for nonmalignant ascites, *Am J Gastroenterol* 79:659-662, 1984.
31. Vacek JL, Wolfe MW, Hightower BM et al: Right heart pseudotumor simulated by ascitic pseudocyst: An unusual complication of peritoneovenous shunting, *Chest* 91:138-139, 1987.
32. Birchard SJ, Gallagher L: Use of pleurodesis in treating selected pleural diseases, *Compend Contin Educ Pract Vet* 10:825-834, 1988.
33. Jerram RM, Fossum T, Berridge B et al: The efficacy of mechanical abrasion and talc slurry as methods of pleurodesis in normal dogs, *Vet Surg* 28:322-332, 1999.

CHAPTER 80

Pyothorax

Eric Monnet

A pyothorax is a septic inflammation of the thoracic cavity. Inflammatory conditions of the pleura may be dry, serofibrinous, pyogranulomatous, or purulent. A purulent pleuritis is called an empyema or a pyothorax. An initial period of *dry pleuritis* often precedes inflammatory pleural effusions and the development of a pyothorax. Pyothorax has been described in both dogs and cats.

Etiology

Dry pleuritis may be caused by bacteria, viruses, or trauma. In humans, a diagnosis of dry pleuritis is suggested by clinical findings of a rapid and shallow respiratory pattern, obscure thoracic pain, nonproductive cough, and auscultation of a pleural friction rub.[1]

Serofibrinous pleuritis is reported with canine hepatitis, canine leptospirosis, canine distemper, and canine and feline upper respiratory viruses. Bacterial pleuropneumonia is also a cause of serofibrinous pleuritis in dogs and cats.[2] Parasitic diseases such as *Aelurostrongylus* in cats and *Spirocerca lupi* in dogs occasionally cause serofibrinous pleuritis.[3,4] Simultaneous rupture of the biliary system and diaphragm and canine tuberculosis are unusual causes of severe serofibrinous pleuritis.[5-8]

Pyogranulomatous pleuritis is commonly associated with feline infectious peritonitis.[9] The effusion results from virus-induced vasculitis affecting all serous membranes. Abdominal effusion, elevated serum globulins, and uveitis are common associated findings.

Purulent pleuritis, also referred to as pyothorax or empyema, is invariably the result of bacterial or fungal sepsis of the pleural space.[2,10-15] Sources of bacterial contamination include penetrating thoracic wounds; extension from bacterial pneumonia; migrating foreign bodies; esophageal perforations; extension of cervical, lumbar, or mediastinal infections; and hematogenous spread. Thoracic bite wounds are commonly implicated in feline pyothorax.[13,16] Inhalation and migration of a grass awn is often suspected in hunting dogs with pyothorax (Figure 80-1).[17] Anaerobic bacteria (e.g., *Fusobacterium*) and *Nocardia asteroides* are most commonly isolated from dogs with pyothorax.[18-20] *Pasteurella multocida* and anaerobes are the most prevalent isolates in cats.[2,13,14,21] Other microorganisms reported include *Chlamydia psittacci*, *Salmonella* spp., *Actinomyces* spp., *Streptococcus* spp., *E. coli*, *Staphylococcus* spp., *Bacteroides* spp., *Klebsiella* spp.,

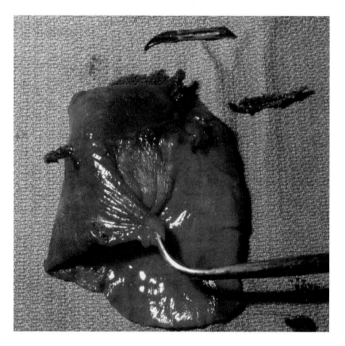

Figure 80-1. *Fragment of plant material found in the pleural cavity and the lung parenchyma of a hunting dog presented for chronic pyothorax.*

Proteus spp., *Corynebacterium* spp., *Enterobacter* spp., *Pseudomonas* spp., *Spirochetes*, *Aspergillus* spp., and *Cryptococcus*.[2,13,14,20,22-26]

Pathophysiology

Inflammation causes pleural effusion by inducing vasodilation and increasing capillary permeability. It allows release of protein rich fluid into the pleural space, which increases the colloid osmotic pressure. More fluid is then pulled into the pleural space. The pleural membrane also becomes thickened because of chronic inflammation, which decreases its ability to absorb fluid.

History

Patients with pyothorax can be presented for lethargy, weakness, weight loss, difficulty breathing, exercise intolerance, and nonproductive cough. Animals with pleuritis and minimal effusion may show pain with coughing or sudden respiratory movement.* Cats from multi-cat households are 3.8 times more likely to develop pyothorax than are cats from single-cat households.[21] Hunting dogs seem to have a higher risk than other breeds to develop pyothorax because of migrating foreign bodies.[18] Hunting dogs often have acute coughing episodes 2 to 3 weeks before presentation with a pyothorax; the initial coughing episode may represent the time that the foreign body was inhaled. The foreign body then migrates through the lung parenchyma, establishes a lung abscess, and finally enters the pleural space. Foreign bodies can also penetrate through the skin and migrate to the thoracic cavity.

Clinical Signs

Pleuritis and pyothorax commonly have an insidious course and presentation is often delayed. Animals can be presented alert and responsive or in shock. The history and clinical signs of patients with pyothorax depend upon the quantity and rapidity of fluid accumulation. Small quantities of effusion are difficult to detect clinically, whereas patients with moderate to large quantities of pleural fluid or air usually present with acute respiratory distress. Chronic pleural effusions associated with slow fluid accumulation are often insidious and escape observation initially. These patients may then suddenly decompensate and present with apparently acute respiratory distress. Animals with pyothorax are usually febrile on presentation, tachycardic, and tachypneic. Femoral pulses are often strong, and mucous membranes are pink with a normal capillary refill time unless the patient is developing septic shock.[1,18,21]

Respiratory distress associated with pyothorax is characteristically restrictive in nature. The presence of pleural fluid reduces functional residual capacity (FRC) and forces the lung to operate on a less compliant portion of the compliance curve. The patient compensates for the increase in respiratory work with a rapid and shallow breathing pattern. Patients may exhibit increased respiratory distress in lateral recumbency (orthopnea), preferring to remain in a sternal recumbent or sitting position. In severe cases, elbows are abducted and the head and neck are extended. Stress associated with handling may cause respiratory arrest because of the limited respiratory reserve.

Diagnosis

PHYSICAL EXAMINATION

Auscultation of animals with pyothorax usually reveals muffling of heart sounds. Breath sounds are variable, often being surprisingly well preserved dorsally but distant or absent ventrally. Pleuritis with minimal pleural effu-

*References 1, 14, 18, 21, 27, and 28.

sion may produce a pleural friction rub, typically heard loudest on inspiration. Systematic percussion of the patient in a standing position may demonstrate a horizontal fluid line. Pleural air produces a characteristic hyperresonant ping on percussion.

RADIOGRAPHY

Thoracic radiographs confirm the presence of pleural effusion, particularly if there are small amounts of fluid, which may be difficult to appreciate on physical examination. As little as 100 ml of pleural fluid may be detected in a medium-sized dog on standard recumbent lateral, ventrodorsal, and dorsoventral views of the thorax.[29,30] Small amounts of pleural fluid are seen on a lateral radiographic view as a fluid-dense triangular wedge that forms at the junction of the sternum and interlobar fissures of the lungs.[29] As fluid accumulates, these wedges coalesce to give the ventral borders of the lungs a scalloped appearance.[29] Large amounts of pleural fluid obscure the cardiac and diaphragmatic silhouettes as well as the cardiophrenic angle. Fluid eventually collects dorsally giving the appearance of floating lungs. The cranial and middle lung lobes may eventually collapse and disappear.

Blunting of the costophrenic angle on the ventrodorsal and dorsoventral view is also a sensitive method of detecting small amounts of pleural fluid.[29,30] Fluid-dense wedges may be visualized at the interlobar fissures of the lungs.[29] On the ventrodorsal view, moderate to large amounts of pleural fluid collect in the paravertebral gutters, obscuring the cardiac silhouette and cardiophrenic angle. A tendency for fluid to accumulate adjacent to the cranial lung lobes gives the cranial mediastinum a widened appearance. Collapse of lung lobes associated with pleural effusion tends to be uniform, causing the partially collapsed lung lobe to retain its original shape. If a fibrinous or fibrous peel develops on the visceral pleura, the lungs become more rounded or irregular in appearance. This finding suggests a chronic inflammatory process, and indicates that the lungs may be difficult to reexpand. For the diagnosis of cranial mediastinal masses or lung lesions, the pleural fluid should be drained before radiography.

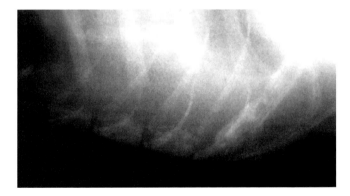

Figure 80-2. *Radiographs of the sternum of a dog with a chronic draining tract caudal to the xyphoid, and a pyothorax. Lesions of osteomyelitis were present.*

Horizontal beam radiography allows gravitational movement of pleural fluid and therefore provides diagnostic information by: (1) demonstrating free versus encapsulated pleural effusion, (2) allowing visualization of thoracic structures by moving fluid away from structures of interest, and (3) detecting small amounts of pleural fluid. The standing lateral and erect ventrodorsal views are sensitive, detecting as little as 50 ml of fluid in a 15-kg animal.[30] The standing lateral view is minimally stressful and may be preferred in orthopneic animals. The lateral decubitus views are useful for detecting small amounts of pleural fluid and allow evaluation of specific lung lobes for intrapulmonary lesions.[29]

It is also important to evaluate the sternum and ribs because the infection may involve these structures. Changes consistent with osteomyelitis may be visible on radiographs (Figure 80-2).

ULTRASONOGRAPHY

The presence of pleural fluid allows visualization of intrathoracic structures. Because the fluid acts as an acoustic window and enhances imaging, ultrasonography should be performed before thoracocentesis. Masses in the cranial mediastinum or lung can then be aspirated under ultrasound guidance to obtain a cytological diagnosis.[31]

THORACOCENTESIS

Once pleural effusion is demonstrated, either clinically or radiographically, thoracocentesis is indicated to remove fluid for diagnostic as well as for therapeutic purposes. The techniques to perform thoracocentesis are described in Chapter 20. Diagnostics performed on the pleural fluid include: (1) preparation of appropriately stained direct smears for cytological examination; (2) submission of fluid for aerobic and anaerobic bacterial culture and sensitivity; (3) determination of physical and biochemical characteristics (e.g., specific gravity, total protein, and clotting characteristics); and (4) determination of total cell counts and preparation of centrifuged cell concentrate smears from fluid anticoagulated with EDTA.[29,32]

Diagnosis of pleuritis or pyothorax is suggested by the presence of an inflammatory or a septic exudate.[9,29,32-35] Inflammatory exudates characteristically exhibit a total protein greater than 3.0 g/dl, a specific gravity greater than 1.018, and a total cell count greater than 3×10^9 cells/L.[9,32,33] Inflammatory exudates may be nonseptic or septic. Nonseptic exudates usually have a serofibrinous or serosanguineous appearance. The distinction between modified transudates and nonseptic effusions may at times be difficult. Feline infectious peritonitis (FIP) produces a nonseptic exudative pleural effusion that appears yellow, translucent, and viscous on gross examination. Total protein values approach serum levels, ranging from 4 to 8 g/dL.[9,32] Electrophoresis reveals an elevated gamma globulin fraction. The predominant cell types in nonseptic exudates are nondegenerative neutrophils and macrophages. Total cell counts are generally not high, ranging from 5 to 15 $\times 10^9$ cells/L.[9,32]

Septic exudates are generally purulent in appearance. The fluid is viscous; opaque; and varies in color between white, yellow, green, and red. The fluid may clot or exhibit fibrinous debris and often has a foul odor. Cell counts are high, ranging from 30 to 200 $\times 10^9$ cells/L, although accurate cell counts are difficult because of extensive cellular degeneration.[33] Degenerate neutrophils predominate and bacteria are often visualized.[9,32] Gram stains may give an early indication of the types of bacteria present. Fluid should be cultured for aerobic and anaerobic bacteria. Macrophages and plasma cells increase as the exudative process becomes longstanding.

Treatment

Treatment of a pyothorax is medical and/or surgical. Surgical intervention is advised for chronic empyema because it has been associated with lower morbidity, recurrence, and complication rates; and shorter hospitalization times than medical treatment.[19,36]

MEDICAL TREATMENT

Medical management of patients with pyothorax includes placement of thoracostomy tubes, fluid therapy, and antibiotherapy. Placement of thoracostomy tubes is required to establish continuous drainage and to permit lavage of the pleural space. Bilateral thoracostomy drains may be required to efficiently drain the pleural space. Broad-spectrum antibiotics should be used initially while the results of culture and sensitivity testing are pending. A combination of ampicillin and enrofloxacin may be used for broad coverage. If the animal is not responding after 2 or 3 days of pleural drainage and lavage and appropriate antimicrobial therapy, a thoracotomy is required.

Arterial blood gases should be performed daily to assess respiratory function. Pyothorax and pleural effusion are associated with atelectasis, which results in an impairment of gas exchange. The alveolar-arterial oxygen tension gradient can be calculated; if the gradient is higher than 20 mm Hg, oxygen therapy may be needed. Evaluating the response to oxygen is also important because it can provide information about the prognosis. An absent or limited response to oxygen is another evaluation of the severity of atelectasis or the presence of other severe pulmonary pathology. Oxygen therapy is required in severely compromised patients even if the response to oxygen is limited.

Response to medical treatment is judged from daily cytology of the pleural fluid (i.e., number of neutrophils per high power field, nature of neutrophils, and bacteria present); the amount of fluid collected every day; and evaluation of a complete blood count. Reduction of the number of neutrophils, reduced proportion of degenerate neutrophils, fewer bacteria, and reduction of the daily volume of fluid collected are all indicators of successful medical treatment. If a lung mass (e.g., abscess or necrotic tumor) is visible on thoracic radiographs, the patient will likely need a thoracotomy to remove the mass and resolve the pyothorax.[19] If *Actinomyces* or *Nocardia* are present, surgery is indicated to try to eliminate the foreign body that is migrating in the thoracic cavity.[19] Cats seem to response more favorably to medical treatment than dogs.[19,21]

PLEURAL DRAINAGE WITH THORACOSTOMY TUBES

A thoracostomy tube (chest tube) is indicated if there is sufficient accumulation of pleural effusion to warrant repeated pleural drainage. Because the fluid can be thick and fibrinous, the large diameter of the chest tube is often necessary to accomplish complete evacuation of the pleural space.[37,38]

A thoracostomy tube may be placed without anesthesia only if the animal is critically ill; local intercostal nerve blocks may be used. A generous portion of the lateral thorax should be clipped, and aseptic technique utilized. A small skin incision in the dorsal one-third of the lateral thoracic wall is made at the level of the tenth to twelfth intercostal space. A tunnel under the latissimus dorsi muscle is then bluntly developed in a cranioventral direction over three or four intercostal spaces. With the aid of a stylet or large hemostatic forceps, the tube is introduced into the seventh or eighth intercostal space with a brisk but controlled thrust directed toward the opposite shoulder. Great care must be exercised when inserting tubes with sharp stylets that extend beyond the end of the tube.

The tube is fed into the cranial ventral pleural space and sutured to the skin with a "Chinese finger cuff" suture pattern. The tube should be covered with a loose bandage and its position confirmed with a thoracic radiograph. The thoracostomy drain is sealed with a three-way stopcock. An extension set and another three-way stopcock or a gate-clamp can be added for better security.

Pleural drainage may be either *intermittent* or *continuous.* Continuous closed suction is indicated when the accumulation rate of fluid or air becomes life threatening.[39] Many commercial systems are now available for continuous pleural evacuation; all are based in principle on the original underwater bottle system. A negative pressure of 10 to 20 cm of water is recommended. Continuous suction has the advantage of keeping pleural surfaces in contact, which can aid in sealing pleuropulmonary fistulas or hemorrhage. Continuous pleural drainage allows reduction of the amount of purulent material in the thoracic cavity, which may improve the efficacy of antibiotic treatment and allow better reexpansion of the lungs. The disadvantage of continuous suction systems is that they require constant monitoring because the tube connecting to the patient is susceptible to removal or damage. Continuous suction systems do not allow measurement of air removed from the pleural cavity. Continuous suction is interrupted during pleural lavage.

Thoracostomy tubes should be removed when they are no longer productive. The amount of fluid produced with a thoracostomy drain is highly variable and depends on the pathology inside the thoracic cavity. In one study, the amount of fluid varied from 0 to 84.5 ml/kg/day (mean 2.1 ml/kg/day) on the first day to a range of 0 to 38 ml/kg/day (mean 1.5 ml/kg/day) the second day.[5]

PLEURAL LAVAGE

Following the diagnosis of a pyothorax, management of these animals needs to be aggressive. After placement of one or two thoracostomy tubes, lavage of the pleural space may begin. Lavage can be performed two to four times daily. An isotonic fluid such as saline is used at room temperature, at 20 ml/kg body weight. The fluid is administered slowly over 10 minutes. If the animal cannot tolerate the total volume of fluid, the frequency of the lavage should be increased, with a lower volume, for the first day. The fluid is left in the thoracic cavity for 1 hour and then drained. Antibiotics are not added to the lavage solution, but instead should be delivered intravenously.

SURGICAL TREATMENT

Surgical treatment requires a complete exploration of the thoracic cavity and resection of the tissue involved in the inflammatory process. Exploration and debridement of the thoracic cavity can be performed with either thoracoscopy or median sternotomy.

Thoracoscopy is a minimally invasive operative procedure for the examination of the pleural cavity and its organs. With the development of high-resolution microcameras, video optics, and fiberoptic light delivery systems, clear magnified images of the surgical field can be transferred to a video screen. Diagnostic and advanced therapeutic procedures are possible, with video-assisted endoscopy in combination with minimally invasive surgical instruments.

Thoracoscopy is indicated for thoracic exploration; and in human medicine, for the treatment of pyothorax.[40-43] In acute cases, debridement of the thoracic cavity is possible, but if the pyothorax is chronic, thoracoscopy is not indicated. After completion of the procedure, a thoracic drain is placed under thoracoscopic control.

A median sternotomy is required to gain full exposure of both the left and right hemithorax (Figure 80-3). The pleural surfaces, lymph nodes, blood vessels, pericardium, trachea, bronchi, and lung parenchyma are evaluated for signs of bleeding, inflammation, air leak, or abnormal masses. Tissue biopsies and samples for microbiological examination are taken for further diagnosis. Thorough inspection and palpation of the lung parenchyma are required to identify a foreign body. It can be difficult to find the foreign material if it is encapsulated in fibrous tissue or because it is small. Debridement of the thoracic cavity requires resection of any tissue incorporated in the inflammatory process (Figure 80-4). Resection of the mediastinum, pericardium, sternebrae, and lung lobes with masses or abscesses may be needed.

Postoperatively, medical treatment is reinstituted as previously described. Patients with a pyothorax are at

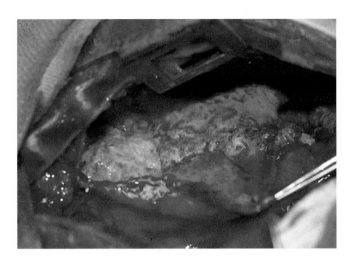

Figure 80-3. *Median sternotomy of a dog with chronic pyothorax. Exposure of both hemithoraces was adequate. The mediastinum and pericardium were involved in the inflammatory process.*

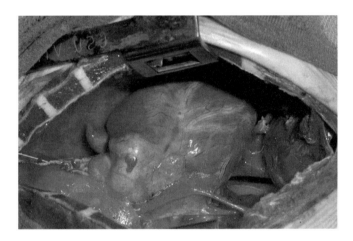

Figure 80-4. *Median sternotomy of the same dog as in Figure 80-3, after debridement of the mediastinum and subtotal pericardectomy.*

high risk to develop septic shock. Therefore, the postoperative patients are monitored intensively to document heart rate and rhythm, systemic arterial pressure, and oxygenation. Fluid therapy with colloids, inotropic support, and antiarrhythmic treatment may be required for 24 to 48 hours. Animals with pyothorax are also at risk for disseminated intravascular coagulation because the inflammatory process can activate the coagulation cascade. Plasma may be required to provide coagulation factors, and heparinization can be considered. Whole blood transfusion may be needed to optimize hematocrit and oxygen delivery. Complete blood counts and cytology of the fluid in the thoracic cavity are performed on a daily basis.

Antibiotherapy is adjusted depending on the results of the cultures taken during surgery. The animals are then discharged with long-term antibiotherapy. Usually 4 to 6 weeks of antibiotic treatment is indicated. If *Actinomyces*

or *Nocardia* have been identified, the patient is kept on antibiotics for 4 months.

The prognosis of dogs and cats treated for pyothorax is guarded for the immediate outcome. However, animals that are discharged from the hospital have a fairly good long-term outcome. In a recent study of 26 dogs with pyothorax by Rooney and colleagues,[19] dogs treated surgically did better (mean disease free interval 209 ± 22.1 days) than dogs treated medically (mean disease free interval 61.8 ± 20.6 days). Dogs with *Actinomyces* or a lung mass responded better to surgical treatment than to medical treatment.[19] In another recent study of 80 cats with pyothorax, the long-term survival rate was 66.1%.[21] Five of those cats underwent surgical treatment because they were not responding to medical treatment or because a lung abscess was suspected on thoracic radiographs. Low heart rate and hypersalivation on presentation have been shown to be associated with a poor prognosis for cats with pyothorax.[21]

REFERENCES

1. Owens MW, Milligan SA: Pleuritis and pleural effusions, *Curr Opin Pulm Med* 1:318-323, 1995.
2. Tomlinson J: Review of pyothorax in the feline, *Fel Pract* 10:26-32, 1980.
3. Geary JC: Chronic pleuritis: A sequela to spirocercosis. A case report, *Auburn Vet* 20:136-138, 1964.
4. Miller BH, Roudebush P, Ward HG: Pleural effusion as a sequela to aelurostrongylosis in a cat, *JAVMA* 185:556-557, 1984.
5. Bellenger CR, Hunt GB, Goldsmid SE et al: Outcomes of thoracic surgery in dogs and cats, *Aust Vet J* 74:25-30, 1996.
6. Liu S, Weitzman I, Johnson GG: Canine tuberculosis, *JAVMA* 177:164-167, 1980.
7. Robins G, Thornton J, Mills J. Bile peritonitis and pleuritis in a dog, *J Am Anim Hosp Assoc* 13:55-60, 1977.
8. Barnhart MD, Rasmussen LM: Pleural effusion as a complication of extrahepatic biliary tract rupture in a dog, *J Am Anim Hosp Assoc* 32:409-412, 1996.
9. Creighton SR, Wilkins RJ: Thoracic effusions in the cat: Etiology and diagnostic features, *J Am Anim Hosp Assoc* 11:66-76, 1975.
10. Crowe DT, Crane SW: Diagnostic abdominal paracentesis and lavage in the evaluation of abdominal injuries in dogs and cats: Clinical and experimental investigations, *JAVMA* 168:700-705, 1976.
11. Robertson S, Stoddart M, Evans RJ et al: Thoracic empyema in the dog: A report of 22 cases, *J Small Anim Pract* 24:103-119, 1983.
12. Holmberg DL: Management of pyothorax, *Vet Clin North Am Small Anim Pract* 9:357-362, 1979.
13. Sherding RG: Pyothorax in the cat, *Comp Cont Ed* 1:247-253, 1979.
14. Withrow SJ, Fenner WR, Wilkins RJ: Closed chest drainage and lavage for treatment of pyothorax in the cat, *J Am Anim Hosp Assoc* 11:90-94, 1975.
15. Noone KE: Pleural effusions and diseases of the pleura, *Vet Clin North Am Small Anim Pract* 15:1069-1084, 1985.
16. Fellenbaum S: A surgical approach to pyothorax in the feline, *J Am Anim Hosp Assoc* 8:259-263, 1972.
17. Frendin J: Pyogranulomatous pleuritis with empyema in hunting dogs, *Zentralbl Veterinarmed A* 44:167-178, 1997.
18. Piek CJ, Robben JH: Pyothorax in nine dogs, *Vet Quat* 22:107-111, 2000.
19. Rooney MB, Monnet E: Medical and surgical treatment of pyothorax in dogs: 26 cases, *JAVMA* 221:86-92, 2002.
20. Walker A, Jang SS, Hirsh DC: Bacteria associated with pyothorax of dogs and cats: 98 cases (1989-1998), *JAVMA* 216:359-363, 2000.
21. Waddell LS, Brady CA, Drobatz KJ: Risk factors, prognostic indicators, and outcome of pyothorax in cats: 80 cases (1986-1999), *JAVMA* 221:819-824, 2002.

22. Love DN, Jones RF, Bailey M: Isolation and characterization of bacteria from pyothorax (empyaema) in cats, *Vet Microbiol* 7:359-362, 1982.
23. Hawkins EC, Feldman BF, Blanchard PC: Immunoglobulin A myeloma in a cat with pleural effusion and serum hyperviscosity, *JAVMA* 188:876-878, 1986.
24. Arizmendi F, Grimes JE, Relford RL: Isolation of *Chlamydia psittaci* from pleural effusion in a dog, *J Vet Diagn Invest* 4:460-463, 1992.
25. Armstrong PJ: Nocardial pleuritis in a cat, *Can Vet J* 21:189-191, 1980.
26. Collins JD, Grimes TD, Kelly WR et al: Pleuritis in the dog associated with actinomyces-like organisms, *J Small Anim Pract* 9:513-518, 1968.
27. Jonas LD: Feline pyothorax: a retrospective study of 20 cases, *J Am Anim Hosp Assoc* 19:865-871, 1983.
28. Holmberg DL: Management of pyothorax, *Vet Clin North Am Small Anim Pract* 9:357-362, 1979.
29. Cantwell HD, Rebar AH, Allen AR: Pleural effusion in the dog: Principles for diagnosis, *J Am Anim Hosp Assoc* 19:227-232, 1983.
30. Lord PF, Suter PF, Chan KF et al: Pleural, extrapleural and pulmonary lesions in small animals: A radiographic approach to differential diagnosis, *J Am Vet Radio Soc* 13:4-17, 1972.
31. Tidwell AS: Ultrasonography of the thorax (excluding the heart), *Vet Clin North Am Small Anim Pract* 28:993-1015, 1998.
32. Prasse KW, Duncan JR: Laboratory diagnosis of pleural and peritoneal effusions, *Vet Clin North Am Small Anim Pract* 6:625-636, 1976.
33. Perman V, Osborne CA, Stevens JB: Laboratory evaluation of abnormal body fluids, *Vet Clin North Am Small Anim Pract* 4:255-268, 1974.
34. Herrgesell JD: Analysis of abnormal chest fluids in clinical practice, *Vet Med Small Anim Clin* 63:246-248, 1968.
35. Christopher MM: Pleural effusions, *Vet Clin North Am Small Anim Pract* 17:255-270, 1987.
36. Powell L, Allen R, Brenner M et al: Improved patient outcome after surgical treatment for loculated empyema, *Am J Surg* 179:1-6, 2000.
37. Frendin J, Obel N: Catheter drainage of pleural fluid collections and pneumothorax, *J Small Anim Pract* 38:237-242, 1997.
38. Munnell ER: Thoracic drainage, *Ann Thorac Surg* 63:1497-1502, 1997.
39. Turner WD, Breznock EM: Continuous suction drainage for management of canine pyothorax: A retrospective study, *J Am Anim Hosp Assoc* 24:485-494, 1988.
40. Silen ML, Naunheim KS: Thoracoscopic approach to the management of empyema thoracis: Indications and results, *Chest Surg Clin N Am* 6:491-499, 1996.
41. Colt HG: Thoracoscopic management of malignant pleural effusions, *Clin Chest Med* 16:505-518, 1995.
42. Grewal H, Jackson RJ, Wagner CW et al: Early video-assisted thoracic surgery in the management of empyema, *Pediatrics* 103:6, 1999.
43. Yim AP, Izzat MB, Lee TW et al: Video-assisted thoracic surgery: A renaissance in surgical therapy, *Respirology* 4:1-8, 1999.

CHAPTER 81

Hemothorax and Sanguineous Effusions

Jennifer Prittie • Linda Barton

Hemothorax is an effusion in the pleural cavity characterized by a packed cell volume (PCV), nucleated cell count/type, total protein, and specific gravity that are at least 25% of peripheral blood.[1] As blood in the pleural space rapidly becomes defibrinated, the pleural fluid appears grossly similar to frank blood but does not clot, in contrast to fresh blood obtained by inadvertent aspiration of a vessel or the heart.[2] The diagnosis of a hemothorax is further supported by cytologic findings of erythrophagocytosis; and the absence of platelets, which quickly aggregate, degranulate, and disappear.

Hemothorax should be distinguished from a sanguineous, or hemorrhagic effusion. Only 5000 to 6000 red blood cells (RBCs)/μL are necessary to give a thoracic effusion a red tint on gross inspection.[1,3] Therefore an effusion may appear bloody but actually have low red blood cell and hemoglobin counts; hemorrhagic effusions rarely contain more than 1 g/dl hemoglobin.[3] Hemorrhagic effusions are most often associated with blood-contaminated thoracocenteses or malignancy, but hemorrhage can complicate many transudates and exudates.[1-3]

Etiology

In companion animals, hemothorax most often occurs secondary to nonpenetrating chest trauma (e.g., motor vehicle collisions, falls, kicks, and sports-related injuries). Hemothorax can also result from coagulopathies, central venous catheter placement, malignancy, traumatic diaphragmatic hernia, lung lobe torsion, pulmonary infarction or abscessation, or recent surgical intervention.[2,4] Infiltrative lesions can erode vessel walls and result in hemorrhage, for example in cases of dirofilariasis or aortic aneurysm caused by *Spirocera lupi*.[4] In humans, direct thoracic trauma (penetrating or blunt) accounts for the majority of hemothoraces. Additional reported etiologies for hemothorax in humans are listed in Box 81-1.[1,5-26]

Spackman and colleagues reviewed records of 267 dogs sustaining injuries from motor vehicle accidents.[27] Thoracic injury was present in 104 (38.9%) of the dogs. Of these, 52 (50%) had pulmonary contusions, 49 (47.1%) had pneumothorax, 26 (25%) had fractured ribs, and 9 (8.7%) had hemothorax.[27] In veterinary patients, hemothorax secondary to chest trauma usually results from damage to small pulmonary or intercostal vessels.[28] Hemorrhage less commonly results from injury to great vessels such as the aorta, the vena cava, and the pulmonary artery, as is occasionally seen in cases of blunt thoracic aortic injury in humans.[29,30] Bleeding from small pulmonary vessels is usually self-limiting. Hemorrhage increases intrapleural hydrostatic pressure, which prevents further bleeding.[28] Intercostal bleeding, or bleeding associated with damage to a great vessel, is less likely to be controlled by intrapleural pressure effects.[10]

Delayed hemothorax following chest trauma has been well documented in humans.[16,29,31] Victims represent hours to days following the initial insult with sudden onset of dyspnea and/or chest pain, and a newly documented hemorrhagic pleural effusion. The majority of these patients sustain multiple or displaced rib fractures during the initial trauma, and the bleeding source is thought to be lacerated pleura over displaced rib fractures with actively bleeding intercostal arteries.

Vitamin K antagonism (secondary to warfarin intoxication or iatrogenic anticoagulant administration) and inherited factor deficiencies can result in hemothorax in humans and companion animals.[21] In humans, drugs such as ticlopidine, an inhibitor of platelet aggregation used in coronary artery and cerebrovascular disease; heparin, utilized in postcoronary angioplasty and in the management of thromboembolism or hemodialysis; and warfarin, a treatment for thrombosis associated with ischemic cardiomyopathy, have been implicated in cases of hemothorax.[14,16,19] Such drugs are thought to prolong spontaneous closure of puncture sites in vessels, result-

ing in active hemorrhage.[24] Hemophilia and von Willebrand disease are heritable disorders that may result in spontaneous hemothorax. Severe thrombocytopenia and disseminated intravascular coagulation (DIC) associated with a variety of primary disease processes may also result in bleeding into the thoracic cavity.

Rarely, placement of central venous catheters, Swan-Ganz catheters, and chest tubes may result in inadvertent laceration of vessels or damage to the lung parenchyma and cause hemothorax. Hemothorax associated with central venous catheter placement in humans has been estimated to occur in less than 0.5% of cases.[9,11] Bagwell and colleagues reviewed 33 life-threatening complications associated with central venous catheter placement in human patients, of which 19 were hemothoraces, resulting in 7 deaths. Other complications included pneumothorax (2), hydrothorax (2), and cardiac tamponade (10).[5] Rupture of the pulmonary artery is a lethal complication associated with flotation of Swan-Ganz catheters, estimated in human patients at 0.001% to 0.47% and carrying up to a 70% mortality rate.[12] Hemoptysis postcatheter placement is a reliable clinical sign, and pulmonary hypertension is a risk factor because sclerotic pulmonary vessels are less compliant and more fragile.[12] Whereas the most common complications associated with tube thoracostomy are empyema formation and residual pneumothorax after chest tube removal, hemothorax secondary to vessel laceration or migration of the tube from the pleural space into lung parenchyma have been documented in human patients.[17]

Spontaneous hemopneumothorax is the accumulation of air and blood within the pleural space in the absence of trauma or another obvious cause. Intrathoracic hemorrhage is estimated to occur in 1% to 12% of cases of spontaneous pneumothorax in humans.[22] Torn adhesions between visceral and parietal pleura associated with apical bullous disease account for the bleeding in up to 82% of the cases.[21] Rupture of vascularized bullae may also cause hemorrhage associated with spontaneous pneumothorax.[22] Although hemopneumothorax is not well-documented in the veterinary literature, breeds predisposed to spontaneous bullae formation may be at increased risk for hemothorax associated with bullous lung disease.[32]

Malignant pleural effusion (MPE) is often bloody in appearance, but true hemothorax is rare in association with neoplasia.[1] When present, possible sources of bleeding into the chest cavity include direct invasion of pulmonary blood vessels, compression or ischemic necrosis of adjacent lung tissues by the tumor, tumor-induced angiogenesis, or rupture of a well-vascularized tumor.[6,20,33] Hemorrhagic or sanguineous effusions typically result from impaired lymphatic drainage of the pleural space.[20] Invasion of lymph nodes, erosion of visceral pleura and disruption of the normal resorptive flow of fluid from the parietal to the visceral surface, embolization or metastatic seeding of parietal and/or visceral pleura, and increased capillary permeability caused by the presence of vasoactive substances may all contribute to lymphatic obstruction.[7,33] Pulmonary embolism, hypoalbuminemia, and complications related to radiation therapy or systemic chemotherapy can also contribute to the development of a sanguineous thoracic effusion.[20] In humans, carcinomas of the lung, breast, ovary, and stomach, and lymphosarcoma account for greater than 80% of MPEs.[20] Lymphosarcoma; primary pulmonary adenocarcinoma; metastatic mammary gland adenocarcinoma; and, rarely, malignant mesothelioma have all been reported to cause hemorrhagic thoracic effusions in dogs and cats.[28,34]

Traumatic diaphragmatic hernia may result in an obstructive and inflammatory hemorrhagic pleural effusion secondary to increased hydrostatic pressure in the lymphatic vessels and/or blood vessels draining the thoracic cavity and/or liver herniations and subsequent constriction of the liver lobe by the diaphragm. Similarly, animals with lung lobe torsion may develop hemothorax secondary to strangulation of the bronchus and associated vascular pedicle and lymphatics, with subsequent impaired venous and lymphatic drainage from the affected lung lobe.[10,28]

Clinical Signs

Clinical signs associated with the development of a hemothorax depend on the primary etiology; the volume; and, more importantly, the rate of blood extravasated into the pleural space.[2] Symptoms may include those referable to anemia (e.g., pallor, changes in mental status, tachycardia, and hyperdynamic pulses); or hypovolemia (e.g., perfusion impairment characterized by weakness/collapse, prolonged capillary refill time, tachycardia, poor pulse quality, and cold extremities).[29] Tachypnea and dyspnea may reflect clinical anemia and decreased pulmonary function secondary to parenchymal compression by the effusion.[29] Cough may be present, although it is more commonly seen in dogs than in cats. Cyanosis, nasal flare, inadequate or abnormal chest wall excursions, perceptible change in thoracic cage conformation, reluctance to lie down, or exercise intolerance may be observed, secondary to altered lung mechanics and gas exchange.[34] Auscultation may reveal quiet to absent lung sounds in the ventral part of the thorax, either unilaterally or bilaterally. In addition, thoracic effusion results in dulling of the percussive vibration.[2,34]

Animals presenting with hemothorax secondary to trauma should be carefully evaluated for additional clinically significant complications such as pulmonary contusions/lacerations, chest wall disruption (e.g., flail chest), diaphragmatic rupture, pneumothorax, or pneumomediastinum.[35] Patients with MPE may be systemically ill, with cancer cachexia characterized by chronic inappetance and weight loss.[20] Bleeding into other body cavities, epistaxis, hematuria, hematochezia, pulmonary hemorrhage, or subcutaneous ecchymosis may accompany coagulopathies.[33] Fever may occur associated with either neoplasia or trauma.[2]

Diagnosis

Pleural effusion often results in inadequate gas exchange caused by lung lobe collapse. Arterial blood gas evaluation is useful in documenting hypoxemia (i.e., PaO_2 less than 60 mm Hg) and hypercapnia (i.e., $PaCO_2$ greater than 45 mm Hg). Pulse oximetry can also be used to monitor for hypoxemia (i.e., SaO_2 less than 92%). A database consisting of a complete blood count, serum chemistry panel, coagulogram, and a urinalysis should be submitted to determine whether there is evidence of RBC regeneration; to screen for underlying hepatic or renal dysfunction (especially if metastatic neoplasia is the suspected primary cause of the effusion); and to evaluate for thrombocytopenia, factor deficiency, and DIC.[2] Cystocentesis and jugular venipuncture should be avoided in animals with suspected bleeding diatheses.

Thoracic radiographs should be obtained when the patient is stable. Costophrenic blunting, pleural fissure lines, separation of lung borders from the thoracic wall, scalloping of lung tangents dorsal to the sternum, masking of the cardiac and diaphragmatic shadows, a widened mediastinum, and tracheal elevation are radiographic findings consistent with the presence of a pleural effusion.[28,34] Radiographs are also valuable in documenting the presence of rib fractures or pneumothoraces in trauma victims; in determining the distribution and size of effusion; and in screening for pulmonary/mediastinal masses, diaphragmatic hernia, or lung lobe torsion.[29] Radiography has previously been determined to have a 67% sensitivity and 70% specificity for confirming the presence of pleural effusion in human patients.[10]

Thoracic computed tomography (CT) is more sensitive than radiography for documenting the presence of effusion and pulmonary contusions, and less sensitive than radiography for evaluation of bony injuries sustained during thoracic trauma.[36] However, use of CT over radiographs has not been associated with improved outcome in human patients, and this imaging modality is not recommended as a routine screening test in the initial work-up of hemothorax.[36] If available, thoracic ultrasonography may be useful for locating loculated pockets of fluid in the pleural space and for differentiating between small amounts of pleural fluid and pleural thickening.[35] Because fluid is an excellent ultrasound-transmitting medium, lesions of the pleura or lungs that were obscured on thoracic radiographs may be visible using ultrasound.[37] Finally, in human medicine, there are reports of using radionuclide-labelled RBCs or angiography to locate the source of thoracic hemorrhage.[26]

Thoracocentesis is necessary for definitive diagnosis of hemothorax or serosanguineous effusion because all types of pleural fluid are radiographically indistinguishable.[35] Relative contraindications to thoracocentesis include bleeding diatheses secondary to anticoagulation, severe thrombocytopenia, and heritable coagulopathy.[35] In dogs and cats, thoracocentesis for pleural fluid is performed at either the seventh or eighth intercostal space at or above the costochondral junction. Most patients will tolerate this procedure with a local lidocaine block (e.g., 2% lidocaine inserted through the intercostal musculature with a small-gauge needle to a depth of 0.5 to 1 cm) or mild sedation. The area should be clipped and surgically scrubbed. Care should be taken to avoid the intercostal vessels located caudal to each rib. A small-gauge butterfly needle, or a small-gauge needle attached to extension tubing, is attached via a three-way stopcock to a syringe. Gentle negative pressure is applied to the syringe after passing the needle between the ribs into the thoracic cavity. Aggressive aspiration will not increase yield and may result in iatrogenic pneumothorax secondary to parenchymal laceration.[35] Often, aspiration of one side of the thorax will drain the contralateral hemithorax because of fluid movement across the mediastinum.[38] If in doubt, thoracocentesis should be performed bilaterally. Use of prophylactic antibiotics is not recommended during this procedure when proper aseptic technique is followed.[38]

The minimum fluid analysis of a hemorrhagic effusion should include pH, specific gravity, protein concentration, packed cell volume, total white count, differential white count, culture (aerobic and anaerobic), and cytologic evaluation.[35] Between 2 and 4 ml of fluid should be placed in a tube with anticoagulant (EDTA) to be used for cell counts and measurement of specific gravity and total protein content.[4,28] Diagnosis of MPE requires the presence of exfoliated malignant cells in the pleural fluid (only 40% to 50% of MPE cytologies are diagnostic[35]); or documentation of malignant cells in pleural tissue by percutaneous pleural biopsy, thoracoscopy, thoracotomy, or necropsy.[20] Hemorrhagic effusions are typically characterized as modified transudates or exudates, and initial bacterial cultures are usually negative.[4,28] Cytologic evaluation reveals RBC counts ranging from 5000 to 50,000 cells/μl, and nucleated cell counts range from 1500 to 4000 cells/μl. Lymphocytes, macrophages, and mesothelial cells are present to varying degrees, and platelets are typically lacking.[2,20] As many as one-third of MPEs have a pH less than 7.3 and a glucose of less than 60 mg/dl.[20] These findings are not specific for malignancy because they also characterize empyema.[7,20]

Treatment

Initial stabilization of companion animals presenting with hemothorax depends on the severity of clinical signs but often includes oxygen supplementation, intravenous catheter placement and intravenous fluid resuscitation, and therapeutic needle thoracocentesis to relieve tamponade and allow lung reexpansion. With severe, acute blood loss, the priority is to replace intravascular volume to support the cardiac output. Some clinicians advocate the use of colloid rather than crystalloid fluids for volume resuscitation following moderate to severe blood loss that accompanies hemothorax but no survival advantage has been demonstrated following colloid fluid resuscitation.[39] In animals with coagulopathies, fresh plasma or whole blood is the colloid of choice, to replace coagulation factors. Alternatively, hetastarch is a synthetic colloid in isotonic saline, available as a 6% solution. Bolus doses of 5 ml/kg hetastarch, administered intravenously to effect or to a total dose of 15 to 20 ml/kg, may be used in conjunction with crystalloid fluids to correct hypovolemia and hypoperfusion associated with acute blood loss into the thoracic cavity. Following resuscitation, hetastarch may be administered as part of the patient's daily fluid requirements as a constant rate infusion at 20 ml/kg/day. Coagulopathy, characterized by mild prolongation of partial thromboplastin time and abnormalities of platelet function, can occur following hetastarch administration but has not been associated with a bleeding diathesis.[39] The glucose polymer, 6% dextran-70 diluted in isotonic saline, is an alternative to hetastarch. This colloidal fluid has been associated with a dose-related induction of bleeding tendencies.[39]

Acute loss of whole blood does not consistently result in a decrease in the hematocrit (HCT) because the relative proportions of plasma and red cell volume are unchanged. Therefore, in the first few hours after the onset of bleeding, a drop in the HCT primarily reflects fluid shifts and fluid resuscitation, not the extent of blood loss. When hemorrhage persists for greater than 8 to 12 hours, the kidneys conserve sodium and water and the HCT drops.[40] In general, an acute drop in PCV to values less than 20% warrants consideration of blood product transfusion; however, many patients with PCVs under 20% remain clinically normal at rest. Therefore the decision to transfuse should be based predominantly on clinical signs. Clinical anemia is characterized by changes in mental status, tachycardia or other arrhythmia, tachypnea or respiratory distress, and/or hyperdynamic femoral pulses. Transfusion with packed RBCs (10 to 15 ml/kg intravenously administered over 4 hours) is appropriate for most animals with anemia resulting from whole blood loss. In the presence of significant coagulopathy, however, fresh whole blood or fresh frozen plasma should be administered (15 to 20 ml/kg IV over 4 hours) to replenish clotting factors. Oxyglobin®, a polymerized hemoglobin solution of bovine origin in a modified Ringer's lactate solution (15 ml/kg in cats, 15 to 30 ml/kg in dogs), is an appropriate alternative to packed RBC transfusion in the absence of coagulopathy. Boluses (5 ml/kg intravenously to effect) of this colloid can be administered in cases with hemorrhage and hypovolemic shock. Autotransfusion is appropriate in cases of massive blood loss or when blood products are in limited supply. Blood should be collected aseptically and administered through appropriate filtering devices and administration sets. Autologous transfusion is relatively contraindicated in cases of suspected malignancy, and will not provide clotting factors in cases of warfarin intoxication.

Needle thoracocentesis is performed diagnostically to collect pleural fluid for subsequent analysis and, in many cases, therapeutically to drain the pleural space. If blood is allowed to remain in the pleural space, autotransfusion occurs rapidly from the pleural cavity via the diaphragmatic lymphatics, resulting in near resolution of hemothorax within several days. The degree of respiratory distress must be weighed against the potential for rapid resorption of blood in determining the amount of blood to be removed by thoracocentesis.[3] If rodenticide exposure is suspected, a prothrombin time (PT) or activated clotting time (ACT) should be evaluated before thoracocentesis.

Following drainage of hemothorax by thoracocentesis, a decision must be made as to whether or not the patient requires emergency surgery or tube thoracostomy for subsequent stabilization. Indications for immediate surgery include diaphragmatic hernia resulting in respiratory distress unresponsive to medical management; or stomach entrapment within the thoracic cavity. Documentation of lung lobe torsion is also an indication for emergency thoracotomy because this condition may result in severe hypotension and respiratory failure. Surgery may also be indicated when drainage is significant and continuous, or if the patient remains in shock despite adequate resuscitative efforts.[10,29]

With large hemothoraces, or in patients requiring multiple thoracocenteses, tube thoracostomy may be necessary.[35] Tube thoracostomy allows monitoring of ongoing blood loss into the thoracic cavity, control of lung compression caused by hemorrhage, and lung reexpansion.[35] Thoracic catheters are specifically manufactured for tube thoracostomy. These tubes have radioopaque depth markers, and end and side ports to facilitate drainage of pleural fluid. The size of tube used depends on the width of the patient's intercostal space and the viscosity of the pleural effusion, and should approximate the size of the patient's mainstem bronchus.[35,38] Placement of a chest tube can often be performed with light sedation and a local lidocaine block in dogs, but usually requires general anesthesia in cats. Radiographs (including at least two views) should be taken to confirm proper positioning of the chest tube. Bilateral chest tubes may be necessary; however, in most dogs and cats the mediastinum is permeable to fluid, allowing a single tube to adequately drain both hemithoraces.[38]

Possible complications associated with tube thoracostomy include hemorrhage, pneumothorax, reexpansion pulmonary edema, pleural shock characterized by bradycardia and/or hypotension, and laceration or perforation of thoracic or abdominal viscera.[35] The thoracic cavity can be evacuated by intermittent manual aspiration of the chest tube or by the application of continuous negative pressure utilizing a commercial continuous suction device or a two- or three-bottle system.[38] The chest tube should be removed when pleural fluid drainage decreases to less than 5 ml/kg/day, a volume that is consistent with that caused by the presence of the tube itself.[38]

In human patients, intrapleural fibrinolysis via tube thoracostomy for clotted hemothorax, loculated empyema, or malignant loculated pleural effusion without lung trapping has been shown to be a viable alternative to thoracotomy or decortication (surgical removal of the fibrous tissue from the visceral pleura). Streptokinase administration through the chest tube into the thoracic cavity degrades a variety of proteins (e.g., fibrin and fibrin blood clots) and has a reported 92% success rate when used to address fibrothorax in people.[41] There is little information available about the use of intrapleural fibrinolysis in companion animals.

Drainage of pleural effusion through intermittent thoracocenteses, obliteration of the pleural space, or placement of a pleuroperitoneal shunt can be attempted as methods of palliation in humans and companion animals with MPE.[7] Thoracotomy with pleurectomy is an invasive surgical procedure with high rates of morbidity and mortality given that the 30-day mortality rate for humans with MPE is reported to be 30% to 50%.[42] Therefore an

additional indication for tube thoracostomy in humans with MPE is the ability to instill a sclerosing agent into the pleural cavity to obliterate the pleural space and allow relief of the respiratory compromise, a procedure referred to as pleurodesis.[42] Before instillation of the sclerosing agent, the pleural space should be drained to prevent dilution of the agent and to allow adequate contact between the visceral and parietal pleura.[20] Complete lung expansion does not appear to be necessary for achievement of successful pleurodesis.[42] A variety of chemical agents have been employed including tetracycline derivatives, bleomycin, and talcum powder. In human patients with MPE, talcum powder has been reported to have the highest success rate (90% to 95%) of the commonly-utilized sclerosing agents, is readily available and inexpensive, and produces minimal side effects (e.g., pleuritic pain and fever).[20] Additional complications that are uncommonly associated with pleurodesis include empyema, arrhythmias, respiratory failure/acute respiratory distress syndrome, and pneumonitis.[20]

Placement of a pleuroperitoneal shunt has also been utilized to palliate humans with MPE. This shunt consists of a pumping chamber (inserted into the subcutaneous tissue) that can transport 1.5 ml fluid per compression; and two one-way valves, one in the chest and one in the abdomen.[13] Compression of the pumping chamber causes movement of fluid from the thorax to the abdomen. The most commonly observed complications associated with this procedure are clogging of the shunt and inadequate drainage of the pleural effusion.[20]

In contrast to humans with MPE, dogs and cats with thoracic malignancy and hemothorax appear to be relatively more resistant to chemical pleurodesis, and limited work has been done with this procedure in veterinary medicine.[33] It has been suggested that companion animals have a more effective pleural fibrinolytic system than other species.[38] Oxytetracycline (20 mg/kg diluted in 50 ml normal saline) was reported to achieve successful pleurodesis in one dog with MPE and in one dog with recurrent chylothorax.[43] Tetracycline causes increased capillary permeability and leakage of clotting proteins into the pleural space, with a resultant inflammatory response. As the inflammation resolves, usually within 7 days, pleural fusion occurs.[43,44]

In human patients, tube thoracostomy has a reported 84% success rate in the management of traumatic hemothoraces and/or pneumothoraces.[45,46] If chest tubes are already in place, indications for thoracotomy include severe hemorrhage into the thoracic cavity, either acutely during chest tube insertion, or persistently over several hours (i.e., when tearing of a great vessel is suspected); or when hemodynamic stability cannot be achieved with tube thoracostomy alone.[29] An additional indication for thoracotomy in humans is for management of residual hemothorax, which occurs in an estimated 2% of cases of hemothorax.[46] Inadequate drainage of fluid from the thoracic cavity via tube thoracostomy may result from malplacement of the tube, migration of the tip of the chest tube away from the site of collection, or obstruction of the tube.[46] In humans, undrained intrathoracic blood can lead to thickened fibrinous layers on the visceral and parietal pleura (fibrothorax) and/or empyema.[29] Management of such cases via thoracotomy allows for liquification of retained blood clots, removal of pleural adhesions, and removal of loculated fluid from within the thoracic space.[29] The significance of residual hemothorax in dogs and cats remains unknown.

More recently in human medicine, the use of video-assisted thoracic surgery (VATS) or thoracoscopy has been advocated in cases of thoracic trauma. Indications include evaluation and control of ongoing hemorrhage in the thoracic cavity, evacuation of retained hemothorax or posttraumatic empyema, evaluation and limited treatment of suspected diaphragmatic injuries, evaluation and treatment of persistent air leaks, and evaluation of mediastinal injuries.[47] In humans, this surgical procedure is minimally invasive; can be performed under local anesthesia or conscious sedation (neuroleptanalgesia); and is associated with decreased morbidity, less postoperative pain, and shorter hospital stays when compared with thoracotomy.[46-49] Contraindications include hemodynamic instability, injury to the heart or the great vessels, inability to tolerate single lung ventilation, obliterated pleural space, and bleeding diatheses.[47] Persistent hemorrhage into the thoracic cavity associated with lung laceration or torn intercostal vessels can be controlled thoracoscopically with electrocautery, endoclips, staples, or suture.[47] Conversion to thoracotomy is required in less than 10% of cases, but it may be necessary if bleeding intercostal vessels are retracted beneath the pleura, or when injured lung parenchymal vessels are located near the hilus.[47] Early (i.e., within 5 days of initial presentation) evacuation of retained hemothoraces via thoracoscopy has been shown to be a successful means of preventing the occurrence and/or progression of empyema and fibrothorax in humans.[48]

Thoracoscopy is also indicated to obtain a diagnosis of malignancy by pleural biopsy when less invasive diagnostic modalities have failed. In human patients with suspected MPE, cytology of the pleural effusion, needle biopsy of pleural tissue, and thoracoscopically-obtained fluid and tissue specimens were compared and had 62%, 44%, and 95% diagnostic sensitivity, respectively.[49,50]

Complications associated with thoracoscopy include cardiac arrhythmias, transient hypertension, hypoxemia, and severe hemorrhage secondary to blood vessel injury. However, with proper training, morbidity is low and mortality is estimated at less than 0.01% in humans.[49]

Prognosis/Outcome

The prognosis associated with hemothorax in dogs and cats depends on the underlying etiology and on appropriate and timely therapeutic intervention. Hemothoraces secondary to thoracic trauma that are not associated with damage to the heart or great vessels, and bleeding into the thoracic cavity secondary to warfarin intoxication, typically carry good prognoses. Hemothorax or hemorrhagic effusion secondary to malignancy, on the other hand, indicates advanced and terminal disease and carries a poor prognosis. Regardless of the etiology, recognition and correction of hypovolemic shock; addressing potential transfusion requirements; documentation and treatment of

hypoxemia; and therapeutic drainage of pleural fluid with needle thoracocentesis, tube thoracostomy, or emergent thoracotomy will improve outcome in the acute stage. The use of pleurodesing agents in the treatment of MPEs in dogs and cats is currently not advocated and warrants further investigation. The role of VATS in veterinary medicine for diagnosis and treatment of hemothorax is undefined, but holds promise as more clinicians become proficient at thoracoscopy.

REFERENCES

1. Johnson RF, Green RA: Pleural diseases. In Baum GL, Wolinsky E, editors: *Textbook of pulmonary diseases,* Boston, 1983, Little, Brown, and Co.
2. Wolf AM: Diseases of the pleural space and mediastinum. In Leib MS, editor: *Practical small animal internal medicine,* Philadelphia, 1997, WB Saunders.
3. Christopher MM: Pleural effusions, *Vet Clin North Am Small Anim Pract* 17:255-269, 1987.
4. Forrester SD, Troy GC, Fossum TW: Pleural effusions: Pathophysiology and diagnostic considerations, *Compendium* 10:121-137, 1988.
5. Bagwell CE, Salzberg AM, Sonnino RE et al: Potentially lethal complications of central venous catheter placement, *J Ped Surg* 35:709-713, 2000.
6. Chou S, Cheng Y, Kao E et al: Spontaneous haemothorax: An unusual presentation of primary lung cancer, *Thorax* 48:1185-1186, 1993.
7. DeCamp MM, Mentzer SJ, Swanson SJ et al: Malignant effusive disease of the pleura and the pericardium, *Chest* 112:291S-295S, 1997.
8. Dhodapkar M, Yale SH, Hoagland HC: Hemorrhagic pleural effusion and pleural thickening as a complication of chronic lymphocytic leukemia, *Amer J Hematol* 42:221-224, 1993.
9. Hagley MT, Martin B, Gast P et al: Infectious and mechanical complications of central venous catheters placed by percutaneous venipuncture and over guidewires, *Crit Care Med* 20:1426-1430, 1992.
10. Ruskin JA, Gurney JW, Thorsen MK et al: Detection of pleural effusion on supine chest radiographs, *Am J Roentgerol* 128:681-683, 1987.
11. Johnson EM, Saltzman DA, Suh G et al: Complications and risks of central venous catheter placement in children, *Surgery* 124:911-916, 1998.
12. Kearney TJ, Shabot MM: Pulmonary artery rupture associated with the Swan-Ganz catheter, *Chest* 108:1349-1352, 1995.
13. Keller SM: Current and future therapy for malignant pleural effusions, *Chest* 103:63S-67S, 1993.
14. Kollef MH, Gronski TJ: Hemothorax and an abdominal hematoma after treatment of ischemic cardiomyopathy with warfarin, *Heart and Lung* 23:125-127, 1994.
15. Pretre R, Murith N, Delay D et al: Surgical management of hemorrhage from rupture of the aortic arch, *Ann Thorac Surg* 65:1291-1295, 1998.
16. Quinn MW, Dillary TA: Delayed traumatic hemothorax on ticlopidine and aspirin for coronary stent, *Chest* 116:257-260, 1999.
17. Resnick DK: Delayed pulmonary perforation: A rare complication of tube thoracostomy, *Chest* 103:311-313, 1993.
18. Reynolds JR, Morgan E: Haemothorax caused by a solitary costal exostosis, *Thorax* 45:68-69, 1990.
19. Robinson NMK, Thomas MR, Jewitt DE: Spontaneous haemothorax as a complication of anti-coagulation following coronary angioplasty, *Resp Med* 89:629-630, 1995.
20. Sahn SA: Pleural diseases related to metastatic malignancies, *Eur Respir J* 10:1907-1913, 1997.
21. Sharpe DAC, Kixon K, Moghissi K: Spontaneous haemopneumothorax: A surgical emergency, *Eur Respir J* 8:1611-1612, 1995.
22. Tatebe S, Kanazawa H, Yamazaki Y et al: Spontaneous hemopneumothorax, *Ann Thorac Surg* 62:1011-1015, 1996.
23. Uchida K, Kurihara Y, Sekiguchi S et al: Spontaneous haemothorax caused by costal exostosis, *Eur Respir J* 10:735-736, 1997.
24. Varan B, Karakayali H, Kutsal A et al: Spontaneous hemothorax in a hemodialysis patient, *Pediatr Nephrol* 12:65-66, 1998.
25. Wagner RB: Massive hemothorax secondary to foreign body and CPR, *Ann Thorac Surg* 59:1241-1242, 1995.

26. Yung CM, Bessen SC, Hingorani V et al: Idiopathic hemothorax, *Chest* 103:638-639, 1993.
27. Spackman CJ, Caywood DD, Feeney DA et al: Thoracic wall and pulmonary trauma in dogs sustaining fractures as a result of motor vehicle accidents, *JAVMA* 185:975-977, 1984.
28. Forrester SD: The categories and causes of pleural effusions in cats, *Vet Med Symposium on Feline Pleural Effusion* 83(9):894-906, 1988.
29. Parry GW, Morgan WE, Salama FD: Management of haemothorax, *Ann R Coll Surg Engl* 78:325-326, 1996.
30. Simon BJ, Leslie C: Factors predicting early in-hospital death in blunt thoracic aortic injury, *J Trauma* 51:906-911, 2001.
31. Simon LJ, Chu Q, Emhoff TA: Delayed hemothorax after blunt thoracic trauma: An uncommon entity with significant morbidity, *J Trauma* 45:673-676, 1998.
32. Kramek BA, Caywood DD, O'Brien TD: Bullous emphysema and recurrent pneumothorax in the dog, *JAVMA* 186:971-974, 1985.
33. Noone KE: Pleural effusions and diseases of the pleura, *Vet Clin North Am Small Anim Pract* 15:1075-1076, 1985.
34. Cantwell HD, Rebar AH, Allen AR: Pleural effusion in the dog: Principles for diagnosis, *J Am Anim Hosp Assoc* 19:227-232, 1983.
35. Bauer T, Woodfield JA: Mediastinal, pleural, and extrapleural diseases. In Etinger SJ, editor: *Textbook of veterinary internal medicine*, ed 4, Philadelphia, 1995, WB Saunders.
36. Marts B, Durham R, Shapiro M et al: Computed tomography in the diagnosis of blunt thoracic trauma, *Amer J Surg* 168:688-692, 1994.
37. Stowater JL, Lamb CR: Ultrasonongraphy of noncardiac thoracic diseases in small animals, *JAVMA* 195:514-520, 1989.
38. Fossum TW, Hulse DA, Johnson AL et al: Surgery of the lower respiratory system: pleural cavity and diaphragm. In Fossum TW, editor: *Small animal surgery*, St Louis, 1997, Mosby-Year Book.
39. Marino PL: Colloid and crystalloid resuscitation. In Marino PL, editor: *The ICU book*, ed 2, Baltimore, 1998, Williams & Wilkins.
40. Marino PL: Hemorrhage and hypovolemia. In Marino PL, editor: *The ICU book*, ed 2, Baltimore, 1998, Williams & Wilkins.
41. Jerjes-Sanchez C, Ramirez-Rivera A, Delgado R et al: Intrapleural fibrinolysis with streptokinase as an adjunctive treatment in hemothorax and empyema, *Chest* 109:1514-1519, 1996.
42. Robinson LA, Fleming WH, Calbraith TA: Intrapleural doxycycline control of malignant pleural effusions, *Ann Thorac Surg* 55:1115-1122, 1993.
43. Laing EJ, Norris AM: Pleurodesis as a treatment for pleural effusion in the dog, *J Am Anim Hosp Assoc* 22:193-196, 1985.
44. Birchard SJ, Fossum TW, Gallagher L: Pleurodesis. In Kirk RW, editor: *Kirk's current veterinary therapy*, vol 10, Philadelphia, 1989, WB Saunders.
45. Mancini M, Smith LM, Nein A et al: Early evacuation of clotted blood in hemothorax using thoracoscopy: Case reports, *J Trauma* 34:144-147, 1993.
46. Velmahos GC, Demetriades D: Early thoracoscopy for the evacuation of undrained haemothorax, *Eur J Surg* 165:924-929, 1999.
47. Lowdermilk GA, Neunheim KS: Thoracoscopic evaluation and treatment of thoracic trauma, *Surg Clin N Am* 80:1535-1542, 2000.
48. Landreneau RJ, Keenana RJ, Hazelrigg SR et al: Thoracoscopy for empyema and hemothorax, *Chest* 109:18-24, 1995.
49. Loddenkemper R: Thoracoscopy: State of the art, *Eur Respir J* 11:213-221, 1998.
50. Loddenkemper R, Grosser H, Gabler A et al: Prospective evaluation of biopsy methods in the diagnosis of malignant pleural effusions: intrapatient comparison between pleural fluid cytology, blind needle biopsy, and thoracoscopy, *Am Rev Resp Dis* 127(suppl 4):114, 1983.

CHAPTER 82

Pneumomediastinum and Pneumothorax

Daniel J. Brockman • David A. Puerto

Definitions and Etiology

Anatomically, the mediastinum is the space between the pleural cavities that is bounded by the axial reflections of the parietal pleura. It contains all of the intrathoracic structures except the lungs. It communicates cranially with the tissue planes of the neck at the thoracic inlet and caudally with the retroperitoneal space via the aortic hiatus. The mediastinum divides the thorax into left and right hemithoracic cavities. The pleural space is a potential space between the parietal pleura of the thoracic cavity and the visceral pleura of the lungs. In the normal animal, only a small volume of pleural fluid occupies the pleural space. This fluid couples the lungs to the thoracic wall so that changes in thoracic volume are accompanied by changes in lung volume.[1]

Pneumomediastinum and pneumothorax are defined as the presence of free air or gas within the mediastinum or pleural space, respectively. Pneumomediastinum is an acquired disease that is usually secondary to accidental or iatrogenic trauma to the lower airways, marginal alveoli, or esophagus.[2-9] Pneumomediastinum has also been recognized as a consequence of sharp penetrating trauma to the pharynx or neck, the presence of mediastinal infection with gas-forming bacteria, and paraquat toxicity.[10,11]

Pneumothorax is also an acquired disease, most commonly associated with accidental blunt or penetrating thoracic trauma.[12-19] Spontaneous leakage of air from pathologically weakened pulmonary tissue is also a well-recognized cause of pneumothorax.[20-27] Iatrogenic sharp thoracic wall trauma and pulmonary barotrauma can cause pneumothorax[3,28,29]; and, as in the mediastinum, the presence of gas-forming organisms within the pleural space could create a pneumothorax.

Four broad categories of pneumothorax can therefore be defined based on etiology:

- *Traumatic,* where the pneumothorax is clearly associated with trauma
- *Spontaneous,* for those pneumothoraces associated with minimal or no trauma
- *Iatrogenic*
- *Infectious*

Traumatic pneumothorax can be usefully subdivided into those in which the thoracic wall has been breached, or is open; and those in which it remains physically intact, or is closed. Finally, when tissue at the site of air leakage into the pleural space is acting as a one-way valve, supra-atmospheric interpleural pressures can be generated, resulting in tension pneumothorax. The categorical designation of a patient with pneumothorax is an important factor that helps guide therapeutic decision-making.

Pathogenesis

PNEUMOMEDIASTINUM

Depending on the underlying etiology, pneumomediastinum may be either self-limiting or progressive. Although most cases of pneumomediastinum are mild and self-limiting, air accumulating within the mediastinum may progress into the pericardial sac; either caudally, to create a pneumoretroperitoneum; or through the thoracic inlet into the tissues of the neck and subcutaneous space, to create subcutaneous emphysema.[8] Commonly, mediastinal air ruptures through the mediastinal tissues, resulting in pneumothorax.[8,9]

TRAUMATIC PNEUMOTHORAX

Accidental trauma can cause pneumothorax by several mechanisms. In open pneumothorax, air may gain direct access to the pleural space across the thoracic wall defect. When the chest remains closed, pneumothorax can be caused by the sharp ends of fractured ribs lacerating the parietal and visceral pleurae, resulting in leakage of air directly from the lung parenchyma. In the absence of rib fractures, compression of the thorax while the glottis is closed can elevate airway pressures, causing barotrauma to the conducting airways or alveoli and resulting in rupture. Finally, rapid acceleration or deceleration of the injured subject (e.g., when hit by a car or in high-rise syndrome) can produce tensile and shearing forces that act on the trachea, mainstem bronchi, or pulmonary parenchyma, resulting in tearing of these structures. Regardless of the pathogenesis, the volume of air that enters the pleural space and the progression of the pneumothorax will be determined predominantly by the size of the defect leaking air, the breathing pattern of the patient, and whether the defect allows unidirectional or bidirectional airflow. It is important to realize that a pneumothorax should not progress to create a pneumomediastinum.

SPONTANEOUS PNEUMOTHORAX

Spontaneous pneumothorax has been associated with leakage of air from sites of pulmonary abscessation, primary and metastatic pulmonary neoplasia, foreign body migration, ruptured intrapulmonary bullae, ruptured subpleural blebs, pneumonia, and feline asthma.[24,27] In addition, parasitic infections (e.g., dirofilariasis, paragonimiasis and *Filaroides osleri*) have been associated with acute pneumothorax in the dog.[30-33]

IATROGENIC PNEUMOTHORAX

Iatrogenic pneumothorax is most commonly seen after needle thoracocentesis, fine-needle lung aspiration, needle biopsy of intrathoracic structures, or thoracostomy tube placement.[28,34] Pneumothorax is also a recognized complication of the lateral approach to the canine thoracolumbar disks.[35] In addition, it can result from barotrauma to the conducting airways or alveoli during anesthesia[3]; or during prolonged periods of mechanically-assisted ventilation, especially in the presence of pulmonary disease that requires the maintenance of high airway pressures such as those created using positive end expiratory pressure (PEEP).[36] Pneumothorax has also been reported as a complication of restraint for jugular venipuncture in the cat.[37]

Pathophysiology

PNEUMOMEDIASTINUM

The effect of a small amount of free gas in the mediastinum alone is usually minimal. In most patients the underlying cause of the pneumomediastinum (e.g., esophageal, tracheal, pharyngeal, or pulmonary injury) influences the pathophysiological derangements in the animal more than the pneumomediastinum per se. Under experimental conditions, accumulation of large amounts of gas in the mediastinum can cause increased mediastinal pressure, resulting in decreased venous return to the heart, a phenomenon termed "airblock." Mediastinal air may also dissect into the pericardium, resulting in pneumopericardium; spread to the interstitium of the lungs, causing decreased pulmonary compliance; and cause subcutaneous emphysema and pneumoretroperitoneum.[38,39] Commonly, however, the most serious potential sequela of massive pneumomediastinum is pneumothorax, the consequences of which are described below.

PNEUMOTHORAX

The effects of pneumothorax have been studied in both conscious and anesthetized normal dogs.[40-46] Several mechanisms appear to help the animal compensate for the deleterious effects of free pleural gas. Once air is introduced into the pleural space, the subatmospheric interpleural pressure is compromised and the elastic rib cage is no longer coupled efficiently to the lungs by the pleural fluid. The immediate effect of pneumothorax, therefore, is partial collapse of the lung(s), a reduced tidal volume during respiration, and an increase in overall thoracic volume caused by the release of the rib cage.[44,45] Lung collapse creates a ventilation/perfusion mismatch that results in a fall in arterial partial pressure of oxygen.[43,44] Intrapulmonary chemoreceptors and mechanoreceptors that detect the fall in alveolar oxygen concentration and alterations in pulmonary stretch, respectively, also influence the respiratory center, via the vagus nerve, to institute compensatory changes.[40,41] In addition, mechanoreceptors in the costovertebral joints and thoracic wall detect the change in thoracic conformation and exert an extravagal influence over the respiratory center.[42,43] The early compensatory response is an increase in respiratory rate accompanied by abolition of expiratory abdominal muscular activity.[41,45] This serves to maintain or increase alveolar ventilation despite a reduced tidal volume.

As the pneumothorax increases, the overall thoracic volume increases but the lung volume decreases. The number of poorly ventilated or completely unventilated alveoli increases, and the ventilation-perfusion mismatch worsens. Vasoactive mediators released locally within the pulmonary circulation cause constriction of pulmonary vessels serving the poorly ventilated areas of lung, reducing the ventilation-perfusion mismatch (hypoxic pulmonary vasoconstriction).[47] Tachypnea is effective in maintaining ventilation such that the arterial partial pressure of carbon dioxide remains within the normal range in all but massive (tension) pneumothorax.[44,45] Lung collapse, ventilation-perfusion mismatch, and intrapulmonary shunting of blood lead to a progressive linear fall in arterial partial pressure of oxygen as the pneumothorax worsens.[45] Hypoxemia detected by the aortic and carotid bodies strengthens the hypoxic ventilatory drive, further stimulating the intercostal and diaphragmatic musculature.[41,42] Activities that increase cardiac output (e.g., anxiety or exercise) will increase the amount of blood shunted through the lungs, exacerbating the hypoxemia. Increased intrathoracic pressure may decrease venous return to the heart and, along with pulmonary artery pressure elevation (secondary to hypoxic pulmonary vasoconstriction and external pressure) and myocardial ischemia, may lead to a fall in cardiac output. If untreated, the hypoxia, hypercapnia, and cardiovascular compromise can be fatal.

The pathophysiological derangements seen in clinical patients with pneumothorax depend not only upon the degree of pneumothorax but also on the presence and severity of concurrent pulmonary, thoracic wall, conducting airway, and abdominal disease. Trauma patients with pneumothorax may have concurrent rib fractures, limb fractures, pulmonary contusion, hemothorax, bronchial or tracheal tears, diaphragmatic rupture, and myocardial contusion, all of which may contribute to the level of cardiovascular and respiratory compromise.

Fortunately, most dogs with spontaneous pneumothorax do not have concurrent systemic diseases.

Tension pneumothorax creates similar initial pathophysiological changes. As supra-atmospheric pressure develops in the pleural space, lung compression becomes more severe and profound hypoxemia develops rapidly. Recent experimental studies on the effect of tension pneumothorax in sheep and pig models suggest that equilibration of pleural pressure with central venous and pulmonary artery pressures (reducing venous return to the heart) is a relatively late event.[48,49] Cardiac output is initially maintained by tachycardia, which increases the myocardial oxygen demand. Ultimately, myocardial oxygen delivery falls short of oxygen demand and the venous return to the heart becomes compromised, further reducing cardiac output. Severe hypoxemia, hypercapnia, and systemic hypotension develop. The progression of tension pneumothorax to a life-threatening state may be very rapid.

Mechanism of Absorption of Entrapped Air from the Pleural Space

Initially, air within the pleural (or mediastinal) space has the same concentrations of oxygen (149 mm Hg), nitrogen (564 mm Hg), and water vapor (47 mm Hg) as humidified air at sea level, adding to a total of 760 mm Hg. The interstitial fluid has a partial pressure of oxygen of 40 mm Hg, carbon dioxide of approximately 40 mm Hg, and nitrogen 572 mm Hg, adding up to a total of 652 mm Hg. Oxygen therefore diffuses out of the cavity along its concentration gradient whereas carbon dioxide and small amounts of nitrogen diffuse into the cavity. Loss of oxygen makes the volume of free gas smaller, with a higher relative concentration of nitrogen. The gases reach equilibrium with carbon dioxide at 40 mm Hg in both the interstitium and the gas cavity, with oxygen at approximately 43 mm Hg in the cavity (40 mm Hg in the interstitium), and with nitrogen at 630 mm Hg in the cavity (572 mm Hg in the interstitium). Saturated vapor pressure in the cavity remains the same at 47 mm Hg. Oxygen and nitrogen are then continually absorbed from the cavity, reducing the volume of free gas and increasing the relative concentration of carbon dioxide and water vapor. Consequently, carbon dioxide and water vapor are absorbed along their concentration gradients until all the gases have left the cavity. Clinically, this process may take several days to several weeks, depending on the initial volume.

Incidence and Prevalence

PNEUMOMEDIASTINUM

The most common cause of pneumomediastinum is trauma. In one study, 8% of cats and dogs with traumatic rib fractures or appendicular fractures were also diagnosed with pneumomediastinum.[17] In the majority of these cases, pneumomediastinum was not the sole injury; other thoracic injuries such as pulmonary contusions and pneumothorax occurred simultaneously and were more common. The prevalence of pneumomediastinum caused by mechanisms other than trauma has not been reported.

TRAUMATIC PNEUMOTHORAX

It has been estimated that 10% of trauma admissions to an urban veterinary emergency practice had thoracic injuries.[50] In addition, reports suggest that between 37% and 57% of dogs and cats with appendicular skeletal injuries have concurrent thoracic injuries.[4-6,12,17] Of these injuries, up to 50% included pneumothorax. In cats with traumatic rib fractures, concurrent pneumothorax was diagnosed in 56% of cases.[12] In a study of thoracic bite wounds, over half (6/11) of the dogs and cats had pneumothorax among their thoracic abnormalities.[16] In high-rise syndrome, thoracic injuries are common, with 63% of cats and 32% of dogs diagnosed with pneumothorax.[13,14]

SPONTANEOUS PNEUMOTHORAX

In the largest study to date, 64 dogs were presented to the University of Pennsylvania because of spontaneous pneumothorax over a 13-year period. During the same period, the total number of emergency room accessions for dogs at the same institution was 59,316, giving an estimated prevalence of 0.11%.

IATROGENIC PNEUMOTHORAX

In a study reporting outcomes for dogs undergoing therapeutic mechanically-assisted ventilation,[36] the prevalence of pneumothorax was 12/41 or 29%. A 31% incidence of pneumothorax has been reported as a complication of transthoracic needle aspiration biopsy of lung pathology in dogs.[28] There are no studies documenting the incidence of pneumothorax after diagnostic or therapeutic thoracocentesis or closed thoracostomy tube placement. Similarly, the frequency with which iatrogenic barotrauma during anesthesia causes pneumomediastinum and pneumothorax is unknown.

Epidemiology and Risk Factors

Although dogs and cats of all sizes and ages may suffer trauma, dogs most at risk for traumatic disease in urban areas were young intact males.[50] In another retrospective study, animals that sustained thoracic injuries as a result of dog fight bite wounds were all either small-breed dogs or cats.[15] Recent retrospective analyses of patients with spontaneous pneumothorax[27,51] revealed that Siberian huskies were at increased risk for pulmonary bullous disease and subpleural blebs. One of these studies[27] that included 21 different breeds suggested that spontaneous pneumothorax was more prevalent among heavier dog breeds. Among mechanically ventilated patients, the most significant risk factor for developing pneumothorax

was the presence of lung pathology serious enough to warrant PEEP.[36]

Traumatic Pneumothorax

HISTORICAL FINDINGS, CLINICAL SIGNS, AND PROGRESSION

Patients with traumatic pneumothorax are usually presented because of the traumatic episode, with a variable degree of respiratory distress, tachypnea, and increased respiratory effort. Mucous membrane color may also vary from pink to pale or cyanotic, depending upon the degree of respiratory and circulatory compromise. Decreased lung sounds may be detected on thoracic auscultation, especially in the dorsal lung fields. The severity of clinical signs is proportional to the volume of air in the pleural space and the extent of the concurrent injuries.

DIFFERENTIAL DIAGNOSIS

Although pneumothorax is the most common cause of respiratory distress in trauma patients, other important conditions should be considered. Pulmonary contusion is a very common consequence of blunt thoracic trauma. Rib fractures, diaphragmatic rupture, traumatic bullae, hemothorax, and hypoperfusion should also be considered.

DIAGNOSTIC TESTS

Assessment of the patient's respiratory status can be made using subjective physical parameters (e.g., respiratory rate, respiratory effort, auscultation, and mucous membrane color). Thoracic auscultation may reveal dull lung sounds in the caudodorsal part of the chest if a pneumothorax is present. Even if there are no respiratory signs, thoracic radiographs should always be made in the veterinary trauma patient to evaluate for the presence of thoracic injuries (Figure 82-1, *A* and *B*). In dyspneic patients with advanced pleural space disease, positioning for radiography may pose an unnecessary risk. In such cases thoracocentesis should be performed before radiography as both a diagnostic and therapeutic maneuver. Objective measurements of lung function (e.g., pulse oximetry and blood gas analysis) can be used once the patient is stabilized.

MANAGEMENT AND MONITORING

All trauma patients should undergo a careful evaluation of their major organ systems, and support should be rapidly provided to ensure adequate performance of vital body functions. In many instances this support will include oxygen supplementation, intravenous fluid therapy, thoracic drainage, and analgesia. Ideally, treatment decisions for all patients with respiratory dysfunction should be influenced most profoundly by the results of arterial blood gas analysis. This is not a practical approach for the majority of animals with traumatic pneumothorax, however, because the restraint required for

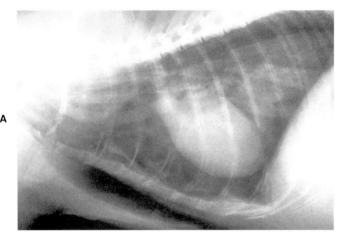

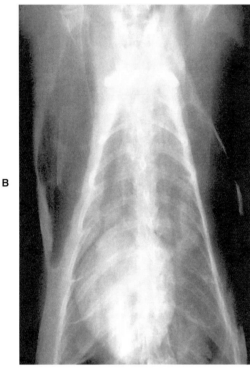

*Figure 82-1. **A,** Lateral and **B,** dorsoventral radiographs of a cat that was hit by a car. There is massive subcutaneous emphysema, pneumomediastinum, and pneumothorax.*

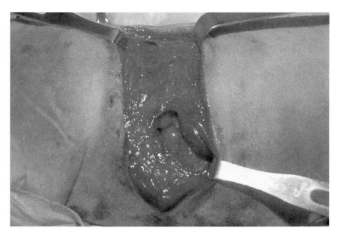

Figure 82-2. A skin incision was made over a small puncture wound on the thorax of this Shih-Tzu that was observed following a fight with a larger dog. The bite wound had penetrated the thorax. The lung can be seen easily through the traumatic thoracotomy.

placement of a durable arterial catheter or for repeated blood sampling by needle puncture of the artery can place the animal at unacceptable risk. Treatment decisions are therefore often based on the type of pneumothorax present and on subjective clinical assessment.

Closed traumatic pneumothorax is best treated conservatively if the subjective and measured objective parameters are minimally affected. Cage rest and frequent observation is required over a 12- to 24-hour period. If unilateral air leakage is suspected, it may be beneficial to place the patient in lateral recumbency with the affected side down.[52] If there is a significant increase in respiratory rate and effort, or evidence of hypoxia or hypoventilation, thoracocentesis should be performed and

supplemental oxygen administered. Repeated thoracocentesis attempts based purely on the apparent radiographic volume of pneumothorax, especially if there is no clinical deterioration of the patient, should be avoided for fear of reopening the fibrin seal over sites of damaged lung and thereby perpetuating leakage of air.

If necessary, thoracocentesis should be repeated, but if thoracocentesis is needed more than three or four times in a 12- to 24-hour period, thoracostomy tube placement should be considered. Thoracostomy tubes allow frequent aspiration of air from the pleural space or application of continuous suction using a pleural drainage system. Thoracostomy tubes are rarely needed to treat traumatic pneumothorax. In order to allow good healing of the site of leakage, strict rest is recommended for 2 weeks following traumatic pneumothorax. Surgery is rarely necessary for successful treatment and resolution of closed traumatic pneumothorax but should be considered in patients with massive uncontrollable leakage, or air leakage that continues for more than 5 days after the trauma.

Open chest wounds require a sterile dressing to prevent further accumulation of air in the chest and contamination of the wound by the environment. Surgical exploration, debridement, thoracic drain placement, and closure of the thoracic defect should be undertaken as soon as the patient has been stabilized. The extent of tissue damage with thoracic bite wounds, in particular, is often quite severe (Figure 82-2).[16] Such patients require intensive supportive care and careful monitoring. The tube thoracostomy is maintained for as long as it is needed to ensure no further leakage of air. An additional benefit of tube thoracostomy is the ability to provide supplemental analgesia using interpleural local anesthetic agents.

Rib fractures may cause pneumothorax by penetration of the lungs, but usually neither the lung laceration nor the rib fractures requires surgical intervention. Severe displacement of fractured rib ends and multiple consecutive rib fractures may represent surgical disease. However, large flail segments experimentally created in the chest wall of normal dogs did not alter arterial blood gas values in spontaneously breathing anesthetized subjects.[53] The authors of that study concluded that the hypoventilation and hypoxemia in patients with rib fractures and flail chest were more likely to be secondary to pain, pleural space disease, and pulmonary contusion, rather than to the rib fractures themselves.[53]

OUTCOME AND PROGNOSIS

The prognosis for patients with traumatic pneumothorax is good, with 90% survival reported in one retrospective study.[54] Factors associated with increased survival were lack of clinical dyspnea, lack of need for thoracocentesis, and longer hospital intensive care stay (i.e., more than 2 days). Nonsurviving patients may be those that are more severely affected and do not stabilize with medical management; those that die of their injuries before treatment; or those that have other serious injuries such as diaphragmatic hernia, severe pulmonary contusion, and abdominal injuries.

Spontaneous Pneumothorax

HISTORICAL FINDINGS, CLINICAL SIGNS, AND PROGRESSION

The most common presenting complaints for dogs with spontaneous pneumothorax are dyspnea, anorexia, tachypnea, cough, and vomiting. Other less common presenting complaints include lethargy, cyanosis, gagging, polyuria/polydipsia, depression, and collapse.[20,26,27] In the largest study to date,[27] the average duration of clinical signs before presentation was 4½ days, and most patients were presented because of a rapid progression of respiratory distress. There are reports of some patients, however, that present with a more chronic history, and clinical signs of greater than 1 week's duration.[20,26,27]

DIFFERENTIAL DIAGNOSIS

The most common cause of spontaneous pneumothorax is a ruptured pulmonary bulla or subpleural bleb, occurring in 36% to 68% of cases.[20,22,26,27] Spontaneous pneumothorax has also been reported to occur secondary to nonbullous disease such as pneumonia, parasitic disease (*Dirofilaria*, *Paragonimus*, and *Filaroides osleri*), and neoplasia.[22,24-27,30,31] Migration of inhaled plant material has also been reported as a cause of spontaneous pneumothorax.[27]

DIAGNOSTIC TESTS

The initial approach to these patients is the same as that outlined for traumatic pneumothorax. A thorough physical examination, complete blood count, chemistry profile, pulse oximetry, and/or blood gas analysis should be performed once the patient has been stabilized. If necessary in the dyspneic patient with a high index of sus-

picion for pneumothorax, diagnostic and therapeutic thoracocentesis can be performed before other diagnostic tests. If the patient is stable enough, thoracic radiographs can be taken to diagnose the pneumothorax, and postthoracocentesis radiographs should be made following drainage of the pleural space. All of the radiographs should be carefully assessed for any underlying cause (e.g., bullae, pneumonia, asthma, or neoplasia). If there is evidence of pneumonia, a tracheal wash for cytology and culture could be considered. If parasitic disease is suspected, serological tests are available for dirofilariasis and paragonimus. Identification of tracheal nodules on radiographs and bronchoscopy, or documentation of larvae in a freshly collected fecal sample by the Baermann technique or in a tracheal wash sample, will provide a diagnosis of *Filaroides osleri* infection. In a recent study, the radiographic description of the presence and location of pulmonary bullae agreed poorly with surgical or postmortem findings.[27] Although there are no reports of the use of computed tomography (CT) scanning in dogs with spontaneous pneumothorax, CT scans have been shown to be more sensitive for the detection of emphysematous changes in human lungs and may prove useful in veterinary medicine.[55]

PATHOLOGICAL AND HISTOPATHOLOGICAL FINDINGS

In one study of spontaneous pneumothorax,[27] a cause for the pneumothorax was identified in 34 of 36 dogs (94.4%) that underwent surgical exploration, and in 2 dogs that underwent necropsy following unsuccessful nonsurgical treatment. Twenty-six (68.4%) dogs had bullous emphysema; 4 dogs (10.5%) had neoplasia (1 each of bronchoalveolar carcinoma, anaplastic carcinoma, multifocal ectatic carcinoma, and metastatic malignant melanoma); 2 dogs (5.2%) had migrating plant material (1 grass awn and 1 pine needle); 2 dogs (5.2%) had pleuritis only; and 1 dog (2.6%) had pulmonary microabscesses with pleuritis. The 2 dogs that were treated non-surgically and subsequently necropsied had bullous emphysema.

MANAGEMENT AND MONITORING

The aim of medical treatment for dogs with spontaneous pneumothorax is to stabilize the patient until diagnostic tests can determine if surgical intervention is indicated. In dogs with spontaneous pneumothorax secondary to pneumonia, dirofilariasis, and paragonomiasis, success has been reported with treatment of the underlying disease.[22] In studies of spontaneous pneumothorax, medical treatment consisting of thoracocentesis or thoracostomy tube drainage combined with rest resulted in a high rate of recurrence and mortality.[26,27]

Early surgical intervention with exploratory thoracotomy via median sternotomy is recommended for patients that do not have identifiable medical disease or diffuse pulmonary disease. Lesions were reported in multiple lung lobes in 37% of cases, and occurred bilaterally in 26% of cases (Figure 82-3).[27] On exploration of the thorax, all of the lung lobes should therefore be ex-

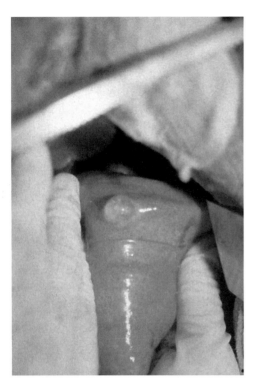

Figure 82-3. The leaking bulla in a dog with spontaneous pneumothorax. The location of the bulla was the dorsal aspect of the right middle lung lobe. Excision of the lobe was curative.

amined for pulmonary bullae, blebs, nodules, pleuritis, or other lesions. The accessory lung lobe must be examined by opening the caudal mediastinum. The lungs can be examined for air leakage by direct inspection and by submersion in saline. Once any lesions have been identified, a complete or partial lung lobectomy is performed. If no lesion is seen, careful sequential occlusion of each lobar bronchus, using atraumatic clamps, can be performed to test for leakage of air (determined by failure to maintain airway pressure) from a closed anesthetic circuit. Such manipulations require careful coordination between the surgeon and anesthetist.

In a small proportion of animals with spontaneous pneumothorax, an obvious site of leakage is not identified at exploratory surgery. Pleurodesis has been suggested as a treatment in circumstances where a site of leakage is not discovered.[56] However, a recent study of several techniques[57] failed to identify a reliable method of pleurodesis, and therefore this treatment cannot be recommended at this time. The authors believe that, as in humans,[58] thoracic omentalization may benefit patients in which a site of leakage is not identified. Theoretically the omentum may adhere to and seal damaged lung sites, but experimental and clinical evidence for this is limited.

Although not commonly available, thoracoscopic techniques have been described for successful treatment of spontaneous pneumothorax.[27,59,60] However, the inconsistent location of pulmonary lesions makes careful examination of all parts of all of the lung lobes necessary

in many cases, which may hinder attempts at thoracoscopic treatment. If CT allows better localization of the site of disease, selection of patients for thoracoscopic exploration and treatment should become easier.

OUTCOME AND PROGNOSIS

The final outcome and prognosis are dependent on the underlying cause for the spontaneous pneumothorax and on the type of treatment. In dogs treated with surgical exploration, there is a recurrence rate of 3.3%, compared with 50% for medically managed dogs.[27] The same was true for mortality rate; surgically managed dogs had 12.1% mortality rate compared with a 53% mortality rate in dogs managed medically.[27] Therefore, after initial stabilization with thoracocentesis or thoracostomy tube placement, surgical exploration is recommended for dogs with spontaneous pneumothorax that do not have identifiable nonsurgical or diffuse pulmonary disease.[22,26,27] Conservative treatment can be offered if surgical exploration is not feasible, but owners should be advised of the higher recurrence and mortality rates.

Iatrogenic Pneumothorax

HISTORICAL FINDINGS, CLINICAL SIGNS, AND PROGRESSION

Patients that undergo thoracocentesis or transthoracic needle biopsy should have thoracic radiographs following the procedure to evaluate the pleural space. Development of tachypnea and respiratory distress after thoracocentesis or transthoracic needle lung biopsy should alert the clinician to the possibility of iatrogenic pneumothorax. Iatrogenic pneumothorax should be considered in patients that are being mechanically ventilated or that are under anesthesia when subcutaneous emphysema or pneumoretroperitoneum (Figure 82-4) develop; or if there is a decrease in pulmonary compliance, oxygen desaturation, tachycardia, or hypotension.

DIFFERENTIAL DIAGNOSIS

Iatrogenic pneumothorax should always be considered in patients that develop respiratory compromise after a procedure that involves anesthesia, or sampling of the lungs or pleural space. However, other causes of respiratory distress should also be remembered, including pleural effusion; hemothorax; pyothorax caused by leakage from an infected lesion during sampling; or bleeding into a bronchus or major airway, causing obstruction. Additional potential causes of worsening respiratory status are aspiration pneumonia, pulmonary thromboembolism, and acute respiratory distress syndrome.

DIAGNOSTIC TESTS

Thoracic radiographs or thoracocentesis will determine whether there is a pneumothorax or if clinical signs are

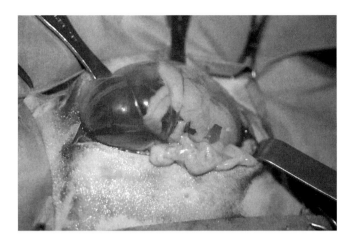

Figure 82-4. *Massive pneumoretroperitoneum in a cat anaesthetized for routine ovarohysterectomy. Such a finding as a sequel to pneumomediastinum indicates either trauma to the trachea by the endotracheal tube or barotrauma involving the lower airways or marginal alveoli.*

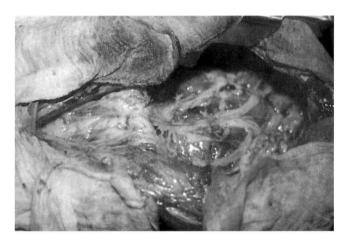

Figure 82-5. *This dog had uncontrollable pneumothorax caused by multiple sites of air leakage from the lung as a result of overzealous aspiration of a chest drain. The omentum has been lengthened and placed across the diaphragm to cover all the sites of lung leakage. Following wound closure, the dog recovered uneventfully.*

caused by another disease process. If tracheal rupture secondary to intubation is suspected, bronchoscopy may aid in diagnosis.

PATHOLOGICAL AND HISTOPATHOLOGICAL FINDINGS

Studies of barotrauma have demonstrated rupture of the marginal alveoli with dissection of air along vascular sheaths, pulmonary interstitial emphysema, and pneumothorax with rupture of the mediastinum or of alveoli in the apex of the lung.[38,39]

MANAGEMENT AND MONITORING

Pneumothorax secondary to thoracocentesis may be managed conservatively if respiratory compromise is minimal. Placing the patient in lateral recumbency with the affected side down may be of benefit even if the patient is being ventilated.[52,61] Thoracocentesis and/or placement of thoracostomy tubes with or without continuous suction may be needed, particularly if the leak is secondary to ventilation using PEEP. Positive pressure ventilation should be discontinued, if possible. Exploratory surgery is reserved for those patients that do not respond to conservative measures. The authors have successfully used thoracic omentalization in a patient with multiple sites of lung leakage following thoracostomy tube mismanagement (Figure 82-5).

OUTCOME AND PROGNOSIS

Most patients with iatrogenic pneumothorax can be successfully treated. Prognosis is dependent on the underlying disease process.

REFERENCES

1. Evans HE, Christensen GC: The respiratory apparatus. In Evans HE, Christensen GC, editors: *Miller's anatomy of the dog*, ed 2, Philadelphia, 1979, WB Saunders.
2. Manning MM, Brunson DB: Barotrauma in a cat, *JAVMA* 205:62-64, 1994.
3. Cimino Brown D, Holt D: Subcutaneous emphysema, pneumothorax, pneumomediastinum, and pneumopericardium associated with positive pressure ventilation in a cat, *JAVMA* 206:997-999, 1995.
4. White RN, Burton CA: Surgical management of intrathoracic tracheal avulsion in cats: Long-term results in 9 consecutive cases, *Vet Surg* 29(5):430-435, 2000.
5. White RN, Milner HR: Intrathoracic tracheal avulsion in three cats, *J Small Anim Pract* 36:343-347, 1995.
6. Hardie EM, Spodnick GJ, Gilson SD et al: Tracheal rupture in cats: 16 cases (1983-1998), *JAVMA* 214:508-512, 1999.
7. Kellagher REB, White RAS: Tracheal rupture in a dog, *J Small Anim Pract* 28:29-38, 1987.
8. Van den Broek A: Pneumomediastinum in 17 dogs: Aetiology and radiographic signs, *J Small Anim Pract* 27:747-757, 1986.
9. Rogers K, Walker MA: Disorders of the mediastinum, *Compend Contin Educ Pract Vet* 19:69-81, 1997.
10. White RAS, Lane JG: Pharyngeal stick injuries, *J Small Anim Pract* 29:13-35, 1988.
11. Kealy K: The thorax. In Kealy K, editor: *Diagnostic radiology of the dog and cat*, ed 2, Philadelphia, 1987, WB Saunders.
12. Kraje BJ, Kraje AC, Rorhbach BW et al: Intrathoracic and concurrent orthopedic injury associated with traumatic rib fracture in cats: 75 cases, *JAVMA* 216:51-54, 2000.
13. Whitney WO, Melhaff CJ: High-rise syndrome in cats, *JAVMA* 191:1399-1403, 1987.
14. Kapatkin AS, Matthiesen DT: Feline high-rise syndrome, *Compend Cont Educ Pract Vet* 1389-1395, 1991.
15. McKiernan BC, Adams WM, Huse DC: Thoracic bite wounds and associated internal injury in 11 dogs and one cat, *JAVMA* 8:959-964, 1984.
16. Shahar R, Shamir M, Johnston DE: A technique for management of bite wounds of the thoracic wall in small dogs, *Vet Surg* 26:45-50, 1997.
17. Tamas PM, Paddleford RR, Krahwinkel DJ: Thoracic trauma in dogs and cats presented for limb fractures, *J Amer Anim Hosp Assoc* 21:161-166, 1985.
18. Selcer BA, Buttrick M, Barstad R et al: The incidence of thoracic trauma in dogs with skeletal injury, *J Small Anim Pract* 28:21-27, 1987.

19. Spackman CJA, Caywood DD, Feeney DA: Thoracic wall and pulmonary trauma in dogs sustaining fractures as a result of motor vehicle accidents, *JAVMA* 185:975-977, 1984.
20. Yoshioka MM: Management of spontaneous pneumothorax in 12 dogs, *J Amer Anim Hosp Assoc* 18:57-62, 1982.
21. Kramek BA, Caywood DD, O'Brien TD: Bullous emphysema and recurrent pneumothorax in the dog, *JAVMA* 186:971-974, 1985.
22. Valentine A, Smeak D, Allen D et al: Spontaneous pneumothorax in dogs, *Compend Contin Educ Pract Vet* 18:53-62, 1996.
23. Berzon JL, Rendano VT, Hoffer RE: Recurrent pneumothorax secondary to ruptured pulmonary blebs: A case report, *J Amer Anim Hosp Assoc* 15:707-711, 1979.
24. Forrester SD, Fossum TW, Miller MW: Pneumothorax in a dog with a pulmonary abscess and suspected infective endocarditis, *JAVMA* 200:351-354, 1992.
25. Dallman MJ, Martin RA, Roth L: Pneumothorax as the primary problem in two cases of bronchioloalveolar carcinoma in the dog, *J Amer Anim Hosp Assoc* 24:710-714, 1988.
26. Holtsinger RH, Beale BS, Bellah JR et al: Spontaneous pneumothorax in the dog: A retrospective analysis of 21 cases, *J Amer Anim Hosp Assoc* 29:195-210, 1993.
27. Puerto DA, Brockman DJ, Lindquist CL et al: Surgical and nonsurgical management of and selected risk factors for spontaneous pneumothorax in dogs: 64 cases (1986-1999), *JAVMA* 220:1670-1674, 2002.
28. Teske E, Stokhof AA, van den Ingh TS et al: Transthoracic needle aspiration biopsy of the lung in dogs with pulmonic diseases, *J Amer Anim Hosp Assoc* 27:289-294, 1991.
29. Stogdale L, O'Conner CD, Williams MC et al: Recurrent pneumothorax associated with a pulmonary emphysematous bulla in a dog: surgical correction and proposed pathogenesis, *Can Vet J* 23:281-287, 1982.
30. Saheki Y, Ishitani R, Miyamoto Y: Acute fatal pneumothorax in canine dirofilariasis, *Jpn J Vet Sci* 43:315-328, 1981.
31. Busch DS, Noxon JO: Pneumothorax in a dog infected with *Dirofilaria immitis*, *JAVMA* 201:1893, 1992.
32. Pechman RD Jr.: Pulmonary paragonimiasis in dogs and cats: A review, *J Small Anim Pract* 21(2):87-95, 1980.
33. Brockman DJ: Unpublished data.
34. Frendin J, Obel F: Catheter drainage of pleural fluid collections and pneumothorax, *J Small Anim Pract* 38(6):237-242, 1997.
35. Bartels KE, Creed JE, Ytrurraspe DJ: Complications associated with the dorsolateral muscle-separating approach for thoracolumbar disk fenestration in the dog, *JAVMA* 183:1081-1083, 1983.
36. King LG, Hendricks JC: Use of positive-pressure ventilation in dogs and cats: 41 cases (1990-1992), *JAVMA* 204:1045-1052, 1994.
37. Godfrey DR: Bronchial rupture and fatal tension pneumothorax following routine venipuncture in a kitten, *J Amer Anim Hosp Assoc* 33:260-263, 1997.
38. Macklin MT, Macklin CC: Malignant interstitial emphysema of the lungs and mediastinum as an important occult complication in many respiratory diseases and other conditions in light of laboratory experiment, *Medicine* 23:281-358, 1944.
39. Macklin CC: Pneumothorax with massive collapse from experimental local overinflation of the lung substance, *Can Med Assoc J* 36:414, 1937.
40. Lee BP, Lin YC, Chiang ST: Role of vagal reflex in maintaining alveolar ventilation during pneumothorax in anaesthetized dogs, *J Formosan Med Assoc* 86:1133-1143, 1987.
41. Hollstien SB, Carl ML, Schelegle ES et al: Role of vagal afferents in the control of abdominal expiratory muscle activity in the dog, *J Appl Physiol* 71:1795-1800, 1991.
42. De Troyer A, Sampson M, Sigrist S et al: Action of costal and crural parts of the diaphragm on the rib cage in dogs, *J Appl Physiol* 54:465-469, 1983.
43. Shannon R: Respiratory pattern changes during costovertebral joint movement, *J Appl Physiol* 48(5):862-867, 1980.
44. Walker M, Hartsfield S, Matthews N et al: Computed tomography and blood gas analysis of anesthetized bloodhounds with induced pneumothorax, *Vet Rad Ultrasound* 34:93-98, 1993.
45. Bennett A, Orton EC, Tucker A et al: Cardiopulmonary changes in conscious dogs with induced progressive pneumothorax, *Am J Vet Res* 50:280-284, 1989.
46. Kern DA, Carrig CB, Martin RA: Radiographic evaluation of induced pneumothorax in the dog, *Vet Rad Ultrasound* 35:411-417, 1994.
47. Fishman, AP: Hypoxia on the pulmonary circulation: How and where it acts, *Circ Res* 38:221-231, 1976.
48. Barton ED, Rhee P, Hutton KC et al: The pathophysiology of tension pneumothorax in ventilated swine, *J Emerg Med* 15(2):147-153, 1997.
49. Hurewitz AN, Sidhu U, Bergofsky EH et al: Cardiovascular and respiratory consequences of tension pneumothorax, *Bull Eur Physiopathol Respir* 22(6):545-549, 1986.
50. Kolata RJ, Johnston DE: Motor vehicle accidents in urban dogs: A study of 600 cases, *JAVMA* 167:938, 1975.
51. Grölinger K, Lorinson D, Wiskocil L et al: Spontaneous pneumothorax caused by bullae pulmonales in four huskies, *Vet Surg* 30:304(Abstract), 2001.
52. Zidulka A, Braidy TF, Rizzi MC et al: Position may stop pneumothorax progression in dogs, *Am J Respir Dis* 126:51-53, 1982.
53. Capello M, Yuehua C, De Troyer A: Rib cage distortion in a canine model of flail chest, *Am J Respir Crit Care Med* 151(5):1481-1485, 1995.
54. Krahwinkel DJ, Rohrbach BW, Hollis BA: Factors associated with survival in dogs and cats with pneumothorax, *J Vet Emerg Crit Care* 9:7-12, 1999.
55. Warner BW, Bailey WW, Shipley RT: Value of computed tomography of the lung in the management of primary spontaneous pneumothorax, *Amer J Surg* 162:39-42, 1991.
56. Birchard SJ, Gallagher L: Use of pleurodesis in treating selected pleural diseases, *Comp Contin Educ Pract Vet* 10(7):826-832, 1988.
57. Jerram RM, Fossum TW, Berridge BR et al: The efficacy of mechanical abrasion and talc slurry pleurodesis in normal dogs, *Vet Surg* 28:322-332, 1999.
58. Kageyama Y, Matsushita K, Kita Y et al: An elderly case of pneumothorax treated with omentopexy, *Kyobu Gecka* 50(13):1152-1155, 1997.
59. Garcia F, Prandi D, Peña T et al: Examination of the thoracic cavity and lung lobectomy by means of thoracopy in dogs, *Can Vet J* 39:285-291, 1998.
60. Liu H, Lin PJ, Hsieh M et al: Thoracoscopic surgery as a routine procedure for spontaneous pneumothorax: results from 82 patients, *Chest* 107:559-562, 1995.
61. Zidulka A: Position may reduce or stop pneumothorax formation in dogs receiving mechanical ventilation, *Clin Invest Med* 10:290-294, 1987.

CHAPTER 83

Diaphragmatic Hernia

Dale E. Bjorling • Gretchen K. Sicard

The diaphragm structurally separates the thorax from the abdomen and also takes an active role in respiration. Despite the passive and active roles of the diaphragm, loss of continuity of the diaphragm itself does not necessary result in the clinical signs commonly associated with a diaphragmatic hernia. Taber's Cyclopedic Medical Dictionary defines a diaphragmatic hernia as the ". . . protrusion of abdominal contents through the diaphragm."[1] Consequently, it is the displacement of viscera that results in morbidity and mortality.

Diaphragmatic hernias can be congenital or acquired. Congenital diaphragmatic hernias result from abnormal embryogenesis. Acquired diaphragmatic hernias are more common than congenital hernias and are usually traumatic in origin.[2] Knowledge of normal anatomy and embryogenesis is important in understanding the pathogenesis of the occurrence and the effects of diaphragmatic hernia.

Anatomy

The diaphragm has two major components: tendinous and muscular.[3,4] The tendinous portion consists of the Y-shaped central tendon, which attaches to the thirteenth rib on either side.[4] It has two layers of concentric fibers that surround the caval foramen.[4] The muscular portion of the diaphragm includes the pars lumbalis, the pars costalis, and the pars sternalis.[4] The pars lumbalis is divided into the medial, intermediate, and lateral portions on each side of the esophageal and aortic hiatus.[4] The tendons of the pars lumbalis arise from vertebral bodies L3 and L4.[4] The pars costalis and sternalis circumvent the central tendon laterally and ventrally.[4] Blood is supplied to the diaphragm by the phrenic arteries, and motor innervation is provided by the phrenic nerves.[4] The phrenic nerves arise from spinal cord segments C5 to C7 in the dog and segments C4 to C6 in the cat.[4-6]

The normal diaphragm has three circular openings (Figure 83-1).[7] The caudal vena cava passes through the caval foramen. The esophageal hiatus contains the caudal esophagus, and support from the diaphragmatic crura and suspensory apparatus forms the caudal esophageal sphincter. The aortic hiatus allows passage of the aorta, azygous vein, hemiazygous vein, and thoracic duct across the diaphragm.

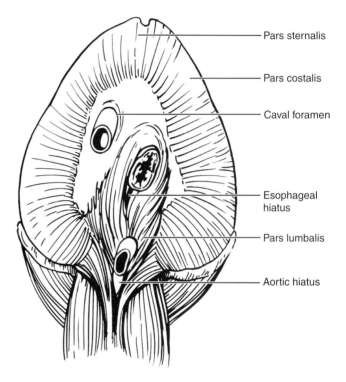

Figure 83-1. *Anatomy of the diaphragm. The ventral portion of the diaphragm is at the top of the illustration.*

- Pars sternalis
- Pars costalis
- Caval foramen
- Esophageal hiatus
- Pars lumbalis
- Aortic hiatus

Embryology

In the embryo, the diaphragm originates as a connective tissue membrane lying opposite the midcervical segments.[8] Myoblasts from the caudal cervical myotomes of cervical segments 4 through 7 migrate onto the diaphragmatic membrane to form the muscular portion of the diaphragm.[8] The origin of the embryonic diaphragmatic membrane near the cervical segments gives rise to the phrenic nerve as the major nerve supply of the musculature of the diaphragm.

Three embryonic structures are the major active contributors to the diaphragmatic membrane.[8] The septum transversum is the ventral component and develops into the central tendon of the diaphragm.[8] The pleuroperitoneal membranes are ingrowths of the body wall that fuse with the mesoesophagus, body walls, and the septum transversum.[8] Fusion of these membranes allows closure of the pleuroperitoneal canals and formation of the pleural cavity.[8] The body wall is thought to allow growth of the diaphragm by incorporation of its tissues circumferentially, although the extent of its contribution is not entirely known.[8] Passive contributors to the diaphragm include the mesoesophagus, the mesonephric remnant with its mesentery, and the mesenchyme around the aorta.[8] These structures contribute to the diaphragm simply because of their proximity to the major components.

Congenital Diaphragmatic Hernias

There are three types of congenital diaphragmatic hernia: pleuroperitoneal, peritoneopericardial, and hiatal.[2] A pleuroperitoneal hernia involves the dorsal tendinous portion of the diaphragm and likely results from incomplete closure of the pleuroperitoneal membranes.[9] Peritoneopericardial hernias result from a defect in the septum transversum in conjunction with anomalous development of the pleuroperitoneal membranes.[8] A hiatal hernia occurs at the point where the esophagus passes through the diaphragm and may result from either incomplete fusion of the pleuroperitoneal membranes and the mesoesophagus, or from an esophageal defect.[8]

PLEUROPERITONEAL HERNIA

Since pleuroperitoneal hernias result from incomplete fusion of the pleuroperitoneal membranes, they create a dorsolateral diaphragmatic defect. The intermediate portion of the left lumbar musculature may be absent, the crura may be absent, and the central tendon may or may not be involved.[10,11] This condition is reported to follow an autosomal recessive mode of inheritance.[11,12] Pleuroperitoneal hernias are uncommonly diagnosed, possibly because of a high neonatal mortality rate.[10] Death often results from fatal respiratory insufficiency as a result of displacement of the stomach, spleen, or small intestine into the thorax.[10]

PERITONEOPERICARDIAL HERNIA

The peritoneopericardial hernia is the most common congenital diaphragmatic hernia in dogs and cats.[12] It involves herniation of abdominal viscera into the pericardial sac through a ventral diaphragmatic defect.[13] It is thought that incomplete closure of the septum transversum occurs prenatally between days 24 and 28 of gestation in animals because of a genetic defect or a teratogen.[14,15] Peritoneopericardial hernia must be congenital in dogs and cats but can be congenital or traumatic in people.[13] Peritoneopericardial hernia can be traumatic in humans because the diaphragm forms one wall of the pericardial cavity, but there is no direct communication between the peritoneal and pericardial cavities in dogs and cats.[13,16] An increased incidence of peritoneopericardial hernia has been reported in weimaraners.[16] There is also a higher incidence in male dogs than in female dogs,

although the sex distribution in cats is equal.[13] Concurrent congenital anomalies are often present, including sternal defects, intracardiac defects, and pulmonary vascular disease.[12,16-19] Concurrent prognathism, portosystemic shunt, and umbilical hernias have also been reported.[16-19]

Viscera that are commonly displaced through a peritoneopericardial hernia include the liver, falciform ligament, omentum, spleen, small intestine, and stomach.[12,13] One study reported that the liver and the intestines herniate most commonly.[13] Clinical signs associated with peritoneopericardial hernia may be nonspecific, including weight loss, abdominal pain, ascites, exercise intolerance, collapse, or shock.[12] Gastrointestinal involvement may result in vomiting, diarrhea, and anorexia or polyphagia.[13,16] Respiratory signs such as coughing, tachypnea, or dyspnea may occur if lung expansion is restricted.[12] Tachypnea and muffled heart sounds were the most common physical examination findings in dogs and cats with peritoneopericardial hernia.[13] This hernia is diagnosed most often as an incidental finding, and one study reported that 60% of cases were found incidentally on routine examination.[13]

Useful diagnostic tools for evaluation of peritoneopericardial hernia include thoracic radiography, contrast radiography, angiography, ultrasonography, and computed tomography.[12,13,16] Thoracic radiographs may reveal an enlarged, round cardiac silhouette or, more specifically, intestinal loops within the cardiac shadow.[12] Although radiography may be useful in diagnosis of the hernia, it is not particularly helpful in determining which organs have herniated.[16] Nonselective angiography may differentiate cardiomyopathy or pericardial effusion from a peritoneopericardial hernia.[12] Peritoneography or a positive contrast study of the upper gastrointestinal tract is often helpful to confirm displacement of the stomach or intestines (Figure 83-2, A and B).[12] Thoracic ultrasound, performed substernally or through the right fifth intercostal space, is highly useful and allows differentiation of fluid and solid structures, with concurrent evaluation of cardiac function.[12,13]

Evidence of incarceration of the liver in a peritoneopericardial hernia warrants further diagnostic evaluation, including liver function tests and a coagulation panel, before surgical correction. Fibrinolysis and associated hepatic hypoxia have been reported in association with incarceration of the liver, and irreversible liver damage is associated with a guarded prognosis.[16]

Early surgical repair of congenital peritoneopericardial hernias is recommended.[13] Clinical outcome of conservatively managed cases, although not widely reported, has been poor.[13] Surgical correction is relatively easy, is associated with few complications, and results in a high rate of success in dogs and cats.[13] The effect of age of the animal on the outcome of surgery is unknown. Adhesions of abdominal viscera to the pericardium or epicardium are uncommon, and a sufficient amount of diaphragmatic tissue is usually available for primary repair. A ventral midline incision is made in the abdomen beginning at the xyphoid and continuing caudally. The edges of the defect are debrided, and the diaphragm is closed with monofilament absorbable or

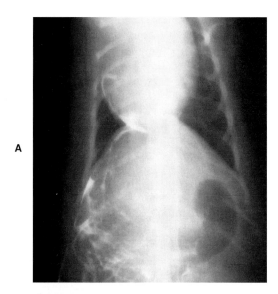

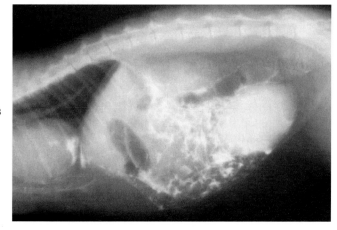

Figure 83-2. **A,** *Ventrodorsal and* **B,** *lateral thoracic radiographs of a cat with a peritoneopericardial hernia. Water-soluble contrast material was placed in the abdominal cavity, and the hindquarters of the cat were elevated to allow the contrast material to migrate into the pericardial sac.*

nonabsorbable suture in a continuous pattern beginning at the most dorsal aspect of the defect. Separate closure of the pericardium is not required, and it may be possible in some animals to close the defect without entering the thoracic cavity.[13] If the thoracic cavity is entered, a thoracostomy tube should be placed before completion of the surgery.

HIATAL HERNIA

A hiatal hernia results from protrusion of abdominal contents through the esophageal hiatus of the diaphragm.[12] Although this particular defect is fairly common in man, it is considered rare in the dog and cat.[20,21] The three types of hiatal hernia described in humans (i.e., sliding hiatal hernia, paraesophageal hiatal hernia, and shortened esophagus) have also been reported in animals.[12,20] A fourth type of hiatal hernia, a combina-

tion of sliding and paraesophageal hiatal hernia, has also been suggested in humans, dogs, and cats.[22]

Sliding hiatal hernias are the most common and involve displacement of the gastroesophageal junction through the hiatus and into the caudal mediastinum.[20] In animals with paraesophageal hiatal hernia, the esophagogastric junction remains fixed and the stomach herniates through a defect in the hiatus along the esophagus.[20] The majority (approximately 60%) of hiatal hernias in dogs and cats occur in animals less than 1 year of age and are considered congenital.[23] A breed predilection has been reported in the Chinese shar-pei.[12,24,25]

Congenital hiatal hernia is thought to result from an inherent weakness of the phrenoesophageal suspensory apparatus, which is the fascial reflection of the diaphragm around the circumference of the esophagus.[26] Although the hernia itself rarely causes clinical signs directly, it may play a major role in the development of gastroesophageal reflux and esophagitis, resulting in clinical signs associated with secondary megaesophagus and esophageal hypomotility.

Hiatal hernia and gastroesophageal reflux often coexist, but hernias are probably an aggravating factor rather than the inciting cause of gastroesophageal reflux. The pathogenesis of gastroesophageal reflux disease is complex but may relate to any of the following factors: function of the caudal esophageal sphincter, esophageal peristalsis, esophageal clearance, composition of the refluxed material, and gastric function.[23,27] Hiatal hernia is assumed to contribute to gastroesophageal reflux by promoting incompetence of the gastroesophageal sphincter.[28] It is thought that the caudal esophagus and the diaphragmatic crura work together to prevent esophageal reflux.[29] Hiatal hernia alters this anatomic relationship, resulting in incompetence of the gastroesophageal sphincter.[28]

Clinical signs associated with hiatal hernia can vary greatly depending on the severity of the esophageal hiatal hernia, and they are usually more severe in animals with a congenital defect. One study of 16 cases of congenital hiatal hernia reported that 7 animals were symptomatic.[23] It is thought that a large number of cases of hiatal hernia remain undetected because they lack clinical signs. If they have clinical signs, most commonly the animals suffer episodes of anorexia, coughing, dysphagia, hypersalivation, and regurgitation.[12,21] Clinical signs may progress to vomiting, hematemesis, and dyspnea. Death can occur secondary to cardiopulmonary compromise or gastric necrosis. Differential diagnoses based on clinical signs should include megaesophagus, esophageal diverticulum, gastroesophageal intussusception, esophageal foreign body, neoplasia, or granuloma.

The diagnosis of hiatal hernia is usually made radiographically (Figure 83-3, *A* and *B*). Thoracic radiographs should be evaluated carefully for the presence of megaesophagus or aspiration pneumonia. If a sliding hiatal hernia results in intermittent signs, positive abdominal pressure may be necessary to induce herniation.[12] Diagnosis of hiatal hernia may require a positive contrast radiographic study of the esophagus and stomach. Done in conjunction with fluoroscopy, this may allow assess-

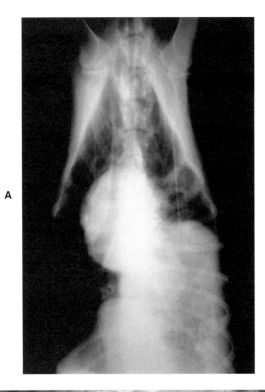

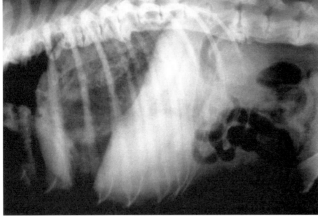

*Figure 83-3. **A,** Ventrodorsal and **B,** lateral radiographs of a dog with a paraesophageal hiatal hernia. The stomach is filled with food and displaced into the thorax.*

ment of esophageal motility, esophageal diameter, and caudal esophageal sphincter function. However, observation of gastroesophageal reflux by radiology or fluoroscopy may not correlate with clinical signs.[12] Endoscopy may allow evaluation of the caudal esophageal sphincter and facilitates detection of lesions consistent with reflux esophagitis (e.g., mucosal hyperemia, erosion, and ulceration); it is performed routinely in humans to determine the severity of disease and, therefore, the course of therapy.[21] However, endoscopy may not be particularly useful for identifying the presence of hiatal hernia or for distinguishing this defect from gastroesophageal intussusception. Other diagnostic tests used in humans include acid clearing tests, 24-hour pH

monitoring, and manometry. These modalities are not widely used in clinical veterinary medicine.

Animals with small sliding hiatal hernias and those with mild clinical signs may benefit from conservative management. Medical therapy is directed at reflux esophagitis, the proposed cause of clinical signs. A low-fat, soft diet may enhance gastric emptying and thereby reduce reflux.[28] Small, frequent (three to five times daily), elevated feedings are recommended if megaesophagus is present.[21] Neutralization and suppression of gastric acid secretion, increased caudal esophageal sphincter tone, and esophageal prokinesis are the goals of drug therapy.[21] H_2-receptor antagonists (e.g., cimetidine, ranitidine, and famotidine) decrease gastric acid, and an increase in gastric pH also increases caudal esophageal sphincter pressure.[21] Metoclopramide increases caudal esophageal sphincter pressure via prokinesis and reduces intragastric pressure by promoting gastric emptying.[28] Sucralfate has been used as a diffusion barrier for peptic digestion and is cytoprotective against acid-induced mucosal injury.[21,28] Omeprazole, a drug used to treat esophagitis in humans, inhibits ATP-dependent exchange of extracellular potassium for intracellular hydrogen ions in the parietal cell.[21] This drug may be useful in animals that do not respond to the antisecretory effects of the H_2-receptor antagonists. Medical therapy alone resulted in improvement of signs in 8 of 15 dogs with hiatal hernia, and complete resolution of clinical signs was observed in some dogs after 30 days of treatment.[21] These results suggest that conservative therapy should be instituted for at least 30 days before consideration of surgical correction of hiatal hernia.

Animals with a paraesophageal hiatal hernia, those with a permanently displaced stomach, and those that fail to respond to conservative management are all candidates for surgical correction.[28] Primary goals of surgical treatment consist of replacement of the stomach and esophagus caudal to the diaphragm, reduction of an enlarged hiatus (hiatal plication), and fixation of the stomach and/or caudal esophageal sphincter within the abdomen (esophagopexy or gastropexy).[28] Antireflux procedures (fundoplication) have also been used to restore caudal esophageal sphincter pressure.[28]

Surgery is performed using a cranial ventral midline abdominal incision. Hiatal plication is performed by incising the ventral phrenoesophageal ligament circumferentially while avoiding the ventral vagal trunk. The caudal esophageal sphincter is retracted into the abdomen, and the diaphragmatic crura are sutured in approximation with 3-0 or 2-0 monofilament nonabsorbable suture to reduce the hiatus to a diameter of 1 to 2 cm. An esophagopexy can be performed by suturing the abdominal esophagus to the diaphragm using the same suture material in an interrupted pattern. Sutures should not penetrate the lumen of the esophagus. A fundic gastropexy can be performed using any of the described techniques (e.g., incisional, belt loop, circumcostal, or tube gastropexy).[12] Current antireflux procedures performed in dogs are modifications of techniques that have been used in humans (e.g., Nissen fundoplication and Belsey fundoplication) and entail wrapping the stomach around the esophagus. Nissen fundoplication is the simplest procedure and the one most commonly used in small animals. A large-bore stomach tube is placed through the esophagus before fundoplication, and umbilical tape or a Penrose drain is used to pull the caudal esophagus into the abdomen. A fold of the cranial wall of the fundus is passed around the esophagus on the right side of the abdomen. Sutures (3-0 or 2-0 monofilament nonabsorbable) are placed, incorporating the esophagus, to approximate the fundus and form a cuff around the caudal 3 to 4 cm of the esophagus.

Hiatal plication alone has not been sufficient for humans with an incompetent lower esophageal sphincter. Therefore gastropexy or an antireflux procedure is generally combined with hiatal plication. The accepted approach to surgical repair of a symptomatic hiatal hernia consists of a combination of hiatal plication, gastropexy, and Nissen fundoplication. However, a study by Prymak and colleagues reported good to excellent results in animals following hiatal plication plus esophageal or gastropexy alone.[24] They advocated the use of an antireflux procedure only if there is primary incompetence of the caudal esophageal sphincter.[24] In a more recent study, Lorinson and Bright reported similar results:[21] they found that 8 of 10 dogs had resolution of signs following hiatal plication, esophagopexy, and gastropexy, whereas fundoplication alone was successful in only 1 of 4 dogs.[21] Based on these results, fundoplication was only recommended in animals that did not respond favorably to esophagopexy.[21]

Potential complications of surgical repair include herniation, esophagitis, vomiting, regurgitation, aspiration pneumonia, dyspnea, and gastric tympani. Development of gastric bloat syndrome (gastric tympani) has specifically been associated with fundoplication. A reduction in the complication rate can be accomplished by using modified fundoplication techniques (loose 360-degree fundoplication) and placement of a gastrostomy tube for decompression. However, the most important factor in reducing complication rate may be careful selection of surgical candidates.

Traumatic Diaphragmatic Hernias

The majority of diaphragmatic hernias are traumatic in origin. In a review of 406 dogs and cats diagnosed with diaphragmatic hernia, 85% were traumatic, whereas 15% were developmental, peritoneopericardial, or esophageal hiatal hernias.[7] Three types of traumatic diaphragmatic hernia have been described: direct, indirect, and iatrogenic.[12] Direct diaphragmatic hernias are caused by direct trauma to the diaphragm (e.g., bite, stab, or gunshot wounds).[12,30] Diaphragmatic hernias caused by direct trauma are relatively rare. Indirect diaphragmatic hernias are more common and are the result of blunt trauma to the abdominal cavity.[31] Automobile accidents are the most common cause of this type of injury, but indirect trauma may also occur from a kick, fall, or fight.[7] Normal pleuroperitoneal pressure gradients vary from 7 cm H_2O

during quiet inspiration to over 100 cm H_2O during maximum inspiration.[32] Indirect trauma resulting in a sudden increase in intraabdominal pressure, in conjunction with an open glottis, may dramatically increase the pleuroperitoneal pressure gradient and lead to a tear in the diaphragm.[31,32] Iatrogenic diaphragmatic trauma can occur during thoracocentesis, chest drain placement, or while making an abdominal incision.[12] Abdominal viscera do not usually pass into the thoracic cavity through a small laceration, and these often heal unremarkably.

Traumatic diaphragmatic tears generally involve the muscular rather than the tendinous portion of the diaphragm because of the relative weakness of muscle.[33,34] Muscular diaphragmatic tears are divided into three general categories based on the location of the damage: circumferential, radial, or a combination of circumferential and radial (Figure 83-4). Two studies reported that approximately 40% of tears were located circumferentially, 40% were located radially, and 20% were combined.[33,34] In a review of 406 cases of diaphragmatic hernia in dogs and cats, right costomuscular tears were observed in 51% of the cases, and left costal tears occurred in 24% of cases.[7] The right diaphragm was lacerated in 13% of the cases, and multiple lacerations were seen in 4% of the cases.[7] The least common lesions involved the central tendon and crura, which made up only 3% of the cases.[7] The decreased incidence of left-sided diaphragmatic hernia may result from the cushioning effect of a gas-filled stomach on the left side of the abdomen because the stomach may act to disperse the intraabdominal forces at impact.[7]

The contents of a diaphragmatic hernia generally correspond to the location of the tear and may significantly impact the clinical outcome of the case. The most common organs found to herniate through a traumatic diaphragmatic hernia were the liver (78% to 88%), the small intestine (64% to 73%), and the stomach (47% to 53%).[7,35] Other organs reported to herniate include the spleen, omentum, pancreas, colon, gall bladder, cecum, kidney, and uterus.[7,12,33] Left-sided traumatic diaphragmatic hernias most commonly contained stomach, spleen, or small intestine, whereas right-sided hernias commonly contained liver, small intestine, and/or pancreas.[33] Because of the force required to create a traumatic diaphragmatic hernia, other injuries are often found.[7] Wilson and Hayes reported that 38% of animals with traumatic diaphragmatic hernia had concomitant traumatic injuries,[7] including hernias at other locations, myocardial and pulmonary contusions, hip luxations, hematomas, and damage to the liver and urinary bladder. Fractured bones are also common, specifically caudal rib fractures and fractures of the pelvis and femur.[12]

CLINICAL CONSEQUENCES OF TRAUMATIC DIAPHRAGMATIC HERNIA

The clinical signs of a diaphragmatic hernia are a summation of the effects of the location of the lesion and the organs that have herniated, as well as accumulation of

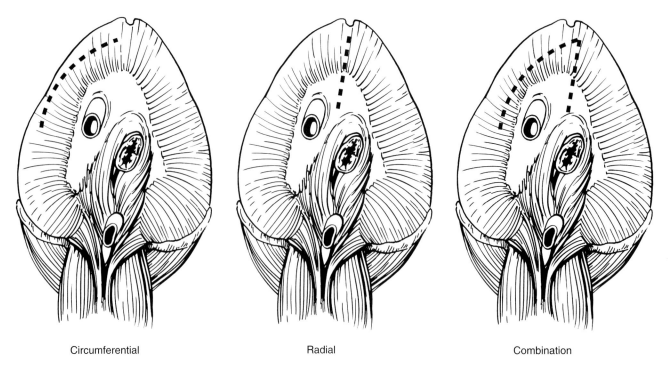

Circumferential   Radial   Combination

Figure 83-4. Diagram depicting the common locations of muscular diaphragmatic tears.

fluid within the thoracic cavity and damage to visceral organs. Respiratory signs including dyspnea and cyanosis are often seen, although the cause of respiratory impairment is not necessarily loss of diaphragm continuity.[2] The cause of dyspnea is often multifactorial and may relate to a combination of shock, chest wall dysfunction, decreased pulmonary compliance, pulmonary contusions, pleural effusion, and cardiovascular dysfunction.[2] Depending on the contents of the hernia, enteric signs may occur alone or in conjunction with respiratory signs. Displacement of enteric organs often results in vomiting, hematemesis, diarrhea, constipation, or anorexia. Entrapment of the stomach within the hernia can result in gastric dilation that can further compromise respiratory function. Prolonged distention of the stomach can result in obstruction of the blood supply leading to gastric necrosis. Other signs reported in conjunction with diaphragmatic hernia include exercise intolerance, dysphagia, weight loss, and depression.

Although the liver is the most common organ found in the thorax as a result of traumatic diaphragmatic hernia, the consequences of its displacement are generally limited.[7] However, if intrahepatic pressure is elevated by 5 to 10 mm Hg, hemorrhagic fluid may exude through the hepatic capsule, resulting in life-threatening fluid accumulation in the thorax or abdomen.[7] There is also the possibility of hepatic infection as a result of colonization with anaerobic and gram-negative aerobic organisms as a result of decreased hepatic bloodflow.[7] On rare occasions, the liver may be strangulated within the hernia, resulting in hepatic necrosis or biliary obstruction, and resection of devitalized liver tissue may be necessary during hernia repair.

DIAGNOSIS

When obvious signs of respiratory distress or enteric pathology are not observed, physical examination may reveal subtle indications of diaphragmatic hernia. The animal may appear gaunt, and abdominal palpation may suggest a lack of viscera within the abdomen. Thoracic auscultation may reveal borborygmus, an apparent lack of lung sounds, or a muffled heartbeat. Thoracic percussion is dull over areas of pleural fluid or displaced abdominal viscera.

The diagnosis of diaphragmatic hernia is made most often by thoracic radiography. If the animal is stable enough, thoracic radiographs should be made with the animal positioned in dorsal recumbency and both right and left lateral recumbency. A high percentage of animals with a diaphragmatic tear have an incomplete diaphragmatic outline on lateral thoracic radiographs (97%), and 67% of these animals have air-filled intestinal loops within the thorax (Figure 83-5, *A* and *B*).[36] Less specific roentgen signs of diaphragmatic hernia include an obscure cardiac outline, increased opacity of the ventral lung fields, pleural fluid, and atelectasis.[33] It may be necessary to remove pleural fluid and obtain additional thoracic radiographs to more clearly differentiate the presence of displaced abdominal viscera from intrathoracic pathology. Ultrasound is often useful to identify abdominal contents within the thorax, especially in the presence of pleural fluid.[37] A positive contrast study of the upper gastrointestinal tract or positive-contrast peritoneography may be useful if a diaphragmatic hernia is suspected and thoracic radiography and ultrasound are nondiagnostic.

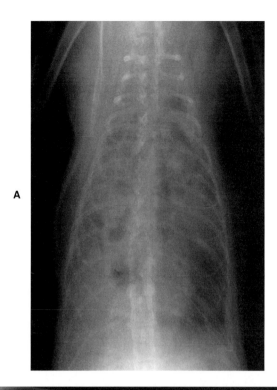

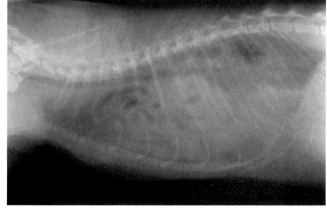

Figure 83-5. A, *Ventrodorsal and* **B,** *lateral thoracic radiographs of a cat with a traumatic diaphragmatic hernia. Note the loss of a distinct outline of the diaphragm. Gas-filled bowel loops are apparent within the thorax.*

MANAGEMENT

Surgical intervention is necessary for resolution of signs. Cardiovascular and pulmonary stabilization is warranted for approximately 1 to 3 days before herniorrhaphy.[38] One report indicates that the mortality rate is highest when surgery takes place within the first 24 hours after diaphragmatic injury.[7] However, this observation may be biased by the fact that surgery is usually performed on the most critically injured animals during this time. Perioperative treatment of pulmonary contusions and pneumothorax can greatly reduce the risks of anesthesia in critically injured hernia patients.[2] It is important that the patient is carefully monitored while being stabilized.

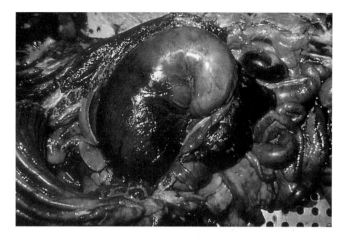

Figure 83-6. *Gastric necrosis is apparent during necropsy of this dog, which had displacement of the stomach through a traumatic diaphragmatic hernia.*

Acute hemorrhage can occur because of organ trauma (particularly from the spleen or liver), and pulmonary compliance may be compromised because of thoracic wall trauma or the presence of fluid or viscera within the thorax. Pulmonary contusions are essentially bruises of the lung and can result in significant ventilation/perfusion mismatch. The full extent of pulmonary contusions may not be apparent for several hours, and arrhythmias resulting from poor myocardial perfusion or contusions may not develop for 24 to 48 hours after trauma. If the animal cannot be stabilized, however, emergency surgery should be performed.[39] Emergency surgery is definitely indicated in animals with acute dilation of a herniated stomach or with strangulated intestines.[2] Whenever the stomach herniates through a diaphragmatic hernia there is a significant risk that it could become severely distended at any time, resulting in acute decompensation of the patient. A distended stomach can compress the caudal vena cava, resulting in decreased venous return, and strangulation can result in bowel necrosis and peritonitis (Figure 83-6).

The goal of herniorrhaphy is to atraumatically reduce the displaced viscera, followed by repair of the diaphragmatic defect.[7] Surgical approaches that have been described for herniorrhaphy include the lateral thoracic, transthoracic, abdominal, and paracostal. Each approach has its own limitations, emphasizing the need for careful planning before surgery. The lateral thoracic approach prevents abdominal viscera from interfering with the closure[7]; however, this approach limits exposure to the ventral midline, the crus, and the costomuscular origins of the diaphragm, and it does not allow thorough exploration of the abdomen.[7] The transthoracic approach allows greater exposure of the ventrolateral diaphragm but exposure of the costal diaphragm is limited.[7] In addition to the anatomical limitations, thoracic approaches can seriously compromise thoracic wall compliance and are therefore not recommended. The abdominal approach is used most commonly and allows thorough exploration of the abdomen and good exposure of all aspects of the diaphragm.[7] The incision can be continued cranially with a median sternotomy or a paracostal incision to provide even greater exposure if necessary.

Thorough examination of the diaphragm during surgery is important to search for multiple diaphragmatic defects. All abdominal organs should be examined to identify concurrent traumatic injuries. Contraction of the diaphragmatic defect may make repositioning organs difficult, especially in chronic cases. Abdominal organs should be gently repositioned into the abdomen without tugging or pulling, and the surgeon should not hesitate to enlarge the primary defect to allow atraumatic replacement of abdominal viscera. In some animals with chronic diaphragmatic hernia, adhesions form between the lungs and abdominal viscera. These can usually be gently broken down with digital pressure. The lungs should be inspected for lacerations that may have occurred during the inciting trauma or as adhesions were divided. Small (i.e., 5 mm or less) superficial lacerations will heal spontaneously, but larger defects should be closed with staples or sutures. Nonviable tissue should be identified and resected if possible.

Debridement of the diaphragm is only necessary if mature scar tissue covers the edges of the defect. Care must be taken to avoid damage to the caudal vena cava, both as the hernia opening is enlarged or debrided and as sutures are placed during closure. It is usually possible to close diaphragmatic defects with available tissue; however, muscle flaps, omentum, autologous fascia, or synthetic materials can be used to close large defects.[2] These procedures should be used judiciously because they may result in additional hemorrhage and increased anesthetic time. Before closure of the defect, a thoracostomy tube should be placed for evacuation of the chest. Closure should begin at the most dorsal aspect (usually the most difficult to reach) of the diaphragmatic defect. The defect in the diaphragm is closed with monofilament absorbable or nonabsorbable suture in a continuous pattern.

According to one study, approximately 15% of diaphragmatic hernia cases die before examination.[34] Of the cases treated for traumatic diaphragmatic hernia, survival rates as high as 78% for dogs and 92% for cats have been reported.[34] In a study comparing survival rates for acute and chronic traumatic diaphragmatic hernia cases, similar survival rates were observed after treatment of acute and chronic diaphragmatic hernias in dogs (72% and 74%, respectively), whereas the survival rate was slightly lower for treatment of acute relative to chronic diaphragmatic hernias in cats (80% and 88%, respectively).[40]

In another study that evaluated the overall survival rate and time of death as a result of diaphragmatic hernia in dogs and cats, the majority of deaths occurred before (16.8%) and following (12.1%) surgery, whereas mortality was relatively low (5.1%) during the surgical procedure.[35] A number of studies report that mortality is greatest for dogs or cats treated for diaphragmatic hernia within the first 24 hours after surgery.[12,33] In dogs, death was most commonly caused by pneumothorax with or without hemothorax, whereas in cats, reexpansion pul-

monary edema was the most common cause of death following diaphragmatic hernia repair.[12]

The most critical intervals during diaphragmatic hernia repair are anesthesia induction and the immediate postoperative period. Some degree of hypoxia is often present in animals with diaphragmatic hernia because of decreased compliance and/or ventilation-perfusion mismatch.[12] Animals should be sedated with cardiovascular sparing drugs to ensure that minimal physical restraint is required during induction of anesthesia.[12] Preoxygenation for at least 2 to 3 minutes before induction is recommended.[12] Minimal doses of induction agents should be used to avoid the hypotensive and respiratory depressant effects of these drugs, and intubation should proceed rapidly after induction, followed by ventilation with oxygen and gas anesthesia.[12]

Reexpansion pulmonary edema can occur in animals with diaphragmatic hernia, particularly when chronic atelectasis is present. The most common cause of reexpansion pulmonary edema in humans is rapid generation of negative intrapleural pressure, resulting in leakage of protein-rich fluid into the alveoli of reexpanded lungs.[41] The pathogenesis is thought to involve the activation of neutrophils and, potentially, the generation of free radicals that leads to increased microvascular permeability.[42-46] The rapidity with which lungs are reinflated is thought to be more important than the duration of collapse.[41] During surgery, peak airway pressures during assisted ventilation should not exceed 20 cm H_2O, and increased end-expiratory pressure should be avoided. As long as the animal is adequately oxygenated, it is not critical that the lungs are fully inflated during surgery, and intrapleural air or fluid can be evacuated slowly over 12 hours via the thoracostomy tube.[7,41] Fortunately, reexpansion pulmonary edema does not occur commonly after diaphragmatic hernia repair. If pulmonary edema develops, prompt treatment should be initiated including oxygen supplementation; positive-pressure ventilation, if necessary; and judicious use of diuretics.[41] The thoracostomy tube should be maintained for at least 12 to 24 hours, and the patient should be monitored carefully postoperatively.[7] The thoracostomy tube is removed when no further air is obtained and the volume of fluid has declined to less than 5 ml/kg/24 hours.

REFERENCES

1. Thomas CL, editor: *Taber's cyclopedic medical dictionary,* Philadelphia, 1993, FA Davis.
2. Bellah JR: Traumatic diaphragmatic hernia. In Bojrab MJ, Ellison GW, Slocum B, editors: *Current techniques in small animal surgery,* ed 4, Baltimore, 1998, Williams & Wilkins.
3. DeTroyer A, Sampson M, Sigrist S et al: The diaphragm: Two muscles, *Science* 213:237-238, 1981.
4. Evans HE, Christensen GC: *Miller's anatomy of the dog,* Philadelphia, 1993, WB Saunders.
5. Bellemare F, Wight D, Lavigne CM et al: Effect of tension and timing of contraction on the bloodflow of the diaphragm, *J Appl Physiol* 54:1597-1606, 1983.
6. Sant'Ambrogio G, Frazier DT, Wilson MF et al: Motor innervation and pattern of activity of cat diaphragm, *J Appl Physiol* 18:43-46, 1963.

7. Wilson GP, Hayes H: Diaphragmatic hernia in the dog and cat: A 25-year overview, *Sem in Vet Med and Surg (Sm Anim)* 1(4):318-326, 1986.
8. Latshaw WK: Mesenteries and compartmentalization. In Latshaw WK, editor: *Veterinary developmental anatomy: A clinically oriented approach*, Philadelphia, 1987, BC Decker.
9. Bellah JR: Congenital diaphragmatic hernia. In Bojrab MJ, Ellison GW, Slocum B, editors: *Current techniques in small animal surgery*, ed 4, Baltimore, 1998, Williams & Wilkins.
10. Valentine BA, Cooper BJ, Dietze AE, et al: Canine congenital diaphragmatic hernia, *JVIM* 2:109, 1988.
11. Feldman DB: Congenital diaphragmatic hernia in neonatal dogs, *JAVMA* 153:942, 1968.
12. Johnson KA: Diaphragmatic, pericardial, and hiatal hernia. In Slatter DH, editor: *Textbook of small animal surgery*, vol 1, Philadelphia, 1985, WB Saunders.
13. Wallace J, Mullen HS, Lesser MB: A technique for surgical correction of peritoneal pericardial diaphragmatic hernia in dogs and cats, *JAAHA* 28:503-510, 1992.
14. Bolton GR, Ettinger S, Rousch JC: Congenital peritoneopericardial diaphragmatic hernia in a dog, *JAVMA* 155:723-730, 1969.
15. Finn JP, Martin CL: Diaphragmatic pericardial hernia, *JSAP* 10:295-300, 1969.
16. Evans SM, Biery DN: Congenital peritoneopericardial diaphragmatic hernia in the dog and cat: A literature review and 17 additional case histories, *Vet Rad* 21(3):108-116, 1980.
17. Bellah JR, Spencer CP, Brown DJ et al: Congenital cranioventral abdominal wall caudal sternal, diaphragmatic, pericardial and intracardiac defects in cocker spaniel littermates, *JAVMA* 194:1741-1746, 1989.
18. Reed CA: Pericardio-peritoneal hernia in mammals with a description in a domestic cat, *Anat Rec* 110:113-119, 1951.
19. Turk MAM, Turk JR, Rantanen NW et al: Necrotizing pulmonary arteritis in a dog with peritoneo-pericardial diaphragmatic hernia, *JSAP* 25:25-30, 1984.
20. Alexander JW, Hoffer RE, MacDonald JM et al: Hiatal hernia in the dog: A case report and review of the literature, *JAAHA* 11:793-797, 1975.
21. Lorinson D, Bright RM: Long-term outcome of medical and surgical treatment of hiatal hernias in dogs and cats: 27 cases (1978-1996), *JAVMA* 213(3):381-384, 1998.
22. Waldron DR, Moon M, Leib MS et al: Oesophageal hiatal hernia in two cats, *JSAP* 31:259-263, 1990.
23. Bright RM, Sackman JE, DeNovo C et al: Hiatal hernia in the dog and cat: A retrospective study of 16 cases, *JSAP* 31:244-250, 1990.
24. Prymak C, Saunders HM, Washabau RJ: Hiatal hernia repair by restoration and stabilization of normal anatomy: An evaluation in four dogs and one cat, *Vet Surg* 18:386-391, 1989.
25. Callan MB, Wahabau RJ, Saunders HM et al: Congenital esophageal hiatal hernia in the Chinese shar-pei dog, *JVIM* 7:210-215, 1993.
26. Eliska O: Phrenoesophageal membrane and its role in the development of hiatal hernia, *Acta Anat* 86:137-150, 1973.
27. Kahrilas PJ, Dodds WJ, Hogan WJ: Effects of peristaltic dysfunction on esophageal volume clearance, *Gastroenterology* 94:73-80, 1988.
28. Prymak C: Esophageal hiatal hernia repair. In Bojrab MJ, Ellison GW, Slocum B, editors: *Current techniques in small animal surgery*, ed 4, Baltimore, 1998, Williams & Wilkins.
29. Boyle JT, Altschuler SM, Nixon TE et al: Role of the diaphragm in the genesis of lower esophageal sphincter pressure in the cat, *Gastroenterology* 88:723-730, 1985.
30. Bellenger CR: Bile pleuritis in a dog, *JSAP* 16:575, 1975.
31. Dronen SC: Disorders of the chest wall and diaphragm, *Emerg Med Clin NA* 1:449, 1983.
32. Marchand P: A study of the forces productive of gastro-oesophageal regurgitation and herniation through the diaphragmatic hiatus, *Thorax* 12:189, 1957.
33. Garson HL, Dodman NH, Baker GJ: Diaphragmatic hernia: Analysis of 56 cases in dogs and cats, *JSAP* 21:469-481, 1980.
34. Bellenger CR, Hunt GB, Goldsmid SE: Outcomes of thoracic surgery in dogs and cats, *Aust Vet J* 74(1):25-30, 1996.
35. Wilson GP, Newton CD, Burt JK: A review of 116 diaphragmatic hernias in dogs and cats, *JAVMA* 159(9):1142-1145, 1971.
36. Sullivan M, Lee R: Radiological features of 80 cases of diaphragmatic rupture, *JSAP* 30:561, 1989.
37. Stowater JL, Lamb CR: Ultrasonography of noncardiac thoracic diseases in small animals, *JAVMA* 195:514, 1989.
38. Boudrieau RJ, Muir WE: Pathophysiology of traumatic diaphragmatic hernia in dogs, *Comp Con Ed* 9:379-385, 1987.
39. Bjorling DE: Management of thoracic trauma. In Birchard S, Sherding S, editors: *Saunders manual of small animal practice*, Philadelphia, 1994, WB Saunders.
40. Downs MC, Bjorling DE: Traumatic diaphragmatic hernias: A review of 1674 cases, *Vet Surg* 16:87, 1987.
41. Stampley AR, Waldron DR: Reexpansion pulmonary edema after surgery to repair a diaphragmatic hernia in a cat, *JAVMA* 203(12):1699-1701, 1993.
42. Gascoigne A, Appleton A, Taylor R et al: Catastrophic circulatory collapse following re-expansion pulmonary oedema, *Resuscitation* 31(3):265-269, 1996.
43. Jackson RM, Veal CF: Re-expansion, re-oxygenation, and rethinking, *Am J Med Sci* 298(1):44-50, 1989.
44. Jackson RM, Veal CF, Alexander CB et al: Re-expansion pulmonary edema: A potential role for free radicals in its pathogenesis, *Am Rev Respir Dis* 137(5):1165-1171, 1988.
45. Jackson RM, Veal CF, Beckman JS et al: Polyethylene glycol-conjugated superoxide dismutase in unilateral lung injury due to re-expansion (re-oxygenation), *Am J Med Sci* 300(1):22-28, 1990.
46. Wilkinson PD, Keegan J, Davies SW et al: Changes in pulmonary microvascular permeability accompanying re-expansion oedema: Evidence from dual isotope scintigraphy, *Thorax* 45(6):456-459, 1990.

CHAPTER 84

Neoplasms of the Cranial Mediastinum and Pleura

Janet K. Carreras • Karin U. Sorenmo

Tumors of the Cranial Mediastinum

The mediastinum is the space located in the central portion of the thorax, between the two pleural cavities, the diaphragm, and the thoracic inlet. Within the mediastinum are many vital structures including the heart, thymus, trachea, esophagus, vagus nerves, great vessels, and many lymph nodes. The mediastinum is subdivided by the heart into three transverse sections: the cranial, middle, and caudal mediastinum. Most primary neoplasia occurs within the cranial mediastinum, which contains the structures positioned in front of the heart.[1] The most common neoplasm of the cranial mediastinum of both dogs and cats is lymphosarcoma. Other types of primary neoplastic processes occurring within the cranial mediastinum include thymoma, ectopic thyroid and parathyroid tumors, and chemodectoma. Lymphangiosarcoma has also been reported in the cranial mediastinum of cats.[2] Metastatic neoplasia also occurs within the mediastinum, including spread of tumors from neighboring structures such as the lungs, or as a sequela of a systemic process.

CRANIAL MEDIASTINAL LYMPHOSARCOMA IN THE DOG

Lymphosarcoma, also called lymphoma, is the most common hematopoietic tumor affecting the dog with an annual incidence of 6 to 24 cases per 100,000 dogs.[3] Lymphosarcoma is a neoplasm of the lymphoreticular system but can affect most other nonlymphoid tissues. This disease entity in the dog parallels Non-Hodgkin's lymphoma in humans. The etiology of lymphosarcoma in dogs remains unknown. Various studies have investigated the potential role of viral etiologies, particularly retroviruses, but no definitive link has been established between exogenous retroviruses and the development of canine lymphosarcoma.[4-6] One study implicated exposure to the chemical 2,4-dichlorophenoxyaceic acid (2,4-D), an herbicide, as a potential risk factor for the development of lymphosarcoma in dogs,[7] but an independent reanalysis of that study did not find a significant association between the use of 2,4-D and the development of lymphosarcoma.[8] Epidemiological studies have placed certain breeds at increased risk for the development of lymphosarcoma, including golden retrievers, Scottish terriers, bassett hounds, German shepherds, poodles, Irish water spaniels, beagles, boxers, briards, and bull mastiffs.[9-12] There are conflicting reports as to whether there is a sex difference in risk for lymphosarcoma. Whereas one study found an increased risk for the development of lymphosarcoma among neutered male and neutered female dogs,[9] a different study found a ratio of males to females of 1.4 to 1,[11] and other reports cite no increased risk based on gender.[13,14] Most dogs affected by lymphosarcoma are middle age to older, but the disease can also affect younger dogs.

The most common clinical presentation of a dog with lymphosarcoma is peripheral lymphadenopathy: greater than 80% of dogs with lymphosarcoma present with multicentric disease that may also involve internal lymph nodes, spleen, and liver. Less common forms of canine lymphosarcoma include alimentary (approximately 7%), cutaneous (approximately 6%), and extranodal sites (uncommon).[15,16] Fewer than 3% of dogs are presented with only a cranial mediastinal mass and no other sites of involvement.[16,17] Most dogs with multicentric lymphosarcoma are presented with no clinical signs, and the finding of a peripheral lymphadenopathy may be an incidental finding by either the owner or veterinarian.[15] Dogs with more advanced disease may be presented with nonspecific signs such as decreased appetite, decreased energy level or weakness, depression, distended abdomen, or signs associated with extranodal sites of involvement (e.g., hyphema in dogs with ocular involvement).

Dogs with cranial mediastinal lymphosarcoma are predisposed to developing hypercalcemia, and these dogs may be presented with signs such as polyuria, polydipsia, vomiting, diarrhea, or signs related to cardiac arrhythmias.[15,18] Other clinical signs may result from secondary pleural effusion or invasion or compression of neighboring structures (e.g., coughing; dyspnea; dysphagia; regurgitation; and edema of the head, neck, and forelimbs caused by compression of the cranial vena cava).[19]

Clinical staging should be performed in dogs diagnosed with cranial mediastinal lymphosarcoma in order to assess other sites of involvement (Table 84-1). Staging should include a thorough physical examination; com-

TABLE 84-1. World Health Organization System for Staging of Canine Lymphosarcoma

Stage	Criteria
I	Involvement limited to single node or lymphoid tissue in single organ excluding bone marrow (includes cranial mediastinum)
II	Regional involvement of two or more lymph nodes, with or without involvement of the tonsils
III	Generalized lymph node involvement
IV	Involvement of liver, spleen or both, with or without generalized lymph node involvement
V	Involvement of blood, bone marrow, or other organs

Substage	
a	No overt clinical signs of illness
b	Overt clinical signs of illness

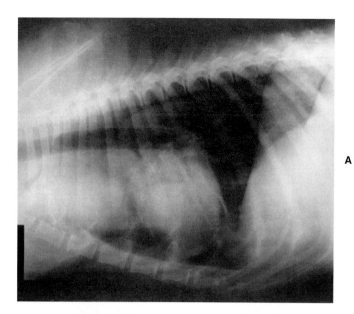

A

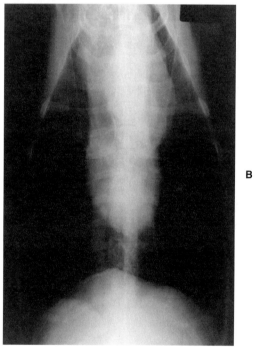

B

Figure 84-1. *A, Left lateral and **B,** ventrodorsal thoracic radiographs from a dog with cranial mediastinal lymphosarcoma.*

plete blood count; serum chemistry screen; urinalysis; imaging studies of the thorax and abdomen (Figure 84-1), as well as any other suspected sites; and aspiration of affected lymphoid tissues and bone marrow. Fine-needle aspiration and cytological evaluation of the cranial mediastinal mass may be diagnostic for canine lymphosarcoma if the cells are lymphoblastic, but biopsy and histopathology may be necessary in cases with small cell lymphosarcoma to rule out thymoma. Further diagnostic tests may include a phenotypic analysis of the lymphosarcoma to determine whether the neoplasm is of B-cell or T-cell derivation. Approximately 75% of canine lymphosarcomas are B-cell phenotype[20,21]; however, lymphosarcomas of the cranial mediastinum may originate in either the thymus or in lymph nodes, and most of these tumors are T-cell phenotype.[22]

Dogs with cranial mediastinal lymphosarcoma may or may not have multicentric disease. For dogs with a localized mediastinal tumor, both chemotherapy and radiation therapy are effective treatment options. Many chemotherapeutic protocols have been reported to induce clinical remission. Combination chemotherapy has been shown to be more efficacious than single-agent chemotherapy; however, the optimal schedule and intensity of treatment have not been determined. Most chemotherapy protocols utilize L-asparaginase, vincristine, prednisone, doxorubicin, and cyclophosphamide for induction chemotherapy.[15] Radiation therapy can be used alone or in combination with systemic chemotherapy for treatment of localized cranial mediastinal lymphosarcoma. Both normal and malignant lymphocytes are extremely radiation sensitive. Radiation therapy can also be useful in alleviating acute clinical signs associated with cranial mediastinal lymphosarcoma including cranial vena caval syndrome. Dogs with evidence of multicentric lymphosarcoma in addition to a cranial mediastinal mass should be treated with systemic chemotherapy with or without radiation therapy.

A complete response to multi-agent chemotherapy can be obtained in 70% to 85% of dogs with lym-

phosarcoma, and a median complete remission duration of approximately 255 days has been reported.[9,23] Some 20% to 40% of dogs with lymphosarcoma and hypercalcemia will have a cranial mediastinal mass.[15,18,24] The presence of a cranial mediastinal mass, hypercalcemia, and lymphosarcoma with a T-cell phenotype have been reported to be poor prognostic indicators.[13,20,21,24] In addition, pretreatment hypoalbuminemia and steroid therapy have also been found to be associated with shorter survival times.[25]

Female dogs had longer survival times in several reports,[9,11,12] but others report no difference in prognosis based on sex.[9,21] According to some investigators, smaller dogs may have a better prognosis than larger dogs,[12] but other reports find no statistical difference in survival based on weight.[9,11,21,25] In most reports, age has not been found to affect remission or survival.* Using the Kiel classification system, dogs with high grade lymphosarcoma had a higher complete response rate than dogs with low grade malignancy, according to one report; but there was no significant difference in complete response rate among the same group of dogs when the working formulation was used to determine grade.[21] Thus according to this and other reports, no significant difference in survival was found based on tumor grade.[20,26] Dogs with Stage V disease have a worse prognosis according to most reports, but studies are inconsistent as to whether there are significant differences in prognosis between other stages of lymphosarcoma.[21,25,26] Reports are also inconsistent with regard to initial illness status (substage) as a prognostic indicator.[13,25,26]

CRANIAL MEDIASTINAL LYMPHOSARCOMA IN THE CAT

Lymphosarcoma is the most common neoplasm in cats.[27] The annual incidence rate is reported as 41.6 to 157 cases per 100,000 cats.[28,29] Infection with the feline leukemia virus (FeLV), a contagious retrovirus of cats, has been considered the cause of virtually all cases of feline lymphosarcoma.[27,29,30] Cats with FeLV-negative lymphosarcoma commonly have a history of exposure to FeLV, suggesting that FeLV may play a role in the development of lymphosarcoma in FeLV-negative cats.[31,32] Truncated FeLV-gag sequences, or FeLV structural proteins have been found within FeLV-negative lymphosarcomas.[29,31,32] Feline oncornavirus-associated cell membrane antigen (FOCMA), an FeLV-associated tumor-specific antigen, has also been found on the surface of tumor cells from both FeLV-positive and FeLV-negative cats with lymphosarcoma. This represents virus-induced neoplastic transformation of lymphocytes.[29,32] Historically it has been reported that FeLV-negative cats with lymphosarcoma tend to be older (median age reported 7 to 12 years) that most commonly suffer from the alimentary form of the disease. In contrast, FeLV-positive cats tend to be much younger at the time of diagnosis of lymphosarcoma (median age 2 to 5 years), and usually suffer from thymic or multicentric lymphosarcoma.[27,29,30,32-38] There has been a shift towards an increasing number of cats with lymphosarcoma testing negative for FeLV. One retrospective analysis evaluating cats with lymphoma treated with chemotherapy between 1988 and 1994 showed that only 11 of 132 cats (8.3%) were FeLV positive,[39] compared with previous studies reporting that approximately 70% of cats with lymphosarcoma are FeLV positive.[27,32,35] The cause for this may be multifactorial, including more recent availability of FeLV vaccines for prevention of FeLV, and improved client education.

Although there are conflicting reports of the prevalence of the various anatomic forms of lymphosarcoma

TABLE 84-2. World Health Organization's International Histological Classification of Lymphoid Neoplasms: Anatomic Forms

Site	Criteria
Multicentric	Disseminated neoplasm of lymphoid organs; usually bilateral involvement of lymph nodes; spleen involvement common; other affected organs include liver, kidney, lungs, heart, gastrointestinal tract, bone marrow
Alimentary	Main lesions in gastrointestinal tract and regional lymph nodes; other most commonly infiltrated organs include liver, kidney, and spleen
Thymic	Main lesion is mass replacing thoracic thymus; may be only site or may involve mediastinal lymph nodes and other organs
Renal	Main lesion is the kidney

in cats, most studies have shown the alimentary form to be the most common.[28,33,34,39-41,43] Other forms of feline lymphosarcoma include central nervous system/spinal and renal lymphosarcoma (Table 84-2). A few reports suggest that male cats may be at higher risk for the development of lymphosarcoma, and Siamese cats have been suggested to be at increased risk compared to other feline breeds.[28,36,37,44] However, other studies have reported no increased risk based on gender or breed.[33]

Mediastinal lymphosarcoma has been reported to represent from 10.5% to 50% of feline lymphosarcoma.* Cats with mediastinal lymphosarcoma are usually presented with clinical signs including dyspnea, cyanosis, depression, lethargy, anorexia, weight loss, vomiting or regurgitation, and fever.[29,35,44] Clinical signs may be referable to compression or shifting of the esophagus, trachea, or other neighboring structures in the mediastinum; malignant hydrothorax secondary to the mediastinal mass; or may be related to the extent of systemic tumor involvement outside the mediastinum. Auscultation of cats with a mediastinal mass and pleural effusion may reveal muffled cardiopulmonary sounds and caudal displacement of the apical heartbeat. Physical examination may reveal decreased compressibility of the anterior thorax.

Cats with mediastinal lymphosarcoma may have disease confined to the chest, or may have additional sites of involvement; therefore all cats diagnosed with lymphosarcoma should be fully staged. Thoracic radiographs should be performed for any cat presenting with dyspnea, after adequate stabilization. If a pleural effusion is suspected, thoracocentesis should be performed, and pleural fluid should be submitted for analysis including cytological evaluation; the presence of malignant lymphoblasts may be diagnostic for lymphosarcoma. Complete clinical staging includes complete blood count, chemistry panel, urinalysis, FeLV and FIV testing, thoracic radiographs, abdominal ultrasound, and bone marrow aspiration or biopsy. If cytology is not diagnostic for lymphosarcoma, an ultrasound-guided needle core biopsy may provide diagnostic samples. If a tru-cut biopsy is not adequate for diagnosis, exploratory thoracotomy may be indicated. Other diagnostic testing may be performed as deemed clinically relevant.

Phenotypical studies of feline lymphosarcoma can be performed, but may offer less prognostic information than that gained from phenotypic analysis in dogs. B- and T-cell phenotypes occur with nearly equal overall frequency, but different anatomical sites are more or less likely to be T- or B-cell. Some 85% to 100% of feline thymic lymphosarcomas have been found to be T-cell.[22,32,45]

The initial treatment of mediastinal lymphosarcoma should be based both on the severity of clinical signs and on the results of staging. Many cats with cranial mediastinal masses are presented with respiratory difficulty because of pleural effusion. In these cats, initial therapy should be directed at relieving acute clinical signs such as respiratory distress. Immediate relief may be possible with thoracocentesis. Chemotherapy is the mainstay of treatment for lymphosarcoma. As in dogs, most protocols utilize first line lymphosarcoma drugs such as prednisone, vincristine, L-asparaginase, cyclophosphamide, and doxorubicin. Evidence suggests that the addition of doxorubicin to induction protocols for feline lymphosarcoma results in prolonged disease-free intervals.[34,41] Radiation therapy may also be effective in cases of lymphosarcoma localized to the cranial mediastinum, particularly if the cat is not initially responsive to chemotherapy.[46] A combination of chemotherapy and radiation therapy may be optimal in cats that are not achieving or maintaining remission with chemotherapy alone.

Thymic lymphosarcoma carries a grave prognosis without treatment[29]; however, a few studies have reported a favorable initial response to therapy in cats with mediastinal lymphosarcoma.[29,47] Cats with mediastinal masses may be FeLV positive. Although FeLV status may not affect response to therapy for lymphosarcoma, multiple studies have shown that FeLV-positive cats have significantly shorter survival times.[34,35,37,39] Other prognostic indicators include response to therapy, a/b substage, and the duration of first remission.[30,34,39]

THYMOMA IN THE DOG

In dogs, thymomas are rare neoplasms that arise in the thymus, a poorly understood lymphatic organ that serves as an environment for T-lymphocyte maturation.[48] Immature lymphocytes travel from the bone marrow to the thymus where they develop into thymic-dependent lymphocytes, T-cells, and cytotoxic T-lymphocytes.[49] This process takes place shortly before birth and lasts for a few months, after which the thymus involutes. The thymus is composed histopathologically of two major cell types, thymic epithelial cells and T-lymphocytes. Thymomas are tumors that arise from the epithelial component of the thymus. Benign lymphoid proliferation accompanies the neoplastic transformation of the epithelial cells. Thymomas are either benign or malignant and have been associated with several paraneoplastic syndromes including myasthenia gravis, polymyositis, hypercalcemia, and increased incidence of nonthymic neo-

plasia.[49-53] Thymomas are uncommon; according to one report, thymomas were found in 15 of 392,744 dogs examined over an 11-year period.[54]

The epidemiology of canine thymoma is not known. Thymomas occur in older dogs but have been reported in dogs as young as 10 months old.[52] The median age of dogs with thymomas is 9 years.[49,54] German shepherds, Labrador retrievers and golden retrievers are overrepresented.[49,52,54] There is disagreement between studies as to whether there is a sex predilection. One study of 15 affected dogs found a 15:6 male to female ratio.[54] Another review of 14 dogs with thymoma found that 85% were female.[53] However, most other studies have determined no significant difference in prevalence based on sex.[49,55]

Many dogs with thymoma lack clinical signs.[56] When present, clinical signs may indicate a space-occupying cranial mediastinal mass or pleural effusion and may include dyspnea, tachypnea, ptyalism, dysphagia, and neck edema secondary to cranial venal cava syndrome.[52-55,57,58] Pleural effusions associated with thymomas may be modified transudates, pseudochylous, or chylous.[51,55] Dogs may also have nonspecific clinical signs such as weight loss, anorexia, and lethargy.[55] In one study of 15 dogs with thymoma, 67% were diagnosed with paraneoplastic syndromes, which may contribute clinical signs such as polyuria/polydipsia, vomiting/regurgitation, coughing, and weakness.[51,54,55] The incidence of myasthenia gravis in dogs with thymoma is reported to be between 7% and 47%.[51,53,54] Aspiration pneumonia may be a sequela to megaesophagus in some dogs with myasthenia gravis.

Staging of dogs with thymoma should include a complete blood count, serum chemistry screen, urinalysis, and thoracic radiographs. Cytological analysis of fine-needle aspirates obtained from a cranial mediastinal mass may provide a presumptive diagnosis of thymoma, but biopsy is often required for definitive diagnosis.[55] Cytology from thymic aspirates often reveals small- to intermediate-sized lymphocytes, and must be distinguished from lymphosarcoma by histopathology. Mast cells, eosinophils, plasma cells, melanocytes, necrosis, and spindle cells can also be seen on cytology.[51,54,55,58,59] Further diagnostic tests should be performed according to clinical and paraneoplastic signs. Thoracic ultrasound, CT, or MRI may be used to assess the invasiveness of the thymic neoplasm. Myasthenia gravis should be suspected in dogs with generalized exercise-induced muscle weakness that improves with rest.[53] Facial muscles and the esophagus may be affected as well. Response to anticholinesterases, EMG testing, and the presence of anti-acetylcholine receptor antibodies contribute to the diagnosis of myasthenia gravis.

The histopathological appearance of thymomas does not correlate well with clinical behavior.[55] The terms malignant thymoma and thymic carcinoma are used interchangeably throughout the veterinary literature.[48] Noninvasive and invasive may be more appropriate terms for benign and malignant thymomas.[56,59] Staging is based on the degree of invasiveness of the thymoma, the presence of distant metastasis, and paraneoplastic signs (Table 84-3).

Metastases from malignant thymomas have been observed in the lungs, diaphragm, pericardium, scapula,

TABLE 84-3. Clinical Staging of Canine Thymoma

Stage	Criteria
I	Growth completely within intact thymic capsule
II	Pericapsular growth into mediastinal fat, adjacent pleura, or pericardium
III	Invasion into surrounding organs or intrathoracic metastasis
IV	Extrathoracic metastasis
P_0	Paraneoplastic syndrome not evident
P_1	Myasthenia Gravis
P_2	Nonthymic malignant tumor

Reproduced with permission from Aronsohn M: Canine thymoma, *Vet Clin North Am Small Anim Pract* 15(4):755-767, 1985.

liver, spleen, kidney, and mediastinal lymph nodes.[49,56] Primary neoplasms that have been reported in conjunction with thymoma in dogs include lymphosarcoma, osteosarcoma, salivary gland adenocarcinoma, chronic lymphocytic leukemia, thyroid adenocarcinoma, hibernoma, bladder polyp, squamous cell carcinoma, mammary neoplasia, pheochromocytoma, astrocytoma, hemangiosarcoma, and primary lung adenocarcinoma.[49,53-56] It has been theorized that the development of the concurrent neoplasms in dogs with thymoma is because of a failure of thymus-dependent immunologic surveillance.[54,55]

Surgery is generally considered to be the treatment of choice for well-encapsulated stage I and stage II thymic tumors[49,51,54,55,59]; however, there are reports of prolonged survival in dogs with thymoma receiving no treatment.[53,55] High morbidity and mortality occurs when surgical excision has been attempted in dogs with concurrent megaesophagus secondary to myasthenia gravis.[55] Thymectomy may result in improvement in clinical signs in 25% to 83% of human patients with thymomatous and nonthymomatous myasthenia gravis.[53] Improvement of clinical signs of megaesophagus secondary to myasthenia gravis, and decrease in serum acetylcholine receptor antibody concentrations, were reported in 1 dog following thymectomy for a thymoma.[60] Clinical signs resolved until the thymoma recurred 6 months postoperatively.[60] Resolution of hypercalcemia following thymectomy has also been reported.[51] Stage III and stage IV tumors are often nonresectable, and radiation therapy or chemotherapy have been recommended both as primary treatments or as adjuvants to surgery in these cases.[17,53] Various chemotherapy agents, most notably prednisone and other first line lymphosarcoma drugs, have been used to treat thymoma, either as the sole treatment or as adjuvants. However, response to therapy may be difficult to gauge because thymomas may be slow-growing tumors, and the decrease in size of a thymic mass may occur due to the cytotoxic effects of prednisone or chemotherapy on thymic lymphocytes rather than an effect against the neoplastic thymic epithelial cells.[53] Prednisone may provide relief of clinical signs in dogs with paraneoplastic syndromes.

Radiation therapy has also been used as primary therapy for thymoma, particularly in cases in which diagnostic imaging has revealed the presence of an invasive thymoma. In these cases, surgical debulking may be difficult and is not recommended.[17] Although there is little correlation between histologic type and response to surgery, it is hypothesized that thymomas with a large lymphocytic component may respond more favorably to radiation therapy because of the high sensitivity of lymphocytes to radiation therapy.[17] According to a recent study, the median survival time for dogs with thymoma treated with radiation therapy was 218 days.[61]

Dogs with stage I thymomas have the best prognosis and may be treated effectively with surgery alone. The presence of myasthenia gravis, cranial venal cava syndrome, and advanced stage (stage III or higher) disease are negative prognostic indicators.[49,55,56] Dogs less than 8 years old that develop thymoma may also have a worse prognosis.[55] Megaesophagus was found to be a significant negative prognostic indicator in a study with 23 cases of thymoma.[55] According to this study, dogs without megaesophagus had a 1-year survival rate of 83% regardless of how they were treated.[55] The median survival time for all dogs (including those with megaesophagus) in the same study was only 13 days, with 30% of dogs alive at 1 year.[55]

THYMOMA IN CATS

Thymoma is a rare neoplasm in the cat. Thymomas most commonly affect older cats, with a median age of 9 years (range 3 to 18 years), and there is no apparent sex or breed predilection.[52,62-64] Cats that develop thymomas usually test FeLV- and FIV-negative.[52,63,65] As in canine thymoma, the etiology of feline thymoma is unknown.

The clinical presentation of cats with thymoma is very similar to that of cats with mediastinal lymphoma. Common presenting complaints include dyspnea, coughing, anorexia, lethargy, vomiting, dysphagia, dysphonia, and weight loss.[27,62-64] Thymoma may also be an incidental finding.[64] Cats with thymomas can suffer from paraneoplastic syndromes including myasthenia gravis, myositis, myocarditis, and exfoliative dermatitis.[52,62,63,65,66] Other clinical signs are likely to be referable to the extent and type of paraneoplastic syndrome.

The histopathological characteristics of thymomas in cats are very similar to the findings in dogs, with the tumor containing a mix of thymic epithelial cells and mature thymic lymphocytes. Either cell type may predominate in a given tumor.[27,52] Necrosis, cysts, mast cells, and eosinophils can also be seen.[62,64] Areas of squamous cell carcinoma within thymomas were reported in 2 cats.[67] Whereas thymomas in cats are predominantly benign, the tumors in these 2 cats behaved very aggressively. One cat developed metastases to the parietal pleura of the thoracic cavity, to the sternal and tracheobronchial lymph nodes, and an occlusive metastasis within the pulmonary artery of the right caudal lung lobe. In the other cat, evidence of vascular invasion was seen at necropsy.[67]

Clinical staging of cats with thymoma should include tests similar to those listed above for dogs. In addition, FeLV and FIV testing should be performed. Thoracocentesis should be performed in cats presenting with

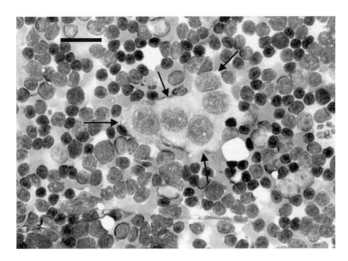

Figure 84-2 *Photomicrograph of a fine-needle aspirate (FNA) of a thymoma from a cat. Most of the cells within the field are small, nonneoplastic lymphocytes, which is typical for FNA of a thymoma. The actual neoplastic cells are the central 5 epithelioid cells (arrows), which are rarely observed in aspirate smears. Bar = 25 μm. (Photomicrographs courtesy of Dr. Patricia McManus, University of Pennsylvania.)*

pleural effusion. The effusion may be chylous, pseudo-chylous, or a modified transudate. Cytological evaluation of pleural fluid and fine-needle aspirations of the thymoma may reveal small- to medium-sized lymphocytes, and differential diagnoses must include thymoma and lymphosarcoma (Figure 84-2).[62] Mast cells may also be seen. Results of FeLV, FIV, and evaluation for systemic neoplasia may help differentiate between thymoma and lymphosarcoma.[17] A biopsy of the mediastinal mass is often needed for a definitive diagnosis.

Surgery is the treatment of choice for thymoma in cats. In one report of 12 cats treated with surgery alone, 2 cats died in the immediate postoperative period, and in the 6 cats available for follow-up, the median survival time was 21 months.[64] The most common surgical complication was hemorrhage.[64] It is unknown whether surgical excision of thymoma will completely ameliorate clinical signs associated with paraneoplastic syndromes. Two cats were reported to develop myasthenia gravis after surgical excision of thymoma.[64] Many authors have suggested that paraneoplastic syndromes associated with thymomas are immune-mediated.[63-66] Therefore, immuno-suppressive agents may be beneficial in reducing clinical signs associated with these syndromes.[63] Local invasion and metastasis to lungs and kidneys have been observed in a minority of cases of thymoma.[68] Owners should be prepared for the potential of a guarded prognosis.

Very little information exists about the use of adjuvant radiation therapy or adjuvant chemotherapy for the treatment of feline thymoma.[27] Because thymomas in cats tend to be clinically benign, adjuvant treatment is not warranted in most cases. If residual microscopic or macroscopic tumor remains following surgery, adjuvant radiation therapy can be utilized with success.[17] According to a recent abstract, the median survival in 7 cats following radiation therapy for thymoma, alone or

as an adjuvant to surgery, was 720 days.[61] As in dogs, cats with thymoma may have prolonged survival if treated with prednisone alone. One cat currently being treated with prednisone and pyridostigmine (for control of myasthenia gravis) by the Oncology Service at the University of Pennsylvania is alive and asymptomatic 14 months after tentative diagnosis of thymoma, based on cytology of the cranial mediastinal mass and the presence of myasthenia gravis.

Neoplasms of the Pleura

Primary neoplasms of the pleura are rare in dogs and cats. Metastatic carcinoma is the most common tumor affecting the pleura in both species. Malignancies affecting the pleura commonly result in the development of pleural effusion, and clinical signs are often similar to other causes of pleural effusion. Potential etiologies of pleural effusion include increased hydrostatic pressure, as occurs in congestive heart failure; increased capillary permeability; decreased oncotic pressure because of hypoalbuminemia; or decreased pleural lymphatic drainage, such as occurs if there is obstruction by a cranial mediastinal mass.[69] The most important causes of neoplastic effusion include increased capillary permeability, secondary to neoplastic or inflammatory disruption of capillary endothelium; and decreased lymphatic drainage because of a mass effect.[69]

CANINE PLEURAL MESOTHELIOMA

Mesotheliomas are rare neoplasms of mesodermal origin, arising from serous membranes including the pleura, pericardium, peritoneum, and the tunica vaginalis of the testes.[66,70,71] In one report, cases of mesothelioma represented 0.2% of necropsy diagnoses over a 20-year period.[72] Mesotheliomas affect older dogs; the median age of affected dogs is 10 years.[72] Because of the paucity of cases reported in the veterinary literature, there is no information regarding gender or breed predilection.[70-72]

Dogs affected with mesothelioma tend to live in urban areas.[73] A significant association has been established between development of mesothelioma in pet dogs and an asbestos-related occupation or hobby of a household member, and with pesticide use.[73] Asbestos has also been found in flea powder, and this may be another potential source of exposure. However, many dogs that develop mesothelioma have no known exposure to asbestos, and asbestos fibers are not seen on evaluation of lung tissue with electron microscopy. Asbestos exposure has also been found to be the predominant causal factor for the development of mesothelioma in humans.[74]

Clinical signs of pleural mesothelioma in dogs are related to the development of pleural effusion and include dyspnea, tachypnea, lethargy, anorexia, and weight loss.[70-72] Mesotheliomas are highly effusive neoplasms. If a pleural effusion is present, thoracocentesis should be performed and samples submitted for fluid analysis and cytological evaluation. In one study of 7 dogs with pleural mesothelioma, hemorrhagic pleural effusions were found in all dogs in which results of thoracocente-

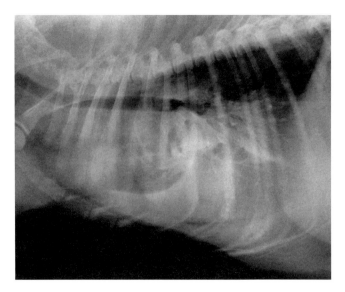

Figure 84-3 *Right lateral thoracic radiograph from a dog with mesothelioma. Notice pneumohydrothorax, a poorly marginated soft tissue mass cranial to heart, and decreased expansion of the lung lobes secondary to pleural disease.*

TABLE 84-4. **Clinical Staging of Malignant Pleural Mesothelioma**	
Stage	**Criteria**
I	Tumor confined to the pleura
II	Tumor involving organs cranial to the diaphragm (e.g., lung or intrathoracic lymph nodes)
III	Tumor involving organs caudal to the diaphragm
IV	Distant hematogenous metastasis

Reproduced with permission from Morrison WB, Trigo FJ: Clinical characterization of pleural mesothelioma in seven dogs, *Comp Cont Ed* 6(4):342-348, 1984.

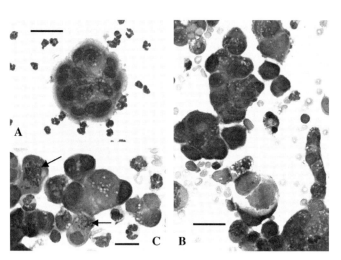

Figure 84-4. A, *Cluster of mesothelial cells detected in an inflammatory exudate from a dog with septic peritonitis. These cells display normal, albeit reactive, morphology. Reactive mesothelial cells are common in dogs with irritating peritoneal and pleural effusions. Reactive mesothelial cells typically display a pink fringe of peripheral cytoplasm, mild to moderate anisocytosis and anisokaryosis, increased cytoplasmic basophilia, and frequent symmetric binucleation. Bar = 25 μm.* **B,** *Clusters of neoplastic mesothelial cells in a pleural effusion from a dog with mesothelioma confirmed at necropsy. The mesothelial cells within this effusion display more extreme pleomorphism compared to reactive mesothelial cells, and there was no evidence of either hemorrhage or inflammation. Bar = 25 μm.* **C,** *A higher magnification of neoplastic cells, same patient as in* **B.** *Arrows point to two atypical mitotic figures. Bar = 10 μm. (Photomicrographs courtesy of Dr. Patricia McManus, University of Pennsylvania.)*

sis were recorded.[70] Other characteristics of the effusions included packed cell volumes from 13% to 22%, specific gravity from 1.014 to 1.023, and nucleated cell counts from 2250 to 24,300 cells/mm.[3,70]

Clinical staging of dogs with pleural mesothelioma should include analysis of the pleural effusion (e.g., cytology, fluid analysis, bacterial culture and sensitivity if appropriate, and biochemistries including triglyceride concentration); complete blood count; chemistry screen; urinalysis; and thoracic radiographs, at a minimum (Figure 84-3). Further evaluation including coagulation testing, abdominal ultrasound, CT, or MRI may be indicated according to the clinical signs. The staging system for canine pleural mesothelioma is described in Table 84-4.

A definitive diagnosis of mesothelioma based on cytological evaluation alone is considered to be very difficult. The effusions are often hemorrhagic, which is a common characteristic of pleural effusions associated with thoracic neoplasms.[70] Abnormal multinucleated mesothelial cells within a pleural effusion are also not necessarily diagnostic for mesothelioma because pleural mesothelial cells undergo hyperplasia and hypertrophy as fluid accumulates within the pleural space. These reactive mesothelial cells may be very difficult to distinguish from malignant mesothelial cells. Reactive mesothelial cells may have several features of malignancy including binucleation or multinucleation. They may contain one or more nucleoli, and mitotic figures can be seen (Figure 84-4).[66] Because of the inability to readily distinguish reactive from malignant mesothelial cells, a definitive diagnosis may require biopsy via exploratory thoracotomy or thoracoscopy. However, even with the benefit of biopsy, misdiagnosis is not uncommon. Metastatic carcinoma may appear very similar to mesothelioma both on gross and histologic evaluation,[71] and special staining techniques can be used to differentiate them. Hyaluronidase digestion of sections stained with toluidine blue or Alcian blue-periodic acid Schiff can be helpful because mesotheliomas produce hyaluronic acid whereas carcinomas do not.[75]

Three histopathologic types of mesothelioma are described in humans including epithelial, sarcomatoid, and mixed (consisting of both epithelial and sarcomatoid components).[74] Epithelial mesotheliomas are the most common variant in both humans and in the dog, and carry a more favorable prognosis than mesotheliomas with a sarcomatoid component.

Treatment of pleural mesothelioma is considered to be only palliative and is aimed at reducing the frequency and amount of pleural effusion produced by the neoplasm. Intracavitary chemotherapy with cisplatin offers the greatest hope of prolonged palliation. With this method, cells on the outer 3-mm surface of the tumor are exposed to cisplatin concentrations 1 to 3 logs higher than the level of exposure achieved after intravenous administration. There is no pharmacokinetic advantage to intracavitary cisplatin versus intravenous administration for cells beneath the 3-mm surface of the tumor.[76] Cisplatin is nephrotoxic; therefore dogs with renal insufficiency should not receive this drug, and appropriate diuresis should be performed even when the drug is used in dogs with normal renal function. Three dogs with pleural mesothelioma treated with intrathoracic cisplatin maintained a response from 129 days to more than 306 days.[76] Only dogs with small tumors are likely to benefit from intracavitary cisplatin, and response to intravenous chemotherapy is poor. Repeated thoracocentesis may be palliative, but the fluid tends to become loculated over time, making drainage uncomfortable and impractical. The prognosis for dogs with mesothelioma is grave.

PLEURAL MESOTHELIOMA IN CATS

Mesotheliomas are more rare in cats than in dogs. Pleural, pericardial, and peritoneal mesotheliomas have been reported.[76-79] As in dogs, diagnosis based on cytology alone is unreliable, and biopsy is warranted for definitive diagnosis. Cisplatin causes fatal pulmonary edema and should not be used for treatment in cats. There is no reported treatment for mesothelioma in cats, and therefore the prognosis is grave.

REFERENCES

1. Miller ME: Thoracic cavity and pleurae. In Evans HE, Christensen GC, editors: *Miller's anatomy of the dog,* ed 2, Philadelphia, 1992, WB Saunders Co.
2. Stobie D, Carpenter JL: Lymphangiosarcoma of the mediastinum, mesentery, and omentum in a cat with chylothorax, *J Am Anim Hosp Assoc* 29(1):78-80, 1993.
3. Rosenthal RC: Epidemiology of canine lymphosarcoma, *Comp Cont Ed* 10:855-860, 1982.
4. Chapman AL, Bopp WJ, Brightwell AS et al: Preliminary report on virus-like particles in canine leukemia and derived cell cultures, *Cancer Res* 27(1):18-25, 1967.
5. Kakuk TJ, Hinz RW, Langham RF et al: Experimental transmission of canine malignant lymphoma to a beagle neonate, *Cancer Research* 28:716-723, 1968.
6. Onions D: RNA dependent DNA polymerase activity in canine lymphosarcoma, *Eur J Cancer* 16:345-349, 1980.
7. Hayes HM, Tarone RE, Cantor KP et al: Case control study of canine malignant lymphoma: positive association with dog owner's use of 2,4-Dichlorophenoxyacetic acid herbicides, *J Natl Cancer Inst* 83:1226-1231, 1991.
8. Kaneene JB, Miller R: Re-analysis of 2,4-D use and the occurrence of canine malignant lymphoma, *Vet Hum Toxicol* 41(3):164-170, 1999.
9. Keller ET, MacEwen EG, Rosenthal RC et al: Evaluation of prognostic factors and sequential combination chemotherapy with doxorubicin for canine lymphoma, *J Vet Intern Med* 7(5):289-295, 1993.
10. Zemann BI, Moore AS, Rand WM et al: A combination chemotherapy protocol (VELCAP-L) for dogs with lymphoma, *J Vet Intern Med* 12:465-470, 1998.
11. MacEwen EG, Hayes AA, Matus RE et al: Evaluation of some prognostic factors for advanced multicentric lymphosarcoma in the dog: 147 cases (1978-1981), *JAVMA* 190(5):564-568, 1987.
12. MacEwen EG, Brown NO, Patnaik AK et al: Cyclic combination chemotherapy of canine lymphosarcoma, *JAVMA* 178(11):1178-1181, 1981.
13. Rosenberg MP, Matus RE, Patnaik AK: Prognostic factors in dogs with lymphoma and hypercalcemia, *J Vet Intern Med* 5(5):268-271, 1991.
14. Valerius KD, Ogilvie GK, Mallinckrodt CH et al: Doxorubicin alone or in combination with asparaginase, followed by cyclophosphamide, vincristine, and prednisone for treatment of multicentric lymphoma in dogs: 121 cases (1987-1995), *JAVMA* 210(4):512-516, 1997.
15. Ogilvie GK, Moore AS: *Managing the veterinary cancer patient,* Trenton, NJ, 1995, Veterinary Learning Systems.
16. Morrison WB: *Cancer in dogs and cats: Medical and surgical management,* Baltimore, 1998, Williams & Wilkins.
17. Meleo KA: The role of radiotherapy in the treatment of lymphoma and thymoma, *Vet Clin North Am Small Anim Pract* 27(1):115-129, 1997.
18. Meuten DJ, Kociba GJ, Capen CC et al: Hypercalcemia in dogs with lymphosarcoma: Biochemical, ultrastructural, and histomorphometric investigations, *Lab Invest* 49:553-562, 1983.
19. Biller DS: Mediastinal disease. In Ettinger SJ, Feldman EC, editors: *Textbook of veterinary internal medicine,* ed 5, vol 2, Philadelphia, 2000, WB Saunders.
20. Greenlee PG, Filippa DA, Quimby FW et al: Lymphomas in dogs: A morphologic, immunologic, and clinical study, *Cancer* 66(3):480-490, 1990.
21. Teske E, van Heerde P, Rutteman GR et al: Prognostic factors for treatment of malignant lymphoma in dogs, *JAVMA* 205(12):1722-1728, 1994.
22. Holmberg CA, Manning JS, Osburn BI: Feline malignant lymphomas: Comparison of morphologic and immunologic characteristics, *Am J Vet Res* 37(12):1455-1460, 1976.
23. Myers NC, Moore AS, Rand WM et al: Evaluation of a multidrug chemotherapy protocol (ACOPA II) in dogs with lymphoma, *J Vet Intern Med* 11(6):333-339, 1997.
24. Weller RE, Theilen GH, Madewell BR: Chemotherapeutic responses in dogs with lymphosarcoma and hypercalcemia, *JAVMA* 181(9):891-893, 1982.
25. Price GS, Page RL, Fischer BM et al: Efficacy and toxicity of doxorubicin/cyclophosphamide maintenance therapy in dogs with multicentric lymphosarcoma, *J Vet Intern Med* 5(5):259-262, 1991.
26. Hahn KA, Richardson RC, Teclaw RF et al: Is maintenance chemotherapy appropriate for the management of canine malignant lymphoma? *J Vet Intern Med* 6(1):3-10, 1992.
27. Hardy WD: Hematopoietic tumors of cats, *J Am Anim Hosp Assoc* 17:921-940, 1981.
28. Dorn CR, Taylor DO, Hibbard HH: Epizootiologic characteristics of canine and feline leukemia and lymphoma, *Am J Vet Res* 28(125):993-1001, 1967.
29. Loar AS: The management of feline lymphosarcoma, *Vet Clin North Am Small Anim Pract* 14(6):1299-1330, 1984.
30. Mooney SC, Hayes AA: Lymphoma in the cat: An approach to diagnosis and management, *Semin Vet Med Surg Small Anim* 1(1):51-57, 1986.
31. Rojko JL, Kociba GJ, Hamilton KL et al: Feline lymphomas: Immunological and cytochemical characterization, *Cancer Res* 49:345-351, 1989.
32. Hardy WD, McClelland AJ, Zuckerman EE et al: Development of virus non-producer lymphosarcomas in pet cats exposed to FeLV, *Nature* 288:90-92, 1980.
33. Meincke JE, Hobbie WV, Hardy WD: Lymphoreticular malignancies in the cat: Clinical findings, *JAVMA* 160(8):1093-1099, 1972.
34. Vail DM, Moore AS, Ogilvie GK et al: Feline lymphoma (145 cases): Proliferation indices, cluster of differentiation 3 immunoreactivity, and their association with prognosis in 90 cats, *J Vet Intern Med* 12:349-354, 1998.
35. Jeglum KA, Whereat A, Young K: Chemotherapy of lymphoma in 75 cats, *JAVMA* 190(2):174-178, 1987.

36. Slaytor MV, Farver TB, Schneider R: Feline malignant lymphoma: Log-linear multiway frequency analysis of a population involving the factors of sex and age of animal and tumor cell type and location, *Am J Vet Res* 45:2178-2181, 1984.
37. Mooney SC, Hayes AA, MacEwen EG et al: Treatment and prognostic factors in lymphoma in cats: 103 cases (1977-1981), *JAVMA* 194(5):696-699, 1989.
38. Francis DP, Cotter SM, Hardy WD et al: Comparison of virus-positive and virus-negative cases of feline leukemia and lymphoma, *Cancer Res* 39: 3866-3870, 1979.
39. Mauldin GE, Mooney SC, Meleo KA et al: Chemotherapy in 132 cats with lymphoma (1988-1994), *Veterinary Cancer Society Proceedings* 15:35-36, 1995.
40. Mahony OM, Moore AS, Cotter SM et al: Alimentary lymphoma in cats: 28 cases (1988-1993), *JAVMA* 207(12):1593-1598, 1995.
41. Moore AS, Cotter SM, Frimberger AE et al: A comparison of doxorubicin and COP for maintenance of remission in cats with lymphoma, *J Vet Intern Med* 10(6):372-375, 1996.
42. Gabor LJ, Canfield PJ, Malik R: Immunophenotypic and histological characterization of 109 cases of feline lymphosarcoma, *Aust Vet J* 77(7):436-441, 1999.
43. Zwahlen CH, Lucroy MD, Kraegel SA et al: Results of chemotherapy for cats with alimentary malignant lymphoma: 21 cases (1993-1997), *JAVMA* 213(8):1144-1149, 1998.
44. Court EA, Watson ADJ, Peaston AE: Retrospective study of 60 cases of feline lymphosarcoma, *Aust Vet J* 75(6):424-427, 1997.
45. Jackson ML, Wood SL, Misra V et al: Immunohistochemical identification of B and T lymphocytes in formalin-fixed, paraffin embedded feline lymphosarcomas: Relation to feline leukemia virus status, tumor site, and patient age, *Cancer J Vet Res* 60:199-204, 1996.
46. Elmslie RE, Ogilvie GK, Gillette EL et al: Radiotherapy with and without chemotherapy for localized lymphoma in 10 cats, *Vet Radiol* 32(6):277-280, 1991.
47. Cotter SM: Treatment of lymphoma and leukemia with cyclophosphamide, vincristine, and prednisone. I. Treatment of dogs. II. Treatment of cats, *J Am Anim Hosp Assoc* 19(2):159-172, 1983.
48. Abdi MM, Elliott HA: Thymic carcinoma with glandular differentiation in a dog, *Vet Rec* 134(6):141-142, 1994.
49. Aronsohn M: Canine thymoma, *Vet Clin North Am Small Anim Pract* 15(4):755-767, 1985.
50. Poffenbarger E, Klausner JS, Caywood DD: Acquired myasthenia gravis in a dog with thymoma: A case report, *J Am Anim Hosp Assoc* 21(1):119-124, 1985.
51. Harris CL, Klausner JS, Caywood DD et al: Hypercalcemia in a dog with thymoma, *J Am Anim Hosp Assoc* 27(3):281-284, 1991.
52. Day MJ: Review of thymic pathology in 30 cats and 36 dogs, *J Small Anim Pract* 38(9):393-403, 1997.
53. Klebanow ER: Thymoma and acquired myasthenia gravis in the dog: A case report and review of 13 additional cases, *JAVMA* 28(1):63-69, 1992.
54. Aronsohn MG, Schunk KL, Carpenter JL et al: Clinical and pathologic features of thymoma in 15 dogs, *JAVMA* 184(11):1355-1362, 1984.
55. Atwater SW, Powers BE, Park RD et al: Thymoma in dogs: 23 cases (1980-1991), *JAVMA* 205(7):1007-1013, 1994.
56. Bellah JR, Stiff ME, Russell RG: Thymoma in the dog: Two case reports and review of 20 additional cases, *JAVMA* 183(3):306-311, 1983.

57. Peaston AE, Church DB, Allen GS et al: Combined chylothorax, chylopericardium, and cranial vena cava syndrome in a dog with thymoma, *JAVMA* 197(10):1354-1356, 1990.
58. Hunt GB, Churcher RK, Church DB et al: Excision of a locally invasive thymoma causing cranial vena caval syndrome in a dog, *JAVMA* 210(11):1628-1630, 1997.
59. Gonzalez M, Rodriguez A, Pizarro M et al: Immunohistochemical study of a non-invasive canine thymoma: A case report, *J Vet Intern Med* 44(7):399-406, 1997.
60. Lainesse MFC, Taylor SM, Myers SL et al: Focal myasthenia gravis as a paraneoplastic syndrome of canine thymoma: Improvement following thymectomy, *JAAHA* 32:111-117, 1996.
61. Smith AN, Wright JC, Brawner WR et al: Radiation therapy in the treatment of canine and feline thymomas: A retrospective study (1985-1999), *J Am Anim Hosp Assoc* 37:489-496, 2001.
62. Carpenter JL, Holzworth J: Thymoma in 11 cats, *JAVMA* 181(3):248-251, 1982.
63. Scott DW, Yager JA, Johnston KM: Exfoliative dermatitis in association with thymoma in three cats, *Feline Practice* 23(4):8-13, 1995.
64. Gores BR, Berg J, Carpenter JL et al: Surgical treatment of thymoma in cats: 12 cases (1987-1992), *JAVMA* 204(11):1782-1785, 1994.
65. Scott-Moncrieff JC, Cook JR, Lantz GC: Acquired myasthenia gravis in a cat with thymoma, *JAVMA* 196(8):1291-1293, 1990.
66. Smith DA, Hill FWG: Metastatic malignant mesothelioma in a dog, *J Comp Pathol* 100(1):97-101, 1989.
67. Carpenter JL, Valentine BA: Squamous cell carcinoma arising in two feline thymomas, *Vet Pathol* 29(6):541-543, 1992.
68. Middleton DJ, Ratcliffe RC, Xu FN: Thymoma with distant metastases in a cat, *Vet Pathol* 22(5):512-514, 1985.
69. Pass HI: Malignant pleural and pericardial effusions. In DeVita VT, Hellman S, Rosenberg SA, editors: *Cancer: Principles and practice of oncology*, ed 5, Philadelphia, 1997, Lippincott, Williams and Wilkins.
70. Morrison WB, Trigo FJ: Clinical characterization of pleural mesothelioma in seven dogs, *Comp Cont Ed* 6(4):342-348, 1984.
71. Thrall DE, Goldschmidt MH: Mesothelioma in the dog: Six case reports, *J Am Vet Radiol Soc* 19(4):107-115, 1978.
72. Harbison ML, Godleski JJ: Malignant mesothelioma in urban dogs, *Vet Pathol* 20(5):531-540, 1983.
73. Glickman LT, Domanski LM, Maguire TG et al: Mesothelioma in pet dogs associated with exposure of their owners to asbestos, *Environ Res* 32(2):305-313, 1983.
74. Antman KH, Schiff PB, Pass HI: Benign and malignant mesothelioma. In DeVita VT, Hellman S, Rosenberg SA, editors: *Cancer: Principles and practice of oncology*, ed 5, Philadelphia, 1997, Lippincott, Williams and Wilkins.
75. Trigo FJ, Morrison WB, Breeze RG: An ultrastructural study of canine mesothelioma, *J Comp Pathol* 91(4):531-537, 1981.
76. Kobayashi Y, Usuda H, Ochiai K et al: Malignant mesothelioma with metastases and mast cell leukaemia in a cat, *J Comp Pathol* 111(4):453-458, 1994.
77. Tilley LP, Owens JM, Wilkins RJ et al: Pericardial mesothelioma with effusion in a cat, *JAVMA* 11(1):60-65, 1975.
78. Andrews EJ: Pleural mesothelioma in a cat, *J Comp Pathol* 83(2):259-263, 1973.
79. Creighton SR, Wilkins RJ: Thoracic effusions in the cat: Etiology and diagnostic features, *J Am Anim Hosp Assoc* 11(1):66-76, 1975.

CHAPTER 85

Pectus Excavatum

Jonathan F. McAnulty

Pectus excavatum (i.e., congenital chondrosternal depression or funnel chest) is a concave deformity of the sternum and associated ventral thoracic wall. Pectus excavatum is rarely reported in animals, although the true incidence of this deformity in the animal population is unknown. In humans, although it remains an unusual occurrence, pectus excavatum is the most commonly reported thoracic wall abnormality.[1]

Genetics

In humans, pectus excavatum is a heritable autosomal dominant trait.[2] In zoo animals, pectus excavatum has been described as a genetic defect related to inbreeding.[3] Pectus excavatum has also been reported in dogs, cats, calves, lambs, and various exotic species, although the heritable nature of this defect in these species has not been determined.[4,5] Pectus excavatum may also occur in conjunction with various lysosomal storage diseases in both humans and animals (e.g., mucopolysaccharidosis type I, congenital cardiac anomalies, and Marfan's syndrome).[6] Because of the potential for genetic heritability of this defect, breeding of animals with pectus excavatum is not advisable.

Pathophysiology

The physical cause of pectus excavatum remains unclear, and specific abnormalities may differ between individual cases. Early theories, such as those ascribing the abnormality to chronic upper respiratory obstruction, have been discredited. More plausible explanations include the presence of a shortened substernal ligament, a short central tendon of the diaphragm, and an effect secondary to abnormal development of the central and anterior muscular portions of the diaphragm.[4] These theories are relevant to treatment of pectus deformities because an occasional case may require that the affected substernal ligament or abnormal diaphragm be incised in order to release the sternum and allow retraction of the affected structures by external splintage. However, this is generally not necessary to obtain a satisfactory outcome.

Clinical Presentation

Animals with pectus excavatum most commonly present with clinical signs attributable to respiratory compromise.[4,5,7-9] The severity of the pectus deformity may vary, and thus the degree of respiratory compromise and clinical signs may range from the most severe to patients with no clinical signs at all. In more severe cases, cardiac compromise may also be evident. Presenting complaints in animals with pectus deformities may vary from mild exercise intolerance to severe respiratory compromise with cyanosis and death. Respiratory distress is primarily caused by decreased thoracic volume, with partial collapse of the lungs combined with altered thoracic wall compliance; this is often exacerbated by pneumonia. Animals with pectus excavatum are more prone to lower airway infections and can present for cough. Clinical signs that have been reported also include vomiting; and animals that are smaller than their littermates, weak, inappetant, or lack weight gain.

Physical Findings and Diagnosis

The concave sternal deformity of pectus excavatum is readily palpable upon physical examination (Figure 85-1). The concavity is created by a dorsal deviation of the affected sternum and the associated costal arches. The deformity involves either the midcaudal or caudal segment of the sternum and not the cranial sternebrae. Midcaudal sternal deformities result in an almost sigmoidal shape to the sternum, with the xiphoid process pointing ventrally or caudoventrally rather than caudally as in the normal animal. Caudal sternal pectus deformities result in the xiphoid process being directed dorsally, giving the appearance of a foreshortened sternum and creating a depression in the cranial ventral abdominal wall. The dorsal deviation of the sternum can be severe enough that the sternebrae appear to be in contact with the vertebral bodies or aorta on lateral thoracic radiographs. Deformities of this degree can result in lateral displacement of the heart and entrapment within the costal arches; or, in severe cases, restriction of the heart muscle, creating a tamponade-like effect. Diagnosis of pectus excavatum is made by physical examination of the defect

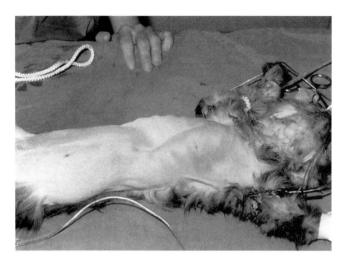

Figure 85-1. *Severe pectus deformity in a cat. The sternal concavity in this case resulted in lateral displacement and entrapment of the heart and apparent contact of the sternum with the aorta and vertebral bodies.*

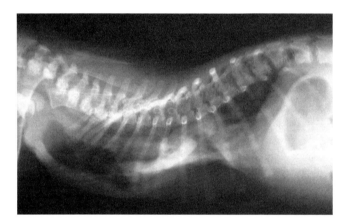

Figure 85-2. *Diagnosis is confirmed with a lateral radiograph of a cat with pectus excavatum. There is a significant decrease in thoracic volume and dorsal deviation of the midcaudal sternebrae.*

and confirmed by thoracic radiographs (Figure 85-2). Radiographic evaluation should also include assessment of the lung fields for pneumonia; lateral displacement of the heart; and examination of the degree of thoracic vertebral lordosis, a finding that may provide clues regarding the presence of shortened substernal or diaphragmatic ligamentous attachments.

Treatment

Treatment of an affected animal is determined by the presence of clinical signs and the severity of the sternal defect. Any animal that presents with cardiac or pulmonary clinical signs, or growth retardation attributable to the pectus deformity should receive treatment. Treatment is best performed when the animal is very young and the affected structures are still pliable.

The severity of the defect can be quantitated from measurements made using radiographs for the calculation of frontosagittal and vertebral indices, as described by Fossum and colleagues.[8] The frontosagittal index is determined by the ratio of the width of the thorax at the tenth thoracic vertebra (on dorsoventral or ventrodorsal radiographs) to the distance measured on lateral radiographs between the sternum and the vertebral body nearest the defect (preferentially used with severe defects) or the tenth vertebral body (in mild defects). The vertebral index is measured on a lateral radiograph and calculated as the ratio of the distance between the center of the dorsal surface of the defect in the sternum to either the nearest vertebral body or the tenth vertebral body and the width of that vertebral body. Normal values for puppies are described as ranging from 0.8 to 1.5 and 11.8 to 19.6 for the frontosagittal index and vertebral indices, respectively. In kittens, the values for the frontosagittal index and vertebral indices are described as normally ranging from 0.7 to 1.3 and 12.6 to 18.8, respectively. These measurements have value for objectively describing the severity of the deformity, and would be useful for assessment of a series of cases and evaluation of the relationship between the severity of the presenting abnormality, the degree of correction, and the clinical outcome.

Severe defects, as described by these measurements, should always be treated, even in the unlikely possibility that such a patient was without clinical signs. However, from a practical clinical standpoint, these measurements may be of limited use in deciding if a patient with a mild-to-moderate chondrosternal depression and no clinical signs should be treated. In such a case, the presence or absence of clinical signs and the age of the animal may play a role in deciding whether repair of the pectus defect is necessary. However, it must be recognized that very young patients may present with mild deformities but that the severity of the defect will increase as the animal grows. If treatment is not elected upon initial presentation, it is important to regularly reexamine the animal and reassess its growth and exercise tolerance until it reaches skeletal maturity. Once the animal reaches skeletal maturity, the sternum and costal arches are less malleable, requiring more invasive and difficult surgery if it becomes necessary to treat the problem.[10] Thus it is always more advantageous to treat pectus deformities in the very young animal, if possible.

The treatment of choice for pectus deformities in the young animal is the application of an external splint affixed to the sternum and costal arches via percutaneous sutures.[7,8] The use of internal struts (K-wires) has also been described for treatment of pectus deformities, but this is a more invasive approach and is technically more difficult to apply. In mature animals with limited flexibility of the sternum and costal arches, costosternal resection has also been described as a treatment.[10]

External Splint Application

Application of an external sternal splint requires general anesthesia. Anesthetic management strategies should

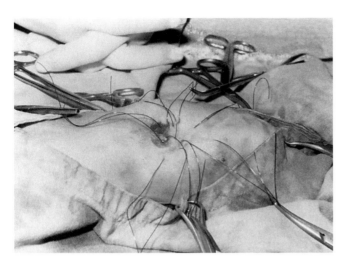

Figure 85-3. Preplacement of circumsternal and circumcostal sutures. Sutures were placed in the periphery of the concavity first and used to retract the sternum away from vital thoracic structures while placing circumsternal sutures in the apex of the defect.

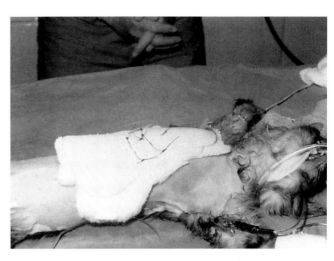

Figure 85-4. External splint molded from thermoplastic splint material. The sutures were passed through a cotton pad and the external splint and then tied with sufficient tension to achieve outward retraction of the sternal defect into a normal thoracic configuration. A gauze square may provide better air circulation under the splint than cotton padding.

assume that some degree of respiratory compromise is present in the affected animal, even if clinical signs were not present before anesthesia. Preoxygenation of the animal before induction of anesthesia may help to reduce the risk of the initial induction and intubation. The patient should be intubated and ventilated by positive pressure ventilation as needed during the anesthetic episode. Because these procedures are most commonly done in the very young animal, hypothermia and hypoglycemia are also pertinent anesthetic risks that should be monitored during anesthesia and after recovery.

The ventral thorax and cranial abdomen are clipped of hair and aseptically prepared for placement of the percutaneous sutures that are used to retract the sternum and costal arches. For small kittens, 1 to 2 ml of air (or more in larger animals) may be injected into each hemithorax at this time to break the surface tension between the lung surface and pleura, create space between the lung and the inner thoracic wall, and reduce the chance of lung damage during suture placement. It is not necessary to remove this air at the end of the procedure. The small degree of pulmonary collapse thereby created may also provide a limited degree of protection against reexpansion pulmonary edema, which can occasionally occur after correction of the pectus defect.[9]

Circumsternal and circumcostal sutures are preplaced before application of the splint (Figure 85-3). The goal of suture placement is to achieve at least two or three circumsternal sutures that are placed within the most severely affected part of the sternal deformity. At least one suture must be placed at the apex of the sternal defect. These sutures will provide sufficient retraction of the most severely affected sternal segment and distribute the tension of the retraction over several sternebrae. In less severe pectus deformities, it may be possible to place the

circumsternal sutures without the necessity for placement of sutures around the costal arches.

In severe defects, circumsternal suture placement within the center of the defect may be difficult or present undue risk for cardiac or aortic trauma. In this situation, it is useful to place circumcostal and circumsternal sutures within the less severely affected area at the periphery of the thoracic depression and use these sutures to retract the pectus deformity away from critical thoracic structures as further sutures are placed within the defect. In this manner, the pectus deformity can be sequentially retracted, working in from the periphery to the central apex of the depression with the least risk for intrathoracic trauma.

Suture placement should be made using monofilament nonabsorbable material (size 0 to 1 material, depending on the size of the animal, is appropriate) swaged onto a taper needle. Cutting needles are not recommended because they may cut through the soft sternal or costal cartilage during needle passage. Circumcostal sutures, if utilized, should be passed from cranial to caudal to reduce the chance of lacerating the intercostal vessels along the caudal rib margin. Care should be taken to avoid levering the needle against the costal arches or sternum. Excess pressure or leverage of the needle can easily fracture these structures in very young animals. Passage of the needle may be made easier by bending the needle into a sharper curve before suture placement. In very small animals where there is limited space between ribs, circumcostal sutures may be more easily placed if the needle is passed around the costal arch at an oblique angle rather than directly perpendicular to the long axis of the costal arch.

The external splint may be constructed of any material that is malleable enough to be conformed to the shape of the normal ventral thorax and allow attachment of the percutaneous sutures (Figure 85-4). Thermoplastic splint materials are particularly well suited to this application because they can be heated and molded to any shape, can be easily trimmed with scissors to remove excess bulk, and can be perforated to allow anchoring of the percutaneous sutures. The external splint should be molded so that it is comfortable for the animal to wear. This author prefers a splint of minimal bulk that contacts, at a minimum, the prominent areas of the ventral thorax around the defect. Larger splints have also been described and work well.[8] The external splint should not impede motion of the forelimbs or inhibit respiration. The splint may also be constructed to extend far enough dorsally to allow lateral compression to the sides of the chest and assist in creating a more normal thoracic configuration, avoiding a barrel-chested configuration. It may also be useful to create a V-shaped keel in the center of the splint to assist in creating a more normal ventral thoracic configuration during treatment. However, if the end result of treatment is a mildly barrel-chested animal, this does not appear to have any negative functional effects but is more of a cosmetic issue.

The splint is attached to the percutaneous sutures by passing the sutures through holes in the splint and tying them with sufficient tension to retract the pectus defect into a normal sternal configuration. This author prefers to pass these sutures through a gauze square before attaching them to the splint. The gauze helps to absorb blood or serum from the suture holes and facilitates keeping the area between the splint and skin dry, reducing the chance of moist dermatitis while the splint is in place. The splint is then covered with a loose bandage that does not inhibit respiration but will prevent the edges of the splint from catching on objects as the animal moves around.

Management After Splint Application

The splint should be left in place until the sternum and costal arches have remodeled into their new position and gained some rigidity. Increased rigidity is difficult to determine but may be assumed if radiographs show increased calcification of the costal arches. The splint is generally left in place for 2 to 3 weeks as long as it is well tolerated and there is no evidence of infection, moist dermatitis, or problems with the splint or sutures. Successful management of pectus excavatum cases has been reported with splint applications lasting between 6 to 33 days.[7,8] In general, the surgeon should plan for the splint to be in place for about 3 weeks but remove it earlier if problems occur.

Animals afflicted with pectus excavatum often experience a growth spurt after retraction of the deformity and attainment of a normal thoracic configuration. Thus these patients should be rechecked at least weekly to make sure that the covering bandage does not become too tight as the animal grows, and that moist dermatitis or infection have not developed under the splint.

Complications

Complications related to treatment of pectus deformities are mostly confined to the perioperative period. It is possible that fatal laceration of the lung, heart, or aorta could occur during suture placement. With careful suture placement, this should be a relatively rare occurrence. Lung laceration may also cause pneumothorax that may be treated by aspiration or thoracostomy tube. Laceration of intercostal vessels may cause bleeding along the suture tract, but this hemorrhage is usually self-limiting. Further, it is possible to cause fracture of the costal arch or sternum during suture placement. A single fracture, although undesirable, will not generally need treatment, and splint application can proceed unhindered. Fatal reexpansion pulmonary edema has been reported after correction of pectus excavatum in one kitten.[9]

After splint application, the animal should be radiographed to evaluate the appropriate retraction of the sternum and if exacerbation of spinal lordosis has occurred. Inability to retract the sternum, or induction of significant lordosis upon sternal retraction, are indications for abdominal exploratory surgery to evaluate and transect substernal or diaphragmatic ligaments. This is seldom necessary.

Complications that may be encountered after discharge from the hospital are primarily limited to development of moist dermatitis and pyoderma of the skin under the splint. Infection of the suture tracts is possible but has not been a significant problem. However, suture tract infection may be one reason for early splint removal if considered to be significant.

Prognosis

The prognosis for treatment of young animals with pectus deformities is guarded to good. A guarded prognosis refers to the possibility of potentially life-threatening complications associated with anesthesia, splint application, and the perioperative period. In spite of the potential risks and young age of these patients, the survival rate of treated animals is very high. If the affected animal survives beyond the perioperative period, the long-term prognosis should be good to excellent for continued growth, a normal life span and normal level of exercise tolerance.

REFERENCES

1. Hebra A: Minimally invasive pectus surgery, *Chest Surg Clin N Am* 10:329-339, 2000.
2. Stoddard EJ: The inheritance of "hollow chest," "cobbler's chest" due to heredity-not occupational deformity, *J Heredity* 30:139-141, 1939.
3. Sedgwick CJ: Pectus excavatum in a Douc langur (Pygathrix nemaeus): One reason for managing genetic variation in zoo animal breeding programs, *J Zoo Anim Med* 12:124-127, 1981.
4. Smallwood JE, Beaver BV: Congenital chondrosternal depression (pectus excavatum) in the cat, *J Am Vet Radiol Soc* 18:141-146, 1977.

5. Pearson JL: Pectus excavatum in the dog, *VM SAC* 68:125-128, 1973.
6. Haskins ME, Jezyk PF, Desnick RJ et al: Animal model of human disease: Mucopolysaccharidosis VI Maroteaux-Lamy syndrome, Arylsulfatase B-deficient mucopolysaccharidosis in the Siamese cat, *Am J Pathol* 105:191-193, 1981.
7. McAnulty JF, Harvey CE: Repair of pectus excavatum by percutaneous suturing and temporary external coaptation in a kitten, *JAVMA* 194:1065-1067, 1989.
8. Fossum TW, Boudrieau RJ, Hobson HP et al: Surgical correction of pectus excavatum, using external splintage in two dogs and a cat, *JAVMA* 195:91-97, 1989.
9. Soderstrom M, Gilson SD, Gulbas N: Fatal reexpansion pulmonary edema in a kitten following surgical correction of pectus excavatum, *J Am Anim Hosp Assoc* 31:133-136, 1995.
10. Bennett D: Successful surgical correction of pectus excavatum in a cat (letter), *VM SAC* 68:936, 1973.

CHAPTER 86

Flail Chest

Mark M. Smith

Flail chest occurs secondary to segmental fracture of 2 or more consecutive ribs. This type of injury is usually related to blunt trauma (e.g., vehicular accidents, kicks, falls, or bites) in dogs and cats.[1-4] In humans and small animals, flail chest is a severe and life-threatening traumatic injury often associated with concomitant intrathoracic injuries.[5-9] Flail chest disrupts thoracic wall integrity, resulting in abnormal or paradoxical movement of the flail chest segment during respiration.[10-13] However, the pathophysiologic effect of this abnormal movement is not as detrimental as the physiologic impact of the associated intrathoracic injuries (e.g., pulmonary contusion, hemothorax, and pneumothorax).[4,10,14]

Clinical Signs and Diagnostic Testing

The clinical diagnosis of flail chest is usually obvious, based on visualizing paradoxical movement of the unstable flail chest segment.[1,5,10] Patients exhibit tachypnea or dyspnea and splinting of the thoracic and abdominal musculature secondary to pain. Crepitus may be palpated in the area of the flail chest segment. Auscultation may indicate harsh bronchovesicular sounds or crackles accompanying pulmonary contusion, or decreased airway sounds secondary to pneumothorax or hemothorax. Thoracic radiography demonstrates the presence of multiple rib fractures (Figure 86-1). Although computed tomography (CT) may provide greater specificity and clarity of rib fractures and chest wall injury compared with parenchymal or mediastinal injury, patients are gener-

ally not suitable anesthetic candidates for this procedure.[15] A delayed diagnosis of flail chest may occur after the patient becomes fatigued, if patient splinting was sufficient to minimize movement of the flail chest segment and thereby obscure the diagnosis.[12] Therefore when thoracic radiographs show multiple rib fractures, patients should be reevaluated for the possibility that a flail chest may be present.

Pathophysiology

The flail chest component moves paradoxically inward during inspiration as a result of negative intrathoracic pressure while the unaffected chest wall is expanding, or moving outward. During expiration, the flail segment moves outward (Figure 86-2). Studies in dogs with experimental flail chest have shown that the abnormal displacement of ribs is primarily determined by the balance between the pleural pressure and the force generated by the parasternal intercostal muscles.[16,17] Dogs with experimental flail chest did not have consistent changes in tidal volume, pleural pressure, breathing frequency, minute ventilation, and arterial $Paco_2$ compared with control values.[18] A small reduction in Pao_2 occurred after inducing flail chest; however, the alteration was inconsistent and not significant. Although performed in anesthetized, spontaneously breathing dogs, these observations underlie the current theory that pain and the associated intrathoracic injuries may be of greater clinical significance than the mechanical impact of partial abnormal thoracic wall movement.[4,10,14]

Both rib fractures and flail chest are known to be associated with severe pain in humans and small animals.

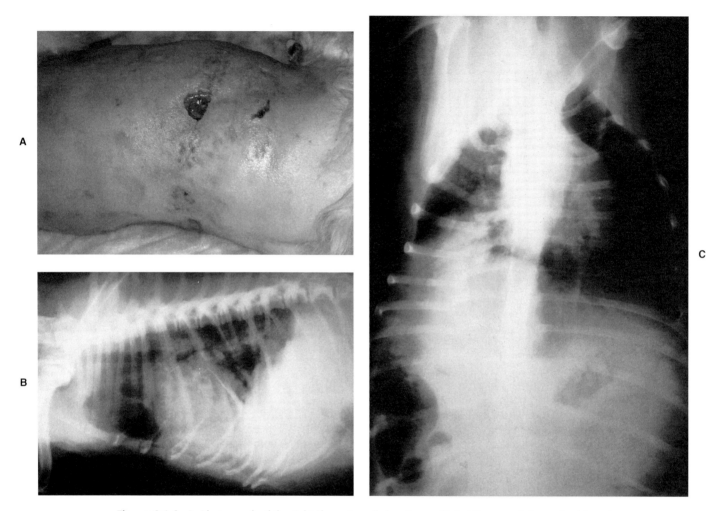

Figure 86-1. A, *Photograph of the right thoracic wall showing multiple bite wounds in a mixed-breed dog.* **B,** *Lateral and* **C,** *dorsoventral thoracic radiographs showing fractures of 5 consecutive ribs, indicative of flail chest.*

In the awake patient, painful stimuli induce a chain of detrimental events including decreased effectiveness of ventilation and coughing, tachypnea, increased pulmonary dead space, and retained secretions.[1,3,8] Pain may contribute to the development of elevated $Paco_2$, decreased Pao_2, and pneumonia.[1,10,11]

Associated intrathoracic injuries (e.g., pneumothorax, hemothorax, and pulmonary contusion) exacerbate pulmonary dysfunction and have been shown to be associated with higher patient mortality compared with patients having only flail chest.[7-9] However, because a significant degree of blunt trauma is necessary to cause flail chest, pulmonary contusion is almost always a concomitant injury.[7] Pulmonary contusion is the extravasation of blood and plasma into the interstitial and alveolar compartments of an area of lung. Fluid accumulation in the extravascular space decreases pulmonary compliance and ventilation while contributing to ventilation/perfusion (V/Q) mismatch and resultant hypoxemia.[1] Further negative sequelae of severe pulmonary contusion and ventilatory deficiencies may include progression to the acute respiratory distress syndrome, a disease process associated with a high mortality rate.

Management

The degree of trauma causing flail chest inevitably impacts intrathoracic structures, resulting in multiple pathophysiologic consequences that make treatment planning complex. Current treatment recommendations deemphasize the flail chest segment and associated mechanical abnormalities, and instead prioritize management of pain and the associated intrathoracic injuries.[4,6,10,11,14]

PAIN MANAGEMENT

Pain management should be instituted rapidly and aggressively as a fundamental component of the treatment plan for flail chest.[1,3,11] Delay in pain management decreases its effectiveness.[11] A minimal analgesic protocol would include local nerve injections. Long-acting local anesthetics should be administered as soon as the pa-

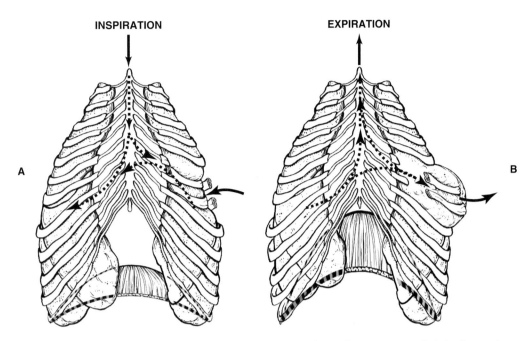

INSPIRATION   **EXPIRATION**

A   B

*Figure 86-2. **A**,* *Depiction of flail chest during inspiration shows the movement of air in the trachea movement of air down the mainstem bronchi, shunting of air from the lung under the flail segment to the opposite hemithorax, position of the diaphragm, expansion of the lungs, and the movement of the flail segment. **B**, Depiction of flail chest during expiration demonstrates the movement of air in the trachea, movement of air out of the lungs and up the main stem bronchi, shunting of air from the lungs of the unaffected hemithorax to the lungs under the flail segment, position of the diaphragm, collapse of the lungs, and the movement of the flail segment.*

tient is initially stabilized. Bupivacaine hydrochloride (0.0625 to 0.125 mg) injections caudal to each fractured rib at the dorsal rib angle, including the caudal and cranial contiguous rib, are recommended.[1] Local nerve injections should be administered every 6 hours or until the effect of other analgesic treatments or surgical stabilization warrant discontinuation of the injections.

An effective, state-of-the-art analgesic combination includes the provision of both local and epidural analgesia, especially for short-term management.[19] A recent study described methods for epidural catheter placement and maintenance for a minimum of 3 days in dogs.[20] Generally, opioids are recommended as the analgesic of choice for epidural administration. This combination of local and epidural analgesia would be appropriate following application of a fentanyl patch, until efficacious blood levels are achieved for more long-term pain control.

Intrapleural administration of local anesthetic agents is not as effective as local nerve injections. Likewise, care should be taken when using systemic opioids because associated respiratory depression may exacerbate hypoventilation. However, appropriate and timely analgesic therapy may decrease respiratory effort to the point where thoracic displacement of the flail chest segment is less prominent, obviating any associated ventilatory compromise.[7] Further, the less painful patient may have improved ventilatory volume and respond more appropriately to pulmonary physiotherapy.

MANAGEMENT OF ASSOCIATED INTRATHORACIC INJURIES

Hemothorax, pneumothorax, and pulmonary contusion are relatively common and predictable injuries associated with flail chest. In contrast, tracheobronchial injury, major pulmonary laceration, cardiac rupture, and aortic or great vessel rupture are unlikely injuries.[7,8] Although the latter, more severe injuries may require operative intervention, it is likely that these animals would not survive transport to a primary care facility.

Current treatment recommendations for flail chest prioritize treatment of pulmonary contusion.[4,10,14] Fluid therapy is an important treatment component of the initial shock associated with the traumatic event causing flail chest. However, fluid therapy should be administered judiciously because the contused portion of lung is susceptible to overhydration and pulmonary edema. Normal parameters for central venous pressure during crystalloid fluid replacement do not necessarily ensure prevention of the progression of pulmonary contusion and edema. In one study, however, colloid solutions had a lung-sparing effect when used at relatively high flow rates to resuscitate shock patients.[21] Monitoring clinical parameters, oxygenation, central venous pressure, urine output, and serial thoracic radiographs provides the clinician with the greatest amount of information to assess fluid therapy in relationship to progressive pulmonary edema associated with contusion.

Furosemide has been shown to decrease pulmonary fluid accumulation in humans with flail chest and associated lung contusion who have received intravenous fluid therapy. By decreasing plasma volume, furosemide decreases the amount of plasma and blood pooling in the contused lung.[1] Care must be taken to avoid excessive decreases of intravascular volume that might result in decreased tissue oxygen delivery, especially in animals that have suffered hypovolemic shock in association with trauma. Current recommendations in small animals include the use of furosemide only following intravenous fluid resuscitation, rather than as an initial therapy for pulmonary contusion. Osmotic diuretics should be avoided unless required for treatment of concurrent intracranial trauma because they may enter the lung through the damaged vascular endothelium of pulmonary vessels and actually worsen the severity of pulmonary contusion or edema.[1]

The effects of corticosteroid administration to promote cell membrane stability and decrease capillary permeability are controversial.[1] Although methylprednisolone sodium succinate may have a protective effect on alveolar type II cells during hypoxic events,[1] this effect must be balanced against the possible negative effects of corticosteroids in the critically ill animal. Maintenance of these surfactant-producing cells may, however, help prevent collapse of alveoli and passage of fluid into the alveolar space, decreasing pulmonary edema.

Associated pneumothorax is treated by thoracocentesis and, if necessary, chest tube placement and closed suction drainage. Hemothorax is usually self-limiting and secondary to the original traumatic event. Ongoing hemorrhage based on comparative packed cell volume (PCV) samples of hemorrhagic pleural effusion and peripheral blood may indicate the need for whole blood transfusion. However, the clinician should be prepared to perform a thoracotomy because ongoing blood loss may be a sign of major pulmonary vessel or aortic laceration.

CONSERVATIVE MANAGEMENT

Clinical studies in humans have shown that early surgical intervention to stabilize flail chest reduces pain; improves ventilatory status; and decreases the need for, and duration of, mechanical ventilatory assistance.[22] However, most clinicians do not consider the mechanical defect of flail chest to be the primary problem.[4,6,7,9-11,14] This viewpoint is based on clinical retrospective studies documenting successful conservative management of flail chest, especially if there are minimal associated intrathoracic injuries. Conservative management emphasizes the treatment of associated intrathoracic injuries, as described previously, while being selective concerning patients that may require surgical intervention.[13]

The decision to provide mechanical (either intermittent or continuous) ventilatory support is based on careful monitoring of arterial blood gases. Intubation is indicated if the Pao_2 is less than 60 mm Hg despite oxygen supplementation, or if the $Paco_2$ is greater than 55 mm Hg when the patient is breathing room air.[13] At one time, intubation and mechanical ventilation was the treatment

of choice for humans with flail chest. Mechanical ventilation and positive end-expiratory pressure (PEEP) provided an "internal" splint of the flail chest segment, limiting movement and associated pain while providing improved ventilation.[10] However, the time interval for intubation and mechanical ventilation was prolonged (14 to 21 days) based on the need for early biological healing of the rib fractures before weaning from the ventilator. This treatment plan also carried a high risk of pneumonia.[9] These latter complications led to studies that evaluated delayed surgical intervention following initiation of intubation and mechanical ventilation. Those studies documented decreased ventilatory time, and a decreased incidence of secondary pneumonia.[9-11,22] Therefore, if intubation and ventilatory assistance are determined to be necessary, based on arterial blood gas analysis, surgical methods should then be employed to stabilize the flail chest in order to decrease the duration of intubation and ventilation and the associated complication of pneumonia. Stabilization of the flail chest may not specifically address pulmonary contusion but will decrease patient pain and discomfort, promoting improved ventilatory function.

SURGICAL MANAGEMENT

Surgical management of flail chest should be performed automatically if thoracotomy or celiotomy is required to treat an associated injury. Interfragmentary wires (18 or 20 gauge) placed in hemicerclage fashion to appose the fractured rib ends is an effective and simple form of internal fixation.[2]

Patients not responding to conservative management and requiring intubation and mechanical ventilation likely have severe intrathoracic injuries and associated pulmonary contusion. These patients are high-risk anesthetic candidates, and equally high-risk thoracotomy patients. Therefore closed, percutaneous surgical methods are recommended to stabilize the flail chest segment as an adjunctive treatment during intubation and ventilatory therapy for hypoxia and hypercapnia.[3,23] These stabilization methods can be performed after injecting a local anesthetic. The hallmark technique common to all closed methods involves passing heavy-gauge suture around each fractured rib segment and securing the rib to a stable device or object attached to the thoracic wall.[3,23] Such objects may include an external aluminum frame; or tongue depressors, which are less cumbersome (Figures 86-3 and 86-4). If a chest tube is not in place, the patient should be monitored for iatrogenic pneumothorax from lung laceration during suture placement. If the patient is being ventilated, a substantial pneumothorax may develop rapidly following lung laceration. The stabilization device should be maintained 3 to 4 weeks because it should be considered the definitive repair method.[3]

External bandaging should not be performed because it may result in decreased effectiveness of already compromised ventilation.[3] However, if a sucking chest wound is associated with the flail chest from a tissue defect communicating with the thoracic cavity, a bandage

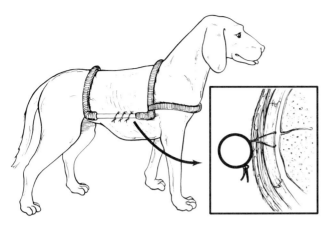

Figure 86-3. *External aluminum frame for stabilization of a flail chest. The ribs are secured to the aluminum frame with circumcostal sutures.*

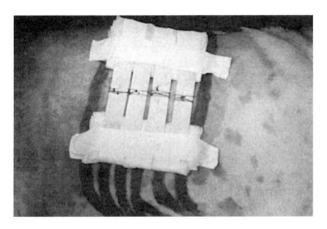

Figure 86-4. *The finished circumcostal suture/tongue depressor stabilization device taped together to prevent shifting of the components. The device is covered by a loose-fitting bandage (stockinette) until the fractures have healed.*

is indicated. Positioning the patient with the flail chest segment ventral or down against a table or cage surface is usually not effective in improving ventilation.

Decision Making

Certainly, the most difficult surgical decision is not to perform surgery. The clinician should avoid the self-doubting thought that conservative management means no treatment. Patient stabilization, including treatment of pulmonary contusion and pneumothorax and institution of an aggressive pain management protocol, are mandatory components in the management of flail chest. In veterinary medicine, it is most appropriate to be selectively aggressive in performing surgical stabilization of the flail chest segment because the procedure

can be performed with the patient receiving only a local anesthetic. Surgical stabilization is especially indicated if an effective pain management protocol cannot be implemented or fails to be effective.[12] Finally, surgical stabilization is preferable to intubation and mechanical ventilation if the flail segment is considered to have a particularly negative effect on patient ventilatory status.

REFERENCES

1. Anderson M, Payne JT, Mann FA et al: Flail chest: Pathophysiology, treatment, and prognosis, *Compend Contin Educ Pract Vet* 15:65-74, 1993.
2. Orton EC: Thoracic wall. In Slatter D, editor: *Textbook of small animal surgery*, ed 2, Philadelphia, 1993, WB Saunders.
3. Bjorling DE: Management of thoracic trauma. In Birchard SJ, Sherding RG, editors: *Saunders manual of small animal practice*, ed 2, Philadelphia, 2000, WB Saunders.
4. Fossum TW: Pleural and extrapleural diseases. In Ettinger SJ, Feldman EC, editors: *Textbook of veterinary internal medicine*, ed 5, Philadelphia, 2000, WB Saunders.
5. Pate JW: Chest wall injuries, *Surg Clin North Am* 69:59-70, 1989.
6. Voggenreiter G, Neudek F, Aufmkolk M et al: Operative chest wall stabilization in flail chest: Outcomes of patients with or without pulmonary contusion, *J Am Coll Surg* 187:130-138, 1998.
7. Ciraulo DL, Elliott D, Mitchell KA et al: Flail chest as a marker for significant injuries, *J Am Coll Surg* 178:466-470, 1994.
8. Kraje BJ, Kraje AC, Rohrbach BW et al: Intrathoracic and concurrent orthopedic injury associated with traumatic rib fracture in cats: 75 cases (1980-1998), *JAVMA* 216:51-54, 2000.
9. Freedland M, Wilson RF, Bender JS et al: The management of flail chest injury: Factors affecting outcome, *J Trauma* 30:1460-1468, 1990.
10. Richardson JD, Mavroudis C: Management of thoracic injuries. In Richardson JD, Polk HC, Flint LM, editors: *Trauma: Clinical care and pathophysiology*, Chicago, 1987, Year Book.
11. Miller HAB, Taylor GA: Flail chest and pulmonary contusion. In McMurtry RY, McLellan BA, editors: *Management of blunt trauma*, Baltimore, 1990, Williams & Wilkins.
12. Glinz W: Shock secondary to chest trauma. In Border JR, editor: *Blunt multiple trauma: Comprehensive pathophysiology and care*, New York, 1990, Marcel Dekker.
13. Wilkins EW: Noncardiovascular thoracic injuries: Chest wall, bronchus, lung, esophagus, and diaphragm. In Burke JF, Boyd RJ, McCabe CJ, editors: *Trauma management*, Chicago, 1988, Year Book.
14. Trinkle JK, Richardson JD, Franz JL et al: Management of flail chest without mechanical ventilation, *Ann Thorac Surg* 19:355-363, 1975.
15. Collins J: Chest wall trauma, *J Thorac Imaging* 15:112-119, 2000.
16. Cappello M, Yuehua C, De Troyer A: Rib cage distortion in a canine model of flail chest, *Am J Respir Crit Care Med* 151:1481-1485, 1995.
17. Cappello M, Legrand A, De Troyer A: Determinants of rib motion in flail chest, *Am J Respir Crit Care Med* 159:886-891, 1999.
18. Cappello M, De Troyer A: Actions of the inspiratory intercostal muscles in flail chest, *Am J Respir Crit Care Med* 155:1085-1089, 1997.
19. Mandabach MG: Intrathecal and epidural analgesia, *Crit Care Clin* 15:105-118, 1999.
20. Gallivan ST, Johnston SA, Broadstone RV et al: The clinical, cerebrospinal fluid, and histopathologic effects of epidural ketorolac in dogs, *Vet Surg* 29:436-441, 2000.
21. Richardson JD, Franz JL, Grover FL et al: Pulmonary contusion and hemorrhage-crystalloid versus colloid replacement, *J Surg Res* 16:330-336, 1974.
22. Ahmed Z, Mohyuddin Z: Management of flail chest injury: Internal fixation versus endotracheal intubation and ventilation, *J Thorac Cardiovasc Surg* 110:1676-1680, 1995.
23. McAnulty JF: A simplified method for stabilization of flail chest injuries in small animals, *J Am Anim Hosp Assoc* 31:137-141, 1995.

Index

Lymphoplasmacytic rhinitis *(Continued)*
 pathological and histopathological findings, 308
 pathophysiology and pathogenesis, 306
Lymphosarcoma, cranial mediastinal, 634-637

M

Magnetic resonance imaging (MRI)
 of pleural space disease, 52
 of pulmonary hypertension, 502
Maltese, 310
Management and treatment
 acute lung injury, 506-507
 acute respiratory distress syndrome, 506-507
 airway obstruction, 5, 38-41
 anticoagulant rodenticide ingestion, 565-566
 aspergillosis, 286-290
 aspiration pneumonia, 426-429
 atelectasis, 470
 bacterial pneumonia, 417-420
 brachycephalic airway syndrome, 312
 bronchiectasis, 378
 bronchoesophageal fistulas, 398-399
 bronchopulmonary dysplasia, 406-409
 canine adenovirus type-2, 438
 canine distemper virus, 435-436
 canine parainfluenza virus type-2, 439
 chronic bronchitis, 384-387
 chylothorax, 600-603
 cough, 45
 cryptococcosis, 291-292
 drowning, 485-486
 endogenous lipid pneumonia, 459
 epistaxis, 33-34
 exogenous lipid pneumonia, 457
 feline bronchial disease, 392-395
 feline calicivirus, 275, 442
 feline herpesvirus-1, 440-441
 fibrosing pleuritis, 603
 fine needle aspiration postprocedure, 136-137
 flail chest, 648-651
 hemothorax, 613-615
 hypoventilation/hypercarbia, 59-60
 iatrogenic pneumothorax, 623
 idiopathic pulmonary fibrosis, 585
 infectious tracheobronchitis, 366-369, 371
 laryngeal trauma, 333-334
 laryngeal tumor, 343
 laryngitis, 337-338
 lung lobe torsion, 560-561
 lymphoplasmacytic rhinitis, 308-309
 nasal discharge, 26-27
 nasal foreign bodies, 304
 nasal neoplasia, 297-298
 nasopharyngeal polyps, 330-331, 331
 neosporosis, 463
 panting, 48
 paraquat ingestion, 568
 parasitic infection, 548-549, 552, 553, 556
 pectus excavatum, 644-646
 pleural space disease, 9, 52
 pleural transudates, 594-596
 pneumocystosis, 464
 pulmonary and bronchial neoplasia, 513
 pulmonary contusion, 475-478
 pulmonary edema, 491-495
 pulmonary hypertension, 502-503
 pulmonary parenchyma, 7-8
 pulmonary thromboembolism, 530-536
 pyothorax, 607-609
 smoke inhalation, 483
 spontaneous pneumothorax, 621-622
 thoracic wall dysfunction, 11
 toxoplasmosis, 462

Management and treatment *(Continued)*
 tracheal collapse, 351-354
 tracheal hypoplasia, 358
 tracheal trauma, 361-363
 tracheal tumor, 343
 traumatic diaphragmatic hernia, 631-632
 traumatic pneumothorax, 619-621
Mast cells, 239, 401
Maxillary sinus, 18
Mechanical ventilation, 59, 209, 218, 255, 477-478, 486. *See also* Ventilation
Mediastinal masses, 84-85
Mediastinal mineralization, 577-579
Medullary neurons, 54-55
Mesenchymal tumors, 107
Methemoglobinemia, 2
Methylxanthine derivatives, 59, 235-238, 385, 418, 531
Metronidazole, 248
Microbiological sampling, 107-108
Microfilariae, 520-521, 524
Mineralization
 definition of, 569-570
 evaluation using alternate imaging techniques, 579-580
 extra-, 570-572
 mediastinal, 577-579
 pleural, 572-573
 pulmonary, 573-577
Morphine, 241
Motor neurons, 54-55
Mouth care during ventilation, 223
Mucociliary scintigraphy, 98, 374-375
Mucoid nasal discharge, 19, 21
Mucokinetics, 242-244
Mucolytics, 243-244, 418
Mucopurulent nasal discharge, 19
Mycoplasmas, 125, 365
Mycotic infection of the nasal cavities, 20

N

N-acetyl-L-cysteine (NAC), 243-244
Nasal cannulation, 494
Nasal cavities
 allergic rhinitis and, 21
 anatomy of, 68
 bacterial infections of, 20
 biopsy of, 103-107
 canine viral infections of, 20
 cultures, 25-26, 143
 cytology of, 25
 diagnosis of diseases related to, 20
 diagnostic imaging of, 23-25
 discharge from, 18-27
 dorsal rhinotomy of, 304
 endoscopy of, 25
 epistaxis into, 19, 22, 26-27, 29-30
 evaluation of, 33
 examination of, 69
 feline upper respiratory tract infection complex and, 20
 foreign bodies in, 22, 302-304
 lymphoplasmacytic rhinitis of, 21
 microbiological sampling of, 107-108
 mycotic infection of, 20-21
 neoplasia of, 20-21, 293-299
 oral disease effect on, 21
 parasitic rhinitis of, 21
 polyps of, 21
 rhinotomy of, 26
 sample collection from, 100-108
 sneezing and, 19
 tissue biopsy, 25
 ventral rhinotomy, 304
Nasal cytology, 144-145

Nasal neoplasia
 biopsies of, 106-107
 diagnostic tests for, 295-296
 differential diagnosis, 295
 epidemiology and risk factors for, 294
 epistaxis caused by, 31
 historical findings, clinical signs, and progression, 294
 lung lobe torsion due to, 561
 management and monitoring, 297-298
 nasal discharge due to, 20-21
 natural history and incidence, 293-294
 outcome and prognosis, 298-299
 pathological and histopathological findings, 296-297
Nasal oxygen administration, 207-208
Nasopharyngeal polyps
 definition and etiology, 328
 epidemiology and risk factors, 329
 historical findings, clinical signs, and progression, 329
 management of, 330-331
 nasal discharge and, 21
 pathophysiology and pathogenesis, 329, 330
 pharyngoscopy for, 109-110
 postoperative care, 331
 prognosis, 331
 surgery for, 330-331
Nasopharyngoscopy, 25
Nasopharynx
 anatomy of, 68
 nasopharyngeal polyps and, 329
 pharyngoscopy of, 109-110
Nebulization, 209-210, 223, 245-246, 386, 418-419
Neoplasia
 bone, 575-576
 cranial mediastinal, 634-639
 nasal, 20-21, 31, 106-107, 293-298, 561
 pleural, 639-641
 pleural effusion and, 593
 pulmonary and bronchial, 508-515
 thymoma, 637-639
Neosporosis, 462-463
Neuromuscular junction disorders, 10
Neuromuscular pedicle grafting/reinnervation, 326
Neuronal control of the respiratory center, 54-55
Newfoundlands, 310, 373
Nitroglycerine, 495
Noncardiac thoracic ultrasonography, 83-87
Noncardiogenic pulmonary edema, 37, 333
Nonsteroidal antiinflammatory drugs (NSAIDs), 240, 260
Noscapine, 241
Nose breathing, 18
Nosocomial infection minimization during ventilation, 224
Nuclear medicine, 93-94
Nutrition
 bronchopulmonary dysplasia and, 407
 tracheal collapse and, 347
 during ventilation, 224

O

Obesity, 358, 381
Ocular irritations, 483
Old English sheepdogs, 294, 373
Olfaction, 18
Olfactory neuroepithelium, 18
Omentalization, 603
Oral cavities, 23, 101, 102
Oral disease and nasal cavities, 21